THE
NATURE
OF DISEASE

Pathology for the Health Professions

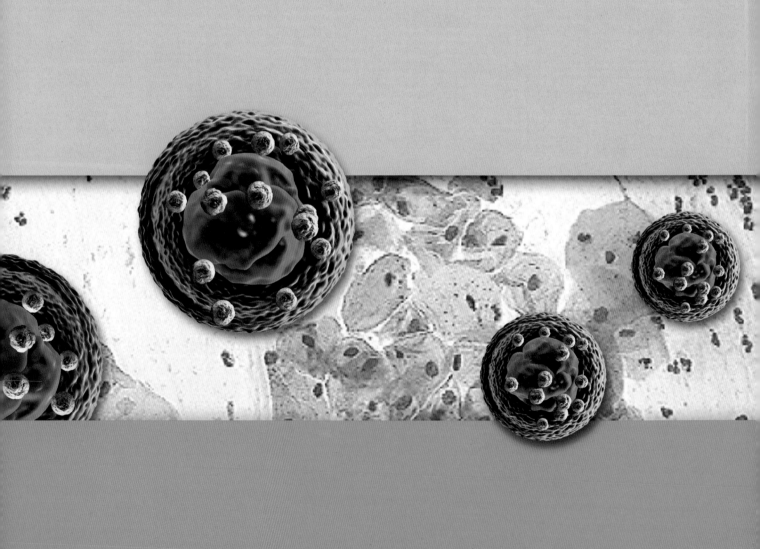

THE
NATURE
OF DISEASE

Pathology for the Health Professions

Thomas H. McConnell, MD, FCAP
Clinical Professor of Pathology
UT Southwestern Medical Center
Dallas, Texas

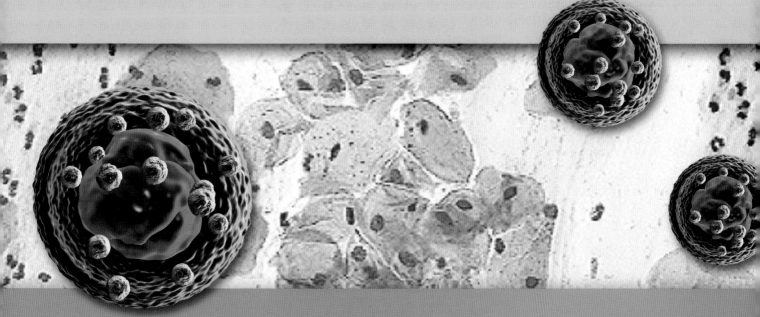

Acquisitions Editor: David B. Troy
Development Editor: Dana L. Knighten
Marketing Manager: Marisa A. O'Brien
Production Editor: Jennifer P. Ajello
Designer: Terry Mallon
Art Direction: Jennifer Clements, LWW; Craig Durant, Dragonfly Media Group
Artists: Rob Fedirko, Rob Duckwall, and Paige Henson, Dragonfly Media Group
Compositor: Maryland Composition, Inc.
Printer: R.R. Donnelley & Shenzhen

Library of Congress Cataloging-in-Publication Data

McConnell, Thomas H.
   The nature of disease : pathology for the health professions / Thomas H. McConnell.
      p. ; cm.
   Includes bibliographical references and index.
   ISBN-13: 978-0-7817-8203-6/0-7817-8203-1 (alk. paper) 1.   Pathology—Textbooks.   I.   Title.
   [DNLM: 1.   Pathology.   QZ 4 M4789n 2007]
   RB111.M21 2007
   616.07—dc22

                                                2006027273

This book is dedicated to:

Hazel and T.H.
for
gifts

Marianne
for
unconditional love

Anne, Allen, Lea, and Jim
for
keeping the faith

Helen
for
pure devotion

Jack, Margot, Andrew, Conner, JuJu, Kate, and Missa
for hope

Charles Ashworth
for
generosity

Vernie Stembridge
for
showing me the way

Adam, Clint, and Jason
for
renewal

Mark and Peggy
for
good example

William Marsh Rice, founder of Rice University
and
the citizens of Texas
for
a rigorous and free education

Preface

The Nature of Disease is a short textbook of pathology, but it took a long time to write. Each sentence has been crafted for a particular audience: students studying for a degree in the health professions.

This text's aim is twofold:

- To present basic normal anatomy and physiology and contrast them with the essential pathology and pathophysiology of the most common and important human diseases.
- To make the material enjoyable and easy to read.

Classroom Vetted

This textbook literally grew out of a classroom. When I joined the academic community after a career in private practice, the classroom was an alien place to me. I puzzled over the fact that the students I taught, who were of the very highest quality, still had trouble grasping the topics. I began to pay more critical attention to the textbooks I had selected for them, and I quickly learned the student perspective of most pathology texts: they are difficult to read.

Most pathology books are compilations written by multiple authors, each with a certain writing style and with differing views about the relative importance of things. The style is generally stilted and formal—the text doesn't flow, and the reading is bare of enjoyment. If I had a hard time with these texts, what about the students?

And so I concluded to write an outline of pathology for them—a simple bullet list of important statements written in declarative sentences that I was sure were clear and easy to understand. This proved a success, but the students wanted more. The demand grew, and my simple outline soon became a self-published, spiral-bound manual. After three editions of this manual, I realized I had the makings of a textbook in my hands. The result is *The Nature of Disease*.

Approach

Having spent much of my professional life communicating with physicians buried in a blizzard of paper, I know that brevity, manner, and style are the essence of written communication. *The Nature of Disease* adopts a deliberately casual, narrative style that served me well in medical practice. It makes reading easier, holds the reader's attention, and enhances understanding and recall of important points without sacrificing scientific relevance.

The Nature of Disease focuses on answering the most important questions that students and patients have about every disease: *what?, why?, where?*, and *how?* It does so by concentrating on the nuts and bolts of human pathology: the causes and the mechanisms of disease, its progress, and its outcome. The science is flavored with a bit of humor to offer a break from the scientific drill. Along the way, the text uses a number of devices to deepen understanding, retain interest, and enhance recall:

- *Much of the molecular and microscopic detail typically found in similar textbooks has been eliminated.* Each chapter focuses on the essentials necessary to build a broad, fundamental understanding, with supporting detail where relevant.
- *Clinical examples from daily life are integrated throughout to explain basic concepts.* For example, fever blisters (cold sores, herpesvirus infection) illustrate the pathology of virus infections. Placing disease in a realistic, familiar context enhances recall and develops insight.
- *Key points and concepts are reiterated where appropriate.* Rather than assume that the reader recalls the details, the text errs (judiciously) on the side of restating the obvious. Experience shows that students benefit from the redundancy.
- *New terms are boldfaced and defined at their first use in the narrative.* This practice alerts the reader to the importance of the new term, which is defined in the same sentence or the one immediately following.
- *Selected important points are italicized for emphasis.* For example, in Chapter 11, Diseases of Blood Cells and Blood Coagulation, the following italicized sentence emphasizes the threat of colon cancer: *Iron deficiency anemia in a man or postmenopausal woman is to be considered bleeding from gastrointestinal cancer until proven otherwise.*

- *The narrative is sprinkled with quotations—serious, whimsical, or humorous—to humanize the material and make the subject matter more memorable.* For example, Chapter 13, Diseases of the Heart, begins with a line from singer Tim McGraw's tune, "Where the Green Grass Grows": "*. . . another supper from a sack, a ninety-nine cent heart attack . . . .*" This snippet of lyric speaks volumes about the American diet and heart disease, and students invariably enjoy and remember it.
- *The* History of Medicine *boxes further humanize the narrative by presenting historical anecdotes that put in its historical perspective.* For example, in Chapter 10, Disorders of Daily Life and Diet, the box titled "French Food, Fast Food, Fat Food" discusses the history of restaurants, the development of fast food in America, and the rise of obesity. The "History of Medicine" box is my favorite feature.

Organization

Although this textbook is unique in many ways, it is organized in a familiar fashion: it presents general aspects of pathology first, with the pathology of organ systems following.

Part 1, General Pathology, opens with a chapter titled *The Nature of Disease*, which discusses the actual nature of disease—that is, the intimate relationship between form and function in both health and sickness. This chapter also emphasizes the difference between the disease itself and the signs and symptoms it produces. The failure of health care professionals and their patients to appreciate this distinction accounts for a great deal of medical misdirection and misunderstanding.

The remainder of Part 1 consists of a series of chapters that deal with pathologic forces that can affect any part of the body: the life and death of cells, inflammation and repair, disorders of fluid balance and blood flow, neoplasia, genetic and pediatric diseases, infectious disease, diseases of diet, workplace and environment, and diseases of the immune system.

Part 1 establishes the foundation, and Part 2, Diseases of Organ Systems, expands understanding by discussing diseases of particular organs and organ systems. Along the way the narrative is stitched together with liberal use of cross-references. In early chapters they are used to steer the reader to more detailed discussion in later chapters. In later chapters they are used to recall earlier discussion of basic concepts. For example, in Chapter 21, Diseases of the Female Genital Tract and Breast, the discussion of dysplasia of the cervix calls on the reader to understand the concept of metaplasia, which was defined and discussed initially in Chapter 2. The cross-reference is presented in the following sentence: "However, during puberty the ectocervix is transformed by metaplasia (Chapter 2) from flat squamous cells into tall, columnar glandular cells."

Art Program

No textbook of human pathology can succeed without an excellent art program. Both photographs and line drawings are necessary for a thorough understanding of the subject. Line art simplifies the structures and concepts depicted by distilling them to their basic, most easily recognizable forms, while photographs show anatomic structures as they appear in real life. *The Nature of Disease* is richly illustrated with both.

More than 600 full-color figures augment the discussions in this book. In keeping with the core notion that anatomic form and function go hand in hand in health and disease, this text contains more pathologic gross photographs of patients and organs than comparable texts do. Each photograph has been chosen to illustrate a critical point and is intended to speak for itself. The guiding principle in developing medical line art is that good art should be understandable at a glance, or with minimal study. The high-quality line drawings in this book have been designed both to be esthetically pleasing and to guide the reader's thought without needing to read a lengthy description.

Chapter Features: A Guided Tour

Think of reading this textbook as a road trip through unfamiliar territory: there is a lot to see, and the driver (reader) needs a roadmap, a short list of the most important things to see, and reference material to study in detail. Each chapter contains a set of consistent chapter opener features; narrative content with supporting features such as sidebar boxes, tables, and figures; and end-of-chapter features to promote retention and comprehension.

CHAPTER OPENER FEATURES

The chapter opener contains several features to help to orient and prepare the reader for the material that follows:

- A brief *overview* of the chapter content provides a thumbnail sketch of what to expect.
- A *chapter outline* of major headings and subheadings serves as a large-scale atlas of the material ahead.

- *Learning Objectives* instruct the reader about the most important learning tasks on a trip through the chapter.
- *Key Terms and Concepts* acquaint the reader with the most important "must see and understand" points of interest on the trip.

CHAPTER FEATURES

The features in the body of each chapter are designed to meet the specific needs of health professions students. Every feature has been carefully crafted to hone critical thinking skills and judgment, build clinical proficiency, and promote comprehension and retention of the material.

Fundamentals

The following features present core concepts that form the foundation of a thorough understanding of pathology. They focus on the essential science necessary to understand each topic.

- *Back to Basics* is a special narrative overview of normal anatomy and physiology, which appears in two chapters in Part 1 (Chapter 5, Disorders of Fluid Balance and Blood Flow, and Chapter 8, Diseases of the Immune System) and at the beginning of all chapters in Part 2. Back to Basics has its own special design to distinguish it from the rest of the chapter, with its text set against a lightly shaded background. This feature not only serves as a refresher of relevant material from students' previous coursework but also provides a basis for comparing and contrasting the abnormal anatomy and function that characterize every disease. For example, it is impossible to understand immune disease without understanding the nature of B and T cells and their role in normal immunity; the *Back to Basics* section in Chapter 8 offers the reader a quick tour of normal immune function before moving on to immune disease.
- *Basics in Brief* boxes expand on the Back to Basics feature and carry a similar design to indicate their relatedness. These boxes offer snippets of basic concepts where specific discussion within a chapter calls for it. For example, in Chapter 13, Diseases of the Heart, it is not possible to understand congenital heart disease without acquaintance with fetal circulation. At the opening of the discussion of congenital heart disease, a Basics in Brief box offers a detailed illustration and discussion of fetal blood flow.
- *Major Determinants of Disease* is a box that occurs in most chapters in Part 1 and in all chapters in Part 2. It consists of a bulleted list of key "rules" that determine why disease occurs and unfolds the way it does.

Each point is brief and written to be remembered. For example, in Chapter 14, Diseases of the Respiratory System, one of the major determinants of disease is: *Smoking is a major cause of lung disease.*

- ⟳ *Key Points* boxes reiterate important points that warrant special emphasis. For example, in Chapter 15, Diseases of the Gastrointestinal Tract, one of these boxes reminds the reader: *The colon is host to more neoplasms than any other organ in the body.*

Clinical Applications

The following features have a practical, real-world focus that teaches students how to apply their learning in clinical situations. They are specifically designed to promote the development of sound clinical judgment and prepare the student to function effectively in his or her chosen health profession.

- ⟳ *The Clinical Side* boxes feature information of several different kinds:
  - Clinical techniques in the diagnosis and management of disease. For example, in Chapter 21, Diseases of the Female Genital Tract and Breast, the box explains the use of the Pap smear in the detection of lesions of the cervix, especially dysplasia and cancer.
  - Therapies as a natural outgrowth of an understanding of basic anatomy and pathophysiology. For example in Chapter 5, Disorders of Fluid Balance and Blood Flow, a box entitled Salt Water Therapy—a discussion of intravenous fluid therapy—is presented in conjunction with a discussion of body water and fluid compartments and how they change with disease.
  - Lifestyle changes and other activities to prevent disease. For example, Chapter 13, Diseases of the Heart, contains a box titled "Lifestyle and Ischemic Heart Disease," which discusses lifestyle habits that cause ischemic heart disease and the changes in lifestyle that will help prevent it.
- The Clinical Side boxes are woven throughout the text and echo relevant basic sciences themes in every instance; they are an integral part of the teaching narrative.
- ⟳ *Lab Tools* feature boxes offer information on common laboratory procedures and results. For example, a box in Chapter 7, Developmental, Genetic, and Pediatric Disease, discusses *Laboratory Diagnosis in Genetic Disease* in simple terms that students can easily grasp.
- ⟳ *Case Studies,* which appear at the end of every chapter just before the chapter review material,

are built from the details of an actual patient's experience. For consistency, each case is organized around the same set of headings. The headings themselves follow the sequence in which events typically unfold in a real-world health care setting:

- *Topics:* Lists the major disease and problems presented by the patient.
- *Setting:* Describes the hospital, clinic, office, and the reader's imagined role in the case.
- *Clinical History:* Tells the patient's story.
- *Physical Examination and Other Data:* Gives the scientific facts.
- *Clinical Course:* Describes what happens.
- *Discussion:* Analyzes the case, with a focus on cause, effect, and outcome.
- *Points to Remember:* Lists the lessons learned.
- *The Road Not Taken—An Alternative Scenario:* Because most of the cases are derived from autopsy material, I have added a twist to some of them, which imagines a better outcome for the patient had the case unfolded in a different way. For example, in Chapter 12, Diseases of Blood Vessels, the case is that of a man found dead from a stroke in his office. The alternative scenario imagines the patient behaving differently—losing weight, taking his blood pressure medicine regularly, exercising, and watching his diet—and living happily ever after.

CHAPTER REVIEW FEATURES

At the end of each chapter are two features that reinforce learning by providing an opportunity to review the material and assess understanding:

- The *Objectives Recap* is a brief narrative explanation of the salient points relating to each chapter objective. More than just a simple chapter outline or bulleted summary of key points, this feature provides a narrative overview of the main points that are directly related to each of the chapter objectives.
- *Typical Test Questions* stimulate recall and give the reader a sense of the kinds of questions to expect on an exam.

OTHER TEXT FEATURES

Several other unique features of this book offer quick access to key information.

- The *Guide to Case Studies* in the front matter lists the titles of cases at the end of every chapter and the topics that each case centers around: diseases, disorders, testing, and other relevant clinical information. Classroom and informal discussions reveal that students enjoy case studies more and learn more from them than from any other aspect of my course, and this guide helps them refer to them easily and quickly.
- The *Index of Case Studies* in the back matter provides another means of accessing useful clinical information in the case studies. It consists of an alphabetical list of the diseases and other topics from the case studies, cross-referenced by case study and text page number.
- The end-of-text *Glossary* contains short definitions of important terms and topics. It includes only terms that are unfamiliar and not easily recalled, that rely especially on precise definition, or that are often misunderstood. These are primarily descriptive terms from the chapters, where all new terms are boldfaced and defined on first encounter. In this respect our glossary is like most, but with a twist: ours includes few disorders or diseases. These are best studied via detailed discussion rather than short definition.

Summary

I trust you will learn by reading my book. But more than that, I hope you will enjoy reading it. I have spent a great deal of time and energy on the latter in the hope that it will improve the former. For example, I have larded the narrative with medical history anecdotes that I hope will entertain and will give disease a human face, and I have salted it with quotations that may add a note of melancholy or humor to the topic.

So, here it is; judge for yourself. And after you have judged, I want you to tell me what you think. This is no idle invitation—please send your comments, suggestions, praise, or criticism to me in care of the publisher at:

Lippincott Williams and Wilkins
351 West Camden Street
Baltimore, MD 21201-2436

Thomas H. McConnell, MD, FCAP
Dallas, Texas, April 15, 2006

Additional Learning Resources

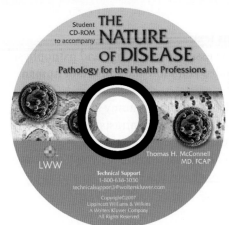

STUDENT CD INCLUDES:

- 250 practice quiz questions to test knowledge and skills
- Animations to reinforce visual learning

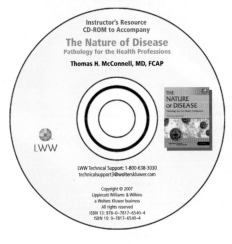

INSTRUCTOR'S RESOURCE CD INCLUDES:

- PowerPoint slides with accompanying lecture notes
- Image bank of figures from the text
- Answers to end-of-chapter review questions in the text
- Test generator with more than 2,000 questions

Everything you need to develop, administer, and present your course!

All of these essential teaching tools are also available on the text's companion website:
http://connection.lww.com/mcconnell

User's Guide

This User's Guide introduces you to the features and tools of The Nature of Disease. Each feature is specifically designed to enhance your learning experience, preparing you for a successful career as a health professional.

Highlights of this text:
- Focuses on the essential pathology and pathophysiology of the most common and important human diseases.
- Presents the basic normal anatomy and physiology of each body system, then contrasts them with the system in disease.
- Provides the conceptual knowledge you'll need as a health professional and teaches you how to apply it in clinical settings.

Chapter Opener Features

Each chapter begins with a two-page chapter opener that previews chapter contents and provides a framework for learning. These features are also handy tools to use when reviewing for tests.

Chapter Overview. Gives a thumbnail sketch of what's covered in the chapter.

Chapter Outline. Serves as a "roadmap" to the material ahead.

Learning Objectives. Preview the most important learning tasks on a trip through the chapter.

Key Terms and Concepts. List the most important terms and concepts in the chapter. These terms appear in bold type the first time they are used. The Glossary also contains a selection of the most important terms and their definitions.

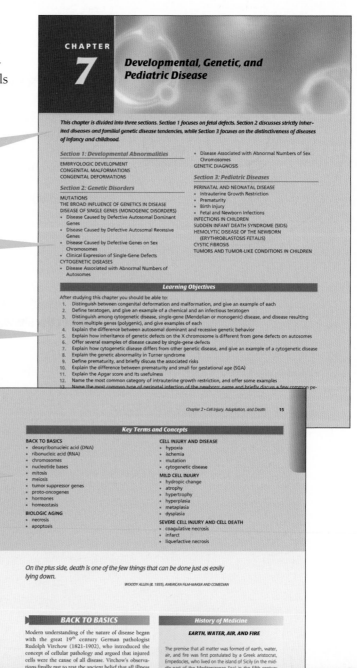

Chapter Features

The following features appear throughout the body of the chapter. They're designed to hone critical thinking skills and judgment, build clinical proficiency, and promote comprehension and retention of the material. They also provide a fun and interesting human perspective on some of the concepts!

FUNDAMENTALS

These features provide an overview, review, or other concise summary of fundamental concepts in anatomy, physiology, and pathology.

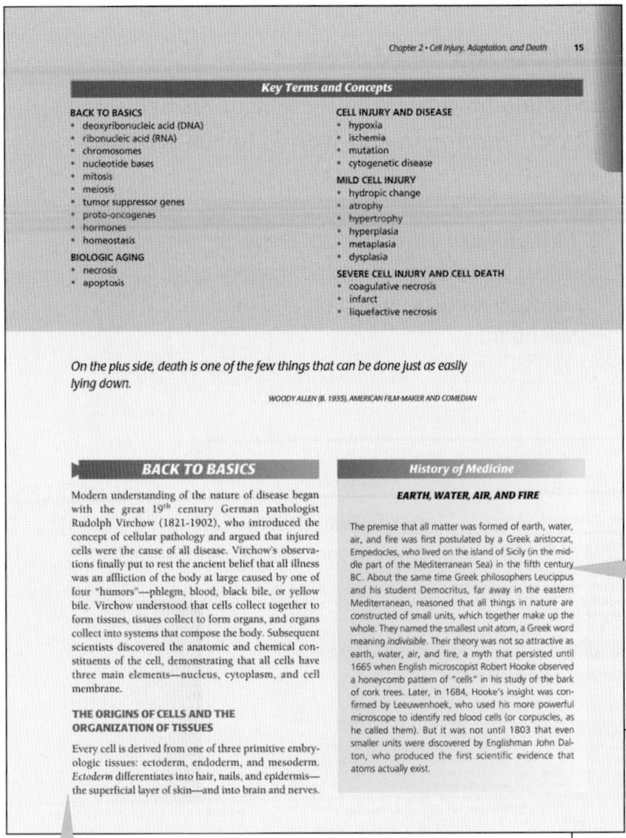

(Sample page content from Chapter 2 and Chapter 6:)

Chapter 2 • Cell Injury, Adaptation, and Death   15

Key Terms and Concepts

BACK TO BASICS
- deoxyribonucleic acid (DNA)
- ribonucleic acid (RNA)
- chromosomes
- nucleotide bases
- mitosis
- meiosis
- tumor suppressor genes
- proto-oncogenes
- hormones
- homeostasis

BIOLOGIC AGING
- necrosis
- apoptosis

CELL INJURY AND DISEASE
- hypoxia
- ischemia
- mutation
- cytogenetic disease

MILD CELL INJURY
- hydropic change
- atrophy
- hypertrophy
- hyperplasia
- metaplasia
- dysplasia

SEVERE CELL INJURY AND CELL DEATH
- coagulative necrosis
- infarct
- liquefactive necrosis

On the plus side, death is one of the few things that can be done just as easily lying down.

WOODY ALLEN (B. 1935), AMERICAN FILM-MAKER AND COMEDIAN

BACK TO BASICS

Modern understanding of the nature of disease began with the great 19th century German pathologist Rudolph Virchow (1821-1902), who introduced the concept of cellular pathology and argued that injured cells were the cause of all disease. Virchow's observations finally put to rest the ancient belief that all illness was an affliction of the body at large caused by one of four "humors"—phlegm, blood, black bile, or yellow bile. Virchow understood that cells collect together to form tissues, tissues collect to form organs, and organs collect into systems that compose the body. Subsequent scientists discovered the anatomic and chemical constituents of the cell, demonstrating that all cells have three main elements—nucleus, cytoplasm, and cell membrane.

THE ORIGINS OF CELLS AND THE ORGANIZATION OF TISSUES

Every cell is derived from one of three primitive embryologic tissues: ectoderm, endoderm, and mesoderm. *Ectoderm* differentiates into hair, nails, and epidermis—the superficial layer of skin—and into brain and nerves.

History of Medicine

EARTH, WATER, AIR, AND FIRE

The premise that all matter was formed of earth, water, air, and fire was first postulated by a Greek aristocrat, Empedocles, who lived on the island of Sicily (in the middle part of the Mediterranean Sea) in the fifth century BC. About the same time Greek philosophers Leucippus and his student Democritus, far away in the eastern Mediterranean, reasoned that all things in nature are constructed of small units, which together make up the whole. They named the smallest unit atom, a Greek word meaning *indivisible*. Their theory was not so attractive as earth, water, air, and fire, a myth that persisted until 1665 when English microscopist Robert Hooke observed a honeycomb pattern of "cells" in his study of the bark of cork trees. Later, in 1684, Hooke's insight was confirmed by Leeuwenhoek, who used his more powerful microscope to identify red blood cells (or corpuscles, as he called them). But it was not until 1803 that even smaller units were discovered by Englishman John Dalton, who produced the first scientific evidence that atoms actually exist.

"History of Medicine" boxes. Put disease in the context of human history—fun and interesting facts help you remember the disease content!

"Back to Basics" section. Previews/reviews the normal anatomy and physiology of each body system. Its shaded background sets it off from the chapter's pathology content—helping you find it fast when you need to review!

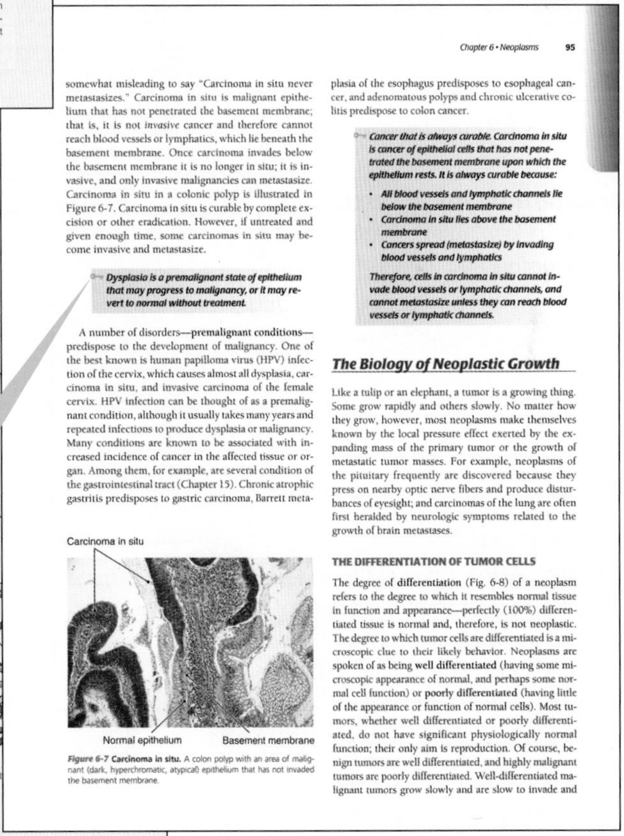

"Key Points" boxes. Repeat the most important points from the narrative, reinforcing learning.

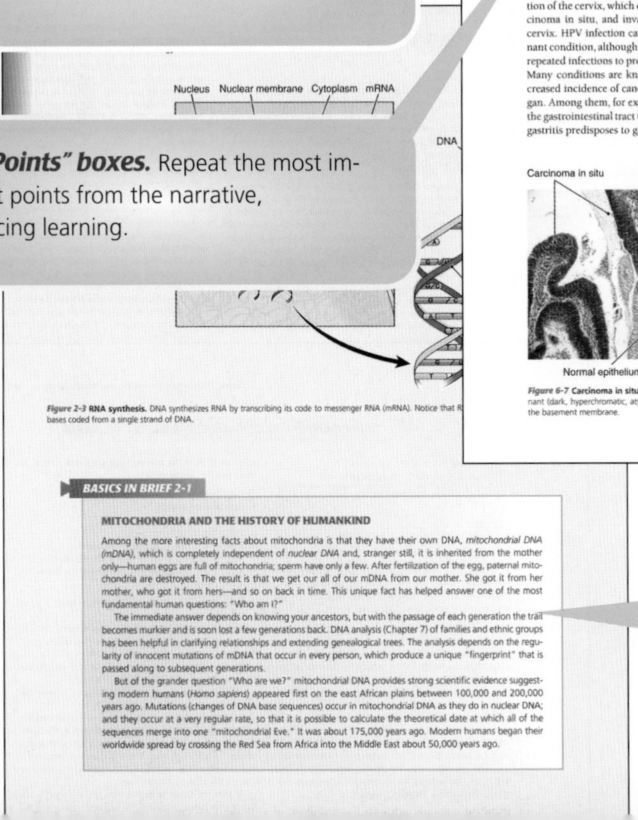

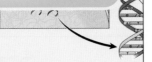

Nucleus   Nuclear membrane   Cytoplasm   mRNA

DNA

Figure 2-3 RNA synthesis. DNA synthesizes RNA by transcribing its code to messenger RNA (mRNA). Notice that R bases coded from a single strand of DNA.

Chapter 6 • Neoplasms   95

somewhat misleading to say "Carcinoma in situ never metastasizes." Carcinoma in situ is malignant epithelium that has not penetrated the basement membrane; that is, it is not invasive cancer and therefore cannot reach blood vessels or lymphatics, which lie beneath the basement membrane. Once carcinoma invades below the basement membrane it is no longer in situ; it is invasive, and only invasive malignancies can metastasize. Carcinoma in situ in a colonic polyp is illustrated in Figure 6-7. Carcinoma in situ is curable by complete excision or other eradication. However, if untreated and given enough time, some carcinomas in situ may become invasive and metastasize.

> *Dysplasia is a premalignant state of epithelium that may progress to malignancy, or it may revert to normal without treatment.*

A number of disorders—premalignant conditions—predispose to the development of malignancy. One of the best known is human papilloma virus (HPV) infection of the cervix, which causes almost all dysplasia, carcinoma in situ, and invasive carcinoma of the female cervix. HPV infection can be thought of as a premalignant condition, although it usually takes many years and repeated infections to produce dysplasia or malignancy. Many conditions are known to be associated with increased incidence of cancer in the affected tissue or organ. Among them, for example, are several condition of the gastrointestinal tract (Chapter 15). Chronic atrophic gastritis predisposes to gastric carcinoma, Barrett meta-

plasia of the esophagus predisposes to esophageal cancer, and adenomatous polyps and chronic ulcerative colitis predispose to colon cancer.

> *Cancer that is always curable. Carcinoma in situ is cancer of epithelial cells that has not penetrated the basement membrane upon which the epithelium rests. It is always curable because:*
>
> - *All blood vessels and lymphatic channels lie below the basement membrane*
> - *Carcinoma in situ lies above the basement membrane*
> - *Cancers spread (metastasize) by invading blood vessels and lymphatics*
>
> *Therefore, cells in carcinoma in situ cannot invade blood vessels or lymphatic channels, and cannot metastasize unless they can reach blood vessels or lymphatic channels.*

The Biology of Neoplastic Growth

Like a tulip or an elephant, a tumor is a growing thing. Some grow rapidly and others slowly. No matter how they grow, however, most neoplasms make themselves known by the local pressure effect exerted by the expanding mass of the primary tumor or the growth of metastatic tumor masses. For example, neoplasms of the pituitary frequently are discovered because they press on nearby optic nerve fibers and produce disturbances of eyesight; and carcinomas of the lung are often first heralded by neurologic symptoms related to the growth of brain metastases.

THE DIFFERENTIATION OF TUMOR CELLS

The degree of **differentiation** (Fig. 6-8) of a neoplasm refers to the degree to which it resembles normal tissue in function and appearance—perfectly (100%) differentiated tissue is normal and, therefore, is not neoplastic. The degree to which tumor cells are differentiated is a microscopic clue to their likely behavior. Neoplasms are spoken of as being **well differentiated** (having some microscopic appearance of normal, and perhaps some normal cell function) or **poorly differentiated** (having little of the appearance or function of normal cells). Most tumors, whether well differentiated or poorly differentiated, do not have significant physiologically normal function; their only aim is reproduction. Of course, benign tumors are well differentiated, and highly malignant tumors are poorly differentiated. Well-differentiated malignant tumors grow slowly and are slow to invade and

Carcinoma in situ

Normal epithelium   Basement membrane

Figure 6-7 Carcinoma in situ. A colon polyp with an area of malignant (dark, hyperchromatic, atypical) epithelium that has not invaded the basement membrane.

BASICS IN BRIEF 2-1

MITOCHONDRIA AND THE HISTORY OF HUMANKIND

Among the more interesting facts about mitochondria is that they have their own DNA, *mitochondrial DNA (mDNA)*, which is completely independent of *nuclear* DNA and, stranger still, it is inherited from the mother only—human eggs are full of mitochondria; sperm have only a few. After fertilization of the egg, paternal mitochondria are destroyed. The result is that we get our all of our mDNA from our mother. She got it from her mother, who got it from hers—and so on back in time. This unique fact has helped answer one of the most fundamental human questions: "Who am I?"

The immediate answer depends on knowing your ancestors, but with the passage of each generation the trail becomes murkier and is soon lost a few generations back. DNA analysis (Chapter 7) of families and ethnic groups has been helpful in clarifying relationships and extending genealogical trees. The analysis depends on the regularity of innocent mutations of mDNA that occur in every person, which produce a unique "fingerprint" that is passed along to subsequent generations.

But of the grander question "Who are we?" mitochondrial DNA provides strong scientific evidence suggesting modern humans (*Homo sapiens*) appeared first on the east African plains between 100,000 and 200,000 years ago. Mutations (changes of DNA base sequences) occur in mitochondrial DNA as they do in nuclear DNA; and they occur at a very regular rate, so that it is possible to calculate the theoretical date at which all of the sequences merge into one "mitochondrial Eve." It was about 175,000 years ago. Modern humans began their worldwide spread by crossing the Red Sea from Africa into the Middle East about 50,000 years ago.

"Basics in Brief" boxes. Feature tidbits of normal anatomy and physiology review, just where you need them!

CLINICAL APPLICATIONS

The hands-on content in these features helps you apply your learning in real-world clinical settings.

"The Clinical Side" boxes. Focus on clinical techniques in diagnosing and managing disease, treatment therapies, and disease prevention.

"Lab Tools" boxes. Explain common laboratory procedures and results.

"Major Determinants of Disease" boxes. List the key "rules" that determine why disease occurs and unfolds the way it does.

Case Studies. Actual cases at the end of every chapter are built from the details of a real patient's illness. The consistent heading structure in every case helps you find the information you need at a glance!

The Road Not Taken. An alternative scenario that imagines how the course of disease might have unfolded differently, with a better outcome for the patient, if certain factors had been changed. (Included in select case studies.)

CHAPTER REVIEW FEATURES

These features help you review chapter content and test yourself before exams.

Objectives Recap. A brief explanation of the chapter's main points related to each chapter objective.

Typical Test Questions. Give you a sense of the kinds of questions to expect on an exam.

---

290   Part 2 • Diseases of Organ Systems

Objectives Recap

1. *Describe the normal functions of endothelial cells:* They control diffusion of substances across the vascular wall into adjacent tissues, and they maintain blood in a smooth, clot-free state.
2. *Classify plasma lipids:* Plasma lipids are classified in two major ways: chemically and by density. Chemically, plasma lipids are either cholesterol or triglyceride, and they circulate attached to a protein (the apoprotein) to form a lipoprotein. Lipoproteins are classified by density into high-density lipoprotein (HDL), low-density lipoprotein (LDL), and very-low-density lipoprotein (VLDL). Each type of lipoprotein contains varying amounts

ous because they tend to be fatty, soft, and unstable. They are prone to ulceration, hemorrhage, and thrombosis. Old atheromas are fibrotic, hard, and sometimes calcified. They are less dangerous and are stable and may cause downstream ischemia, but they are not prone to thrombosis and sudden occlusion.
9. *Name the two main components that determine blood pressure:* Peripheral resistance and cardiac output.
10. *Name and define the two major types of hypertension:* Essential (primary) hypertension is not associated with any identifiable underlying causative

---

Chapter 12 • Diseases of Blood Vessels   291

Typical Test Questions

1. Which one of the following is associated with increased risk of atherosclerosis?
   A. HDL cholesterol <40 mg/dL
   B. LDL cholesterol <100 mg/dL
   C. VLDL cholesterol <30 mg/dL
   D. Triglyceride <150 mg/dL
2. Which one of the following is the site of the initial arterial injury in atherosclerosis?
   A. Endothelial cell
   B. Basement membrane
   C. Muscular wall (media)
   D. Adventitia
3. Which one of the following is the lowest pressure that qualifies as stage 3 (severe) hypertension?
   A. Blood pressure 135/85 mm Hg
   B. Blood pressure 175/105 mm Hg
   C. Blood pressure 185/110 mm Hg
   D. Blood pressure 205/125 mm Hg
4. Which one of the following explains most aneurysms?
   A. Cystic medial necrosis of the wall of the aorta
   B. Atherosclerotic weakening of the vascular wall

C. Anatomic weakness in the wall of arteries at a branching point
   D. Vasculitis of large arteries
5. Which one of the following is true about thrombophlebitis?
   A. Most instances occur in varicose veins
   B. Most instances occur in the anus and esophagus
   C. Most instances occur in small superficial veins of the legs
   D. Most instances occur in deep veins of the legs
6. True or false? Blood pressure is determined mainly by heart rate.
7. True or false? The innermost part of a blood vessel is the basement membrane.
8. True or false? Plasma lipids circulate attached to C-reactive protein.
9. True or false? Atherosclerosis begins around age 30.
10. True or false? Most aneurysms occur in the abdominal aorta.

Index of Case Studies

The table below is a quick-reference key to the common diseases and disorders discussed in the case studies that appear at the end of each chapter. It is arranged alphabetically by disorder, with cross-references to the case studies that contain information about the condition.

Disease/Disorder	Related Case Study	Page
AIDS	Case 8-1, "I'm afraid I have AIDS."	173
Amniotic fluid embolism	Case 5-1, "She's gone."	83
Angina pectoris	Case 10-1, "My chest feels funny."	229
Barrett metaplasia of the esophagus	Case 2-1, "This heartburn is killing me."	31
Blood glucose testing	Case 1-2, How High Is Up?	12
Bronchopneumonia	Case 9-1, "I knew she was sick when she didn't want a cigarette."	201
Cancer of the cervix	Case 21-1, "I can't get pregnant."	576
Carcinoma of the breast	Case 21-2, "I have a lump in my breast."	578
Carcinoma of the colon	Case 15-1, "I'm in great shape."	384
Cholelithiasis	Case 17-1, "He drinks; I don't."	443
Chronic obstructive pulmonary disease	Case 14-1, Cigarette Asthma	349
Chronic salpingitis	Case 21-1, "I can't get pregnant."	576
Cigarette smoking, effects of	Case 9-1, "I knew she was sick when she didn't want a cigarette."	201
	Case 14-1, Cigarette Asthma	349
Colon cancer	Case 11-1, "I'm tired and short of breath all the time."	266
Diabetes mellitus	Case 4-1, "You'd think I'd know better."	62
	Case 1-2, How High Is Up?	12
Dysplasia	Case 2-1, "This heartburn is killing me."	31
Fibromyalgia	Case 22-1, "The doctor told me I was being poisoned."	609
Glaucoma	Case 25-1, "I'm having a different kind of migraine."	700
Glomerulonephritis, acute	Case 19-1, "His water looks like Coca-Cola."	506
Hepatitis C infection	Case 16-1, "I didn't give it a second thought."	418
Hostility, patient	Case 3-1, "My doctor thinks I'm crazy."	48
Hypertension	Case 12-1, A man found dead in his office	288
Hypothyroidism	Case 18-1, "I'm running out of gas."	475
Infant small for gestational age	Case 7-1, "I thought it would go away."	140
Infertility	Case 21-1, "I can't get pregnant."	576
Influenza	Case 9-1, "I knew she was sick when she didn't want a cigarette."	201

Other Useful Features

The Nature of Disease contains several other unique features that offer quick access to key information.

Index of Case Studies. An alphabetical list of diseases and other clinical topics from the case studies. Cross-referenced by case study and text page number for quick access!

Glossary

This glossary is intended to serve as a quick reference to many of the most important words and phrases commonly encountered in the study of pathology. It does not include all of the boldfaced terms in the text but instead focuses on terms that are often misunderstood or unfamiliar. It also includes some terms that are not boldfaced in the text, especially ones that may be unfamiliar. Definitions of boldfaced terms not included here can be located by referring to the comprehensive main index at the end of this book.

abnormal A measurement or observation not falling into the usual range
abortion Interruption of pregnancy before 20 weeks or 500 grams fetal weight
abrasion Injury to skin that scrapes away epidermis
acetylcholine A neurotransmitter; a molecule released at the ends of nerve fibers that carries the nerve signal across the synapse to cause action on the other side
achalasia Painful esophageal muscle spasms
acid-fast stain A laboratory dye to stain tuberculosis bacilli for diagnosis
acidosis Blood pH that is lower (more acid) than normal
ACTH See *adrenocorticotrophic hormone*
actin One of the two contractile proteins in muscle cells

adrenocorticotrophic hormone (ACTH) The hormone released by the pituitary that stimulates the adrenal cortex to produce and release cortisol and other hormones
aerobic Requiring oxygen for metabolism
afferent arteriole The arteriole bringing blood into the glomerulus
agammaglobulinemia Absence of plasma gamma globulins; an immunodeficiency
agent An infective bacterium, virus, prion, or other object that causes infectious disease
agglutinin Naturally occurring blood group antibodies; anti-A and anti-B
agranulocytosis Marked decrease in the number of blood granulocytes
AIDS Acquired immunodeficiency syndrome
albumin The most abundant blood protein, made by the liver; accounts for most plasma osmotic pressure
aldosterone An adrenocortical hormone that stimulates kidney retention of sodium and water, thereby increasing vascular volume and cardiac output; also stimulates kidney excretion of potassium
alkalosis Blood pH that is higher (more alkaline) than normal
allele One gene of a pair that controls a given trait; one allele inherited from the father, one from the mother

Glossary. Contains definitions of the most important terms and topics discussed in the text.

Acknowledgments

There was a time when I paid little attention to Acknowledgments pages in books. That was then; this is now, and I have an unimagined appreciation for the contributions of people whose name is not on the cover.

This textbook is largely an accident that would not have occurred but for a chain of unlikely events that led me into academia after a career as a practicing pathologist. It began in June 1997 when I answered the phone to hear the voice of Lynn Little, a former employee I'd not heard from in years. He was calling in his capacity as Chairman of the Medical Laboratory Sciences department in the UT Southwestern Allied Health Sciences School. Lynn asked if I would be interested in teaching the required pathology course for health professions students. Being somewhat at loose ends at the time, and having narrowly chosen private practice over academia 30 years earlier, I leapt at the chance.

Almost immediately, I began to worry if I would be accepted in the Department of Pathology or by the Chairman, Errol Friedberg, whom I scarcely knew and who had succeeded my mentor, Vernie Stembridge. To their everlasting credit, Errol and his colleagues graciously accepted me in my teaching role and encouraged this project in every way.

Then came the task of assembling course materials. Beni Stewart, chief guru in the photography lab, guided me through a huge collection of images and in short order helped me assemble the rudiments of a course. In the succeeding years I have called on her time and again as those images began to find their way into this book.

Once I began creating my first outline of pathology for students, pathology residents Reade Quinton and Trey Martin agreed to help by taking new photographs. When the outline grew into a compact textbook, I took the raw project to a pathology department colleague, Jim Richardson, a master teacher, for his advice. His patient, detailed notes on that early manuscript set me on the correct course.

As word spread and other programs began using my materials, I soon found myself in the business of self-publishing. This proved to be so time-consuming that I decided to mail copies of my ring-bound textbook and companion CD to about two dozen editors. A copy landed on John Goucher's desk at Lippincott Williams and Wilkins. It was my lucky day. Several other publishers were interested, but it didn't take long for John and Lippincott to rise to the top of the heap by virtue of plainly evident professionalism.

Then came the formal editorial process, completely new to me, which has proven to be one of the best educational experiences in a lifetime of learning. I fancied myself good with words until I got into the hands of professional editors. It's especially hard on someone with an ego as big as mine, especially about language and literature, to have my carefully crafted sentences disassembled with surgical precision and denuded of excess. David Troy, senior acquisition editor who succeeded John Goucher, oversaw our collective effort. Dana Knighten, senior development editor, presided over the editorial development process with admirable maturity borne of long experience. She answered technical and procedural questions, listened patiently to my rants about politically correct language, kept me on schedule, and offered sound advice and new ideas. Lonnie Christiansen edited the raw manuscript. Her consistent grammatical and structural insights were invaluable. Lastly, Bev Shackelford, copy editor, did far more than merely clean up and coordinate: she spotted critical shortcomings, and her knowledge of medicine, history, grammar, and literary style added gloss to the final product.

Jim McCulley, Chairman of Ophthalmology at UT Southwestern, and his staff furnished many of the photographs of eye disease. A note of thanks is also due to several physician friends in the private sector, each of whom brings an academic mindset to the private practice of medicine. Alan Menter, dermatologist and athlete, allowed me to troll through his collection of dermatology photographs, which constitute the bulk of images in the chapter on skin disease. Bob Kramer, a long-time friend and pediatrician colleague, critiqued the text from his unique perspective. Dee Dockery, radiologist and philosopher, assisted by providing some useful radiographs.

Finally, Sean Hussey, chief pathology resident at UT Southwestern and Parkland Memorial Hospital, agreed to help me with this project. As the project grew, he not only provided some wonderful photographs, but he also read chapters for scientific accuracy and currency. Sean has a way with words, too, and his editorial advice has been invaluable.

Thomas H. McConnell, MD, FCAP
Dallas, Texas

Reviewers

We gratefully acknowledge the generous contributions of the reviewers whose names appear in the list that follows. These instructors were kind enough to read the proposal or the manuscript, or in some cases both, and make thoughtful suggestions for improvement. Their comments determined much of the direction for this text and helped us shape the content to meet the specific needs of health professions students. We hope they will be pleased with the results of their hard work.

Karen Bawel, PhD
University of Southern Indiana
Evansville, Indiana

Carie Braun, PhD
College of St. Benedict/St. John's University
St. Joseph, Minnesota; Collegeville, Minnesota

Patricia Brewer
University of Texas Health Science Center at San
   Antonio
San Antonio, Texas

Bridget Calhoun, MHP, PA-C
Duquesne University
Pittsburgh, Pennsylvania

Linda Ludovico, MS
Tyler Junior College
Tyler, Texas

Kathryn Robinson, MS
University of Texas Health Sciences Center at San
   Antonio
San Antonio, Texas

Barbara Sawyer
Texas Tech University Health Sciences Center
Lubbock, Texas

Margaret Schmidt, EdD, CLS
Duke University
Durham, North Carolina

Terry Powell, BS
Shoreline Community College
Shoreline, Washington

Henry Wormser, PhD
Wayne State University
Detroit, Michigan

Contents

Dedication v

Preface vii

Additional Learning Resources xi

User's Guide xii

Acknowledgments xvi

Reviewers xvii

Guide to Case Studies xxvi

PART 1   GENERAL PATHOLOGY

1   The Nature of Disease: How to Think about Illness 2

2   Cell Injury, Adaptation, and Death 14

3   Inflammation: The Reaction to Injury 34

4   Repair: Recovery from Injury 51

5   Disorders of Fluid Balance and Blood Flow 65

6   Neoplasms 86

7   Developmental, Genetic, and Pediatric Disease 110

8   Diseases of the Immune System 144

9   Infectious Disease 176

10   Disorders of Daily Life and Diet 205

PART 2   DISEASES OF ORGAN SYSTEMS

11   Diseases of Blood Cells and Blood Coagulation 234

12   Diseases of Blood Vessels 270

13   Diseases of the Heart 292

14   Diseases of the Respiratory System 324

15   Diseases of the Gastrointestinal Tract 354

16   Diseases of the Liver and Biliary Tract 389

17   Diseases of the Pancreas 422

18   Diseases of Endocrine Glands 448

19   Diseases of the Kidney 479

20   Diseases of the Lower Urinary Tract and Male Genitalia 509

21   Diseases of the Female Genital Tract and Breast 536

22   Diseases of Bones, Joints, and Skeletal Muscle 581

23   Diseases of the Nervous System 612

24   Diseases of the Skin 648

25   Diseases of the Eye and Ear 677

Glossary 704

Index of Case Studies 723

Index 725

Expanded Contents

Dedication / v
Preface / vii
Additional Learning Resources / xi
User's Guide / xii
Acknowledgments / xvi
Reviewers / xvii
Guide to Case Studies / xxvi

PART 1 GENERAL PATHOLOGY

1   **The Nature of Disease: How to Think about Illness** / 2
The Nature of Disease / 3
Bodily Structure and Function in Disease / 5
Healthy Is Not the Same as Normal; Sick Is Not the Same as Abnormal / 6
Defining Normal / 6
    The Extent of Abnormality / 8
    Test Sensitivity and Specificity / 8
The Usefulness of Tests in Diagnosis / 8
    The Effect of Disease Prevalence on Test Usefulness / 10
    Initial Tests and Follow-up Tests / 10
Disease and Diagnosis / 11

2   **Cell Injury, Adaptation, and Death** / 14
Back to Basics / 15
    The Origins of Cells and the Organization of Tissues / 15
    The Nucleus / 16
    The Cytoplasm / 17
    The Cell Membrane / 20
    The Cell Cycle / 20
    Cellular Communication / 23
Biologic Aging / 24
Cell Injury and Disease / 24
Mild Cell Injury / 26
    Intracellular Accumulations / 26
    Adaptations of Cell Growth and Differentiation / 28
Severe Cell Injury and Cell Death / 29

3   **Inflammation: The Reaction to Injury** / 34
The Inflammatory Response to Injury / 35
The Cellular Response in Inflammation / 36
The Vascular Response in Inflammation / 39
Molecular Mediators of Inflammation / 40
Acute Inflammation / 41
    The Pathogenesis of Acute Inflammation / 41
    The Anatomic Characteristics of Acute Inflammation / 42
    The Consequences of Acute Inflammation / 43

Chronic Inflammation / 44
    The Pathogenesis of Chronic Inflammation / 44
    The Anatomic Characteristics of Chronic Inflammation / 45
    The Consequences of Chronic Inflammation / 45
Distant Effects of Inflammation / 46
    Lymphangitis, Lymphadenitis, and Lymphadenopathy / 46
    Systemic Effects of Inflammation / 46
The Inflammatory Response to Infection / 46

4   **Repair: Recovery from Injury** / 51
Definitions / 52
Replacement of Injured Cells / 52
    The Importance of Tissue Structure / 55
    The Control of Cell Reproduction and Tissue Growth / 56
Wound Healing and Fibrous Repair / 56
    Cell Migration into the Wound / 57
    The Growth of New Blood Vessels / 57
    Scar Development / 57
    Healing by First Intention / 58
    Healing by Second Intention / 59
Abnormal Wound Healing / 61
    Host Factors Interfering with Wound Healing / 61
    Pathologic Wound Healing / 61
Overview of Injury, Inflammation, and Repair / 62

5   **Disorders of Fluid Balance and Blood Flow** / 65
Back to Basics / 66
    Blood Pressure / 66
    Osmotic Pressure / 67
    The Circulation of Blood and Lymph / 68
    The Anatomy of Blood Vessels and Lymphatics / 69
    Body Water and Fluid Compartments / 69
Edema / 72
    Low-protein Edema / 73
    High-protein Edema / 74
    Clinical Aspects of Edema / 74
Hyperemia and Congestion / 74
Hemorrhage, Thrombosis, and Embolism / 75
    Hemorrhage / 75
    Thrombosis / 76
    Embolism / 79
Blood Flow Obstruction / 80
    Infarction / 80
    The Development of an Infarct / 81
The Collapse of Circulation: Shock / 81
    Types of Shock / 81
    Stages of Shock / 82

6   Neoplasms / 86
The Language of Neoplasia / 87
Types of Neoplasms / 89
The Molecular and Genetic Basis of Neoplasia / 90
     Mutations / 90
     Cell Growth Control Genes / 90
     DNA Repair / 91
The Causes of Cancer / 91
The Structure of Neoplasms / 92
     The Gross Anatomy of Neoplasms / 92
     The Microscopic Anatomy of Neoplasms / 93
Premalignant States and Conditions / 94
The Biology of Neoplastic Growth / 95
     The Differentiation of Tumor Cells / 95
     Clones of Cells / 96
     The Speed of Tumor Growth / 96
     The Nourishment of Tumors / 97
     Tumor Cell Variation / 98
The Spread of Neoplasms / 98
The Immune Defense Against Neoplasia / 99
The Epidemiology of Cancer / 100
The Clinical Picture of Cancer / 101
Clinical and Laboratory Assessment of Neoplasms / 101
     Clinical History / 101
     Obtaining Tissues and Cells for Diagnosis / 102
     Grading and Staging of Malignancies / 103
     Early Detection of Cancer / 105
     Tumor Markers / 106

7   Developmental, Genetic, and Pediatric Disease / 110

Section 1: Developmental Abnormalities / 111
Embryologic Development / 112
Congenital Malformations / 114
Congenital Deformations / 115

Section 2: Genetic Disorders / 116
Mutations / 118
The Broad Influence of Genetics in Disease / 118
Disease of Single Genes (Monogenic Disorders) / 119
     Disease Caused by Defective Dominant Autosomal
        Genes / 120
     Disease Caused by Defective Recessive Autosomal
        Genes / 121
     Disease Caused by Defective Genes on Sex Chromo-
        somes / 122
     Clinical Expression of Single-Gene Defects / 122
Cytogenetic Diseases / 125
     Disease Associated with Abnormal Numbers of Au-
        tosomes / 126
     Disease Associated with Abnormal Numbers of Sex
        Chromosomes / 129
Genetic Diagnosis / 130

Section 3: Pediatric Diseases / 132
Perinatal and Neonatal Disease / 132
     Intrauterine Growth Restriction / 134
     Prematurity / 134
     Birth Injury / 136
     Fetal and Newborn Infections / 136
Infections in Children / 136
Sudden Infant Death Syndrome (SIDS) / 137

Hemolytic Disease of the Newborn
     (Erythroblastosis Fetalis) / 137
Cystic Fibrosis / 138
Tumors and Tumor-like Conditions of Children / 139

8   Diseases of the Immune System / 144
Back to Basics / 145
     Nonimmune Defense Mechanisms / 145
     The Normal Immune System / 147
     Immunity in Blood Transfusion / 152
Classification of Immune Disease / 153
Mechanisms of Immune Reaction / 153
     Type 1 Immune Reaction: Immediate
        Hypersensitivity / 154
     Type 2 Immune Reaction: Cytotoxic
        Hypersensitivity / 154
     Type 3 Immune Reaction: Immune-complex Hyper-
        sensitivity / 154
     Type 4 Immune Reaction: Cellular (Delayed) Hyper-
        sensitivity / 158
Hypersensitivity Disease / 159
     Allergic Disease / 159
     Autoimmune Disease / 159
Immunity in Organ and Tissue Transplantation / 164
Immunity in Blood Transfusion / 165
Amyloidosis / 167
Immunodeficiency Diseases / 167
     Inherited Immunodeficiency Diseases / 167
     Acquired Immunodeficiency Syndrome (AIDS) / 168
Malignancies of Immune Cells / 172

9   Infectious Disease / 176
Back to Basics / 177
Infection / 182
Contagion / 184
The Spread of Organisms in Tissue / 185
Mechanisms of Microbiologic Injury / 186
The Inflammatory Response to Infection / 186
Infections of Organ Systems / 186
     Respiratory Infections / 186
     Gastrointestinal Infections / 188
     Genitourinary Infections / 189
     Skin Infections / 191
Infections by Pyogenic Bacteria / 191
Infections by *Clostridium* Organisms and Other Necrotizing
     Agents / 193
Opportunistic and AIDS-related Infections / 193
Tropical, Vector-borne, and Parasite Infections / 194
     Vector-borne Infections / 195
     Parasitic Infections / 195
The Natural Course of an Infection / 197
Signs and Symptoms of Infection / 199
Laboratory Tools / 199

10   Disorders of Daily Life and Diet / 205
Injury Resulting from Trauma / 207
Injury Resulting from Extremes of Temperature / 208
     Thermal Burns / 208
     Cold Injury / 209
     Heat Cramps, Heat Exhaustion, and Heat
        Stroke / 209

Pollution and Occupational Disease / 210
Exposure to Toxic Materials / 211
   Chemicals / 211
   Adverse Reactions to Therapeutic Drugs / 213
   Radiation / 215
   Inhalant Lung Disease / 215
Tobacco, Alcohol, and Drugs / 216
   Cigarette Smoking / 216
   Alcohol Abuse / 217
   Drug Abuse / 219
Nutritional Disease / 221
   Malnutrition / 221
   Obesity / 222
   The Metabolic Syndrome / 227

PART 2 DISEASES OF ORGAN SYSTEMS

11   **Diseases of Blood Cells and Blood Coagulation** / 234

   Section 1: Diseases of Blood Cells / 235
   Back to Basics / 235
      Normal Blood Production (Hematopoiesis) / 236
      Cell Compartments and Life Span / 236
      Laboratory Assessment of Blood Cells / 237
   Too Little Hemoglobin (Anemia) / 240
      The Anemia of Hemorrhage / 240
      Anemia of Red Cell Destruction
         (Hemolytic Anemias) / 241
      Anemia of Insufficient Red Cell Production / 245
   Too Many Red Cells—Polycythemia / 248
   Too Few White Cells—Leukopenia and
      Agranulocytosis / 249
   Too Many White Cells—Benign and Malignant Disorders of
      Leukocytes / 249
      Peripheral Leukocyte Responses to Infection or
         Injury / 250
      Lymph Node Response to Injury or Infection / 251
      Lymphoid Neoplasms / 252
      Myeloid Neoplasms / 257
   Disorders of the Spleen and Thymus / 260

   Section 2: Bleeding Disorders / 260
   Back to Basics / 260
   Bleeding Disorders / 263
      Vascular or Platelet Deficiency / 264
      Coagulation Factor Deficiency / 264
      Disseminated Intravascular Coagulation (DIC) / 265
   Thrombotic Disorders / 266

12   **Diseases of Blood Vessels** / 270
   Back to Basics / 271
      The Normal Vascular System / 271
      Regulation of Blood Pressure / 273
      Lipid Classification and Metabolism / 275
      Desirable Plasma Lipid Concentrations / 275
   Nomenclature of Blood Vessel Disease / 277
   Atherosclerosis / 277
      The Causes and Consequences of
         Atherosclerosis / 277
      The Pathogenesis of Atherosclerosis / 278
      Risk Factors for Atherosclerosis / 279

      The Pathologic Anatomy of Atherosclerosis / 280
      Clinical Manifestations of Atherosclerosis / 281
   Hypertension / 282
      Types of Hypertension / 283
      Pathogenesis of Hypertension / 283
      The Pathology of Hypertension / 283
      Clinical Aspects of Hypertension / 284
   Aneurysms and Dissections / 285
   Vasculitis / 286
   Raynaud Phenomenon / 286
   Diseases of Veins / 287
   Tumors of Blood and Lymphatic Vessels / 287

13   **Diseases of the Heart** / 292
   Back to Basics / 293
      The Normal Heart / 293
      The Coronary Circulation / 294
      The Cardiac Cycle / 295
   Arrhythmias / 297
   Congestive Heart Failure / 298
      Pathophysiology / 298
      Etiology / 300
      Clinical Features / 300
   Ischemic Heart Disease (Coronary Artery Disease) / 302
      Epidemiology of Ischemic Heart Disease / 302
      Causes of Coronary Ischemia / 303
      Angina Pectoris / 304
      Myocardial Infarction / 304
      Chronic Myocardial Ischemia / 307
      Sudden Cardiac Death / 308
   Hypertensive Heart Disease / 309
   Valvular Heart Disease / 309
      Rheumatic Heart Disease / 309
      Calcific Aortic Stenosis / 310
      Myxomatous Degeneration of the Mitral Valve / 312
   Endocarditis / 312
      Nonbacterial Thrombotic Endocarditis / 312
      Infective Endocarditis / 313
   Primary Myocardial Diseases / 314
      Myocarditis / 314
      Cardiomyopathies / 314
   Congenital Heart Disease / 315
      Malformations With Shunts / 315
      Malformations With Obstruction to Flow / 318
      Pericardial Disease / 319

14   **Diseases of the Respiratory System** / 324
   Back to Basics / 325
      The Normal Respiratory Tract / 325
      Lung Volume, Air Flow, and Gas Exchange / 328
   Diseases of the Upper Respiratory Tract / 330
   Atelectasis (Collapse) / 330
   Obstructive Lung Disease / 331
      Asthma / 331
      Chronic Obstructive Pulmonary Disease (COPD) / 332
   Restrictive Lung Disease / 335
      Interstitial Fibrosis without Granulomatous Inflam-
         mation / 336
      Interstitial Fibrosis with Granulomatous
         Inflammation / 336

Vascular and Circulatory Lung Disease / 336
    Pulmonary Edema / 337
    Pulmonary Thromboembolism / 337
    Pulmonary Hypertension / 337
    Adult Respiratory Distress Syndrome / 338
Pulmonary Infections / 339
    Pneumonia / 339
    Lung Abscess / 341
    Pulmonary Tuberculosis / 341
    Pulmonary Fungus Infections (Deep Mycoses) / 345
    Other Lung Infections / 346
Lung Neoplasms / 347
    Bronchogenic Carcinoma / 347
    Bronchial Carcinoid Tumor / 349
Diseases of the Pleura / 349

15   Diseases of the Gastrointestinal Tract / 354
Back to Basics / 355
    The Mouth and Esophagus / 358
    The Stomach / 358
    The Small Intestine / 358
    The Large Bowel / 359
    Intestinal Bacteria / 359
Intestinal Bleeding / 359
Intestinal Obstruction and Ileus / 361
Diseases of the Oral Cavity / 361
Diseases of Salivary Glands / 365
Diseases of the Esophagus / 365
Diseases of the Stomach / 367
    Gastritis / 367
    Gastric and Duodenal Ulcers / 367
    Carcinoma of the Stomach / 369
Nonneoplastic Diseases of the Small Bowel and Large
    Bowel / 369
    Congenital Anomalies / 369
    Vascular Diseases / 370
    Diarrheal Diseases / 371
    Malabsorption Syndromes / 374
    Inflammatory Bowel Disease / 374
    Colonic Diverticulosis and Other Conditions / 377
Peritonitis / 379
Neoplasms of the Large and Small Bowel / 379
    Nonneoplastic Polyps / 380
    Neoplastic Polyps (Adenomas) / 380
    Carcinoma of the Colon / 381
Diseases of the Appendix / 384

16   Diseases of the Liver and Biliary Tract / 389
Back to Basics / 390
    Liver Anatomy / 392
    Liver Function / 392
The Liver Response to Injury / 394
    Anatomic Patterns of Liver Injury / 394
    Functional Patterns of Liver Injury / 394
Cirrhosis / 397
    Anatomic Types of Cirrhosis / 398
    The Pathophysiology of Cirrhosis / 398
    Clinical Features of Cirrhosis / 398
Viral Hepatitis / 401
    Clinicopathologic Syndromes / 402
    Hepatitis A Virus (HAV) Infection / 402
    Hepatitis B Virus (HBV) Infection / 404

    Hepatitis C Virus (HCV) Infection / 406
    Hepatitis D Virus (HDV) Infection / 406
    Hepatitis E virus (HEV) Infection / 406
    The Anatomic Pathology of Hepatitis /407
Autoimmune Hepatitis / 407
Liver Abscess / 408
Toxic Liver Injury / 408
Alcoholic Liver Disease / 408
    Fatty Liver / 409
    Alcoholic Hepatitis / 410
    Alcoholic Cirrhosis / 410
Inherited Metabolic and Pediatric Liver Disease / 410
    Hemochromatosis / 410
    Wilson Disease / 412
    Hereditary Alpha-1 Antitrypsin Deficiency / 412
    Neonatal Cholestasis, Biliary Atresia, and
        Hepatitis / 412
    Reye syndrome / 412
Disease of Intrahepatic Bile Ducts / 413
    Primary Biliary Cirrhosis / 413
    Primary Sclerosing Cholangitis / 413
Circulatory Disorders / 413
Tumors of the Liver / 414
    Primary Carcinomas of the Liver / 414
    Cholangiocarcinoma / 415
Diseases of the Gallbladder and Extrahepatic Bile
    Ducts / 415
    Diseases of the Gallbladder / 415
    Diseases of Extrahepatic Bile Ducts / 417

17   Diseases of the Pancreas / 422
Back to Basics / 423
    The Digestive (Exocrine) Pancreas / 423
    The Hormonal (Endocrine) Pancreas / 424
Diseases of the Digestive (Exocrine) Pancreas / 427
    Pancreatitis / 427
    Carcinoma of the Pancreas / 431
Diseases of the Hormonal (Endocrine) Pancreas / 433
    Diabetes Mellitus / 433
    Pancreatic Endocrine Neoplasms / 442

18   Diseases of Endocrine Glands / 448
Back to Basics / 449
    Homeostasis / 449
    The Pituitary Gland / 450
    The Thyroid Gland / 452
    The Parathyroid Glands / 453
    The Adrenal Glands / 454
Diseases of the Pituitary Gland / 455
    Diseases Affecting the Anterior Pituitary / 455
    Disease of the Posterior Pituitary / 458
Diseases of the Thyroid Gland / 459
    Overactivity of the Thyroid Gland
        (Hyperthyroidism) / 459
    Underactivity of the Thyroid Gland
        (Hypothyroidism) / 462
    Goiter / 463
    Thyroiditis / 463
    Neoplasms of the Thyroid Gland / 464
Diseases of the Parathyroid Glands / 465
    Overactivity of the Parathyroid Glands (Hyper-
        parathyroidism) / 465

Underactivity of the Parathyroid Glands (Hypoparathyroidism) / 467
Diseases of the Adrenal Gland / 468
    Diseases of the Adrenal Cortex / 468
    Diseases of the Adrenal Medulla / 474

19 Diseases of the Kidney / 479
Back to Basics / 480
    Renal Function / 480
    The Normal Glomerulus / 483
    Formation of the Glomerular Filtrate / 484
    Tubular Processing of the Glomerular Filtrate / 485
The Language of Renal Disease / 486
Normal Urine and Urinalysis / 487
Clinical Syndromes of Renal Disease / 490
Inherited, Congenital, and Developmental Disease / 493
Glomerular Disease / 494
    The Initiation and Progression of Glomerular Disease / 494
    Glomerulonephritis / 494
    Secondary Glomerular Disease / 498
Diseases of Renal Vasculature / 498
Acute Tubular Necrosis / 499
Tubulointerstitial Nephritis / 500
    Obstruction, Reflux, and Stasis / 500
    Pyelonephritis and Urinary Tract Infection / 500
    Drugs, Toxins, and Other Causes of Tubulointerstitial Nephritis / 503
Renal Stones / 503
Tumors of the Kidney / 505

20 Diseases of the Lower Urinary Tract and Male Genitalia / 509
Back to Basics / 510
Diseases of the Lower Urinary Tract / 514
    Congenital Anomalies / 514
    Urinary Obstruction, Reflux, and Stasis / 514
    Infection and Inflammation / 515
    Neoplasms / 516
Diseases of the Male Genitalia / 517
    Erectile Dysfunction and Infertility / 517
    Diseases of the Penis and Urethra / 517
    Diseases of the Scrotum and Groin / 518
    Diseases of the Testis and Epididymis / 519
    Diseases of the Prostate / 520
Sexually Transmitted Disease / 525
    Syphilis / 525
    Gonorrhea / 530
    Nongonococcal Urethritis / 531
    Genital Herpes and Other Sexually Transmitted Diseases / 531

21 Diseases of the Female Genital Tract and Breast / 536

Section 1: Diseases of the Female Genital Tract / 537
Back to Basics / 537
    The Pituitary-Ovarian Cycle / 540
    Ovulation / 540
    The Menstrual Cycle / 542
Menopause / 543
Sexually Transmitted Disease / 544
Vaginitis and Other Vaginal Conditions / 545

Vulvar Disease / 545
Diseases of the Cervix / 546
    Ectropion, Polyps, and Cervicitis / 548
    Dysplasia and Carcinoma of the Cervix / 549
Diseases of the Endometrium and Myometrium / 554
    Abnormal Endometrial Bleeding / 555
    Endometriosis / 555
    Endometrial Polyps, Hyperplasia, and Adenocarcinoma / 556
    Other Conditions of the Uterus and Pelvis / 558
Diseases of the Fallopian Tube / 560
Diseases of the Ovary / 560
    Nonneoplastic Ovarian Cysts / 560
    Tumors of the Ovary / 561
Diseases of Reproduction / 565
    Infertility / 565
    Ectopic Pregnancy and Abortion / 565
    Placental Disease / 566

Section 2: Diseases of the Breast / 568
Back to Basics / 568
Inflammatory Disease / 569
Fibrocystic Change / 569
Benign Tumors / 571
Breast Cancer / 571
    Types of Breast Cancer / 572
    Factors Affecting the Risk of Developing Breast Cancer / 573
    Prognostic Factors for Patients with Breast Cancer / 574
    Clinical Presentation and Behavior / 574
    Diagnosis and Treatment / 575
Diseases of the Male Breast / 576

22 Diseases of Bones, Joints, and Skeletal Muscle / 581

Section 1: Diseases of Bone / 582
Back to Basics / 582
Skeletal Deformities and Disorders of Bone Growth / 585
Fractures / 585
Bone Infection / 587
Bone Infarct / 589
Osteoporosis / 589
Osteomalacia / 591
Bone Tumors / 591
    Bone-forming Tumors / 592
    Cartilage-forming Tumors / 593
    Fibrous Tumors and Tumor-like Conditions / 593
    Other Tumors of Bone / 594

Section 2: Diseases of Joints and Related Tissues / 594
Back to Basics / 594
Osteoarthritis / 595
Rheumatoid Arthritis / 596
Spondyloarthropathies / 599
Other Types of Arthritis / 600
Injuries to Ligaments, Tendons, and Joints / 601
Periarticular Pain Syndromes / 601
Tumors and Tumor-like Lesions of Joints / 602

Section 3: Diseases of Skeletal Muscle / 603
Back to Basics / 603
Muscle Atrophy / 605
Muscular Dystrophy / 606

Myositis and Myopathy / 606
Myasthenia Gravis / 607
Tumors and Tumor-like Lesions of Soft Tissue / 608

23   Diseases of the Nervous System / 612
Back to Basics / 613
    The Central Nervous System / 613
    Vascular Supply / 618
    The Peripheral Nervous System / 618
    The Autonomic Nervous System / 619
    Cells of the Nervous System / 620
    Nerve Cell Connections and Signals / 622
Congenital and Perinatal Disease / 624
Increased Intracranial Pressure / 624
Intracranial Hemorrhage / 627
    Bleeding on the Surface of the Brain / 627
    Bleeding Directly Into the Brain / 630
Ischemia and Infarction / 630
Brain and Spinal Cord Trauma / 633
Infections of the Central Nervous System / 633
    Infections of the Meninges and Cerebrospinal
        Fluid / 634
    Infections of Brain Parenchyma / 636
Degenerative Diseases / 637
    Degenerative Diseases of Gray Matter / 637
    Degenerative Diseases of White Matter / 639
Metabolic and Toxic Disorders / 639
Neoplasms / 640
Diseases of Peripheral Nerves / 642
    Neuropathies / 643
    Neoplasms / 643

24   Diseases of the Skin / 648
Back to Basics / 649

Section 1: Nonneoplastic Diseases of Skin / 651
The Uniqueness of Skin Disease / 651
General Conditions of Skin / 652
    The Effects of Sunlight / 652
    The Effects of Pregnancy / 652
    Disorders of Hair Growth / 652
The Skin in Systemic Disease / 654
Diseases of the Epidermis / 656
    Disorders of Pigmentation / 656
    Other Diseases of the Epidermis / 658

Diseases of the Basement Membrane Zone / 659
Diseases of the Dermis / 660
    Noncontact Dermatitis / 660
    Contact Dermatitis / 661
Inflammatory Diseases of Subcuticular Fat / 663
Acne / 663
Infections and Infestations / 664

Section 2: Neoplasms of Skin / 665
Tumors of the Epidermis / 665
    Keratoses / 666
    Malignant Tumors of the Epidermis / 668
Tumors of Subepidermal Tissue / 669
Tumors of Melanocytes / 670
    Nevi / 670
    Malignant Melanoma / 671

25   Diseases of the Eye and Ear / 677

Section 1: Diseases of the Eye / 678
Back to Basics / 678
    The Anterior Segment / 679
    The Posterior Segment / 680
Disorders of Alignment and Movement / 682
Disorders of Refraction / 682
Disorders of the Orbit / 684
Disorders of the Eyelid, Conjunctiva, Sclera, and
    Lacrimal Apparatus / 684
Disorders of the Cornea / 685
Cataract / 686
Disorders of the Uveal Tract / 687
Disorders of the Retina and Vitreous
    Humor / 689
Disorders of the Optic Nerve / 692
Glaucoma / 693
Neoplasms / 695

Section 2: Diseases of the Ear / 696
Back to Basics / 696
Disorders of the External Ear / 697
Disorders of the Middle Ear / 698
Disorders of the Inner Ear / 699
Deafness / 699

Glossary / 704
Index of Case Studies / 723
Index / 725

Guide to Case Studies

Case studies bring the chapter to life. The case studies in this book are built from the details of actual patients' experiences. By demonstrating hands-on application of concepts, case studies give a realistic glimpse of work in a clinical setting. The following guide is a handy chapter-by-chapter reference that shows at a glance the topics that each case centers around: diseases, disorders, testing, and other relevant clinical considerations.

At the end of this text, the **Index of Case Studies** provides another way to locate cases quickly. It is arranged alphabetically by the topics listed below and is located immediately before the main index.

Chapter 1	The Nature of Disease: How to Think About Illness
Case Study 1-1	A Diagnosis Missed and a Diagnosis Made
	<u>Topics</u>: Acute otitis media, acute meningitis, and test sensitivity and specificity
Case Study 1-2	How High Is Up?
	<u>Topics</u>: Test sensitivity and specificity, blood glucose testing, diagnosis of diabetes mellitus

Chapter 2	Cell Injury, Adaptation, and Death
Case Study 2-1	"This Heartburn is Killing Me"
	<u>Topics</u>: Metaplasia, dysplasia, Barrett metaplasia of the esophagus

Chapter 3	Inflammation: The Reaction to Injury
Case Study 3-1	"My Doctor Thinks I'm Crazy"
	<u>Topics</u>: Hostile reactions in patients, polymyalgia rheumatica

Chapter 4	Repair: Recovery from Injury
Case Study 4-1	"You'd Think I'd Know Better"
	<u>Topics</u>: Diabetes mellitus, peripheral vascular disease, wound healing

Chapter 5	Disorders of Fluid Balance and Blood Flow
Case Study 5-1	"She's Gone"
	<u>Topics</u>: Shock, amniotic fluid embolism

Chapter 6	Neoplasms
Case Study 6-1	"I Have a Chest Cold That Won't Go Away"
	<u>Topics</u>: Lung cancer, paraneoplastic syndrome

Chapter 7	Developmental, Genetic, and Pediatric Disease
Case Study 7-1	"I Thought it Would Go Away"
	<u>Topics</u>: Uterine infection, premature birth, infant small for gestational age, respiratory distress syndrome of the newborn

Chapter 8	Diseases of the Immune System
Case Study 8-1	"I'm Afraid I Have AIDS"
	<u>Topics</u>: AIDS, opportunistic infections

Chapter 9	Infectious Diseases
Case Study 9-1	"I Knew She Was Sick When She Didn't Want a Cigarette"
	<u>Topics</u>: Effects of cigarette smoking, influenza, bronchopneumonia

Chapter 10	Disorders of Daily Life and Diet
Case Study 10-1	"My Chest Feels Funny"
	<u>Topics</u>: Angina pectoris, obesity, metabolic syndrome

Chapter 11	Diseases of Blood Cells and Blood Coagulation
Case Study 11-1	"I'm Tired and Short of Breath All the Time"
	<u>Topics</u>: Intestinal bleeding, iron deficiency anemia, colon cancer

Chapter 12
Case Study 12-1
Diseases of Blood Vessels
A Man Found Dead in His Office
Topics: Hypertension, stroke, patient compliance with health care directions

Chapter 13
Case Study 13-1
Diseases of the Heart
"He's Been Having a Lot of Heartburn Lately"
Topic: Acute myocardial infarction

Chapter 14
Case Study 14-1
Diseases of the Respiratory System
Cigarette Asthma
Topics: Chronic obstructive pulmonary disease, effects of cigarette smoking, pneumonia, nosocomial infection

Chapter 15
Case Study 15-1
Diseases of the Gastrointestinal Tract
"I'm in Great Shape"
Topic: Carcinoma of the colon

Chapter 16
Case Study 16-1
Diseases of the Liver and Biliary Tract
"I Didn't Give it a Second Thought."
Topic: Hepatitis C infection

Chapter 17
Case Study 17-1
Diseases of the Pancreas
"He Drinks; I Don't"
Topics: Cholelithiasis, acute pancreatitis
Case Study 17-2
"I Don't Know What's Come Over Him; He's Acting Crazy"
Topics: Diabetes, diabetic ketoacidosis

Chapter 18
Case Study 18-1
Diseases of Endocrine Glands
"I'm Running Out of Gas"
Topic: Hypothyroidism

Chapter 19
Case Study 19-1
Diseases of the Kidney
"His Water Looks Like Coca-Cola"
Topics: Streptococcal pharyngitis, acute glomerulonephritis

Chapter 20
Case Study 20-1
Diseases of the Lower Urinary Tract and Male Genitalia
"A Spider Bit Me"
Topic: Syphilis

Chapter 21
Case Study 21-1
Diseases of the Female Genital Tract and Breast
"I Can't Get Pregnant"
Topics: Infertility, sexually transmitted disease, chronic salpingitis, cancer of the cervix
Case Study 21-2
"I Have a Lump in My Breast"
Topic: Carcinoma of the breast

Chapter 22
Case Study 22-1
Diseases of Bones, Joints, and Skeletal Muscle
"The Doctor Told Me I was Being Poisoned"
Topic: Fibromyalgia

Chapter 23
Case Study 23-1
Diseases of the Nervous System
"Something Doesn't Seem Right in My Head"
Topic: Stroke

Chapter 24
Case Study 24-1
Diseases of the Skin
"She Fries Easier Than Bacon"
Topic: Malignant melanoma

Chapter 25
Case Study 25-1
Diseases of the Eye and Ear
"I'm Having a Different Kind of Migraine"
Topic: Glaucoma
Case Study 25-2
"JuJu Has a Fever"
Topic: Otitis media

General Pathology

The chapters in Part 1 focus on the pathology of basic physiologic processes and conditions that can affect any tissue, organ, or system of organs.

Chapter 1 The Nature of Disease: How to Think About Illness
Discusses the different meanings of the words "healthy" versus "normal" and "sick" versus "abnormal." Explains how to use clinical, laboratory, and other information to determine who is sick and who is not.

Chapter 2 Cell Injury, Adaptation, and Death
Discusses the natural and pathologic life and death of cells and how they change with disease.

Chapter 3 Inflammation: The Reaction to Injury
Explores the body's reaction to tissue damage (injury), which is the cause of all disease.

Chapter 4 Repair: Recovery from Injury
Focuses on how cells regenerate to replace damaged tissue, or mend tissue if regeneration is not possible.

Chapter 5 Disorders of Fluid Balance and Blood Flow
Reviews osmotic pressure, blood pressure, the movement of blood and other fluids in the body. Discusses the causes and consequences of abnormal accumulations of fluid and the causes and consequences of interruptions of blood flow.

Chapter 6 Neoplasms
Discusses how neoplasms are named, their molecular basis, the control and loss of control of normal cell growth, and the growth and biology of neoplasms as well as their diagnosis and clinical behavior.

Chapter 7 Developmental, Genetic, and Pediatric Disease
Focuses on fetal defects; strictly inherited diseases and familial genetic disease tendencies; and the distinctiveness of diseases of infancy and childhood.

Chapter 8 Disease of the Immune System
Reviews the normal, protective immune system; discusses the immune system's overreaction to outside agents (allergy), the anti-self reactions of autoimmune diseases, the acquired immunodeficiency syndrome (AIDS) and other immune defects, and malignancies of the immune system.

Chapter 9 Infectious Disease
Reviews the different varieties of infectious agents and discusses their spread and effects in the body, their spread from person to person, and the clinical nature and diagnosis of infection.

Chapter 10 Disorders of Daily Life and Diet
Discusses the adverse effects of habits, workplace conditions and activities, environment, and improper nutrition.

CHAPTER 1

The Nature of Disease: How to Think about Illness

This chapter discusses the different meanings of the words "healthy" versus "normal" and "sick" versus "abnormal." It also explains how to use clinical, laboratory, and other information to determine who is sick and who is not.

THE NATURE OF DISEASE
BODILY STRUCTURE AND FUNCTION IN DISEASE
HEALTHY IS NOT THE SAME AS NORMAL; SICK IS NOT
   THE SAME AS ABNORMAL
DEFINING NORMAL
* The Extent of Abnormality
* Test Sensitivity and Specificity

THE USEFULNESS OF TESTS IN DIAGNOSIS
* The Effect of Disease Prevalence on Test Usefulness
* Initial Tests and Follow-up Tests
DISEASE AND DIAGNOSIS

Learning Objectives

After studying this chapter you should be able to:
1. Define the following terms: disease, etiology, pathogenesis, lesion, and pathophysiology
2. Explain the difference between anatomic and clinical pathology
3. Describe the relationship between structure and function
4. Differentiate between a symptom and a sign
5. Explain the meaning of normal, abnormal, healthy, and sick
6. Describe the differences among true positive, false positive, true negative, and false negative tests
7. Explain the meaning of normal range as it relates to medical tests
8. Explain the meaning of test sensitivity and test specificity
9. Explain the concept of the predictive value of test results
10. Discuss why sensitive tests should be used first in the diagnostic process
11. Differentiate between prevalence and incidence
12. Explain why it is usually futile to test for disease in a population in which the prevalence of disease is very low

Be careful about reading health books. You may die of a misprint.

MARK TWAIN (SAMUEL LANGHORNE CLEMENS) (1835–1910), AMERICAN NOVELIST AND HUMORIST

The Nature of Disease

Webster's Online Dictionary (2004) defines "nature" and "disease" as follows:

Nature (noun): The essential qualities or characteristics by which something is recognized.

Disease (noun): An impairment of health or a condition of abnormal functioning.

True to its title, this textbook focuses on the essential characteristics of impaired health.

The nature of impaired health (disease) is revealed best by contrasting it with normal anatomy and physiology. With this in mind, every chapter in this book includes a review of the anatomy and physiology of health, in order to contrast it with disease. Most chapters open with a special feature called *Back to Basics,* a narrative overview of normal anatomy and physiology. Where this is impractical, normal anatomy and physiology basics are woven into the narrative along with the pathology. Another special feature in many chapters is

the *Basics in Brief* box, a brief, focused description of basic concepts that will help in understanding the specific pathology discussed within a chapter.

All **disease** occurs as a result of injury; disease is, therefore, an unhealthy state caused by the effects of injury. All disease is either acute or chronic. **Acute disease** arises rapidly, is accompanied by distinctive symptoms, and lasts a short time. For example, a bacterial infection in a child's middle ear, *acute otitis media* (Chapter 25), begins suddenly, is accompanied by specific signs and symptoms: ear pain and fever, and lasts a few days. **Chronic disease** usually begins slowly, with signs and symptoms that are difficult to interpret, persists for a long time, and generally cannot be prevented by vaccines or cured by medication. For example, the onset of wear and tear arthritis (osteoarthritis, Chapter 22) begins with vague stiffness or aches in certain joints, progresses slowly, cannot be cured (but can be treated), and lasts a lifetime.

Pathology is the study of changes in bodily *structure* and *function* that occur as a result of disease. The purpose of the discipline of pathology is to discover the etiology (cause) of the injury (disease), understand the **pathogenesis** (natural history and development), explain the **pathophysiology** (the manner in which the incorrect function is expressed), and describe the **lesion** (the structural abnormality produced by injury). If etiology is unknown, the disease is said to be **idiopathic**. If the disease is a byproduct of medical diagnosis or treatment it is said to be **iatrogenic** (from Greek *iatros*, for physician).

For example, the etiology of sunburn is excessive exposure to sunlight. The pathogenesis of sunburn is absorbtion of high-energy ultraviolet (UV) rays, which injure skin. The pathophysiology is characterized by blood vessel dilation and increased blood flow, both of which are part of the reaction to the injury. The lesion is red, swollen, hot, painful skin. Case Study 1-1 at the end of this chapter, "A Diagnosis Missed and a Diagnosis Made," illustrates these concepts in an actual case history.

Anatomic pathology is the study of structural changes caused by disease. Assessment of tissue speci-mens, such as biopsy or autopsy material, by the unaided eye is **gross examination**; assessment of magnified images of small structures is **microscopic examination**. The most extensive and basic gross examination is an **autopsy**, an after-death (post mortem) dissection of a body to determine the cause of death and other facts about the condition of the patient at the time of death. On a smaller scale, microscopic study of tissues and cells in a breast biopsy or Pap smear also is an anatomic pathology procedure. Refer to the nearby Lab Tools box to see how tissue specimens are prepared for study.

Clinical pathology is the study of the functional aspects of disease by laboratory study of tissue, blood, urine, or other body fluids. Examples include blood glucose measurement to diagnose diabetes or culture of urine to detect bacterial infection. Clinical pathology extends from the lab to the bedside, too. A pathologist who supervises the performance of a laboratory test, such as a blood aldosterone assay, and consults with another physician about the results is practicing clinical pathology.

LAB TOOLS

What Happens Before a Biopsy Specimen Slide Goes Under the Microscope?

Microscopic study requires very thin slices of tissue; thin enough to be transparent, usually less than one cell thick. In such thin slices there is not enough pigment present to give cells color, just as a glass of water from the deep blue sea is almost colorless. Cells have natural color to the unaided eye: muscle is reddish brown, brain is grey and white, red blood cells are red, liver is brown, and so on. Nevertheless, in very thin slices for microscopic study, color must be added to make cells visible.

Consider a specimen from a breast biopsy. The surgeon puts the raw lump of tissue in formaldehyde to cure it (somewhat like leather) and kill any bacteria that might cause decay during lab processing. A 1-cm to 2-cm sample is selected by the pathologist for further processing and is placed in a series of chemicals to soak out the fat and water, both of which render tissue fuzzy and blurry under the microscope. Next, the piece is immersed in hot paraffin wax, which soaks into the specimen to take the place of the missing fat and water. The paraffinized piece is chilled and becomes hard enough for very thin slicing by a highly precise instrument. A slice is laid flat on a slide and dipped in a se-ries of chemicals to remove the paraffin, leaving behind on the slide surface an exceedingly thin layer of waterless, fat-free tissue; all that remains is protein, carbohydrate, and minerals. This is then dipped in a series of chemicals that stain cell nuclei blue and cytoplasm red. Collagen, calcium, and other interstitial materials stain red or blue or reddish blue depending on individual characteristics. Places where fat and water used to be are empty and colorless.

Pathologists, or other specialists with microscopic expertise, study the tissue searching for patterns of disease—inflammation, degeneration, peculiar-looking cells, and so on.

In addition to ordinary microscopic study, special techniques can highlight certain cell characteristics and make them microscopically visible. An example is detection of estrogen-receptor molecules in breast cancer cells. The presence or absence of estrogen receptors is important in crafting the best therapy for breast cancer. The technique requires treating a thin slice of raw tumor tissue with antibodies and chemicals, the combination of which causes a colored precipitate to accumulate in breast cancer cells if estrogen receptors are present in them.

Bodily Structure and Function in Disease

Structure and function are intimately related in health and in disease—alteration of one results in alteration of the other. A **structural disorder**, or defect in form, leads to a **functional disorder**. For example, bacterial infection of the mitral heart valve may eat a hole (a structural abnormality) in the valve (Fig. 1-1). With each ventricular contraction the hole allows backflow of blood into the left atrium. This inefficiency causes the heart to perform extra work to move the required amount of blood. This extra labor can lead to heart exhaustion (congestive heart failure), a functional disorder discussed in Chapter 13.

Likewise, a functional disorder may lead to structural change. For example, high blood pressure is a functional disorder that puts excessive strain on heart muscle, which enlarges like any other muscle subjected to hard work. The abnormally enlarged heart muscle is a structural disorder that has arisen from a functional disorder (Fig. 1-2).

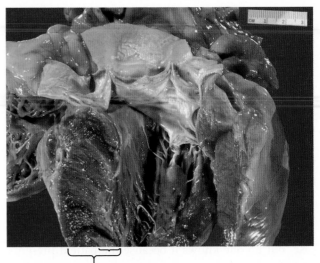

Thickened heart muscle
⎵ = Normal thickness

Figure 1-2 **Initial functional disorder.** High blood pressure is the initial functional disorder. Pumping against abnormally high pressure puts excess strain on the left ventricle. The result is thickening of heart muscle—a structural disorder.

Holes in mitral valve

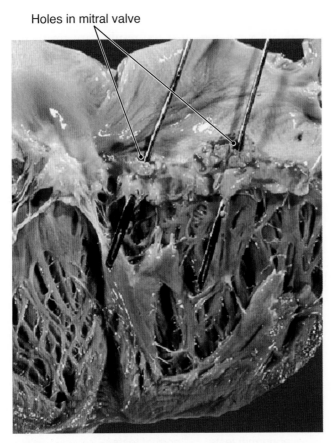

Figure 1-1 **Initial structural disorder.** Holes eaten in the mitral valve by bacteria are the initial structural defect. The result is regurgitation (backflow) of blood into the atrium—a functional disorder.

With the notable exception of many psychiatric disorders, all disease is associated with structural or functional abnormality. Our inability to demonstrate a chemical or anatomic defect in, for example, schizophrenia, does not necessarily reflect the actual state of things in the brain, but rather the limits of current science—patients with mental disorders have diseased brains in ways that are largely invisible to science.

Diseases present themselves by causing observable and measurable changes in the appearance (form) or performance (function) of cells, tissues, and organs. Alterations of form (a mass in the neck) and function (difficulty breathing) are assessed by recording a medical history, performing a physical examination, and collecting scientific data by laboratory tests, x-rays, and other means.

Symptoms are complaints reported by the patient or by someone else on behalf of the patient and are a part of the medical history. **Signs** are direct observations by an examiner (e.g., nurse, physician assistant, physician). For example, diarrhea reported by the patient is a symptom, whereas diarrhea observed by the examiner is a sign. Scientific data are a third way in which disease may make itself known. A collection of clinical signs, symptoms, and data is a **syndrome**. A particular syndrome may be caused by different diseases. For example, Cushing syndrome results from excess steroids, which may be caused by medical treatment, adrenal hyperplasia, or pituitary tumor.

Healthy Is Not the Same as Normal; Sick Is Not the Same as Abnormal

Sickness (disease) and **health** (wellness) are words that refer to the actual presence or absence of disease and do *not* refer to symptoms, signs, laboratory test results, x-rays, or scientific studies. That is to say, a person is either healthy or sick according to whether or not disease is *actually* present. For example, a person with an early lung cancer may be free of signs and symptoms and have a completely normal physical exam, chest radiographs, and laboratory tests. Such a person has a disease, but no one knows it because the patient presents with no signs or symptoms; that is, no structural or functional defect is *detectable*.

To the contrary, **normal** and **abnormal** describe the results of *measurements* or *observations* (physical examination, history, tests) used to determine whether disease is present. Most sick patients have abnormal (unusual) measurements or observations produced as a result of the disease, while most healthy patients have normal (usual) measurements or observations. For example, most patients with untreated diabetes have abnormally high fasting blood glucose levels, and most healthy persons without diabetes have normal (neither too high nor too low) blood glucose levels. However, *sometimes sick patients have normal test results and sometimes healthy patients have abnormal test results.* Figure 1-3 depicts these concepts.

Tests for a particular disease are often referred to as *positive* if abnormal and *negative* if normal. Presuming

> **Abnormal but Not Sick.** By any standard, shoe size 17 EEE is big. It may be normal for a 6′ 10″, 350 lb. man, but for a 5′ 2″ 105 lb. woman it would be highly abnormal. However, even in a small woman, such a foot, though very abnormal, is not necessarily sick; it may function normally and be perfectly healthy.

we know by other means whether the patient is sick or well, test results for a particular disease are referred to as **true positive** if the test is positive and the patient actually has the disease. Conversely, the test is referred to as **false positive** if the test is positive but the patient does *not* have the disease. That is to say, a true positive test correctly indicates that disease is present, whereas a false positive test incorrectly suggests disease is present when, in fact, it is not. Likewise, in regard to a particular disease, negative results are referred to as **true negative** or **false negative**, depending on whether the test result correctly or incorrectly indicates that disease is absent. These combinations are depicted in grid form in Table 1-1.

Defining Normal

Laboratory, x-ray, and other test results vary greatly for healthy people just as do height, weight, foot size, and other physical features. As offered in the nearby Key Points example of a small woman with an extremely large shoe size, some healthy people may have unusually low or high results that do not signify disease—the abnormal results merely reflect variation among indi-

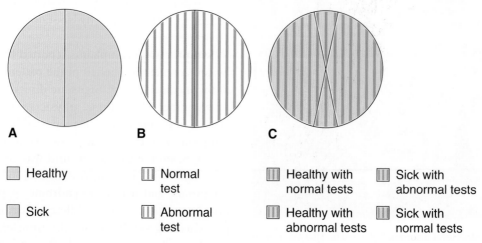

Figure 1-3 **Healthy or sick, normal or abnormal, and how they combine. A.** All patients are either healthy or sick. **B.** All measurements (tests) are either normal or abnormal. **C.** Some healthy patients have abnormal test results, and some sick patients have normal test results.

Table 1-1	**Test Results: True and False, Positive and Negative**	
	Normal Test	**Abnormal Test**
HEALTHY	Healthy patient with normal test result: **True negative**	Healthy patient with abnormal test: **False positive**
Example: People without diabetes	Normal fasting blood glucose level: *Diagnosis—no diabetes*	High fasting blood glucose level: *Perhaps patient not really fasting*
SICK	Sick patient with normal test result: **False negative**	Sick patient with abnormal test result: **True positive**
Example: People with untreated diabetes	Normal fasting blood glucose level: *Perhaps lab error*	High fasting blood glucose level: *Diagnosis—diabetes*

viduals. These variations of normal require that we establish a definition of normal. For our purposes "normal" means "the usual result in health."

A **normal range** (*reference range*) is established for quantitative tests that have numerical results. At the low end is the *lower limit of normal*; at the upper end is the *upper limit of normal*. For example, the normal (reference) range for blood glucose levels in most laboratories is 70–110 mg/dL. Results outside of this range are considered to be abnormally low or high.

For qualitative results there is no need for a range: the test is either positive (abnormal) or negative (normal). For example, if a patient has clinical evidence of liver disease, a test for hepatitis virus may be done. If the test is positive, the virus is present (an abnormal condition); if the test is negative, the virus is absent (the normal condition), and decisions can be made accordingly about the cause of the patient's apparent liver disease.

To deal with the natural variability of test results, a normal range is established by testing a large number of *presumably healthy* people selected for study because they have no evidence of the disease. The results are averaged to determine the normal **mean**. Statistical formulas are applied to the data to determine the **standard deviation**, a measure of the degree of natural variability of results. In this instance the variation is from one normal person to another. When test results cluster tightly around the mean, the standard deviation is small. The test for blood calcium levels, for example, is a test that has a small standard deviation because the body tightly controls blood calcium, and levels vary little from one person to another. On the other hand, when test results are widely scattered above and below the mean, as they are with blood glucose levels, the standard deviation is large.

By widespread agreement, the lower limit of normal is set at two standard deviations below the mean and the upper limit at two standard deviations above the mean. A graphic display of a hypothetical normal range study for blood glucose is shown in Figure 1-4. When normal is defined this way, the lowest 2.5% and highest 2.5% of results in presumably healthy persons are not included in the normal range. Thus, by definition, *5% of presumably healthy people will have an abnormal test result.*

For example, 100 presumably healthy young adults are asked to volunteer to submit to a blood glucose test. Those with signs or symptoms that suggest diabetes or those with a family history of diabetes are rejected, and the others are instructed not to eat or drink anything for four hours before the test. A blood glucose test is performed on each person, and the mean (average) and standard deviations are calculated for the group. If the

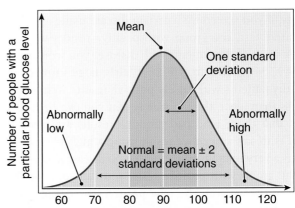

Figure 1-4 **A normal distribution curve.** Among healthy people who do not have diabetes, the greatest numbers of blood glucose levels are near the mean (90 mg/dL). A few people will have a blood glucose level below 70 mg/dL or greater than 110 mg/dL.

average glucose in our group is 90 mg/dL, and one standard deviation (SD) is 10 mg/dL, then the normal range for fasting blood glucose levels would be 70–110 mg/dL, as is shown in Figure 1-4. By definition it follows, therefore, that 5% of healthy, nondiabetic, fasting people will have abnormal blood glucose levels. Some levels will be abnormally high; others will be abnormally low. However, none of these people is necessarily unhealthy.

THE EXTENT OF ABNORMALITY

If a test is abnormal, the *degree* of abnormality is important—markedly abnormal results are more significant than are mildly abnormal ones. Disease is a continuum from mildly ailing to desperately ill, and test results vary accordingly. The greater the degree of abnormality, the more likely it is that the result means disease is present (the test is truly positive). For example, if the upper limit of normal blood glucose levels is 110 mg/dL, a patient with fasting blood glucose level of 190 mg/dL is much more likely to have diabetes than is a patient with a fasting blood glucose level of 120 mg/dL.

TEST SENSITIVITY AND SPECIFICITY

The ability of a test to be positive in the presence of disease is test **sensitivity**. For example, a test is 99% sensitive if it is positive in 99 of 100 patients *known to have the disease*. Similarly, **specificity** is the ability of a test to be negative in the absence of the disease. A test is said to be 99% specific if it is negative in 99 of 100 persons known *not* to have the disease.

There is a trade-off between sensitivity and specificity. *Highly sensitive tests* are likely to be positive in disease (truly positive), but they also have a tendency to be positive (falsely positive) in healthy people, too. That is to say, if you screen for a certain disease using a highly sensitive test, the group with positive results will include most of the patients with disease (you won't miss many), but mixed in will be a fairly large number of healthy patients with falsely positive results. While this is less than ideal, the flip side is that you can be confident that those who had negative results are healthy. That is to say, a negative result using a highly sensitive test is a very reliable indicator that no disease is present. In the group with positive tests, you can sort out the false positives from the true positives by doing additional tests.

On the other hand, the opposite is true for *highly specific tests*—they are likely to be negative in health (truly negative), but they may be negative in some patients with disease; that is, to be falsely negative. If you screen a group of patients using a highly specific test, you can be confident that those with positive tests have the disease. However, the group with negative results will include some patients with disease, whom you can identify by further testing later.

This is the rule: highly sensitive tests are not very specific; and highly specific tests are not very sensitive. As is illustrated in Figure 1-5, some tests are more sensitive and others more specific. For example, imagine a cowboy on a Texas horse ranch who can hear a thundering herd beyond the trees before he can see them. Hearing is a more sensitive "test" than is sight in this instance. Hearing is not very specific—the thundering herd could be horses, cows, or zebras. The cowboy expects that the herd is horses (after all, he works on a horse ranch) but to be absolutely certain he must use a more specific "test," eyesight. As the herd emerges from behind the trees, he applies the "sight test," which is highly specific, to determine if there are cows, horses, or zebras in the herd.

By way of further example, consider home burglar alarms as a test for burglars. Alarms are very sensitive but not very specific. If operating properly, they do not miss many burglars. Although burglar alarms have lots of false positives, they have few false negatives. By contrast, having a personal observer at home is much more specific but less sensitive. Rarely would an observer falsely accuse someone of being a burglar, but if the observer is working in the garden, the burglar might miss detection. Case Study 1-1 at the end of the chapter offers another example of the relationship between sensitivity and specificity.

The Usefulness of Tests in Diagnosis

The purpose of testing is to determine who has disease and who does not. A useful test has high **predictive value**; that is, it accurately predicts who has and who does not have disease. If a test has many true positives and few false positives, the predictive value of a positive test is high. Likewise, if a test has a great number of true negatives and few false negatives, the predictive value of a negative test is high.

For example, cardiac troponin I, a heart muscle protein that increases in blood as a result of a heart attack, normally circulates in blood in small amounts. Therefore, in a patient with chest pain and possible heart attack, increased cardiac troponin I is considered a positive test for cardiac muscle damage and a reliable sign of heart attack. Normal levels of cardiac troponin suggest no cardiac muscle damage has occurred, and the cause

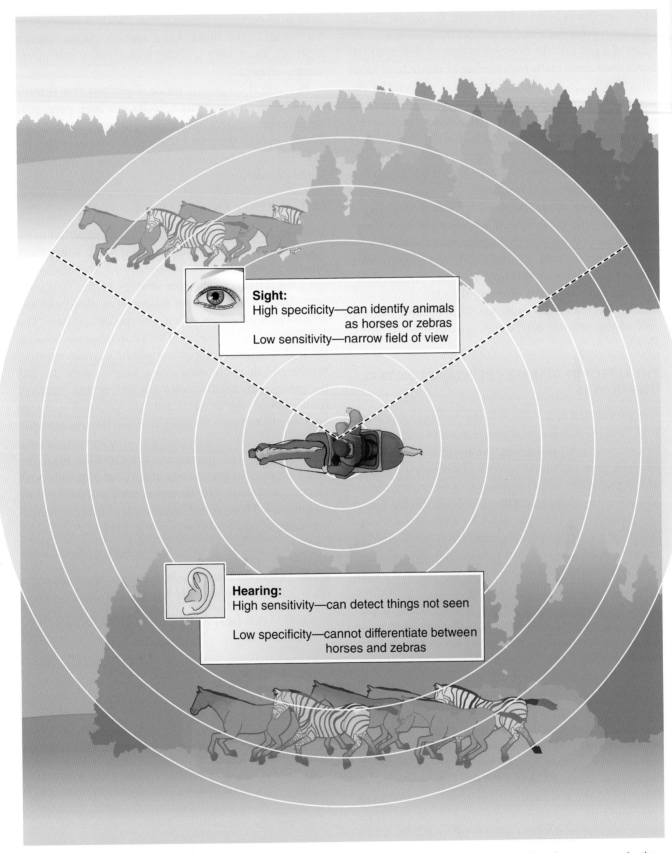

Figure 1-5 Sensitivity versus specificity. Hearing is more sensitive than sight but less specific—the cowboy can hear but cannot see the thundering herd until it emerges from the trees. Sight is more specific than hearing but less sensitive—the herd can be identified as horses, cows, or zebras as it emerges from behind the trees.

of the pain must be found elsewhere. Diagnostic use of cardiac troponin as a tool to predict the presence or absence of heart muscle damage has proven that most patients with abnormally high cardiac troponin have heart muscle damage. Conversely, the great majority of patients with normal cardiac troponin do not have heart muscle damage. Thus, the predictive value of cardiac troponin I as an indicator of possible heart muscle damage is high for both positive and negative tests, making cardiac troponin a very widely used diagnostic test when heart muscle damage is suspected.

As discussed above, the degree of test abnormality is important—the greater the abnormality the more likely is it that the result correctly suggests that disease is present. This means that a patient with very high cardiac troponin is much more likely to have heart muscle damage (and more extensive damage) than is a patient with mildly elevated cardiac troponin. Case Study 1-2 at the end of the chapter offers another example to think about.

THE EFFECT OF DISEASE PREVALENCE ON TEST USEFULNESS

The **prevalence** of a disease is the number of persons who have the disease *at any given moment* and is not to be confused with **incidence**, the number of *new cases* per year. How well a test performs (whether it has high or low predictive value) depends to a surprising degree on how many cases exist (the prevalence) in the group being tested. For example, consider a blood test for evidence of a heart attack. The number of people having an acute heart attack is near zero among asymptomatic persons entering a shopping mall. Any positive test in such a group is very likely a false positive. On the other hand, the same test will be much more useful if performed in patients who present with chest pain to an emergency room. In the emergency room population a positive result is much more likely to be truly positive.

Referring back to Figure 1-5 and our example of the ranch hand on a Texas horse ranch: The cowboy hears the thunder of hoof beats and makes a quick and reasonable diagnosis of "horses" because the prevalence of horses on Texas horse ranches is high and the prevalence of zebras is very low. Alternatively, if the observer is a Masai warrior on the Serengeti Plain in East Africa, the test method (listening) and the result (pounding hooves) will be the same as on the Texas ranch, but the conclusion will be different—the Masai will expect zebras, not horses. The test and the result are the same in Africa and in the United States, but the conclusion is different because the circumstances are different. However, in both instances in order to an-

swer with certainty the question "What is causing the hoof beats?" the ranch hand and the Masai warrior must rely on a more specific, less-sensitive test mechanism—eyesight.

In medical diagnostic terms, a positive test is more likely to be truly positive (to have a high predictive value; to be a correct indication of disease) if there are a lot of people in the tested population who have the disease; that is, if the prevalence of disease is high in the tested population.

INITIAL TESTS AND FOLLOW-UP TESTS

So far we have been talking about single tests, but in reality patients are subjected to many tests, some more sensitive and others more specific for the disease in question. The most effective strategy is this: *first use a very sensitive test, and then follow-up on those who test positive by testing them with a very specific test* (see "The Clinical Side" box nearby). This strategy works because the highly sensitive initial test produces many positive results and does not miss many patients with disease; the group with positive tests is a mix of true positives (patients with the disease) and false positives (patients who do not have the disease). Because the test is highly sensitive, it is safe to conclude that very few people with a negative test have the disease. On the other hand, the positive group of patients includes a lot of people with disease, and these can be tested with a second, more specific test. Those tested and found positive by the second test are very likely to have the disease.

 THE CLINICAL SIDE

SENSITIVE TESTS FIRST, SPECIFIC TESTS LATER

In testing for disease by any method—blood tests, x-rays, physical examination, you name it—use the *most sensitive* tests first. By screening with a highly sensitive test, you will collect a lot of suspects (those with positive tests) and will not miss many sick patients. Then you can test the suspects with highly specific tests to sort out the people with true-positive results (those actually sick) from those with false-positive results (healthy patients with positive tests). Pap smears are an example—they are highly sensitive; that is, they miss few cases of cancer. However, they are not specific enough alone to warrant surgery, irradiation, or chemotherapy. Biopsy is a much more specific test and must be performed to separate the true-positive smears (cancer) from false-positive smears (not cancer).

Disease and Diagnosis

Disease spans a scale from very sick to almost well. Diagnostic tests, medical history, and physical findings determine where each patient fits. The information can be misleading, however: Diseased patients may have normal tests, unremarkable history, and normal physical exam. A patient with a small lung cancer may be normal by every conceivable measure and have no physical signs or symptoms. The opposite is also true: The history in healthy patients may be misleading, abnormal test results may be statistical flukes or errors. In short, there may be some medical conditions we cannot diagnose correctly at a given time. We can improve the accuracy of diagnosis by sensible test selection, careful physical examination, and thorough history. Ultimately, however, we may have to wait for disease to reveal itself.

CASE STUDY 1-1   A DIAGNOSIS MISSED AND A DIAGNOSIS MADE

TOPICS
Acute otitis media
Acute meningitis
Test sensitivity and specificity

THE CASE

Setting: As medical officer of the day you are seeing after-hours outpatients at a military hospital.

Clinical history: Coming to the next cubicle you see "fever" written on the chalkboard. Inside you find an anxious mother and her 21-month-old girl. The mother tells you the child became feverish during the day and has been tugging on her left ear and crying.

Physical examination and other data: You find that the baby has a temperature of 103°F and a perforated left eardrum with pus in the external auditory canal. The remainder of the exam is unremarkable—there is no rash, the chest is clear, the neck is not stiff, and the anterior cranial fontanelle is flat and soft. You write "acute otitis media" in the chart, swab the pus for culture, and prescribe an antibiotic.

Clinical course: The next evening you pick up the phone to hear the mother telling you the child is still feverish and seems sleepy and "jumpy" at the same time. You tell her to meet you in the emergency room, where you find that the child's neck is stiff and the fontanelle is tense and bulging. A spinal tap produces fluid with many white blood cells and bacteria. A call to the laboratory reveals that the initial ear culture is growing a pure culture of the bacterium *Haemophilus influenzae*. The diagnosis now is acute bacterial meningitis. The child is admitted to the hospital and placed on high doses of intravenous antibiotics. She makes a prompt recovery.

DISCUSSION

The child's disease was a bacterial infection that evolved from acute otitis media into acute bacterial meningitis. The etiology was *H. influenzae*. The pathogenesis was acute bacterial infection that invaded the blood stream and seeded the meninges. The pathophysiology included fever, irritability, and drowsiness, all three of which were related to altered brain function. The lesion was acute inflammation of the middle ear and meninges.

This child initially developed symptoms of illness reported by the parent: fever and tugging at an ear. Initial signs included high body temperature, a red, bulging eardrum, and pus in the ear canal. Later symptoms included drowsiness and irritability, and later signs were a stiff neck and bulging fontanelle. You were careful and correct in your initial evaluation, and you checked for signs of meningitis: neck flexibility and the shape and tension of the anterior fontanelle. Both were normal because they were not sufficiently sensitive to detect the early meningitis, which in retrospect must have been present in a very early stage on the initial visit. In other words, the neck-flexion test and fontanelle shape and tenseness tests were negative (false negative) because they were not sensitive enough to detect meningeal inflammation in the early stage of bacterial meningitis. In this instance the predictive value of fontanelle palpation and neck manipulation was poor. The next day the same tests were abnormal (true positive) because the disease was more fully developed, and test sensitivity and predictive value improved accordingly. The final test, a spinal tap, was a much more specific test and confirmed the suspected diagnosis.

POINTS TO REMEMBER
- Medical tests—laboratory tests, radiographs, physical findings, and other data—are not perfect predictors of disease.
- The interpretation of medical tests and other data is strongly influenced by clinical history and clinical findings.

CASE STUDY 1-2 *HOW HIGH IS UP?*

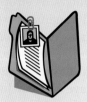

TOPICS
Test sensitivity and specificity
Blood glucose testing
Diabetes mellitus

THE CASE
Setting: You work for a city health department and are assigned to a team charged with developing a screening program for diabetes among patients coming to a free city clinic.

The problem: At the first meeting you are given the task of recommending criteria for the diagnosis of diabetes. Your research reveals widespread agreement about the normal range for fasting blood glucose levels: 70–110 mg/dL. You also learn that the American Diabetes Association and the World Health Organization consider diabetes to be present if the fasting blood glucose level is 126 mg/dL or more. Your task seems easy, until a senior and highly respected physician on the committee calls you to discuss the matter. He is critical of the 1997 American Diabetes Association decision to lower their fasting blood glucose standard for diagnosis of diabetes from 140 mg/dL to 126 mg/dL. He argues that the 126 mg/dL standard makes the test too sensitive and will result in too many false-positive diagnoses of diabetes, with "disastrous" consequences to the patient for future health insurance premiums and the ability to find employment. He further argues that health department funds are limited and that it will be expensive to deal with the large number of patients that are going to test "abnormal" using the 126 mg/dL standard. He says, "I think we should spend our money on patients who are much more likely to be diabetic; we can't afford to go on a wild goose chase after every patient who *might* have diabetes."

DISCUSSION
More people will be diagnosed as having diabetes using the 126 mg/dL standard, and fewer will be diagnosed using the 140 mg/dL standard. In other words, the 126 mg/dL standard is more sensitive but less specific, so it produces more false-positive results and fewer false-negative results. By contrast, the 140 mg/dL standard is less sensitive but more specific. It produces more false-negative results and fewer false-positive results. The predictive value of a positive result is higher for the 140 mg/dL standard: a result of 140 mg/dL or higher is more likely to identify diabetes than is a value from 126 to 140 mg/dL. However, by using the higher standard, you will likely miss some cases.

So, which standard would you choose? How high is too high? Are you willing to miss some cases of diabetes in order not to falsely label other patients as having diabetes and subject them to unnecessary treatment and insurance and employment problems? If so, choose the 140 mg/dL standard. Would you rather diagnose the disease early and get treatment started at the expense of falsely labeling some patients as having diabetes when they do not? Early control of blood glucose levels can prevent or delay heart attack, stroke, and other long-term complications of diabetes. On the other hand, health insurance premiums could go up and identified individuals might not be able to get insurance or find work in the future.

What are you going to recommend to the committee at the next meeting?

POINTS TO REMEMBER
- Test sensitivity and specificity depend on definitions of "normal," "positive," "abnormal," "diseased," and similar terms.
- There is a trade-off between test sensitivity and specificity.
- Health care decisions are often difficult and may have far-reaching and sometimes unanticipated consequences.

Objectives Recap

1. *Define the terms: disease, etiology, pathogenesis, lesion, and pathophysiology:* Disease is defective biologic function. Etiology is the cause of disease. Pathogenesis is the natural history and development of disease. Lesions are the anatomic abnormalities of disease. Pathophysiology is the abnormal functionality of disease.
2. *Explain the difference between anatomic and clinical pathology:* Anatomic pathology is the study of

structural change; clinical pathology is the study of functional change.
3. *Describe the relationship between structure and function:* Structure and function are intimately related; abnormal structure often produces abnormal function and vice versa.
4. *Differentiate between a symptom and a sign:* Symptoms are complaints reported by the patient or by someone else and are a part of the medical

history. Signs are direct observations by the examiner (e.g., nurse, PA, physician).

5. *Explain the meaning of normal, abnormal, healthy, and sick:* Normal and abnormal are terms applied to observations (e.g., blood tests, physical findings, history, radiographs). Healthy and sick are terms applied to the underlying disease (diseased structure or function) or lack of disease.

6. *Describe the differences among true positive, false positive, true negative, and false negative tests:* These terms characterize test results according to whether or not the test correctly points to a healthy or diseased state. Most patients with a disease have abnormal results (tests that are true positives); most healthy patients have normal test results (tests that are true negatives). False-positive tests are abnormal tests in healthy patients. False-negative tests are normal tests in patients with disease.

7. *Explain the meaning of normal range as it relates to medical tests:* A normal range is established for tests that have numerical results. Normal range is defined by statistical methods to include 95% of test results in a population of healthy persons. It follows that 5% of healthy persons will have abnormal results.

8. *Explain the meaning of test sensitivity and test specificity:* The ability of a test to be positive in the presence of disease is test sensitivity. For example, a test is 99% sensitive if it is positive in 99 of 100 patients *known to have the disease.* Similarly, specificity is the ability of a test to be negative in the absence of the disease. A test is said to be 99% specific if it is negative in 99 of 100 persons known not to have the disease.

9. *Explain the concept of the predictive value of test results:* The purpose of testing is to determine who has disease and who does not. A useful test has high predictive value; that is, it accurately predicts who has and who does not have disease. If a test has many true-positive results and few false-positive results, the predictive value of a positive test is high. Likewise, if a test has many true-negative results and few false-negative results, the predictive value of a negative test is high.

10. *Discuss why sensitive tests should be used first in the diagnostic process:* Positive results with a highly sensitive test include almost all people with disease plus some that are healthy; it misses few who have disease. This positive group can then be tested in follow-up by a highly specific test.

11. *Differentiate between prevalence and incidence:* The prevalence of a disease is the number of individuals per 100,000 who have the disease at any given time. Incidence is the number of new cases appearing each year.

12. *Explain why it is usually futile to test for disease in a population in which the prevalence of disease is very low:* Most positive results will be false-positive results.

Typical Test Questions

1. Which of the following is an example of clinical pathology?
   A. Study of a breast biopsy specimen
   B. Study of blood glucose level patterns
   C. An autopsy

2. Which of the following is a functional disorder?
   A. Myocardial infarct
   B. Bacterial endocarditis
   C. Congestive heart failure

3. Which of the following is the more sensitive test? One that has
   A. Relatively large number of false-positive results
   B. Low number of positive results
   C. High number of false-negative results

4. True or false? Healthy people may have abnormal test results.

5. True or false? The prevalence of a disease is the number of new cases that appear each year.

6. True or false? The best way to use diagnostic tests is to start with sensitive tests and follow with specific tests.

CHAPTER

2

Cell Injury, Adaptation, and Death

This chapter discusses the natural and pathologic life and death of cells and how they change with disease, covering biologic aging as well as distinguishing between mild and severe cell injury.

BACK TO BASICS
- The Origins of Cells and the Organization of Tissues
- The Nucleus
- The Cytoplasm
- The Cell Membrane
- The Cell Cycle
- Cellular Communication

BIOLOGIC AGING
CELL INJURY AND DISEASE
MILD CELL INJURY
- Intracellular Accumulations
- Adaptations of Cell Growth and Differentiation
SEVERE CELL INJURY AND CELL DEATH

Learning Objectives

After studying this chapter you should be able to:
1. Offer a brief description of the basic organization of a cell and of the organization of tissues, organs, and organ systems
2. Explain how the genetic code is written into DNA
3. Explain the role of messenger RNA
4. Explain the role of mitochondria
5. Explain how DNA replicates during cell division (mitosis)
6. Differentiate between apoptosis and necrosis
7. Explain the relationship between injury and disease
8. Explain the relationship of genes and environment in the pathogenesis of disease
9. Name the most common cause of cell injury
10. Name one cell reaction resulting from mild acute cell injury and one resulting from mild chronic injury
11. List at least two causes of cell atrophy
12. Differentiate between hypertrophy and hyperplasia
13. Define dysplasia
14. Define metaplasia and offer an example
15. Name the consequence of severe, irreversible cell injury
16. Name the most common cause of necrosis and the most common type of necrosis

Key Terms and Concepts

BACK TO BASICS
- deoxyribonucleic acid (DNA)
- ribonucleic acid (RNA)
- chromosomes
- nucleotide bases
- mitosis
- meiosis
- tumor suppressor genes
- proto-oncogenes
- hormones
- homeostasis

BIOLOGIC AGING
- necrosis
- apoptosis

CELL INJURY AND DISEASE
- hypoxia
- ischemia
- mutation
- cytogenetic disease

MILD CELL INJURY
- hydropic change
- atrophy
- hypertrophy
- hyperplasia
- metaplasia
- dysplasia

SEVERE CELL INJURY AND CELL DEATH
- coagulative necrosis
- infarct
- liquefactive necrosis

On the plus side, death is one of the few things that can be done just as easily lying down.

WOODY ALLEN (B. 1935), AMERICAN FILM-MAKER AND COMEDIAN

BACK TO BASICS

Modern understanding of the nature of disease began with the great 19th century German pathologist Rudolph Virchow (1821-1902), who introduced the concept of cellular pathology and argued that injured cells were the cause of all disease. Virchow's observations finally put to rest the ancient belief that all illness was an affliction of the body at large caused by one of four "humors"—phlegm, blood, black bile, or yellow bile. Virchow understood that cells collect together to form tissues, tissues collect to form organs, and organs collect into systems that compose the body. Subsequent scientists discovered the anatomic and chemical constituents of the cell, demonstrating that all cells have three main elements—nucleus, cytoplasm, and cell membrane.

THE ORIGINS OF CELLS AND THE ORGANIZATION OF TISSUES

Every cell is derived from one of three primitive embryologic tissues: ectoderm, endoderm, and mesoderm. *Ectoderm* differentiates into hair, nails, and epidermis—the superficial layer of skin—and into brain and nerves.

History of Medicine

EARTH, WATER, AIR, AND FIRE

The premise that all matter was formed of earth, water, air, and fire was first postulated by a Greek aristocrat, Empedocles, who lived on the island of Sicily (in the middle part of the Mediterranean Sea) in the fifth century BC. About the same time Greek philosophers Leucippus and his student Democritus, far away in the eastern Mediterranean, reasoned that all things in nature are constructed of small units, which together make up the whole. They named the smallest unit *atom*, a Greek word meaning *indivisible*. Their theory was not so attractive as earth, water, air, and fire, a myth that persisted until 1665 when English microscopist Robert Hooke observed a honeycomb pattern of "cells" in his study of the bark of cork trees. Later, in 1684, Hooke's insight was confirmed by Leeuwenhoek, who used his more powerful microscope to identify red blood cells (or corpuscles, as he called them). But it was not until 1803 that even smaller units were discovered by Englishman John Dalton, who produced the first scientific evidence that atoms actually exist.

Endoderm differentiates into the internal lining (mucosa) of the intestinal and respiratory tracts and into the liver and pancreas. *Mesoderm* differentiates into the deep layer of skin (dermis), bone, skeletal muscle, blood vessels, smooth muscle—including the muscular wall of the gastrointestinal tract—pleura, peritoneum, pericardium, and the urinary system and gonads.

With the exception of skin, bone, muscle, and ductless glands (endocrine glands), all organs can be conceived of as hollow tubes surrounded by tissue. Even the brain and spinal cord are hollow, tubular structures. The ventricles and canals are in the center; however, the hollow space is small compared to total organ mass. Similarly, the liver and other ducted glands can be conceived of as a network of small, hollow tubes—ducts—to which a large number of specialized cells are attached.

Epithelium is a sheet of cells that covers a body surface or lines the hollow interior of an organ or its ducts. Epithelium rests on a **basement membrane**, a thin film of non-cellular tissue. There are two types of epithelial cells: *columnar* (tall and thin) and *squamous* (like fish scales; from Latin *squama*, for scale). Gland ducts (such

as pancreatic or breast ducts) and the intestine are hollow tubes lined by a shoulder-to-shoulder layer of columnar epithelial cells. Conversely, squamous epithelial cells are layered, shingle-like to form the covering layer (epidermis) of skin, and they line the vagina, oral cavity, and esophagus.

The specialized cells of an organ form the **parenchyma** (e.g., hepatocytes in the liver, or neurons in the brain). Parenchymal cells are held together by a supporting network of **stroma**—fibrocytes and collagen and elastin fibers—whose purpose is to maintain structural integrity and to provide space through which blood vessels and nerves can travel.

THE NUCLEUS

The critical parts of a cell are illustrated in Figure 2-1. Every living cell has a nucleus, with the exception of red blood cells (RBC), which expel their nucleus upon entering the circulation in order to have maximum room for hemoglobin to carry oxygen. The nucleus is organized into a round mass floating in the middle of each

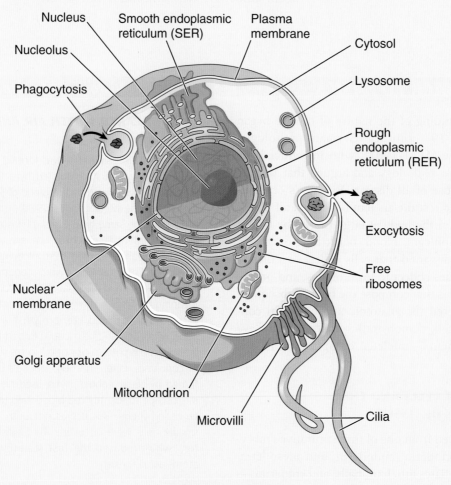

Figure 2-1 **The normal cell.**

cell and is composed of nuclear **proteins**, which are large molecules composed of multiple amino acids. The proteins of the nucleus are **deoxyribonucleic acid (DNA)** and **ribonucleic acid (RNA)**. DNA has two purposes: 1) to duplicate itself during cell division and 2) to code for proteins to be synthesized by elements of the cytoplasm. RNA carries DNA messages from the nucleus into the cytoplasm, the fluid part of the cell surrounding the nucleus.

DNA is constructed of building blocks known as *nucleotide bases*, small molecules that are strung together in a long chain. A **gene** is a segment of DNA with a specific task: to code for a protein to be made by a cell. Many genes are combined to form a **chromosome** (Fig. 2-2). There are 46 chromosomes, 23 from the ovum and 23 from the sperm. In humans this parental set of 23 is referred to as the **haploid** number. People with a normal haploid set from each parent are said to be genetically **diploid**, or **euploid** (chromosomally normal). *Each gene governs production of a single protein or variations of that protein*; these proteins in turn influence every molecular event in life. For example, a gene on chromosome 9 governs major blood group type, determining whether a person is blood type A, B, AB, or O (Chapter 8).

DNA is a very, very long molecule composed of sequences of four small molecules, the **nucleotide bases**: adenine (A), thymine (T), guanine (G), and cytosine (C). *The sequence of these bases is the genetic code.* A short sequence might be . . . AAACGTGCGATC . . . ; however, the actual code is thousands of bases long. Two strands of these molecules are twisted together like a rope to form the complete DNA molecule. As is illustrated in Figure 2-2, each nucleotide base has a "handshake" link with a matched companion base on the *other* strand of DNA—guanine (G) and cytosine (C) always link together, while thymine (T) is always matched to adenine (A) on the other side.

DNA sends its commands to the cytoplasm by synthesizing RNA. RNA is composed of the same nucleotide bases as DNA, with one exception: in RNA uracil (U) replaces the thymine (T) found in DNA. Furthermore, RNA is a single molecular strand, not a twisted double strand like DNA. There are several types of RNA, one active in the nucleus, the others active in the cytoplasm. As is illustrated in Figure 2-3, DNA synthesizes RNA and transcribes its code into it. This initial RNA is *messenger RNA* (mRNA), which carries the code across the nuclear membrane and into the cytoplasm, where it requires the help of *transfer RNA* (tRNA) to pass the code to ribosomes composed of *ribosomal RNA* (rRNA), which are where proteins are made.

THE CYTOPLASM

Elements of the cytoplasm are illustrated in Figure 2-1. The fluid component of cytoplasm is the **cytosol**, com-

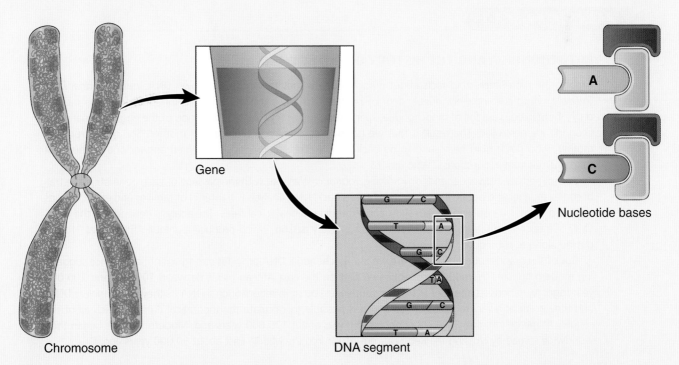

Figure 2-2 **Subdivisions of a chromosome.** Chromosomes are composed of genes, genes are composed of DNA, and DNA is composed of two very long, intertwined spiral strands of four nucleotide bases: adenine (A), cytosine (C), guanine (G), and thymine (T). The bases on one strand link across to the other strand: adenine (A) always connects across to thymine (T), and cytosine (C) always connects across to guanine (G).

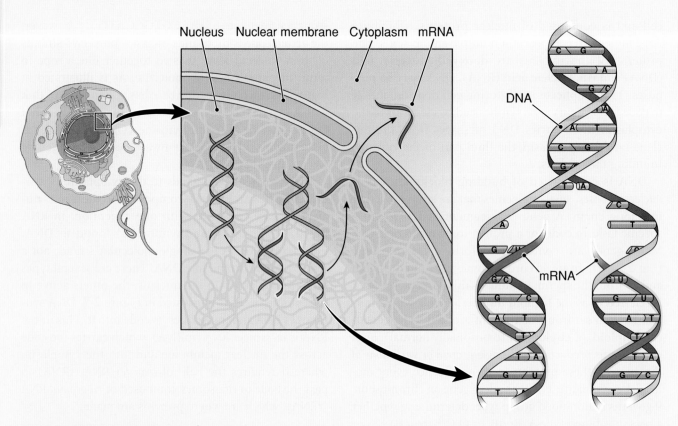

Figure 2-3 RNA synthesis. DNA synthesizes RNA by transcribing its code to messenger RNA (mRNA). Notice that RNA is only a single strand of bases coded from a single strand of DNA.

BASICS IN BRIEF 2-1

MITOCHONDRIA AND THE HISTORY OF HUMANKIND

Among the more interesting facts about mitochondria is that they have their own DNA, *mitochondrial DNA (mDNA)*, which is completely independent of *nuclear DNA* and, stranger still, it is inherited from the mother only—human eggs are full of mitochondria; sperm have only a few. After fertilization of the egg, paternal mitochondria are destroyed. The result is that we get our all of our mDNA from our mother. She got it from her mother, who got it from hers—and so on back in time. This unique fact has helped answer one of the most fundamental human questions: "Who am I?"

The immediate answer depends on knowing your ancestors, but with the passage of each generation the trail becomes murkier and is soon lost a few generations back. DNA analysis (Chapter 7) of families and ethnic groups has been helpful in clarifying relationships and extending genealogical trees. The analysis depends on the regularity of innocent mutations of mDNA that occur in every person, which produce a unique "fingerprint" that is passed along to subsequent generations.

But of the grander question "Who are we?" mitochondrial DNA provides strong scientific evidence suggesting modern humans (*Homo sapiens*) appeared first on the east African plains between 100,000 and 200,000 years ago. Mutations (changes of DNA base sequences) occur in mitochondrial DNA as they do in nuclear DNA; and they occur at a very regular rate, so that it is possible to calculate the theoretical date at which all of the sequences merge into one "mitochondrial Eve." It was about 175,000 years ago. Modern humans began their worldwide spread by crossing the Red Sea from Africa into the Middle East about 50,000 years ago.

posed mainly of water, in which are floating small structures—*cytoplasmic organelles*. The main organelles are mitochondria (see Basics in Brief 2-1), ribosomes, endoplasmic reticulum, the Golgi apparatus, and lysosomes. Also, some cells have specialized cytoplasmic organelles; for example, glandular cells contain secretory vacuoles, and muscle cells contain contractile protein filaments.

Mitochondria *produce the energy required for all metabolic processes*. They are shaped somewhat like elongated, intracellular bacteria. Mitochondria are formed of an external membrane with many internal folds, and they are packed with enzymes that consume oxygen and

chemical foodstuffs (glucose, fatty acids, and amino acids) to create the chemical energy that powers metabolism. In the process, carbon dioxide, water, and heat are produced. The latter accounts for body temperature.

Ribosomes are tiny granules composed of ribosomal RNA (rRNA). As is illustrated in Figure 2-4, ribosomes manufacture amino acids and string them together to form proteins. Each amino acid component of a protein is coded by sequential sets of three nucleotide bases (that is, by a particular sequence of A, C, T, or G). The DNA code for the amino acid methionine is TAC, and for glycine the code is CCG. Therefore, a protein con-

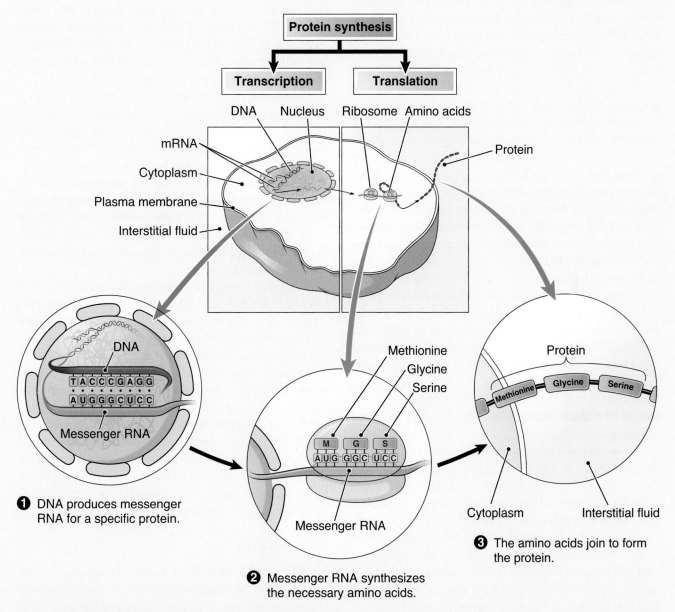

Figure 2-4 **Protein synthesis.** In the nucleus, the genetic code from DNA is transcribed into messenger RNA (mRNA), which carries the code to ribosomes, where the code is translated into amino acids. The amino acids are joined together in a particular sequence to form a specific protein, which is then used internally or exported from the cell into interstitial fluid.

taining methionine attached to glycine would originate with the DNA base sequence TACCCG. In this way a protein composed of a long string of amino acids is originally coded by a long set of DNA bases, transferred by matching sequences of messenger RNA, which carries the code to ribosomes that use it to synthesize protein.

The **endoplasmic reticulum** is a folded network of membranes that connect with the nucleus on one side and the cytoplasmic membrane on the other. *Rough (granular) endoplasmic reticulum (RER)* has ribosomes attached to its surface. RER accepts messenger RNA from the nucleus and delivers packets of synthesized proteins into either the cytoplasm or into the extracellular space (the interstitial fluid) for further distribution to nearby cells or into blood. For example, insulin is synthesized by the rough endoplasmic reticulum of the beta cells of the pancreatic islets of Langerhans (Chapter 17) and is secreted into blood for distribution throughout the body as a key ingredient in cellular glucose metabolism. One of the two main types of diabetes is caused by a deficiency of cellular insulin synthesis.

Smooth endoplasmic reticulum (SER) has a number of complex functions, the two most important of which are synthesis of steroids and the metabolic breakdown of drugs and other molecules. Liver cells have a large amount of SER because they degrade and excrete drugs and products of metabolism in other parts of the body.

The **Golgi apparatus** is a hollow metabolic cytoplasmic organelle somewhat like a balloon collapsed upon itself into multiple folds. It accepts packets of protein from the endoplasmic reticulum, biochemically modifies them, stuffs them into packets, and releases them into the cytoplasm. These free-floating, intracellular packets may 1) remain in the cytoplasm as packets of enzymes (*lysosomes*) or storage vesicles; 2) be incorporated into the cell membrane; or 3) be expelled from the cell into the extracellular space. For example, lipoproteins (Chapter 12) are formed in the Golgi complex of liver cells and are expelled from the cell and absorbed into blood.

Lysosomes are packets of lytic (digestive) enzymes surrounded by a membrane. They originate from the Golgi complex and may remain in the cell, either to destroy foreign material ingested by the cell or to metabolize foodstuff molecules for further cell metabolism. Lysosome activity is exemplified by neutrophils, a type of white blood cell that accumulates quickly in injured tissue (Chapter 3). Neutrophil cytoplasm contains lysosomes, which by conventional microscopy are a neutral (pale) tan, hence the name. Neutrophils are phagocytes (they ingest things) that swallow bacteria and foreign material to kill or digest it.

THE CELL MEMBRANE

The **plasma membrane** (cell membrane) is illustrated in Figure 2-5. It forms the outer surface of the cell and controls interaction between the cell and its environment. Just as skin separates and protects the body's inner parts from the environment, the cell membrane keeps cell cytoplasm separated from the interstitial fluid. Rupture of the membrane usually results in cell death (necrosis). Because most of the cytoplasm and interstitial fluid is composed of water, the membrane is composed mainly of lipids (lipid means "fat soluble"), which allow limited passive diffusion of small molecules. Large molecules require active transport, controlled by membrane proteins that act as channels through which some proteins leave the cell. Additional proteins lie on the outer surface of the cell membrane and act as receptors, latching onto molecules that regulate cell activity. Other surface proteins are enzymes that speed up reactions on the cell surface.

In addition to the molecular-scale (microscopic) activities described above, the cell membrane engages in larger-scale (macroscopic) actions. Phagocytosis and exocytosis are bulk transfer mechanisms. **Phagocytosis** (Fig. 2-1) is the ingestion of bacteria and similarly large bits of outside material through the membrane and into cytoplasm. **Exocytosis** is the reverse—passage of packets of material from the cytoplasm into the extracellular fluid. Material expelled by exocytosis can be the remains of ingested material or substances synthesized in the cell.

A cell membrane may contain specialized structures. **Microvilli** are tiny, closely packed, short, hair-like projections of cell membrane on cells that need increased surface area for absorptive purposes—the internal margin of intestinal epithelial cells is an example. **Cilia** are much larger than microvilli and are long hair-like structures that project from the cell membrane and sway together with cilia of nearby cells in waves to move material from one point to another in hollow organs. Cilia of cells lining the bronchi and trachea move mucus and inhaled particles up the tracheobronchial tree, where they can be coughed out or swallowed; and cilia in the fallopian tube move ova (fertilized or unfertilized) down the tube to the uterine cavity.

THE CELL CYCLE

Mitosis (see Basics in Brief 2-2) is the division of one cell into two identical daughter cells. During mitosis chromosomes line up single-file around the equator of the parent cell. The two strands of DNA unravel, and one strand goes to each daughter cell. Figure 2-6 illus-

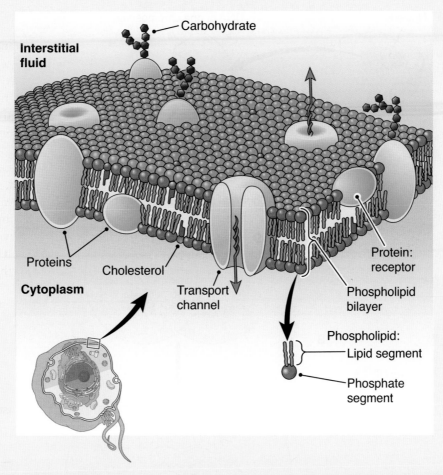

Figure 2-5 The plasma membrane. This membrane consists primarily of phospholipid molecules oriented so that the lipid segment is in the center of the membrane, and the phosphate (water-soluble) segment faces interstitial fluid on the outside and cytoplasm on the inside. The membrane also contains proteins, carbohydrates, and cholesterol, which serve special functions.

BASICS IN BRIEF 2-2

MITOSIS VERSUS MEIOSIS

Mitosis is cell division of the type that occurs in somatic (non-germ) cells, the cells that compose every organ in the body except some of the cells in the gonads. In mitosis every chromosome (all 46 of them) divides, half going into one cell, half into the other, so that each new cell contains 46 chromosomes.

Meiosis is cell division of the type that occurs only in ovarian and testicular germ cells (the precursor cells of ova and sperm). In meiosis chromosomes line up in matched pairs and one of each goes into the new cells. For example, both number 21 chromosomes line up side by side—one entire chromosome destined for one offspring ovum or sperm, the other destined for the other. Ova and sperm, therefore, contain 23 chromosomes, not 46. Thus, when one ovum and one sperm combine fertilization the new conceptus has a normal complement of 46 chromosomes.

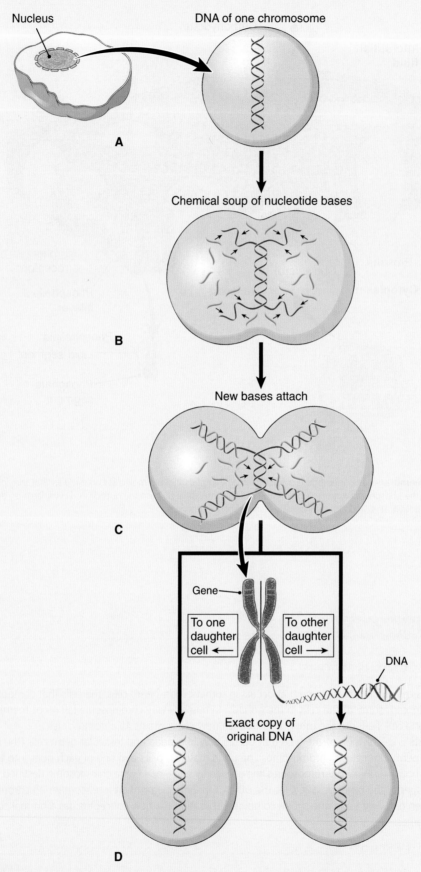

Figure 2-6 DNA replication. A. DNA before division. **B.** DNA begins to unravel, with each strand attracting new nucleotide bases. **C.** Cell division continues as new nucleotide bases attach to each strand to form a coil of new DNA. **D.** Cell division is complete. Each new cell contains an exact copy of the parent chromosome's DNA.

trates the process. After unraveling, the nucleotide bases in each strand capture a partner base in the "chemical soup" of the cytoplasm—glycine (G) grabs onto to a cytosine (C) molecule, and adenine (A) to a new thymine (T), and so on. These newly captured nucleotides then link sideways to one another to form a new strand of DNA identical to the strand lost to the new daughter cell. The result is a newly formed DNA chain with two intertwined strands of nucleotide bases. The original DNA molecule has thus become two; one in each new daughter cell. The DNA in each daughter cell is identical to the DNA of the parent cell, which ensures perpetuation of the original genetic code from one generation of cells to another.

Cell reproduction is either promoted or restrained by pro- or anti-growth genes. Anti-growth genes synthesize growth inhibition proteins and are called **tumor suppressor genes** because unsuppressed cell growth may grow uncontrollably into a tumor. A very important tumor suppressor is the **p53 gene**. Over 50% of all cancers contain an ineffective, mutated (abnormal) p53 gene, which fails to suppress cell growth. Conversely, some genes that stimulate cell growth (**proto-oncogenes**) are capable of mutation into genes (**oncogenes**) that promote uncontrolled cell overgrowth and the formation of tumors.

Cells differ in their ability to proliferate. Some cells (*labile* cells) reproduce continuously; some (*stable* cells) are quiet and reproduce very slowly until stimulated (by injury, for example); and others (*permanent* cells) never divide—they must last a lifetime. Cells of the epidermis and epithelial cells lining the GI tract are labile cells, and they divide continuously and are renewed every few days, a feature that ensures a constant supply of fresh cells to face the harshness of the outside environment and intestinal lumen. Liver, kidney, and pancreas cells, stable cells, divide slowly but can reproduce rapidly in response to injury. Brain and muscle cells are permanent cells and cannot reproduce.

CELLULAR COMMUNICATION

Normal function requires that cells influence one another. As is illustrated in Figure 2-7, influence is communicated by chemicals known as **hormones**. There are

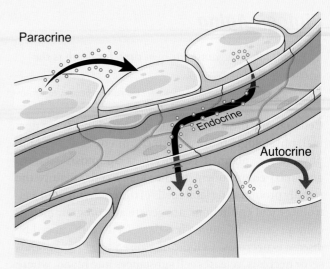

***Figure 2-7* Hormones.** Cells influence one another by producing hormones. Autocrine hormones act on the cell from which they arise. Paracrine hormones act on adjacent or nearby cells. Blood transports endocrine hormones to act on cells at a distant site.

three varieties of hormones: autocrine, paracrine, and endocrine. Autocrine hormones act on the cell that produced them; paracrine hormones diffuse through interstitial fluid to act on nearby cells; and **endocrine** hormones are transported by blood to act on other organs at a distant site.

Hormones are essential in the maintenance of cells, tissues, organs, and organ systems in a balanced, steady state of equilibrium known as **homeostasis**, a word derived from Greek *homoios* (steady) and *stasis* (state). External events may upset this equilibrium or move it to a faster or slower rate for some period of time, during which a new steady state may exist for a while; for example, running increases the heart rate. However, such deviations are temporary and cannot be maintained indefinitely without injury. If demand exceeds adaptive capacity, an injurious imbalance may occur. For example, if blood sugar rises, the pancreas secretes insulin into blood to reduce it by enabling cells to use more. However, if the patient is diabetic and lacks enough functioning beta cells in the islets of Langerhans, demand for insulin may exceed the ability of the pancreas to respond, and diabetic acidosis or coma may occur.

Biologic Aging

We all labour against our own cure, for death is the cure of all diseases.

SIR THOMAS BROWNE (1605–1682), ENGLISH PHYSICIAN AND AUTHOR

Cells age and die like every other living thing. It is a normal, physiologic process distinct from disease. Natural, physiologic, planned cell death is **apoptosis**—a programmed commitment to die. Many cells, mainly the rapidly proliferating labile cells of the epidermis and gastrointestinal epithelium, are genetically programmed to commit "suicide" after a few days. Cell death caused by *disease* is **necrosis**. Cell death, caused by either apoptosis or necrosis, releases cell substances into blood, where their concentration can be measured by laboratory tests.

It is also clear that as cells age they, like we, function with less efficiency. Just as a 70-year-old person cannot run as far or as fast as a teenager can, old cells do not function as well as young ones do. Old cells burn energy less efficiently and do not make DNA and proteins as well as young ones can. Cell nuclei, mitochondria, and other cell parts become deformed and less functional in old cells. As a result we and our cells adapt less effectively to environmental stress. For example, as we age our heat muscle loses some of its contractile power, our kidneys are less efficient at filtering waste, and nerve conduction (reflexes, for example) is slower. Interestingly, modern medicine has improved the *average* life span of humans, but the *maximum* life span has not changed. It has been about 100 years for centuries.

How cells age is not completely clear, but genes play an important role. In tissue culture normal cells do not continue to divide much beyond 50 doublings (generations). However, cancer cells, which have abnormal DNA, divide endlessly. An interesting feature of DNA that appears to play an important role in cell aging is the **telomere**, a cap of nucleotide bases on the end of each strand of DNA that does not reproduce with each cell division. Instead, it loses a few nucleotide bases with each cell replication. Telomeres are, in effect, genetic debit cards preloaded with a certain number of ticks. Reproduction stops when the account is emptied, and the cell dies.

That genes are important in aging is also clear from the study of patients with *progeria* and *Werner syndrome*. Both are rare genetic diseases associated with early aging and short life span. Early in life these patients develop gray hair, cataracts, atherosclerosis, diabetes, wrinkled skin, and other attributes of old age, and they die very young.

Cell Injury and Disease

All disease occurs because of injury. Severe injury causes cell death (necrosis). Mild injury or stress, however, induces cells to alter and adapt without dying. Cellular adaptations may occur in cells pushed to physiologic extremes by unusual physiologic demand. Regardless of the cause, cell adaptations return to normal once the stress or injury is relieved. The process of cell injury or stress and reactions to it are depicted in Figure 2-8.

☞ **All disease is caused by injury.**

Injury may occur at the molecular level or any level above it—at the level of cells, tissues, or organs. Cancer is an example of injury that arises at the molecular

---

LAB TOOLS

Detecting Cell Death with Blood Tests

When a cell dies some of its contents are swept away into the blood, where they can be detected in increased amounts by laboratory tests (enough cells die naturally that blood normally contains small amounts of cell contents). The most common and useful tests for escaped cell contents are tests for cell enzymes and other proteins.

For example, when heart muscle cells die in a heart attack (myocardial infarct), the dead cells release cardiac troponin, a protein not found in any other organ. If you are suspecting a heart attack, finding an increased amount of cardiac troponin in blood is concrete evidence that your suspicion is correct.

Or, if you suspect liver disease, finding an increased amount of liver enzyme in blood is confirmation that liver cells are injured or dying.

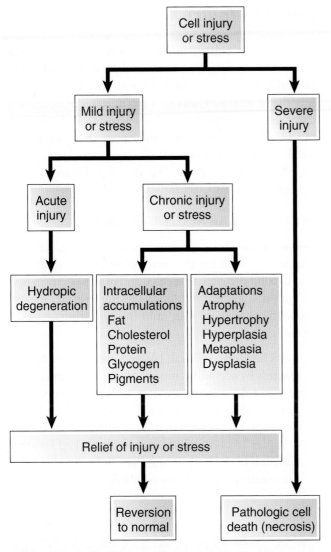

Figure 2-8 Cell reactions to injury or stress. Cells react in similar ways to mild chronic injury or unusual physiologic demand (stress).

level—injured DNA is the root cause of cancer. However, injury is not confined to the level of molecules and cells, as anyone with a broken bone can testify.

Our genes influence how we react to injury. Some people are more predisposed than others to develop severe disease from a given injury. Genes may be thought of as the soil in which the seed of injury is planted; some soil is fertile to certain seeds and less fertile to others. Some persons (very few) can eat all the cheeseburgers they want and not develop high cholesterol (Chapter 12), but others (most of us) cannot remain healthy and eat a lot of fatty foods because our cholesterol rises and we develop atherosclerosis. Genes account for much of the difference between those who develop atherosclerosis and those who do not.

Disease may result from the injury itself or from the repair process that follows. Fatal hemorrhage from a gun-

shot wound is disease resulting directly from injury. On the other hand, the new blood vessel growth and scar formation that occurs as the body tries to repair an injured cornea can impair vision long after the original injury is resolved.

Cells can be injured in several ways:

- *Inadequate oxygenation* (**hypoxia**): Hypoxia is the most common cause of cell injury and is usually caused by insufficient arterial blood flow (**ischemia**). Ischemia usually affects a local block of tissue supplied by a single artery. However, generalized hypoxia may be produced by lung disease, some kinds of poison, and other conditions. Hypoxia initiates a series of chemical and acid-base imbalances that may be reversible if blood flow or oxygenation is restored; however, prolonged hypoxia produces cell death.
- *Direct physical action:* *Mechanical force* disrupts organ tissues on a large scale, altering their structure; hemorrhage and ischemia are major consequences. Ingested *acids* or *alkalis* may so profoundly alter blood pH that death ensues. Acids, alkalis, or *heat* may cause necrosis of skin, cornea, or mucosal surfaces. Low temperature may freeze cell water in skin (frostbite), from which cell necrosis occurs when ice crystals rupture cell membranes. *Low body temperature* may cause cardiac arrest subsequent to slowing of the heart's intrinsic pacemaker.
- *Ionizing radiation:* Ionizing radiation is radiation strong enough to break (ionize) water (H_2O) into H^+ (hydrogen ion) and OH^- (hydroxyl ion). In *acute* radiation injury the hydroxyl ion attaches to DNA and prevents cell reproduction. For brain cells (permanent cells, which do not divide) and liver cells (stable cells, which divide slowly) this is of little consequence; however, for the bone marrow and gastrointestinal epithelium (rapidly dividing labile cells, which must be replaced daily), it is a disaster. In acute radiation injury, intestinal lining cells stop reproducing, and the lining sloughs away. The white blood cell count falls dramatically because white blood cells live only a few days and must be replaced daily. Loss of intestinal epithelium and decreased white blood cell count leave the body vulnerable to infection. *Chronic* radiation injury causes DNA mutations that may result in neoplasia.
- *Toxic molecular injury:* Virtually any natural or synthetic molecule can cause injury. Depending on the chemical, injury may occur in different organs and by different mechanisms. For example, heavy metals such as mercury and lead cause direct toxic injury to enzymes necessary for cell health. The effect of most

toxic molecules is dose related; fatal overdose of heroin is an example.

- *Microbes*: Bacteria often produce toxins that interfere with cell protein synthesis or cell oxygen utilization. For example, *Staphylococcus aureus* growing on unrefrigerated food produces a toxin that may cause food poisoning. The ingested toxin damages intestinal epithelial cells. The cell wall of some bacteria contains substances that are released into blood when the bacteria die. Typically these toxins cause vascular collapse (shock) or widespread blood clotting inside of blood vessels (Chapter 5). Viruses invade cells and kill from within: They disrupt the cell or nuclear membrane or incite an immune system (Chapter 8) response that, while aimed at the virus, kills the cell.
- *Inflammatory and immune reactions*: Inflammation and immune reactions are the result of cell injury, but they may in turn cause injury themselves. The neutrophils of acute inflammation (Chapter 3) release digestive enzymes designed to neutralize foreign agents, but they also digest nearby tissue. Immune reactions injure cells directly by several mechanisms, discussed in Chapter 8. A common example is an autoimmune disease such as rheumatoid arthritis, in which the immune system is fooled into believing that the body's own cells (joint cells, in the case of rheumatoid arthritis) are foreign and must be attacked.
- *Nutritional imbalance*: Too much or too little nutrition can cause disease. Obesity is an epidemic in the developed world. About 65% of Americans are overweight, and about half of these are frankly obese. Obesity is associated with cardiovascular disease, cancer, diabetes, and dozens of other ills. Excess intake of animal fat leads to atherosclerosis. Conversely, cells may not receive enough energy (calories) or building blocks (protein). Protein-calorie deficiency is a major cause of illness and death worldwide. Specific vitamin and mineral deficiencies may induce cell injury by interfering with metabolic reactions necessary for cell health. Nutritional disease is discussed in Chapter 10.
- *Genetic defects*: There are two main types of genetic defects: mutations and cytogenetic abnormalities. A **mutation** is a permanent change in DNA represented by an abnormal sequence of nucleotide bases. **Cytogenetic disease** is large-scale change in chromosomes and is characterized by extra or missing whole chromosomes or parts of chromosomes. Genetic diseases are discussed in detail in Chapter 7.
- *Aging*: Cell aging is a progressive, mild injury that ultimately leads to cell death directly or renders cells less able to withstand other injury.

Mild Cell Injury

Normally the cell membrane maintains intracellular sodium at a lower concentration than in the extracellular fluid, a job that requires expenditure of energy. Injury that is mild and lasts for a few minutes or hours may damage this mechanism and allow intracellular sodium to rise, which attracts water and causes the cytoplasm to swell. The result is **hydropic change** (vacuolar degeneration), as can be seen in Figure 2-9. Substances other than water can also accumulate in cells.

INTRACELLULAR ACCUMULATIONS

Not all intracellular accumulations are attributable to cell injury. Some are the result of phagocytosis (ingestion of solid material by a cell), and others occur in normal physiology. Accumulations owing to injury usually occur in association with mild injury lasting at least a few weeks.

- *Fat*: The kidney (Fig. 2-10) and the liver often react to stress by accumulating fat. Most fat accumulates as triglyceride, which appears as clear cytoplasmic globules (Fig. 2-11). Injured liver cells are particularly apt to accumulate fat. Chronic alcoholism (Chapter 16) is notable for causing marked fat accumulation in the liver because alcohol (ethanol) interferes with triglyceride metabolism.

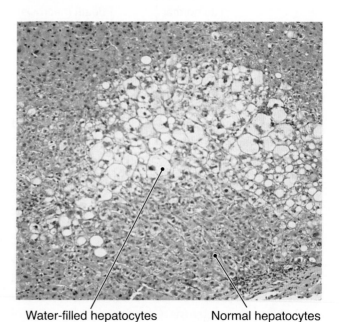

Water-filled hepatocytes   Normal hepatocytes

Figure 2-9 **Hydropic change in liver cells.** This microscopic study is from a patient with toxic liver injury. Injured hepatocytes are enlarged and filled with water. (Reprinted with permission from Rubin E. Pathology. 4th ed. Philadelphia. Lippincott, Williams and Wilkins, 2005.)

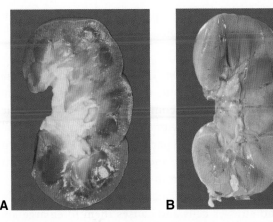

A   **B**

Figure 2-10 **Fatty change in the kidney.** Mildly injured cells can accumulate fat. **A.** Normal kidney. **B.** Fatty change in a patient with toxic injury to the kidney.

- *Cholesterol*: The most extensive and most damaging intracellular accumulation is cholesterol, deposited in the cells of arteries in atherosclerosis (Chapter 12). Cholesterol first appears in macrophages and smooth muscle cells in the arterial wall and later accumulates into large, extracellular pools in the arterial wall.
- *Protein*: Protein accumulations can occur in cells. An important feature of normal proteins is that they are long molecules that must be folded into correct shape for normal function. Microscopically visible cytoplasmic accumulations of misfolded or otherwise abnormal proteins occur in a variety of diseases.
  - Alpha-1 antitrypsin deficiency is a heritable disorder (Chapter 14) associated with protein clumps in hepatocytes.

- Alcoholic liver disease (Chapter 16) is associated with cytoplasmic protein clumps known as *Mallory bodies*.
- Several brain diseases (Chapter 23) are associated with abnormal accumulations of protein in cells. Among the most notable is Alzheimer disease.
- *Glycogen*: Glycogen is a long chain of glucose molecules formed and stored in liver and muscle as a glucose reserve. Glycogen synthesis is regulated by blood glucose concentration. For example, patients with diabetes (Chapter 17); have high blood glucose levels, and, as a consequence, hepatocytes and kidney cells in people with diabetes are often stuffed with glycogen.
- *Pigments*: The most widely occurring cell pigment accumulation is **lipofuscin**, a "wear-and-tear," golden brown substance most notable in brain neurons and myocardial muscle cells, both of which are permanent, non-reproducing cells, and in hepatocytes, which are slow-dividing, stable cells. *Melanin* is a dark-brown compound that gives skin its color (Chapter 24). It is synthesized by melanocytes in the epidermis and deposited in the cytoplasm of cells in the basal layer of the epidermis. Inhaled *carbon particles* from cigarette smoke or polluted air are ingested by macrophages of bronchial lymph nodes (Fig. 2-12) and remain permanently with little damage. *Hemosiderin* and *ferritin* are brownish pigmented normal iron-storage compounds important in iron and hemoglobin metabolism (Chapter 11).

Liver cell with fat:
— Nucleus
— Cytoplasm

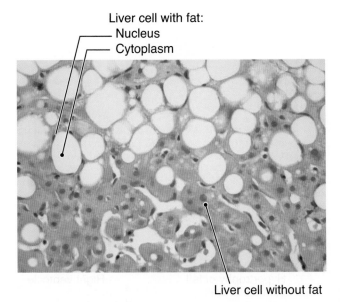

Liver cell without fat

Figure 2-11 **Fatty change in liver cells.** This microscopic study is from a patient with alcoholic liver disease.

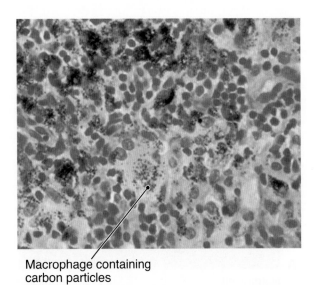

Macrophage containing carbon particles

Figure 2-12 **Intracellular accumulation of carbon pigment.** This photomicrograph shows phagocytosis of carbon particles by macrophages in a bronchial lymph node of a smoker.

ADAPTATIONS OF CELL GROWTH AND DIFFERENTIATION

In addition to hydropic degeneration and intracellular accumulations, cellular response to persistent stress or chronic mild injury may include a change in size (atrophy or hypertrophy), an increase in number (hyperplasia), or alteration into another type of cell (metaplasia).

Atrophy is decreased size and function of a cell. It is an adaptive response to decreased demand or to increased stress; the cell shuts down its metabolic processes to conserve energy. Cells atrophy for several reasons:

- *Reduced functional demand.* For example, muscle atrophy occurs in a limb encased in a cast.
- *Inadequate blood supply (ischemia).* For example, atherosclerosis of the renal artery can impair blood flow enough to cause atrophy of a kidney.
- *Absent or reduced neural or hormonal support.* For example, to remain healthy, skeletal muscle cells must be continually stimulated by intact nerves; interruption of nerve supply leads to muscle atrophy (Chapter 23). Other cells require hormonal support, as do thyroid and adrenal glands, which atrophy if they do not receive hormonal support from the pituitary gland.
- *Chronic inflammation associated with chronic injury.* For example, chronic inflammation of the stomach lining is associated with a condition known as *chronic atrophic gastritis* (Chapter 15), which causes the lining to become atrophic and very thin.

Hypertrophy is the opposite of atrophy—an increased *size* and functional capacity of a cell. It can be caused by:

- *Hormonal stimulation.* Cells depend on hormonal support. Too little and they wither; too much and they enlarge and become overactive. For example, following delivery, women's breasts enlarge and become temporarily hyperfunctional in order to produce milk, a change induced by secretion of prolactin (a hormone) from the pituitary.
- *Increased functional demand.* Increased functional demand stresses cells and causes them to enlarge and increase their activity. For example, a heart under the constant strain of high blood pressure increases in size because the individual cardiac muscle cells increase in size (Fig. 2-13).

Hyperplasia is the enlargement of a tissue or organ owing to an increase in the *number* of cells, as opposed to an increase in the cell *size*. It is cause by:

- *Hormonal stimulation.* For example, the increase of estrogen in female puberty causes an increase in the number of endometrial cells.
- *Increased functional demand.* For example, low atmospheric oxygen stimulates bone marrow production of RBC to carry oxygen. It is for this reason that people living at high altitude have increased numbers of circulating red blood cells (RBC).
- *Chronic stress or injury.* For example, the stress of exceptionally high blood pressure (Chapter 12) on small arteries in the kidney causes cells in the arterial

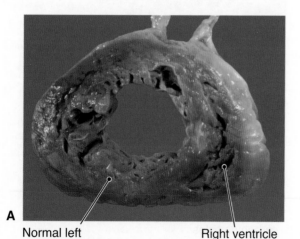
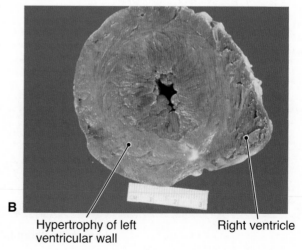

A Normal left ventricular wall   Right ventricle

B Hypertrophy of left ventricular wall   Right ventricle

Figure 2-13 **Hypertrophy. A.** Normal left ventricle. **B.** Hypertrophic left ventricle in a patient with severe, chronic hypertension. Ventricular wall is markedly thickened as a result of the increased size of individual muscle cells.

wall to divide and accumulate in layers, an effect called "onionskin" hyperplasia, illustrated in Figure 2-14.

As a rule, tissues whose cells are capable of dividing enlarge by undergoing both hyperplasia and hypertrophy. But tissues composed only of permanent cells (which cannot divide) can respond to increased demand only by cell enlargement (hypertrophy). Heart muscle is an example: All enlarged hearts occur because the *size*, not the *number*, of cardiac muscle cells increases.

Dysplasia a premalignant change of cells discussed in more detail in Chapter 6. Dysplasia typically occurs in previously normal epithelium, which features an orderly arrangement of cells of uniform size, shape, and appearance. In dysplastic epithelium this bland appearance is replaced by a disorderly overgrowth of cells with enlarged, dark, irregular nuclei. Dysplasia is a milepost on the way to malignancy; however, it is reversible and not yet malignant.

As is illustrated in Figure 2-15, **metaplasia** is a reversible change of one cell type into another. It is most common in epithelium, because epithelial cells are short-lived and are always being replenished from special cells (*stem cells*) that reside all along the basement membrane (see Case Study 2-1 at the end of this chapter). Normally epithelial stem cells mature into the usual cell type, but when injured or stressed they mature into

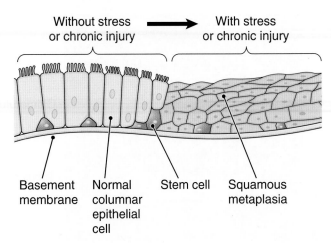

Figure 2-15 Metaplasia. Stress or chronic injury stimulates stem cells to produce squamous cells (*right*) instead of normal columnar epithelial cells (*left*). Columnar cells on the left have cilia and are not layered; squamous cells on the right have no cilia and are flat and layered.

a different type of cell more suitable to existing conditions. For example, the normal endocervix is lined by tall, columnar, mucinous cells, but when chronically inflamed it changes into squamous epithelium, a simpler, more durable epithelium better suited to defend against the agents causing the chronic inflammation. Metaplastic epithelium usually reverts to normal when the injury stops.

Severe Cell Injury and Cell Death

As discussed above, *necrosis* is the pathologic death of cells and is one of the most common of pathologic findings in disease. It is to be distinguished from *apoptosis*, the programmed, normal death of cells. Necrosis usually occurs in blocks of cells forming a collective mass fed with blood from a single artery. For example, a heart attack is the death of a group of heart muscle cells fed by a single blocked coronary artery. Similarly, an **abscess** is a group of liquefied cells killed by localized bacterial infection. However, in certain circumstances selected groups of cells die because they are of a certain type in a certain organ. For example, in patients in shock from blood loss, kidney blood flow falls dramatically because blood vessels to the kidney and other abdominal organs constrict in order to conserve blood for the brain, heart, and lungs. In this circumstance, certain kidney cells are vulnerable to necrosis because they are metabolically very active and require more oxygen than does the remainder of the kidney.

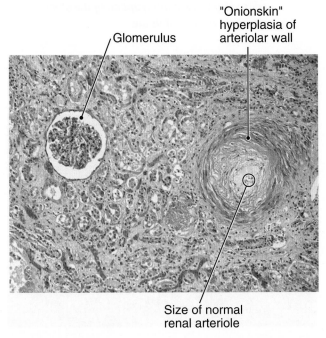

Figure 2-14 Hyperplasia. This is a microscopic study of the kidney from a patient with severe chronic hypertension. Blood pressure stress on renal arterioles stimulates multiplication (hyperplasia) and "onionskin" layering of cells in the arteriolar wall.

> **Apoptosis is normal, physiologic, planned cell death. Necrosis is pathologic cell death.**

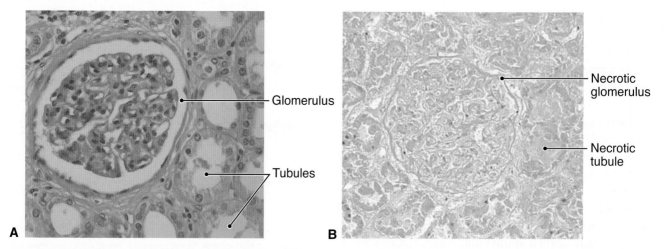

A **B**

Figure 2-16 **Coagulative necrosis.** This microscopic study shows kidney tissue. **A.** Normal renal glomerulus and tubules. **B.** Coagulative necrosis. "Ghost" outline of normal anatomy remains visible in the dead tissue.

There are four types of necrosis:

- **Coagulative necrosis** is the most common type and is a gel-like change in blocks of freshly dead cells in which cell anatomy remains visible. The word *coagulative* derives from the most common use of the word *coagulate*—to convert fluid into a soft, solid mass, as when blood coagulates from fluid into a jelly-like consistency. In this case, the intracellular and extracellular fluid of the dead tissue is temporarily converted into a gel. The hallmark of coagulative necrosis is that the cells die in place, without anatomic disruption, so tissue architecture is preserved. Microscopic study reveals a ghostly outline of cells and tissues, as is seen in Figure 2-16. As discussed above, ischemia (insufficient arterial blood flow) is the most common cause of coagulative necrosis.

- An **infarct** is the ischemic death of a group of cells fed by an artery. *It is the most common cause of coagulative necrosis.* In an infarct, cells die and remain undisrupted and unrepaired for some time because the repair process (Chapter 4) must creep in from nearby living tissue that has a normal blood supply. For example, a heart attack is caused by blockage of a coronary artery, which deprives cardiac muscle tissue of oxygen; the dead muscle shows coagulative necrosis and remains a ghostly image of itself until the repair process can clean up the site. Figure 2-17 shows a liver with numerous infarcts and coagulative necrosis that resulted from occlusion of multiple small hepatic arteries.

- **Liquefactive necrosis** is cell death in which the dead tissue dissolves into fluid. Liquefaction occurs because dead cells are disrupted (not left intact as in

coagulative necrosis) and dissolved by the injury at a rate faster than the repair process (Chapter 4) can clean it up. The most frequent type of liquefactive necrosis is an abscess produced by bacterial infection.

- **Caseous necrosis** is a special type of necrosis caused by tuberculosis infection. Caseous means cheesy and the dead tissue is off-white, soft, pasty, and clumpy, like some varieties of cheese. All cellular detail is obliterated.

> 🔑 ***An infarct is an area of coagulative necrosis caused by sudden interruption of the blood supply to a block of tissue.***

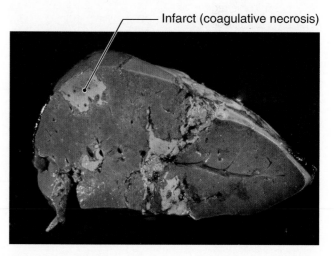

Figure 2-17 **Infarction.** This is a liver with multiple infarcts that occurred after embolic thrombi from the heart occluded hepatic arteries. The light-colored blocks of necrotic liver tissue showed coagulative necrosis on microscopic examination.

In addition, **fat necrosis**, a specialized necrosis of fatty tissue, is usually found in retroperitoneal fat around the pancreas in cases of pancreatitis (Chapter 17). Sometimes fat necrosis occurs in subcutaneous or breast fat as a result of trauma. Triglycerides from disrupted fat cells are digested, and free fatty acids are released and precipitated as calcium soaps, which accumulate around the edges of the dead fat. The associated calcium deposits are microscopically distinctive and may be large enough to be visible on radiographic exam. On mammograms, calcium in fat necrosis can mimic calcium deposits in breast cancer (Fig. 2-18).

Fat necrosis is not the only cause of tissue calcium deposits. The calcium deposits in fat necrosis are but one type of **dystrophic calcification**, a type of calcification that may occur in any inflamed or necrotic tissue, particularly in cases of chronic injury and scarring. To the naked eye, calcium deposits appear as gritty white flecks, often visible on radiographic study.

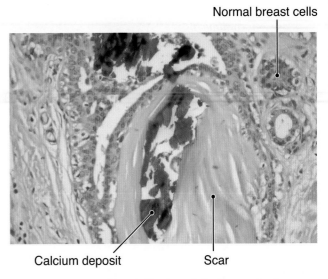

Normal breast cells

Calcium deposit   Scar

Figure 2-18 **Dystrophic calcification of the breast.** Routine mammography detected a small calcified breast scar. In this biopsy study the scar is pale, pink, acellular fibrous tissue, and the calcium is stained purple. Compare with the normal breast cells labeled here.

CASE STUDY 2-1 "THIS HEARTBURN IS KILLING ME"

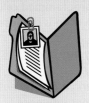

TOPICS
Metaplasia
Dysplasia
Barrett metaplasia of the esophagus

THE CASE

Setting: Your job is to do initial interviews on new patients and see some regular patients on follow-up visits in the office of a gastroenterologist on the faculty of a medical school. Today you are accompanying the gastroenterologist to a "difficult case" presentation in the department conference room, where he is to present the case of a patient you know well because he was one the first patients you saw on your first day at work a little over a year ago. While waiting for the conference to begin, you study the chart.

Clinical history: Rod B. is a 42-year-old man who was referred from his primary care physician with a diagnosis of "severe heartburn." The physician had been treating him with limited success for several years and referred him for consultation when the problem became more severe. The first entry in his chart is your handwritten quote of his main complaint, "This heartburn is killing me."

The chart is thick and crammed with notes, imaging reports, and lab results about the problem, which subsequent

workup by the gastroenterologist proved to be caused by stomach acid refluxing upward into the lower esophagus (gastroesophageal reflux disease). Direct examination of his esophagus with a flexible endoscope revealed that the lower end of his esophagus was inflamed and showed evidence of Barrett metaplasia, which the gastroenterologist explained to you is a change of the lining cells of the lower esophagus from flat squamous cells, which normally are not bathed in acid, to tall, columnar mucus cells identical to those in the stomach, which tolerate acid much better. A variety of oral medicines helped relieve some of the symptoms, but altogether the results have been disappointing, and the gastroenterologist is seeking other opinions about how to proceed.

The gastroenterologist presents the case to the assembled physicians, residents, and others in the conference room. After a lengthy discussion about different medicines and possible surgery, the group agrees that the patient needs a biopsy of the lower esophageal mucosa in the area of metaplasia because there is an increased risk for esophageal cancer in patients with Barrett metaplasia.

Several weeks later a biopsy is obtained through an endoscope. The diagnosis on the pathology report is, "Severe chronic esophagitis, with gastric (Barrett) metaplasia. Moderate dysplasia is present in the metaplastic epithelium. No malignancy is present." ▶

[Case 2-1, continued]

DISCUSSION

Metaplasia is a reversible change of one cell type into another. Dysplasia is a reversible, *premalignant* change of epithelium, which can progress to cancer. In this instance esophageal squamous epithelium was being flooded by gastric acid regurgitated upward from the stomach, which stimulated esophageal epithelial stem cells to mature into gastric-type mucus cells that were resistant to the effect of gastric acid. The injury was long standing and severe, enough to cause precancerous change.

Dysplasia is a well-known risk of Barrett metaplasia. Dysplasia is a mile-post on the road to malignancy, but it is not fully malignant, nor is it irreversible. However, if the chronic injury and dysplasia persist, the dysplastic epithelium can become frankly malignant, invade and spread widely.

This patient needed vigorous treatment, perhaps including surgery, to stop the acid reflux into his esophagus and remove or destroy the dysplastic epithelium.

POINTS TO REMEMBER

- Chronic injury can cause cells to change from one type to another.
- Chronic injury can cause cells to change from benign to malignant.
- Barrett metaplasia is a premalignant condition.

Objectives Recap

1. *Offer a brief description of the basic organization of a cell and of the organization of tissues, organs, and organ systems:* A cell consists of a nucleus that is surrounded by cytoplasm, which is contained within a cell membrane. The nucleus is composed of DNA, which is organized into the genetic code, and which controls all cell activity. The cytoplasm carries out the metabolic instructions of nuclear DNA. Cells are organized into tissues, which are organized into organs, which are organized into organ systems.

2. *Explain how the genetic code is written into DNA:* The code is very long sequence of four specialized molecules, the DNA bases—adenine (A), thymine (T), guanine (G), and cytosine (C). The order in which these molecules occur is the genetic code.

3. *Explain the role of messenger RNA:* Messenger RNA (mRNA) carries a copy of the genetic code from DNA in the nucleus to ribosomes in the cytoplasm, where the code is used to synthesize the protein coded by the DNA.

4. *Explain the role of mitochondria:* Mitochondria produce the energy required for metabolic processes.

5. *Explain how DNA replicates during cell division (mitosis):* During mitosis chromosomes line up single-file around the equator of the parent cell; one strand of DNA goes to one daughter cell; the other strand to the second daughter cell. To do this DNA unravels from the end into two strands like a frayed rope—one strand destined for each new daughter cell. Bases in each unraveled strand create a "handshake" with complementary bases from the "chemical soup" of the cytoplasm to form a second, new strand of DNA—glycine (G) forms a loose bond across to a new cytosine (C), and adenine (A) to a new thymine (T), and so on. These handshakes steady the new ATCG (base) sequences so that they can bind laterally up and down the chain to form a new helix intertwined with the other to form a new DNA molecule.

6. *Differentiate between apoptosis and necrosis:* Apoptosis is natural, physiologic, programmed cell death; necrosis is pathologic death of cells because of injury.

7. *Explain the relationship between injury and disease:* All disease is caused by injury.

8. *Explain the relationship of genes and environment in the pathogenesis of disease:* Genes influence how we react to injury. Some people are more disposed, others less disposed, to develop severe disease from a given injury.

9. *Name the most common cause of cell injury:* Hypoxia; usually secondary to ischemia (low blood flow).

10. *Name one cell reaction resulting from mild acute cell injury and one resulting from mild chronic injury:* Acute mild injury—hydropic (vacuolar) change; chronic mild injury—intracellular accumulations of fat, cholesterol, protein, glycogen or pigments.

11. *List at least two causes of cell atrophy:* Reduced functional demand, inadequate blood supply, lack of hormonal or neural support, chronic injury, cell aging.

12. *Differentiate between hypertrophy and hyperplasia:* Hypertrophy is tissue enlargement resulting from an increase in the size of individual cells. Hyperplasia is tissue enlargement resulting from increased number of cells.

13. *Define dysplasia:* Dysplasia is a premalignant change of cells typically seen in epithelium, in which the orderly arrangement of normal cells is replaced by a disorderly overgrowth of cells with enlarged, dark, irregular nuclei.

14. *Define metaplasia and offer an example:* Metaplasia is the change of one cell type into another following stress or chronic mild injury; for example, the change of endocervical glandular epithelium into squamous epithelium as a result of chronic inflammation of the cervix (cervicitis).

15. *Name the consequence of severe, irreversible cell injury:* Necrosis.

16. *Name the most common cause of necrosis and the most common type of necrosis:* Coagulative necrosis is the most common type of necrosis; it is most often caused by ischemia (inadequate blood flow).

Typical Test Questions

1. Which of the following is composed of nucleotide bases?
   A. DNA
   B. mRNA
   C. tRNA
   D. rRNA
   E. All of the above

2. Which of the following is characteristic of apoptosis?
   A. It is reversible
   B. It is natural
   C. It is caused by injury
   D. It features fat accumulation in cells

3. Which of the following is the most common cause of cell injury?
   A. Physical action
   B. Toxic molecular injury
   C. Ionizing irradiation
   D. Hypoxia

4. True or false? Hemosiderin is a normal iron storage molecule that may accumulate in cells.

5. True or false? Hypertrophy is increased number of cells.

6. True or false? Metaplasia is a reversible change of cell type.

Inflammation: The Reaction to Injury

This chapter explores the body's reaction to tissue damage (injury), which is the cause of all disease. It discusses acute and chronic inflammation, as well as inflammation that occurs beyond the site of injury. It ends with an examination of several of the various forms of inflammation caused by infection.

THE INFLAMMATORY RESPONSE TO INJURY
THE CELLULAR RESPONSE IN INFLAMMATION
THE VASCULAR RESPONSE IN INFLAMMATION
MOLECULAR MEDIATORS OF INFLAMMATION
ACUTE INFLAMMATION
- The Pathogenesis of Acute Inflammation
- The Anatomic Characteristics of Acute Inflammation
- The Consequences of Acute Inflammation

CHRONIC INFLAMMATION
- The Pathogenesis of Chronic Inflammation
- The Anatomic Characteristics of Chronic Inflammation
- The Consequences of Chronic Inflammation
DISTANT EFFECTS OF INFLAMMATION
- Lymphangitis, Lymphadenitis, and Lymphadenopathy
- Systemic Effects of Inflammation
THE INFLAMMATORY RESPONSE TO INFECTION

Learning Objectives

After studying this chapter you should be able to:
1. Describe the purpose of inflammation
2. Describe the main cell types in acute and chronic inflammation
3. Contrast acute and chronic inflammation
4. Describe the sequence of events in acute inflammation
5. Name the four classic clinical signs of inflammation
6. Name the three gross anatomic types of inflammatory exudate
7. Name the four possible outcomes of acute inflammation
8. Name the usual causes of chronic inflammation and offer an example of each
9. Define granulomatous inflammation
10. Name the outcomes of chronic inflammation
11. Name the distant effects of inflammation
12. Name two important reactant proteins found in the blood in inflammation
13. Discuss the inflammatory response to various types of infectious agents

Key Terms and Concepts

THE INFLAMMATORY RESPONSE TO INJURY
- inflammation
- chronic inflammation
- acute inflammation

THE CELLULAR RESPONSE IN INFLAMMATION
- macrophages
- granulocytes
- phagocytosis
- eosinophils
- lymphocytes
- monocytes

THE VASCULAR RESPONSE IN INFLAMMATION
- capillary
- endothelial cell

MOLECULAR MEDIATORS OF INFLAMMATION
- clotting system
- complement system
- kinin system
- cytokines

ACUTE INFLAMMATION
- edema
- inflammatory exudate
- pyogenic

CHRONIC INFLAMMATION
- angioneogenesis
- fibrosis
- chronic inflammatory cells
- lymphocytes
- macrophages
- granulomatous inflammation

DISTANT EFFECTS OF INFLAMMATION
- lymphangitis
- lymphadenopathy
- C-reactive protein
- leukocytosis
- erythrocyte sedimentation rate

Dreading that climax of all human ills,
The inflammation of his weekly bills.

GEORGE GORDON, LORD BYRON (1788–1824), ENGLISH POET, DON JUAN (III.xxxv)

The Inflammatory Response to Injury

All disease is caused by injury, and **inflammation** is the body's reaction to injury. It is a combined response of local blood vessels, blood cells, plasma proteins, and cells in the surrounding tissue. Figure 3-1 illustrates the vascular, blood, and tissue elements of the inflammatory response. **Acute inflammation** is the result of short-term injury and lasts a few hours or days; **chronic inflammation** is the result of longer term injury and lasts weeks to years.

The purpose of inflammation is to limit the extent and severity of injury, eliminate or neutralize the offending agent, and initiate the repair process (Chapter 4). Any type of cell can be damaged by any injury—physical trauma, chemical toxin, vascular ischemia, radiation, or infection.

Inflammation is a chain of events involving white blood cells, blood vessels, special blood proteins, and molecules released from injured tissue. Injured cells release substances into the damaged area and bloodstream to attract white blood cells and to cause blood vessels to dilate and become "leaky." Gaps appear between the endothelial cells lining the vessel and allow plasma to ooze into injured tissue, bringing proteins and molecules to influence the reaction. Depending on the degree and duration of injury, tissue swells with fluid and blood and becomes distended, red, warm, and painful. Figure 3-2 illustrates the chain of events in inflammation.

Thus, *inflammation is the collective cellular and vascular response to injury.* It is initiated by injury and maintained by hormones released by injured cells, by local hormones released from white blood cells that migrate to the site, and by substances from blood that ooze into the site.

Inflammation precedes and is intimately linked to the repair process (Chapter 4). Repair begins as the immediate effects of injury begin to fade. In acute injury inflammation continues until the damaged tissue is repaired or replaced by scar tissue. However, in the case of chronic inflammation, the injury is ongoing—injury, inflammation, and repair often coexist, sometimes indefinitely, as is the case of joints inflamed by chronic arthritis.

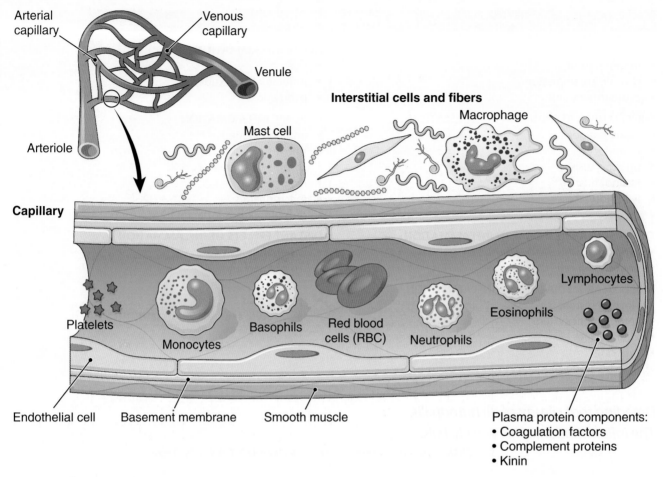

Figure 3-1 Elements of the inflammatory response. This figure shows the microcirculation and the blood and tissue elements of the inflammatory response. Collectively, the neutrophils, eosinophils, and basophils are known as *granulocytes*.

The Cellular Response in Inflammation

Blood contains two compartments: plasma and formed elements (Table 3-1). Plasma is the fluid; formed elements are the red and white blood cells and platelets (fragments of cytoplasm from bone marrow mega-karyocytes). Water is the main component of plasma; the remainder is protein (mainly albumin) and other small but very important molecules such as calcium, glucose, and hormones.

All blood cells are derived from a single type of bone marrow ancestor stem cell, which gives rise to two lines of cells—lymphocytic cells and myelocytic (Chapter 11). The lymphocytic line develops into lymphocytes; the myelocytic line develops into granulocytes, monocytes, red blood cells, and megakaryocytes. Blood cells are grouped into two main categories, red and white, based on their natural color. Red blood cells give blood its color; white blood cells give pus its color.

Lymphocytes from the lymphocytic line and granulocytes and monocytes from the myeloid line are known as **white blood cells** (WBC, also called **leukocytes**) and participate in the inflammatory process. Red blood cells transport oxygen and carbon dioxide between lungs and tissues. White blood cells are made and stored in the bone marrow until they are released into the blood. Normal circulating blood contains about 5,000-10,000 WBC per cubic millimeter (microliter) of whole blood.

As is illustrated in Figure 3-1 and detailed in Table 3-1, the three types of white blood cells are: granulocytes, lymphocytes, and monocytes.

- **Granulocytes** have large, cytoplasmic granules and are involved mainly in *acute* inflammation. Lymphocytes and monocytes do not have cytoplasmic granules and are mainly involved in chronic inflammation. Granulocytes are made in the bone marrow and constitute about 70% of circulating WBC. There are three types of granulocytes—*neutrophils, eosinophils, and basophils*—each having within their cytoplasm

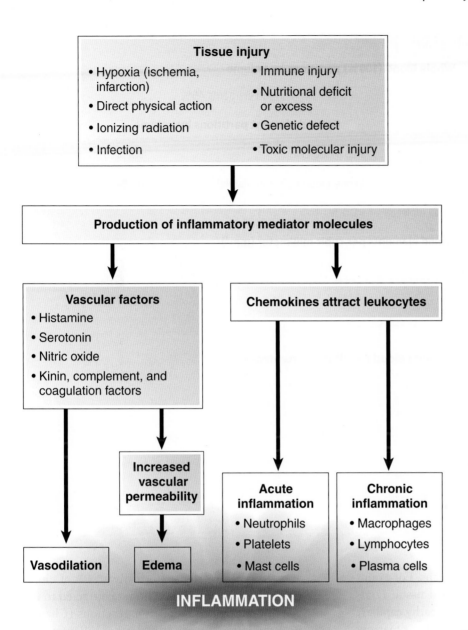

Figure 3-2 Chain of events in inflammation. This figure illustrates the sequence of events that occurs from initial tissue injury to inflammation.

special packages, called lysosomes, enclosed in which are specific digestive enzymes, or granules. The granulocytes are named according to the color imparted to their specific cytoplasmic granules by a standard laboratory dye (stain)—*hematoxylin* (the "basic" dye, which is blue-purple) and *eosin* (a red, "acidic" dye).

- **Neutrophils** have neutral (tan) granules and a segmented, multilobed (2–5 lobes) nucleus. As discussed in the nearby History of Medicine box, neutrophils are sometimes called *polymorphonuclear leukocytes, polys,* or *segs.* Normally, about 65% of circulating WBCs are neutrophils, which are the main inflammatory cells in *acute* inflammation.

Their main task is **phagocytosis**—the engulfment and digestion of tissue debris and foreign material. For capture and ingestion of bacteria and other foreign material to occur, cell membrane receptors must couple with antibody (Chapter 8) and complement molecules (a type of attack protein) that have previously attached to the bacterial wall (Fig. 3-3). Neutrophils then release the contents of their cytoplasmic granules (**degranulation**) to flood the ingested material with oxidants and enzymes, destroying and digesting it. Neutrophils also produce chemical messenger molecules (hormones) that communicate to nearby cells or enter the blood as

Table 3-1	The Components of Blood*

Whole Blood (100%) partitions by volume

Plasma 55%	Formed elements 45%

Plasma partitions by volume		**Formed element partitions by volume**	
Water	90%	Red blood cells	99.9%
Proteins	10%	White blood cells and platelets	<0.1%
Glucose, hormones, minerals, fats, other small molecules	<0.1%		

Formed elements per cubic millimeter (mm³)

Red blood cells	5,000,000
Platelets	250,000
White blood cells	7,500

White Blood Cell (WBC) percentages

Granulocytes	70%
Neutrophils	65%
Eosinophils	3%
Basophils	<1%
Lymphocytes	25%
Monocytes	5%

*Figures are approximate and vary by age and sex.

messenger molecules to distant organs. For example, substances released in inflamed tissue 1) attract more white blood cells from nearby capillaries; 2) circulate in blood to stimulate bone marrow to release and produce additional neutrophils; and 3) act on the brain to increase body temperature (fever) and cause a feeling of malaise, drowsiness, and other familiar symptoms associated with inflammation.

- **Eosinophils** have red cytoplasmic granules (named for their affinity for the red dye eosin) and a bilobed nucleus. Normally about 3% of circulating WBC are eosinophils. Eosinophil granules have anti-parasite properties and are the principal inflammatory cell in parasitic infections, such as intestinal worm infestation. They also are attracted in large numbers to allergic reactions (such as hay fever) by basophils, but their role in allergic reactions is not completely clear.
- **Basophils** have deep blue-purple granules (named for their affinity for the basic dye hematoxylin)

and a bilobed nucleus. Normally < 1% of circulating WBC is basophils. They are attracted to tissue injured by certain allergic reactions (Chapter 8). Basophils, in turn, attract other inflammatory cells, including large numbers of eosinophils. Basophil granules contain large amounts of *histamine*, which is responsible for the local signs of allergic reactions: swelling, itching, congestion, and mucus production. A closely related cell is the **mast cell**. Mast cells look and react like basophils but are less numerous and are located in tissue, not in blood.

- **Lymphocytes** do not have cytoplasmic granules and are made in the bone marrow. They migrate to and mature in other lymphoid organs such as the spleen, thymus, tonsils, and lymphoid patches in the respiratory and gastrointestinal tracts. They normally make up about 25% of circulating WBCs and have a single relatively large nucleus and a small amount of cytoplasm. They are the main cell of the immune system (Chapter 8) and are the principal reactive cell in *chronic* inflammation. There are two types of lymphocytes—B and T—named according to their origin and function, but they look identical, except for a variant of the B lymphocyte, the **plasma cell**, which is a stimulated B cell with a distinctive appearance.

- **Monocytes** have small, inconspicuous cytoplasmic granules, are made in the bone marrow, and normally account for about 5% of circulating WBCs. They are closely related to granulocytes and are large, phagocytic cells with a single nucleus and abundant cytoplasm. Like neutrophils, they ingest and digest foreign material; however, unlike neutrophils they capture foreign proteins (antigens) for presentation to lymphocytes as a vital step in certain chronic reactions (Chapter 8) and are mainly associated with chronic inflammation. Monocyte-like cells (**macrophages**) are permanent residents of many organs, where they have acquired special names; in the liver, for example, they are called *Kupffer cells*; in the brain they are known as *microglia*.

Collectively, lymphocytes, plasma cells, monocytes, and macrophages are spoken of as **chronic inflammatory cells**; neutrophils are often called **acute inflammatory cells.**

The Vascular Response in Inflammation

The walls of large vessels are composed of multiple layers. However, as vessels branch into smaller sizes, the outer layers become thinner and disappear, until at the smallest level (capillaries) only endothelial cells remain. Blood vessels of virtually any size, capillaries included, may dilate in order to deliver more blood to a site as a response to injury or to provide more oxygen. Dilation is controlled partially by the autonomic nervous system (Chapter 23) and partially by hormones and other substances.

Capillaries are the smallest blood vessels and are the principal vessels involved in inflammation. The main job of any blood vessel is to convey life's essential substances to tissues and to carry away waste products of metabolism. To control this process blood must remain separated from tissue and must flow smoothly. Important in this process is the **endothelial cell**, which internally lines all blood vessels (Chapter 12) and the heart chambers and is the sole cell forming the wall of a capillary. Endothelial cells are joined together securely at their edges to prevent leakage of cells or plasma into tissues, but they are metabolically busy. By becoming more or less permeable, they act as gatekeepers in the

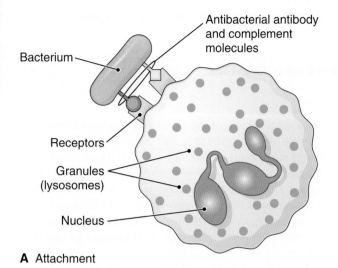

Bacterium

Antibacterial antibody and complement molecules

Receptors

Granules (lysosomes)

Nucleus

A Attachment

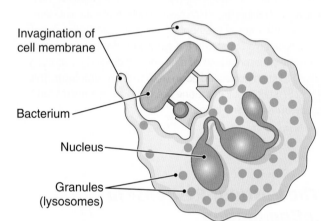

Invagination of cell membrane

Bacterium

Nucleus

Granules (lysosomes)

B Phagocytosis

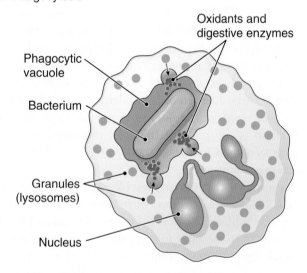

Oxidants and digestive enzymes

Phagocytic vacuole

Bacterium

Granules (lysosomes)

Nucleus

C Degranulation

Figure 3-3 **Phagocytosis.** The figure shows ingestion, digestion, and destruction of foreign particulate matter (a bacterium, in this example). **A.** Cell membrane receptors bind to antibody and complement molecules previously attached to the bacterial surface. **B.** The cell membrane creeps around the bacterium and envelopes it. **C.** The bacterium is trapped in a special space, the phagocytic vacuole, into which lysosomes discharge oxidants to kill it and digestive enzymes to dissolve it.

flow of oxygen, carbon dioxide, hormones, proteins, nutrients, and other essentials into and out of the bloodstream and tissues. Additionally, in the inflammatory process endothelial cells change their character and become "sticky" by activating adhesion molecules, which bind with related molecules on the surface of passing neutrophils and platelets, causing them to attach to both the endothelial cells and to other neutrophils and platelets. After injury, gaps appear in the seams between endothelial cells, allowing passage of red cells, white cells, platelets, and plasma components into extravascular tissue.

It is important in both inflammation and healing (Chapter 4) that endothelial cells are stable cells (Chapter 2). That is, they do not divide frequently unless they are stimulated by stress or injury, at which time they can grow rapidly and branch into new blood vessels—a process called **angioneogenesis** (sometimes called *angiogenesis*). Angioneogenesis occurs in the healing process and in chronic inflammation. It is also the mechanism by which tumors grow their own blood supply (Chapter 6).

Molecular Mediators of Inflammation

Inflammation is a complex process that requires extensive cell-to-cell molecular signaling by plasma-derived and cell-derived mediators. Three groups of *plasma proteins* are important mediators of inflammation: the clotting (coagulation) system, the complement system, and the kinin system, each of which is an interlocking chain of reactions. Much like a row of falling dominoes, one reaction powers the next to generate new products that influence the inflammatory process.

The *plasma-derived* mediators of inflammation are:

• The **clotting system** (Chapter 5) is a set of about a dozen proteins that interact with one another in a complex cascade to cause blood to clot, a necessity in control of hemorrhage associated with injury. Activation of the clotting system also stimulates the kinin system and complement systems, enhancing their activity.

• The **complement system** is a set of about two dozen proteins that react with one another in a chain reaction initiated by the immune system or by the presence of certain products derived from microbes. The products of complement interactions cause vasodilation, attract WBCs, and directly attack and destroy microbes.

- The **kinin system** is closely related to the clotting system and consists of more than a dozen blood proteins that interact to generate molecules that cause vasodilation and increased endothelial cell permeability.

The *cell-derived* molecular mediators are:

- *Vasoactive amines* are small, preformed molecules that are stored in granulocyte cytoplasmic lysosomes and act to cause local capillaries to dilate and become "leaky." **Histamine** is released from the cytoplasm of mast cells, basophils, and platelets. **Serotonin** has similar actions and is derived from platelets.
- *Cell membrane factors* are formed from phospholipids in the cell membranes (Chapter 2) of injured cells and act as local hormones to attract leukocytes and cause vasodilation.
- **Cytokines** are hormone-like protein molecules secreted by cells that act to enhance immune reactions by attracting leukocytes, stimulating phagocytosis, and causing vasodilation. **Chemokines** are a subset of cytokines that cause leukocytes to migrate toward the site of injury, a process known as **chemotaxis**.
- *Reactive oxygen compounds*: 1) **Nitric oxide** (NO) causes vasodilation and also has bactericidal properties; 2) *oxygen superoxide* (O_2^-) is generated in injured tissue and is bactericidal.

Collectively, these plasma-derived and cell-derived substances govern the inflammatory reaction.

Acute Inflammation

Acute inflammation follows *brief* injury and lasts a few hours or days. It is characterized by vascular dilation, accumulation of fluid, and infiltration of neutrophils. It usually resolves without scarring (Chapter 4) and is usually a result of one of the following:

- *Microbial infections*: caused by bacteria especially; less often by viruses or other organisms
- *Physical or chemical injury*: such as thermal or chemical burns
- *Immune injury*: such as the skin rash of poison ivy (although most immune injury produces chronic, rather than acute, inflammation)

THE PATHOGENESIS OF ACUTE INFLAMMATION

The vascular response in inflammation is an *active* process of vascular dilation that is distinct from *passive* congestion (Chapter 5), associated with obstruction of venous outflow, or sluggish blood flow, caused by other factors, such as heart failure. Inflammation is an overlapping sequence of events that occur in a predictable order following injury until a full inflammatory response has developed. Figure 3-4 graphs the timing and duration of these events. Figure 3-5 presents a detailed look at the steps in the sequence:

- *Before injury* (Fig. 3-5A): Blood flows rapidly and smoothly; most white blood cells flow in the center of the stream. Endothelial cells are snugly fitted together.
- *Injury occurs; vasodilation follows immediately* (Fig. 3-5B): Blood vessels dilate to bring more blood *volume* to the injured tissue; however, even as more blood is being delivered, it is flowing at a slower *speed* because the dilated vessels are so enlarged: blood cells tend to "settle out" or "sludge" along the edges of the stream.
- *The vascular wall changes* (Fig. 3-5C): Endothelial cells become "sticky" and "leaky." Gaps appear between endothelial cells, plasma seeps into the injured site, and neutrophils adhere to "sticky" capillary walls and crawl into the injured site through gaps between endothelial cells.
- *Fluid (edema) accumulates* (Fig. 3-5D): **Edema** is a collection of excess fluid in tissue or a body space. It accumulates from plasma leaking through the vascular wall.
- *Neutrophils accumulate* (Fig. 3-5E): Neutrophils continue to migrate into injured tissue, swimming upstream against the gradient of local hormones (*chemokines*) and other molecules that spread outward from the injured site.

Plasma collecting as edema fluid begins to clot (Chapter 5), initiating the kinin and complement system reactions that produce additional and longer lasting

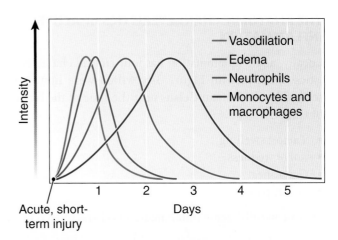

***Figure 3-4* Timing of acute inflammatory events.** The graph shows both intensity and duration for vasodilation, edema, neutrophils, and monocytes and macrophages.

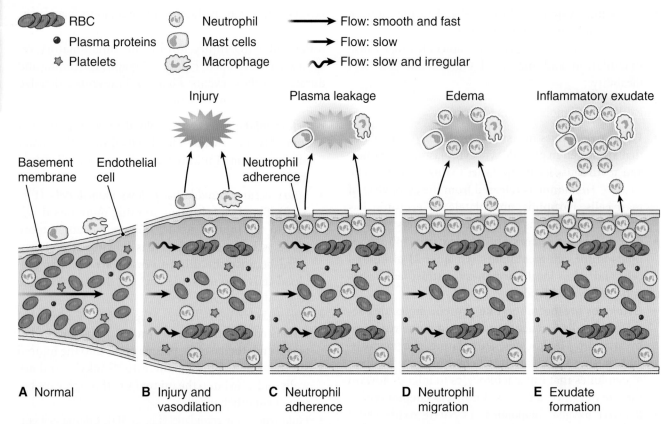

RBC
Plasma proteins
Platelets
Neutrophil
Mast cells
Macrophage
Flow: smooth and fast
Flow: slow
Flow: slow and irregular

Injury
Plasma leakage
Edema
Inflammatory exudate

Basement membrane
Endothelial cell
Neutrophil adherence

A Normal
B Injury and vasodilation
C Neutrophil adherence
D Neutrophil migration
E Exudate formation

Figure 3-5 **Sequence of events in acute inflammation. A.** Normal capillary, blood cells, and adjacent tissue. **B.** After injury, capillaries dilate and the volume of blood flow increases. However, speed of flow is slow at the edges of the stream. Tissue macrophages and mast cell migrate toward the injury. **C.** Injured endothelial cells become "sticky" and "leaky." Plasma begins to leak into the injury site, and neutrophils and platelets begin to adhere to the endothelium. **D.** Plasma collects as edema fluid, and white blood cells migrate through the capillary wall toward the injury site. **E.** An inflammatory exudate is formed of edema and inflammatory cells.

vasodilation and other effects that sustain the inflammatory reaction. At all stages of inflammation, multiple derivatives are synthesized by injured cell membranes. The synthesis of these derivatives is blocked by aspirin, which accounts for some of its therapeutic effect.

THE ANATOMIC CHARACTERISTICS OF ACUTE INFLAMMATION

Locally, acute inflammation has four *clinical* characteristics, illustrated in Figure 3-6, which were first described by the Roman Celsus near the time of the birth of Christ:

- *Tumor*: swelling
- *Rubor*: redness
- *Calor*: heat
- *Dolor*: pain

Microscopically, acute inflammation is characterized by:

- *Injured cells* in various stages of reaction to injury—hydropic degeneration, necrosis, or other changes (Chapter 2)

- *Dilated capillaries* gorged with blood
- An *accumulation of neutrophils*, which may be either sparse or dense according to the severity of injury (Fig. 3-7). An exception is acute allergic reactions, which are characterized by dense accumulations of eosinophils, a few basophils, and lesser numbers of neutrophils.

Red blood cells may or may not be present, according to whether or not injury has damaged blood vessels severely enough for red cells to escape.

The accumulation of fluid and white blood cells at the injured site is the **inflammatory exudate**, which may accumulate in several *gross anatomic patterns*:

- **Serous inflammation** is a pattern seen in mild, short-term inflammation. It is characterized by copious amounts of watery fluid that is *relatively* low in protein compared to other inflammatory exudates and contains relatively few inflammatory cells. Examples include second-degree thermal skin burn—the fluid in burn blisters is a serous inflammatory exudate. Other serous fluids are the joint effusions of active rheumatoid arthritis, and the inflammatory reactions

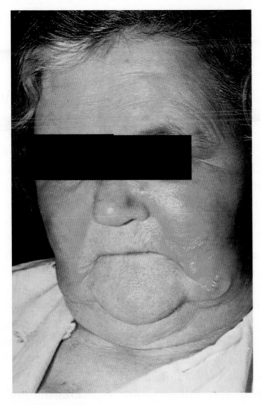

Figure 3-6 **Acute inflammation.** This patient has erysipelas (an acute bacterial skin infection). Intense inflammation (rubor) and moderate edema (tumor) are visible. It is easy to imagine the heat (calor) and pain (dolor).

matory fluid, such as in the tissues of the feet of patients with varicose veins (Chapter 5).

- **Fibrinous inflammation** follows a somewhat more severe injury. It is characterized by greater vascular permeability and exudation of plasma, which gives it higher protein content than is found in serous inflammatory fluid. Much of the protein is from coagulation proteins that leak into the fluid and clot to form fibrin, which gives the process its name. Fibrinous inflammatory fluid usually contains more inflammatory cells than serous fluid. Examples of fibrinous inflammation include the crust (scab) of superficial skin injuries, and inflammations of mesothelial surfaces such as the lining of the pericardium, pleura, or peritoneum (Fig. 3-8).
- **Suppurative (purulent, pyogenic) inflammation** occurs with severe acute injury and is associated with liquefactive necrosis, characterized by a creamy fluid (**pus**) composed of fluid, necrotic debris, and overwhelming numbers of neutrophils. Certain bacteria, such as *Staphylococcus aureus*, are especially prone to form pus. A collection of pus in a body cavity is an **empyema.** For example, a patient with an abscess in the pleural space is said to have a pleural empyema.

THE CONSEQUENCES OF ACUTE INFLAMMATION

Acute inflammation is followed by: 1) resolution; 2) scarring; 3) abscess; or 4) chronic inflammation.

of most viral infections such as pharyngitis or rhinitis. Serous exudates, however, are higher in protein than the fluid that accumulates in most non-inflam-

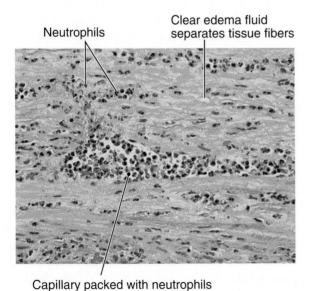

Figure 3-7 **Acute inflammation.** In this microscopic study of the wall of an inflamed appendix, the capillary in the center is dilated and packed with neutrophils, which have also spread into the surrounding tissue.

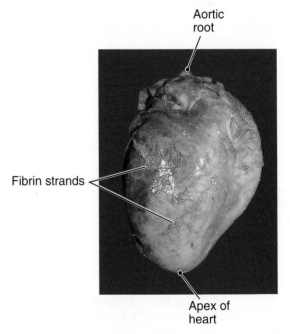

Figure 3-8 **Acute fibrinous inflammation.** In this case of acute fibrinous pericarditis, the heart remains in the pericardial sac, which is covered externally by an exudate containing a stringy film of fibrin strands.

Complete resolution is the usual outcome because most acute inflammation is associated with limited, short-term injury—sunburn, for example. Mildly injured tissue regenerates, molecular mediators are washed away, necrotic debris from severely injured cells is digested or phagocytized, blood vessels contract, and fluid is drained away by the lymphatic system.

Scarring may occur with severe or repeated acute inflammatory episodes if substantial tissue destruction occurs beyond the capacity of tissue to regenerate. A severe (third-degree) burn (Chapter 10) is an example—it is always associated with scarring.

An *abscess* may develop. An **abscess** is a local accumulation of edema, necrotic debris, and dead white blood cells (pus). It is characterized by a central core of pus composed of necrotic tissue, edema fluid, and a great number of neutrophils surrounded by hyperemic, edematous tissue, and it occurs when the pace of local inflammation and liquefactive necrosis outstrips the ability of the inflammatory process to remove the material.

Chronic inflammation may develop if the injury (the cause of the inflammation) persists.

Chronic Inflammation

Chronic inflammation is caused by *persistent* injury that lasts for weeks or years and in which continuing injury, inflammation, and repair proceed simultaneously. As is depicted in Figure 3-9, the main inflammatory cells are lymphocytes, macrophages, and plasma cells (stimulated B lymphocytes). Persistent injury and chronic inflammation, as in chronic viral hepatitis (Chapter 16), are characterized by **fibrosis** (scarring) and ingrowth of new blood vessels (**angioneogenesis**).

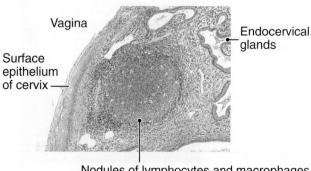

Vagina

Endocervical glands

Surface epithelium of cervix

Nodules of lymphocytes and macrophages (large clear cells in center)

Figure 3-9 **Chronic inflammation.** In this microscopic study of the female cervix, a nodule of lymphocytes and macrophages has accumulated in response to persistent injury.

THE PATHOGENESIS OF CHRONIC INFLAMMATION

Chronic inflammation is usually caused by one of the following:

- *Persistent infection by certain microorganisms:* While any infection can become persistent, certain microbes are less toxic than others, tend to invoke a particular type of immune reaction called delayed immunity (Chapter 8), and therefore tend to invoke chronic inflammation. This group includes *Mycobacterium tuberculosis*, the agent of tuberculosis (Chapter 14), *Treponema pallidum*, the agent of syphilis (Chapter 20), most parasites and fungi, and some viruses.
- *Autoimmune disease:* Autoimmune diseases (Chapter 8) are those in which the immune system mistakenly attacks "self" tissues. An example is rheumatoid arthritis, which is caused by the immune system's attack on the patient's own joints. All autoimmune disease is chronic, and most, but not all, autoimmune reactions cause a chronic inflammatory cell response. A few autoimmune reactions are intense and elicit acute inflammation, especially autoimmune blood vessel inflammation (arteritis).
- *Persistent exposure to injurious agents:* For example, chronic inflammation occurs in response to daily cigarette smoking, or inhalation of silica (rock dust) that lodges in the lungs and cannot be eliminated.

Persistence of the injury is the most important aspect of chronic inflammation. An initial injury may evoke short-term acute inflammation, but if the injury persists chronic inflammation will evolve. If a wood splinter enters skin, it produces immediate, mild acute inflammation. If, however, it is contaminated with bacteria and is not removed, an abscess likely will occur. Furthermore, if it remains longer than a week, the abscess will resolve by antibiotic therapy, rupture, or natural defenses. Nevertheless, if the splinter is not removed, chronic inflammation will develop around it, and the initial infiltrate of neutrophils will be replaced by an accumulation of lymphocytes, macrophages, new blood vessels, and scar tissue.

In most instances, chronic inflammation is not preceded by acute inflammation and appears de novo as the initial inflammatory response. Most autoimmune diseases, such as rheumatoid arthritis (Chapter 22), appear in this manner, and the initial cellular infiltrate is composed of lymphocytes and macrophages. The lymphocytes in chronic inflammation attack foreign material, usually microbes, or, in the case of autoimmune disease (Chapter 8), attack material that *appears* to be foreign. Lymphocytes are helped by macrophages, which ingest cell debris and foreign material. Moreover, macrophages can transform into fibroblasts to produce scar tissue, or endothelial cells to form new blood vessels. In chronic parasite infection and certain chronic allergic reactions, large numbers of eosinophils emerge to do their unique anti-parasitic and immune work (Chapter 8).

THE ANATOMIC CHARACTERISTICS OF CHRONIC INFLAMMATION

Chronic inflammation is less intense than is acute inflammation, and therefore is usually not as hot, swollen, red, and tender. Moreover, some chronically inflamed tissue may be shrunken by scar, atrophy, or necrosis. For example, muscle involved by chronic inflammation often becomes atrophic.

The cells of chronic inflammation are often called "**mononuclear cells**" or "**chronic inflammatory cells.**" The name is a misnomer, however, because all cells have a single nucleus. By contrast, to early observers the neutrophils of acute inflammation appeared to have multiple nuclei because, as we now know, the nucleus is segmented into small lobes connected by a strand of nuclear chromatin too small for early observers to detect.

Macrophages are the most important cells in chronic inflammation. They arise in the bone marrow and circulate in blood as **monocytes**, which have a life span of a few days. They migrate into tissue where they evolve into larger cells called **macrophages**, which have a lifespan of many months or years and are known by various names according to the tissue in which they reside. Macrophages are **phagocytes**—cells that ingest material and either digest it or prepare it for presentation to lymphocytes of the immune system (Chapter 8). They also secrete a wide variety of cytokines that include enzymes, coagulation factors, special proteins that facilitate immune reactions, and other factors that aid cells in their tasks.

Lymphocytes and **plasma cells** represent the immune system at the injured site. There are two types of lymphocytes, which act in different ways to attack foreign agents. **T lymphocytes** (which originate in the *thymus*) govern the *cellular immune system* and attack foreign agents directly. **B lymphocytes** (which originate in the *bone marrow*) represent the *humoral immune system* and secrete antibodies, which circulate in the blood as special proteins known as *immunoglobulins*. Immunoglobulins can attack foreign material far away from the cells at which they were made. When stimulated by

antigen, B lymphocytes change appearance and are known as **plasma cells**.

Granulomatous inflammation is a special type of chronic inflammation that is the hallmark of tuberculosis but may also occur in some other conditions. It features massive accumulations of macrophages (and some lymphocytes), which aggregate to form inflammatory nodules (**granulomas**) with distinctive microscopic features: sheets of macrophages gathered around a central point and the fusion of many macrophages to form huge cells with dozens of nuclei—**multinucleated giant cells** (Fig. 3-10).

THE CONSEQUENCES OF CHRONIC INFLAMMATION

The two consequences of chronic inflammation are: 1) resolution to *scar* or 2) *persistent chronic inflammation*. The process may be normal fibrous repair, in which fibroblasts and collagen (scar tissue) replace lost parenchymal cells, or the inflammation may persist, in which case the site remains a mixture of new blood vessels, inflammatory cells, edema fluid, and scar tissue.

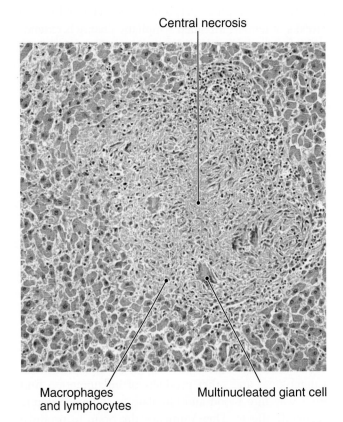

Figure 3-10 **Granulomatous inflammation.** In this microscopic study of tuberculosis of the liver, macrophages and lymphocytes form a nodular mass. Some of these cells have coalesced to form multinucleated giant cells.

Distant Effects of Inflammation

Inflammation, whether acute or chronic, has effects beyond the site of injury: the regional lymphatic system can become involved, and cytokines and other cell products find their way into blood to produce general effects on the body.

LYMPHANGITIS, LYMPHADENITIS, AND LYMPHADENOPATHY

The *lymphatic system* may become involved by inflammation. All parts of the body except the brain are drained by the lymphatic system, a delicate network of endothelial channels that in inflammation serve as a one-way drain from tissue to blood for inflammatory fluid, microbes, and debris. Normally, a small amount of interstitial fluid and protein flows into the lymphatic system to be filtered through lymph nodes as it is being returned to the bloodstream via a network of progressively larger lymph channels, which empty into a large vein in the upper chest. Lymph nodes trap and destroy bacteria and other foreign material and delay the spread of cancer cells that invade the lymphatic system.

Lymphangitis is inflammation, usually because of infection, of lymph vessels and is characterized by red streaks of tender, inflamed lymphatic channels extending centrally from the infected site. For example, a bacterial infection of the hand may be accompanied by red streaks extending up the arm, a sign very frightening to the general public, who equate it with "blood poisoning." While lymphangitis is not to be disregarded, it is not as dire as often imagined; it resolves with treatment of the primary infection.

Likewise, lymph nodes draining an injured or infected site may become infected (**lymphadenitis**); affected lymph nodes are usually enlarged or tender or both. Often the lymph node is not infected; rather, it is reacting to inflammatory products draining away from the infection or injury, a condition known as *reactive hyperplasia* (Chapter 11). *Clinically*, the term **lymphadenopathy** is applied to enlarged or tender lymph nodes irrespective of suspected diagnosis, be it malignancy or infection or other benign reaction.

SYSTEMIC EFFECTS OF INFLAMMATION

Chemokines and other products of inflammation find their way into blood and circulate to induce systemic (general) effects. They influence the brain to produce fever, malaise, drowsiness, and poor appetite. By other means they cause blood pressure to fall, suppress liver production of albumin, and cause the liver to produce certain proteins, **reactant proteins**, in response to the inflammation. Reactant proteins can be assayed by simple laboratory tests, as the accompanying Lab Tools box outlines, and are a very useful diagnostic tool. Each of these changes may occur to varying degree with acute or chronic inflammation depending on intensity. Acute infections produce the most severe systemic effects.

Among the more important acute reactant proteins is **C-reactive protein** (CRP), made by the liver. An increased level of blood CRP is a reliable marker for inflammation, and CRP is elevated with even minor degrees of inflammation. An elevated level of blood CRP is a useful differential tool for separating "sick" from "well," as was discussed in the opening pages of this textbook; that is to say, to sort out those who have some kind of tissue damage and inflammation somewhere in the body, as opposed to those who do not have tissue damage but have medical complaints; fibromyalgia (Chapter 22) is one such condition. And it is now clear that significant inflammation is associated with atherosclerosis, cancer, obesity, and Alzheimer disease. For example, an elevated level of CRP in an otherwise apparently healthy, non-obese patient has a strong association with atherosclerosis.

Inflammatory cytokines also stimulate the liver to manufacture other proteins, notably **fibrinogen**, the coagulation protein that polymerizes into the meshwork of fibrin in a blood clot. A peculiar but useful effect of increased fibrinogen is that it causes red blood cells to settle rapidly in their own plasma, an effect measured by the **erythrocyte sedimentation rate** (ESR). ESR and CRP are useful laboratory tools, as Case Study 3-1 at the end of this chapter demonstrates. Products of inflammation also circulate to act on the bone marrow to produce **leukocytosis**, an increased number of white blood cells (WBC) in circulating blood.

The Inflammatory Response to Infection

It is a common mistake to think that infection (Chapter 9) is the sole cause of inflammation, leukocytosis, fever, and other general symptoms of inflammation. Inflammation and the symptoms that accompany it can be caused by any type of tissue injury, including infarction, autoimmune disease, trauma, toxin. However, inflammation caused by infection may be dramatic and may take many forms.

Leukocytosis is a common feature of acute inflammatory reactions, especially in bacterial infections. Most bacteria produce a blood neutrophilic leukocyto-

Laboratory Indicators of Inflammation

Increased erythrocyte sedimentation rate (ESR) or C-reactive protein (CRP) indicates that inflammation is present somewhere in the body. Occasionally they may be the only indicators of inflammation.

ESR is a time-honored test widely used in office practice or in locations where easy access to laboratory services is not available. This old, simple, sensitive, cheap, and reliable test is performed by collecting whole blood in an anticoagulant, putting it into an upright standardized narrow tube and measuring how fast the red blood cells settle to the bottom. Persons with an increased ESR have inflammation of some kind somewhere, the extent roughly proportional to the degree of ESR increase. However, it may be increased by a very long list of non-inflammatory conditions including pregnancy, anemia, and malignancy. Furthermore, despite apparent simplicity it is easy to produce erroneous results. For example, even the slightest vibration or tilting of the tube will produce falsely high results. Use of ESR has declined in recent years as improved CRP testing has become available, although ESR remains a useful diagnostic tool.

CRP rises and falls more quickly than ESR after an acute inflammatory event. CRP is, therefore, a better indicator of current inflammation. Additionally, it is a much more sensitive test, detecting inflammation that ESR may miss. For example, low-grade inflammation occurs in the fatty deposits in patients who are obese, and is reflected by increased CRP in obesity. Inflammation also plays an important role in the pathogenesis of atherosclerosis, and CRP is elevated in patients with atherosclerosis (Chapter 12). What's more, CRP tends to rise in advance of the development of type II diabetes mellitus (Chapter 17). CRP detects this inflammatory reaction and therefore correlates with risks for obesity, atherosclerosis, and the development of type II diabetes. As a result, elevated CRP parallels increasing risk of heart attack, stroke, peripheral vascular disease and diabetes. However, CRP also may be increased by a long list of non-inflammatory conditions including high blood pressure, alcohol use, smoking, coffee consumption, and estrogen therapy.

---

sis (*neutrophilia*). On the other hand, allergic and parasitic reactions produce an *eosinophilia* (increased numbers of eosinophils in blood), and viral infections, such as measles, generally produce *lymphocytosis* (increased numbers of lymphocytes in blood). It is worth noting that bacterial infection of the bloodstream (sepsis, septicemia) has a toxic effect on bone marrow and may be associated with low peripheral blood WBC count (*leukopenia*); viral infections also may depress the total white cell count.

Bacteria usually produce a neutrophilic, acute, pyogenic (suppurative, purulent) inflammation. For example, staphylococci commonly cause abscesses filled with pus.

Other types of bacteria may produce other reactions. For example, *syphilis* and *Lyme disease* are infections caused by slender, corkscrew-shaped bacteria (spirochetes) that evoke a chronic inflammatory reaction. Because they are less acutely toxic and better able to defeat body defense mechanisms, they tend to produce chronic infections. *Tuberculosis* evokes a special type of chronic inflammatory reaction, granulomatous inflammation. In the stomach and duodenum, *Helicobacter pylori* causes ulcerative destruction of the gastric and small bowel intestinal mucosa (peptic ulcer, Chapter 15), which is accompanied by acute or

chronic inflammation depending on whether the ulcer is fresh or old. *Clostridium perfringens*, the agent of gas gangrene, cannot grow in the presence of oxygen (it is *anaerobic*). It produces direct tissue necrosis by secretion of toxins, lives in the dead tissue, and causes little inflammation.

Most *parasites* invade tissue, attracting eosinophils and stimulating an outpouring of eosinophils from the bone marrow, thus causing increased numbers of eosinophils to appear in blood (eosinophilia). However, protozoan parasites usually do not invade tissue and cause acute, superficial mucosal inflammation. For example, *Trichomonas vaginalis* infection of the vagina and *Giardia lamblia* infection of the gastrointestinal tract do not invade below the vaginal and intestinal mucosa and produce superficial, acute inflammation.

Most *viral* infections evoke a lymphocytic reaction; for example, influenza, the common cold, and infectious mononucleosis (Chapter 9). However, some viruses cause direct tissue *necrosis* with acute inflammation. For example, herpesvirus infection (oral cold sores) causes cell necrosis and acute inflammation. On the other hand, some chronic infections are notable for the *scarring* they produce. Chronic hepatitis B and chronic hepatitis C infections can cause severe fibrosis of the liver (cirrhosis, Chapter 16). ∎

CASE STUDY 3-1 "MY DOCTOR THINKS I'M CRAZY"

TOPICS
The hostile patient
Polymyalgia rheumatica

THE CASE

Setting: You work in a county hospital system in a large metropolitan area doing psychiatric interviews on patients referred from outlying primary care clinics.

Clinical history: The referral note is brief and almost illegible, but clearly printed at the end are "*Demanding!*" and "*Hostile!*" With some difficulty you read that Jane T. is a 43-year-old woman referred with a diagnosis of "possible depression." The chart reveals that on her first visit several months earlier she named a long list of vague complaints—she "hurt all over," and she said her "eyes are sore." She answered nearly every question about possible symptoms with "sometimes" and "maybe." Physical exam, urinalysis, blood tests, and other lab studies were unremarkable. Several follow-up visits were much the same: she complained of aches and pains but had no physical or lab abnormalities.

You find her in the interview room perched tensely on the edge of a chair, arms folded across her chest. You introduce yourself, but she pays no attention to your courtesy and says, "I suppose you think I'm crazy, too; wouldn't surprise me in the least. All of you are in league with one another." Taken aback, you wonder if the referring physician just wanted to get her out if his hair and referred her away.

In the interview she admits to family and work stress and says, "The doctor that sent me over here thinks I'm crazy, but he's the one that's nuts. I know this is where they send the mental cases, but I'm telling you it's not just 'in my head,' as they say. *Something* is wrong with me." You listen patiently and begin to question her in detail. She says she does not sleep well, has lost a few pounds, feels tired, and has "fevers" but has not taken her temperature. She complains of stiffness in her neck and shoulders, so much that she has trouble combing her hair. She says her lower back "aches all the time," and her joints are stiff each morning when she wakes up. There is no history of muscle weakness or tenderness, and she reports no visual, skin, or neurologic problems.

Physical examination and other data: She looks tired and glum, and as you examine her she is jumpy and tender at almost every point of touch on her neck, shoulders, and lower back. The physical exam is otherwise unremarkable, and you specifically note that she has no evidence of joint disease in her hands, knees, or feet.

Outside the examination room you collect your thoughts and admit that she is hostile, demanding, and cynical—a thoroughly unpleasant patient. As you are pondering a graceful way to get rid of someone so upsetting and unlikable, you recall a psychiatry lecture about hostile patients—it is normal for caregivers to become angry with some patients. The anger must be recognized and managed, and it must not hamper judgment or conduct because it can interfere with good patient care. Clearing your head, you take a deep breath and study the chart again, trying to think anew before sending her to a psychiatrist—and you note that the results of previous laboratory tests for rheumatoid factor (RF) (for rheumatoid arthritis) and antinuclear antibodies (ANA) (for autoimmune diseases) were negative. However, much to your surprise, there is no record that she had an erythrocyte sedimentation rate (ESR) test or a C-reactive protein (CRP) test. You order both and decide to repeat RF and ANA tests. You also request a test for creatine kinase (CK) (for increased muscle enzyme in blood) and several other laboratory tests and give her an appointment to return in a week.

The next day the ESR and CRP are reported as markedly elevated; and the RF, ANA, CK, and other laboratory results are unremarkable.

DISCUSSION

History, lab tests, and physical exam ruled out anemia, malignancy, pregnancy, and other non-inflammatory conditions known to increase ESR and CRP. The negative RF test and lack of visible joint disease eliminated a diagnosis of rheumatoid arthritis. The negative ANA test and lack of joint or skin disease eliminated diagnoses of systemic lupus erythematosus and other major autoimmune processes. The normal CK result excluded polymyositis, an inflammatory disease of muscle. However, the elevated ESR and CRP indicated that there was inflammation somewhere in the body, proving that your patient's illness was not "in her head."

The diagnosis was *polymyalgia rheumatica (PMR)*, a syndrome of pain and stiffness located around joints in the shoulder and pelvic area. Evidence suggests that this is a type of arthritis not severe enough to cause radiographic abnormalities or joint deformities. It affects women more often than men; most patients are over 60, and many of them are depressed or under other emotional stress. Typical PMR patients have no objective signs of disease except abnormal ESR and CRP—no joint or other abnormalities are evident. Some PMR patients develop *temporal arteritis*, a serious inflammatory disease of the temporal artery (Chapter 12) that can cause blindness if the optic artery becomes involved.

Polymyalgia rheumatica is mainly a diagnosis of exclusion after other, more serious illnesses (e.g., systemic lupus erythematosus, rheumatoid arthritis, and other autoimmune ▶

[Case 3-1, continued] diseases) have been ruled out. A diagnosis of *fibromyalgia* can be made for patients with aches and complaints similar to those of polymyalgia rheumatica but with *no* laboratory abnormalities or other objective findings of disease—that is, patients with normal ESR and CRP levels and normal physical examination and radiographic results. Fibromyalgia is seen predominately in young adult women who are depressed or under emotional stress and responds best to anti-depression drugs.

Polymyalgia rheumatica can be treated effectively with low-dose steroids, which may need to be continued for years. Aspirin and other non-steroidal anti-inflammatory drugs are not helpful.

POINTS TO REMEMBER
- Angry, hostile patients deserve good medical care.
- Inflammation causes distinct changes in blood proteins, which are detectable by laboratory tests.

Objectives Recap

1. *Describe the purpose of inflammation:* The purpose of inflammation is to limit the extent and severity of injury, eliminate or neutralize the offending agent, and to initiate the repair process.

2. *Describe the main cell types in acute and chronic inflammation:* The cells of acute inflammation are neutrophils; those of chronic inflammation are lymphocytes, monocytes (macrophages), and plasma cells.

3. *Contrast acute and chronic inflammation:* Acute inflammation occurs with short-term injury and lasts a few hours or a week or so. It features a cell infiltrate of neutrophils. Chronic inflammation occurs with persistent injury and lasts weeks or years. It features an infiltrate of lymphocytes and monocytes (macrophages) and sometimes plasma cells.

4. *Describe the sequence of events in acute inflammation:* Vasodilation, edema, neutrophil infiltration, monocyte and macrophage infiltration, resolution.

5. *Name the four classic clinical signs of inflammation:* Tumor (swelling), rubor (redness), calor (heat), dolor (pain).

6. *Name the three gross anatomic types of inflammatory exudate:* Serous, fibrinous, and purulent.

7. *Name the four possible outcomes of acute inflammation:* Complete resolution, scar, abscess, chronic inflammation.

8. *Name the usual causes of chronic inflammation and offer an example of each:* Persistent infection (tuberculosis), autoimmune disease (rheumatoid arthritis), persistent exposure to injurious agents (daily cigarette smoking).

9. *Define granulomatous inflammation:* It is a special form of chronic inflammation characteristic of tuberculosis but also seen in a few other conditions. It features large nodules of macrophages, some of which merge to form giant cells with dozens of nuclei.

10. *Name the outcomes of chronic inflammation:* Scar and persistent chronic inflammation.

11. *Name the distant effects of inflammation:* Involvement of lymphatics and lymph nodes, and systemic effects such as fever, malaise, leukocytosis, and poor appetite, and the production of reactant proteins, such as fibrinogen and C-reactive protein.

12. *Name two important reactant proteins found in the blood in inflammation:* C-reactive protein; and fibrinogen, which accounts for elevated erythrocyte sedimentation rate (ESR).

13. *Discuss the inflammatory response to various types of infectious agents:* Bacteria usually produce a neutrophilic, acute, pyogenic (suppurative, purulent) inflammation; however, syphilis and other spirochetes cause chronic inflammation (mostly lymphocytes). Parasites usually evoke an infiltrate of eosinophils. Viruses usually evoke an infiltrate of lymphocytes.

1. Acute injury is characterized by which one of the following?
    A. Lymphocytic cellular infiltrate
    B. Immune reaction
    C. Neutrophilic cellular infiltrate
    D. Scarring

2. The principal job of neutrophils in inflammation is which one of the following?
    A. Phagocytosis
    B. Apoptosis
    C. Secretion of histamine and serotonin
    D. The production of fever

3. Edema in acute inflammation is mainly the result of which one of the following?
    A. Accumulation of neutrophils
    B. Plasma leaking from capillaries
    C. Fluid liberated from dead cells
    D. Increased fibrinogen

4. Pyogenic inflammation is characterized by which one of the following?
    A. Dense infiltrates of lymphocytes
    B. Accumulations of pus
    C. Marked angioneogenesis
    D. Scar formation

5. The most important cell in chronic inflammation is which one of the following?
    A. Macrophage
    B. Lymphocyte
    C. Giant cell
    D. Eosinophil

6. True or false? Acute inflammation occurs with short-term injury.

7. True or false? Chronic inflammation is characterized by an infiltrate of macrophages and lymphocytes.

8. True or false? Macrophages control most of the exchange of substances between blood and tissue.

9. True or false? Parasites that invade tissue usually produce an eosinophilic reaction.

10. True or false? Persistent infection by microorganisms is one cause of chronic inflammation.

Repair: Recovery from Injury

This chapter focuses on repair, the process by which the body attempts to restore normal structure and function to the site of injury. It discusses how cells regenerate to either replace damaged tissue or mend tissue if regeneration is not possible.

DEFINITIONS
REPLACEMENT OF INJURED CELLS
- The Importance of Tissue Structure
- The Control of Cell Reproduction and Tissue Growth
WOUND HEALING AND FIBROUS REPAIR
- Cell Migration into the Wound
- The Growth of New Blood Vessels

- Scar Development
- Healing by First Intention
- Healing by Second Intention
ABNORMAL WOUND HEALING
- Host Factors Interfering with Wound Healing
- Pathologic Wound Healing
OVERVIEW OF INJURY, INFLAMMATION, AND REPAIR

Learning Objectives

After studying this chapter you should be able to:
1. Distinguish among repair, regeneration, and healing
2. Name the two main elements of the repair process
3. Name the types of cells according to their ability to regenerate
4. Explain the importance of the basement membrane and extracellular matrix in the repair process
5. Define "wound"
6. List in sequence the component steps in fibrous repair (scarring)
7. Define angioneogenesis
8. Define granulation tissue
9. Discuss what is meant by "healing by first and second intention" by contrasting the two
10. Discuss some obstacles to normal repair
11. Name and discuss two examples of pathologic wound repair

Can honour set to a leg? No. Or an arm? No. Or take away the grief of a wound? No.

WILLIAM SHAKESPEARE (1564–1616), ENGLISH PLAYWRIGHT, *HENRY IV, PART 1* (V.i)

Definitions

After injury (Chapter 2) and inflammation (Chapter 3) comes repair. As is illustrated in Figure 4-1, **repair** is the body's collective attempt to restore normal structure and function to the injured site. Repair consists of two processes: *regeneration* and *healing*.

- **Regeneration** is the complete or nearly complete restoration of normal anatomy and function by the regrowth of normal functional cells (**parenchyma**) and supporting tissue (**stroma**); little or no scarring occurs in regeneration. Regeneration usually follows relatively mild injury.
- **Healing** is a broader process that occurs when regeneration is partial or not possible, and tissue that cannot be replaced "good as new" by regeneration must be mended by scar (fibrous) tissue, a process called **fibrous repair** (scarring).

Replacement of Injured Cells

Normal cells are classified according to their ability to regenerate themselves. In other words, they either can, or they cannot, regenerate. As is illustrated in Figure 4-2, all normal adult tissue is composed of one of three types of cells, *labile, stable,* or *permanent*:

- **Labile cells** are capable of regeneration. They have a short life span and are replaced from a reserve of continuously reproducing **stem cells**, which are primitive, multipotent cells that possess a unique method of reproduction: At cell division one daughter cell becomes a new stem cell to replenish the stem cell population, and the other differentiates into a functional cell to replace lost or injured cells. Basics in Brief 4-1 explains more about stem cells. Bone marrow cells, intestinal epithelial cells, bronchial epithelial cells, and epidermal cells (of skin) fall into this category. There is good reason for this design: skin, bronchial epithelium, and gastrointestinal epithelium are in constant contact with bacteria and other harmful environmental elements and need continual replacement. Likewise, white blood cells are consumed daily defending the body and repairing damage. Similarly, red blood cells have a normal life span of about 120 days, and fresh cells are needed daily to ensure O_2 delivery to tissue and CO_2 return to the lungs.
- **Stable cells** are also capable of complete regeneration. They have a life span of months to years and reproduce slowly unless injured. They are in protected

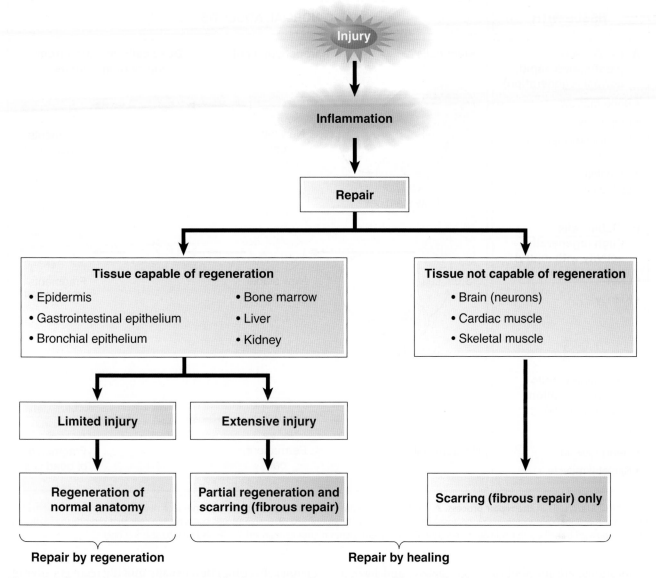

Figure 4-1 The repair process. In tissues capable of regeneration (those with stem cells), repair of mild injury takes place by means of regeneration of new functional (parenchymal) cells and the restoration of normal anatomy. Repair of severe injury occurs by means of regeneration of new functional cells and partly by scarring (fibrous repair). In tissues not capable of regeneration (without stem cells), repair of injury takes place only by scarring.

STEM CELLS

The realization that stem cells can regenerate tissue is one of the most exciting topics in modern medicine. The thing that makes stem cells so unusual is their potential to evolve into every type of tissue.

Not all stem cells are the same; some have a broader ability to differentiate into new tissue than others. *Embryonic stem cells* are the most flexible; however, adult bone marrow contains *adult stem cells* that can differentiate into cells as varied as hepatocytes and neurons. *Tissue stem cells* are those that reside in organs or tissues other than bone marrow and have the narrowest potential.

TISSUE WITH	NORMAL ADULT TISSUE		

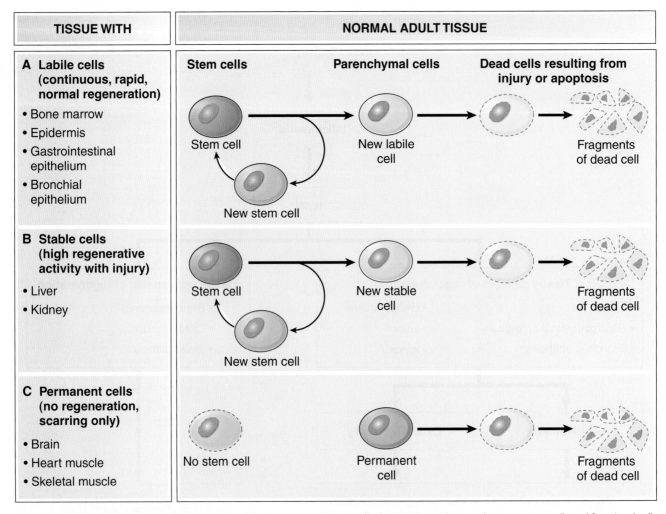

A Labile cells (continuous, rapid, normal regeneration)
- Bone marrow
- Epidermis
- Gastrointestinal epithelium
- Bronchial epithelium

B Stable cells (high regenerative activity with injury)
- Liver
- Kidney

C Permanent cells (no regeneration, scarring only)
- Brain
- Heart muscle
- Skeletal muscle

Stem cells — Parenchymal cells — Dead cells resulting from injury or apoptosis

Stem cell / New stem cell → New labile cell → Fragments of dead cell

Stem cell / New stem cell → New stable cell → Fragments of dead cell

No stem cell → Permanent cell → Fragments of dead cell

***Figure 4-2* Stem cells in the repair process. A.** Labile tissues contain stem cells that continuously reproduce new stem cells and functional cells to replace functional cells lost to injury (necrosis) or natural cell death (apoptosis). **B.** Stable tissues contain stem cells that reproduce rapidly only when stimulated by cell death resulting from injury. **C.** Permanent tissues do not contain stem cells and heal by scarring only.

locations, are metabolically very active, and have a reserve of stem cells that can be activated by stress or injury to replace dead or defective cells. Liver cells (hepatocytes) and renal tubular epithelial cells fall into this category.

- **Permanent cells** are not capable of regeneration. Permanent cells are at an end stage of specialization (differentiation) and are thus not capable of regeneration after injury. Tissues composed of permanent cells do not have a reserve of stem cells capable of regeneration. Permanent cells cannot reproduce and must last a lifetime. Cardiac and skeletal muscle cells and neurons fall into this category.

Tissues composed of each cell type respond differently to injury; differences that are clinically important. For example, wounds such as skin cuts are usually repaired quickly because epidermal cells are in a perpetual state of renewal from stem cells. The same is true of bone—it reconstitutes completely after fracture. In like manner, liver function usually quickly recovers after injury because hepatocytes are labile cells that normally do not reproduce but are famously capable of regeneration after injury. An example is pediatric liver transplant using part of an adult liver to replace an entire child's liver. The adult donor's liver quickly regenerates to near-normal size. However, the opposite is true for brain or myocardial cell necrosis (stroke or heart attack), each of which always results in scarring because brain and myocardial cells are permanent cells incapable of regeneration.

> ☞ *The manner in which tissues repair depends on the cell type of the injured tissue—labile cells (epidermis and mucosa), stable cells (liver and kidney) or permanent cells (brain, heart, and skeletal muscle). Labile cells regenerate easily and stable cells less easily; permanent cells cannot regenerate.*

THE IMPORTANCE OF TISSUE STRUCTURE

Although labile and stable tissues are capable of regeneration, restoration of normal anatomy is not always successful. It must be organized correctly, and organized regeneration requires an intact supporting stromal framework upon which regenerating cells can grow. The two elements of the stromal framework are the basement membrane and the extracellular matrix.

- The **basement membrane** (Fig. 4-3) is a thin, filmy membrane that underlies all epithelium (for example, epidermis, bronchial, and gastrointestinal epithelium). An intact basement membrane provides the surface upon which epithelial cells grow normally and regrow after injury. Basics in Brief 4-2 highlights the critical role basement membrane plays in cancer development.
- The **extracellular matrix** is a mixture of collagen, elastin fibers, and other elements synthesized by fibroblasts and other cells to create a structural meshwork to support cell regrowth.

The basement membrane and extracellular matrix provide the scaffolding upon which regenerating cells grow in an orderly manner to redevelop normal anatomy and function. Without their support, tissues cannot return to normal, and scarring occurs. The more severe the injury, the more likely it is that the stromal framework will be too damaged for regeneration of normal anatomy.

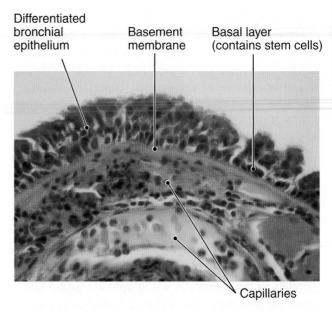

Differentiated bronchial epithelium

Basement membrane

Basal layer (contains stem cells)

Capillaries

Figure 4-3 **Basement membrane in normal bronchial mucosa.** An intact basement membrane provides the surface upon which epithelial cells grow normally and regrow after injury. This microscopic study is of bronchial epithelial cells, which are labile cells that have a short life span and require daily replacement by stem cells located on the basement membrane.

The repair of skin burns is instructive. Epidermis is a labile tissue resting on a basement membrane. First-degree burns (erythema only) or second-degree burns (blisters) may be repaired perfectly and without scarring because in first-degree and second-degree burns the epidermal basement membrane is intact and the epidermis regrows in an orderly manner. Scarring is absent. On the other hand, in third-degree burns the injury destroys the epidermis, the basement membrane, and at least some of the dermis. Therefore, an intact basement membrane and other structures are missing, which could otherwise guide epidermal regeneration. As a result, scarring always occurs.

THE CONTROL OF CELL REPRODUCTION AND TISSUE GROWTH

Repair requires cells to divide and multiply. Cell growth is governed in normal and in injured tissue by **proto-oncogenes** (Chapter 6), which stimulate the production of multiple **growth factors** derived from leukocytes, platelets, endothelial cells, and fibroblasts (proto-oncogenes are also important in cancer biology, Chapter 6). Growth factors are small protein molecules that govern cell regeneration and scar production; they stimulate increased vascular permeability, attract cells into the site, and stimulate them to divide. Two of the most important growth factors are *epidermal growth factor* and *vascular endothelial growth* factor. **Epidermal growth factor** is derived from platelets and macrophages and stimulates epidermal cells and fibroblasts to migrate into a skin wound and multiply. **Vascular endothelial growth factor** is derived from mesenchymal cells (e.g., fibrocytes, muscle cells), and it increases vascular permeability and stimulates endothelial cells to divide.

The action of growth factors and related hormones is influenced by the **extracellular matrix**, which is a mix of fibers (collagen and elastin) and soluble proteinaceous molecules mixed with water. Coupled with basement membranes, it provides a structural lattice for cell growth. Moreover, it sustains the repair process, binds cells together, provides cushioning and viscosity, and serves as a medium for migration of cells and diffusion of growth factors and other molecules.

Wound Healing and Fibrous Repair

For this discussion of the repair process, a **wound** is defined as an injury resulting from short term injury at a discrete site; for example, a surgical skin incision. Most wounds are minor—a skin scratch or a bruise, for example—and heal without treatment. However, some wounds require medical management. How wound care has improved in the last century is illustrated in the nearby History of Medicine box, which recounts the wound care given to 20th United States President, James Garfield (1831–1881) after he was shot in an assassination attempt.

History of Medicine

THE WOUNDS OF PRESIDENT JAMES A. GARFIELD

On July 2, 1881, less than four months after inauguration, United States President James A. Garfield was shot twice at point blank range by a frustrated office-seeker using a .44 pistol. One bullet caused a superficial arm wound; the other, however, entered his back at the right lower side of his ribs, passed in front of his spine and lodged in the retroperitoneum slightly below the pancreas—facts established later at autopsy; only the entry wound could be detected at the time.

Unfortunately for Garfield, he lived during a period when medicine had not fully accepted that microbes could cause disease—surgical gloves, antiseptics, masks, antibiotics, and sterile instruments did not exist. The first physician on the scene inserted an unsterile metal probe into the wound in an attempt to find the bullet. Within days the wound was obviously infected and oozing pus. Later, almost all of the dozen or more physicians who attended Garfield probed the wound with their bare fingers and gadgets, opening it further in an attempt to find the bullet or in order to drain accumulations of pus. By the time Garfield died on September 19th, eighty days after being shot, the original wound, which probably would have healed on its own if left alone, had been enlarged to a 20 inch gash that extended around his flank and ended near his right groin.

Modern wound care is completely different and depends on rigorously sterile procedures, antibiotics, good drainage, proper dressing for protection from the environment, and an understanding that some bullets are best left alone.

The cause of Garfield's death is not certain. He complained suddenly of chest discomfort and died not long thereafter. It is reasonable to speculate that he died of a heart attack or pulmonary embolus, either of which could have been prompted in several ways by awful consequences of his wound. At the time death, he had wasted from robust good health at 210 lb to a near skeleton of 130 lb.

Ideal repair is complete restoration of normal anatomy and function by **regeneration** of the anatomy and specialized functional (parenchymal) cells of the organ. In contrast, **healing** is a process that occurs when regeneration is not possible or is incomplete and additional mending of the site is required by **fibrous repair**—the production of a scar. Fibrous repair occurs under the following circumstances:

- The damage to tissue is so extensive that the supporting framework is destroyed; third-degree thermal burns of skin are an example.
- The injured tissue is composed of permanent cells, such as myocardium, skeletal muscle, or brain.

As is illustrated in Figure 4-4, fibrous repair evolves from injury and inflammation and may coexist with chronic inflammation. The evolution of fibrous repair occurs in the following sequence:

- *Fibrocyte migration and proliferation*—to provide raw material for repair
- *Angioneogenesis*—the growth of new blood vessels to nourish the process
- *Scar development*—the synthesis of extracellular matrix proteins and deposition of collagen followed by contraction (shrinking), reshaping (remodeling), and strengthening of the fibrous tissue

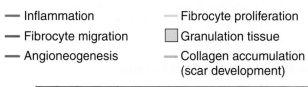

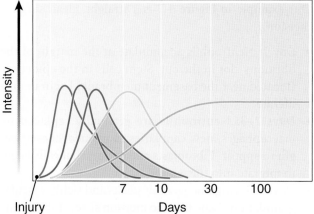

Figure 4-4 **Fibrous repair (scarring).** After injury and inflammation, fibrocytes migrate into the wound and begin proliferating as inflammation fades. New blood vessels sprout and form a rich fibrovascular mix called granulation tissue, which fades as collagen deposited by fibrocytes accumulates as a scar.

CELL MIGRATION INTO THE WOUND

The healing process begins within hours of injury as leukocytes limit the damage and begin clearing the site of debris and foreign material. Leukocytes attracted to the site produce cytokines that stimulate migration and proliferation of fibroblasts into the injury site. At the same time, endothelial cells from nearby blood vessels begin to sprout angioblasts, which form into new capillaries. Fibroblasts proliferate to fill space not occupied by regenerating parenchymal cells, synthesize collagen fibers to knit back together the disrupted tissue, and provide the permanent structure to support additional cell growth. Later these collagen fibers slowly contract to tighten the wound into a firm bond.

THE GROWTH OF NEW BLOOD VESSELS

Angioneogenesis is the growth of new blood vessels into the wound. Vascular endothelial growth factor and other factors stimulate new vessels to sprout from existing vessels. Angioneogenesis occurs in several smooth, interrelated steps, as is depicted in Figure 4-5:

- *Normal capillary with intact basement membrane and endothelial cells*
- *Dissolution of the basement membrane of the parent vessel(s) in the injured site by proteolytic enzymes released by inflammatory cells*
- *Migration and proliferation of angioneoblastic endothelial cells through the defect and up the gradient of cytokines released by inflammatory cells and injured cells*
- *Organization of a new capillary branch as the tube of endothelial cells generates a basement membrane*

Later in the healing process, angioneogenesis continues as blood vessels enlarge in order to convey nutrients, cytokines, and hormones to the site.

SCAR DEVELOPMENT

Scar development follows angioneogenesis and occurs in several related and overlapping steps, listed below, which deposit a network of collagen and other fibers to bind together the edges of the wound.

- *Migration and proliferation of fibroblasts and new blood vessels into the injured site*
- *Deposition of an extracellular matrix of collagen and other supportive proteins*
- *Maturation, remodeling (remolding), contraction, and strengthening of the fibrous tissue*

The initial phase in scar development is a highly vascular mixture of capillaries, fibroblasts, residual edema,

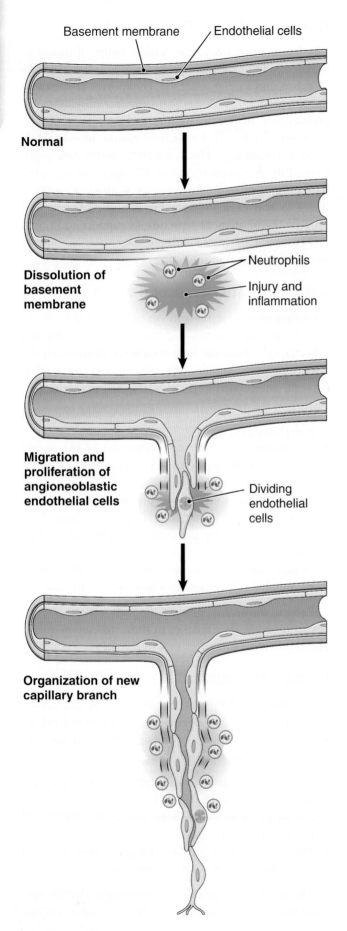

Normal

Dissolution of basement membrane

Neutrophils

Injury and inflammation

Migration and proliferation of angioneoblastic endothelial cells

Dividing endothelial cells

Organization of new capillary branch

and small numbers of leukocytes collectively known as **granulation tissue** (Fig. 4-6A), a phase that persists from a few days to several weeks depending on the size of the wound. As the process unfolds, fibroblasts contract, pulling the edges of the wound inward, decreasing the volume to be healed. As the wound edges are pulled inward, fibroblasts produce collagen and other extracellular components to bind the wound firmly and give it strength. Gradually fluid is resorbed, inflammatory cells disappear, and the site becomes occupied by a less cellular, more collagenous tissue. Finally, blood vessels shrink or disappear as workload decreases. Similarly, as more collagen accumulates to bind the wound tightly, fibroblasts shrink and disappear. The result is a dense, relatively bloodless scar, as depicted in Figure 4-6B. Finally, the scar is reshaped (remodeled) as mechanical forces pull it into a configuration that eases stress on the wound. A fresh scar is tense and produces a noticeable sensation of tightness or deformity. However, after complete remodeling, a scar fits comfortably in the site, molded in conformity to surrounding tissue.

The fundamentals of wound healing are the same in every wound; however, it is instructive to compare the differences between the healing of narrow and broad skin wounds, which are depicted in Figure 4-7. Narrow wounds with closely approximated edges heal by what is called **first intention**; surgical incisions are an example. Broad wounds with widely separated margins heal by **second intention**; for example, deep skin burns, or ulcers. The healing process is similar in sites other than skin: An incision of liver or kidney heals by first intention; and a gastric ulcer heals by second intention.

HEALING BY FIRST INTENTION

Our example in Figure 4-7 is a straight, clean surgical incision.

- *Day 1*: Neutrophils accumulate at the margin of the fibrinous clot in the cut. Stem cells in the epidermis (located near the basement membrane) begin to proliferate.
- *Days 2–3*: Neutrophils are gradually replaced by macrophages; new capillaries (angioneogenesis) begin to appear. Fibroblasts and endothelial cells begin to migrate into the wound.
- *Days 3–7*: Angioneogenesis peaks and richly vascular granulation tissue fills the incision space. Fibroblasts

Figure 4-5 **Angioneogenesis.** The basement membrane of injured capillaries dissolves, and endothelial cells migrate through the defect and into the injury, where they form a new capillary.

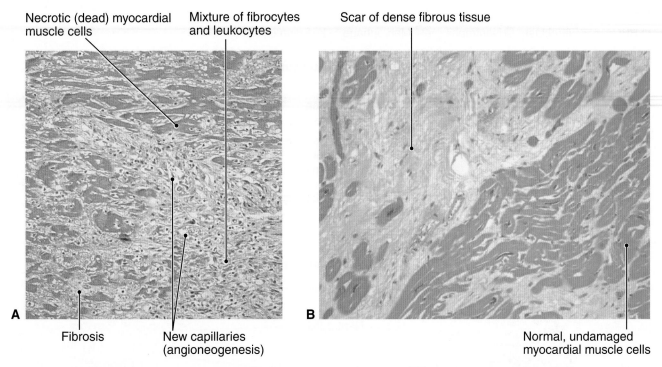

Necrotic (dead) myocardial muscle cells

Mixture of fibrocytes and leukocytes

Scar of dense fibrous tissue

A

B

Fibrosis

New capillaries (angioneogenesis)

Normal, undamaged myocardial muscle cells

Figure 4-6 **Granulation tissue in a healing myocardial infarct. A.** Ten days after infarct, some dead muscle cells remain; others have been replaced by a mixture of inflammatory cells, edema, fibrous tissue, and new blood vessels (granulation tissue). **B.** Healed myocardial infarct, months or years old. Dead muscle cells (which cannot regenerate) have been removed and replaced by dense scar tissue. Nearby are normal, undamaged cardiac muscle cells.

produce large amounts of collagen to bridge the space between the edges of the wound. Growth of epidermal stem cells has produced a thin layer of epithelium to cover the wound.

- *Second week*: Fibroblastic proliferation continues and collagen accumulates. Inflammatory cells, edema fluid, and blood vessels are disappearing rapidly.
- *End of first month*: A pink (vascularized) scar is present. It is composed largely of collagen, is devoid of inflammatory cells, has a declining number of blood vessels, and is covered by normal epidermis. The tensile strength of the wound continues to improve as fibroblasts contract and continue to add collagen.
- *After several months or a year*: A narrowed, white, fitted scar is present. Skin tensile strength has returned to near normal.

A freshly sutured wound has about 70% of normal tensile strength if sutures are placed correctly. After suture removal at one week, tensile strength is about 10%. Strength improves to about 75% at three months and after a year has returned to near normal.

HEALING BY SECOND INTENTION

Healing by second intention (also Fig. 4-7) is much the same as healing by first intention: inflammation first, followed by macrophage clean-up, neovascularization and scarring. However, the volume of necrotic tissue to be removed is greater, and reepithelialization of the surface is slower because the wound is wider. Healing by second intention is characteristic of ulcers, infarcts, abscesses, or other wounds where the defect is large and wound edges are not close together. A greater volume of necrotic and inflammatory debris must be removed, and a large amount of granulation tissue is required to fill the gap. The granulation tissue is replaced by scar tissue, which in turn contracts so that the final volume of the scar may be as little as 10% of the original defect. In tissue covered by epithelium, new epithelial cells advance inward from the edges, first forming a thin membrane of immature cells that rest on underlying granulation tissue and then differentiate into mature epithelium as the wound below matures into scar.

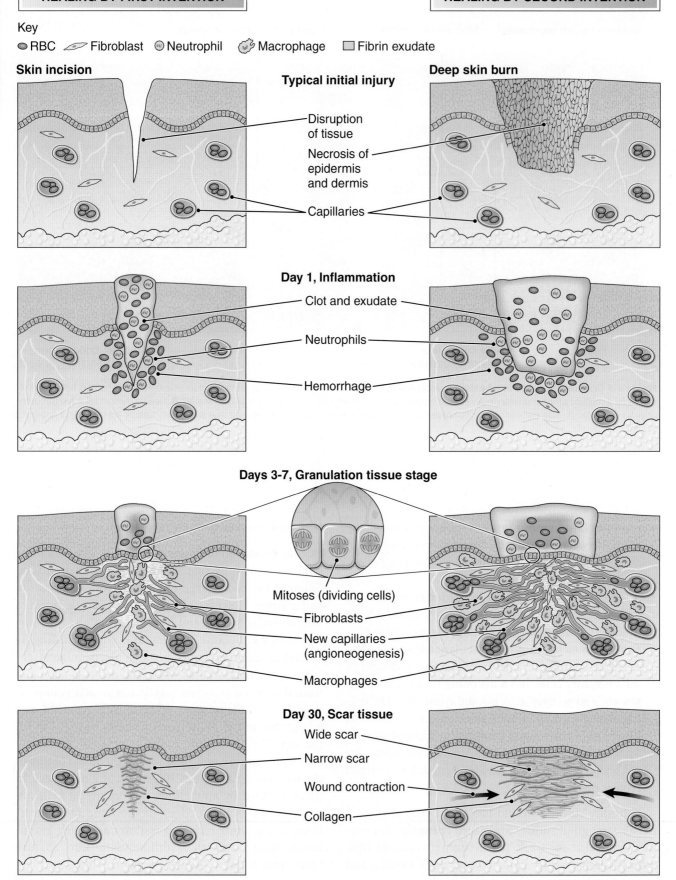

Key
● RBC   ✎ Fibroblast   ⊚ Neutrophil   🦠 Macrophage   ☐ Fibrin exudate

Skin incision

Deep skin burn

Typical initial injury

Disruption of tissue

Necrosis of epidermis and dermis

Capillaries

Day 1, Inflammation

Clot and exudate

Neutrophils

Hemorrhage

Days 3-7, Granulation tissue stage

Mitoses (dividing cells)

Fibroblasts

New capillaries (angioneogenesis)

Macrophages

Day 30, Scar tissue

Wide scar

Narrow scar

Wound contraction

Collagen

Figure 4-7 **Healing by first and second intention.** Small, narrow wounds heal by first intention (*left*), usually in less than a week, and leave a small scar. Large wounds heal by second intention (*right*), have more inflammatory tissue, take several weeks to heal, and leave a larger scar.

Abnormal Wound Healing

Wound healing may be impaired by local or systemic factors or it may be pathologic. Local factors include Infections and retained foreign bodies; systemic factors include vascular disease and poor nutrition. For example, wounds in patients with diabetes are notably slow to heal because of the vascular disease from which most patients with diabetes suffer. Also, the repair process may become abnormal; that is, it may become pathologic. Case Study 4-1 at the end of this chapter illustrates the problem of impaired wound repair.

HOST FACTORS INTERFERING WITH WOUND HEALING

Local and general host factors may prevent a wound from healing normally.

- *Infection:* The most frequent cause of abnormal wound healing is infection, which prolongs the injury and interferes with healing at the same time.
- *Poor nutrition:* Deficiency of vitamin C or protein inhibits collagen synthesis. For example, elderly people are often poorly nourished because they may be poor, forgetful, or unable to feed themselves properly.
- *Steroid drugs:* Anti-inflammatory glucocorticoids, widely used in therapy of autoimmune disease and other conditions, slow the growth of fibroblasts and production of collagen, which binds wound edges together. An example is a surgical wound from joint surgery in a patient with severe arthritis who is on long-term steroid therapy.
- *Poor blood supply:* Blood brings nutrition to the site and poor blood flow impairs healing. For example, patients with long-standing diabetes usually have diseased small blood vessels, especially in the feet and legs. As a result, diabetic wounds heal slowly, especially those in the feet. Something as seemingly harmless as an ingrown toenail can be very difficult to treat in a patient with diabetic vascular disease.
- *Foreign bodies:* Pieces of metal, wood, glass, or bone may obstruct the tight closure of a wound and produce continued irritation and inflammation that may also encourage infection.
- *Mechanical factors:* Increased pressure or torsion may stress the wound so that a tight closure does not occur.

Wounds that do not heal properly may rupture (**dehiscence**) or may ulcerate. Dehiscence is most common in abdominal wounds and occurs when high tension is placed on the abdominal wall case by body motion.

Sitting up or turning over in bed, coughing, vomiting, or sneezing may be enough to rupture a dehisced wound.

Additionally, wounds may ulcerate, especially if wound repair is not proceeding normally. Wound edges may not knit together and consequently can pull apart or the epithelium may not regenerate, leaving the surface without an epithelial covering. Ulceration exposes wounds to infection, dehiscence, and other problems.

PATHOLOGIC WOUND HEALING

Certain intrinsic abnormalities may cause wound repair to deviate from normal. That is, wound repair may create a problem rather than solving one. There are two main types of pathologic repair: formation of a *keloid* or accumulation of *excess granulation tissue*, both of which may be thought of as non-neoplastic, exuberant overgrowths of otherwise normal tissue.

A **keloid**, pictured in Figure 4-8, is a hyperplastic scar that is prominent, raised, or nodular and contains excess collagen. Some patients, especially people of African heritage, have a genetic predisposition to keloid formation. Despite the fact that keloids may appear quickly and grow rapidly, they are not neoplastic, and are rarely anything more than a cosmetic problem.

The second type of aberrant wound repair is a localized, highly vascular collection of persistent granulation tissue called **pyogenic granuloma**, an anomaly that represents a repair process halted in its most vascular stage. Often these nodules of vascular tissue have lost their inflammatory infiltrate and edema fluid, giving them an exceptional vascularity that makes them look like a benign vascular tumor (hemangioma). One of the most noticeable sites for pyogenic granuloma is in the

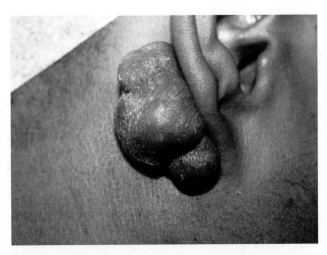

Figure 4-8 Keloid of the ear lobe. A keloid is hyperplastic scar. This one was successfully removed with good cosmetic effect and did not recur.

healing umbilicus of newborns, where it appears as a fleshy bleeding nodule that can appear alarming to the child's parents.

Overview of Injury, Inflammation, and Repair

In Chapter 2 we discussed *injury,* in Chapter 3 *inflammation,* and in this chapter we have studied *repair.* Inflammation and repair occur in a smooth continuum after acute injury and lead to one of three possible outcomes: 1) complete repair by regeneration; 2) repair by a mixture of regeneration and fibrosis; or 3) repair by fibrosis only. The outcome is dependent on the degree and extent of injury and the type of cells composing the injured tissue—labile, stable, or permanent.

Complete restitution of normal anatomy and function by *regeneration* is common in minor skin and mucosal defects in the mouth, vagina, bronchi, and gastrointestinal tract and may occur in the liver in some circumstances. On the other hand, *healing* by *fibrous repair* is much more common and while imperfect provides a permanent patch that allows continued function. In some circumstances the scar may impair function—corneal scars impair vision and some scars after myocardial infarction interfere with heart rhythm and contraction to such a degree that they are a permanent liability and may require excision.

Finally, persistent injury is associated with chronic inflammation and continued attempted repair, which results in a mixture of chronic inflammation and microscopic scarring (**fibrosis**), a combination that occurs in a variety of chronic diseases such chronic viral hepatitis, rheumatoid arthritis, systemic lupus erythematosus, or other autoimmune diseases (Chapter 8). Moreover, chronic inflammation and the fibrosis it causes is important in the development of atherosclerosis (Chapter 12), cirrhosis of the liver (Chapter 16), chronic pancreatitis (Chapter 17), interstitial pulmonary fibrosis (Chapter 14), interstitial nephritis (Chapter 19), and many other disorders. ■

CASE STUDY 4-1 *"YOU'D THINK I'D KNOW BETTER"*

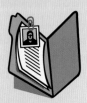

TOPICS
Diabetes mellitus
Peripheral vascular disease
Wound healing

THE CASE

Setting: You work in a wound care clinic seeing a group of regular patients for periodic visits. Most are diabetic and have foot wounds; many are amputees.

Clinical history: R.H., a retired 69-year-old priest, has had diabetes for thirty years. Despite careful diet, proper medication, and close monitoring of his blood glucose levels he experienced increasing health problems related to diabetes. For the last few years his visits to your clinic have been focused on the poor circulation and numbness in his feet and lower legs. Infected ingrown toenails have been a recurring problem, requiring constant foot care and repeated antibiotic treatment. Six months ago the toes on his right foot began to blacken with dry gangrene, and his foot and part of his lower leg were amputated at mid-calf. The surgical wound did not heal well, requiring bandages and additional

wound care until a month ago when he was judged well enough to accept a trial prosthesis. He has returned to clinic today because he fell and injured his stump while trying to hop from one spot to another on his remaining leg because he did not want to put on his prosthesis. Trying his best to be upbeat, he greets you with a grin, holding up his bloody stump and saying, "You'd think I'd know better." You can't help but laugh and admire his courage in the face of such difficulty.

Physical examination and other data: Your mood changes as you examine his injury. The skin over the stump is atrophic and tissue-paper thin; it is very fragile and rests on a bed of beet-red granulation tissue. The fresh wound consists of a large area of denuded skin, which has peeled away to expose a bed of raw granulation tissue.

Clinical course: You carefully cleanse the wound, débride scraps of dead tissue and skin fragments, and apply a fresh dressing. You ensure that he has a supply of fresh dressings at home, renew his insulin prescription, and ask him to return in a week. You see him regularly for the next six months, during which the wound heals slowly and he begins to wear his prosthesis regularly. ▶

[Case 4-1, continued]

DISCUSSION

Wounds in people with diabetes heal poorly and tend to become infected. This is particularly true in the lower legs, because with diabetes blood circulation is especially affected by a combination of atherosclerosis of the iliac, femoral, and popliteal arteries, and by the microvascular disease that is unique to the disease (Chapter 17). Poor circulation may lead to poor wound healing, an impaired ability to resist infection, and to gangrene of toes, foot, or lower leg.

POINTS TO REMEMBER
- Patients with diabetes often have severe peripheral vascular disease.
- Wounds in patients with diabetes heal slowly.
- Wound care is a very important aspect of the management of patients with long-standing diabetes.

Objectives Recap

1. *Distinguish among repair, regeneration, and healing:* Repair is the body's collective attempt to restore normal structure and function to the injured site. Regeneration is one type of repair and is the complete or nearly complete restoration of normal anatomy and function by the regrowth of normal parenchymal cells and supporting tissue; little or no scarring is present. Healing is another type of repair that occurs when regeneration is partial or not possible; some scarring is always present.

2. *Name the two main elements of the repair process:* Regeneration and fibrous repair (scarring).

3. *Name the types of cells according to their ability to regenerate:* Labile cells, which divide continuously from a pool of stem cells; stable cells, which have a reserve of stem cells, and which divide very slowly until stimulated by injury, after which they divide rapidly; and permanent cells, which are highly specialized and have no reserve of stem cells, and which are incapable of division and regeneration.

4. *Explain the importance of the basement membrane and extracellular matrix in the repair process:* They provide structure upon which regenerating cells grow in an orderly manner.

5. *Define "wound":* A wound is the injury resulting from short-term injury at a discrete site.

6. *List in sequence the component steps in fibrous repair (scarring):* Fibrocyte migration, angioneogenesis, and scar development.

7. *Define angioneogenesis:* Angioneogenesis is the growth of new blood vessels into a wound.

8. *Define granulation tissue:* Granulation tissue is a mixture of new blood vessels, fibrous tissue, and residual edema and leukocytes that is at its peak a few days into wound healing.

9. *Discuss what is meant by "healing by first and second intention" by contrasting the two:* Wounds with closely approximated edges heal by first intention; surgical incisions are an example. Wounds with widely separated margins heal by second intention; for example, skin or intestinal ulcers. Healing by second intention is much the same as healing by first intention: inflammation first, followed by macrophage clean-up, neovascularization, and scarring. However, the volume of necrotic tissue to be removed is greater, and reepithelialization of the surface is slower because the wound is wider.

10. *Name some obstacles to normal repair:* Infection is the most common obstacle to normal repair. Other obstacles include poor nutrition, steroid drug medication, diabetes, poor vascular supply, foreign body, and mechanical forces that pull apart the wound.

11. *Name and discuss two examples of pathologic wound repair:* Keloid formation and granulation tissue (pyogenic granuloma). A keloid is a hyperplastic scar that is prominent, raised, or nodular and that contains excess collagen. Pyogenic granuloma is a localized, highly vascular collection of persistent granulation tissue.

Typical Test Questions

1. Which one of the following is composed of permanent cells incapable of regeneration?
   A. Heart
   B. Epidermis
   C. Liver
   D. Gastrointestinal epithelium

2. Which one of the following wounds can be completely repaired by regeneration?
   A. Myocardial infarct
   B. Second-degree skin burn
   C. Surgical incision
   D. Brain injury

3. Which one of the following occurs first in fibrous repair?
   A. Angioneogenesis
   B. Collagen deposition
   C. Cell migration and proliferation
   D. Remodeling

4. Which one of the following is the most common cause of impaired wound healing?
   A. Poor nutrition
   B. Poor blood supply
   C. Mechanical factors
   D. Infection

5. True or false? Stem cells are found in labile tissue but not in stable and permanent tissue.

6. True or false? Cell growth factors originate mainly from blood plasma.

7. True or false? The main components of granulation tissue are capillaries and fibroblastic tissue.

8. True or false? A surgical wound obtains its maximum repaired strength by the end of the first month.

Disorders of Fluid Balance and Blood Flow

This chapter reviews osmotic pressure, blood pressure, and the movement of blood and other fluids in the body. It also discusses the causes and consequences of abnormal accumulations of fluid and the causes and consequences of interruptions of blood flow.

BACK TO BASICS
- Blood Pressure
- Osmotic Pressure
- The Circulation of Blood and Lymph
- The Anatomy of Blood Vessels and Lymphatics
- Body Water and Fluid Compartments

EDEMA
- Low-Protein Edema
- High-Protein edema
- Clinical Aspects of Edema

HYPEREMIA AND CONGESTION

HEMORRHAGE, THROMBOSIS, AND EMBOLISM
- Hemorrhage
- Thrombosis
- Embolism

BLOOD FLOW OBSTRUCTION
- Infarction
- The Development of an Infarct

THE COLLAPSE OF CIRCULATION: SHOCK
- Types of Shock
- Stages of Shock

Learning Objectives

After studying this chapter you should be able to:

1. Explain the difference between hemodynamic pressure, hydrostatic pressure, and osmotic pressure.
2. Describe the origin and flow of lymph fluid
3. Briefly discuss body water compartments and body water balance
4. Define edema; discuss the types of edema, and separate them into high- and low-protein groups
5. Explain why hydrostatic edema usually occurs in the legs
6. Explain how proteinuria causes edema
7. Explain the difference between congestion and hyperemia
8. Define hemostasis, and name the three elements of hemostasis that act to stop bleeding
9. Explain why bleeding is a problem for patients with disseminated intravascular coagulation (DIC)
10. Classify hemorrhages by size
11. Contrast thrombosis and clotting
12. Define embolus, and name the most common type of embolus
13. Define ischemia and infarct, and explain the difference between white and red infarcts
14. Explain why arterial occlusion is not always followed by infarction and why infarction may occur without arterial occlusion
15. Name the types and stages of shock

Key Terms and Concepts

BACK TO BASICS
- hemodynamic pressure
- hydrostatic pressure
- osmotic pressure
- semipermeable membrane
- osmosis
- endothelium
- interstitial space

EDEMA
- edema
- hydrostatic edema
- transudate
- exudate
- osmotic edema

HYPEREMIA AND CONGESTION
- hyperemia
- congestion

HEMORRHAGE, THROMBOSIS, AND EMBOLISM
- hemostasis
- coagulation
- disseminated intravascular coagulation
- petechiae
- purpura
- ecchymosis
- hematoma
- thrombus
- thrombophlebitis
- embolus

BLOOD FLOW OBSTRUCTION
- ischemia
- infarct

THE COLLAPSE OF CIRCULATION: SHOCK
- shock
- sepsis

Of William Harvey, the most fortunate anatomist, the blood ceased to move on the third day of the Ides of June, in the year 1657, the continuous movement of which in all men, moreover he had most truly asserted ...

FROM AN OBITUARY OF WILLIAM HARVEY (1578–1657), ENGLISH PHYSICIAN, WHO DISCOVERED THAT BLOOD CIRCULATES CIRCULARLY AND CONTINUOUSLY

BACK TO BASICS

Jupiter has its moons; Saturn has its rings; and Mars is "the red planet." It is not for nothing that Earth is called "the water planet," for, alone among the planets, Earth has water. Life is not possible without water: it is the major ingredient in every cell, every tissue, and every fluid in the body. For example, blood is about 90% water. Water must move from one place to another to sustain life: to carry nutrients, oxygen, and other essentials to cell, and to carry waste away. The movement of water requires waterways—blood and lymph vessels—and pressure—blood pressure and osmotic pressure.

BLOOD PRESSURE

Blood circulates through arteries because it is under highest pressure as it is forced from the left ventricle. Pressure gradually falls in the circulatory path until it is near zero in the right atrium. Blood flows into tissues under the continued force of left ventricular contraction and the squeeze of the aorta and great vessels. Blood in veins flows from tissues back to the heart by the massaging action of muscles and one-way valves in veins, which prevent backflow. **Hemodynamic pressure**, also called **blood pressure**, is the pressure associated with moving blood through the vascular tree. In medical science blood pressure is expressed as the number of millimeters upward it can force a column of mercury (Hg), which is about 13 times heavier than water. Normal *average* arterial blood pressure in the upper arm can force a column of mercury upward to about 100 mm (about 4 inches), which is expressed as 100 mm Hg.

Blood pressure is determined by two variables: 1) the flow rate (cardiac output) and 2) vascular resistance to flow (Chapter 12). Blood pressure is governed by the following equation:

Blood pressure = cardiac output × vascular resistance

Cardiac output is determined by heart rate and blood volume. Vascular resistance is governed by the collective size of small peripheral arteries (arterioles), which increase resistance (and pressure) by constriction or decrease resistance (and pressure) by dilation.

History of Medicine

DOES BLOOD EBB AND FLOW LIKE THE TIDE? OR RUN ONE-WAY LIKE A STREAM?

The answer, we now know, is neither—it runs in a circle. In the second century AD Greek physician Galen postulated blood was made by the liver and the heart and spread outward to tissues where it was consumed, a doctrine that survived nearly 2000 years until it was refuted by English physician William Harvey (1578–1657). Harvey postulated that blood moved in a circle, flowing away from the heart in arteries and returning to it by veins, though he could not understand how blood passed from arteries into veins.

Harvey was an energetic anatomist, and by dissecting humans and animals he made an observation that had escaped others for centuries. He observed that the human heart could contain about 2 ounces (60 ml) of blood, and coupling this figure with the number of beats the heart makes in a day, he calculated that the volume of blood moved was many, many times the volume of the average person.

Another Harvey observation, critical to his conclusion about the circular nature of blood flow was his observation of the behavior of superficial veins of the forearm after simple occlusion by finger pressure, something curious children may do. The vein above the occlusion collapses; the vein below remains filled with blood. If occluded at two points, the vein will refill only from below. Harvey reached his conclusions in 1615 but waited until 1628 to publish his immortal paper, "On the movement of the heart and blood in animals." Why did he wait so long? He was afraid of upsetting established belief. Despite his genius, it was another 200 years before Harvey's insight was widely accepted in medicine.

Therefore, blood pressure is increased by increased heart rate or blood volume, or constriction of peripheral arterioles; and blood pressure is decreased by decreased heart rate or blood volume, or dilation of peripheral arterioles.

Another type of blood pressure is important. **Hydrostatic pressure** is the force exerted on blood vessel walls by the *weight* of a column of fluid (blood). In most circumstances hydrostatic pressure is low and has a negligible effect on blood pressure. There is an exception, however; in a human standing absolutely still and, therefore, not massaging blood upward by muscular action on veins with their one-way valves, a column of blood about four feet high (equivalent to about 90 mm Hg) adds its weight to pressure in the legs. This added pressure has most potential effect in veins, where pressure is normally very low. Certain pathologic conditions affect blood flow and hydrostatic pressure to produce disease; for example, varicose (dilated) veins, which occur mainly in the legs.

> ☞ **Blood pressure has two important functions:**
>
> • **to move blood through blood vessels; and**
> • **to aid in the diffusion of fluid across blood vessel walls from blood into tissues.**

OSMOTIC PRESSURE

Blood and all other body fluids possess another type of pressure, **osmotic pressure**. To understand osmotic pressure requires understanding semipermeable mem-branes and osmosis and the distinction between *solvent* and *solute*. A solvent is the fluid in which the solute is dissolved. For example, in human plasma, water is the solvent, and all of the things dissolved in it are the solutes: protein, salts, and so on. A **semipermeable membrane** allows some molecules to cross *passively* (no energy required), but others can cross only if *actively* transferred from one side to the other. Cell membranes are semipermeable, including the endothelium that lines blood vessels. Water crosses these membranes passively; but other molecules cannot cross unless aided by a membrane "pump," which requires energy.

As is illustrated in Figure 5-1, **osmosis** is the passage of water from a region of high *water* concentration (low-solute concentration) across a semipermeable membrane to a region of low *water* concentration (high-solute concentration). For example, if two saltwater solutions are separated by a semipermeable membrane, water passes from the less salty side (the side with a low solute concentration) across the membrane to the saltier side, where water concentration is lower and the salt (dissolved solid) concentration is higher. If allowed to continue unopposed, osmosis of water continues until the water and salt concentrations are equalized on both sides of the membrane. Cells must spend energy to keep concentrations different.

Osmotic pressure is the amount of *hydrostatic* or *hemodynamic* pressure that must be applied on the side with low water concentration to prevent water from passing into the saltier side. In Figure 5-1, water could be prevented from moving across the membrane from

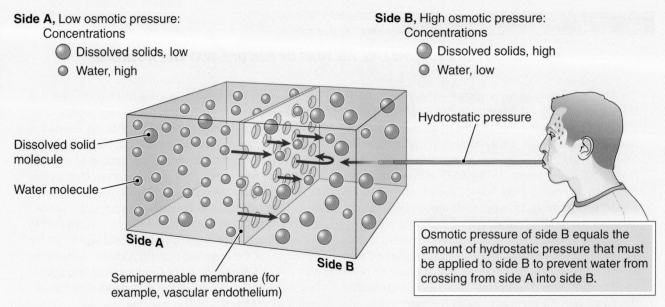

Side A, Low osmotic pressure:
Concentrations
- Dissolved solids, low
- Water, high

Side B, High osmotic pressure:
Concentrations
- Dissolved solids, high
- Water, low

Hydrostatic pressure

Dissolved solid molecule

Water molecule

Side A

Side B

Semipermeable membrane (for example, vascular endothelium)

Osmotic pressure of side B equals the amount of hydrostatic pressure that must be applied to side B to prevent water from crossing from side A into side B.

Figure 5-1 Osmosis. Water moves across a semipermeable membrane (for example, the vascular endothelium) according to the balance of osmotic and hydrostatic pressures. In this example, the fluid on the left (side A) has a low concentration of dissolved solids (red), low osmotic pressure, and high concentration of water (blue). Fluid on the right side (side B) has a high concentration of dissolved solids, high osmotic pressure, and low water concentration. If hydrostatic pressure is equal on both sides, water flows from the side with low osmotic pressure (side A) to the side with high osmotic pressure (side B). The *osmotic* pressure of side B is equal to the amount of *hydrostatic* pressure that must be applied to side B to keep water from crossing the membrane from side A into side B. However, flow across the membrane is influenced by hydrostatic pressure, too. Most osmotic pressure in blood is caused by plasma albumin and sodium.

the less salty side to the saltier side by applying hydrostatic pressure on the saltier side. Conversely, the rate of osmosis can be increased by increased hydrostatic pressure on the side with high water concentration.

A convenient way of thinking about osmotic pressure is to remember that solutions with high concentrations of solute have high osmotic pressure—*high osmotic pressure attracts water, expanding the volume; low osmotic pressure allows water to escape, decreasing the volume.*

> 🔑 *For solutions with differing concentrations of dissolved substances on different sides of a semipermeable membrane:*
>
> - *Solutions with high content of dissolved substances, such as salt, have high osmotic pressure and attract water across the membrane from solutions with low content of dissolved substances.*
> - *Solutions with low content of dissolved substances have low osmotic pressure and favor loss of water across the membrane into solutions with a high content of dissolved substances.*

THE CIRCULATION OF BLOOD AND LYMPH

Health depends in part on smooth, unobstructed flow of blood within the vascular system (Chapters 12 and 13) and normal flow lymph in the lymphatic system.

The heart is a two-sided pump that powers blood through two vascular circuits, which are connected end to end in a larger circuit. The general (systemic, peripheral) circuit begins in the left ventricle and carries blood out to the body through the aorta and large arteries. As blood passes through the microcirculation (Fig. 5-2), hemodynamic pressure (blood pressure) and osmotic pressure combine to cause the flow of a small amount of fluid from blood into the interstitial space, where some of it enters the lymphatic system. The remainder is reabsorbed into blood from interstitial tissue for return to the right ventricle. From the right ventricle blood passes into the pulmonary circuit as it enters the pulmonary artery, and moves through the lungs and down the pulmonary veins into the left ventricle, where it begins another round trip.

In health about 5,000 mL of blood leaves and returns to the heart each minute. As Figure 5-2 indicates, almost all of it returns through veins; however, a small volume (2 ml/min, or 3 liters/day) of fluid returns via the lymphatic system. The balance of blood pressure and osmotic pressure forces a small amount of water out of capillaries and into the interstitial space, where it replenishes interstitial fluid and is collected by the lymphatic system. The collected fluid empties into a large vein in the chest through the terminal lymph channel—the thoracic duct. In doing so, the flow of interstitial fluid sweeps microbes and other

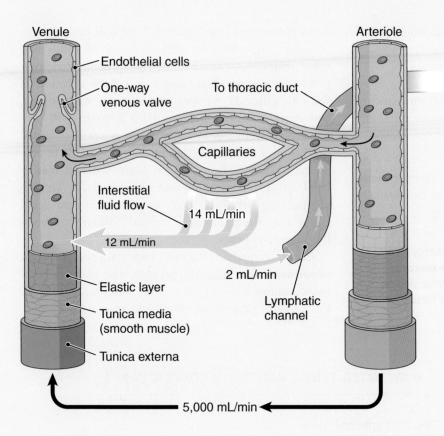

Venule

Arteriole

- Endothelial cells
- One-way venous valve

To thoracic duct

Capillaries

Interstitial fluid flow

14 mL/min

12 mL/min

2 mL/min

- Elastic layer
- Tunica media (smooth muscle)
- Tunica externa

Lymphatic channel

5,000 mL/min ←

Figure 5-2 **Fluid flow in the microcirculation.** Arteries and veins are connected by capillaries composed of a single layer of endothelial cells. Total normal cardiac output, about 5,000 mL/min, passes through the microcirculation. About 14 mL/min crosses the endothelium into interstitial space. Of this 14 mL/min, about 2 mL/min enters the lymphatic system as lymph fluid; the remaining 12 mL/min is reabsorbed into blood for return to the heart.

foreign material into lymph nodes for immune reaction or destruction.

THE ANATOMY OF BLOOD VESSELS AND LYMPHATICS

Arteries and veins are tubes with walls formed of multiple layers of tissue and a central, hollow core (the lumen). Innermost are endothelial cells, the **endothelium**, the lining of all blood vessels, which controls the exchange of substances between blood and tissue. Arteries have thick, rubbery walls with multiple layers and carry oxygenated blood under high pressure away from the heart to the body. Veins are pliable and relatively underfilled, much like a balloon partially filled with water, have thin walls, and carry low pressure, deoxygenated blood from the body back to the heart.

As arteries extend further from the heart, they branch into progressively smaller channels, and blood pressure decreases. In capillaries, pressure is low, and capillary walls are composed solely of endothelial cells, which control the exchange of O_2, CO_2, water, and other molecules between blood and tissues.

Lymphatics are a low-pressure system that collect fluid (*interstitial fluid*) from between cells and deliver it into blood via a delicate network of lymph vessels. In contrast to blood, fluid flow in lymphatics is one way—away from tissues and into the chest, where it spills into

blood. The walls of lymph capillaries, like capillaries elsewhere, are formed of a single layer of cells. However, in contrast to capillaries, small lymphatics have openings between the cells to allow collection of protein and particulate matter such as bacteria. As a result, normal lymph fluid is high in protein. Small lymph vessels merge into larger lymph vessels that connect to lymph nodes, which filter lymph fluid, removing bacteria and other foreign matter. All lymphatic vessels ultimately empty into the final lymph vessel, the thoracic duct, which connects with general circulation by the left subclavian vein.

> *Endothelial cells separate blood from tissue and act as a semipermeable membrane, allowing passage of some substances from blood into tissues and blocking others.*

BODY WATER AND FLUID COMPARTMENTS

Water is the primary constituent of body cells, and it moves into and out of several body water compartments:

- The intravascular space, which consists of
  - The formed elements of blood—red cells, white cells, and platelets, which contain a small fraction of total body water.

- The fluid portion of blood—plasma, which is 90% water.
- The extravascular space, which consists of
  - Intracellular space—fluid within cells
  - Extracellular space—has two sub-compartments: the **interstitial space**, fluid between cells, and fluid in other spaces such as the cerebrospinal fluid and secretions in gland ducts.

Water moves into and out of these compartments and acts as a medium for the movement of dissolved O_2, CO_2, nutrients, minerals, and electrolytes.

> ⚷ *Interstitial space is the space outside of blood vessels and between cells. It is the source of lymph fluid. Everything that is exchanged between blood and tissue must pass through it.*

As is illustrated in Figure 5-3, 60% of body weight is water; the remaining 40% is dissolved solids and other materials—carbohydrate, fat, protein, and minerals. On average, body water is a 0.9% solution of sodium, chloride, potassium, calcium, bicarbonate, and other ions, that also contains a mixture of proteins, fats, and carbohydrates. Most water is obtained from food and drink, although a tiny amount is produced by metabolic reactions. Body water is lost in stool, urine, perspiration, and respiratory air. The accompanying Lab Tools box contains additional detail about measurements and normal volumes of body fluid compartments.

Clinically, perhaps the most important compartment in intravascular fluid—blood cells and plasma. Total blood volume is about 7% of body weight: a normal 70 Kg (155 lb.) person has about 5 liters of whole blood,

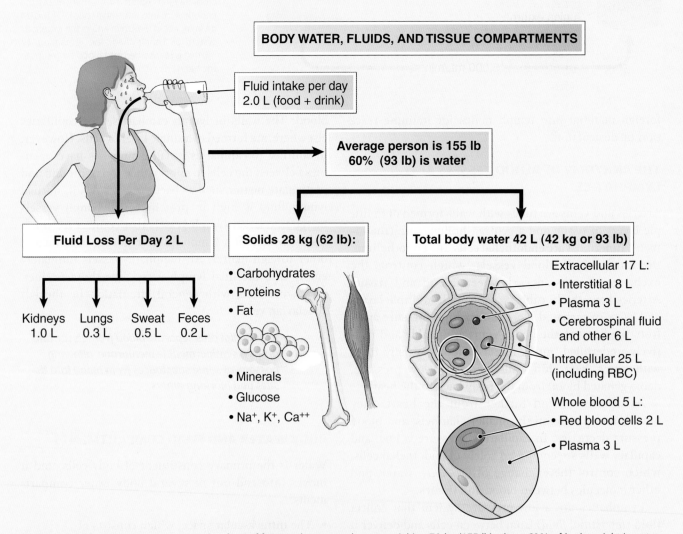

BODY WATER, FLUIDS, AND TISSUE COMPARTMENTS

Fluid intake per day
2.0 L (food + drink)

Average person is 155 lb
60% (93 lb) is water

Fluid Loss Per Day 2 L

Kidneys	Lungs	Sweat	Feces
1.0 L	0.3 L	0.5 L	0.2 L

Solids 28 kg (62 lb):
- Carbohydrates
- Proteins
- Fat
- Minerals
- Glucose
- Na^+, K^+, Ca^{++}

Total body water 42 L (42 kg or 93 lb)

Extracellular 17 L:
- Interstitial 8 L
- Plasma 3 L
- Cerebrospinal fluid and other 6 L

Intracellular 25 L (including RBC)

Whole blood 5 L:
- Red blood cells 2 L
- Plasma 3 L

Figure 5-3 **Body water compartments, intake and loss.** In the average human weighing 70 kg (155 lb), about 60% of body weight is water. Daily average oral intake is about 2 liters per day, which is lost through urine (1 liter), respiratory evaporation (0.3 liter), sweat (0.5 liter), and feces (0.2 liter). In the body, water resides in various fluid compartments: intravascular and extravascular; intracellular and extracellular, are subdivided into smaller compartments.

LAB TOOLS

Mixing Blood and Water

It may be useful to measure the total amount of fluid in body compartments. The table below displays the fluid volume of various body compartments. The method used is the **indicator-dilution principle**.

Let's say we want to measure the amount of water in a pond. Doing so is easier than you might think. All that is necessary is to take a known volume of deeply colored dye (the *indicator*), pour it into the water, and wait a few days for it to disperse, then collect a sample of pond water and measure how much the color of the dye has been diluted. If the dye in the pond water is one-millionth as intensely colored as the indicator, the pond holds one million times the volume of dye poured into the pond.

This principle can be used to measure the volume of fluid in body compartments by injecting a material that will remain confined to the space you are interested in measuring. For example, red blood cells injected intravenously will stay in the vascular space. A small volume of radioactively labeled red cells is injected. After time for mixing and diluting in the vascular space, a specimen of blood is collected and the degree of dilution determined.

Clinically, the most useful body compartment measurement is **total blood volume**—an important measurement

in patients who may have unusually high numbers of red blood cells.

Body Fluid Volumes, 70-Kg (155 lb) person†	Approximate Normal Fluid Volume (liters)
Intravascular (total blood volume)	5
Red cell	2
Plasma	3
Extravascular volume	39
Intracellular*	25
Interstitial	8
Others: cerebrospinal fluid (CSF), joint fluid, glandular secretions and others	6
*Extracellular volume	17
Plasma	3
Interstitial fluid	8
Others: cerebrospinal fluid, etc.	6

†Volumes sum to more than total body water because dissolved substances such as protein and minerals expand volume.

most of which is water. Of this 5 liters, about 2 liters are red blood cells and 3 liters are plasma. Because blood is collected and transfused in 500 mL "units" of whole blood, total blood volume is about 10 "units". More than 90% of plasma is water, which contains sodium, potassium, bicarbonate, and other electrolytes. The remaining 10% of plasma is protein, mainly albumin. Small but important volumes of fat (cholesterol and triglyceride) and carbohydrate (glucose and other sugars) are also present in plasma. Understanding body fluid compartments and their contents is clinically important; for example, in the emergency room restoring intravascular volume after severe hemorrhage often depends initially on intravenous water and electrolyte infusions while waiting for transfusion blood to arrive, as the accompanying box The Clinical Side explains.

Too much water, or **overhydration**, may cause cerebral edema or compound other pathologic conditions, such as congestive heart failure (discussed below and in Chapter 13)—too much water adds to vascular volume and can further burden a failing heart. **Dehydration**, or too little water, may be a problem, even a fatal one, or may complicate other conditions such as extensive burns. Burn patients lose large amounts of water, protein, and electrolytes through burned skin, a loss that can be great enough to cause shock (below).

THE CLINICAL SIDE

EMERGENCY SALT WATER THERAPY

Maintaining blood *volume* is physiologically critical. For example, severe hemorrhage depletes oxygen-carrying capacity because red blood cells are lost; but of equal or more importance is that blood volume (and, therefore, cardiac output) is also reduced. Merely having enough red cells to sustain life is of little value if there is not enough volume of blood to carry red cells and oxygen to tissues. Therefore, in severe hemorrhage it is important to restore:

1. blood volume, and
2. oxygen carrying capacity

When seconds count, blood for transfusion may not be immediately available, but saltwater solutions (0.9% sodium chloride or osmotically similar solutions, such as Ringer's lactate) may be handy. These can be life-saving because they have the same osmolarity as plasma and expand blood volume. Expansion of blood volume increases cardiac output, which raises blood pressure and aids diffusion of essential substances from blood into tissues. Patients in shock may require multiple drugs for various reasons, but the simple expedient of rapid IV infusion of an electrolyte solution can temporarily replenish blood volume. Even though oxygen-carrying capacity is not increased, oxygen delivery to tissue is improved because cardiac output is increased.

MAJOR DETERMINANTS OF DISEASE

- Fluid moves into and out of body compartments according to the balance of osmotic and hemodynamic pressures.
- Injury causes increased blood flow to the injured part.
- Blood remains inside blood vessels because of the physical integrity of vessel walls and the normal function of blood coagulation factors and platelets.
- Coagulation is a normal process that occurs normally only outside of blood vessels; intravascular coagulation is always pathologic.
- Thrombosis is always intravascular and always pathologic.
- Obstruction to arterial blood flow usually causes death of downstream tissue (infarction).
- Normal blood flow requires adequate blood pressure.

Edema

Water remains in the intravascular space or leaves it according to the balance of pressure and osmotic force inside and outside the vascular space. Water is constantly leaving and reentering the vascular space to transport nutrients, hormones, electrolytes, and other essentials to and from cells. Pressure tends to push water out, and the physical integrity of the vascular wall resists. Plasma osmotic pressure also plays a role. Plasma osmotic pressure, which is relatively high, tends to hold water in the intravascular space, countering the blood pressure force. In some pathologic conditions, abnormally low plasma osmotic pressure or increased intravascular pressure causes water to escape into the interstitial space or a body compartment, such as the peritoneal or pleural space.

Edema is a shift of water from the vascular space into another compartment. Severe, generalized edema is termed **anasarca**. Local edema is named according to the site of fluid accumulation. In the feet it is called pedal edema (or dependent edema) because the fluid is accumulated in the lowest part of the body. Fluid in the abdominal cavity (peritoneal space) is **ascites**; fluid in the pericardium is *hydropericardium*, and fluid in the pleural space is *hydrothorax*; however, clinically the word "**effusion**" is commonly used to describe these accumulations, as in "pericardial effusion" or "pleural effusion."

Two basic types of edema fluid occur: that with low protein content and that with high protein content. Low-protein edema is called a **transudate** (Figure 5-4) and accumulates when there is excess venous pressure (**hydrostatic edema**) or low plasma osmotic pressure (**osmotic edema**), each of which allows water to leave the vascular space and accumulate in tissues or body spaces. One type of high-protein edema is **inflammatory edema**, which is formed by plasma that leaks from capillaries into an area of inflammation (inflammatory **exudate**, Chapter 3). A less common type of high-protein edema is **lymphedema**, which is caused

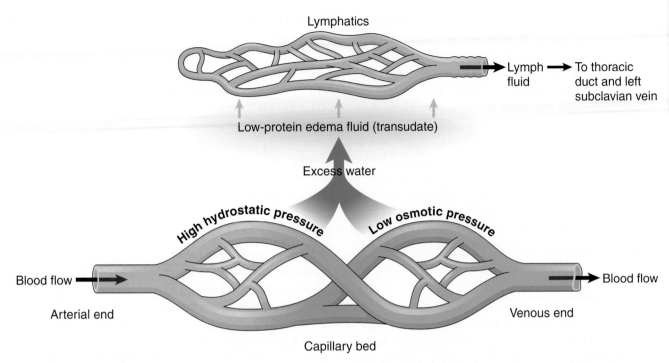

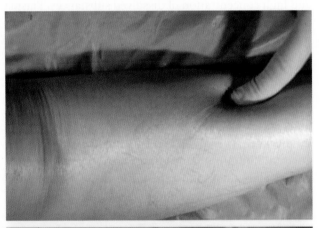

Figure 5-4 The formation of low-protein edema (transudate). Edema accumulates as a result of abnormally high venous hydrostatic pressure or abnormally low plasma osmotic pressure, either of which allows escape of water from blood plasma into interstitial tissue or body spaces.

by lymphatic obstruction and is high in protein because lymph fluid is naturally high in protein.

LOW-PROTEIN EDEMA

Tissue swollen by an accumulation of low-protein hydrostatic or osmotic edema fluid "*pits*" to finger pressure, as is illustrated in Figure 5-5. That is to say, gentle pressure with a finger squeezes water from the tissue, like from a sponge, and the indentation (pit) remains until water slowly returns. High-protein accumulations of edema fluid do not "pit," an important clinical test to distinguish between low-protein edema and high-protein edema.

Hydrostatic Edema

A common clinical accumulation of low-protein fluid is the edema seen in the feet and lower legs of patients with varicose veins, where high hydrostatic venous pressure forces water out of the vascular space and into tissues. The hydrostatic pressure of venous blood is greatest in the feet because the feet are normally the lowest part of the body and have a tall column of blood in veins above them. Hydrostatic pressure would be much higher in the feet except that one-way valves in the large veins of the legs prevent backflow and constrain downward hydrostatic pressure. However, if

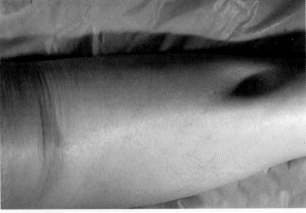

Figure 5-5 Pitting of low-protein edema (transudate). Gentle finger pressure leaves an impression.

these valves are incompetent, as they are in patients with **varicose veins**, hydrostatic pressure increases markedly, veins bulge, and edema results. Another important cause of increased venous hydrostatic pressure is **congestive heart failure** (Chapter 13), a condition in which the heart is incapable of ejecting the blood delivered to it—intravenous hydrostatic pressure increases as blood "dams up" in veins as it tries to get into the right side of the heart. The result is increased hydrostatic pressure and edema, usually in the lower extremities. Similarly, in left heart failure (Chapter 13) blood may "dam up" in the lungs, raising intravascular pressure, which causes water to leave the vascular space and enter the alveoli, a condition known as **pulmonary edema**.

Osmotic Edema

Osmotic edema is a type of low-protein edema that accumulates when there is low plasma osmotic pressure.

As explained above, **osmotic pressure** is a force that moves water across a semipermeable membrane from a fluid with high concentration of water and low concentration of dissolved substances (such as sodium or albumin) into an area with low concentration of water and high concentration of dissolved substances. Plasma albumin is the most important element determining plasma osmotic pressure. If albumin is abnormally low, plasma water concentration becomes relatively high (low osmotic pressure) and allows water to escape from the intravascular space into the interstitial space. Low plasma albumin (*hypoalbuminemia*) is the most common cause of osmotic edema. Because albumin is made by the liver, liver disease is often associated with decreased albumin and resultant osmotic edema. Low plasma albumin also may be the result of albumin loss associated with renal glomerulus disease (Chapter 19), which allows albumin to leak into urine.

Sodium also plays an important role in the formation of osmotic edema. First, low plasma sodium lowers intravascular osmotic pressure, allowing water to escape from the vascular space. Second, low plasma sodium stimulates the kidney to retain sodium, causing retention of excess body water, much of which escapes the vascular space to form edema. Salty food or drink causes water retention, which may produce edema or exaggerate existing edema.

HIGH-PROTEIN EDEMA

The most common cause of high-protein edema is the fluid that accumulates with inflammation. **Inflammatory edema** accumulates when "leaky" capillaries release water and plasma protein into the interstitial space at a site of injury.

Edema resulting from lymphatic obstruction is termed **lymphedema**. Like inflammatory edema, lymph fluid has high protein content. The skin is tense and does not pit to finger pressure, and skin pores are exaggerated and have a *peau d'orange* (orange peel) appearance. Lymphedema usually occurs in an extremity, the breast, or genitalia and is most often attributable to metastatic tumor or other anatomic obstruction of lymph channels.

CLINICAL ASPECTS OF EDEMA

Edema is always the result of underlying disease. For example, edema of the lower leg may be a key diagnostic observation pointing to heart, kidney, or liver disease, or to venous obstruction. Edema is usually mild, as it is, for example, with the pedal edema associated with varicose veins. On the other hand it can be severe: patients with certain types of kidney disease lose so much plasma protein into urine that they develop generalized edema (anasarca); patients with liver disease can accumulate large amounts of peritoneal fluid (ascites). Edema can be fatal. Cerebral edema may prove fatal because the swollen brain has no place to expand, and increased pressure may cause brain tissue to herniate through cranial openings (Chapter 23), causing direct pressure necrosis and venous obstruction and hemorrhage. Pulmonary edema may fatally impair gas transport, or it may encourage bacterial growth and pneumonia.

Hyperemia and Congestion

Hyperemia and *congestion* are terms that describe an increased volume of blood in an affected part of the body. **Hyperemia** (Chapter 3), associated with inflammation or with increased metabolic activity of the affected part, is an *active* process of engorgement with bright red, oxygenated blood recruited by signals from the injured site. For example, sunburned skin is hyperemic because of inflammation, and skin becomes hyperemic after exercise because it disseminates body heat by bringing blood to the surface for heat loss. **Congestion**, on the other hand, is a *passive* process associated with impaired venous outflow. The affected part is passive, has not signaled a need for blood, and is gorged with bluish, poorly oxygenated blood; for example, the arm below an inflated blood pressure cuff. **Chronic passive congestion** is a fairly common occurrence, especially in the liver, as is depicted in Figure 5-6. The most common

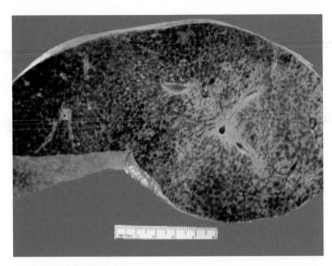

Figure 5-6 **Chronic passive congestion.** In this cross-section of liver from a patient with severe congestive heart failure, the red spots are congested central veins.

cause of chronic passive congestion of the liver is chronic right heart failure, in which the right ventricle is unable to eject the blood delivered to it. The blood "dams up" in the vena cava, increasing venous pressure and causing the liver to become congested with sluggish, poorly oxygenated blood. Liver damage can result.

Hemorrhage, Thrombosis, and Embolism

Hemorrhage is the escape of blood from a blood vessel into tissue. Blood and blood vessels are designed to stop hemorrhage. Collectively, this protective mechanism is called **hemostasis** and refers to processes that 1) maintain blood in a smooth, clot-free state inside blood vessels and 2) stand ready to stop bleeding if hemorrhage occurs. Hemostasis is maintained by a combination of three elements: factors inherent in blood vessels (vascular factors), platelets, and plasma coagulation (clotting) factors.

Blood **coagulation** (clotting) is a natural process that occurs in two circumstances—when blood comes into contact with extravascular tissue, or when it comes into contact with a foreign material such as the plastic of a blood collection tube or the material in an artificial heart valve. Normally, coagulation occurs only outside of blood vessels—*clotting inside blood vessels is always pathologic.*

Hemostasis depends on intact, normally functioning blood vessels and endothelial cells, collectively referred to as *vascular factors*. *Platelets* play a key role in hemostasis. When hemorrhage occurs, platelets release sub-

stances that promote clotting and in small vessels adhere to one another to form a plug in the defect to stop the hemorrhage.

The coagulation process is a cascade of "falling dominos," a chain reaction of various blood coagulation proteins (factors), most of which are produced by the liver. The coagulation process produces **fibrin**, an elastic, insoluble protein that becomes woven into a network of fibers to trap blood cells and plasma and create a gelatinous mixture (**clot**) that obstructs blood flow and stops hemorrhage.

HEMORRHAGE

Hemorrhage is the escape of blood from a blood vessel. Hemorrhage occurs in one of two ways: from large vessels (arterioles or larger) or from capillaries. Large vessel bleeding occurs as a result of a coagulation factor defect (Chapter 11), trauma, the rupture of an atherosclerotic aneurysm (Chapter 12), or erosion of an artery by inflammation or tumor. On the other hand, bleeding from small blood vessels is usually associated with platelet abnormalities or vascular factor defects.

Hemorrhages confined to tissue are classified according to size.

- **Petechiae** (Fig. 5-7) are the smallest hemorrhages, about one millimeter, and are often visible in skin or mucous membranes. Buccal or conjunctival mucosal petechiae are usually associated with platelet disorders, especially **thrombocytopenia** (low platelet count).
- Slightly larger hemorrhages (less than 1 cm) are called **purpura**
- Hemorrhages greater than 1 cm are called **ecchymoses** (Fig. 5-8)
- **Hematomas** are large collections of blood that usually are the result of trauma and are usually not life-threatening. Some, however, such as intracranial hematoma (Chapter 23), can be fatal.

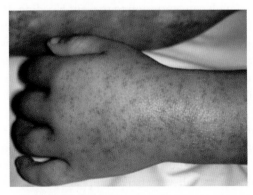

Figure 5-7 **Petechiae.** These tiny skin hemorrhages occurred in a child with low platelet count (thrombocytopenia).

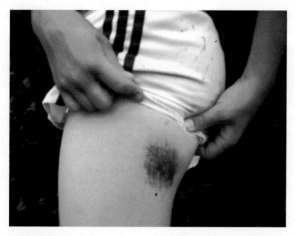

Figure 5-8 **Ecchymosis.** A hemorrhage larger than 1 cm is known as an ecchymosis.

Bleeding from large vessels (arterioles or larger) is usually consequent to trauma or a coagulation factor deficiency and tends to produce the largest and most serious hemorrhages. Bleeding from small vessels presents as skin or mucosal petechiae, nosebleed, or urinary bleeding (hematuria, Chapter 19). It can be quite serious if it occurs in the brain. Capillary bleeding most often results from a low platelet count; less often, it stems from vascular factor defects. Hemorrhage related to coagulation-factor problems (Chapter 11) is common. Most *types* of coagulation defects are caused by genetic conditions—hemophilia, for example. However, most *cases* of coagulation factor defect result from a single condition—acquired liver disease (because the liver makes most coagulation factors).

Ironically, sometimes clotting can lead to hemorrhage. Clotting that occurs within blood vessels is always pathologic. When widespread and severe it is called **disseminated intravascular coagulation** (DIC). DIC clots obstruct small blood vessels, but, paradoxically, the most serious consequence is hemorrhage, which occurs because coagulation factors and platelets are consumed by the clotting process and no longer exist in enough concentration to prevent bleeding. Hence, DIC is sometimes described as a **consumptive coagulopathy** or **hemorrhagic diathesis**. DIC is always secondary to some other pathologic process; for example, bacterial infection of the bloodstream (septicemia) that stimulates generalized *intravascular* clotting (Chapter 11).

Platelet abnormalities, either low platelet count (**thrombocytopenia**) or defective platelet function, can cause bleeding, too. Platelet-related bleeding usually occurs from small vessels and appears as petechiae in skin or mucous membranes. Thrombocytopenia may be the result of a low production of platelets (for example,

bone marrow disease such as leukemia), or platelets may be destroyed in the spleen. Although the spleen normally removes platelets at the end of their usual life span, an overactive spleen (hypersplenism) can cause increased platelet destruction.

Other than trauma, few bleeding problems result solely from *vascular factors*. Bleeding that can be attributed to specific vascular factor defects is uncommon. Vitamin C deficiency damages the intercellular cement between endothelial cells and may cause bleeding gums and other minor hemorrhages. Some people bruise easily, especially the elderly, but the reasons are not clear and may relate to weak supporting connective tissue around the vessels.

THROMBOSIS

A clot and a thrombus are not the same, but the terms are often confused because clinicians, even pathologists, sometimes use them interchangeably. A **thrombus** is a collection of the solid elements of blood (platelets, white blood cells, and red blood cells) that forms when there is abnormal blood flow or local vascular injury, or sometimes because of other factors. As is illustrated in Figure 5-9, a thrombus begins as aggregates of platelets and white blood cells that adhere to the vascular wall in a pattern that creates a *visible internal architecture*—layers of WBC and platelets that form distinct layers, the *lines of Zahn*. Thrombosis is *never normal*, always the result of a *pathologic process*, and is always *intravascular*. Conversely, clotting is a *normal* process that occurs *extravascularly* and does *not* have the internal architecture that distinguishes a thrombus.

Figure 5-9 illustrates the formation of a thrombus in a vein. Formation of a thrombus requires some combination of 1) endothelial injury, 2) abnormal local blood flow (either stasis or turbulence), and 3) hypercoagulability, a tendency of blood to have more than the normal tendency to clot. As is depicted in Figure 5-10, injured endothelium can disturb local blood flow and promote hypercoagulability, and abnormal blood flow, such as turbulence or stasis, can cause endothelial injury. For example, after a heart attack (myocardial infarct, Chapter 13) a thrombus can form within a heart chamber (Fig. 5-11) because dead heart muscle and damaged endocardial cells attract platelets from blood in the chamber. The platelets adhere to the chamber wall, the next step in the process. Typically, however, thrombi form in veins, especially large veins in the legs, or on the walls of large arteries that have been damaged by atherosclerosis.

The formation of a thrombus does not depend *initially* on the coagulation process; thrombi begin with-

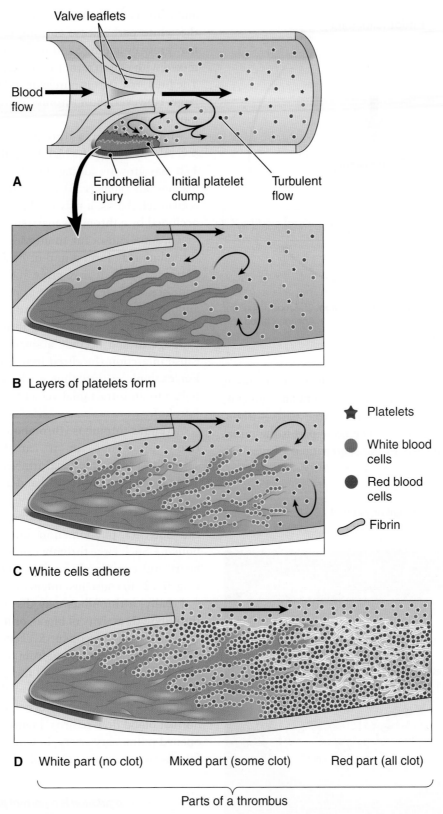

Figure 5-9 **Formation of a thrombus. A.** Platelets separate and agglutinate as a result of turbulent flow and endothelial injury in the valve pocket. **B.** Further platelet agglutination forms platelet layers. **C.** White blood cells adhere to platelet layers. **D.** A clot adds volume as the thrombus grows.

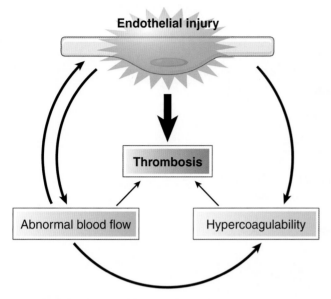

Endothelial injury

Thrombosis

Abnormal blood flow

Hypercoagulability

Figure 5-10 **Factors in thrombus formation.** The most important factor in thrombus formation is endothelial injury. Abnormal blood flow and hypercoagulability of blood also play a role.

out coagulation. However, once a thrombus forms it can grow by *adding* a clot. Small thrombi have no clot; however, a large thrombus has three parts—*white, mixed,* and *red* (Fig. 5-9D). The *white* part is the initial thrombus and consists of the aggregations of platelets

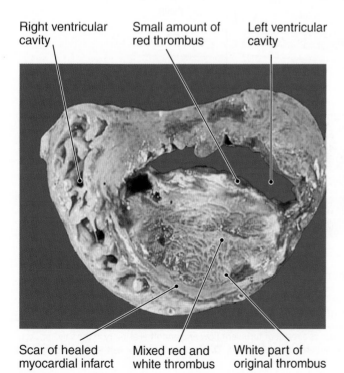

Right ventricular cavity

Small amount of red thrombus

Left ventricular cavity

Scar of healed myocardial infarct

Mixed red and white thrombus

White part of original thrombus

Figure 5-11 **Large intracardiac thrombus.** This thrombus is situated on the internal lining of the heart over muscle damaged by a myocardial infarction. It occupies most of the volume of the left ventricle.

and white cells stuck to the vascular wall. As platelets in the white part release clotting factors, the thrombus may grow by adding additional platelets and white cells mixed with clot to form the *mixed* part of the thrombus. The final, *red,* part is pure clot and may grow to be very large. However, most thrombi are relatively small (a few mm or cm).

After formation, a thrombus may evolve in one of several ways, each of which has different consequences: 1) it may grow by adding clot; 2) it may break loose and become an *embolus*; 3) it may dissolve; or 4) it may rechannel; that is, it may be "bored out," and the vessel occluded by a thrombus may reopen slowly.

Thrombi can occur in arteries or veins. An arterial thrombus may form a non-occlusive mass on the wall of an artery, or it may grow suddenly by adding clot and then occlude the artery to produce local ischemia and necrosis. An arterial thrombus also can break loose and embolize, traveling through the arterial tree to lodge in and occlude a smaller, distant artery and cause infarction (localized tissue necrosis, Chapter 2). For example, a thrombus in the aortic arch may embolize to an intracranial vessel to cause a brain infarct (stroke).

A venous thrombus (**thrombophlebitis**) can be relatively innocuous, or it can be life-threatening. Thrombosis of a superficial arm vein is usually not a serious matter; on the other hand a thrombus in a deep vein of the leg is very dangerous because it can grow very large, break loose, and embolize to another part of the body (a phenomenon known as **thromboembolism**). Such large thrombi can be washed through the heart and completely occlude the pulmonary artery (Fig. 5-12) to cause instantaneous death.

Finally, a thrombus may dissolve through normal thrombolytic activity of blood, or it may rechannel; that is, it may slowly reopen. *Rechanneling* occurs as repaired blood vessels sprout from the internal wall of the vein and work their way into the thrombus. Ultimately they connect with the lumen of the vein and enlarge enough so that the vessel becomes unobstructed and normal blood flow returns. Figure 5-13 illustrates a reopened pulmonary artery, in which only a few bands of fibrous tissue remain to identify the previous thrombus.

- *Coagulation is a normal process that typically occurs outside of the vascular space. Intravascular coagulation is always pathologic.*
- *Thrombosis is always a pathologic process and is always intravascular.*

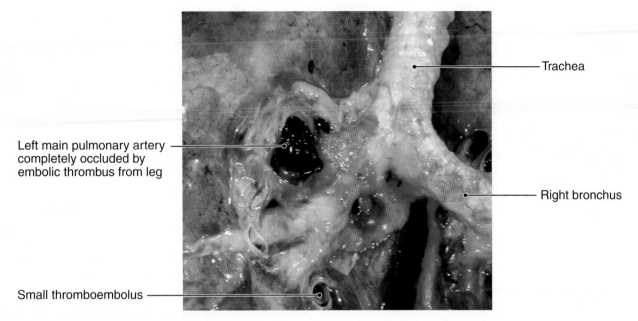

Trachea

Left main pulmonary artery completely occluded by embolic thrombus from leg

Right bronchus

Small thromboembolus

Figure 5-12 **Fatal pulmonary thromboembolus.** This large thrombus arose in a leg vein and embolized through the heart to completely occlude the pulmonary artery. Instantaneous death occurred.

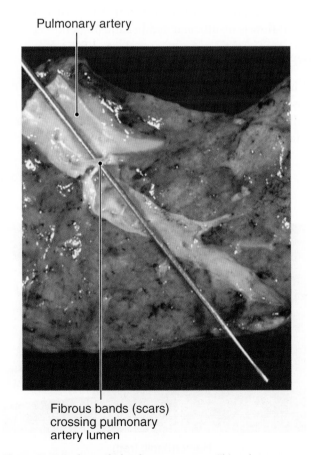

Pulmonary artery

Fibrous bands (scars) crossing pulmonary artery lumen

Figure 5-13 **Rechanneled pulmonary artery.** This pulmonary artery was occluded by a thromboembolus and rechanneled (reopened), leaving only remnant fibrous bands. The probe passes under bands that cross the vessel lumen.

EMBOLISM

An **embolus** is an intravascular object that travels in the bloodstream from one place to another. The main danger of an embolus is obstruction of blood flow. Sources of emboli include:

- *Thrombi,* usually from large veins of the legs or pelvis, called *thromboemboli.* The main danger of thromboemboli is vascular occlusion: a piece of a thrombus on the wall of an aneurysm of the aortic arch can embolize to the brain to cause brain infarction (stroke); or a thrombus that embolizes to the lung from a leg vein can cause a pulmonary infarct. A very large embolus can cause complete obstruction of the pulmonary artery and instant death.
- *Atherosclerotic debris* from ulcerated atheromas, which may embolize to cause vascular occlusion and infarction in any organ.
- *Marrow fat* from the bone marrow of broken bones, which sometimes may prove fatal when fat globules lodge in small brain or lung vessels. An additional hazard is that the fat may initiate DIC.
- *Air (mainly nitrogen),* as in *decompression sickness (the bends),* associated with rapid ascent from prolonged deep-water diving.
- *Amniotic fluid* may embolize (rarely) in pregnancy, with fatal results (also rarely), as is related in Case Study 5-1 at the end of this chapter and as is illustrated in Figure 5-14.

Bronchiole   Alveolus

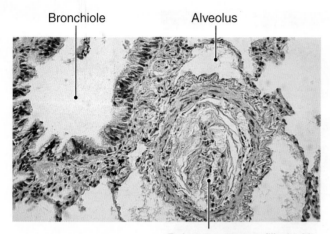

Pulmonary artery filled with
cellular amniotic debris (fetal
skin cells, amnion cells)

Figure 5-14 **The lung in amniotic fluid embolism.** A pulmonary arteriole is filled with cells from fetal skin and amniotic lining.

Emboli are more frequent than might be imagined. At autopsy they are commonly an incidental finding in the lungs. Small thromboemboli are especially common; and bits of bone marrow fat are frequently found in the lungs of patients subjected to chest compression for cardiopulmonary resuscitation (CPR).

Blood Flow Obstruction

Ischemia is a lack of oxygen supply to tissue and is almost always caused by obstruction of blood flow. A few minutes of complete arterial obstruction may be harmless, but longer periods usually result in an **infarct**. A heart attack is caused by obstruction of coronary artery blood flow, which deprives heart muscle of oxygen and produces coagulative necrosis in the tissue fed by the artery. However, sometimes infarction may occur without complete vascular occlusion. For example, despite having normal cerebral arteries, survivors of near-drowning or of carbon monoxide poisoning (Chapter 10) may suffer infarction of the cerebral cortex when oxygenation of blood becomes compromised. However, most infarcts are caused by thrombotic or embolic complete occlusion of an artery.

Rarely, infarcts may result from torsion (twisting) of mobile tissue around the arterial vessel supplying it, as in infarction of the small bowel occurring following torsion of the bowel around the superior mesenteric artery. Vasospasm (contraction of smooth muscles in the vascular wall) can narrow the lumen and cause an infarct. Cocaine is well known for its ability to induce coronary vasospasm and sudden death in drug abusers.

Sometimes, however, venous obstruction may also produce infarction if the obstruction is so severe that the stasis prevents arterial perfusion. For example, occlusion of the hepatic vein by tumor or thrombus produces such a severe degree of liver congestion that normal arterial blood flow is insufficient and hepatic infarction occurs.

INFARCTION

White infarcts (bloodless infarcts) form when arterial obstruction occurs in dense, solid tissue, such as the kidney, heart, or liver, as is depicted in Figure 5-15. **Red infarcts** (hemorrhagic infarcts, Fig. 5-15B) are bloody

Pulmonary artery   Thromboembolus from
deep veins of leg

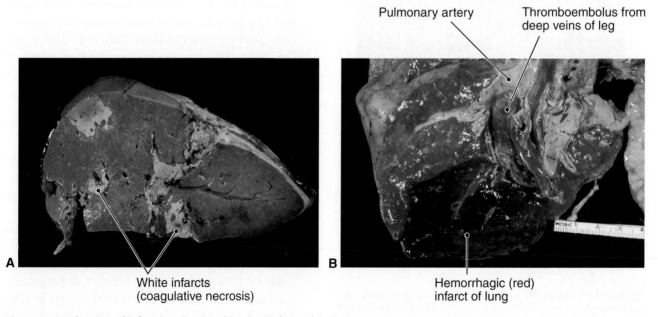

A

White infarcts
(coagulative necrosis)

B

Hemorrhagic (red)
infarct of lung

Figure 5-15 **Ischemia and infarction. A.** White (bloodless) infarcts of the liver owing to sudden arterial occlusion by thromboemboli from cardiac valves. **B.** Red (hemorrhagic) infarcts in the lung owing to venous thromboembolism from the legs.

because venous or arterial obstruction occurs in loose, spongy tissue or tissue with a dual blood supply, notably the lung (which has blood supply from the right ventricle through the pulmonary artery and from the left ventricle via the bronchial artery branches from the aorta). In these organs, occlusion of one supply can cause infarction, but the other supply continues to pump blood into the dead tissue.

THE DEVELOPMENT OF AN INFARCT

As mentioned above, *infarction does not always follow vascular occlusion. Conversely, infarction can occur without vascular occlusion.* Factors influencing the development of an infarct include 1) whether the organ has a single or dual vascular supply; 2) the rate at which the obstruction develops; 3) the sensitivity of downstream tissue to oxygen deprivation; and 4) the oxygen content of blood.

The dual vascular supply in the lungs and liver make these organs resistant to infraction. In the lungs, alveolar tissue depends mainly on oxygenated arterial blood from bronchial artery branches of the aorta. However, enough oxygen is provided by venous blood from the pulmonary arteries and from inhaled air so that the lung is resistant to infarction from bronchial artery occlusion. Most lung infarcts result from venous embolic thrombi from large veins of the pelvis or legs that are washed into the pulmonary arterial tree. A similar dual vascular supply exists in the liver. The portal vein brings venous blood from the bowel, but the liver depends on arterial supply from the hepatic artery. At the opposite end of the spectrum, the kidney is especially sensitive to vascular insufficiency and infarction (Chapter 19). Its arteries have few interconnections with other vessels. Thus, if occlusion occurs there is no alternative route of blood (oxygen) supply.

Occlusion of an artery can be sudden, as in occlusion from an embolus, or slow, as in the development of atherosclerotic obstruction. Slow occlusion over several years may provide enough time for alternative (collateral) circulation to develop, so that complete occlusion may not produce an infarct. For example, slow total occlusion of a carotid artery by atherosclerosis may not cause stroke, because the basilar arteries provide an alternative supply of blood (oxygen) via the circle of Willis.

Some tissues become infarcted quickly after a short period of ischemia. Brain neurons are the best example; they are exquisitely sensitive to hypoxia and die if deprived of oxygen for 3 or 4 minutes. Most other tissues are much more tolerant of ischemia: myocardial cells, for example, die after about 20 minutes of hypoxia, whereas fibroblasts may tolerate many hours of hypoxia without damage.

The oxygen content of blood is also an important determinant of infarction. All other things being equal, low blood oxygen content may facilitate transformation of ischemia into infarction. For example, a patient who is hypoxic from severe lung disease is at greater risk than usual for stroke or heart attack owing to cerebral or coronary atherosclerosis.

The Collapse of Circulation: Shock

Shock, or circulatory collapse, is a state of systemic low blood flow (hypoperfusion) when cardiac output is reduced or *effective* blood volume (that is, either blood is lost or the vascular space dilates) is decreased. Shock may be the final stage of a number of clinical conditions, including severe hemorrhage, overwhelming bacterial sepsis, catastrophic allergic reaction, burns, severe myocardial infarction, or trauma with extensive soft tissue damage. Whatever the cause, the end result of shock often is multi-organ failure and death.

TYPES OF SHOCK

Shock may be classified into three categories, cardiogenic shock, hypovolemic shock, and septic shock.

Cardiogenic shock (pump failure) often occurs with myocardial infarction or other myocardial disease. In such cases, cardiac muscle simply lacks the mechanical power to maintain perfusion pressure.

Hypovolemic shock results from an underfilled vascular space, usually the result of hemorrhage. Hypovolemic shock also may be caused by fluid loss following burns or severe diarrhea. Surprisingly, hypovolemic shock also may occur without loss of blood. In such situations, marked *vasodilation* may expand the vascular space to such a degree that the *effective* blood volume is insufficient to maintain perfusion pressure. For example, severe allergic reaction may cause systemic vasodilation, shock, and death.

Septic shock, which associated with systemic bacterial infection (sepsis) by organisms that release bacterial endotoxin, is somewhat more complicated. Gram-negative bacteria are the usual culprits. **Endotoxins** are bacterial-wall molecules (lipopolysaccharides) that induce shock by a combination of three mechanisms:

- peripheral vasodilation, which results in an underfill of the vascular tree
- decreased myocardial contractility
- endothelial cell damage, which can initiate DIC, the presence of which severely complicates and prolongs the original underlying clinical condition

STAGES OF SHOCK

Unless hemorrhage is massive and immediately fatal, as in a ruptured aortic aneurysm, shock may progress through three overlapping stages: non-progressive, progressive, and irreversible shock.

As is illustrated in Figure 5-16 the initial stage of shock is a *nonprogressive* stage, characterized by reflex actions to reestablish perfusion. Low blood pressure stimulates the sympathetic nervous system: tachycardia increases cardiac output, and systemic vasoconstriction

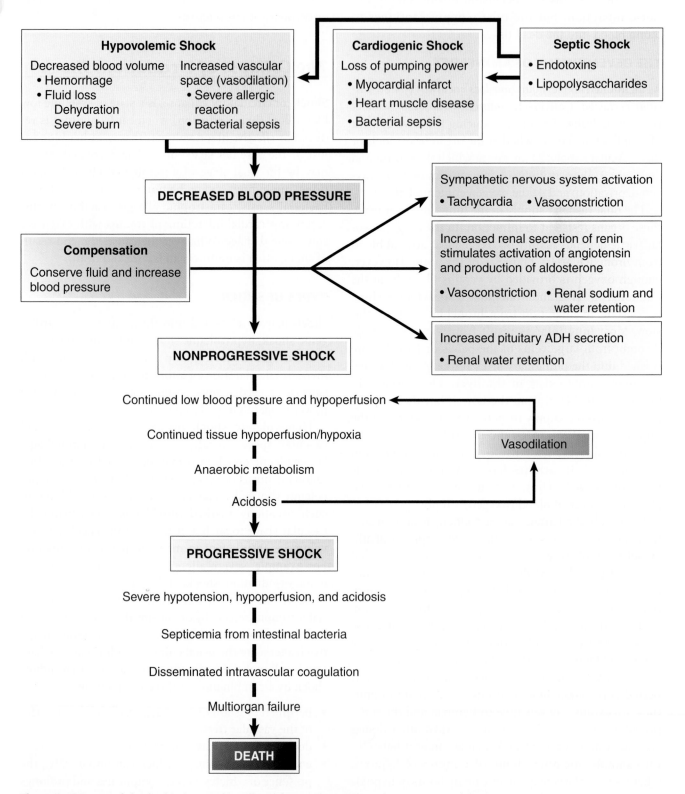

Figure 5-16 **Stages of shock.** This diagram shows the etiology, pathogenesis, and consequences of shock.

(mainly in the skin and extremities) increases peripheral resistance, both of which act to raise blood pressure to maintain tissue perfusion. Low blood pressure and blood flow to the kidneys stimulate 1) the renin-angiotensin-aldosterone system, which induces peripheral and renal vasoconstriction and stimulates the kidney (Chapter 12) to retain sodium and water, and thereby decreases urine output and expands blood volume; and 2) stimulates the pituitary to increase release of antidiuretic hormone (Chapter 18), which also causes renal retention of water and decreased urine output.

The second stage is a *progressive stage,* characterized by more severe hypoperfusion and metabolic imbalances caused by hypoxia. Insufficient oxygen shifts energy metabolism to the anaerobic cycle, producing lactic acid excess (lactic acidosis), which in turn results in vasodilation and pooling of blood. The result is low blood pressure, decreased tissue perfusion, further hypoxia, and more acidosis, a vicious circle that often results in the final, irreversible, stage of shock.

Without effective intervention a final, *irreversible stage* supervenes. This is characterized by 1) progressively severe hypotension, hypoperfusion, and acidosis; 2) decreased myocardial contractility; 3) leakage into blood of cytokines and enzymes from dying cells, which spread widely and further compound the metabolic difficulties; and 4) invasion of the bloodstream by intestinal bacteria (septicemia) as hypoxic intestinal mucosa is overwhelmed. Finally, multi-organ failure leads to death. ■

CASE STUDY 5-1 *"SHE'S GONE"*

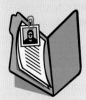

TOPICS
Shock
Amniotic fluid embolism

THE CASE

Setting: You are employed as Case Manager for the Problem Pregnancy Unit at a large metropolitan hospital.

Clinical history: R. B., a 40-year-old woman in her fourth pregnancy, is admitted in active labor at term after a carefully supervised pregnancy. She had one live birth from her first pregnancy, a daughter now 8 years old, born by caesarian section for breech presentation. Two later pregnancies ended prematurely in spontaneous abortions.

Physical examination and other data: Physical examination, laboratory studies, and ultrasound images reveal no abnormalities.

Clinical course: Labor progresses smoothly, and a healthy infant is delivered. Immediately after delivery there is brisk bleeding, but the placenta does emerge. Suddenly the patient develops dusky skin color (cyanosis) and shortness of breath (dyspnea); her blood pressure falls to 55/25 mm Hg (hypotension), and her heart rate rises to 120 (tachycardia). Vasoconstrictor medications and large volumes of electrolyte solution are given intravenously without apparent effect. Vaginal bleeding continues, and manual exploration of the uterus reveals an embedded placenta (placenta accreta, Chapter 21) and a large tear in the low, anterior uterus.

Hypotension, tachycardia, dyspnea, and cyanosis continue and vital signs eventually become undetectable. Cardiopulmonary resuscitation (CPR) is begun, and the abdomen is surgically opened. No intra-abdominal bleeding is discovered, and the uterus is removed while at the same time transfusions of blood and plasma are given. CPR and other heroic measures continue for an hour before the chief obstetrician says, "She's gone," and the patient is pronounced dead.

DISCUSSION

Perinatal maternal death is very rare, especially in women with careful prenatal care, and in most jurisdictions a medicolegal autopsy is mandatory. The autopsy in this case confirmed placenta accreta and revealed a uterine tear in the caesarian section scar. Microscopic study of lung tissue obtained at autopsy revealed cellular debris in pulmonary arterioles, as is illustrated in Figure 5-14, a conclusive finding for the diagnosis of amniotic fluid embolism.

An important question in this case is: Should women with prior caesarian section be allowed to deliver vaginally in a later pregnancy? The rate of complications is low for women delivering vaginally after caesarean section, about 1%; when complications occur they are rarely fatal. Experts agree that vaginal delivery after caesarean section is a valid choice for fully informed patients with careful prenatal care. The uterine tear may have contributed to amniotic fluid embolism; however, amniotic fluid embolism is very rare, uniformly fatal, unpredictable, and very much a mystery—why it occurs is difficult to explain.

POINTS TO REMEMBER

- Pregnancy is an important medical condition that deserves careful management.
- Sometimes even the best medical care does not produce a favorable outcome.
- Cardiovascular collapse (shock) is an extremely dangerous and usually fatal condition.

Objectives Recap

1. *Explain the difference between hemodynamic pressure, hydrostatic pressure, and osmotic pressure:* Hemodynamic pressure is the pressure associated with moving blood through the vascular tree. Hydrostatic pressure is the force exerted on blood vessel walls by the weight of a column of fluid (blood). Osmotic pressure is a function of the amount of dissolved solids in water. Osmotic pressure is expressed as the amount of hydrostatic pressure that must be applied to fluid on one side of a membrane, the side with the lower water concentration (higher concentration of dissolved substances, such as salt), to prevent water from crossing the membrane from the side with the higher concentration of water (lower concentration of dissolved substances).

2. *Describe the origin and flow of lymph fluid:* In capillaries the balance of blood pressure (hemodynamic pressure) and osmotic pressure forces a small amount of water out of blood vessels and into the interstitial space, where it replenishes interstitial fluid and enters the lymphatic system.

3. *Briefly discuss body water compartments and body water balance:* Body water exists in several compartments, some of which are overlapping: intravascular and extravascular; and intracellular and extracellular. For example, intravascular water is the main component of plasma, which is an extracellular fluid; and most of the water in cells exists in extravascular tissues. Almost all water is obtained from food and drink and is lost in stool, urine, perspiration, and respiratory air. Clinically, the most important compartment is intravascular fluid—blood cells and plasma. More than 90% of plasma is water; the remaining 10% of plasma is protein, mainly albumin.

4. *Define edema, discuss the types of edema, and separate them into high-protein groups and low-protein groups:* Edema is a shift of water from the vascular space into another compartment. The types of edema are: inflammatory, hydrostatic, osmotic, and the edema of lymphatic obstruction (lymphedema). Hydrostatic and osmotic edemas have low protein content; inflammatory and lymphatic edemas have high protein content.

5. *Explain why hydrostatic edema usually occurs in the legs:* Most edema occurs in the legs because hydrostatic pressure is highest there (i.e., the column of fluid—blood—above the lower leg is higher than at any other point in an erect patient).

6. *Explain how proteinuria causes edema:* Proteinuria (albuminuria) can cause protein to be wasted faster than it can be replaced by the liver; the result is low blood albumin (hypoalbuminemia).

Albumin accounts for most of the osmotic pressure in blood plasma. Low albumin, therefore, causes low intravascular osmotic pressure, which allows water to cross the vascular endothelium (a semipermeable membrane) into the interstitial space.

7. *Explain the difference between congestion and hyperemia:* Congestion is a passive accumulation of excess blood in vessels resulting from hydrostatic forces. Hyperemia is the active accumulation of excess blood in vessels owing to inflammation.

8. *Define hemostasis, and name the three elements of hemostasis that act to stop bleeding:* Hemostasis refers to the combination of forces that maintain blood normally in a smooth, clot-free state and also stand ready to stop bleeding when it occurs. The elements that act to stop bleeding depend on the interaction of vascular factors, platelets, and coagulation factors.

9. *Explain why bleeding is a problem for patients with DIC:* In DIC intravascular clotting consumes coagulation factors and platelets faster than the body can replace them, leaving the blood without a sufficient supply of either; spontaneous hemorrhage is the result.

10. *Classify hemorrhages by size:* Petechiae are the smallest hemorrhages, about one millimeter; next larger in size are purpuric hemorrhages (purpura), which are a few millimeters; hemorrhages a few centimeters across are ecchymoses. Largest are hematomas, which are usually several centimeters across and contain a volume of blood large enough to form a pool.

11. *Contrast thrombosis and clotting:* Clotting is a normal process designed to stop hemorrhage. Under normal circumstances clotting occurs only outside of blood vessels; however, it may occur within blood vessels as part of a pathologic process. A clot is formed of fibrin and entrapped blood cells, and it has no internal architecture. Thrombosis is never normal. It is always the result of a *pathologic* process and always occurs intravascularly. A thrombus is initially formed by pathologic aggregation of the formed elements of blood, in which platelets and white cells aggregate in layers, giving a thrombus its distinctive internal architecture.

12. *Define embolus, and name the most common type of embolus:* An embolus is a detached intravascular mass (solid, liquid, or gas) carried by blood to a distant site. Thrombi are the most common emboli.

13. *Define ischemia and infarct, and explain the difference between white and red infarcts:* Ischemia is a lack of oxygen supply to tissue and is almost always caused by obstruction of blood flow. Severe ischemia can cause tissue death (an infarct). A

white infarct is a bloodless infarct, one that contains few RBCs. These usually occur in ischemia in dense, solid tissue such as myocardium or kidney. A red infarct is a hemorrhagic infarct. These usually occur in loose, spongy tissue or in tissue with a second blood supply that continues to pump blood into the dead tissue.

14. *Explain why arterial occlusion is not always followed by infarction and why infarction may occur without arterial occlusion*: If vascular occlusion develops slowly and if collateral circulation is sufficient, complete occlusion of an artery may not produce an infarct because oxygenated blood can arrive by a secondary route. Conversely, if blood flow is low, or blood is not carrying sufficient oxygen, infarction may occur in tissues supplied by patent vessels, especially if the tissue is metabolically very active.

15. *Name the types and stages of shock*: There are three types of shock: cardiogenic (pump failure), hypovolemic (an underfilled vascular space created by hemorrhage or marked vascular dilation), and septic. The latter is usually associated with bacterial endotoxins released during severe systemic infection. The three stages of shock are non-progressive, progressive, and irreversible.

Typical Test Questions

1. Which one of the following is an example of osmotic edema? Edema in association with:
   A. Inflammation
   B. Lymphatic obstruction
   C. Severe proteinuria
   D. Varicose veins

2. Which one of the following is an example of hyperemia? Excess blood in vessels because of:
   A. Varicose veins
   B. Inflammation
   C. Congestive heart failure
   D. Low osmotic pressure

3. Which one of the following is found in a thrombus but not in a clot?
   A. Fibrin
   B. Red blood cells
   C. Internal architecture
   D. Edema

4. True or false? Thrombi are always pathologic.

5. True or false? Necrosis always follows arterial occlusion.

6. True or false? Cardiogenic shock is characterized by blood loss or vasodilation.

This chapter discusses how neoplasms are named, their molecular basis, the control and loss of control of normal cell growth, and the growth and biology of neoplasms. It also examines their diagnosis and clinical behavior.

THE LANGUAGE OF NEOPLASIA
TYPES OF NEOPLASMS
THE MOLECULAR AND GENETIC BASIS OF NEOPLASIA
• Mutations
• Cell Growth Control Genes
• DNA Repair
THE CAUSES OF CANCER
THE STRUCTURE OF NEOPLASMS
• The Gross Anatomy of Neoplasms
• The Microscopic Anatomy of Neoplasms
PREMALIGNANT STATES AND CONDITIONS
THE BIOLOGY OF NEOPLASTIC GROWTH
• The Differentiation of Tumor Cells
• Clones of Cells

• The Speed of Tumor Growth
• The Nourishment of Tumors
• Tumor Cell Variation
THE SPREAD OF NEOPLASMS
THE IMMUNE DEFENSE AGAINST NEOPLASIA
THE EPIDEMIOLOGY OF CANCER
THE CLINICAL PICTURE OF CANCER
CLINICAL AND LABORATORY ASSESSMENT OF
   NEOPLASMS
• Clinical History
• Obtaining Tissues and Cells for Diagnosis
• Grading and Staging of Malignancies
• Early Detection of Cancer
• Tumor Markers

Learning Objectives

After studying this chapter you should be able to:
1. Define the difference between benign and malignant neoplasms
2. List in descending order the three leading causes of cancer death in men and women
3. Name several types of carcinogenesis, and give some examples
4. Discuss the gross and microscopic characteristics of malignant tumors
5. Define dysplasia and contrast it with carcinoma in situ, and offer several examples of premalignant clinical conditions
6. Explain the concept of doubling time and the growth of tumors
7. Explain the importance of tumor growth fraction
8. Explain why the cells in a tumor that are most likely to survive are those that are the most malignant
9. Name several ways by which malignant tumors may spread
10. Explain why patients with immunodeficiency have an increased risk for cancer
11. Explain paraneoplastic syndromes and give an example
12. Explain the difference between histologic grading and clinical staging
13. Name two tumor markers found in blood, and explain their use

Key Terms and Concepts

THE LANGUAGE OF NEOPLASIA
- oncology
- neoplasm
- tumor
- cancer
- sarcoma
- carcinoma
- adenocarcinoma

TYPES OF NEOPLASMS
- benign
- malignant

THE MOLECULAR BASIS OF NEOPLASIA
- aneuploid
- proto-oncogenes
- tumor suppression genes

CARCINOGENESIS
- mutagenic

THE STRUCTURE OF NEOPLASMS
- poorly differentiated
- well differentiated

PREMALIGNANT STATES AND CONDITIONS
- dysplasia
- carcinoma in-situ

THE BIOLOGY OF NEOPLASTIC GROWTH
- clone
- tumor growth fraction

THE SPREAD OF NEOPLASMS
- invasiveness
- metastasis

THE IMMUNE DEFENSE AGAINST NEOPLASIA
- immune surveillance

THE CLINICAL PICTURE OF CANCER
- paraneoplastic syndromes

CLINICAL AND LABORATORY ASSESSMENT OF NEOPLASMS
- cancer grading
- cancer staging
- tumor markers

The same people who tell us that smoking doesn't cause cancer are now telling us that advertising cigarettes doesn't cause smoking.

ELLEN GOODMAN (B. 1941), U.S. POLITICAL COLUMNIST, AS QUOTED IN NEWSWEEK MAGAZINE, P. 17 (JULY 28, 1986)

Cancer is second only to cardiovascular disease as a cause of death in the United States. Figure 6-1 shows the *incidence* (number of *new* cases per annum) of new cancer cases and new cancer deaths in the United States for 2003 (skin cancers excluded). Lung cancer is the most common cause of cancer death in both sexes. In females, breast cancer is the second most common fatal cancer. In males, prostate cancer fatality is second to lung cancer. Note that prostate cancer is the most common of all cancers; however, although 221,000 men developed prostate cancer in 2003, only 29,000 died of it because prostate cancer is not as aggressively lethal as some other cancers. In contrast, note that in both men and women there were 15,000 new cases each of pancreatic cancer and 15,000 deaths because pancreatic cancer is uniformly and quickly lethal.

> *Two statistics are important in understanding the occurrence of disease in a population—incidence and prevalence:*
>
> - *Incidence is the number of new cases per year.*
> - *Prevalence is the number of existing cases at any moment in time.*

The Language of Neoplasia

Oncology is the study of neoplasms. Some of the most important definitions that apply to neoplasms are:

- **Benign**: not capable of metastasizing and usually not capable of causing death

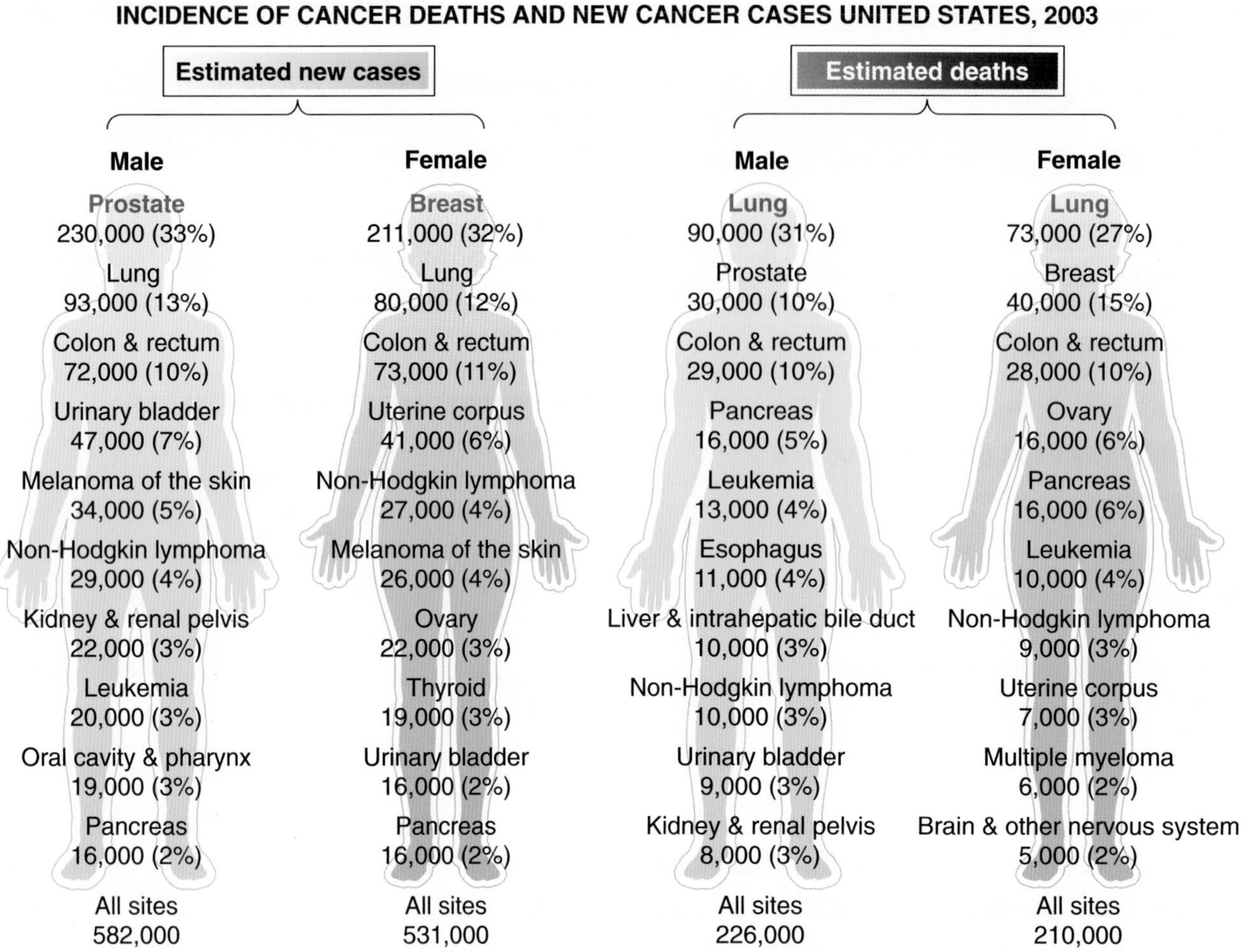

INCIDENCE OF CANCER DEATHS AND NEW CANCER CASES UNITED STATES, 2003

Estimated new cases		Estimated deaths	
Male	**Female**	**Male**	**Female**
Prostate 230,000 (33%)	Breast 211,000 (32%)	Lung 90,000 (31%)	Lung 73,000 (27%)
Lung 93,000 (13%)	Lung 80,000 (12%)	Prostate 30,000 (10%)	Breast 40,000 (15%)
Colon & rectum 72,000 (10%)	Colon & rectum 73,000 (11%)	Colon & rectum 29,000 (10%)	Colon & rectum 28,000 (10%)
Urinary bladder 47,000 (7%)	Uterine corpus 41,000 (6%)	Pancreas 16,000 (5%)	Ovary 16,000 (6%)
Melanoma of the skin 34,000 (5%)	Non-Hodgkin lymphoma 27,000 (4%)	Leukemia 13,000 (4%)	Pancreas 16,000 (6%)
Non-Hodgkin lymphoma 29,000 (4%)	Melanoma of the skin 26,000 (4%)	Esophagus 11,000 (4%)	Leukemia 10,000 (4%)
Kidney & renal pelvis 22,000 (3%)	Ovary 22,000 (3%)	Liver & intrahepatic bile duct 10,000 (3%)	Non-Hodgkin lymphoma 9,000 (3%)
Leukemia 20,000 (3%)	Thyroid 19,000 (3%)	Non-Hodgkin lymphoma 10,000 (3%)	Uterine corpus 7,000 (3%)
Oral cavity & pharynx 19,000 (3%)	Urinary bladder 16,000 (2%)	Urinary bladder 9,000 (3%)	Multiple myeloma 6,000 (2%)
Pancreas 16,000 (2%)	Pancreas 16,000 (2%)	Kidney & renal pelvis 8,000 (3%)	Brain & other nervous system 5,000 (2%)
All sites 582,000	All sites 531,000	All sites 226,000	All sites 210,000

Figure 6-1 **New cancer cases and deaths, 2003.** Skin cancers are not included because they are very common but rarely fatal (the exception is malignant melanoma, which is uncommon but sometimes fatal). (Data rounded upward to next whole thousand. Modified from American Cancer Society, Inc. Surveillance Research, Cancer Facts & Figures 2003. Atlanta, GA. American Cancer Society, 2003.)

- **Malignant**: capable of metastasizing and capable of causing death
- **Neoplasm**: an uncontrolled growth of new cells, benign or malignant
- **Tumor**: literally, a mass; however, in everyday language, a neoplasm
- **Cancer**: any kind of malignant neoplasm
- **Carcinoma**: a malignant neoplasm of epithelial cells
- **Sarcoma**: a malignant neoplasm of mesenchymal tissue

It is important to note that "benign" and "malignant" are defined by *behavior*, not by microscopic appearance. Microscopic appearance is a good guide to probable behavior, but in the end it is behavior that matters most. However, the usefulness of microscopic diagnosis of neoplasms lies in the close correlation that exists between microscopic appearance and clinical behavior. A notable exception to this rule is brain neoplasms (Chapter 23), which may appear innocuous microscopically but can cause death by virtue of critical location.

Table 6-1 is a short listing of various types of tissues and the benign and malignant tumors that arise from them. Tumors are usually named according to the cells from which they arise, and for every benign tumor there is a matching malignant variety. For example, a benign tumor of a gland is usually called an *adenoma* (from Greek, *aden* for gland, *oma* for swelling). Other benign tumors are similarly named; for example, a benign tumor of fibrous tissue is a fibroma.

Malignant tumors are similarly named but add **carcinoma** (from Greek *carcinoma* for cancer) if the tumor is of epithelial origin (breast duct epithelium, prostate

Tissue of origin	Benign	Malignant
Table 6-1	**The Naming of Tumors**	
Fibrous	Fibroma	Fibrosarcoma
Fat	Lipoma	Liposarcoma
Bone	Osteoma	Osteosarcoma
Cartilage	Chondroma	Chondrosarcoma
Blood vessels	Hemangioma	Hemangiosarcoma
Blood cells Granulocytes Lymphocytes		Leukemia Leukemia, if in blood Lymphoma, if in lymph nodes or organs
Muscle Skeletal Smooth	Rhabdomyoma Leiomyoma	Rhabdomyosarcoma Leiomyosarcoma
Epithelium Epidermis Gland ducts Bronchi Hepatocytes	Squamous cell papilloma Adenoma, papilloma Bronchial adenoma Hepatoma	Squamous cell carcinoma Adenocarcinoma Bronchogenic carcinoma Hepatocarcinoma
Melanocytes	Nevus	Malignant melanoma

Types of Neoplasms

A **neoplasm** (from Greek, *neo* for *new*, and *plasm* for *form*) is a new formation, a new growth, of cells. Of course, the body normally and constantly grows new cells that are not neoplastic—the epidermis, for example, sheds dead cells daily and grows new ones. So what is the difference between normal and neoplastic cells? A neoplasm is an *uncontrolled* growth of new cells. Cell growth is governed by so-called "go" and "stop" signals controlled by genes. If the "go" switch is stuck in the "on" position, or if the "stop" switch does not work, a neoplasm results. In addition, neoplasms may grow or fail to grow because of the adequacy or inadequacy of their vascular supply or the availability of hormones and nutrients they must obtain from the host (the patient).

Benign neoplasms grow slowly and are usually not fatal, whereas malignant neoplasms grow rapidly and are capable of causing death. As with all rules, there are exceptions: some neoplasms fall somewhere in between; that is, they may be locally aggressive and destructive but do not spread widely. How do we know which neoplasm is benign and which is malignant? As with human behavior, past tumor behavior is the best predictor of future behavior—a lesion that has behaved as malignant is not going to behave benignly in the future. However, waiting invites disaster; we must try to predict how the tumor will behave so we can treat it early, while it is most curable. The best way to predict

epithelium, bronchial epithelium, and so on), or **sarcoma** (from Greek *sarcoma*, meaning fleshy) if the tumor arises from mesenchymal tissue (bone, cartilage, fat, muscle, or fibrous tissue). Thus, a malignant tumor of gland epithelial cells is an **adenocarcinoma** (from Greek *aden*, for gland), and a malignant tumor of fibrous tissue is a **fibrosarcoma**.

Typically, malignant tumors are named first by the type of malignant tissue they produce, second for their site of origin. For example, a malignant growth of squamous cells in the lung might have the following formal diagnostic line on the pathology report of a lung biopsy: "Lung biopsy: Squamous cell carcinoma."

Unfortunately, some names do not follow convention so neatly—**lymphoma**, for example, is a malignant tumor of lymphoid tissue, and **melanoma** is a malignant tumor of melanocytes, the pigment-producing cells in skin.

HISTORY OF MEDICINE

THE ONLY AMERICAN PRESIDENT TO DIE OF CANCER

The only U.S. president to die of cancer was Ulysses S. Grant (1822–1885), who gained fame during the American Civil War (1861–1865) and was appointed by Lincoln to be general-in-chief of the Union Army in 1864. He served as President of the United States from 1869 though 1877 and succumbed to a tumor of the throat, a point worth noting because Grant loved cigars and whiskey—tobacco *use* and alcohol *abuse*, especially together, are associated with carcinomas of the mouth, tongue, pharynx, larynx, and esophagus.

Lincoln heard "Grant is a drunkard" from politicians so often and heard so little praise for the damage he was inflicting on the Confederates that he is said to have replied on one occasion, ". . . you just find out, to oblige me, what brand of whiskey Grant drinks, because I want to send a barrel of it to each one of my generals."

tumor behavior is to study it with the naked eye (**gross examination**) and with a microscope (**microscopic examination**). The gross and microscopic findings are described using the language of neoplasia.

MAJOR DETERMINANTS OF DISEASE

- Damaged DNA is the root cause of all neoplasms.
- Neoplasms are living things that require nutrients and adequate blood supply.
- Neoplasms take many years to grow to a clinically detectable size.
- The transformation of cells from benign to malignant is slow.
- Malignant cells have a distinctive appearance and behavior.
- Malignant cells do not spread unless they are able to invade lymphatic channels or blood vessels.
- The immune system plays an important role in cancer prevention.

The Molecular and Genetic Basis of Neoplasia

The root cause of all cancer is damaged (mutant) DNA, which causes the normal cycle of cell reproduction (Chapter 2) to go awry. Almost all mutations are defects in *somatic* cells, not the reproductive (*germ*) cells of the ovary or testis (Chapter 7). Somatic cell DNA defects are acquired after birth and are the result of the effects of age, viruses, chemicals, or radiation. They affect only the neoplastic cells, and they are not inheritable. However, some mutations involve the germ cells of the ovary or testis and can be inherited. In such instances, the defective gene is present in every cell in the body, but not every cell becomes malignant because the defective gene has a narrowly focused function. An example of an inheritable cancer gene is the *RB* gene, which is responsible for a certain type of familial eye tumor.

☞ *The cause of all cancer is damaged DNA.*

MUTATIONS

Because DNA is organized into segments called genes (Chapter 2), the damaged DNA is always part of a particular gene. It is important to understand that mutant (damaged) genes associated with cancer are first discovered and named because they are associated with a particular cancer; hence the name given to the gene usually is related to the abnormal (defective, cancer-causing) form of the gene, not the normal gene or its usual function. This often leads to the mistaken assumption that the abnormal gene is the only one that exists. For example, the *BRCA* gene, associated with breast cancer, is named for the cancer with which it is associated. We know little of the normal function of the undamaged gene in healthy people.

The most common genetic defect in human cancer is mutation or complete loss of the *p53* gene, a gene that normally commands apoptosis (natural cell death) of cells with damaged DNA. About half of all cancers have a defective *p53* gene, but it is especially prevalent in cancers of the breast and colon. Without the *p53* gene to command apoptosis, cells with damaged DNA remain alive and on the road to malignancy. Loss of the ability of *p53* to command apoptosis has important therapeutic implications. Much of the effectiveness of chemotherapeutic agents lies in their ability to induce apoptosis, and they depend upon *p53* to aid them in this task. The loss of p53 reduces the effectiveness of chemotherapy by making cells less sensitive to chemotherapy-induced signals for apoptosis.

Mutations of single genes are not the only defect in cancer cells. In healthy cells the nucleus contains one set of normal chromosomes; however, as tumors evolve they can acquire extra chromosome or sets of chromosomes as a result of faulty DNA reproduction. Normal cells are said to be **euploid** (Chapter 2); that is, they have a normal set of 46 chromosomes, a **haploid** set of 23 from the sperm and ovum of each parent, organized into a nucleus that is relatively small and has a smooth, uniform appearance. Tumor cells with more than the normal set of chromosomes—most cancers—are said to be **aneuploid** and have enlarged, dark nuclei, reflecting the increased amount of DNA.

CELL GROWTH CONTROL GENES

All cells contain genes that function as "go" or "stop" switches, stimulating or restraining cell growth. Normally, the effect of growth-stimulating and growth-suppressing genes is in balance. The "go" genes are **proto-oncogenes**. The normal function of proto-oncogenes is to produce growth-promoting proteins that stimulate normal cell division. However, if they are converted by mutation into **oncogenes** (cancer genes), their function becomes one of stimulating uncontrolled cell division.

Growth-suppressor genes are the opposite of to proto-oncogenes—they are "stop" switches, **tumor suppression genes**, which produce proteins that inhibit cell division. If a growth-suppressing gene suffers injury and loses its ability to function, it leaves cell growth uninhibited. An example of this phenomenon is familial retinoblastoma, an eye tumor of infants and children, which is caused by a *defective RB* gene, a defective growth-suppressor gene.

DNA REPAIR

DNA injury can cause nucleotide base sequences (Chapter 2) to be out of order; that is, the sequence of bases can be "misspelled." To correct these errors there is a **DNA repair system**, which can be thought of as a "spell-checker" for DNA nucleotide sequences. For example, if the DNA sequence should be AAACCGT but is misspelled ACACCGT, the DNA repair system corrects the error. If, however the DNA repair system itself is damaged, the misspelled DNA remains defective and prone to promote cancer. For example, *xeroderma pigmentosa*, a skin disorder with predisposition to development of skin cancers, is caused by a faulty DNA repair apparatus that allows defective DNA to proceed to malignancy.

The Causes of Cancer

As is illustrated in Figure 6-2, cancer is caused by a transformation of cells (**carcinogenesis**) that follows injuries that produce direct damage to DNA (mutagene-

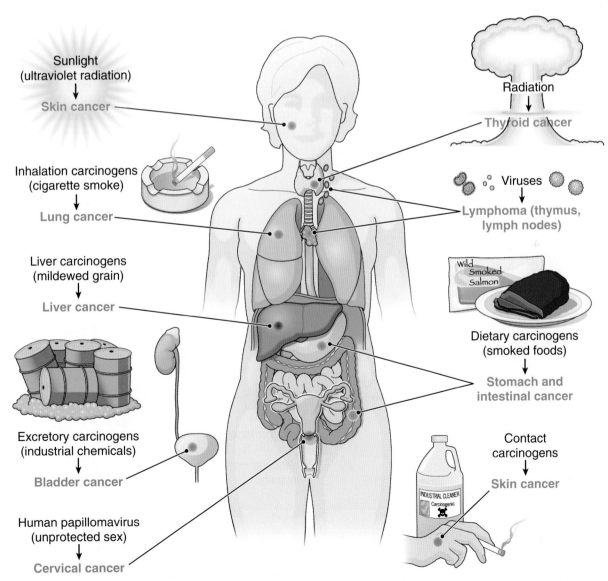

Figure 6-2 **The causes of cancer.** Cancer is caused by transformation of cells (carcinogenesis) following injuries that directly damage DNA (mutagenesis).

sis). Chemicals, ionizing radiation, and viruses can be responsible.

The list of *chemical* carcinogens is very long. In addition to Sir Percival Pott's linking of scrotal cancer to soot exposure in 18th century chimney sweeps, modern examples include links between: 1) the chemical content of cigarette smoke and lung cancer; 2) certain dyes and bladder cancer in the dye and rubber industry; and 3) aflatoxin in improperly stored food grains (produced by a mold, *Aspergillus*) and the development of hepatocellular carcinoma in parts of Africa and the Far East.

Ionizing radiation also may induce carcinogenesis. For example, survivors of the atomic bomb blasts at Hiroshima and Nagasaki, Japan, at the end of World War II have a marked increase of leukemia, and miners of uranium have a marked increase of lung cancer. Very common, but not as well appreciated, is the **mutagenic** effect of ultraviolet light in ordinary sunlight. At greatest risk are light-skinned people who get a lot of sun exposure. The lower lip, the forehead, and the back of the neck are particularly susceptible to development of skin cancers, including malignant melanoma.

Viruses also may cause cancer. Human papilloma virus (HPV, Chapter 21) causes most carcinoma of the cervix, Epstein-Barr virus (EBV) is implicated as the cause of some lymphomas, and hepatitis B virus (HBV) is important in the genesis of hepatocellular carcinoma.

Finally, certain conditions are well known as forerunners of malignancy. The mechanism of the carcinogenesis in some of these **premalignant conditions** is not clear, but others are well known. One such condition is Barrett esophagus (Chapter 15), an inflammatory condition of the lower esophagus caused by gastric acid reflux, which is associated with an increased risk for development of esophageal cancer.

The Structure of Neoplasms

Understanding how neoplasms are structured—their gross and microscopic anatomy—is critical to understanding their behavior. As is depicted in Figure 6-3 and listed in Table 6-2, benign and malignant neoplasms grow in very different ways and have very different appearances.

THE GROSS ANATOMY OF NEOPLASMS

The gross shape and structure of a neoplasm are important. Benign neoplasms tend to be slow growing and have a rounded, smooth outline with a rim of compressed fibrous tissue at the edge (a fibrous capsule). The cut surface is smooth and uniform, with a regular consistency and appearance throughout. Malignant neoplasms, on the other hand, tend to be irregular, with

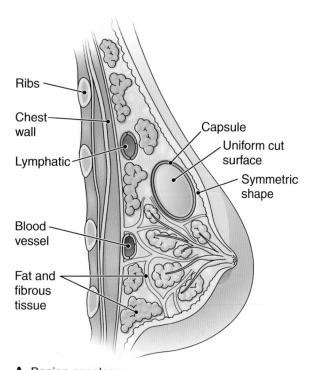

A Benign neoplasm

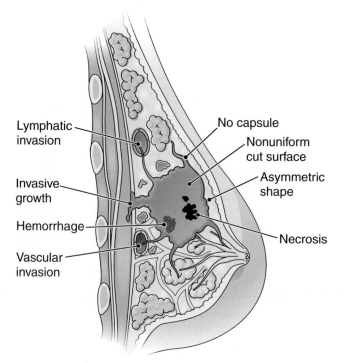

B Malignant neoplasm

Figure 6-3 **The gross structure of neoplasms.**

Table 6-2	Characteristics of Benign and Malignant Tumors	
Characteristic	**Benign**	**Malignant**
Tissue differentiation (specialization)	Well differentiated; structure fairly close to tissue of origin	Poorly differentiated; little structural resemblance to tissue or origin
Nuclear atypia	Minimal atypia; nuclei small and uniform	Substantial atypia; nuclei large, dark, irregular
Local growth	Slow growth; cut surface uniform; regular expansion compresses surrounding tissue into a fibrous capsule	Rapid growth; cut surface variegated; irregular growth at margins; infiltration of adjacent tissue
Metastasis	None	Frequent

fingers of tumor invading adjacent tissue, and the cut surface has a varied appearance, with areas of necrosis, hemorrhage, calcification, or other irregularities.

Tumors, both benign and malignant, may be described by their shape. Some grow as a **polyp**, a mass that protrudes from an epithelial surface. Others may grow as a **papilloma**, which grows in a fern- or finger-like pattern with prominent folds like a head of broccoli and rises above the epithelial surface, like a polyp. Likewise, both benign and malignant tumors may be cystic; that is, they may have a hollow center, and the feature is incorporated into the name. For example, cystadenoma and cystadenocarcinoma are two types of tumors commonly found in the ovary.

THE MICROSCOPIC ANATOMY OF NEOPLASMS

As is depicted in Figure 6-4, all neoplasms have two basic components: 1) the *parenchyma*, which is the neoplastic tissue, and 2) the *stroma*, a non-neoplastic supporting network of blood vessels and fibrous tissue. Most microscopic diagnostic and descriptive phrases relate to the parenchyma.

The microscopic appearance of a neoplasm correlates much better with tumor behavior than does gross appearance. Neoplasms may be either completely benign or extremely malignant, and their microscopic appearance varies accordingly. Benign neoplasms may reproduce tissue recognizably close to normal tissue, but very aggressive tumors fail to reproduce a semblance of the normal tissue.

Malignant nuclei are large and dark because of the presence of excess DNA, a feature called **hyperchromatism** because of the excess number of chromosomes in malignant nuclei. **Atypia** refers to the degree to which

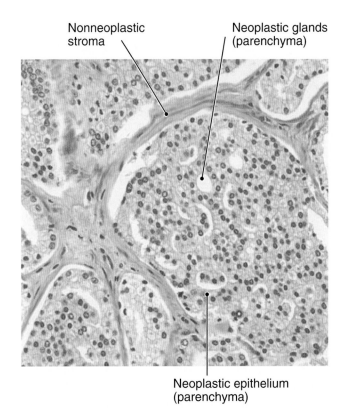

Nonneoplastic stroma

Neoplastic glands (parenchyma)

Neoplastic epithelium (parenchyma)

Figure 6-4 The microscopic structure of neoplasms. All tumors are formed of the neoplastic supporting stroma of fibrous tissue and blood vessels

individual neoplastic *nuclei* fail to resemble normal nuclei by microscopic examination. If the tumor is growing rapidly, cells are dividing rapidly and numerous **mitotic figures** (cells caught in the act of dividing) are present. Figure 6-5 illustrates the microscopic features of a highly malignant tumor.

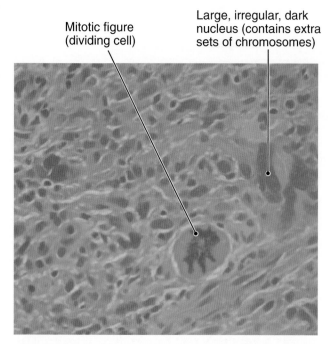

Mitotic figure (dividing cell)

Large, irregular, dark nucleus (contains extra sets of chromosomes)

Figure 6-5 **Nuclear atypia in malignant neoplasms.** The nuclei of malignant neoplasms are large, dark (hyperchromatic), and irregular because of the presence of extra sets of chromosomes. Mitotic figures (dividing cells) are common. Although this tumor arose from skeletal muscle, no normal muscle is present, indicating that the tumor is highly anaplastic.

Premalignant States and Conditions

As is depicted in Figure 6-6, neoplasms do not leap into existence in an instant. They evolve over time from normal tissue and go through recognizable stages along the way. **Dysplasia** refers to a pre-malignant state of tissue (usually epithelium) that is atypical and clearly abnormal but not yet malignant; that is, it is on the way to malignancy. It is critical to understand that *dysplasia does not always progress to malignancy*: it may revert to normal even without treatment, and with proper treatment dysplasia is curable. However, dysplasia cannot be disregarded; it warrants careful investigation and action. For example, mild dysplasia of the cervix usually regresses to normal without treatment. On the other hand, dysplasia can progress to **carcinoma in situ**, a tissue state that is literally cancer "in place." It is true but

Figure 6-6 **The development of an epithelial malignancy (carcinoma). A.** Normal epithelium resting on basement membrane. Lymphatics and blood vessels are below the basement membrane. **B.** Dysplasia. Nuclei of cells with injured DNA are large and atypical but not yet malignant. **C.** Carcinoma in situ. Further DNA injury transforms the cells into a malignancy that has not crossed (invaded) the basement membrane and, therefore, cannot metastasize because it has not reached into blood vessels or lymphatics. **D.** Early invasive carcinoma. Additional injury produces malignant cells that penetrate the basement membrane. **E.** Invasion of blood vessels or lymphatics with distant metastasis.

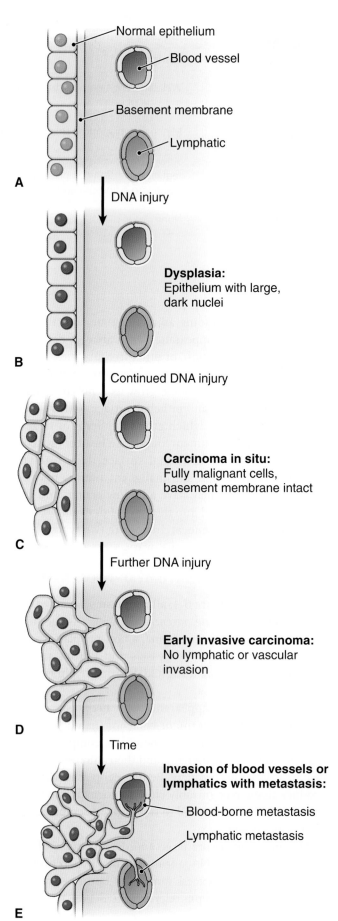

Normal epithelium
Blood vessel
Basement membrane
Lymphatic

A

DNA injury

Dysplasia: Epithelium with large, dark nuclei

B

Continued DNA injury

Carcinoma in situ: Fully malignant cells, basement membrane intact

C

Further DNA injury

Early invasive carcinoma: No lymphatic or vascular invasion

D

Time

Invasion of blood vessels or lymphatics with metastasis:
Blood-borne metastasis
Lymphatic metastasis

E

somewhat misleading to say "Carcinoma in situ never metastasizes." Carcinoma in situ is malignant epithelium that has not penetrated the basement membrane; that is, it is not *invasive* cancer and therefore cannot reach blood vessels or lymphatics, which lie beneath the basement membrane. Once carcinoma invades below the basement membrane it is no longer in situ; it is invasive, and only invasive malignancies can metastasize. Carcinoma in situ in a colonic polyp is illustrated in Figure 6-7. Carcinoma in situ is curable by complete excision or other eradication. However, if untreated and given enough time, some carcinomas in situ may become invasive and metastasize.

> **Dysplasia is a premalignant state of epithelium that may progress to malignancy, or it may revert to normal without treatment.**

A number of disorders—**premalignant conditions**—predispose to the development of malignancy. One of the best known is human papilloma virus (HPV) infection of the cervix, which causes almost all dysplasia, carcinoma in situ, and invasive carcinoma of the female cervix. HPV infection can be thought of as a premalignant condition, although it usually takes many years and repeated infections to produce dysplasia or malignancy. Many conditions are known to be associated with increased incidence of cancer in the affected tissue or organ. Among them, for example, are several condition of the gastrointestinal tract (Chapter 15). Chronic atrophic gastritis predisposes to gastric carcinoma, Barrett meta-plasia of the esophagus predisposes to esophageal cancer, and adenomatous polyps and chronic ulcerative colitis predispose to colon cancer.

> **Cancer that is always curable. Carcinoma in situ is cancer of epithelial cells that has not penetrated the basement membrane upon which the epithelium rests. It is always curable because:**
> - **All blood vessels and lymphatic channels lie below the basement membrane**
> - **Carcinoma in situ lies above the basement membrane**
> - **Cancers spread (metastasize) by invading blood vessels and lymphatics**
>
> **Therefore, cells in carcinoma in situ cannot invade blood vessels or lymphatic channels, and cannot metastasize unless they can reach blood vessels or lymphatic channels.**

The Biology of Neoplastic Growth

Like a tulip or an elephant, a tumor is a growing thing. Some grow rapidly and others slowly. No matter how they grow, however, most neoplasms make themselves known by the local pressure effect exerted by the expanding mass of the primary tumor or the growth of metastatic tumor masses. For example, neoplasms of the pituitary frequently are discovered because they press on nearby optic nerve fibers and produce disturbances of eyesight; and carcinomas of the lung are often first heralded by neurologic symptoms related to the growth of brain metastases.

THE DIFFERENTIATION OF TUMOR CELLS

The degree of **differentiation** (Fig. 6-8) of a neoplasm refers to the degree to which it resembles normal tissue in function and appearance—perfectly (100%) differentiated tissue is normal and, therefore, is not neoplastic. The degree to which tumor cells are differentiated is a microscopic clue to their likely behavior. Neoplasms are spoken of as being **well differentiated** (having some microscopic appearance of normal, and perhaps some normal cell function) or **poorly differentiated** (having little of the appearance or function of normal cells). Most tumors, whether well differentiated or poorly differentiated, do not have significant physiologically normal function; their only aim is reproduction. Of course, benign tumors are well differentiated, and highly malignant tumors are poorly differentiated. Well-differentiated malignant tumors grow slowly and are slow to invade and

Carcinoma in situ

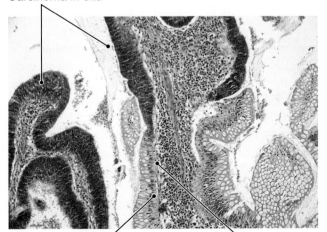

Normal epithelium   Basement membrane

Figure 6-7 **Carcinoma in situ.** A colon polyp with an area of malignant (dark, hyperchromatic, atypical) epithelium that has not invaded the basement membrane.

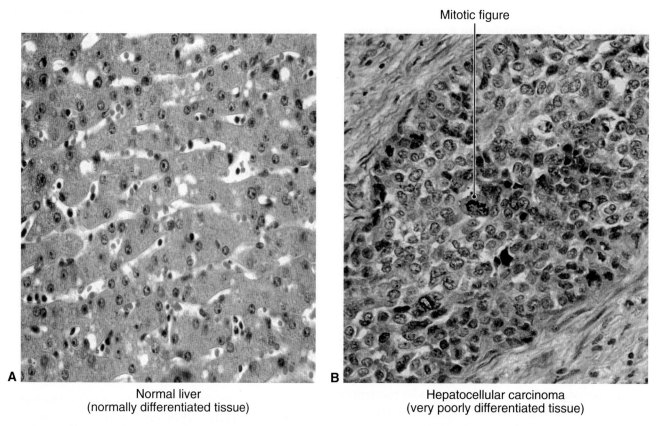

A
Normal liver
(normally differentiated tissue)

B
Mitotic figure

Hepatocellular carcinoma
(very poorly differentiated tissue)

Figure 6-8 **Differentiated versus undifferentiated tissue. A.** Normal liver (microscopic view). The cells are perfectly well differentiated (normal). **B.** Malignant tumor of liver. The cells are so poorly differentiated that no hint of normal liver cells remains.

metastasize; poorly differentiated malignant tumors grow rapidly, invade aggressively, and metastasize early.

CLONES OF CELLS

Tumor cells reproduce by forming a **clone** (Fig. 6-9), a set of identical cells descended from a single ancestor. All tumors are monoclonal; that is, they arise from a single cell and grow as expanding generations of that cell. Malignancy evolves in this way: 1) slow transformation of a normal cell line (clone) into a malignant clone; 2) uncontrolled proliferation of the descendants (clonal expansion); 3) local infiltration of adjacent tissues; 4) invasion of lymphatics or blood vessels, and, finally, 5) metastasis to distant sites.

THE SPEED OF TUMOR GROWTH

It takes far longer for a normal cell to become malignant than for any other stage of tumor growth. Cells must divide for a tumor to grow. A single malignant cell divides into two, these two double to form four, these four double again to form eight, and so on until the mass of cells

is large enough to be detected. A single cell is about one-billionth of a gram, so it takes about 30 generations, about 30 doublings, for a tumor mass to grow large enough, about the size of a grape (about one gram), to be detectable. As is depicted in Figure 6-9, this takes time, usually many years: a malignant neoplasm has lived most of its life *before* it becomes large enough to be detectible. It takes far more time for a tumor to grow from the tiny size of a cell to the size of a grape than it does for one the size of a grape to grow into one the size of a football.

In most tumors most of the cells are resting and only some of them are dividing. How rapidly a neoplasm grows depends primarily upon the *fraction* (percent) of cells that are dividing at any moment, a figure known as the **tumor growth fraction**, depicted in Figure 6-10. For example, if 40% of cells in a tumor are dividing, it will grow four times as rapidly as a tumor in which 10% of cells are dividing. How *rapidly* cells are dividing (for example, once a day versus once a week) is much less significant. This is important clinically because cancer chemotherapy drugs typically exert their effect by inter-

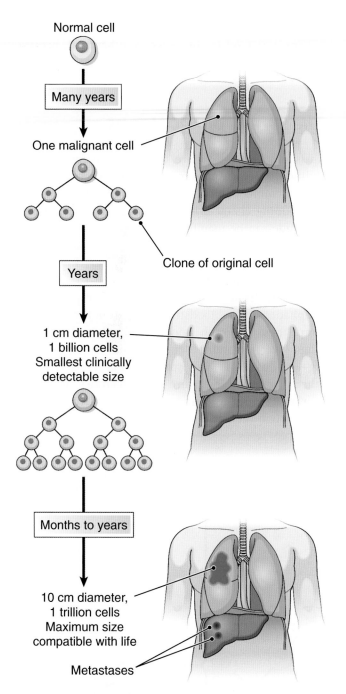

Figure 6-9 Tumor doubling time. Tumors arise as a single cell and are composed of cells (a clone) derived from a single ancestor. One cell divided into two, two into four, four to eight, and so on, doubling in roughly the same amount of time. It takes far more time for a normal cell to become cancerous than for the tumor to grow large enough to be detectable, and it takes even less time for a tumor to grow large enough to cause death.

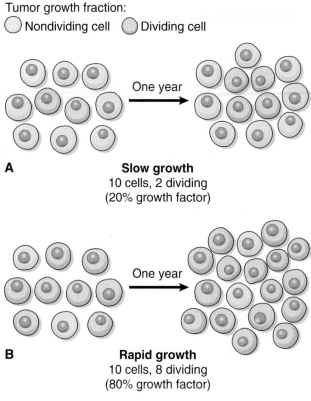

Figure 6-10 Tumor growth fraction. A. Low (slow) growth fraction. In this example, 20% (the growth fraction) of tumor cells are dividing at any given time, and the tumor grows relatively slowly. **B.** High (rapid) growth fraction. In this example, 80% of the cells are dividing at any given time, and the tumor grows much faster than the one shown in part A.

rupting or slowing the growth cycle of dividing cells; therefore, tumors with a high growth fraction are most affected by chemotherapy. Lymphomas and leukemias grow more rapidly than most other tumors because they have high growth fractions, not because the cells are dividing more frequently than other neoplasms. Lymphomas and leukemias are, therefore, usually sensitive to chemotherapeutic drugs.

THE NOURISHMENT OF TUMORS

Like other tissues, neoplasms must have nourishment from the bloodstream. Because neoplasms are new growths, they must develop their own network of blood vessels—a neoplasm without a blood supply would never become larger than a few cells. Neoplasms develop their own blood supply by the process of **angioneogenesis** (Chapter 4). Angioneogenesis is as necessary for the growth of neoplasms as damaged DNA is necessary for their creation. Early in their development most dysplastic or malignant cells do not stimulate angioneogenesis; thus, they remain dysplastic or in situ for years before becoming invasive. What's more, the degree of tumor angioneogenesis affects the ability of malignant tumors to metastasize: tumors with rich vascular networks are more prone to metastasize than are those with fewer blood vessels, because blood vessels are more abundant and accessible for invasion.

TUMOR CELL VARIATION

As a tumor grows, the clone of cells diverges into lines with different characteristics; some tumor cell variants have mutations of one kind, others have mutations of a different kind. As is illustrated in Figure 6-11, **tumor cell heterogeneity** (variation from one cell to the next) is important in a Darwinian "survival of the fittest" sense: some cells are sturdier, more capable of defeating natural defenses or surviving attack by therapeutic anticancer drugs. In other words, the most malignant cells survive; the less malignant ones do not. For example, tumor cells that require hormone support are vulnerable to therapy that reduces hormone availability. An example is prostate cancer: it thrives on testosterone and its growth is slowed if the testicles are removed or antitestosterone drugs are administered. Tumor cells that do not have such needs are less vulnerable and better able to survive to kill the host. Likewise, tumor cells

that produce large amounts of angioneogenesis factor (Chapter 4) tend to thrive where others fail, because they are more effective in growing their own blood supply.

The Spread of Neoplasms

As is depicted in Figure 6-12, **invasiveness** is the ability of a neoplasm to invade tissues, especially basement membrane, blood vessels, and lymphatics, and is the defining characteristic of malignancy. This ability to invade can be manifest clinically by mechanical effect; for example a bronchial carcinoma may obstruct airflow in the bronchi. Often, however, invasion is manifest clinically by **metastasis** (Fig. 6-13), the ability to skip from one place to another, especially via lymphatics or the bloodstream; say from the breast via lymphatics to lymph nodes, or via blood to bone, lungs, liver, or brain. Metastases may occur by **seeding**—by floating in body space from one surface to another. For example, Figure 6-14 illustrates seeding of ovarian carcinoma to the surface of the liver by floating through the peritoneum.

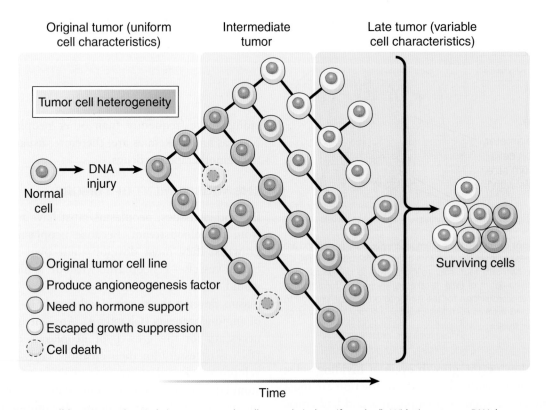

Figure 6-11 **Tumor-cell heterogeneity.** Early in tumor growth, cells are relatively uniform (red). With time, tumor DNA becomes unstable and gives rise to mutant cell offspring whose DNA is different from that of the parent cell (other colors). For example, tumor cells (orange) that have no need of hormone support survive antihormone therapy. Tumor cells (green) that produce large amounts of angioneogenesis factor are more capable of growing their own blood supply and become more numerous. Some tumor cells (yellow) escape natural cell growth control mechanisms and also become more numerous. As a result, late stage tumors (right) are composed of a varied (heterogeneous) mix of cells that have special characteristics and that outnumber cells of the unchanged original tumor line.

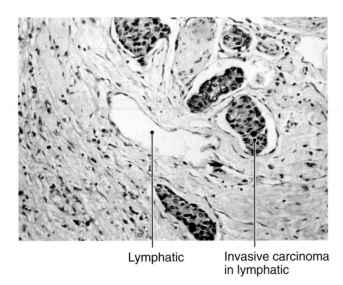

Lymphatic   Invasive carcinoma
                 in lymphatic

Figure 6-12 Invasive carcinoma in lymphatics. Shown are nests of malignant cells present in lymphatic channels. Metastases were present in lymph nodes fed by these lymphatics.

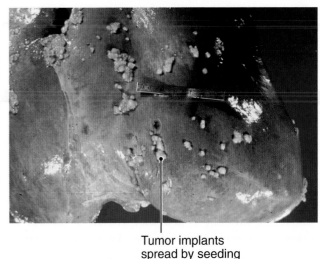

Tumor implants
spread by seeding

Figure 6-14 Metastasis by seeding. Gross study of the peritoneal surface of the liver with ovarian carcinoma implants seeded into the peritoneal space.

The most feared feature of any malignancy is its ability to spread by direct invasion of blood vessels, because vascular invasion can cause spread of tumor to any site in the body. By contrast, spread through lymphatic channels is often stopped by lymph nodes; however, if not detected and removed, lymphatic spread ultimately enters the bloodstream via the thoracic duct. Once a tumor has metastasized by blood, it is beyond surgical correction, although chemotherapy and other therapies may be effective.

Sarcomas have a propensity for vascular invasion and widespread metastasis. Carcinomas, on the other hand, tend to invade lymphatics first and metastasize to local lymph nodes, where they make themselves known by lymph node enlargement (lymphadenopathy). Lymph nodes enlarged by metastatic carcinoma may be detected and removed surgically, offering some hope that the tumor has been caught before moving further up the lymphatic chain to be emptied into blood for spread throughout the body. Carcinomas may invade blood vessels directly, too, but much less frequently than sarcomas do. Veins are more susceptible to invasion than arteries are. For example, carcinoma of the colon commonly spreads via the portal venous system into the liver. Because all venous blood must pass through the sieve of the lungs, the lungs are a very common site of tumor metastasis.

> **The clinical hallmark of malignancy is the spread of the tumor from the primary site to distant sites, usually via the lymphatic system or bloodstream.**

The Immune Defense Against Neoplasia

With the exception of identical twins, all of us are genetically unique: our DNA is ours alone and is unlike anyone else's. It is useful, therefore, to think of a person's DNA and the proteins produced under DNA command as "self" and all other proteins as alien, or nonself. It is the job of the immune system (Chapter 8) to attack things that are made of nonself protein. To protect

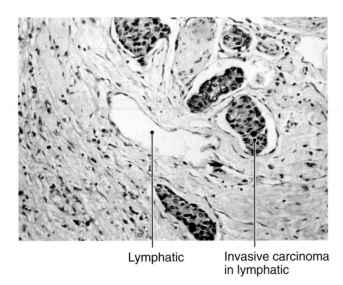

Metastatic tumor   Normal liver

Figure 6-13 Metastatic cancer. This cross-section of liver shows multiple blood-borne nodules of metastatic colon cancer.

against infection, the immune system attempts to destroy the invading nonself protein of the invading microbe. For example, the measles virus and other microorganisms are bundles of alien, nonself proteins that are attacked by the immune system whenever they enter the body. The same is true for organ transplants, which are alien to the recipient; hence the need for immunosuppressive therapy to prolong the life of transplanted organs.

As is illustrated in Figure 6-11, as neoplasms grow, their cells become increasingly abnormal. Eventually, they become so abnormal that they are viewed as nonself by the immune system and, therefore, subject to attack, as a microbe would be. This anti-neoplastic function of the immune system is referred to as **immune surveillance**. Once DNA is changed by injury (mutation), it becomes nonself DNA and subject to immune attack. Therefore, in healthy people mutant cells that otherwise might develop into malignancy are eliminated by the immune system. Sometimes, however, mutant cells escape to perpetuate themselves as neoplasms.

Logic suggests that immunodeficient patients should suffer from more neoplasms than those with normal immune systems; and they do—AIDS patients and patients on immunosuppressive therapy for organ transplants or other reasons also have a higher than expected occurrence of malignant neoplasms.

The Epidemiology of Cancer

Epidemiology is the study of the patterns and causes of diseases (or other health-related conditions) in certain populations. As is illustrated by the nearby History of Medicine box, much of our knowledge about the causes and behavior of malignancies comes from our understanding of its epidemiology. Some links are clear—smoking and lung cancer, or excess sun exposure and skin cancer, for example. More often, however, the links between disease and behavior or environment are less clear.

Age and *sex* are important. Older people have more malignancies than younger people do. Although the reasons are not clear, year-by-year accumulation of cell mutations probably plays a role. Differences in cancer rates among males and females are attributable largely to malignancies of sex organs—women have a high incidence of breast cancer, and men have a high incidence of prostate cancer.

Genetics and heredity are also important. Most neoplasms have at least some element of genetic predisposition, but clear genetic linkage is rare. One example of clear linkage is **retinoblastoma**, an inherited malignant tumor of the retina in children, which is linked to the *RB* gene. Breast, ovarian, and colon cancer show some degree of clustering in certain families, but inheritance patterns are usually not clear in any given case. Breast cancer is illustrative: about 10% of women with breast cancer have a mother, daughter, or sister with breast cancer; and of these about one fourth (3%) have a specific gene defect—the *BRCA* gene. However, 90% of breast cancer is episodic; that is, no cause can be identified. Table 6-3 lists some cancers and their genetic relationships, but most cancers are episodic.

History of Medicine

Rx: TAKE A BATH ONCE A WEEK

The first example of cancer epidemiology and of chemical carcinogenesis occurred in 1775 when surgeon Sir Percival Pott noted that chimney sweeps developed carcinoma of the scrotal skin and correctly concluded it was associated with accumulated soot caked in the groin. The good doctor prescribed bathing at least once per week, which was effective.

In the 20th century it became clear that cigarette smoking causes lung cancer. Especially noteworthy is that lung cancer was rare in women until World War II when "Rosie the Riveter" abandoned crib and kitchen to build tanks and trucks and took up smoking, which had been a man's habit until then.

Environmental influences are common but rarely are as clear as these two examples are.

Table 6-3	**Genetic Inheritance and Cancer**
Gene	**Cancer**
colspan selected	**Selected specific gene-associated, autosomal dominant inheritable cancers**
RB	Retinoblastoma (malignant tumor of the retina in infants)
APC	Hereditary colon polyposis and colon cancer
BRCA	Hereditary breast and ovarian cancers
	Cancers with some familial clustering of cases*
n/a	Breast, ovarian, and pancreatic cancers

*Most cases of these cancers are episodic and not associated with specific gene defects.

The Clinical Picture of Cancer

The American Cancer Society lists the following warning signals of cancer, the first letters of which cleverly spell C-A-U-T-I-O-N:

- **C**hange in bowel or bladder habits (colon or bladder cancer)
- **A** sore that doesn't heal (skin cancer, especially malignant melanoma)
- **U**nusual bleeding or discharge (breast, intestinal, cervical, or uterine cancer)
- **T**hickening or lump in the breast or elsewhere (breast or other cancer)
- **I**ndigestion or difficulty swallowing (throat or esophageal cancer)
- **O**bvious change in a wart or mole (malignant melanoma)
- **N**agging cough or hoarseness (lung or laryngeal cancer)

Another warning sign is unintended weight loss (visceral cancer, lymphoma, or leukemia).

Signs and symptoms of cancer are systemic or local. The most important local symptom is a mass, which may be visible or palpable or may produce symptoms related to its location. For example, intestinal bleeding or bowel obstruction is often the first sign of a tumor of the intestine; tumors of the bronchi may produce coughing, wheezing, or shortness of breath; and brain tumors may cause epileptic seizures.

Sometimes the direct effect of a tumor mass can create severe clinical problems even if the tumor is benign. For example, some benign tumors of the pituitary may cause blindness by pressing on the optic nerves, a leiomyoma (benign smooth muscle tumor) of the stomach may cause massive gastric bleeding, or a uterine leiomyoma may cause abnormal endometrial bleeding.

Although benign tumors are far more common than are malignant ones, almost any mass requires biopsy and microscopic diagnosis. There are some notable exceptions, especially in skin (Chapter 24),where the clinical look and feel of subcutaneous lipomas (benign tumors of fat) and certain cysts are so unmistakable that a biopsy is not necessary. On the other hand, *every* breast mass must be investigated.

Some neoplasms, either benign or malignant, may produce far-reaching effects on the body that are distinct from the direct mass effect of the primary tumor or its metastases. These effects are **paraneoplastic syndromes**. Case Study 6-1 at the end of this chapter offers a clinical example. Paraneoplastic syndromes usually stem from tumor production of hormones that fall into two categories: 1) hormones native to the normal tissue from which the tumor arose, and 2) hormones that produce substances not normally produced by the tissue from which the tumor originated. An example of a tumor that produces native hormone is *pheochromocytoma*, a tumor of the adrenal medulla (Chapter 18) that secretes epinephrine and norepinephrine and is associate with severe surges of dangerously high blood pressure. An example of a tumor that produces non-native hormone is lung cancer that produces adrenal hormones in quantities large enough to produce striking clinical findings of adrenocortical hormone excess (Cushing syndrome, Chapter 18). Dozens of paraneoplastic syndromes have been identified that cause mental aberration, neurologic disease, hypercalcemia, enlargement of male breasts (gynecomastia), Cushing disease and other endocrine syndromes, very low plasma sodium, and other problems. Tumors most commonly causing paraneoplastic syndrome are carcinoma of the lung, renal cell carcinoma, and tumors of endocrine glands.

Sometimes malignancies may produce general effects that cannot be linked directly to known substances. An example is **cachexia**, a wasting of body fat and muscle (Fig. 6-15) that affects many patients with advanced cancer. Decreased appetite may cause some of the weight loss, but most of the loss is attributable to a high metabolic rate induced by the tumor. Another poorly understood paraneoplastic syndrome is the tendency of some patients to develop deep vein thrombi and inflammation (thrombophlebitis), usually in leg or pelvic veins. The appearance of otherwise unexplainable thrombophlebitis will prompt experienced diagnosticians to search for hidden cancer.

Clinical and Laboratory Assessment of Neoplasms

The assessment of neoplasms, especially malignant ones, is an exercise that involves obtaining a thorough clinical history, doing a complete physical examination, obtaining medical images and laboratory data, and microscopic study of tissues and cells.

CLINICAL HISTORY

Would that C-A-N-C-E-R could be spelled out on the surface of each malignant cell, and the only thing for a pathologist to do was to "read the slide." Not so. In practice, this point can be notoriously difficult to appreciate. The importance of context—*clinical history*—in pathologic, radiologic, or clinical diagnosis cannot be over-

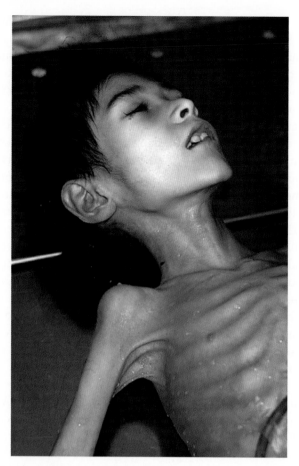

Figure 6-15 **Cachexia of malignancy.** This photo is of a patient with pancreatic carcinoma. The wasting away of body tissue is not entirely a matter of lost appetite.

a photograph of a man in a ski mask standing at the counter holding a shotgun, and you are told nothing of the circumstances. Based solely on what you see, the most reasonable conclusion is that a robbery is about to take place, and you will agree that the police should have been called. On the other hand, you will probably reach a different conclusion if you are told that members of the cast of a gangster movie being filmed around the corner frequently come into the store in costume, and the "shotgun" is merely a cleverly carved and painted piece of wood. The point is this: To act solely on microscopic appearance and without taking clinical history into account is to risk, for example, amputating a leg for a benign bone condition that has a misleading microscopic appearance, or not doing an amputation on a malignant bone tumor that has deceptively bland microscopic features.

A microscopic slide sent for pathologist diagnosis is nothing more than a picture frozen in time, much like the snapshot in our example. The story—the clinical history—is extremely important if a correct conclusion is to be reached.

OBTAINING TISSUES AND CELLS FOR DIAGNOSIS

Cytology is the diagnostic study of individual cells for evidence of cancer or other abnormality. The nearby Lab Tools box offers more information about cytology. The best known cytology procedure for cancer diagnosis is the Papanicolaou (**Pap**) **smear** (Chapter 21) of the female cervix, depicted in Figure 6-16 and named after Dr. Georges Papanicolaou, who perfected the technique

stated. Clinical history is essential for bedside diagnosis; but it is just as critical for pathologic or radiologic diagnosis, a fact even experienced practitioners sometimes forget. For example, a microscopic slide taken from a healing bone fracture can look amazingly similar to a slide taken from some types of malignant bone tumor, so much so that even the savviest pathologist can be fooled without knowing the history of the fracture. If the same microscopic slide is presented to another pathologist who is told (misleadingly) that the biopsy specimen is from a bone mass of the femur of a fifteen-year-old boy, then a mistaken diagnosis of malignancy might be made.

Although knowing the history of a patient changes nothing on the slide, that very history (context) can make an immense difference in the story the slide tells us. History and context—these are the framework. The significance we attach to everything we see, be it in medicine or on the street, is determined by history and context. Consider the following example: Imagine yourself reviewing security camera snapshots of a convenience store cash register counter. You are presented

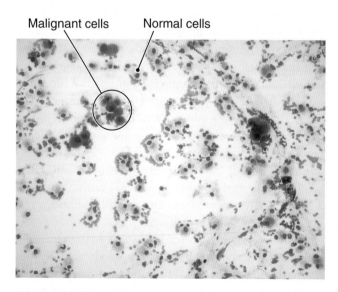

Figure 6-16 **Pap smear of the cervix.** Many normal cells are present, which have small, uniform nuclei. Also present are clumps of malignant cells, which have large, dark nuclei.

LAB TOOLS

Cytologic Diagnosis

Cytology is the diagnostic microscopic study of collections of cells, usually with the intent to see if any of them appear to be malignant or premalignant. It is in contrast with the microscopic study of intact pieces of tissue obtained by biopsy or at autopsy. The best known cytology study is the Pap smear (Chapter 21), which consists of cells scraped from the female cervix and smeared on a slide for microscopic diagnosis. However, cells for cytologic exam can also be gathered by

- Collecting sputum, cerebrospinal fluid, urine, joint fluid, or fluid from other body cavities, such as ascitic fluid from the peritoneal cavity
- Washing a hollow organ, such as a bronchus, with a small amount of fluid and recollecting it
- Aspirating cells from a solid mass (a breast tumor, for example) or organ (the thyroid, for example) by use of a very thin needle

Specimens collected by scraping or needle aspiration are often spread directly on clear glass slides, which are passed through a series of chemicals and dyes to ready them for microscopic study similar to the method for biopsy specimens (Chapter 1). On the other hand, cells in fluids are usually first concentrated by centrifugation or collected by filtration before being placed on a slide.

A cytology specimen found to contain malignant cells is reliable: As a "test" it is very nearly 100% specific (Chapter 1); that is, very few false-positive results occur. On the other hand, false-negative results (negative cytology studies from patients later proven to have cancer) can occur despite the most careful and correct procedures. Most false-negative results occur because even the most carefully collected specimen may not capture malignant cells even though they are present in the patient's tissue. That false-negative results occur with regularity is one of the main reasons that annual pap smears are recommended for most adult women.

In any circumstance, a woman who has had an abnormal smear must be followed carefully.

in the 1930s by study of cells scraped from the cervices of female lab rats. The technique was adopted in the 1940s and is now universally practiced. It is accepted as having been instrumental in a dramatic reduction of deaths from cervical cancer since its inception.

Another technique for obtaining specimens for diagnosis is **fine needle aspiration** of cells. A thin (fine) needle is inserted into the lesion, sometimes under radiologic guidance, and clusters of cells are aspirated and spread onto a slide for examination. This technique has made possible the accurate diagnosis of some lesions without the necessity of open surgical biopsy.

Biopsy is the collection of tissue for diagnosis by surgical excision or large bore needle to "core out" a cylinder of tissue. For example, prostate biopsies are usually obtained by needle biopsy technique. After collection the specimen must be carefully preserved, usually in a formaldehyde solution, and properly transported. Careful attention to specimen handling is paramount: careless handling can result in dried, lost, poorly preserved, or otherwise ruined specimens, and improper paperwork can result in Jane being mistakenly diagnosed with breast cancer if Mary's cancer biopsy specimen goes to the lab with Jane's paperwork.

GRADING AND STAGING OF MALIGNANCIES

Cancers are graded and staged (Fig. 6-17) in order to treat them appropriately. An overview of treatments is listed in Table 6-4. **Cancer grading** (Fig. 6-17A) is a *pathologic* exercise—the microscopic assessment of the degree of differentiation (cell specialization), atypia, and other microscopic features of malignancy. According to widely accepted practice, cancers are graded into categories according to their microscopic appearance. Practices vary somewhat from one type of malignancy to another and one pathologist to another: some tumors are graded on a scale of I to IV, others I to III. Typically *grade I* cancers (low grade) are those with the least aggressive microscopic appearance—tumors that are well differentiated and have little nuclear atypia. *Grade II* cancers are intermediate, and *grade III* (high-grade) cancers are those that appear to be the most aggressive—poorly differentiated and highly atypical. The Gleason system for grading prostate cancer (Chapter 20) is an example—well-differentiated cancers with little atypia are scored as grade I; poorly differentiated, very atypical tumors are scored as grade 5.

Cancer staging (Fig. 6-17B) is a *clinical* exercise—an evaluation of *behavior* by assessing the size of the pri-

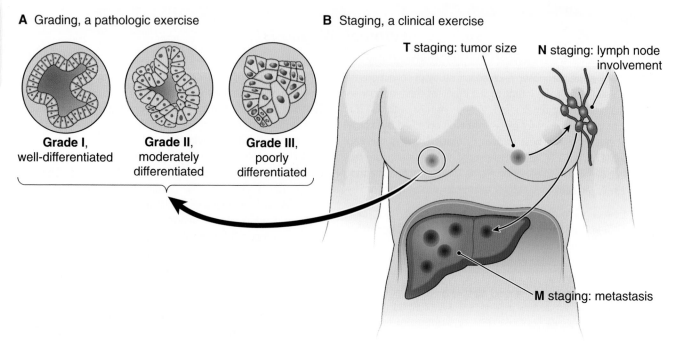

A Grading, a pathologic exercise

Grade I, well-differentiated

Grade II, moderately differentiated

Grade III, poorly differentiated

B Staging, a clinical exercise

T staging: tumor size

N staging: lymph node involvement

M staging: metastasis

Figure 6-17 **Grading and staging of malignancies. A.** Grading is a pathologic exercise that classifies tumors according to their microscopic characteristics. **B.** Staging is a clinical exercise that classifies tumors according to their size, invasiveness, and spread. Tumors are staged according to the TNM system (T, tumor size; N lymph node involvement; M, metastasis to distant organs). Schemes for TNM classification vary according to tumor type and organ involved.

mary tumor and its spread, either local or metastatic, as assessed by physical examination, history, and pathologic and diagnostic imaging. Staging is a much better guide than is grading for making decisions about therapy and for determining prognosis. It's like your mother said, "It's not what you say but what you *do* that counts"—

what tumors *do*, not what they look like, is most important. Think of grading as what the cancer looks like and staging as what the cancer is actually doing.

As is illustrated in Figure 6-17B, a common clinical staging convention in popular use is the **TNM system**— T for the size of the *primary* tumor, N for the extent, if

Table 6-4	*Cancer Treatments*
Treatment	**Purpose**
Surgery	Physical removal of all or most of primary tumor; may involve removal of nearby lymph nodes that may contain tumor metastases. Example: excision of breast cancer and axillary lymph nodes
Radiation	Kill tumor cells by concentrated doses of ionizing radiation
External	Radiation source is outside of body; beam of rays focused on tumor. Example: radiation of brain cancer
Internal	Radiation source is inside body; capsules, seeds, or needles of radioactive material placed in tumor. Example: radioactive seeds placed in prostate gland to treat prostate cancer
Systemic	Selective tumor absorption of radioactive material. Example: radioactive iodine is selectively absorbed by some thyroid cancers
Chemotherapy	Interferes with cancer cell reproduction, cancer-cell hormone use, or tumor blood vessel growth (angio-neogenesis) Example: oral or IV administration of drugs in leukemia and lymphoma
Immunotherapy	Use of immune methods to stop or slow tumor cell growth by stimulating the body's natural antitumor substances (such as cytokines) by administering synthetic antibodies targeted at tumor antigens or by vaccinating the patient with tumor antigen to stimulate immune system production of antitumor antibodies.

any, of *local* lymph node involvement, and M for *distant* metastases beyond local lymph nodes. TNM stages are closely correlated with survival data and are a valuable guide to prognosis and therapy. Each feature of the malignancy—size, local nodes, distant metastasis—is assessed according to certain criteria.

Staging breast cancer is a good example.

- Primary tumor (T)
  - T1: Tumor 2.0 cm or less
  - T2: Tumor 2–5 cm
  - T3: Tumor larger than 5 cm
  - T4: Any tumor, regardless of size, that invades chest wall or skin
- Local lymph nodes (N)
  - N0: No lymph node metastasis
  - N1: Axillary lymph node metastases in nodes that are moveable
  - N2: Axillary lymph node metastases that are fixed to one another or to the chest wall
  - N3: Metastasis to internal mammary lymph nodes (beneath sternum)
- Distant metastasis (M)
  - M0: No distant metastases
  - M1: Distant metastases beyond axillary or internal mammary nodes

For example, a patient with a 3-cm primary tumor, moveable positive axillary lymph nodes, and metastasis in bone would be staged T2, N1, M1. Other malignancies have different and equally detailed staging criteria.

EARLY DETECTION OF CANCER

In an ideal world we would be able to test (screen) everyone with a cheap, convenient, painless technique to detect all cancers early enough to cure them. The best example is Pap smear screening for cervical cancer (Chapter 21), which has resulted in a marked decline of deaths from cancer of the cervix. But early detection is no guarantee of cure. For example, experimental, highly sensitive radiographic techniques can find lung cancer at a very early stage; however, detecting these very early cancers appears not to result in a decrease in the number of lung cancer deaths. Nevertheless, early detection of every cancer is a worthy goal. The question is this: How do we detect and identify cancers before they metastasize? Barnett Kramer, MD, of the National Institutes of Health, put it this way: "Finding a cancer early is sometimes like being tied to a railroad track and given a pair of binoculars: you can see the train coming from further way, but you haven't done anything to change when the train is going to hit you."

Approaches vary, but everyone agrees that people with a positive family history of cancer benefit most from screening tests to detect cancer early.

- *Lung cancer* (Chapter 14): There is no good screening test. Chest radiographs using current technology are not sensitive enough to detect lesions early enough for surgical cure, and false positives necessitate unnecessary, hazardous lung surgery. Early detection, discussed immediately above, is not saving lives.
- *Prostate cancer* (Chapter 20): Screening is somewhat controversial because experts disagree on many of the details regarding the usefulness of testing blood for elevated levels of prostate-specific antigen (PSA), a prostate protein that is increased in many prostate diseases, including prostate cancer. The best policy seems to be annual blood test for PSA and an annual digital rectal exam beginning at age 50 to feel the prostate. The prostate can be felt through the anterior wall of the rectum, and many prostate cancers are hard and feel different from normal prostate. Men with a family history of prostate cancer should have exams beginning at age 40.
- *Breast cancer* (Chapter 21): The consensus recommendation is for breast examination by a qualified health professional every 3 years between ages 20 and 39 and annual examination with mammogram beginning at age 40. Rapid progress is being made with imaging techniques, so the recommendation may very likely change in a few years. Breast self-examination does not seem to detect cancers early enough to save lives; however, early detection by mammography has reduced the death rate from breast cancer in the United States about 25% since 1990.
- *Cervical cancer* (Chapter 21): Cervical cancer screening with Pap smears should begin approximately 3 years after the onset of vaginal intercourse, but no later than age 21, and should be done annually until age 30, after which screening may continue every 2 to 3 years for those women who have had three consecutive negative results. Women over 70 may choose to cease screening if they have had three consecutive negative pap smears and also no abnormal Pap smears within the prior 10 years.
- *Colorectal cancer* (Chapter 15): Beginning at age 50, adults at average risk should have an annual fecal occult blood test (FOBT) because almost all colon cancers arise from pre-existing polyps, which take many years to become malignant and tend to bleed. Annual FOBT may be supplemented by direct visual examination (flexible sigmoidoscopy) of the rectum and sigmoid colon every 5 years. Another alternative is

complete examination of the colon every five or ten years by imaging technique (barium enema) or colonoscopy. People with a history of adenomas (adenomatous polyps) of the colon or a family history of colon polyps or cancer should be screened more intensely.

TUMOR MARKERS

Tumor markers are substances produced by normal or neoplastic tissue and may appear in blood at increased levels in the presence of a neoplasm. However, these markers are usually not useful for the *early detection* of cancer. The holy grail of cancer detection is a simple blood test that will detect a cancer early enough for cure. The problem is that tumor markers do not appear in blood early enough or in high enough concentration to be useful in *early* cancer detection; that is, the tests are frequently falsely negative—in most instances the tumor is far advanced by the time tumor marker concentration is high enough for detection. Furthermore, markers may be elevated in non-cancerous conditions; that is, the tests are falsely positive. Rather than detecting cancer, these markers may be useful to confirm diagnosis or monitor therapy. For example, a falling level of blood tumor marker may validate the effectiveness of cancer therapy or surgery.

The first tumor marker discovered was **carcinoembryonic antigen** (CEA), which for a while seemed to show promise for early detection of colon cancer. However, experience revealed that CEA is elevated in many different diseases, both benign (cirrhosis of the liver) and malignant (carcinoma of the colon, pancreas, and other organs), and it reaches abnormal levels too late and too inconsistently to be useful as a screen for cancer. Nevertheless, CEA is useful as a guide to the effectiveness of therapy in monitoring tumor regression or progression.

Alpha-fetoprotein (AFP) is another marker that may be produced by neoplasms and appear in blood, but abnormal levels are also associated with other conditions. For example, when elevated in amniotic fluid, AFP has a positive association with neural tube defects; when low, it has a correlation with Down syndrome (Chapter 7).

Prostate-specific antigen (PSA), a third example, initially seemed to offer promise as a screen for early prostate carcinoma (Chapter 20). Perhaps its greatest advantage, when compared to other markers, is that it is not expressed by any tissue other than prostate. Nevertheless, PSA also may be increased in benign prostatic hyperplasia, so that it, too, has proven not to have either the specificity or sensitivity for use as a *sole* screening test. Another way to detect prostate cancer, perhaps the best, is by digital rectal palpation of the gland because most prostate cancers grow in the posterior part of the gland and are easily palpable through the anterior wall of the rectum.

Many prostate cancers are discovered by finding elevated levels of PSA; however, evidence suggests they could have been discovered *earlier* by digital rectal exam. On the other hand it is true that some early prostate cancers are detected by PSA in patients who have a normal digital rectal exam. The best strategy is to combine the evaluation of PSA levels with annual digital rectal examination in men over 50; those with a family history of prostate cancer should begin at age 40.

Other examples of markers include elevated blood levels of immunoglobulins in certain tumors of the immune system (e.g., multiple myeloma, Chapter 8), elevated hormones produced by tumors of the adrenal glands or other endocrine glands, and a variety of specific markers that are produced by ovarian, colon, pancreatic, and breast cancers, such as the CA-15-3 marker that circulates in the blood of some patients with breast cancer. ∎

CASE STUDY 6-1 *"I HAVE A CHEST COLD THAT WON'T GO AWAY"*

TOPICS
Lung cancer
Paraneoplastic syndrome

THE CASE

Setting: You are employed by a group of internists to do initial history and physical examinations on new patients before they see a physician.

Clinical history: A 52-year-old female dress-shop owner who consulted a dermatologist because of an increasing amount of dark facial hair is referred to your clinic for further workup.

When you ask why she is in your office today, she does not mention facial hair, and between coughs, she says, "I have a chest cold that won't go away." You also learn that she smoked two packs of cigarettes a day from the time she was a teenager until her divorce 4 years ago, when she stopped smoking. After the divorce she also changed ▶

[Case 6-1, continued] her diet, lost weight, took up yoga, and began to focus on her growing small business. She pronounces herself "back in charge of my life." Further questioning reveals that in the last several months her dress size has changed because of the amount of weight she has gained.

Physical examination: Her vital signs are unremarkable except for mild hypertension, 140/90. She is anxious and appears depressed and slightly overweight, with most of her bulk in the abdomen; her limbs are thin. As proof that she used to be in much better shape, she offers a picture of herself from a year ago. You note that in addition to new, dark hair, her face has changed dramatically from thin and angular to very round. The remainder of the physical examination is unremarkable except for purplish "stretch marks" on her abdomen and thighs.

Clinical course: You order routine blood and urine intake tests and add a chest radiograph because of the cough and smoking history. The physician who sees her after your initial workup orders a urine cortisol test and a skull radiograph and tells the patient to return in a week for further evaluation. All of her lab tests are unremarkable except for two: urine cortisol levels are markedly elevated, and the urine is positive for glucose. The skull radiograph is normal, but the chest radiograph shows a baseball-size mass in the right lung. The radiologist also diagnoses osteoporosis of the spine. Bronchoscopy is performed, and a biopsy specimen is taken from the mass for evaluation. The pathologic diagnosis is "small cell carcinoma."

DISCUSSION

This patient had a paraneoplastic syndrome—hypercortisolism (Cushing syndrome, Chapter 18) owing to secretion of the pituitary hormone adrenocorticotrophic hormone (ACTH) by small cell carcinoma of the lung. The normal skull radiograph ruled out a pituitary tumor, and special studies of the biopsy tissue demonstrated ACTH in the tumor.

Cushing syndrome is characterized by a rounded, "moon" face, obesity, hypertension, glucose intolerance or diabetes, skin striae (stretch marks), osteoporosis, decreased muscle mass, a "buffalo hump" of fat at the base of the neck, and menstrual abnormalities. This patient had all of them except for menstrual abnormalities and a buffalo hump, neither of which were mentioned in the record.

Cushing syndrome is caused by cortisol (hydrocortisone) excess. The most common cause is steroid therapy for chronic inflammatory disease, especially rheumatoid arthritis and related diseases. Sometimes, however, it may be caused by pituitary disease or tumor (in this case small cell carcinoma of the lung) secretion of ACTH, the hormone normally secreted by the pituitary to stimulate the adrenal cortex to increase cortisol output.

Of all lung cancers, small cell carcinoma has the strongest relationship to cigarette smoking and is the deadliest. It is uniformly fatal, usually within a year. Among lung cancers it is the most likely to produce a paraneoplastic syndrome. This case also illustrates that smoking risks linger after the patient stops smoking. This patient smoked two packs a day for over 30 years (in excess of 60 pack-years), so she had accumulated substantial risk. Risk returns to near normal after about 10 to 15 years without smoking, but for our patient it was "too little, too late."

POINTS TO REMEMBER
- Smoking causes lung cancer.
- Some neoplasms secrete hormones that have important clinical effects.

Objectives Recap

1. *Define the difference between benign and malignant neoplasms:* Benign neoplasms grow slowly, do not metastasize, and usually are not capable of causing death; malignant ones grow rapidly and are capable of causing death.

2. *List in descending order the top three causes of cancer death in men and women:* Men: Lung cancer, prostate cancer, colon cancer, and rectal cancer. Women: Lung cancer, breast cancer, colon cancer, and rectal cancer.

3. *Name several types of carcinogenesis, and give some examples:* The types of carcinogenesis with examples: chemical (cigarette smoke), radiation (x-ray or other ionizing radiation), or viral (human papillomavirus) damage, each of which can alter DNA to such an extent that the affected cell becomes malignant.

4. *Discuss the gross and microscopic characteristics of malignant tumors:* Benign neoplasms have a round or smooth outline with a rim of compressed fibrous tissue at the edge (a fibrous capsule). The cut surface is smooth and uniform, with a regular consistency and appearance throughout. Malignant neoplasms tend to be irregular, with fingers of tumor invading adjacent tissue, and the cut surface is variegated and may have areas of necrosis, hemorrhage, calcification, or other irregularities of composition.

Microscopically, malignant tissue looks little like normal tissue: The growth is disorganized, and normal structures are absent. Malignant nuclei are large and dark, owing to excess DNA, a feature called hyperchromatism because of the excess number of chromosomes in malignant nuclei. Atypia refers to the degree to which individual neoplastic *nuclei* fail to resemble normal nuclei by microscopic examination. If the tumor is growing rapidly, cells are dividing rapidly and numerous mitotic figures (cells caught in the act of dividing) will be present. Figure 6-5 illustrates the microscopic features of a highly malignant tumor.

5. *Define dysplasia and contrast with carcinoma in situ, and give several examples of premalignant clinical conditions:* Dysplasia refers to a pre-malignant state of tissue (usually epithelium) that is atypical and clearly abnormal but not yet malignant; that is, it is on the way to malignancy but not completely autonomous. Carcinoma in situ is malignant epithelium that has not penetrated the basement membrane, cannot reach blood vessels or lymphatics, which are on the other side of the basement membrane, and therefore cannot metastasize. Invasive carcinoma is a carcinoma that has invaded through the basement membrane. Some premalignant clinical conditions are human papillomavirus infection of the cervix, Barrett metaplasia of the esophagus (in reflux esophagitis), adenomatous polyps of the colon, and chronic ulcerative colitis.

6. *Explain the concept of doubling time and the growth of tumors:* A single malignant cell divides into two, these two double to form four, these four double again to form eight and so on, until the mass of cells is large enough to be detected. A single cell is about one-billionth of a gram, so it takes about 30 generations, about 30 doublings, for a tumor mass to grow large enough, about the size of a grape (about one gram), to be detectable. This takes time, usually many years: a malignant neoplasm has lived most of its life *before* it becomes large enough to be detectible. It takes far more time for a tumor to grow from the tiny size of a cell to the size of a grape than it does for one the size of a grape to grow into one the size of a football.

7. *Explain the importance of tumor growth fraction:* Tumor growth fraction is the percentage of tumor cells that are dividing. Tumors with high growth fraction grow more rapidly than do those with low growth fraction.

8. *Explain why the cells in a tumor that are most likely to survive are those that are the most malignant:* As the tumor grows, some tumor-cell variants develop mutations of one kind; others develop mutations of a different kind. This variation (heterogeneity) of tumor cells is important in a Darwinian "survival of the fittest" sense: Some cells are sturdier, more capable of defeating natural defenses (for example, the immune system, discussed below) or surviving attack by therapeutic anti-cancer drugs. In other words, the most malignant cells survive; the less malignant ones do not.

9. *Name several ways by which malignant tumors may spread:* Malignant cells extend locally by direct invasion, they may metastasize to distant sites by lymphatic or vascular invasion, or they may spread by seeding a body fluid and spreading throughout the space involved (e.g., intraperitoneal spread of ovarian carcinoma).

10. *Explain why patients with immunodeficiency have an increased risk for cancer:* Normal DNA and the proteins it encodes are recognized as self by the immune system and are therefore not subject to immune attack. Injured DNA and its proteins become nonself and are subject to immune attack. Therefore, most mutated cells are eliminated by the immune system. People with an immune deficiency lack the ability to eliminate mutated cells and as a result are more likely to develop neoplasms. Even in normal people, some mutant cells escape this mechanism and perpetuate themselves as tumors.

11. *Explain paraneoplastic syndromes and give an example:* Neoplasms may produce a general effect apart from the direct mass effect of the primary tumor or its metastases. The effect is usually the result of production of hormones by the tumor. An example is small cell carcinoma of the lung. This tumor produces a variety of hormones, one of which, ACTH, stimulates adrenal hyperplasia and Cushing syndrome.

12. *Explain the difference between histologic grading and clinical staging:* Histologic grading is microscopic (pathologic) assessment of the appearance of malignant cells. Staging is a clinical exercise that assesses the size, location and degree of spread (if any) of the tumor from its original site.

13. *Name two tumor markers found in blood, and explain their use:* Prostate-specific antigen (PSA) and carcinoembryonic antigen (CEA) are tumor markers often found in blood in association with prostate (PSA) and colon (CEA) cancer. These markers are not good *sole* screening tests for cancer because they are not very sensitive, that is, too often the test result is negative in early disease (that is, the test result is a false negative). Additionally, blood levels of markers may be increased in non-neoplastic diseases. However, markers may be useful for monitoring treatment or detecting recurrence of tumor.

Typical Test Questions

1. Which one of the following is closest to the correct definition of neoplasm?
   A. Cancer
   B. Sarcoma
   C. Malignant
   D. Tumor
   E. Carcinoma

2. Which one of the following is a condition of abnormal cells?
   A. Having oncogenes
   B. Being aneuploid
   C. Having the *p53* gene
   D. Having tumor suppression genes

3. Which of the following terms describes a tumor most likely to be aggressive?
   A. Well differentiated
   B. Euploid
   C. Grade I
   D. Very atypical nuclei

4. Which one of the following takes the most time?
   A. Normal cell to malignant cell
   B. Malignant cell to detectable malignant mass
   C. Detectable malignant mass to death of patient

5. Which one of the following provides the best information to guide prognosis and therapy in patients with malignancy?
   A. Mitotic figure count
   B. TNM classification
   C. Grade of tumor
   D. Degree of differentiation (specialization)

6. True or false? Blood levels of carcinoembryonic antigen are a useful screening test for cancer of the colon.

7. True or false? A Pap smear positive for cancer cells is highly reliable; few false positives occur.

8. True or false? Defective *BRCA* gene is responsible for most breast cancers.

9. True or false? Patients with immune deficiency have more neoplasms than do normal people.

10. True or false? Carcinomas tend to invade lymphatics before they invade blood vessels.

Developmental, Genetic, and Pediatric Disease

This chapter is divided into three sections. Section 1 focuses on fetal defects. Section 2 discusses strictly inherited diseases and familial genetic disease tendencies, while Section 3 focuses on the distinctiveness of diseases of infancy and childhood.

Section 1: Developmental Abnormalities

EMBRYOLOGIC DEVELOPMENT
CONGENITAL MALFORMATIONS
CONGENITAL DEFORMATIONS

Section 2: Genetic Disorders

MUTATIONS
THE BROAD INFLUENCE OF GENETICS IN DISEASE
DISEASE OF SINGLE GENES (MONOGENIC DISORDERS)
* Disease Caused by Defective Autosomal Dominant Genes
* Disease Caused by Defective Autosomal Recessive Genes
* Disease Caused by Defective Genes on Sex Chromosomes
* Clinical Expression of Single-Gene Defects
CYTOGENETIC DISEASES
* Disease Associated with Abnormal Numbers of Autosomes

* Disease Associated with Abnormal Numbers of Sex Chromosomes
GENETIC DIAGNOSIS

Section 3: Pediatric Diseases

PERINATAL AND NEONATAL DISEASE
* Intrauterine Growth Restriction
* Prematurity
* Birth Injury
* Fetal and Newborn Infections
INFECTIONS IN CHILDREN
SUDDEN INFANT DEATH SYNDROME (SIDS)
HEMOLYTIC DISEASE OF THE NEWBORN
   (ERYTHROBLASTOSIS FETALIS)
CYSTIC FIBROSIS
TUMORS AND TUMOR-LIKE CONDITIONS IN CHILDREN

Learning Objectives

After studying this chapter you should be able to:
1. Distinguish between congenital deformation and malformation, and give an example of each
2. Define teratogen, and give an example of a chemical and an infectious teratogen
3. Distinguish among cytogenetic disease, single-gene (Mendelian or monogenic) disease, and disease resulting from multiple genes (polygenic), and give examples of each
4. Explain the difference between autosomal dominant and recessive genetic behavior
5. Explain how inheritance of genetic defects on the X chromosome is different from gene defects on autosomes
6. Offer several examples of disease caused by single-gene defects
7. Explain how cytogenetic disease differs from other genetic disease, and give an example of a cytogenetic disease
8. Explain the genetic abnormality in Turner syndrome
9. Define prematurity, and briefly discuss the associated risks
10. Explain the difference between prematurity and small for gestational age (SGA)
11. Explain the Apgar score and its usefulness
12. Name the most common category of intrauterine growth restriction, and offer some examples
13. Name the most common type of perinatal infection of the newborn; name and briefly discuss a few common pediatric infections

14. Briefly list some of the epidemiologic characteristics of sudden infant death syndrome (SIDS)
15. Explain the pathogenesis of erythroblastosis fetalis
16. Explain the nature of the metabolic defect in patients with cystic fibrosis

Key Terms and Concepts

Section 1: Developmental Abnormalities

- congenital

CONGENITAL MALFORMATIONS
- congenital malformation

CONGENITAL DEFORMATIONS
- congenital deformation

Section 2: Genetic Disorders

- germ cell
- somatic cell
- autosome
- sex chromosome
- monogenic
- cytogenetic

MUTATIONS
- mutation

THE BROAD INFLUENCE OF GENETICS IN DISEASE
- polygenic

DISORDERS OF SINGLE GENES (MONOGENIC DISORDERS)
- allele
- homozygous
- heterozygous
- dominant
- recessive
- Mendelian

CHROMOSOMAL ABNORMALITIES (CYTOGENETIC DISEASES)
- cytogenetic
- karyotype
- Down syndrome
- meiosis

GENETIC DIAGNOSIS
- amniocentesis

Section 3: Pediatric Diseases

PERINATAL AND NEONATAL DISEASE
- premature
- gestational age
- small for gestational age
- intrauterine growth restriction
- respiratory distress syndrome

HEMOLYTIC DISEASE OF THE NEWBORN
- hemolytic disease of the newborn

Teach your children well, . . .
And feed them on your dreams
The one they pick's the one you'll know by.
GRAHAM NASH (B. 1942), OF CROSBY, STILLS & NASH, AMERICAN ROCK GROUP, *TEACH YOUR CHILDREN* (1970)

Section 1: Developmental Abnormalities

"Find out the cause of this effect,
Or rather say, the cause of this defect,
For this effect defective comes by cause"
WILLIAM SHAKESPEARE (1564–1616), ENGLISH PLAYWRIGHT, *HAMLET* (II,ii)

Congenital means "present at birth," although a congenital defect may not reveal itself for many years. Congenital **malformations** are conditions stemming from intrinsically abnormal embryologic development, which are usually *genetic* defects. Congenital **deformations**, on the other hand, are caused by extra-fetal (maternal) *mechanical* factors that distort the fetus.

MAJOR DETERMINANTS OF DISEASE

- Most congenital defects result from faulty development of the embryo.
- The fetus is especially vulnerable to injury during weeks 3–9 of embryologic development, when fetal organs are forming.
- Some congenital disease results from an inherited genetic defect and may not be apparent at birth.

About 3% of newborns have significant cosmetic or functional defects, and the figure is higher if minor abnormalities are included. Each year about 250,000 infants are born with a serious birth defect; the cause is unknown in most. Chromosome abnormalities account for a minority of newborn birth defects; however, studies reveal that about half of spontaneously aborted fetuses have chromosome abnormalities, indicating that most inborn chromosome defects are lethal. In developed nations, congenital defects are responsible for about half of newborn and childhood deaths; by contrast, in underdeveloped nations, infectious diseases, malnutrition, and other environmental factors are responsible for the great majority of newborn and childhood deaths.

Embryologic Development

Understanding developmental abnormalities requires understanding the basics of embryologic and fetal development.

The combination of ovum and sperm creates a single-cell conceptus (fertilized ovum), which within a few days divides first into two, then four, then eight primordial cells that are not programmed to develop into a particular tissue or organ. Loss of one of these primitive cells does not cause adverse consequences; however, as more divisions occur, cells differentiate (specialize) and are programmed to develop into particular tissues or organs, such as brain or heart. Loss or damage to cells at this stage can result in spontaneous abortion (Chapter 21) or de-

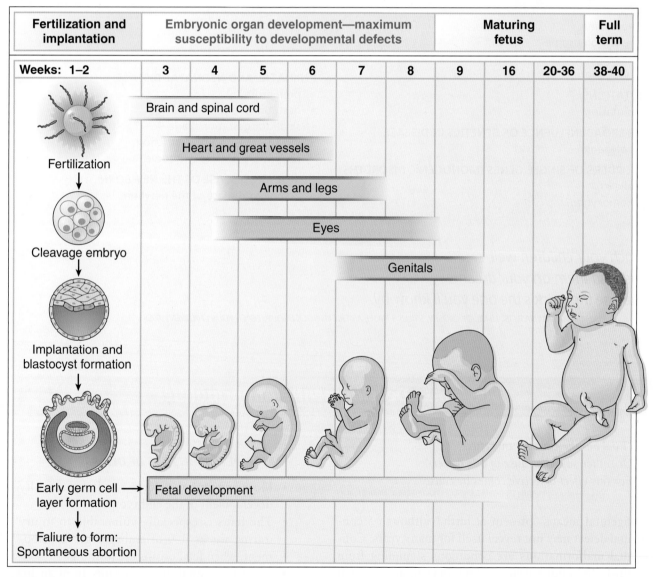

Figure 7-1 Critical stages of embryo development. Important congenital malformations are most likely to occur in early pregnancy (weeks 3–9), when organs are first developing. Maternal exposures to microbes, usually virus infection, and chemical abuse (drugs and alcohol) are the most common identifiable causes. Serious exposures before or near the time of endometrial implantation usually lead to spontaneous abortion. Exposures to infections, toxins, and other forces have less effect after the 9th week.

velopmental abnormality. As is illustrated in Figure 7-1, beginning about two weeks after conception the embryo begins a period of **organogenesis**, during which time it is susceptible to injury that can result in fetal *malformation*.

The embryo forms first as a hollow sphere that grows, stretches, and folds into a series of chambers (the heart and the cerebral ventricles, for example) and tubes (the intestines, bronchi, gland ducts, and spinal canal, for example). Many of these spaces begin originally as grooves, which become tubes as the groove rims grow over and join to form an enclosed space. Some of these spaces do not lead to development of an adult structure but may persist as a congenital malformation. For those spaces that lead to an adult structure, a congenital malformation occurs if the space fails to close normally. Some organs form by dividing from one another, and malformations occur if separation does not occur. Finally, tissues or organs may fail to develop;

that is, they may fail to appear or may develop incompletely. Some examples are:

- *Failure of space to close properly.* The vertebral column is a bony tube containing the meninges and spinal cord. If the embryonic neural tube fails to close, the bony vertebral arch remains open posteriorly, usually in the lower back, and the result is **spina bifida** (Fig. 7-2) and related conditions (Chapter 23). Occult spina bifida, or spina bifida occulta (Fig. 7-2B), is common and innocuous. However, in more severe defects (Figure 7-2C, D, and E), the meninges or spinal cord protrude through the defect in the spinal column and are associated with infection and neurologic defects, especially paralysis in the legs and loss of bowel and bladder control. In the severest form of spina bifida, the brain and entire spinal cord fail to form, a condition known as **anencephaly**.

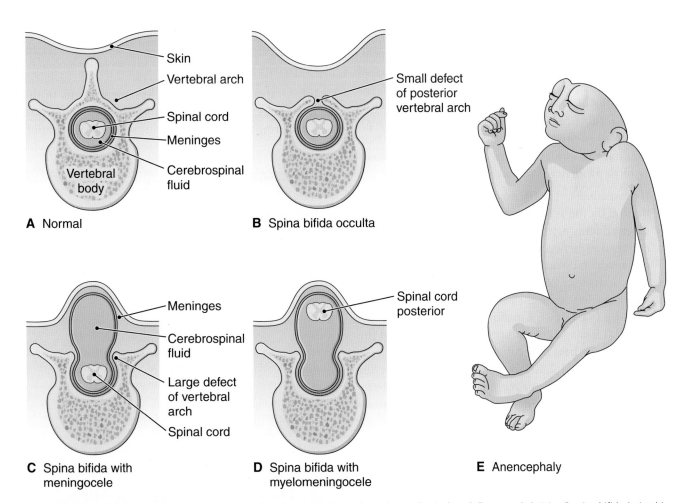

Figure 7-2 **Neural tube defects.** Cross-section studies of spine. **A.** Normal vertebra and spinal cord. **B.** In occult (minimal) spina bifida (spina bifida occulta) the posterior vertebral arch fails to form. It is usually asymptomatic. **C.** In spina bifida with meningocele, the meninges protrude through the defect. **D.** In spina bifida with myelomeningocele, the meninges and spinal cord protrude through the defect. **E.** In anencephaly, almost all of the brain and spinal cord fail to form.

Adding folic acid supplement to the maternal diet sharply reduces the number of these defects

- *Failure of tissue to divide.* Fingers and toes must divide from one another; if division is erroneous, digits may be fused (*syndactyly*) or may be too numerous (*polydactyly*).
- *Failure of an embryologic structure to disappear normally.* The thyroid gland is formed by cells budding from a temporary embryonic duct that arises from the base of the tongue (the thyroglossal duct). If the duct fails to involute normally, it may accumulate fluid to form a *thyroglossal duct cyst.*
- *Failure of tissue or organ to differentiate or grow (agenesis):* The drug thalidomide, a sedative no longer prescribed for pregnant women, prevents normal limb development in children of mothers taking the drug.

There are many other congenital malformations in other organs, some of which are discussed below.

Congenital Malformations

Congenital malformations are associated with flawed embryologic development. The cause of most congenital malformations is unknown, but it is clear that good nutrition and prenatal care significantly reduce the number of malformed fetuses. Some congenital malformations result from genetic defects (DNA mutations); others from environmental factors. The most common congenital malformations are listed below (approximate birth incidence is in parentheses):

- Hypospadias (~1:300), an abnormal opening of the urethra on the ventral surface of the penis
- Patent ductus arteriosus (~1:600), a persistent open connection between the pulmonary artery and the aorta, which normally closes at birth
- Ventricular septal defect (~1:900), an opening between the left and right ventricles of the heart
- Cleft lip (~1:1,100), a malformation of the upper lip that features a slit extending from the margin of the lip up to the base of the nose
- Spina bifida (~1:2,100), an opening in the posterior (dorsal) arch of one or more of the spinal vertebrae, through which meninges or spinal cord structures may protrude
- Anencephaly (1:3,200), a failure of the brain to develop
- Atrial septal defect (1:5,900), an opening between the right and left atria of the heart, which should close shortly after birth

Deformed fetuses are said to be *teratoid* (from Greek *teras*, for monster). A **teratogen** is an agent, such as a chemical or virus, capable of inducing congenital fetal malformation. Teratogens include infectious agents, drugs, chemicals, and ionizing radiation. That ionizing radiation can damage fetal or ovarian DNA and induce birth defects became clear as defects soared in the aftermath of the atomic bomb explosions in Hiroshima and Nagasaki, Japan, which ended World War II. There are many chemical teratogens but the most important is alcohol.

Alcohol abuse in pregnancy accounts for the **fetal alcohol syndrome**, consisting of intrauterine fetal growth restriction, central nervous system abnormalities, and distinctive facial characteristics. The full-blown syndrome occurs in about 1 in 1,000 live births in the general population, usually to a mother who is a chronic alcoholic. However, a more common result is less severe maternal alcohol abuse that causes mild childhood mental deficiency and emotional problems.

The most common infectious teratogens are the so-called **TORCH teratogens**:

- *Toxoplasmosis*
- *Rubella*
- *Cytomegalovirus*
- *Herpesvirus*

Infection occurs in 1–5% of live-born infants in the United States. The greatest damage results if infection occurs during weeks 3–9, the critical period of gestation

THE CLINICAL SIDE

PREVENTING BIRTH DEFECTS

The cause of most birth defects is unknown, but birth defects are associated with smoking, alcohol or other drug abuse, poor nutrition, poorly controlled diabetes, and a wide variety of other maternal factors. Pregnant women should not smoke, use drugs, or take any medication without supervision. Alcohol should be avoided. Diabetes, if present, should be tightly controlled.

Because *folic acid* is important for normal embryologic development in the first few weeks after conception, there is universal agreement that women of childbearing age should take daily multivitamin containing folate *before* becoming pregnant. Despite dramatic benefit, only about 25% of women do so. Daily consumption of the usual amount of folate (folic acid) in most multivitamin tablets reduces by about 60% the number of infants born with neural tube defects such as spina bifida. In the United States, certain basic food products (enriched flour, for example) have supplemental folic acid added.

when fetal organs are formed. Infection before three weeks induces abortion; later infections produce milder disturbances, including mental impairment. TORCH infections are usually not distinguishable from one another and produce a set of signs and symptoms (the **TORCH syndrome**). Affected infants exhibit some, but not all, of the following characteristics, which are illustrated in Figure 7-3: microcephaly (small skull), mental retardation, brain calcifications, microphthalmia (small eyeballs), cataracts (opacified lenses), chorioretinitis (inflammation of the retina and iris) and conjunctivitis, congenital heart defects, pneumonia, hepatitis and jaundice, splenomegaly (enlarged spleen), and skin hemorrhages.

Infection by cytomegalovirus or herpesvirus may produce severe fetal damage even as late as the third trimester. Congenital rubella infection can be prevented by maternal vaccination. A vaccine for herpes is gaining acceptance, but there are no vaccines for other TORCH infections.

Congenital Deformations

Congenital deformations are caused by maternal mechanical factors that distort the fetus. The two most common deformations are listed below. Approximate birth incidence is in parentheses.

- Clubfoot (~1:400), a twisting inward or outward of the foot so that the sole is not flat to the ground
- Hip dislocation (~1:1,100), a failure of the head of the femur to rest in its socket in the pelvis

Deformations usually arise in the 35th–38th weeks of pregnancy, when the growth of the fetus exceeds the growth of the uterus, filling it to the point that there is not enough amniotic fluid surrounding the fetus to provide cushioning and room for movement. Maternal factors include a malformed uterus owing to large leiomyomas (benign tumors of the uterine wall, Chapter 21), the crowding of multiple pregnancy, and oligohydramnios (decreased amniotic fluid).

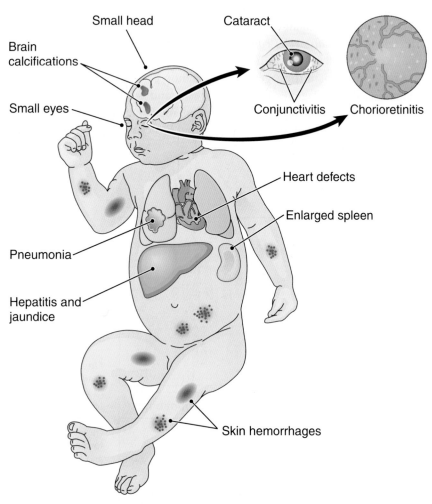

Figure 7-3 **TORCH infections.** Fetuses infected in the first trimester by *Toxoplasma, rubella, cytomegalovirus, herpesvirus,* or other microbes have similar clinical findings as those illustrated in this figure.

Section 2: *Genetic Disorders*

Insanity is hereditary; you get it from your children.
SAM LEVENSON (1911-1980), AMERICAN COMEDIAN

MAJOR DETERMINANTS OF DISEASE

- Almost every disease is influenced to some degree by multiple, subtle genetic variations that confer vulnerabilities to environmental influences. The inheritance of these characteristics is not strictly predictable.
- Strictly genetic disease is caused by DNA mutations inherited in a predictable manner.

Genetic disease, or genetic tendency to develop disease, is transmitted from parent to child by genes in the germ cells of ova or sperm.

Genetically, the normal body has two types of *cells*: **germ cells** in the ovary and testis, which produce ova and sperm, and **somatic cells**, which form all other tissues and organs. *Germ cells and somatic cells contain identical sets of chromosomes*, but chromosomes in somatic cells are not capable of transmitting genetic defects. For example, smoking damages genes in lung (somatic) cells to cause lung cancer, but the cancer is not transmissible to offspring because it occurs in somatic cells; germ cells are unaffected. **Autosomes** are those chromosomes that are not sex chromosomes. **Sex chromosomes** are specialized chromosomes that determine sex, but they also influence other characteristics.

> **Normal hereditary traits and inheritable disease can be passed on only if the affected genes occur in *germ* cells of the testis and ovary. Acquired genetic defects, the type that arise in *somatic* cells as a cause of cancer, are not inheritable. Rarely, however, acquired genetic defects occur in germ cells and become inheritable.**

There are two types of sex chromosomes, X and Y. Males have one X and one Y; females have two X chromosomes. Normal somatic and germ cells contain 44 autosomes plus two sex chromosomes (either X and Y, or two Xs). *The shorthand notation for normal males is 46,XY; normal females are designated 46,XX.* The genetic makeup of a person is called the **genotype**; the physical traits produced by the genotype are called the **phenotype**. For example, XX is the genotype for the female phenotype. The relationships and differences between germ and somatic cells and their chromosomes are explained in greater detail later in this chapter in the box titled Basics in Brief 7-1. Figure 7-4 illustrates a normal

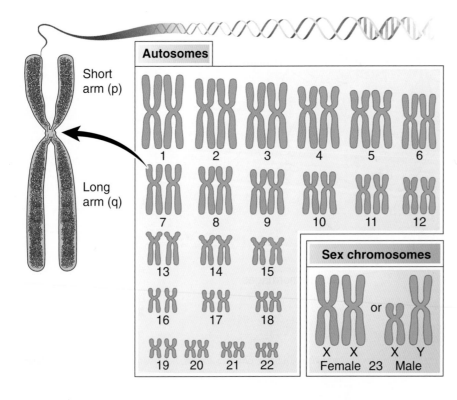

Figure 7-4 **A set of normal chromosomes (karyotype).** There are 46 total chromosomes, of which 44 are autosomes (pairs 1-22 in the figure; non-sex chromosomes) and two are sex chromosomes (pair 23 in the figure; two X chromosomes for a female, or one X and one Y for a male). The shorthand for a female is 46,XX and for a male, 46,XY. In each pair one is from the male (blue) and one is from the female (pink parent). Genes are short segments of DNA and are located either on the short (p) arm of the chromosome above the waist or the long (q) arm below it.

Table 7-1	Types and Examples of Genetic Disease	
Type of Genetic Defect	**Chromosomal Abnormality**	**Disease**
Polygenic	Multiple genes affected; identity unknown	Type II diabetes
Monogenic (single-gene defect)	Mutation in gene 19 at locus p13	Familial hypercholesterolemia
Cytogenetic	Extra chromosome 21	Down syndrome

set of chromosomes displayed in a manner called a **karyotype**, a photographic display of chromosomes.

All disease is either genetic or environmental or a combination of the two:

- *Genetic* disease is transmitted to a subsequent generation only by genetic defects (mutations) in germ cells, not by genetic defects in somatic cells. Germ cell genetic defects cause **familial** (**hereditary**) disease.
- On the other hand, some diseases are almost purely *environmental*. Lung cancers, for example, are tumors of somatic cells acquired by inhaling cigarette smoke. The genes in lung cancer cells typically have many genetic and chromosomal abnormalities, but they are not transmissible because the patient's germ cells are not affected.
- Some diseases are a *mixture* of environmental effect and genetic influence. Type 2 (adult onset diabetes,

Chapter 17), for example, is associated with obesity (an environmental influence) and a strong familial (hereditary) tendency.

In people with normal *numbers* of chromosomes, traits or diseases that occur because of defects in a *single gene* are called **monogenic** (Table 7-1). Analysis of DNA has led to the identification of thousands of diseases caused by single-gene defects, each of which is characterized by specific and predictable abnormalities. Sickle cell disease and red-green color blindness are examples. **Polygenic** genetic diseases are those conditions associated with the influence of multiple genes.

A third category of genetic disorder is **cytogenetic disease**, caused by extra or absent *whole chromosomes*, or large-scale structural dislocations of chromosome parts, such as pieces of one chromosome that become attached to another. Most cytogenetic disorders occur

HISTORY OF MEDICINE

AN ACORN WITH A PURPOSE

The great Greek thinker Aristotle (384–322 BC) reasoned that oak trees spring from acorns because the acorn contains a "plan" or a "purpose," that is to say, something within that was meant to be fulfilled, which we now know is DNA. The unraveling of this mystery took two millennia.

That living things were composed of cells was discovered by Englishman Robert Hooke in 1665, as he studied the microscopic structure of the bark of cork trees. Nearly two hundred years passed before another Englishman, Charles Darwin, published *Origin of the Species* in 1859 and opened an era of intense scientific investigation of biologic phenomena. In 1866 Scotsman Robert Brown, of "Brownian motion" fame to legions of high school science students, was studying the microscopic anatomy of orchids when he noticed that every cell contained a nucleus. Shortly thereafter German medical researcher Friedrich Meischer discovered that nuclei contained a new molecule, which he called nuclein. Other investigators discovered that nuclein (DNA) was composed of four simple chemicals, but the scientific establishment resisted the idea that such sim-

ple molecules could be responsible for all of life's complexities.

Then in the 1920s English bacteriologist Fred Griffith discovered that bacteria contained a mysterious substance that could carry behavior from one bacterium to another, and in the 1940s American scientist Oswald Avery discovered that the substance was DNA.

In the early 1950s English scientist Rosalind Franklin discovered that DNA had a corkscrew structure. At the same time, two other English scientists, James Watson and Francis Crick, were trying to build physical models of DNA but could not find one that explained the experimental data. They learned of Franklin's corkscrew idea and took a critical conceptual step, theorizing that DNA was composed of *two intertwined* corkscrews. The structure they built perfectly explained the experimental data and was widely adopted. Watson and Crick were awarded the Nobel Prize in 1962, by which time Rosalind Franklin had died. Inasmuch as the Nobel Prize can be awarded only to living recipients, Franklin was not honored, a sore point to her many supporters.

spontaneously in the fertilization process. Because they are not related to defective chromosomes in germ cells, they are not inheritable. For example, Klinefelter syndrome, discussed later in this chapter, is caused by an extra X chromosome: the patient, who would otherwise be a normal male (XY), has an extra X, and his genotype is XXY.

Mutations

A **mutation** is a permanent change in DNA. The DNA of each gene is composed of long sequences of four nucleotide bases: adenine (A), thymine (T), guanine (G), and cytosine (C). It is convenient to think of DNA as a very long sentence spelled with only four letters: A, T, G, and C. A very short sequence might be . . . GATACGATCCCAGT . . . but the entire "sentence" extends thousands of letters in both directions. Sometimes there are typographic mistakes, called mutations. Any force, either chemical or radiologic, that induces DNA mutation is said to be **mutagenic** (causing mutations) or **carcinogenic** (causing cancer). Mutations can occur in germ cells (reproductive cells of the ovary or testis) or somatic cells (all other cells). *Germ cell mutations are transmissible from one generation to the next; somatic cell mutations are not.* For example, mutation of sperm DNA is transmissible, but mutation in the DNA of lung cancer cells is not.

DNA damage can occur in utero. Mutations in embryonic *somatic* cell genes may produce congenital defects, which are not inheritable. An example is a first trimester maternal rubella virus infection that damages embryonic somatic cell genes and produces severe congenital abnormalities.

Sometimes the germ cell gene defect results from an error in a single point, a **point mutation** (Fig. 7-5). Thus, a sequence that should read *CTC* becomes *CAC*. This defect, the substitution of adenine (A) for thymine (T) at a certain point in the gene that controls hemoglobin synthesis, is responsible for sickle cell anemia. In the production of normal hemoglobin A the affected segment of DNA normally codes for *glutamic acid*. In the presence of the sickle mutation, thymine is substituted for adenine, causing the production of the amino acid *valine* and the synthesis of abnormal hemoglobin, which we call hemoglobin S. Although most germ cell mutations are inherited from one or both affected parents, some can arise spontaneously in the ovaries or testes of people not previously affected. This new mutation does not cause disease in the parent in whom it developed, but it can be passed to succeeding generations.

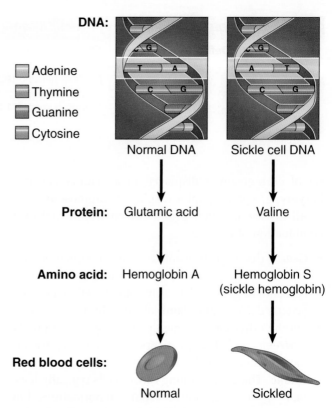

Figure 7-5 The DNA mutation in sickle cell disease. In the gene for hemoglobin synthesis, the DNA contains adenine at a certain point, which causes production of normal hemoglobin (hemoglobin A), containing glutamic acid. In sickle cell disease this segment of DNA in the gene undergoes a mutation in which thymine (T) is substituted for the adenine (A), which reverses the T/A pair to A/T and produces an abnormal hemoglobin (hemoglobin S) that contains valine instead of glutamic acid at a certain point. Hemoglobin S has physical characteristics that cause it to crystallize and deform red blood cells.

The Broad Influence of Genetics in Disease

Most human characteristics (traits) result from effects of multiple genes (they are **polygenic**): hair and eye color, height, weight, intelligence, facial features, and so on. While polygenic influences play a role in many human diseases, they are usually not solely responsible—the environment also plays an important role. Polygenic influence confers vulnerability to disease that becomes evident only with the presence of environmental influences that exceed a certain threshold. For example, a patient may have a familial tendency toward diabetes, but the disease will not occur until the patient's weight exceeds a certain amount.

Defects involving a single gene are inherited according to strict rules, but the inheritance risk in polygenic disorders can only be estimated and usually equates to an approximate 5–10 percent increase in risk for the disease in question. Lower inheritance risk is associated with mild disease, higher inheritance risk with more severe disease. Notable examples of inheritable polygenic risk are cleft lip, hypertension, atherosclerosis, adult-onset (type 2) diabetes, gout, mental retardation, and schizophrenia.

When more than one gene influences the development of disease, it is difficult to identify the individual genes responsible. Nevertheless, evidence of their influence can be seen when certain disease tendencies occur in families and the tendency toward disease is passed from one generation to another. Think of inheritable polygenic risk in this way: in affected people, genes create a fertile field for the seeds of environmental injury—if it rains cheeseburgers and French fries a flood of obesity and diabetes may sprout in fertile genetic soil. In other people the genetic soil is less fertile, and a flood of cheeseburgers and fries may not produce obesity or diabetes. There is at least some degree of genetic influence in almost every disease.

Disease of Single Genes (Monogenic Disorders)

Of every pair of chromosomes, one is from the father and carries the genetic code for his traits, and one is from the mother and carries the genetic code for her traits. All normal chromosomes from each parent are structurally similar, each carrying a particular gene for a particular trait on a particular chromosome. The matching genes, say for eye color, are called **alleles** of one another, somewhat like matching earrings, one a gift from the father and one from the mother. The alleles are said to be **homozygous** if they are identical; that is, if they code for exactly the same trait, say brown eyes. However, if the alleles are not identical, the condition is said to be **heterozygous**. For example, if one allele codes for brown eyes and its partner codes for blue, the condition is heterozygous.

Either allele may behave in a dominant or in a recessive (submissive) manner. **Dominant genes** have greater power of expression than do **recessive genes**. Thus, if a person has one dominant and one recessive gene for the same characteristic, the trait carried by the dominant gene is expressed. If a dominant *healthy* allele from one parent is paired with a defective recessive allele from the other parent, the dominant trait is expressed, and the patient is healthy but carries the trait. This principle can be observed in the inheritance of normal eye color: the gene for brown eyes is dominant over the gene for blue eyes, which is recessive. If one of the allele pair is brown and the other blue, the brown gene overpowers the

recessive blue gene, and the person has brown eyes. The same is true in disease: if the dominant allele is normal and its allele (partner) is mutant, then the recessive mutant (disease-carrying) allele is overpowered, and no disease occurs. A phenotypically normal (physically unaffected) person with a recessive genetic defect is a **carrier** but does not have the disease.

The inheritance mechanisms for single-gene characteristics are illustrated in Figure 7-6. They were first worked out in the 1860s by Austrian monk Gregor Mendel and are called **Mendelian** patterns or Mendel's laws.

As initially described by Mendel, genetic makeup and genetic traits are characterized as follows:

- **Autosomal dominant** (Fig. 7-6A): A trait or disease expressed physically (phenotypically) if only one allele (partner gene) in one autosome of a set of two autosomal chromosomes is present. No identical allele (partner gene) on the companion autosomal chromosome is required. Familial hypercholesterolemia (Chapter 7) is an example.
- **Autosomal recessive** (Fig. 7-6B): A trait or disease expressed physically (phenotypically) only if both alleles (partner genes) are present, one on each chromosome pair. Sickle cell disease (Chapter 11) is an example.
- **Sex-linked recessive**: A trait or disease expressed physically (phenotypically) only if the allele (gene) is present on the X chromosome of a male (XY) or on both X chromosomes of a female (XX). Trait or disease occurs almost exclusively in males (XY) because *X and Y share no alleles*, that is, there are no partner genes on X for Y and vice versa, and the X allele is expressed because in males there is no normal allele on Y to compensate for the X defect. Females (XX) very rarely may express the trait if, by chance, both copies of X have the same mutant allele. Classic hemophilia (hemophilia A, Chapter 11) is a sex-linked recessive disease. The same rules apply to genes on the Y chromosome, but Y-related defects are rare and are related mainly to sperm production. Certain types of infertility are linked to Y chromosome gene defects.

It is also important to keep in mind that although a particular gene codes a particular trait, that trait may be expressed in various ways, a qualitative characteristic called **expressivity**. That is to say, the *type* of disease can somewhat from patient to patient. For example, some patients with cystic fibrosis, discussed later in this chapter, suffer primarily from lung disease; others suffer chiefly from pancreatic and intestinal problems. The

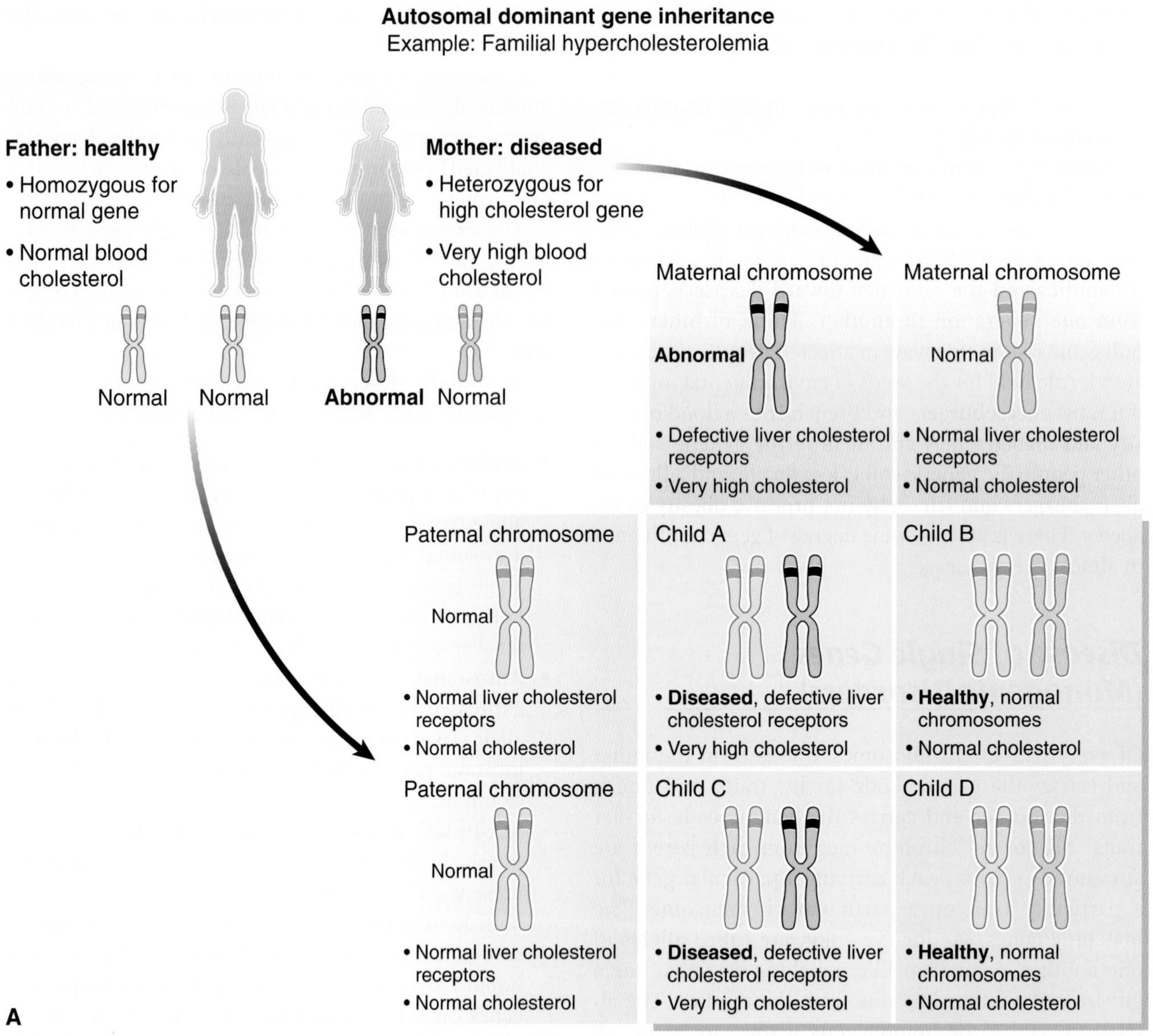

Autosomal dominant gene inheritance
Example: Familial hypercholesterolemia

Father: healthy
- Homozygous for normal gene
- Normal blood cholesterol

Normal   Normal

Mother: diseased
- Heterozygous for high cholesterol gene
- Very high blood cholesterol

Abnormal   Normal

Maternal chromosome

Abnormal
- Defective liver cholesterol receptors
- Very high cholesterol

Maternal chromosome

Normal
- Normal liver cholesterol receptors
- Normal cholesterol

Paternal chromosome

Normal
- Normal liver cholesterol receptors
- Normal cholesterol

Child A
- **Diseased**, defective liver cholesterol receptors
- Very high cholesterol

Child B
- **Healthy**, normal chromosomes
- Normal cholesterol

Paternal chromosome

Normal
- Normal liver cholesterol receptors
- Normal cholesterol

Child C
- **Diseased**, defective liver cholesterol receptors
- Very high cholesterol

Child D
- **Healthy**, normal chromosomes
- Normal cholesterol

A

Figure 7-6 **Patterns of gene inheritance. A.** Autosomal dominant inheritance. The dominant gene is present in one affected, unhealthy (diseased) parent. Half of the children will be affected. **B.** Autosomal recessive inheritance. A recessive gene is present in each healthy, carrier parent. Half of the children will be healthy but carry the gene defect (Hgb SA, sickle cell trait); one fourth will be genetically and clinically normal (Hgb AA); and one fourth will have sickle cell disease (Hgb SS).

degree of abnormality, the *severity* of disease, is a quantitative characteristic called **penetrance**. That is, some genes are relatively weak (they have low penetrance), and the resulting disease is less severe than would be a disease resulting from genes with higher penetrance. For example, some patients with cystic fibrosis have severe lung disease, but others may have mild lung disease.

Over 5,000 Mendelian (single-gene) disorders have been identified, and new ones are discovered regularly. They occur in about 0.5% of the population and account for about 1% of hospital admissions. Most humans carry about 6–8 defective genes, almost all of them recessive and therefore are not expressed.

DISEASE CAUSED BY DEFECTIVE AUTOSOMAL DOMINANT GENES

An autosomal dominant trait is expressed by a gene located on one of the 44 autosomes. Being autosomal dominant, this trait is dominant over its recessive partner (allele) on the copy of the gene inherited from the other parent.

As is illustrated in Figure 7-6A, the rules of autosomal dominant disease inheritance are:

- The gene is physically expressed if only one copy of it is present in a pair of chromosomes
- An affected parent has a 50% chance of passing the gene to a child

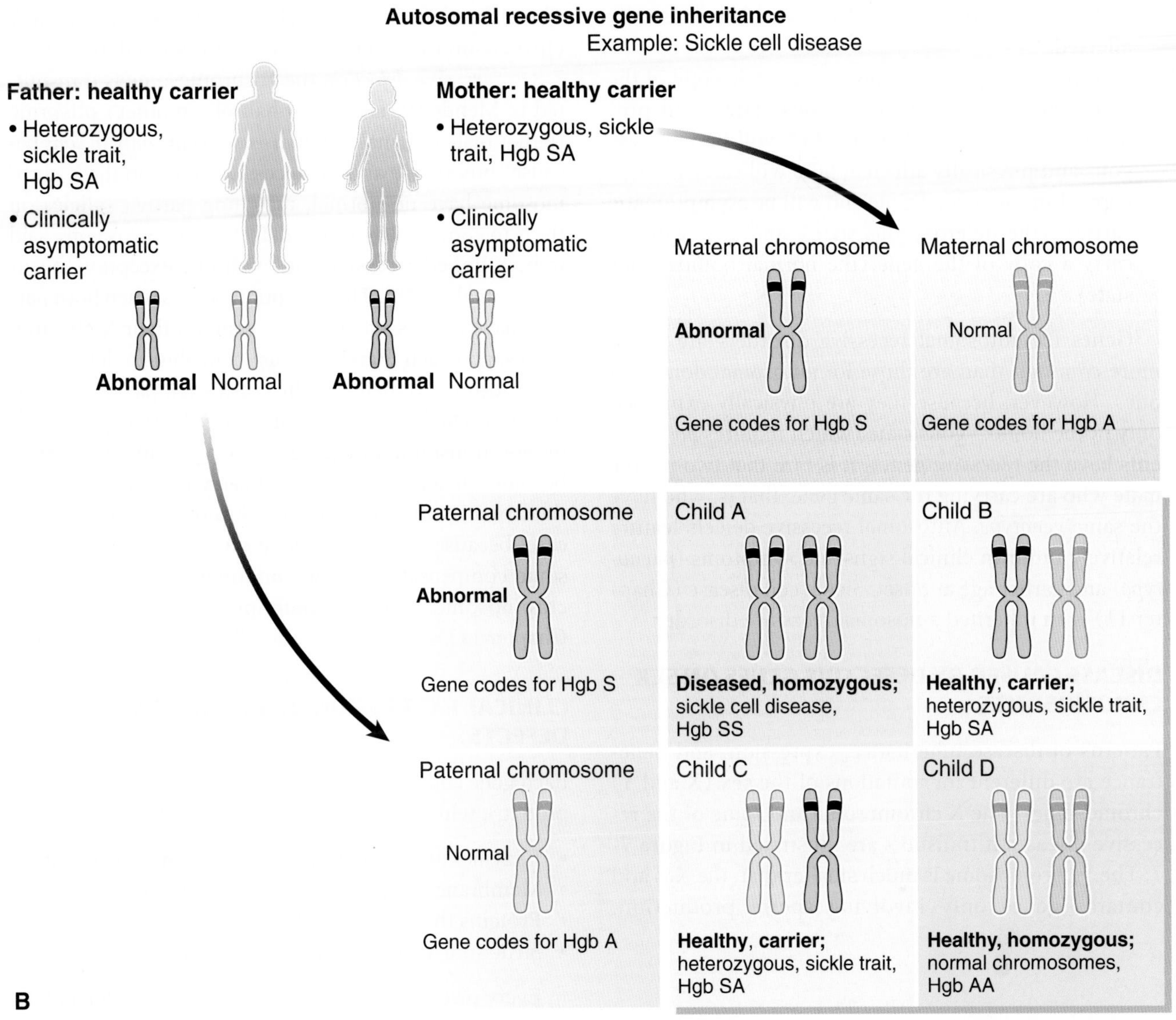

Autosomal recessive gene inheritance
Example: Sickle cell disease

Father: healthy carrier
- Heterozygous, sickle trait, Hgb SA
- Clinically asymptomatic carrier

Mother: healthy carrier
- Heterozygous, sickle trait, Hgb SA
- Clinically asymptomatic carrier

Abnormal Normal   **Abnormal** Normal

Maternal chromosome

Abnormal

Gene codes for Hgb S

Maternal chromosome

Normal

Gene codes for Hgb A

Paternal chromosome

Abnormal

Gene codes for Hgb S

Child A

Diseased, homozygous; sickle cell disease, Hgb SS

Child B

Healthy, carrier; heterozygous, sickle trait, Hgb SA

Paternal chromosome

Normal

Gene codes for Hgb A

Child C

Healthy, carrier; heterozygous, sickle trait, Hgb SA

Child D

Healthy, homozygous; normal chromosomes, Hgb AA

B

Figure 7-6 (continued).

- Inheritance of the defective gene ensures physical expression of the defect
- Healthy children are not carriers of the defective gene

Not all mutant genes are inherited from prior generations; some arise as a *new* mutation in the germ cells of the ovary or testis of a parent and are then passed down the generations as a new defect. For example, about half of all new cases of neurofibromatosis (multiple tumors of nerves, Chapter 23) occur when new mutations arise in chromosome 17 in the germ cells in the ovary or testis of a parent.

DISEASE CAUSED BY DEFECTIVE AUTOSOMAL RECESSIVE GENES

An autosomal recessive trait requires two copies of the defective gene: one from the mother and one from the father. Recall the example above regarding eye color: Brown is dominant over blue, and blue eyes result only if a person inherits a recessive blue gene from *both* parents. One brown-eye gene from either parent guarantees brown eyes.

As is illustrated in Figure 7-6B, the rules of autosomal recessive inheritance are:

- The gene is physically expressed only if both chromosomes of a pair carry a copy of the gene (the homozygous state).
- If a patient carries two copies of the gene, each parent must have had at least one copy each of the gene.
- A parent with two copies of the gene (the abnormal homozygous state) mated with a parent not having the gene (the normal homozygous state) will produce offspring 50% of whom will be carriers of the abnor-

mal gene, but none of the offspring will be physically affected.

• Two parents, each of whom has a single copy of the abnormal gene (the heterozygous state), will produce the following offspring: 25% will be homozygous and physically affected; 50% will carry a single copy of the abnormal gene and will be asymptomatic carriers (the heterozygous state), and 25% will not carry a copy of the gene (the normal homozygous state).

Genes for autosomal recessive disorders are much more common than are those for autosomal dominant ones. However, because they are physically expressed only in the homozygous state (which requires *both* parents have the recessive gene), it is rare that two people mate who are carrying the same gene; that is, who have the same *genotype*. Autosomal recessive defects feature relatively uniform clinical signs and symptoms (*phenotype*) and earlier age at onset. Sickle cell disease (Chapter 11) is an inherited autosomal recessive disorder.

DISEASE CAUSED BY DEFECTIVE GENES ON SEX CHROMOSOMES

Patterns of disease inheritance, expression, and penetrance are different for mutations of the sex (X and Y) chromosomes. The X chromosome and some of the recessive diseases it transmits are illustrated in Figure 7-7. The Y chromosome is much smaller than the X is and contains genes only involving sperm production.

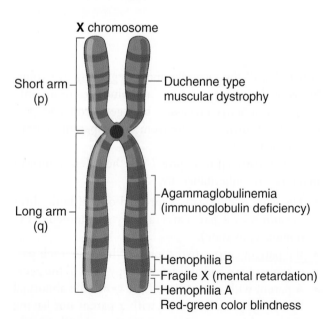

Figure 7-7 The X chromosome. Inherited diseases linked to the X chromosome are displayed.

Therefore, there are no matching alleles between X and Y chromosomes. Therefore, as is illustrated in Figure 7-8, a recessive *defect* on the X chromosome is transmitted in Mendelian fashion to half of a mother's offspring (either male or female), but *disease occurs only in sons* because sons are XY and the recessive genes on the X chromosome have no normal, matching partner (allele) on the Y to compensate for the defect. Such diseases are said to be **X-linked recessive** and, with rare exception, occur only in males (XY). The exception occurs when both parents have a recessive defective gene on their X chromosomes, and each therefore must contribute a defective X chromosome to their daughter. An example of X-linked disease is Duchenne muscular dystrophy (Chapter 23), a disease transmitted by mothers to sons only. Daughters become carriers. Females (XX) carry the trait on one of their two X chromosomes but do not have clinical disease, because the normal gene on the partner chromosome compensates for the abnormal gene on the other chromosome. Classic hemophilia (hemophilia A, Chapter 11) is inherited as a sex-linked recessive disease.

CLINICAL EXPRESSION OF SINGLE-GENE DEFECTS

Each gene codes for a single protein (or variations of that protein), which may be one of four types:

• Enzymes and proteins that regulate enzyme activity
• Membrane receptor and transport proteins
• Proteins that regulate cell growth
• Structural, coagulation, and other proteins

Every disease resulting from a single-gene defect falls into one of these categories.

Disease of Enzymes and Proteins Regulating Enzyme Activity

Enzymes are proteins that promote chemical reactions but are not consumed in the reaction. They act on a substance called a substrate and convert it into a product. Therefore, enzyme defects cause either an accumulation of upstream (substrate) raw material or a deficit of an end (downstream) product, much like a dam on a stream results in an accumulation of water upstream and a lack of it downstream.

Gaucher disease is an example of an autosomal recessive disease caused by accumulation of unmetabolized substrate. It results from a defect in the gene that codes for an enzyme that metabolizes glucocerebroside. Unmetabolized glucocerebroside accumulates in macrophages throughout the body, especially in the brain, bone marrow, lymph nodes, and spleen.

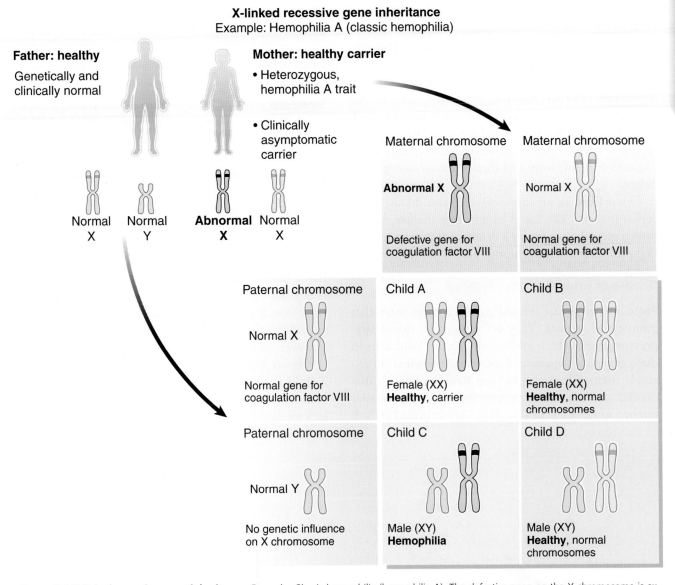

Figure 7-8 **X-linked recessive gene inheritance.** Example: Classic hemophilia (hemophilia A). The defective gene on the X chromosome is expressed in males only because the Y chromosome contains no matching normal gene (allele) to offset the effect of the defective X gene.

Sometimes deficiency of an end product is the cause of disease. **Glycogen storage disease** is a genetic disease in which the affected enzyme normally converts muscle glycogen into glucose. The defect deprives muscle of glucose and results in severe muscle cramps and necrosis.

Alpha-1 antitrypsin (AAT) deficiency is an autosomal recessive genetic disorder of enzyme regulatory proteins. AAT, a blood protein synthesized by the liver, permeates tissues to protect against *excess* effect of proteolytic enzymes released by neutrophils recruited to sites of tissue injury and inflammation. Deficiency of AAT is associated with excessive tissue digestion by inflammatory reactions. This is particularly noticeable in the lungs of affected patients, especially smokers. The inflammatory reaction caused by cigarette smoke results in severe autodigestion of alveoli, which in turn results in emphysema.

Disease of Membrane Receptor and Transport Proteins

Some proteins are designed to attach to other molecules. When they hold the molecule in place, such proteins are called **receptors**, and when they attach to and move a molecule from one place to another, they are called **transport proteins**. For example, receptors in the liver capture and hold low-density lipoprotein during the process of excreting cholesterol into bile. Thus, a genetic defect resulting in too few low-density lipoprotein receptors would manifest with high levels of blood cholesterol. **Familial hypercholesterolemia** (Fig. 7-9) is a result of such a genetic defect. It is an autosomal-dominant defect of liver receptor proteins for low-density lipoprotein (LDL) and is the most common Mendelian disorder, affecting about one of every 500 people. It assumes special significance because high LDL cholesterol levels in blood are associated with accelerated atherosclerosis. However, most cases of high cholesterol result from bad dietary habits, not genetic defect.

Cystic fibrosis, an autosomal recessive disease of receptor proteins, discussed later in this chapter, results from a gene that codes for a defective transport protein that enables transfer of chloride across cell membranes.

Disease of Growth Control Proteins

Proto-oncogenes are normal growth control genes that promote cell growth. They are opposed by **tumor suppressor genes**, which inhibit cell growth. Mutations in these genes are the cause of some malignancies. For example, **neurofibromatosis (von Recklinghausen disease)** is an autosomal dominant disorder of a particular tumor suppressor gene that allows uncontrolled growth of certain cells. Patients with neurofibromatosis have peripheral nerve tumors that may become malignant.

Disease of Structural, Coagulation, and Other Proteins

Structural proteins provide support for tissue. For example, fibrillin, a structural protein synthesized by fibroblasts, is an important component of the extracellular matrix. A genetic defect of fibrillin synthesis produces **Marfan syndrome** (Figs. 7-10 and 7-11), an autosomal dominant disease characterized by defects in: 1) the skeleton (very long legs and fingers, a high, arched palate, and hyperextensible joints); 2) the eyes (dislocation of the lens resulting from stretched ligaments), and 3); the cardiovascular system (lax aortic tissue that produces aneurysms and aortic valvular incompetence). Marfan disease is rare, affecting about 1 in 10,000. Because of his tall, lanky habitus, it has been speculated that Abraham Lincoln had Marfan disease; however, most experts think it unlikely.

Classic hemophilia (hemophilia A) (Fig. 7-8) is an X-linked recessive disorder of factor VIII, an important blood coagulation protein. Males with hemophilia A lack enough factor VIII for normal clotting.

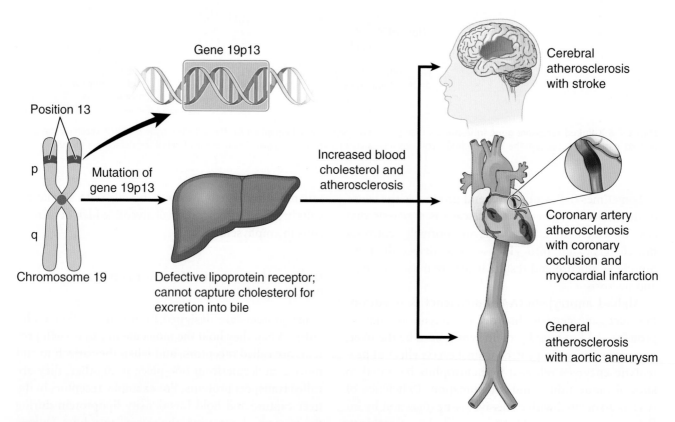

***Figure 7-9* Familial hypercholesterolemia.** A defective gene at position 13 on the short (p) arm of chromosome 19 causes defective liver cholesterol metabolism, leading to high levels of blood cholesterol and causing accelerated atherosclerosis.

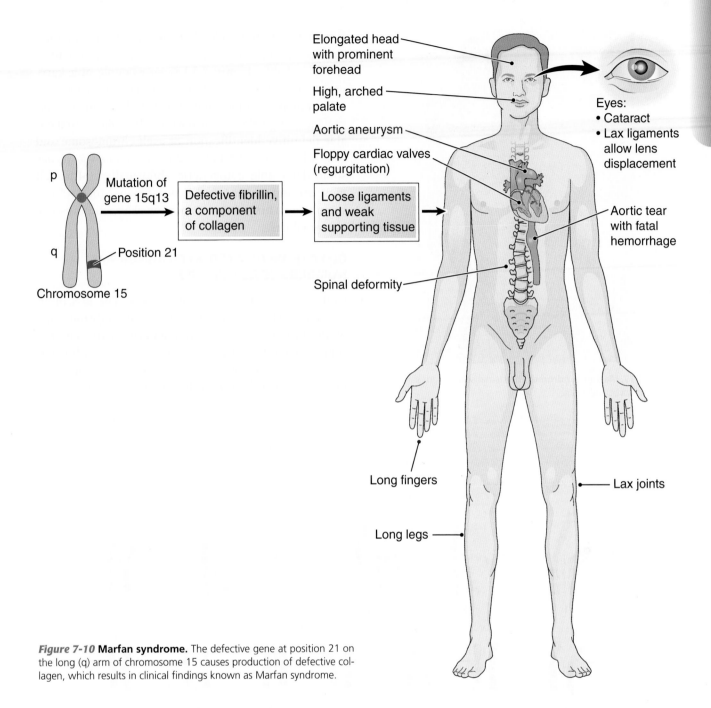

Elongated head with prominent forehead

High, arched palate

Aortic aneurysm

Floppy cardiac valves (regurgitation)

Spinal deformity

Eyes:
• Cataract
• Lax ligaments allow lens displacement

Aortic tear with fatal hemorrhage

Long fingers

Long legs

Lax joints

p

Mutation of gene 15q13

Defective fibrillin, a component of collagen

Loose ligaments and weak supporting tissue

q — Position 21

Chromosome 15

Figure 7-10 **Marfan syndrome.** The defective gene at position 21 on the long (q) arm of chromosome 15 causes production of defective collagen, which results in clinical findings known as Marfan syndrome.

Cytogenetic Diseases

Cytogenetic disease results from large-scale chromosome abnormalities involving large parts or entire chromosomes and arising *in the process of producing ova and sperm* from ovarian and testicular germ cells. By contrast, the mutations discussed above involve only a few genes or a tiny fraction of the DNA in a single gene.

Cytogenetic diseases are characterized by: 1) one or more extra chromosomes, 2) a missing chromosome, or 3) structural abnormalities of chromosomes, such as missing parts (deletion), parts that have been moved from one chromosome to another (translocation), or parts that detach and reattach upside down (inversion). Cytogenetic disorders may affect any chromosome.

The basic tool of cytogenetic investigation is the **karyotype**—a photographic display of chromosomes arranged in matched pairs (one maternal, one paternal) in descending order of length—the largest labeled number 1, the smallest number 22, with the X chromosome

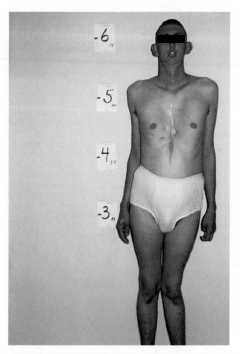

Figure 7-11 Marfan syndrome. The sternal scar is from surgical repair of an aortic aneurysm.

(large) and Y (tiny) added at the end. By this method extra or missing chromosomes and other abnormalities are identifiable. Figure 7-12 is an example of a karyotype of a female patient with Down syndrome. Additionally, chromosomes also may be stained to reveal patterns of alternating dark and light bands that enable definitive identification of each chromosome and some of its internal detail. About 1 in 200 newborns has some detectable cytogenetic abnormality (although most are innocuous), and it is estimated that 50% of spontaneous first trimester abortions have chromosome abnormalities.

DISEASE ASSOCIATED WITH ABNORMAL NUMBERS OF AUTOSOMES

Non-sex chromosomes are autosomes. The loss of an autosome, which leaves the embryo with only one copy of the chromosome instead of the normal pair, is **monosomy**, a condition that is not compatible with life and results in spontaneous abortion. An extra copy of an autosome, so that the patient has three copies of a partic-

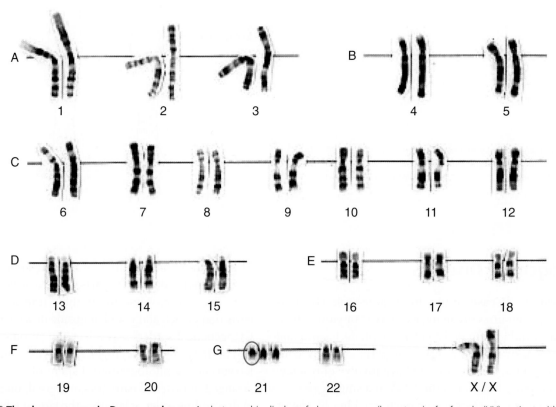

Figure 7-12 The chromosomes in Down syndrome. A photographic display of chromosomes (karyotype) of a female (XX) patient with Down syndrome reveals three copies of chromosome 21 (trisomy 21) instead of the normal two.

ular chromosome, not two, is **trisomy**. Most autosomal trisomy results in spontaneous abortion; however, some fetuses survive, especially those with trisomies of chromosomes number 13, 18, or 21, each of which is associated with severe mental and physical problems.

Trisomy 21 (**Down syndrome**) is the most common cytogenetic disorder in the United States and the single most common cause of mental retardation. Strongly influenced by maternal age, Down syndrome occurs about 1 in every 1,500 births to women under age thirty and about 1 in 25 births to women over 45 years old. A Down syndrome fetus possesses three copies of chromosome 21 (Fig. 7-12), rather than the normal two. The usual cause is a defective ovum that contains two number 21 chromosomes, rather than one; fertilization by sperm adds the third copy.

To understand how an ovum could have an extra 21 chromosome, recall that *germ cell division* (reduction division) in the ovary (and testis) is different than in other cells. In somatic cell division each of 46 chromosomes divides in half, one half going to one new daughter cell, the other half to the other daughter cell. However, in ovarian and testicular germ cells, chromosomes gather in matched pairs—one whole chromosome goes to one new cell (ovum or sperm), and its twin goes to another cell. This process is known as **meiosis**, a special type of cell division that occurs only in the gonads and produces ova and sperm with 23 chromosomes each, instead of the 46 in somatic cells. Basics in Brief 7-1 explains meiosis in more detail. Rarely, however, a mistake occurs and both 21 chromosomes go into one new ovum or sperm, and the other ovum or sperm gets none. If such an ovum is fertilized, the sperm brings a copy of 21 to make a total of three. Thus, the conceptus has three copies of chromosome 21, not two. In cytogenetic shorthand the combination for females is 47,XX,+21; in males the combination is expressed 47,XY,+21. Even though the pathogenesis of every case of Down syndrome is not understood, its close association with maternal age suggests that most cases involve an error in ovarian meiosis.

Infants with Down syndrome are mentally retarded and have a flat face with epicanthal folds and abnormalities of the hands and feet, as can be seen in Figures 7-13 and 7-14. They also may have cardiac and intestinal malformations, as well as immune deficiencies and associated infections, and are at an increased risk of leukemia. With correct care many patients live beyond

---

▶ BASICS IN BRIEF 7-1

MEIOSIS: FROM 46 CHROMOSOMES TO 23 AND BACK AGAIN

Sperm and ova are different from all other cells because they contain half the number of chromosomes present in all other cells—all other cells contain 46 chromosomes; ova and sperm contain only 23.

Mitosis is the way **autosomes** (chromosomes of somatic—non-germ—cells) divide: each of the 46 chromosomes is duplicated in the two new offspring cells. In mitosis, chromosomes line up at the cell equator, and each chromosome splits into two parts, half going to one daughter cell and half to the other. For example, as skin cells are shed daily and replaced, the new cells are exact copies of the parent cell—each has 46 chromosomes, including the two sex chromosomes. However, in germ cells of the gonads, the process is much different.

Gonadal **germ cells**, which also contain 46 chromosomes, undergo **meiosis** (or reduction division) to form **gametes** (ova and sperm) with 23 chromosomes each. In meiosis, chromosomes line up in *pairs* (for example, both number 21 chromosomes pair up), and one *whole* chromosome of each pair goes to each new gamete, so that the number of chromosomes in the gamete is half that of the parent germ cell. Each ovum and each sperm, therefore, contain 22 autosomes and one sex chromosome. The new ova have 22 autosomes plus an X sex chromosome; and the new sperm have 22 autosomes, plus an X or a Y sex chromosome. Half of sperm get an X, and the other half get a Y. At conception the total number of chromosomes returns to 46,XX or 46,XY: the ovum contributes 22 autosomes and an X sex chromosome; the sperm contributes 22 autosomes and either an X (and the fertilized egg becomes female) or a Y (and male).

Sometimes, however, meiosis is defective, and *both* of a pair of chromosomes go into one gamete, which when fertilized has 47 chromosomes; the other gamete does not get one and when fertilized has 45 chromosomes. Fertilization with such defective gametes is the cause of most cytogenetic disorders.

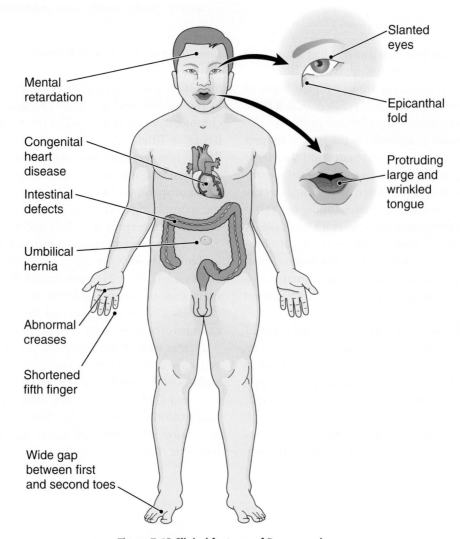

Mental retardation

Congenital heart disease

Intestinal defects

Umbilical hernia

Abnormal creases

Shortened fifth finger

Wide gap between first and second toes

Slanted eyes

Epicanthal fold

Protruding large and wrinkled tongue

Figure 7-13 Clinical features of Down syndrome.

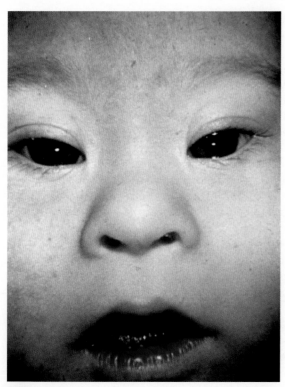

Figure 7-14 **Facies of Down syndrome.** The face is flat, the eyes are wide-set, the bridge of the nose is low, the eyes have epicanthal folds, and the mouth is usually partially open to accommodate an enlarged tongue.

age thirty, but often they develop early Alzheimer disease.

DISEASE ASSOCIATED WITH ABNORMAL NUMBERS OF SEX CHROMOSOMES

The most common cause of sex chromosome cytogenetic disease is *faulty meiosis*. In the ovary one ovum gets both of the X chromosomes and the other gets none and is designated O; in the testis one sperm gets both the X and the Y and the other gets none and is designated O. Combinations are depicted in Figure 7-15. If

abnormal ovarian meiosis produces an ovum with two X chromosomes and it is fertilized by a normal Y sperm the result is 47,XXY, which is recognized clinically as **Klinefelter syndrome** (Fig. 7-16). A typical patient is tall and effeminate, with long arms and legs, a small penis and atrophic testicles, scant pubic hair, no beard, and female-like hip shape. Many also have enlarged breasts (gynecomastia).

With abnormal meiosis in the testis, one sperm get both the X and the Y, and the other gets no sex chromosome. If the sperm with no sex chromosome fertilizes a

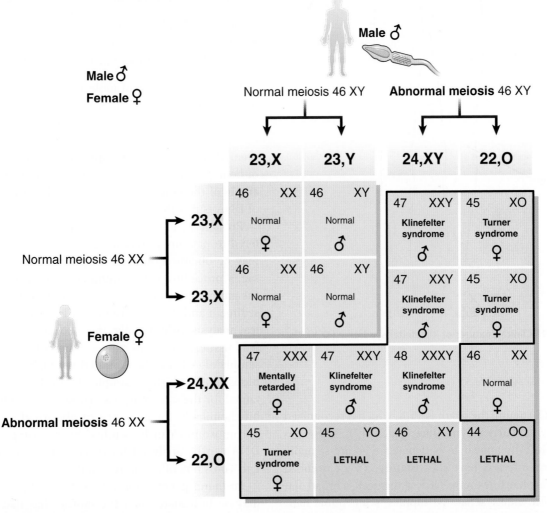

Figure 7-15 Sex chromosomes in cytogenetic disease. Some combinations of sex chromosomes are caused by faulty germ cell division (meiosis). On the top left, note that normal ovarian germ cell meiosis produces two ova, each with an X chromosome. At the bottom left note that abnormal ovarian meiosis produces one ovum with two X chromosomes (XX) and one with none (O). Across the top, note on the left that normal testicular germ cell meiosis produces one sperm with an X chromosome and one with a Y chromosome. To the right, note that abnormal testicular meiosis produces one sperm with both the X and Y chromosomes (XY) and one with none (O). The grid displays genetic combinations (genotypes) and clinical syndromes (phenotypes) that result from fertilization of these defective ova and sperm.

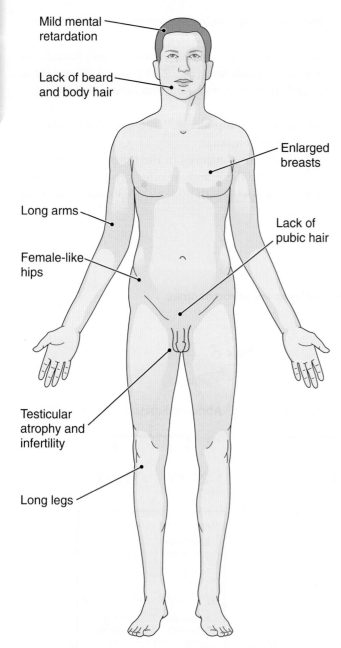

Mild mental retardation

Lack of beard and body hair

Enlarged breasts

Long arms

Lack of pubic hair

Female-like hips

Testicular atrophy and infertility

Long legs

Figure 7-16 **Clinical features of Klinefelter syndrome (47,XXY).**

Other combinations, such as 49, XXXXY, may occur. Mental retardation is common, and severity roughly parallels the number of X chromosomes. The processes involved are beyond the scope of this discussion.

Genetic Diagnosis

Prenatal genetic diagnosis is important for many reasons: 1) genetic diseases are transmissible down the generations; 2) they can create lifelong burdens for parents, families, and the affected child, and 3) they consume large amounts of health resources per patient. Diagnosis of genetic disorders usually requires expert advice by a geneticist and laboratory examination of maternal and/or fetal chromosomal material.

Below are some indications for genetic study:

- Mother 35 years or older
- Parents who have a child with known genetic disease
- Other family history of genetic problems

Prior to the arrival of molecular techniques, genetic diagnosis was made by clinical study or by detection of abnormal accumulations of substances in blood, urine, or tissue. Observation of mental retardation in phenylketonuria is an example of the former; detection of hemoglobin S by a sickle cell test on blood is an example of the latter. Now, however, direct examination of DNA is possible.

Prenatal genetic diagnosis (Fig. 7-18) should be offered to patients at risk for genetic disease. Fetal cells may be obtained by needle aspiration of the amniotic sac, a procedure called **amniocentesis**. Fetal cells line the amniotic sac and can be collected from centrifuged sediment and subjected to molecular, genetic, or chemical analysis. Additionally, the placenta is composed of fetal tissue, and by inserting a catheter into the cervix a sample of cells can be aspirated for analysis (**chorionic biopsy**). After birth, a sample of cord blood can be obtained for the same purpose. These cells can be studied biochemically for evidence of abnormal substances, chromosomes can be studied by karyotype, and the DNA can be analyzed for defects (the accompanying Lab Tools box offers more detail).

Postnatal genetic analysis of fetal or parental cells may be indicated when the mother has had multiple spontaneous abortions or a child is born with multiple congenital anomalies, Down syndrome, or other recognizable clinical cytogenetic or genetic disease. Infertile patients also may require genetic diagnosis.

normal (X) ovum, the result is 45,X, which is recognized clinically as **Turner syndrome** (Fig. 7-17). These patients clinically appear to be females who are sexually immature, infertile, have short stature, a wide, webbed neck, a low hairline on the back of the neck, a broad, flat chest with widely separated nipples, scant pubic hair, multiple pigmented skin lesions (nevi, Chapter 24), and no breast development. They do not have menstrual periods, and their ovaries are rudimentary streaks. Congenital cardiac malformations are common.

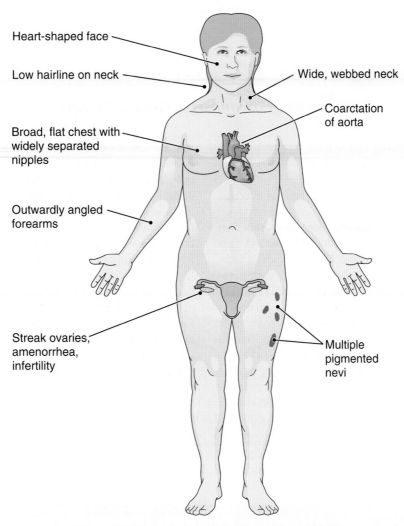

Heart-shaped face

Low hairline on neck

Wide, webbed neck

Coarctation
of aorta

Broad, flat chest with
widely separated
nipples

Outwardly angled
forearms

Streak ovaries,
amenorrhea,
infertility

Multiple
pigmented
nevi

Figure 7-17 **Clinical features of Turner syndrome (46,X).**

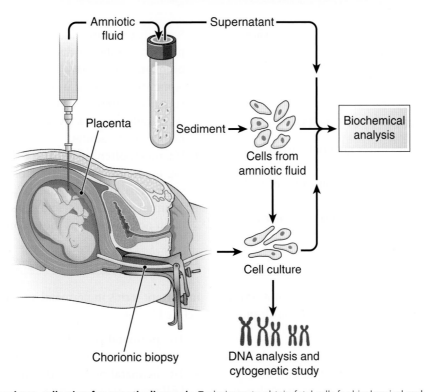

Amniotic
fluid

Supernatant

Placenta

Sediment

Biochemical
analysis

Cells from
amniotic fluid

Cell culture

Chorionic biopsy

DNA analysis and
cytogenetic study

Figure 7-18 **Prenatal specimen collection for genetic diagnosis.** Techniques to obtain fetal cells for biochemical and genetic study (karyotype or DNA analysis).

Laboratory Diagnosis in Genetic Disease

Laboratory cytogenetic diagnosis requires construction of a karyotype, as discussed nearby and demonstrated in Figures 7-4 and 7-12.

On the other hand, laboratory investigation of disorders resulting from single-gene (monogenic) defects depends on other techniques. First is **polymerase chain reaction (PCR)**, in which a very small amount of DNA is artificially multiplied into an amount large enough to study, a technique widely used in criminal investigations. Second is **restriction fragment length polymorphism (RFLP)**, a technique of DNA analysis also used in criminal investigations, as well as in genealogy studies and in paternity testing.

Despite its formidable name, the principle of RFLP is simple. *Restriction enzymes* are known to break DNA at a specific base sequence, wherever it occurs, thus shredding long chains of DNA into a collection of shorter fragments of varying length. For example, a certain enzyme might break DNA at every GAC base sequence; another might break it at every TCA sequence. These enzymes break DNA into fragments of recognizable length, forming a reproducible pattern for any given individual, based on that person's unique DNA sequences of bases (Chapter 2). The value of RFLP in genetic *disease* investigation rests on the fact that mutations alter the base sequences. For example, TCA sequences might appear where they had not previously existed and alter the breaking points so that the abnormal DNA has a pattern of fragment lengths different from those of normal DNA.

To understand RFLP, think of people as custom-built houses. RFLP analysis is like taking apart a custom-built house and sorting the lumber into sets according to length. Each house has a distinctive pattern. Identical homes can be disassembled into identical sets of boards time after time, just as DNA—normal or abnormal—can be disassembled into identical restriction fragments each time. However, if a rogue architect changes the plan, causing a mutation, so to speak, in the lengths of boards used to build some areas of the house, the disassembled lumber would reveal the change.

Section 3: *Pediatric Disease*

Train up a child in the way he should go: and when he is old he will not depart from it.
THE CHRISTIAN BIBLE, PROVERBS 22:6 (KJV)

MAJOR DETERMINANTS OF DISEASE

- Pediatric diseases differ materially from adult diseases.
- Genetic defects are a common cause of pediatric disease.
- Maternal factors are the cause of many fetal and neonatal disorders.

Children are not little adults—not mentally, not physically, not physiologically. Pediatrics is not adult medicine in miniature because:

- Genetic disease is more often a problem in children than adults. For example, sickle cell disease and cystic fibrosis are serious and common diseases that appear first in children.

- Some diseases are unique to childhood. For example, hyaline membrane disease is a condition unique to premature newborns
- Some diseases take a distinctive form when occurring in children. For example, meningitis in children is usually caused by different microbes than is meningitis in adults.
- Diagnosis often relies on specialized laboratory testing that is not widely available. For example, blood specimens are small and require special skill and equipment to collect, and tests done on children are often not the same as those done on adults.

Perinatal and Neonatal Disease

Important terms in perinatal and neonatal medicine are defined below:

- The **perinatal** period is the time from the 28th week of pregnancy to the seventh day after birth.
- The **neonatal** period is the first month after birth.
- **Full term** pregnancy is 38–40 weeks (after the end of the 37th week).

- **Normal birth weight** is 3,500 grams.
- **Post-term** infants are those born after 42 weeks.
- **Premature** infants are those born before the end of the 37th week; sometimes these infants are called **preterm**.
- **Low birth weight** infants weigh less than 2,500 grams (5.5 lb)

Determining **gestational age** (length of time in the womb) by counting from the first day of the mother's last menstrual period is a useful technique because women recall it easily. In reality, however, it is about two weeks more than the actual length of gestation because fertilization usually occurs about two weeks after the first day of the last menstrual period.

Duration of gestation, birth weight, and organ maturity go hand-in-hand in normal pregnancy (Fig. 7-19). Most term infants have normal birth weight and have organs that are appropriately mature and ready for life outside the womb. As a rule, infants with low birth weight have shorter gestational age, have less mature organs, and have higher mortality and morbidity than do term infants with normal birth weight and mature organs. However, this is not always the case, and newborn in-

fants are classified according to a system that takes into account both birth weight and gestational age:

- **Small for gestational age (SGA)** infants are those weighing less than predicted for any given gestational age.
- **Appropriate for gestational age (AGA)** infants are those weighing as much as expected at any given gestational age.
- **Large for gestational age (LGA)** infants are those weighing more than expected at any given gestational age.

For example, according to Figure 7-19, an infant born at 32 weeks should weigh near 1,500 grams. An infant born at 32 weeks that weighs 2,500 grams is large for gestational age (LGA) but is very premature. It is sure to have immature organs and is at high risk for complications of prematurity, especially respiratory distress syndrome (discussed below). However, an infant born at 36 weeks and weighing 1,500 gm, though small for gestational age (SGA), is at relatively less risk for complications because its organs are more mature.

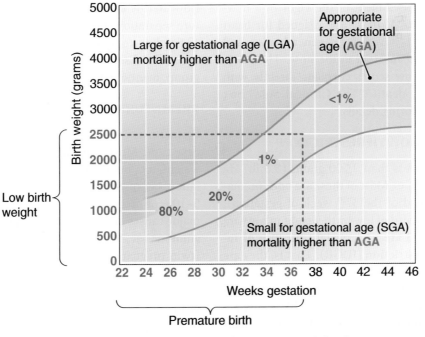

Figure 7-19 Neonatal mortality risk. Fetal death rate (percent) as a function of birth weight and gestational age. Normal gestation is 38–40 full weeks. Prematurity is gestational age less than 37 full weeks. For example, the mortality is <1% for term infants that weigh appropriately for gestational age (AGA), but it is about 20% for infants born weighing under 1,500 grams and born at about 30 weeks gestational age.

THE CLINICAL SIDE

CLINICAL EVALUATION OF NEWBORN INFANTS: THE APGAR SCORE

Assessment of newborn infant vigor correlates closely with infant survival. Practices vary, but typically infants are scored at 1 minute or 5 minutes after birth. Infants with low scores have higher morbidity and mortality than do infants with higher scores. For example:

- Infants with a five minute score of 0–1 have a 50% mortality rate.
- Mortality is very close to zero for infants scoring 7 or better.

The Apgar Scoring System for Newborns

Sign	Apgar Points		
	0	1	2
Heart rate	Absent	Below 100	Over 100
Respiratory effort	Absent	Slow, irregular	Good, crying
Muscle tone	Limp	Some flexion of extremities	Active motion
Response to catheter inserted in nostril	No response	Grimace	Cough or sneeze
Color	Blue, pale	Body pink, extremities blue	Completely pink

A very useful tool in newborn care is the **Apgar score**, named after its originator, pediatric anesthesiologist Virginia Apgar. A numerical assessment of an infant's condition immediately after birth, it is a useful method for clinical assessment of the vigor of a newborn infant. Points (0, 1, or 2) are assigned for heart rate, respiratory effort, muscle tone, general color, and response to a catheter inserted in the nose. The maximum score is ten. Low scores correlate directly with neonatal illness and death. "The Clinical Side" box above presents the scoring details.

INTRAUTERINE GROWTH RESTRICTION

Newborns weighing less than 2,500 grams (5.5 lb) are **low birth weight** infants. Most of these are born prematurely (before the end of the 37th week of gestation); however, about one third of low birth weight infants are born at full term and are underweight because of **intrauterine growth restriction (IUGR)**. That is, they are SGA, rather than premature.

Often the cause of IUGR is not known, but *maternal factors* are the most common identifiable causes—hypertension of pregnancy (toxemia, Chapter 21), malnutrition, drug or alcohol abuse, and heavy cigarette smoking. **Fetal alcohol syndrome**, a common cause of IUGR, is characterized by a history of maternal alcohol abuse and an SGA infant with a small head (micro-

cephaly), mental retardation, atrial septal defect (Chapter 13), and a characteristic facial appearance.

Placental factors can also cause IUGR. Examples include insufficient placental blood flow, placenta previa (low uterine implantation of the placenta), and premature separation (placental abruption).

Fetal factors include genetic disease, congenital anomalies diseases, and infections (mainly the TORCH group, mentioned above).

PREMATURITY

Prematurity is birth before the end of the 37th week of gestation. Most premature infants are of low birth weight, too, but the most critical aspect is length of gestation, because it takes time for organs to mature. About 5–10% of pregnancies produce premature infants. The major causes of prematurity are preterm rupture of the amniotic sac, intrauterine infection, multiple gestation (twin pregnancy), and structural abnormalities of the uterus, cervix, or placenta (such as leiomyomas of the uterine wall), placental hemorrhage, abnormal location of the placental implantation in the wall of the uterus, or a relaxed cervix that opens too early.

Premature infants have immature organs regardless of birth weight and are at substantial risk for brain, liver, and lung disease. Those that are SGA are at even greater risk.

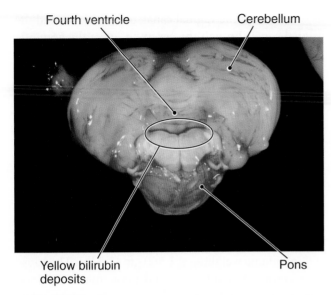

Fourth ventricle   Cerebellum

Yellow bilirubin   Pons
deposits

Figure 7-20 Kernicterus. Cross-section of newborn midbrain at the level of the fourth ventricle. Sustained high blood bilirubin has caused bilirubin to be deposited in the floor of the third ventricle. Severe neurologic damage results.

The *brain* is the least mature of all organs at birth, whether premature or full term. It is especially vulnerable to birth-related hemorrhage as the skull is molded into somewhat of an elongated shape as it passes through the birth canal. Intracranial hemorrhage can occur without skull fracture or bruised or torn brain tissue, and can lead to severe neurologic impairment or death.

The newborn *liver* is not fully capable of processing bilirubin until about two weeks of age, and almost all healthy newborns experience a normal period of nontoxic **physiologic jaundice** (Chapter 16) shortly after birth. However, in prematurity the liver is even less capable of handling the normal physiologic load, and bilirubin can rise to toxic levels, resulting in **kernicterus**, a syndrome of severe brain damage characterized by deposits of bilirubin in the floor of the third ventricle (Fig. 7-20). Thanks to modern prenatal and neonatal care, kernicterus is now very rare in developed nations.

High levels of bilirubin can be treated in two ways. For most infants, *phototherapy* is sufficient. For a few hours a day the infant is exposed to intense light, which penetrates deep enough into skin to interact with bilirubin in superficial blood vessels and converts bilirubin into a form more easily handled by the infant's immature liver. In *exchange transfusion*, necessary for more severe cases, small amounts of infant blood are repeatedly withdrawn and replaced each time with fresh donor blood or plasma that, of course, has little bilirubin in it.

The *lungs* do not reach full maturity until 6–8 years after birth. In utero they undergo rapid evolution between 28–32 weeks, as type II pneumocytes begin secreting *surfactant*, a slick, soapy fluid that decreases surface tension of intra-alveolar fluid and decreases the effort required to keep alveoli open and filled with air after birth. **Respiratory distress syndrome (RDS)** of the newborn (also known as **hyaline membrane disease**) stems from a lack of surfactant in immature infant lungs (see Case Study 7-1 at the end of this chapter).

Respiratory distress syndrome is a disease of prematurity that affects about 25% of infants born between 32–36 weeks and more than 50% of those born before 28 weeks. The absence of surfactant makes alveoli difficult to keep open, and they collapse, preventing gas exchange. Keeping alveoli open requires intense respiratory effort, and some infants die because they suffocate as their muscles tire. A typical case is a premature, low birth weight infant whose weight is appropriate for gestational age (AGA), and a mother who has diabetes or some other complication of pregnancy. Shortly after delivery, the infant's breathing becomes difficult, with grunting respirations and sternal and lower rib retraction from the severe effort. Within a few hours after birth, blood oxygen levels fall (hypoxia) and the infant turns blue (cyanosis). Hypoxia causes alveolar and pulmonary vascular damage, and fluid (exudate) accumulates in the alveoli. Protein in the exudate cannot be absorbed, and in time the protein condenses to glue-like consistency that forms a thick membrane (the hyaline membrane, Fig. 7-21) coating alveolar walls, further impairing oxygen transfer. Surviving infants may suffer

Hyaline membrane

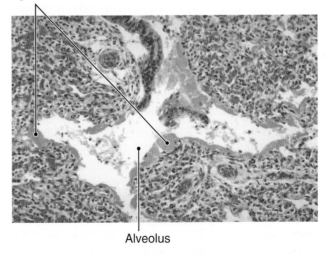

Alveolus

Figure 7-21 Pulmonary hyaline membranes. Respiratory distress syndrome (hyaline membrane disease) of the newborn. Note the thick alveolar membranes, which impair oxygenation.

hypoxic brain damage. Oxygen and surfactant inhalation may be effective treatments.

Oxygen therapy can be life saving. However, in newborns it must be administered with special care because inhalation of high concentrations of oxygen can result in *retinopathy of the newborn* ("oxygen blindness"), associated with toxic effect of oxygen on the neonatal retina, or in *bronchial dysplasia*, associated with a similar toxic effect of oxygen on bronchial mucosa. Oxygen blindness is rare, but bronchial dysplasia occurs in about half of infants weighing less than 1,000 gm who are treated with oxygen. Pathologically it is characterized by bronchial and lung scarring (fibrosis).

BIRTH INJURY

About 1 in 5,000 live-born infants is born with an injury directly traceable to the birth process. Considering the contortions and forces of vaginal passage, it is surprising that infants are not injured more often. LGA infants are injured more often than others because greater force is necessary to push the fetus through the birth canal. The most common injuries are, in descending order: fractured clavicle, facial nerve injury with facial paralysis, brachial plexus injury with paralysis of the upper extremity, skull fracture or intracranial injury, and fracture of the humerus. Intracranial hemorrhage is the most severe injury and can produce immediate problems or death; or it may become manifest later as cerebral palsy.

Cerebral palsy (see Chapter 23, Figure 23.11) is a broad clinical term for a non-progressive syndrome of infant brain damage. About 75% of cerebral palsy cases arise from *unknown* prebirth conditions. About 15% of cases arise from damage suffered after birth: brain or meningeal infections, hyperbilirubinemia, automobile accidents, falls, or child abuse. Cerebral palsy is characterized by varying degrees of motor difficulty including paralysis, uncontrollable movements, and inability to coordinate body movements, which may not be evident at birth but assert themselves as development progresses. Because brain development continues during the first two years of life, cerebral palsy can result from brain damage that occurs in utero or before age two. Neonatal risk factors for cerebral palsy include prematurity, low birth weight, and intrauterine growth retardation (Chapter 7).

FETAL AND NEWBORN INFECTIONS

Some maternal infections cross the placenta to infect the fetus, notably the TORCH infections discussed earlier in this chapter. However, most infections are from vaginal bacteria. Sometimes infection is acquired as the fetus passes through the vaginal canal; or bacteria ascend the vaginal canal through the cervix to infect the amniotic fluid (amnionitis), usually late in pregnancy, and particularly if there is an amniotic fluid leak. Infected amniotic fluid is inhaled by the fetus and may cause premature labor and pneumonia or other infections.

Herpesvirus may be a serious fetal threat if a pregnant woman suffers an outbreak of genital herpes at the time of delivery. The threat is so serious that caesarean section may be required in mothers with active genital herpes to avoid exposing the infant to the risk of infection by vaginal delivery.

Necrotizing enterocolitis, a severe inflammatory condition of the gastrointestinal tract, occurs in about 10% of infants weighing <1,500 gm (3.3 lb). The cause is unknown, but infection and poor intestinal blood flow are suspected. The findings are distinctive: intestinal mucosal hemorrhage with bloody diarrhea and shock. Surgical excision of affected bowel is often required. Mortality is high.

Infections of Children

The most common pediatric infections are viral; many of them cause acute upper respiratory illnesses featuring fever, cough, and rhinorrhea.

Respiratory syncytial virus (RSV) causes a pediatric syndrome of acute bronchitis, bronchiolitis, and bronchopneumonia.

Measles (rubeola) is a highly contagious respiratory virus best known for the skin rash it produces. In well-nourished, healthy children it is usually not much more than a rite of passage, but in malnourished children it can cause fatal pneumonia, accounting for over one million deaths per year worldwide.

Rubella (German measles, three-day measles) is caused by the rubella virus and presents as sore throat, skin rash, and enlarged lymph nodes. It is much shorter in duration and is a less serious condition than rubeola is. Rubella infection of the fetus, however, can cause especially severe and deforming disease or fetal death (Chapter 7).

Mumps virus causes acute inflammation of the parotid salivary gland (parotitis), and it occasionally causes orchitis (inflammation of the testes), pancreatitis, or encephalitis. It has been virtually eliminated by vaccination.

Infectious mononucleosis is a self-limited (it disappears without treatment), mild syndrome of fever, sore throat, listlessness, lymphocytosis, and splenomegaly, which typically occurs in late adolescence or in college-age youths (Chapter 11). It is caused by the *Epstein-*

Barr virus (EBV) and almost always is passed in saliva during kissing. Transmission by sexual contact and shared eating and drinking utensils is rare. Diagnosis requires finding distinctive large lymphocytes (atypical lymphocytes) in the peripheral blood and characteristic antibodies (called *heterophil antibodies*) in blood.

Chickenpox is caused by the *varicella-zoster virus*, which causes an acute febrile illness characterized by vesicular skin eruptions that may leave unsightly scars.

One of the most common bacterial diseases of children is **acute otitis media**, discussed in detail in Chapter 25. *Streptococcus pneumoniae* and *Haemophilus influenzae* are the most common bacteria involved.

Bronchiolitis, a viral infection of the small airways, is usually caused by the *respiratory syncytial virus (RSV)*. It occurs most often as winter epidemics in infants and children. It presents clinically with low-grade fever, wheezing respiration, and shortness of breath. Secondary bacterial pneumonia may develop, but most cases resolve in 7–10 days with supportive therapy.

Whooping cough is caused by *Bordetella pertussis*, a Gram-negative bacillus that produces a highly contagious syndrome of intense inflammation in the larynx, trachea, and bronchi, and which can cause fatal asphyxia. Whooping cough gets its name from severe spasms of coughing and the sharp, inspiratory barking sound (stridor, or whoop) that is characteristic of the disease. Whooping cough is usually mild in older children, but may cause death in infants. Vaccination programs have made it uncommon in the United States, but it causes hundreds of thousands of deaths annually in unvaccinated children in developing nations.

Croup is an illness of children, usually age 3 or younger, resulting from influenza A or B virus infection. It can cause inflammation of the larynx, trachea, or bronchi. The most dangerous aspect is laryngitis, which features laryngeal edema that causes a hoarse, brassy, barking cough and a crowing sound (*stridor*) on inspiration. Most cases resolve spontaneously, but a neglected case can cause fatal suffocation.

Diphtheria is caused by a gram-positive bacillus, *Corynebacterium diphtheriae*, which produces a pharyngitis and laryngitis associated with a thick, obstructive inflammatory membrane that can cause death by suffocation. Moreover, the bacillus secretes an exotoxin that can damage the heart, kidney, and brain. Diphtheria now has been almost eliminated in developed nations by effective vaccinations.

Acute bacterial **epiglottitis** is a disease of school age children caused by *H. influenzae* and marked by hoarseness and painful swallowing. The epiglottis and nearby pharyngeal tissues are severely inflamed, narrowing the airway and sometimes causing critical airway obstruction.

Sudden Infant Death Syndrome (SIDS)

The cause of **sudden infant death syndrome (SIDS)**, sometimes referred to as crib death, is unknown and is best characterized by its epidemiology:

- 90% of victims are under 6 months of age
- Most victims routinely sleep in the prone position
- There is a higher than usual history of prematurity or low birth weight
- Males outnumber females
- Mothers are often less than 20 years old, are unmarried, are smokers or drug abusers, and have low socioeconomic condition
- African-American infants are more often affected than other ethnic groups (genetic? socioeconomic?)

Pathologic findings at autopsy are scant, but a few patients may have minor microscopic abnormalities in structures related to respiratory control: the carotid body, vagus nerve, or part of the brain. A very small number of cases prove to be homicide rather than SIDS, and the index of suspicion rises dramatically with a second case in the same family.

HEMOLYTIC DISEASE OF THE NEWBORN (ERYTHROBLASTOSIS FETALIS)

Hemolytic disease of the newborn is anemia resulting from destruction of fetal red blood cells (hemolysis) by maternal antibodies that cross the placenta and enter the fetal circulation. Thanks to modern maternal and neonatal care, it is now very rare in the United States, but it will be discussed in detail because the pathogenetic mechanisms are instructive. In hemolytic disease of the newborn the mother becomes immunized against fetal red blood cells during a pregnancy; then in a *subsequent* pregnancy the antibodies cross the placenta to attack (hemolyze) red blood cells of the fetus.

Fetal red cells leak into the maternal bloodstream in normal pregnancy, usually without ill effect. However, the red cell membrane contains many proteins, some of which are highly antigenic, and if mother and fetus have certain differences in blood type, the mother may develop antibodies against fetal red cells. One of the most potent antigens is the Rh D antigen (Chapter 8)—often referred to as the "Rh factor"—which is present in the red blood cells of 85% of the United States population.

Although major blood group (A, B, and O) differences between mother and fetus are common, they rarely cause problems. However, Rh D differences can be very serious. If an Rh D-*negative* mother receives a large dose of Rh D-*positive* fetal RBCs, she can become immunized against Rh D protein; in other words, the mother becomes primed to produce a flood of antibodies against Rh D fetal RBCs the *next* time she is pregnant with a fetus having *Rh D positive* RBCs.

The ill effect on the fetus is directly proportional to the degree of fetal red-cell destruction. Affected infants are anemic because their red cells are destroyed faster than they can be replaced. Destruction of RBCs releases large amounts of hemoglobin, which is metabolized into more bilirubin than the fetal liver can excrete (Chapter 16). Very high blood bilirubin causes bilirubin deposits in the brainstem, producing a clinical condition known as *kernicterus* (Fig. 7-20). Severe anemia causes high-output congestive heart failure (Chapter 13), and impairs the liver's ability to produce albumin, resulting in generalized osmotic edema (Chapter 5). The combination of heart failure and osmotic edema produces severe generalized fetal edema, known as **hydrops fetalis** (Fig. 7-22). Those most severely affected fetuses may be stillborn or die shortly after birth.

Preventive therapy is very effective and has dramatically reduced the number of cases. ABO and Rh D characteristics of mothers should be determined early in pregnancy. Rh D-negative mothers are given a prophylactic injection of anti-Rh D antibody because there is a high chance that the infant is Rh D positive. A second dose is given immediately after delivery. The injected anti-Rh D antibody attaches to Rh D protein on any Rh D-positive fetal cells in the maternal circulation, masking the fetal Rh D protein from the maternal immune system and preventing maternal production of anti-Rh D antibodies that could cause a problem for a subsequent pregnancy with an Rh D-positive infant.

Cystic Fibrosis

Cystic fibrosis is the most common lethal genetic disease of Caucasians, affecting about 1 in 2,000 live births. The genetic defect affects the transport of chloride (Cl^-) across epithelial cell membranes of gland ducts, resulting in decreased chloride in glandular secretions. Because sodium and chloride are transported across the cell membrane together, secretions have *decreased* sodium (and chloride) and low osmotic pressure and are unable to attract water. The result is very thick mucus that obstructs bronchial and intestinal mucus gland ducts, pancreatic ducts, hepatic bile ducts, and the vas deferens.

Accumulations of this thick mucus in pancreatic ducts prevents digestive enzymes from reaching the GI tract. The result is chronic pancreatitis, gastrointestinal malabsorption (Chapter 15), and malnourishment. Obstruction of hepatic bile ducts causes chronic inflammation and widespread liver scarring (cirrhosis, Chapter 16). Obstruction of the vas deferens causes low sperm count and infertility. Thick mucus from bronchial glands obstructs small bronchi, impairs respiration, and promotes infection (Fig. 7-23). In the fetus or newborn, intestinal mucus may be so thick that it causes intestinal obstruction, which is known as *meconium ileus.*

In sweat gland ducts the chloride transport defect has the opposite effect: sweat chloride is high, a diagnostic finding characteristic of patients with cystic fibrosis. The Lab Tools box below explains the **sweat chloride test** and other lab diagnostic tests for cystic fibrosis.

The clinical manifestations of CF vary in severity and in the organs affected. The diagnosis is made early in some patients; in others the disease may not manifest itself for many years. In certain patients intestinal malabsorption symptoms predominate, and patients have large, fatty, smelly stools, malnutrition, and abdominal distention. However, in most patients severe bronchitis and recurrent pneumonia are the biggest problems. Pulmonary infections account for the great majority of CF deaths. Median life expectancy is about 30 years.

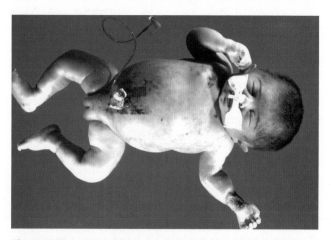

Figure 7-22 **Hydrops fetalis.** Hemolytic disease of the newborn (erythroblastosis fetalis). Some infants with severe erythroblastosis fetalis have blood red cell counts so low that it causes hypoxic injury to the heart and liver. Liver failure impairs synthesis of albumin, which causes low blood albumin levels and osmotic edema, which, combined with heart failure, causes generalized edema (hydrops).

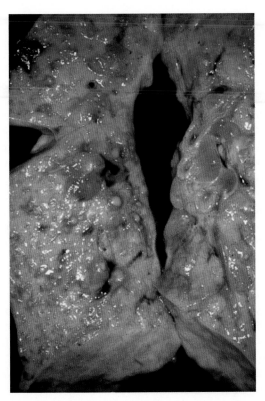

Figure 7-23 **The lungs in cystic fibrosis.** Bronchi are dilated and filled with thick, infected mucus.

Tumors and Tumor-like Conditions in Children

Malignant neoplasms in children are uncommon, but nevertheless they are the second most common cause of death; only fatal accidents are more common. Benign tumors and tumor-like masses are much more common than are malignant ones.

A common and innocuous tumor-like (but non-neoplastic) condition is **choristoma**. Choristomas are *normally formed* tissue in an *abnormal* location. For example, a fairly common choristoma is a patch of embryologically misplaced but otherwise normal pancreas found in the stomach wall. On the other hand, **hamartomas** are local collections of *abnormally formed* normal tissue in a *normal* location. They are best thought of as somewhat of a benign neoplasm and somewhat of a congenital malformation. A good example is bronchial hamartoma. Normal bronchi contain cartilage, epithelium, blood vessels, and lymphoid tissue. A bronchial hamartoma may contain one or all of these tissues, but arranged as a small, nodular mass, not as a normal bronchus. Some experts believe **congenital hemangiomas**, which are common and may be quite large, are hamartomatous collections of small blood vessels and are not neoplastic.

Acute leukemia is the most common malignant neoplasm of children. Other common tumors include lymphoma (Chapter 11) and tumors of the brain and kidney. As compared to adult malignancies, those in children are more often associated with genetic abnormalities, congenital malformations, and a tendency to spontaneously regress or mature into less malignant tissue. They have a better survival rate, often because they are more responsive to therapy. ■

LAB TOOLS

Laboratory Testing for Cystic Fibrosis

Patients with cystic fibrosis have high levels of sweat sodium and chloride, the exact opposite of the low sodium and chloride content of thick, water-deprived secretions of bronchial glands and the pancreas that account for most of the clinical symptoms. Patients also have abnormal DNA that can be analyzed for a telltale defect, and high levels blood trypsin, a pancreatic digestive enzyme that "backs up" in the blood because pancreatic ducts are plugged with viscous mucus.

Sweat chloride is the most widely applied laboratory test for cystic fibrosis. Specialized apparatus not often found in adult medical settings is required to collect and analyze sweat in patients suspected of having cystic fibrosis. The test entails applying a weak solution of pilocarpine, a drug that stimulates sweating, to a small area of skin, usually on an ex-

tremity, which is then stimulated by a weak electrical current for about five minutes. The skin is then cleaned, and an absorbent patch is applied to the area for 30 minutes. The sweat is weighed and analyzed for chloride concentration. Two specimens should be collected, one from each arm or leg, and the results averaged.

CF patients also have high sweat sodium. Most laboratories now perform both sodium and chloride assays on collected sweat. Abnormally high sweat chloride or sodium levels are very reliable indicators that CF is present.

Sweat collection is very difficult in infants less than six weeks old. In these patients a drop of blood may be collected on paper and analyzed for an abnormally high level of trypsin. A similarly small amount of blood may be subjected to analysis of DNA for the genetic defect of CF.

CASE STUDY 7-1 "I THOUGHT IT WOULD GO AWAY"

TOPICS
Uterine infection
Premature birth
Infant small for gestational age
Respiratory distress syndrome of the newborn

THE CASE

Setting: You are the sole health care provider in a remote west Texas town whose hospital closed years ago. You and an assistant are the only staff at a walk-in clinic in what used to be the emergency room. You take care of routine matters on most patients and consult by phone with medical staff at the hospital fifty miles away, and you refer complex cases to this hospital.

History: KLC, a 21-year-old obese woman who is obviously pregnant and in labor, is brought to the clinic by a friend. You ask a few questions and establish that KLC is about 28 weeks pregnant and has had no prenatal care. She says her water broke 48 hours earlier, but she did not seek care because "I thought it would go away." When fever and cramping began, she became frightened and asked her friend to bring her to the clinic.

You look in the old records and find her chart, which reveals a history of heavy smoking, occasional drug use, and missed clinic appointments. A prior pregnancy was complicated by excessive weight gain, high blood pressure, and spontaneous abortion.

Physical examination and other data: You do a quick evaluation and find temperature 101° F, respirations 14, heart rate 96, and blood pressure 145/95. She has noticeable edema in her feet and a yellowish vaginal discharge. You detect faint, irregular fetal heart sounds. A quick "dipstick" test of a urine sample reveals moderate proteinuria.

Clinical course: You are concerned not only about the fetus but also about the mother's very high blood pressure and proteinuria; she clearly has preeclampsia (Chapter 21). You call for an ambulance and then seek advice from a physician at the referral hospital, who gives you instructions to start an IV containing anti-hypertensive medication and diuretics. You ride in the ambulance with the patient and speculate privately that if she had not been forced to come to the clinic, and her high blood pressure had continued untreated, her uncontrolled hypertension probably would have provoked seizures, stroke, or some other calamity. Within minutes of arriving at the hospital, she delivers a 626 gm (1 lb, 6 oz) male infant with Apgar score 5 at one minute and 6 at five minutes. Measurements of head circumference and body length suggest that gestation is between 25–28 weeks.

Immediately after birth the infant develops respiratory distress with sternal retractions. Administration of pulmonary surfactant fails to improve respiratory status, and respiratory assistance is initiated. Chest radiograph reveals hazy opacification of both lungs. On the next day, seizures occur, and the infant dies. At autopsy the important gross findings include lungs that are heavy and airless, intraventricular brain hemorrhage, and heavy meconium staining of the amniotic sac. (The placenta is available for study because hospital personnel have saved it.). Microscopic study shows widespread acute inflammation in the lungs (acute pneumonia) and the amniotic membranes (acute amnionitis).

DISCUSSION

This woman developed preeclampsia, a syndrome of hypertension, proteinuria, and pedal edema in pregnancy. It can be fatal, especially if not recognized and treated early. The cause is unknown. Delivery of the infant is curative.

This infant was premature by menstrual history and birth weight. Body measurements suggest the gestation was at least 25 weeks; the infant weighed 626 grams, indicating he was also small for gestational age (SGA). Premature labor and SGA are likely attributable to the mother's heavy smoking, drug use, obesity, and high blood pressure.

The fetal membranes of the placenta were stained green by meconium (meconium is fetal intestinal contents), a sign of fetal distress. These findings were supported by faint, irregular fetal heart sounds on admission and low Apgar scores after birth. Microscopic examination of the membranes revealed acute inflammation, strongly suggesting ascending infection from the vagina, a finding supported by the vaginal exudate and the 48-hour delay between the time when the mother's water broke and her appearance at the emergency room. The fetal lungs showed bronchopneumonia, indicating the infection spread to the infant, through inhalation of amniotic fluid (a fetus inhales amniotic fluid until birth).

The intraventricular hemorrhage in the brain was consistent with the terminal seizures. Such hemorrhages are associated with prematurity and hypoxia, both of which were present in this infant.

POINTS TO REMEMBER

- Women who do not receive prenatal care tend to have complicated pregnancies, including preeclampsia and premature birth.
- Women who smoke or abuse drugs or alcohol are at increased risk for delivering infants who are sick and premature.
- Premature infants have high rates of illness and death.

CASE STUDY 7-1 THE ROAD NOT TAKEN—AN ALTERNATIVE SCENARIO

For all sad words of tongue or pen,
The saddest are these: "It might have been."
JOHN GREENLEAF WHITTIER (1807–1892),
AMERICAN QUAKER POET AND REFORMER, *MAUD MULLER*

THE CASE
With a bit of imagination, we can speculate how this case might have had a happier ending.

Setting: You are employed by a charitable trust that operates a maternal-care and pediatric clinic near a hospital in a medium-size city. Your clinic serves a very large and sparsely populated area in the United States Northwest.

History: KLC is a 24-year-old woman referred to you by a clinic in a small town 50 miles away because she is pregnant and has no insurance. She is accompanied by an older woman who introduces herself as the wife of the foreman of the ranch where KLC works as a cook. "She doesn't have anyone but us," she says. "We don't know where the father went; he left last week when her urine test came out positive."

You question KLC about her past medical history, which is remarkable for a pregnancy three years earlier in another state that was complicated by "high blood pressure" and excessive weight gain and which ended with a spontaneous abortion. You learn that she smokes and drinks "a few beers" on the weekends. According to her menstrual history, she is about 12 weeks pregnant.

Physical examination and other data: Vital signs are normal except for blood pressure 138/88. Physical examination is unremarkable except for obesity and slight pedal edema. An ultrasound study reveals that the fetus is of normal size for the estimated gestational age, and fetal heartbeat is normal. Blood studies are normal; urinalysis shows a trace of protein.

Clinical course: When you call her to your office for counseling before sending her home, she asks if the foreman's wife can sit in. In the interview you emphasize to both of them that the patient should:

- Stop smoking
- Stop drinking alcohol
- Not use illegal drugs
- Watch her weight very carefully
- Take a multi-vitamin containing folic acid
- Take the blood pressure medicine you will prescribe
- Return for care according to the schedule you lay out for them

The patient agrees, but says, "Stopping smoking is going to be hard."

You agree, but insist she must try, and if she cannot quit completely, then she should smoke as few cigarettes as possible.

"I'll do my best," she says. "I don't want to get into the mess I was when I got pregnant the first time."

"I'll help her," the foreman's wife says. "I think she learned a lot from that first pregnancy."

As the pregnancy develops, you are very pleased by her progress. She keeps all of her appointments and actually loses a few pounds. She stops consuming alcohol but smokes "a few" cigarettes now and then. Her blood pressure remains under control, and fetal monitoring suggests that the baby is growing normally.

At term she delivers a healthy little girl who weighs 7 lb 8 oz. At her final post-partum checkup both mother and the baby are doing well.

DISCUSSION
The critical difference between this scenario and the previous one was the emotional support this young woman got from the ranch foreman's wife. The good medical advice and care she got supplemented the emotional support, and the combination produced the desired result: a healthy mother and newborn infant.

Objectives Recap

1. *Distinguish between congenital deformation and malformation, and give an example of each:* Congenital malformations are caused by intrinsic abnormalities of the embryologic developmental process. Deformations, on the other hand, are caused by intrauterine mechanical factors. For example, spina bifida is a malformation; clubfoot is a deformation.

2. *Define teratogen, and give an example of a chemical teratogen and an infectious teratogen:* A teratogen is an agent capable of inducing abnormal embryologic development to produce a fetal malformation. The most common teratogens are chemicals and viruses. Of chemicals, the most common teratogen is alcohol abuse by the mother, which produces fetal alcohol syndrome. Of infec-

tious teratogens, the most common are the so-called TORCH group, of which rubella is one agent.

3. *Distinguish among cytogenetic disease, single-gene (Mendelian or monogenic) disease, and disease resulting from multiple genes (polygenic), and give examples of each:* Cytogenetic disorders result from the absence or duplication of an entire chromosome or to large-scale structural dislocations of parts of a chromosome. Down syndrome (three instead of the normal two copies of chromosome 21) is a cytogenetic disorder. Single-gene (monogenic) disorders result from a defect of one gene and are inherited according to Mendelian principles. Sickle cell disease is an example. Polygenic influence on the development of disease is associated with multiple genes, not usually identifiable. Type II diabetes mellitus is a disease with clear polygenic (hereditary) influences. Polygenic influence is much more common than are cytogenetic or single-gene defects.

4. *Explain the difference between autosomal dominant and recessive genetic behavior:* An autosomal dominant genetic characteristic requires only one copy of the gene (from either mother or father) for the characteristic to be physically expressed. An autosomal recessive trait requires two copies of the gene, one from each parent.

5. *Explain how inheritance of genetic defects on the X chromosome is different from gene defects on autosomes:* The principal difference is that a *single* defective *recessive* gene is expressed as disease when it occurs on an X chromosome. Recessive genes are not expressed when they occur on autosomes unless *both* copies of the autosome carry the same defective gene.

6. *Offer several examples of disease caused by single-gene defects:* Gaucher disease, familial hypercholesterolemia, neurofibromatosis (von Recklinghausen disease), Marfan syndrome, hemophilia A (classic hemophilia).

7. *Explain how cytogenetic disease differs from other genetic disease, and give an example of a cytogenetic disease:* A cytogenetic disorder is one in which there is 1) one or more extra chromosomes, 2) a missing chromosome, or 3) large scale structural abnormalities such as missing parts (deletion), parts that have been transposed (translocation) to another chromosome, or parts that detach and reattach upside down (inversion). By contrast, other genetic diseases are caused by abnormalities in single genes. Down syndrome (trisomy 21) is a cytogenetic disease.

8. *Explain the genetic abnormality in Turner syndrome:* With abnormal meiosis in the testis, one sperm get both the X and the Y, and the other gets no sex chromosome. If the sperm with no sex chromosome fertilizes a normal (X) ovum, the result is 45,X, which is recognized clinically as **Turner syndrome.**

9. *Define prematurity, and briefly discuss the associated risks:* An infant is premature if it is born before 37 full weeks of gestation. Premature infants are especially at risk for respiratory distress syndrome, because their lungs are not mature, and for severe hyperbilirubinemia, which can cause kernicterus, a syndrome of severe brain damage characterized by deposits of bilirubin in the floor of the third ventricle.

10. *Explain the difference between prematurity and small for gestational age (SGA):* Prematurity is a condition in which the newborn infant is born before the end of the 37th full week of pregnancy. SGA is a condition in which the newborn infant weighs less than predicted for any given gestational age.

11. *Explain the Apgar score and its usefulness:* It is a numerical assessment of an infant's vigor immediately after birth. Points (0, 1, or 2) are awarded for heart rate, respiratory effort, muscle tone, color, and response to a catheter inserted in the nose. The maximum score is ten. Vigorous (high-scoring) infants have low perinatal morbidity and mortality; the opposite is true of low-scoring infants.

12. *Name the most common category of intrauterine growth restriction, and offer some examples:* Most causes are maternal and include toxemia of pregnancy, chronic hypertension, malnutrition, drug or alcohol abuse, and heavy cigarette smoking.

13. *Name the most common type of perinatal infection of the newborn; name and briefly discuss a few common pediatric infections:* Most perinatal infections are bacterial and occur as the infant passes through the vaginal canal, or they are caused by ascending infection from the vagina into the amniotic sac. The most common pediatric infections are viral; many of them cause acute upper respiratory illnesses featuring fever, cough, and rhinorrhea. Some examples of viral infections are measles, rubella, chickenpox, bronchiolitis, and croup. Bacterial infections include whooping cough, diphtheria, and epiglottitis.

14. *Briefly list some of the epidemiologic characteristics of sudden infant death syndrome (SIDS):* SIDS occurs disproportionately with age under 6 months, prone sleeping position, prematurity, low birth weight, male sex, unmarried mothers less than 20 years old, smoking, drug abuse, low socioeconomic condition, and African American ethnicity.

15. *Explain the pathogenesis of erythroblastosis fetalis:* It is an immune hemolytic anemia in infants that occurs in Rh D-negative mothers who have developed anti-Rh D antibodies from a prior pregnancy

with an Rh D-positive infant. Any *subsequent* pregnancy with an Rh D-positive infant runs the risk that her antibodies will attack the infant's red blood cells, causing hemolytic anemia in the infant.

16. *Explain the nature of the metabolic defect in patients with cystic fibrosis:* Cystic fibrosis patients have a defect in the transport of chloride across epithelial cell membranes in ductal glands and in respiratory and gastrointestinal mucus glands. Low chloride in ductal secretions fails to attract sodium; low sodium fails to attract water by osmosis. The result is dehydrated, viscous mucus that obstructs gland ducts and creates a seductive environment for infections.

Typical Test Questions

1. Which one of the following is an example of teratogenesis?
   A. Hyaline membrane disease
   B. Fetal rubella infection at 6 weeks
   C. Acute leukemia
   D. Neonatal pneumonia

2. An autosome is which one of the following?
   A. A somatic cell chromosome
   B. A sex chromosome
   C. A defective gene
   D. A recessive gene

3. The heterozygous state is which one of the following?
   A. Both parents have a gene defect
   B. The patient has one copy of a recessive gene
   C. Half of offspring are affected
   D. Gene expression is high

4. Which of the following is the perinatal period?
   A. The first month after birth
   B. From the 28th week of pregnancy to day 7 of infant life
   C. From conception to delivery
   D. From conception to one month of newborn life.

5. Intrauterine growth restriction is usually caused by which one of the following?
   A. Infection
   B. Fetal factors
   C. Maternal alcohol abuse
   D. Maternal factors

6. True or False? Most term, AGA infants have a brief period of increased blood bilirubin shortly after birth.

7. True or False? Hyaline membrane disease (respiratory distress syndrome) is mainly a disease of prematurity.

8. True or False? Sudden infant death syndrome is usually accompanied by diagnostic changes in brain neurons.

9. True or False? ABO blood group incompatibility is the cause of most hemolytic disease of the newborn.

10. True or False? Intestinal and bronchial gland secretions in cystic fibrosis have low sodium and chloride content.

8

Diseases of the Immune System

This chapter reviews the normal, protective immune system. It also discusses the immune system's overreaction to outside agents (allergy), the antiself reactions of autoimmune diseases, the acquired immunodeficiency syndrome (AIDS) and other immune defects, and malignancies of the immune system.

BACK TO BASICS
- Nonimmune Defense Mechanisms
- The Normal Immune System
- Immunity in Blood Transfusion

CLASSIFICATION OF IMMUNE DISEASE

MECHANISMS OF IMMUNE REACTION
- Type 1 Immune Reaction: Immediate Hypersensitivity
- Type 2 Immune Reaction: Cytotoxic Hypersensitivity
- Type 3 Immune Reaction: Immune-complex Hypersensitivity
- Type 4 Immune Reaction: Cellular (Delayed) Hypersensitivity

HYPERSENSITIVITY DISEASE
- Allergic Disease
- Autoimmune Disease

IMMUNITY IN ORGAN AND TISSUE TRANSPLANTATION

IMMUNITY IN BLOOD TRANSFUSION

AMYLOIDOSIS

IMMUNODEFICIENCY DISEASES
- Inherited Immunodeficiency Diseases
- Acquired Immunodeficiency Syndrome (AIDS)

MALIGNANCIES OF IMMUNE CELLS

Learning Objectives

After studying this chapter you should be able to:

1. Define immunity and autoimmunity
2. Name the two principal nonimmune defense systems
3. Define antigen and antibody
4. Describe the two main types of immune cells
5. Classify antibodies by type of protein, and briefly contrast the differing roles of IgG and IgM in response to antigen challenge
6. Briefly describe the immune reaction in type 1 hypersensitivity disease
7. Explain the principal difference between type 4 hypersensitivity reaction and the other three types
8. Explain the difference between allergic and autoimmune disease
9. Explain what is meant by "molecular mimicry"
10. Briefly discuss the immune mechanism and clinical finding in systemic lupus erythematosus
11. Explain why persons with type A blood cannot be safely transfused with type B blood
12. Explain how B and T cells are affected in AIDS
13. Name the most common AIDS risk groups in developed nations
14. Briefly discus the phases of HIV infection and the appearance of AIDS
15. Explain the role of infections and AIDS-defining neoplasms in HIV infection
16. Name the three main types of malignancies of immune cells

Key Terms and Concepts

BACK TO BASICS
- immune
- antigen
- antibody
- B cell
- T cell
- autoimmune
- immune paint
- immunoglobulin
- Rh positive
- Rh negative

CLASSIFICATION OF IMMUNE DISEASE
- hypersensitivity

MECHANISMS OF IMMUNE HYPERSENSITIVITY
- anaphylaxis
- cytotoxic reaction
- immune complex
- delayed hypersensitivity

HYPERSENSITIVITY DISEASE
- allergen
- atopy
- systemic lupus erythematosus
- antinuclear antibodies
- rheumatoid arthritis

IMMUNITY IN BLOOD TRANSFUSION
- Crossmatch

IMMUNODEFICIENCY DISEASES
- AIDS (acquired immunodeficiency syndrome)
- human immunodeficiency virus (HIV)

MALIGNANCIES OF IMMUNE CELLS
- lymphoma
- lymphocytic leukemia

Immune: Having the capacity to withstand, impervious, insusceptible, proof, resistant, resistive, unsusceptible.

ROGET'S II: THE NEW THESAURUS, THIRD EDITION, 1995

BACK TO BASICS

To be **immune** is to be protected. *Immune* is derived from Latin *im* (without) + *munus* (duty), has been part of the English language for 500 years, and is generally used to indicate exempt status. However, it was not a medical term until the 1880s, when, nearly 100 years after Edward Jenner discovered the principle of vaccination (see the nearby History of Medicine box), the term "immune" began to be used to describe resistance to contagious disease that is conferred by vaccination or previous infection.

In modern medicine "immune" refers to the special function of lymphocytes and macrophages that defends the body against alien ("nonself," foreign) threats, mainly microbes. However, the immune system is not the body's only defense against the environment.

NONIMMUNE DEFENSE MECHANISMS

Nonimmune systems are also important in defending the body against microbes and other environmental threats (Fig. 8-1). The first line of defense is **physical barriers**, each of which has special features:

- *Skin:* Although microbes populate every square inch of skin, skin is not a place where they can grow easily: the epidermis is dry, the surface is composed of dense, indigestible keratin, and the pH is acidic. Disruption of the skin's physical integrity, however (e.g., by needle stick, burn, insect bite), may allow microorganisms to penetrate. Moist skin is more susceptible than is dry skin to invasion by agents such as HIV and syphilis.
- *Sclera:* The white of the eye is washed by tears, which have antibiotic qualities, and wiped clean every few seconds by blinks.
- *Respiratory tract:* With each breath, we inhale at least a few microorganisms, most of which are trapped by nasal and bronchial mucus. Those that reach the bronchi are swept upward to the throat by the bronchial cilia and are swallowed. Some microbes reach the alveoli, where alveolar macrophages ingest and dispose of them. Anything that interferes with these mechanisms promotes respiratory infection.

EDWARD JENNER'S JOY

The joy I felt at the prospect before me of being the instrument destined to take away from the world one of its greatest calamities (smallpox) was so excessive that I found myself in a kind of reverie.

EDWARD JENNER (1749–1823), ENGLISH SURGEON, UPON REALIZING THAT COWPOX VACCINATION COULD PREVENT SMALLPOX.

Smallpox is an infectious viral disease known since antiquity—the mummified remains of Egyptian pharaoh Ramses IV (d. 1156 BC) bears evidence of the disease. As recently as 1967 two million people died of smallpox; however, a massive vaccination effort by the World Health Organization led to elimination of the disease: the last recorded case was in Somalia in 1977. The only remaining smallpox viruses are believed to be in two tightly guarded laboratories, one in Russia the other in the United States.

Jenner is often credited with discovering the principle of vaccination (immunization); however, in a certain sense it is not true. In ancient China and India it was known that purposeful infection of healthy people with "matter" taken from patients with a mild case of smallpox would prevent the recipient from ever becoming infected again. Jenner's contribution—one of the most important in the history of medicine—is that inoculation (vaccination) of people with "matter" from innocuous cowpox infections could prevent smallpox infection.

The tale of Jenner's discovery is well known. In May of 1796, Jenner found a young dairymaid, Sarah Nelmes, with fresh cowpox sores. He collected some of the fluid from her lesions and on May 14 inoculated James Phipps, an eight-year-old boy. The youngster became mildly ill for a few days but quickly recovered, and on July 1 Jenner inoculated the boy with smallpox matter. No disease developed. Over the next two years Jenner repeated his experiment on more patients and was always successful. He published his results in 1798, the practice spread around the world, and smallpox infections and deaths plunged.

For example, alcohol impairs the sweeping motion of the bronchial cilia so that chronic alcoholics are prone to bacterial pneumonia; cigarette smoke has much the same effect. In cystic fibrosis (Chapter 7) the viscosity of the bronchial mucus is so great that it cannot be moved effectively by the cilia, and severe pulmonary infections result.

- *Gastrointestinal tract*: The intestinal tract is defended by multiple mechanisms, including a protective layer of mucus, gastric acid, pancreatic enzymes, and detergent bile salts. Gastrointestinal epithelial cells are shed daily, making it difficult for organisms or particles to gain a strong grip. Moreover, countless nonpathogenic bacteria—the normal intestinal flora—make their home in the intestinal lumen, and any pathogen must out-compete them for nutrients to gain an infective foothold. Alteration of the flora (by antibiotics, for example) may allow pathogens to establish residence or allow minor populations of normal flora to cause disease by overwhelming growth.
- *Genitourinary tract*: Urine is normally sterile because it is acidic and flushed constantly by a system designed to avoid retrograde flow. However, stagnant urine associated with urinary obstruction encourages bacterial growth. Once infection is established, it tends to spread upward. For example, infection of the bladder or prostate may ascend to infect the kidney.

In addition to these physical barriers, body fluids are sifted and flushed regularly through various filtering apparatuses, each of which can capture and dispose of infective agents. Blood constantly passes through the spleen and bone marrow so that blood is filtered thousands of times a day. Furthermore, lymph nodes are populated with a variety of immune and nonimmune cells to destroy alien material, and lymph fluid is continuously collected from all tissues and passed through them on its way to remixing with blood via the thoracic duct.

In addition to physical barriers, there are several **innate (nonimmune) cellular and molecular defenses**.

- *Phagocytosis*: Through their engulfing function, macrophages and white blood cells ingest, digest, and dispose of bacteria, viruses, and other foreign material. Macrophages inhabit virtually every organ of the body: Kupffer cells in the liver, alveolar macrophages in the lungs, monocytes and granulocytes in the circulating blood and in the bone marrow, microglia in the brain, and dense accumulations of macrophages in the spleen and lymph nodes.
- *Natural killer cells*: Natural killer cells are so named because of their innate ability to kill cancer cells or virus-infected cells. Natural killer cells reside in lymph nodes, spleen, and other collections of lymphoid tissue.

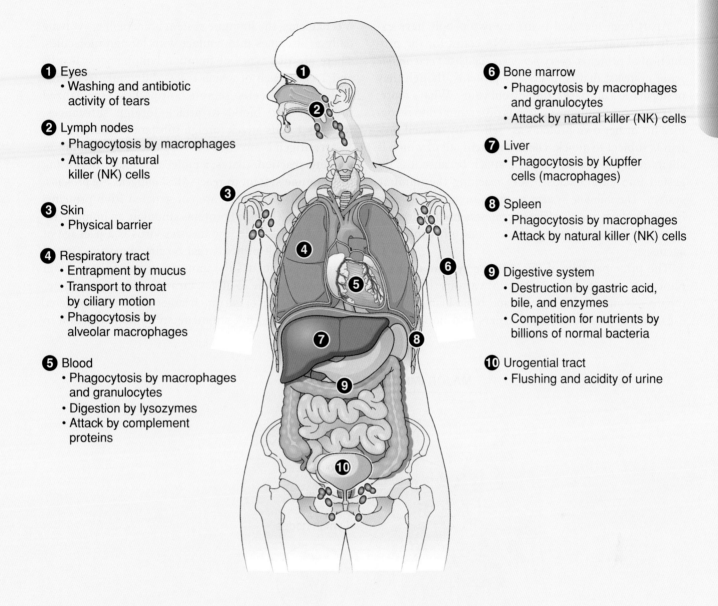

1 Eyes
- Washing and antibiotic activity of tears

2 Lymph nodes
- Phagocytosis by macrophages
- Attack by natural killer (NK) cells

3 Skin
- Physical barrier

4 Respiratory tract
- Entrapment by mucus
- Transport to throat by ciliary motion
- Phagocytosis by alveolar macrophages

5 Blood
- Phagocytosis by macrophages and granulocytes
- Digestion by lysozymes
- Attack by complement proteins

6 Bone marrow
- Phagocytosis by macrophages and granulocytes
- Attack by natural killer (NK) cells

7 Liver
- Phagocytosis by Kupffer cells (macrophages)

8 Spleen
- Phagocytosis by macrophages
- Attack by natural killer (NK) cells

9 Digestive system
- Destruction by gastric acid, bile, and enzymes
- Competition for nutrients by billions of normal bacteria

10 Urogential tract
- Flushing and acidity of urine

Figure 8-1 **Nonimmune antimicrobial protective mechanisms.** The numbered areas show the functions of various organs and systems that defend against bacteria and other microbes.

- *Lysozymes*: The intracellular digestive enzymes of some cells, notably granulocytes in the peripheral blood such as neutrophils, kill and digest foreign agents.
- *Complement system*: A group of about 20 proteins generates a *membrane attack complex* that digests the cell membranes of microbes, stimulates white blood cell activity, and increases vascular permeability at the site of infection, ensuring delivery of other body cellular defense elements

THE NORMAL IMMUNE SYSTEM

The immune system differs from innate defenses in a key way: the immune system is *programmable* to defend against and attack a specific target; innate defenses are not. Think of innate defenses as a medieval castle surrounded by a moat. The moat is a passive, general defense that will slow or stop horse, ox, or human. The immune system is like archers defending the castle by shooting from the walls: the archers can aim for specific targets.

Apart from identical twins, no two people have exactly the same DNA. Because DNA codes for the production of proteins, *every person is composed of a unique set of proteins*; that is to say, my proteins, though they perform the same tasks, differ from yours. What's more, every person's immune system is programmed to recognize his or her own proteins as "self." Any nonself protein is subject to attack. Dietary protein, all of which is alien, does not invoke immune attach because it is digested into amino acids before reaching the immune system. *The immune system is, therefore, a programmable, molecularly specific defense against nonself molecules,* especially against bacteria, viruses, and other infective agents.

The principal cells of the immune system are lymphocytes, which are located in various lymphoid organs—lymph nodes, spleen, and bone marrow (Fig. 8-2). In contrast to surface barriers and nonimmune mechanisms, the immune system is adaptable, evolving daily as it comes into contact with foreign molecules. There are two types of immune lymphocytes: B cells and T cells, each of which reacts differently to foreign molecules. **B cells** secrete antibodies (specialized proteins) into blood to attack foreign substances, whereas **T cells** attack foreign substances directly.

An **antigen** is any molecule capable of stimulating an immune reaction; that is, a molecule capable of causing the immune system to react. *Most antigens are proteins.* Because all of our cells are constructed from proteins, only nonself (foreign) proteins stimulate an immune reaction. For example, the measles virus is a package of foreign, nonself proteins that on first exposure (initial infection) stimulates the immune system to reprogram itself permanently to attack measles virus forevermore. A transplanted liver is a much larger package of antigens, antigens that did not stimulate an immune reaction in

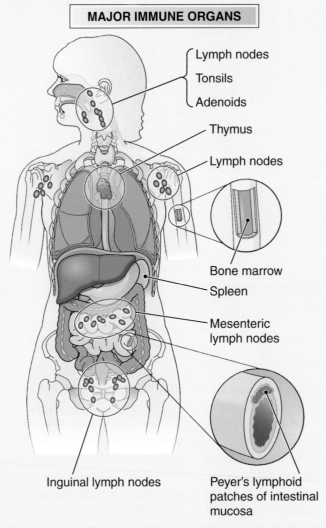

MAJOR IMMUNE ORGANS

Lymph nodes
Tonsils
Adenoids
Thymus
Lymph nodes
Bone marrow
Spleen
Mesenteric lymph nodes
Inguinal lymph nodes
Peyer's lymphoid patches of intestinal mucosa

Figure 8-2 **The immune system.** The anatomic locations of major immune organs are shown here. Bone marrow and all lymph nodes contain B cells, T cells, macrophages, and other immune cells.

the donor because they were self but that become non-self the moment they are transplanted. Keeping in mind liver transplants as an example, *it is important to remember in our discussion that when the word "antigen" is used it does not necessarily mean "foreign" or "nonself." All proteins are antigens, but they are foreign only to someone else. We will refer repeatedly to the normal proteins that make up all "self" cells, including immune cells, and we will often call them antigens.*

In addition to nonself protein, some otherwise harmless, *small, nonprotein* can stimulate an immune reaction by combining with a self-protein in such a way that the *combination becomes nonself.* Molecules that behave in this way are called **haptens.** For example, the skin rash of poison ivy is an immune reaction caused by a hapten.

Immune reactions demonstrate their effect through the production of **cytokines,** which are small, soluble molecules that promote and sustain inflammation and other effects to neutralize or destroy the target.

Programming the Immune System

The immune system is composed of two types of cells: lymphocytes and macrophages.

There are two types of *lymphocytes—B cells* and *T cells—*each of which reacts differently to nonself antigens. Some antigens incite T-cell immunity; others incite B-cell immunity. When stimulated by nonself antigen, **B cells** (**B lymphocytes**) release programmed attack proteins, **antibodies,** into the circulation. Antigenically stimulated B lymphocytes are microscopically distinctive and are called **plasma cells.** Antigenic stimulation of **T cells** (**T lymphocytes**) causes programming and release of attack cells (**cytotoxic T cells**). B-cell antibodies and cytotoxic T cells are *anti*-antigens, which attack the protein (antigen) of nonself microbes, cells, and pollens, and kill them directly or incite an inflammatory reaction (Chapter 3) to neutralize and eliminate them.

In the fetus, B cells are developed by the *bone* marrow and T cells by the *thymus.* In the embryonic stage, many B cells and T cells *initially* are capable of reacting with self, but after passing through the bone marrow and thymus cells capable of reacting with self are eliminated; that is, the immune system is purged of cells capable of reacting with self. However, there are two important exceptions: a few B and T cells capable of reacting with self remain alive but are held in check by the immune system. The reason for this exception is not clear. It is helpful to think of these exceptions as potential immune "time bombs," which sometimes attack self antigens. Attack by such cells is *one* of several mechanisms for the production of **autoimmune** disease—disease in which

the immune system attacks self, the body's own proteins, instead of foreign (nonself) proteins.

The interaction of antigen with B and T cells and the consequences are depicted in Figure 8-3. There are two main types of immune reactions:

- *normal* protective immune reactions, in which T and B cells react to attack and destroy foreign antigens
- *autoimmune* reactions, in which the T-cell and B-cell reactions are against self tissue

Macrophages play an important role in the immune system: they digest, prepare, and present foreign antigens to T cells, as is depicted in Figure 8-3. Macrophages have on their surface certain self proteins that act as *receptors* to capture, hold, and present *foreign* antigen to T lymphocytes. For historical reasons these normal receptor proteins are popularly known as **human lymphocyte antigens (HLA).** HLA antigens are also known as major histocompatibility complex antigens (MHC antigens) because they are coded by a large family of genes known as the **major histocompatibility complex (MHC)** and because MHC antigens are a major cause of tissue transplant rejection by the immune system. Basics in Brief 8-1 explains the clinical importance of HLA antigens.

B lymphocytes: The Humoral Immune System

B cells react directly with freely circulating antigen and secrete antibodies into the circulation, where they combine with antigens. Because of this feature, the B-cell system is termed **humoral immunity** after the old term for mythical substances, called humors, thought to be circulating in the blood as the cause of all disease. However, *B-cell function is critically dependent on the T-cell system.* Certain T cells help or suppress B-cell activity. These relationships are depicted in Figure 8-3.

B cells are initially processed and programmed in the fetal bone marrow and then spread to other lymphoid organs. They constitute about 10–20% of circulating lymphocytes and are also found in lymph nodes, bone marrow, tonsils, spleen, and lymphoid patches of the bronchial and gastrointestinal mucosa (Peyer patches, or mucosa associated lymphoid tissue, MALT). Bronchial and intestinal mucus contains high concentrations of a certain type of antibody—the mucosal "**immune paint**"—which provides special protection for the gastrointestinal and respiratory mucosa, both of which are exposed to very high numbers of environmental microbes and other antigens. Antibodies are a prime defense mechanism against bacterial infection, but are less effective against other microbes.

Not all B cells produce antibody; some are programmed as **memory B cells,** which linger in the body,

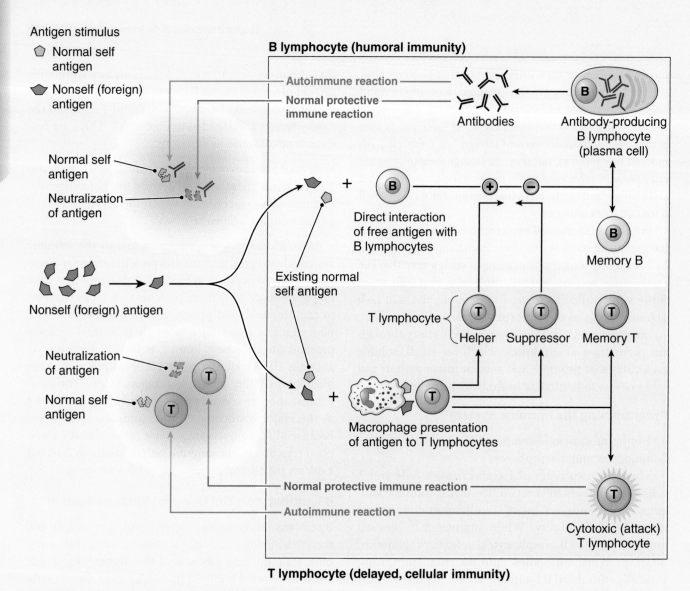

Antigen stimulus

⬠ Normal self antigen

⬟ Nonself (foreign) antigen

B lymphocyte (humoral immunity)

Autoimmune reaction
Normal protective immune reaction
Antibodies
Antibody-producing B lymphocyte (plasma cell)

Normal self antigen
Neutralization of antigen

Direct interaction of free antigen with B lymphocytes

Memory B

Existing normal self antigen

Nonself (foreign) antigen

T lymphocyte
Helper Suppressor Memory T

Neutralization of antigen
Normal self antigen

Macrophage presentation of antigen to T lymphocytes

Normal protective immune reaction
Autoimmune reaction

Cytotoxic (attack) T lymphocyte

T lymphocyte (delayed, cellular immunity)

Figure 8-3 **Sequence of immune reactions.** In normal protective immune reactions, an alien (nonself) antigen stimulates T and B cells, which react to neutralize it. In autoimmune reactions, self antigen stimulates T- and B-cell reactions against itself for reasons that are usually unknown.

BASICS IN BRIEF 8-1

HLA ANTIGENS

HLA antigens (also known as major histocompatibility complex, MHC antigens) are present on the surface of every cell except red blood cells. On macrophages they serve the critical task of capturing and holding nonself antigens for presentation to T lymphocytes in order to program the immune system. However, they have two other critical roles in medicine.

First, HLA antigens are the prime reason tissue transplants are rejected. As "self" antigens they are capable of inciting an immune reaction in *another* person if they are transplanted. For example, the HLA antigens in a transplanted heart are "nonself" to the recipient and incite the recipient's immune system to attack HLA antigens in the transplanted heart much the same as it does to the measles virus or any other alien antigen.

Second, HLA antigens tend to be associated with certain diseases. HLA antigens vary from person to person. Each human has a different set, but they also share common features that allow them to be sorted into subtypes. Certain HLA subtypes are associated with certain diseases, especially autoimmune genetic diseases. For example, people with HLA-B27 subtype have a much higher prevalence of rheumatic diseases. As a result HLA typing can be used as a diagnostic tool in the investigation of some diseases.

ready to react quickly the next time the antigen appears. The production of memory B cells is the scientific foundation for vaccinations against infection. A vaccine stimulates B cells to produce antibodies, but it also stimulates the production of memory B cells that are ready to respond quickly to later exposure to the infective agent.

Antibodies (Immunoglobulins)

Antibodies are formed from a type of protein known as **immunoglobulin**, which is made by lymphocytes and constitutes about 20% of blood protein. Each immunoglobulin is composed of two *heavy chain* molecules and two *light chain* molecules. There are five types of immunoglobulins, each with a different molecular structure and different role in immune reactions—immunoglobulins G, A, M, D, and E (abbreviated IgG, IgA, and so on). Immunoglobulins are named after the heavy chain component; thus, IgG contains G-type heavy chain. Immunoglobulins are part of the *gamma globulin* fraction of blood protein (Chapter 11).

Most immunity arises from endogenous (internal) production of antibodies by the person's own immune system. However, antibodies can be transferred passively (**passive immunity**) to confer temporary immunity, as in the case of antibody injections (gamma globulin injections) to prevent infection. Additionally, fetuses and newborn infants gain temporary immunity by passive transfer of antibody from mother to infant across the placenta and in breast milk.

The immune system produces each type of immunoglobulin for a particular purpose. **IgM antibodies** are formed quickly after antigen challenge and constitute the immediate response of the immune system to provide quick, short-term protection. IgM antibodies have a short life span and are replaced after a few weeks or months by IgG antibodies that confer long-term protection (Fig. 8-4). IgM, because it is the largest and heaviest type of immunoglobulin molecule, is also known as **macroglobulin**.

IgG antibodies are the most abundant immunoglobulin in blood; they appear after IgM antibodies and confer long-term immunity. For example, after measles vaccination, long-lasting anti-measles IgG type antibodies are produced.

IgA antibodies are heavily concentrated in breast milk, and in respiratory tract and gastrointestinal mucus, where they form a mucosal "immune paint," discussed above, that protects those systems from inhaled and ingested foreign infective agents.

IgD and IgE do not circulate in blood but are confined to tissues and inflammatory cells. IgD helps B cells in their immune role. IgE is important in tissue reactions to pollens and other non-bacterial antigens (allergies).

Antibodies achieve their effect by attaching to the target foreign antigen, which is often part of a tissue or microbial cell membrane. They achieve their effect by 1) blocking the function of the antigen; 2) rupturing the cell membrane to cause cell death; 3) inciting an inflammatory reaction to neutralize or digest the cell or

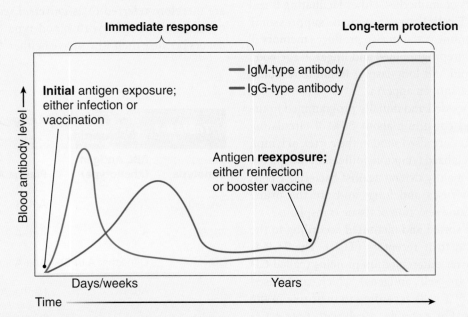

Figure 8-4 **Antibody response to antigen exposure.** On initial antigen exposure IgM-type antibody is produced first, providing quick protection but no permanent immunity. IgG-type antibody levels soon rise and provide additional immune defense and permanent immunity. On re-exposure IgG antibody rises quickly to prevent infection.

microbe; or 4) making the cell or microbe more suscep-tible to phagocytosis.

An antibody may attach to freely circulating antigen to form an **antigen-antibody complex (immune complex)**. These complexes may lodge in tissues and injure them by inciting an inflammatory reaction. Antibodies and immune complexes in blood can be de-tected by diagnostic laboratory tests. For example, pa-tients with rheumatoid arthritis usually have in their blood an immune complex known as rheumatoid factor (Chapter 22), which can be detected by a simple labo-ratory test.

T Lymphocytes: The Cellular Immune System

The T-cell system is termed **cellular immunity** because, when stimulated by nonself antigen, T cells are pro-grammed and released into the circulation to attack antigen directly (no antibodies are produced). T cells are "blind" to free antigen; they do not react to freely circulating foreign antigen as B cells do. T cells react only to antigen presented to them by macrophages or related cells. Because the reaction takes longer to de-velop than B-cell reactions, usually a few days, T-cell reactions are also termed **delayed immunity**.

T cells have two main roles in immunity. First, they can be programmed to recognize and attack a specific nonself antigen. Such cells are called **cytotoxic T cells** (or killer T cells) and attach to the antigen using a re-ceptor on their cell membrane, the **T-cell receptor (TCR)**. Second, certain T cells modulate B cells in their role as producers of antibodies, either facilitating B-cell activity (**helper T cells**) or restraining it (**suppressor T cells**). T-cell immune reaction also produces **memory T cells**, which are preprogrammed and linger in the body to produce a rapid and long-lasting immune response the next time the antigen appears.

T cells are processed and initially programmed in the fetal thymus and constitute about 80% of circulating lymphocytes. They are also found in the cortex of lymph nodes and in specialized lymphoid follicles in the spleen. Whereas B cells mainly defend against bacteria, T cells defend against viruses and fungi and are the prime mediator in immune rejection of tissue transplants.

T cells can be sorted and identified according to the type of protein in their receptors (TCR). The TCR is composed of cluster differentiation proteins (called **CD antigens**, which are "self" antigens), which can be used to classify types of T cells according to their role in the immune process. For example, a cell with type 4 CD antigen is designated CD4+. Most helper T cells are CD4+; most cytotoxic T cells are CD8+.

IMMUNITY IN BLOOD TRANSFUSION

RBC **major blood groups** (A, B, O) are determined by specific genes: a set that codes for the A and B blood group proteins on red cells. Often, however, the genes are null: they do not code for a protein. The null state is called O.

Children receive one A or B gene from each parent, so that the *genetic* combinations (the *genotypes*) are AA, AB, BB, AO, BO, and OO. The A and B genes are Mendelian dominant (Chapter 7), therefore the geno-types and clinical blood groups (the phenotypes) are as follows (genotype listed first, *clinical blood group [the phenotype]* in parentheses): AA (*clinical type A*), AB (*clinical type AB*), BB (*clinical type B*), AO (*clinical type A*), BO (*clinical type B*), and OO (*clinical type O*). The result is that there are four major A-B clinical blood groups: A, B, AB, and O.

Additionally, blood groups have naturally occurring plasma **agglutinins** (naturally occurring antibodies), capable of clumping (agglutinating) RBCs. Table 8-1 lists the various combinations of genes and resulting blood groups and agglutinins. Clinical type A blood contains anti-B plasma agglutinin, capable of clumping clinical type B blood. Type B blood has anti-A plasma agglutinin. Clinical blood type O has both anti-A and anti-B plasma agglutinins, and clinical type AB blood has neither anti-A nor anti-B plasma agglutinin. Therefore, patients with type AB blood can receive blood of any type (A, B, or O) because they have neither anti-A nor anti-B agglutinins in their plasma to aggluti-nate the A or B antigens of any other blood type. They are therefore referred to as *universal recipients*. On the other hand, persons with blood type O are *universal donors* because their RBCs have neither A nor B antigens

Table 8-1	Red Blood Cell Antigens and Agglutinins	
Genotype	**RBC Antigen (Phenotype)**	**Plasma Agglutinin**
AA, AO	A	Anti-B
BB, BO	B	Anti-A
OO	O (neither A or B)	Anti-A and Anti-B
AB	AB	Neither Anti-A nor Anti-B
Rh D positive	Rh D positive	No Rh agglutinin
Rh D null	Rh D negative	No Rh agglutinin

to be agglutinated by the anti-A or anti-B in other blood types.

In addition to A, B, and O groupings, every person's red blood cells have an **Rh type**, so named for the *Rhesus* monkeys in which they were first discovered. Multiple Rh genes and antigens exist, but only Rh D has enough antigenic strength to be of clinical importance. Patients who have the Rh D gene have Rh D antigen on their red blood cells and are said to be **Rh positive**; patients without Rh D antigen are said to be **Rh negative**. About 85% of the United States population is Rh D positive. No naturally occurring anti-Rh agglutinins exist. However, anti-Rh antibodies may be created in some clinical circumstances.

One of the most important consequences of Rh differences among people is that Rh-*negative* mothers may develop anti-Rh antibodies if they become sensitized (immunized) by carrying an Rh-*positive* fetus. These antibodies can attack Rh-positive *fetal* RBC in subsequent pregnancies, a condition known as *erythro-blastosis fetalis* (Chapter 7). Maternal sensitization can be prevented by drug therapy; therefore, newborn and maternal Rh blood typing is standard practice.

There are hundreds of **minor blood groups** classified according to weak antigens on the RBC cell membrane, including antigens such as *Lewis*, *Kell*, and *Duffy*. They are not potent and rarely cause clinical transfusion problems. They do not figure in transfusion calculations unless antibodies against them are present in the plasma of a patient who needs a transfusion. These minor blood group antibodies develop at the time of a *prior* blood transfusion with red cells containing a minor blood group antigen for which the recipient is negative. For example, a *Lewis*-negative person may have previously been transfused with Lewis-positive RBCs and developed anti-*Lewis* antibodies. Prior to a subsequent transfusion, the potential recipient's blood is screened for such antibodies. If antibodies are detected, the patient is transfused with blood that does not have the antigen in question.

MAJOR DETERMINANTS OF DISEASE

- The immune system attacks microbes and related threats from the environment.
- Immune deficiency is associated with infection.
- The immune system monitors tissues to eliminate cells with precancerous changes.
- Immune deficiency is associated with increased risk of malignancy.
- The immune system may over-react (allergy, hypersensitivity) to certain foreign molecules (antigens).
- The immune system may attack the body's own tissue (autoimmunity).
- Autoimmune and allergic reactions cause tissue damage and inflammation
- Immune cells can become malignant.

Classification of Immune Disease

There is no completely satisfactory system for categorizing immune disease. The big picture is best described by the following classification:

1. **Hypersensitivity disease** is an *exaggerated* immune reaction to certain antigens or other molecules. Most hypersensitivity diseases are **autoimmune** disease and allergy. An **allergy** is an exaggerated immune reaction to an environmental substance (**allergen**), usually from a plant or, less commonly, microorganisms or metal. Allergens have no detectable effect on non-allergic people.
2. *Miscellaneous immune conditions,* such as transfusion and tissue transplant reactions and other conditions.
3. **Immunodeficiency** disease, such as infection by the human immunodeficiency virus (HIV), in which immune defenses are defective and infection is the most common consequence.
4. *Malignancy* of immune cells, such as lymphoma, leukemia, and related tumors (Chapter 11).

Mechanisms of Immune Reaction

Every *hypersensitivity disease* (whether an allergy or an autoimmune disease) involves one of four basic immune mechanisms.

- B-cell reactions
  - Type I, immediate hypersensitivity
  - Type 2, cytotoxic hypersensitivity
  - Type 3, immune complex hypersensitivity
- T-cell reaction
  - Type 4, cellular (delayed) hypersensitivity

TYPE 1 IMMUNE REACTION: IMMEDIATE HYPERSENSITIVITY

Type 1 immune reaction (immediate hypersensitivity, Fig. 8-5) is an immediate (within minutes) reaction that occurs when antigen combines with *preformed* antibody that is attached to mast cells (tissue basophils). The preformed antibody is created by a previous exposure (the initial, sensitizing exposure) to the antigen. The sensitizing exposure produces no symptoms, but it sets the stage for a rapid reaction on subsequent exposure.

On *initial, sensitizing* exposure to the antigen, IgE antibodies are produced by B cells and attach to mast cells, coating the mast cell with programmed, specific antibody against the invading antigen. On *subsequent* exposure the antigen combines with IgE antibody already present on the surface of mast cells and triggers an instant reaction: inflammatory and vasoactive substances are released from mast cell granules, causing vasodilation, increased capillary permeability and accumulation of edema, an influx of eosinophils and other inflammatory cells into the site, and increased numbers of eosinophils in blood (eosinophilia). Typical type I reactions include "hay fever" (allergic rhinitis), hives, and some cases of asthma

Anaphylaxis (from Greek, *ana*, away from, + *phylaxis*, protection) is an especially a severe type I reaction that results in immediate and widespread release of inflammatory and vasoactive substances from mast cells, provoking widespread vasodilation and edema. Vasodilation causes flushing, low blood pressure, and fainting or shock, and accumulation of edema can cause swelling of skin, puffy eyes, or airway obstruction caused by laryngeal edema. In some cases smooth muscle spasm can occur and cause severe bronchial restriction (bronchospasm).

Immediate hypersensitivity may be local or generalized depending on the route of exposure. For example, anaphylactic reaction to an intravenous drug is more likely to be general and may include high blood count of eosinophils, skin erythema and hives, copious bronchial and nasal mucin production, laryngeal edema, and bronchospasm. Death can occur because of vascular collapse or to asphyxiation from laryngeal edema or bronchospasm. In local reactions the eosinophilic inflammation occurs at the site of antigen contact and includes the nose (hay fever), the bronchi (some asthma), and the skin (allergic eczema, Chapter 24).

TYPE 2 IMMUNE REACTION: CYTOTOXIC HYPERSENSITIVITY

As is illustrated in Figure 8-6, a **type 2 immune reaction** (cytotoxic hypersensitivity) is one in which an *antibody attaches directly to an antigen in the target tissue*, usually a cell membrane. The antibody-coated cell membrane is susceptible to rupture (cytolysis) and phagocytic destruction by other cells. It is not clear why cell membranes sometimes lose their "self" identity and become alien and incite a reaction against self.

Two types of cytotoxic reactions occur. The first type (Fig. 8-6A) results in death of the target cell—the cell is coated by antibodies, which render it susceptible to destruction by macrophages or inflammatory cells. Immune hemolytic anemia (Chapter 11) results from direct red cell destruction (lysis) by cytotoxic antibodies. In the second type of cytotoxic reaction (Fig. 8-6B), IgG antibodies bind to target-cell membrane receptors and block receptor function. For example, in *myasthenia gravis* (Chapter 23) an autoimmune antibody attaches to acetylcholine receptors on the muscle side of the neuromuscular connection, preventing transmission of the nerve signal to muscle.

TYPE 3 IMMUNE REACTION: IMMUNE-COMPLEX HYPERSENSITIVITY

Type 3 immune reaction (immune complex hypersensitivity) is an immune reaction in which antigen and antibody combine to form an **immune complex**. Formation of these complexes is the cause of most *autoimmune* disease. As is illustrated in Figure 8-7, immune complexes form in one place and circulate to be deposited elsewhere. They incite an inflammatory reaction and activation of the *complement system*, one of the nonimmune defense mechanisms mentioned earlier in this chapter. These complexes often circulate in blood and deposit in blood vessels to produce vasculitis (Chapter 12) and other effects at sites far from the point at which they combined, or they may remain at the point of formation and cause a local reaction.

In *distant* (or disseminated) type 3 reactions the complexes circulate away from the site of their formation and deposit in kidneys, joints, skin, heart, serosal surfaces, or small blood vessels (Fig. 8-7A). For example, deposition of immune complexes in various organs causes the manifestations of systemic lupus erythematosus.

In *local* type 3 reactions (Fig. 8-7B), the immune complexes remain in situ at the site of antigen introduction and do not circulate in blood. For example, inhaled hay mold (a fungus) may lodge in the lung and stimulate production of antifungus antibody that combines locally with the inhaled antigen to cause autoimmune pneumonia. The antibodies combine with mold trapped in the alveoli to form an immune complex, which activates the complement system and causes

TYPE 1 IMMUNE REACTION (IMMEDIATE HYPERSENSITIVITY)

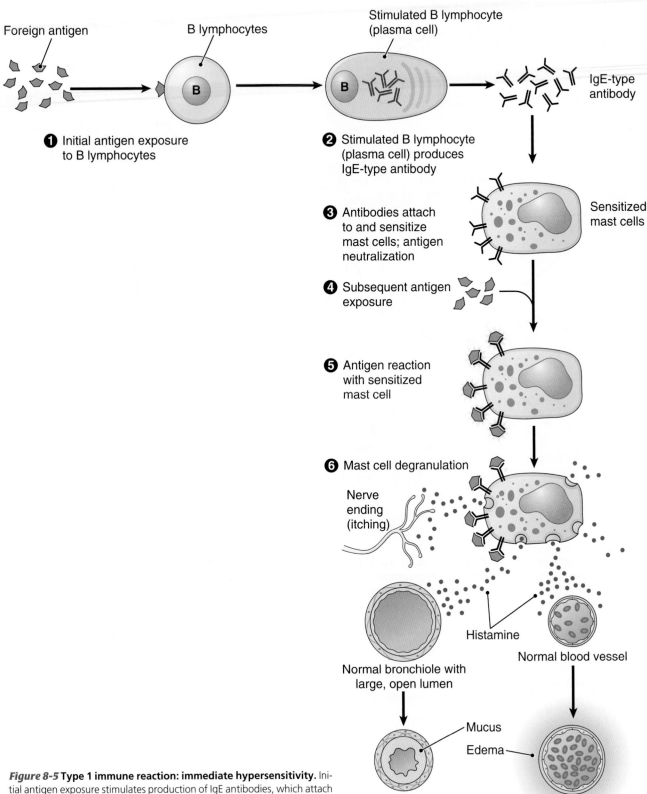

Figure 8-5 **Type 1 immune reaction: immediate hypersensitivity.** Initial antigen exposure stimulates production of IgE antibodies, which attach to the surface of mast cells. On subsequent exposure the antigen combines with antibody on the mast cell surface to stimulate immediate release of histamine from mast cell cytoplasmic granules, which causes itching; bronchospasm, wheezing, and shortness of breath; and vasodilation and edema formation with low blood pressure, weakness, and tissue swelling.

TYPE 2 IMMUNE REACTION (CYTOTOXIC HYPERSENSITIVITY)

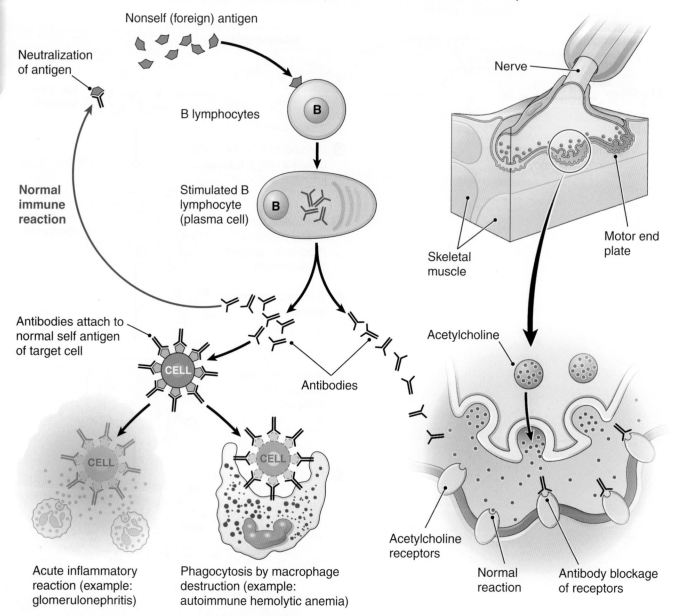

A **Autoimmune reaction:** Inflammation or target cell death

B **Autoimmune reaction:** Interference with target cell function (example: motor end plate of nerves in myasthenia gravis)

Figure 8-6 **Type 2 immune reaction: cytotoxic hypersensitivity. A.** Antibodies attach to target cell, which is destroyed by phagocytosis or inflammation. **B.** Antibodies attach to target-cell receptors and interfere with target-cell function, as in the blockage of signal transmission from nerve to muscle in myasthenia gravis.

TYPE 3 IMMUNE REACTION (IMMUNE COMPLEX HYPERSENSITIVITY)

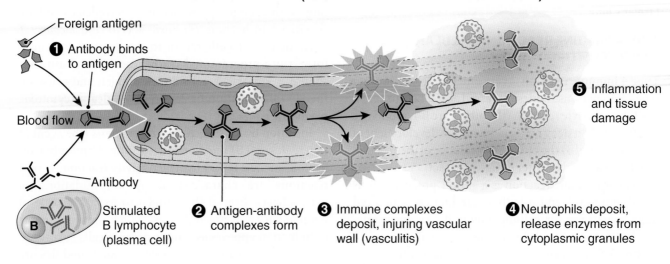

A Autoimmune reaction: Circulating immune complex reaction

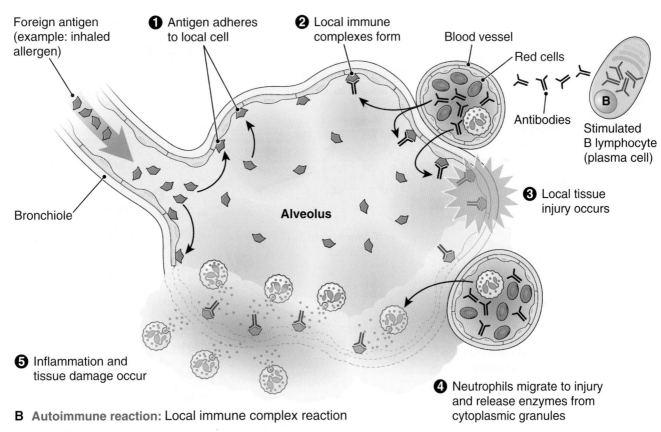

B Autoimmune reaction: Local immune complex reaction

Figure 8-7 **Type 3 immune reaction: immune-complex hypersensitivity.** Antigen and antibody bind together to create an immune complex. **A.** In circulating (distant, or disseminated) autoimmune reactions, immune complexes cause vasculitis and widespread tissue damage. **B.** In local autoimmune reactions, immune complexes form and remain locally to cause damage (as with allergic pneumonia caused by inhaled antigens).

local inflammation, a type of pneumonia known as *farmer's lung.*

TYPE 4 IMMUNE REACTION: CELLULAR HYPERSENSITIVITY

Type 4 immune reaction is very different from the other types of hypersensitivities discussed above because: 1) it is a T-lymphocyte reaction (the others are B-lymphocyte reactions); 2) it does not depend on the development of antibodies; and 3) the clinical appearance of the reaction is delayed a few days after antigen contact.

Type 4 immune reaction is a slower process than is B-cell immunity, and it is therefore known as **delayed hypersensitivity** (or **cellular immunity** because it depends on direct attack by T cells). As is illustrated in Figure 8-8, antigen is captured by macrophages for presentation to T lymphocytes. T lymphocytes react only to the antigen presented by macrophages and are sensitized to become *cytotoxic T cells* and *memory T cells.* Memory T cells return to the immune system to form a pre-programmed ready reserve for future response. Cytotoxic T cells attack antigen and cause either 1) inflammation or 2) direct cell death (cytotoxic reaction).

Infection by *Mycobacterium tuberculosis* (the agent of tuberculosis; TB) and some deep fungus and other infections incite a type 4 hypersensitivity reaction. Type 4 reactions are characterized by accumulations of macrophages around the antigen to form a nodule of lymphocytes and macrophages, which on microscopic examination appears as a mass of large cells surrounding a central area of tissue necrosis. Such nodules are

TYPE 4 IMMUNE REACTION (DELAYED, CELLULAR HYPERSENSITIVITY)

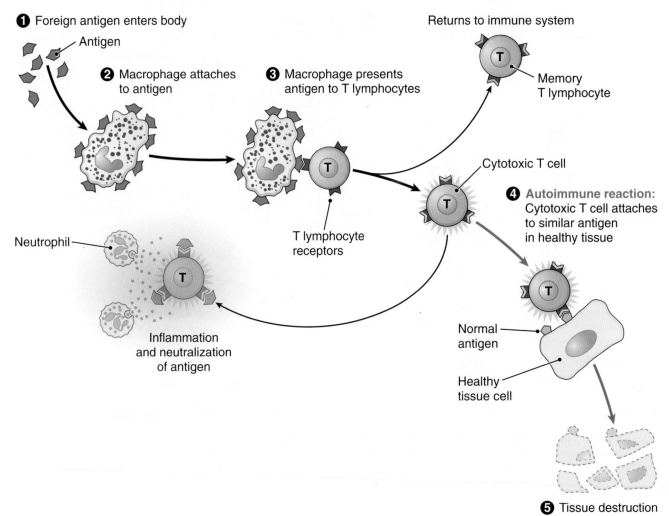

Figure 8-8 **Type 4 immune reaction: cellular hypersensitivity.** Macrophages capture antigen and present it to T lymphocytes, thus programming (sensitizing) them. Some lymphocytes become cytotoxic T cells that attack the antigen wherever it is found; others become memory T cells and return to the immune system to be ready for prompt response in the future.

called **granulomas** (Chapter 3), and they are particularly characteristic of the chronic inflammatory immune reaction to the TB bacillus. Type 4 immune inflammation is the basis for a TB skin test, the *Mantoux test*. Antigen from TB bacilli is injected into skin; a positive reaction takes 48 hours to appear.

Cytotoxicity is the mode of type 4 hypersensitivity T-cell reaction that is important in tissue transplant rejection. However, the most common cytotoxic T-cell reaction is contact dermatitis, caused by poison ivy, rubber gloves, metallic jewelry, and other substances. The skin reaction to these substances does not appear clinically for 2–3 days after exposure.

Hypersensitivity Disease

Many diseases are the result of a hypersensitivity reaction, but the two most important types are:

- **Allergy**, which is an exaggerated immune sensitivity to certain environmental compounds, usually plants, or, less commonly, microorganisms, metals, and other materials. Examples are poison ivy skin rash, seasonal rhinitis from airborne pollens, and reactions to certain foods. *Most allergic disease is caused by a type I immune reaction.*
- **Autoimmune** disease, which is an immune reaction to the body's own (self) tissues. Rheumatoid arthritis is an example. *Most autoimmune disease is caused by type 3 immune reaction.*

> **Inflammation is the main consequence of an autoimmune reaction.**

ALLERGIC DISEASE

Allergy is exaggerated immune reactivity (hypersensitivity) to certain environmental substances (**allergens**) that normally have little effect on most people. The hypersensitivity is established on initial exposure to the allergen (the sensitizing "dose"); subsequent exposure causes the hypersensitivity reaction. Most allergic reactions are mediated by the type I (anaphylaxis) immune mechanism. Allergic disease is fundamentally different from autoimmune disease. In allergy the reaction is an exaggerated but otherwise normal immune response against foreign antigen, whereas in autoimmune disease the immune system attacks self antigens.

Atopy (from Greek, meaning out of the way or unusual) is a hereditary predisposition toward developing certain hypersensitivity reactions, such as hay fever, asthma, or chronic urticaria, upon exposure to specific allergens. *Hay fever* (seasonal allergic rhinitis) is caused by wind-borne pollens from trees, grasses, and weeds. It is characterized by sneezing, runny nose (rhinorrhea), and nasal congestion and usually occurs in spring or fall. *Allergic conjunctivitis* is caused by similar allergens, often occurs at the same time as hay fever, and is characterized by sclera and eyelid congestion, tearing, edema, and itching. *Atopic dermatitis* (atopic eczema, endogenous eczema, Chapter 24) is the most common type of dermatitis, affecting about 5–10% of the United States population, and frequently it occurs in patients with other atopic disease. The lesions are usually very itchy, and usually wax and wane with symptoms of hay fever or other allergies.

Acute systemic anaphylaxis is an explosive, generalized type I immune reaction that can cause fatal vascular collapse from systemic vasodilation (vascular relaxation) or bronchospasm and sometimes occurs when the offending allergen finds its way into the general circulation. The most common causative agents are injectable therapeutic drugs, blood (transfused) or blood products, insect stings, and some foods. Very small amounts of allergen can precipitate acute systemic anaphylaxis; in some cases the amount is so small that the agent and the route of exposure are unknown.

Urticaria (hives) is an acute superficial skin allergy characterized by local swelling and itching. *Angioedema* is similar but involves deeper tissues and mucus membranes. The most common causes are drugs, certain foods, and insect stings or bites.

Food allergy is sometimes postulated to explain almost any imaginable human ailment, including obesity, depression, fatigue, childhood hyperactivity, and arthritis. Virtually all such claims are unverifiable scientifically. However, allergy to peanuts and a few other foods is established fact. Allergic patients suffer vascular collapse from clear anaphylactic symptoms, which can generalized and fatal. Scientific evidence supports the thesis that some cases of irritable bowel syndrome and ulcerative colitis (Chapter 15) may be caused by food allergy.

Some cases of bronchial asthma and a few uncommon pulmonary diseases (Chapter 14) may be caused by allergic reaction.

AUTOIMMUNE DISEASE

The immune system exists to defend the body from foreign (nonself) agents. It does so by reacting against the proteins (antigens) that the agent contains. But in autoimmune disease it is our own tissues, composed in large part by our own antigens, that become the enemy. In the quotation below, Walt Kelly was speaking of environmental pollution in his immortal comic strip,

Pogo, but the sentiment he expressed applies to auto-immune disease:

We have met the enemy and he is us.
POGO, A POSSUM WITH AN ACID WIT;
CREATED BY WALT KELLY (1913–1973), AMERICAN CARTOONIST

Historically, autoimmune diseases have been called collagen-vascular diseases or connective tissue diseases because blood vessels and connective tissues are often the immune target. In this discussion we will focus on the most common diseases, such as lupus erythematosus and rheumatoid arthritis; however, autoimmunity may cause disease of any organ or system. Table 8-2 lists the most common autoimmune diseases.

What is it that goes so terribly wrong with our own tissues that our "self" becomes alien and is attacked by the very immune system that is designed to protect us? In most instances, it is not "self" that changes, but the immune system. Some patients are genetically susceptible to faulty immune system antigen identification and to misidentifying self as nonself. There is clear evidence that microbes initiate the process in some instances.

Loss of Self-Tolerance

Tolerance of self refers to the normal lack of immune responsiveness to one's own tissue antigens; normal people do not develop antibodies to their own tissue. This normal tolerance of self can be lost in three ways.

First, *the antigens on some infectious agents or other foreign proteins share common antigenic features with "self,"* a phenomenon called **molecular mimicry**. Antibody to the foreign antigen is therefore capable of reacting with self (Fig. 8-9). Post-streptococcal rheumatic carditis (Chapter 13) is a good example. Some

Table 8-2   *Autoimmune Diseases*

Systemic Diseases	Organ-specific Diseases
Systemic lupus erythematosus	Multiple sclerosis (brain)
Rheumatic fever	Hashimoto thyroiditis (thyroid)
Rheumatoid arthritis	Autoimmune hemolytic anemia (red blood cells)
Systemic sclerosis (dermatomyositis)	Glomerulonephritis (kidney)
Polyarteritis nodosa	Primary biliary cirrhosis (liver) Dermatomyositis (skin) Myasthenia gravis (skeletal muscle)

streptococci have antigens similar to those found in human heart and kidney, and strep infection produces anti-streptococcal antibodies that react with cardiac or renal antigens to cause carditis or nephritis.

Second, *antigen that has always been hidden from contact with immune cells may become unmasked and attacked because they were never initially designated as self in the embryo.* Sympathetic ophthalmitis is an example. During normal embryogenesis, some ocular antigens are never processed by the immune system to be recognized as self. Ocular trauma or disease may expose these antigens to the immune system, thereby stimulating production of antibodies that attack antigen in *both* eyes. It is the threat of autoimmune ophthalmitis in the *other* eye that prompts removal of sightless eyes that are severely diseased or traumatized.

Third, *helper T-cell or suppressor T-cell activity may become abnormal.* Recall that in the embryo some lymphocytes capable of reacting with self are not eliminated by the thymus and bone marrow. **Suppressor T cells** keep these cells under control; however, if this suppressor function is lost, these antiself lymphocytes become free to attack self, and autoimmune disease is the result. Also, normal B-cell function requires assistance from **helper T cells**, which, if they become overactive, may stimulate B cells to such an extent that autoimmune disease is the result.

Genetic and Microbial Factors in Autoimmunity

Genetic makeup influences the tendency to develop autoimmune diseases. Some autoimmune disease occurs in clusters of people in family groups, and several autoimmune diseases are associated with the inheritance of certain HLA (MHC) antigens. For example, the presence of HLA-B27 antigen is closely linked to certain rheumatoid diseases.

It is clear that some autoimmune diseases are induced by *microbes* (Fig. 8-9). A prime example is the autoimmune myocarditis and arthritis (rheumatic fever, Chapter 13) that occurs in some patients after streptococcal throat infections. Evidence suggests that other microbes, Epstein-Barr virus (EBV), for example, may be the initiating agent for other autoimmune diseases.

Systemic Lupus Erythematosus (SLE)

SLE (lupus) is a multisystem autoimmune disease caused by type 3 (immune complex) hypersensitivity reaction. It has strikingly diverse manifestations that may affect any organ or tissue, especially the skin, serosal membranes, heart, kidney, and joints. It is unpredictable

MOLECULAR MIMICRY

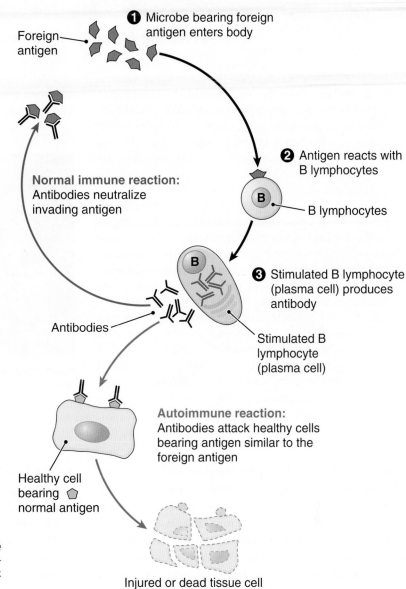

Figure 8-9 Molecular mimicry. Antigens on some microbes have features similar to self antigen. Antibodies produced to attack foreign antigen also attack normal self antigens

by nature, waxing and waning in intensity and manifestation. SLE is characterized by a multitude of antibodies to various organs and tissue components, but it is associated in particular with **antinuclear antibodies (ANA)**, antibodies that target DNA or RNA. The disease is fairly common, affecting about one in 2,500 people; ninety percent of patients are female, most of them 15–30 years old.

Etiology and Pathogenesis

SLE self tolerance is lost probably following loss of suppressor T-cell activity that keeps in check the antiself lymphocyte immune "time bombs" (discussed earlier) that remain from embryologic development of the im-

mune system. ANAs are the laboratory hallmark of SLE; the accompanying Lab Tools box explains one way in which autoimmune antibodies are detected. The detection of ANA in a patient's blood is a very *sensitive* test for the presence of an autoimmune disease, but it is not highly *specific*. That is to say, almost every SLE patient has a positive ANA, but positive ANA may be seen in other autoimmune disease.

In addition to antibodies against DNA, other antibodies are often present and include antibodies to red blood cells, platelets, and lymphocytes. Antibodies also may form against certain substances used in some blood tests for syphilis, hence *false-positive test results for syphilis are regularly found in SLE.* Some antibodies found in lupus also interfere with certain blood coagu-

Detecting Autoimmune Antibodies

The antinuclear antibodies (ANA) characteristic of systemic lupus erythematosus are but a few of the hundreds of antibodies that occur in autoimmune disease and can be detected by laboratory methods, one of which is fluorescent microscopy. The key to understanding this test is to keep in mind that human *antibodies* (immunoglobulins) are *antigens* to other animals.

A fluorescent microscopy test typically begins by incubating patient plasma with mouse kidney cells. If the patient's plasma contains anti-nuclear (anti-DNA) antibodies, they attach to the DNA in mouse cell nuclei. The second stage of the test requires a reagent containing antibody against human immunoglobulin. Like the Coombs reagent discussed in the Lab Tools box later in this chapter, antibodies are obtained by injecting a goat with human immunoglobulin, collecting the anti-antibodies produced (goat anti-human antibodies), and tagging them with a fluorescent dye. Because all antibodies in humans, including ANAs, contain immunoglobulin, the goat anti-human immunoglobulin antibody attaches to the human immunoglobulin in the antinuclear antibodies attached to the mouse cell nuclei. As is

depicted in the accompanying illustration, the fluorescent tag glows green under the microscope when examined in fluorescent light.

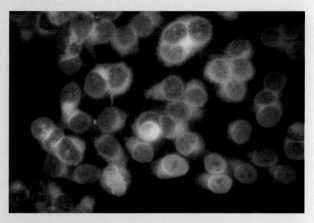

Positive test for blood antinuclear antibodies. The presence of antibodies is indicated by green fluorescence of test nuclei (see text for details).

lation tests, falsely suggesting that patients have a coagulation defect. Actually, the contrary is true: SLE patients can be plagued with venous and arterial thromboses, thrombocytopenia, and miscarriages.

Other factors are also important in the pathogenesis of SLE. There is clear evidence of genetic influence—the high concordance rate in identical twins is a good example; that is, there is a very high chance that if one twin has SLE, the other will also. Sex hormones are also important: nine of ten cases occur in women. Chronic administration of some drugs, most notably procainamide (a cardiac antiarrhythmic drug) and hydralazine (an anti-hypertensive drug), which induce SLE in 15–20% of cases.

Clinical and Pathologic Features

Figure 8-10 depicts the clinical findings in patients with SLE, which can affect virtually any tissue or organ. The following anatomic lesions are most common:

- *Acute necrotizing vasculitis* (Chapter 12) in any organ. Blood vessels in any organ may be involved, explaining the sometimes remarkable variety of signs and symptoms of SLE

- *Skin lesions*, which may be exacerbated by exposure to sunlight (photosensitivity, Chapter 24)
- *Serous effusions and fibrinous exudates* of the pericardium and pleurae
- *Myocarditis and cardiac valvular vegetations*
- *Glomerulonephritis* (Chapter 19), which is common and often severe
- *Arthritis* (Chapter 22), which may be clinically striking, though deforming lesions are rare
- *Brain involvement*, which is common and includes microinfarcts and organic psychosis or dementia

The diagnosis is obvious in a young woman with a photosensitive butterfly rash on the face, fever, pleuritic chest pain, and multi-joint arthritis or other symptoms. However, the presentation may not be as obvious in a male (Fig. 8-11) with fever of unknown origin, a bit of protein in the urine, and psychosis. SLE is a notorious masquerader.

The clinical course of SLE is variable. Some patients have minimal problems, but others are seriously affected. Thirty percent die in the first ten years after diagnosis. Sooner or later renal disease becomes a problem in most patients. Death often results from renal failure, infections, or diffuse CNS involvement.

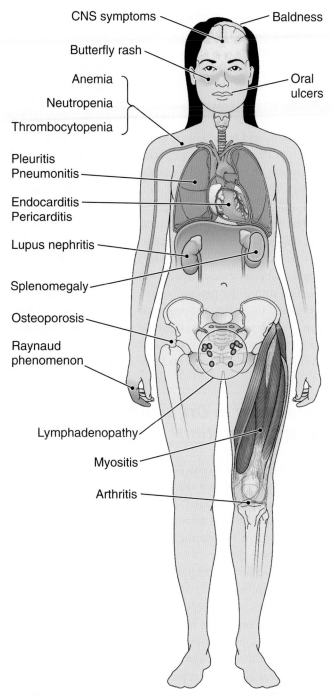

CNS symptoms — Baldness

Butterfly rash —

Anemia ⎤
Neutropenia ⎬
Thrombocytopenia ⎦

— Oral ulcers

Pleuritis
Pneumonitis —

Endocarditis —
Pericarditis

Lupus nephritis —

Splenomegaly —

Osteoporosis —

Raynaud
phenomenon —

Lymphadenopathy —

Myositis —

Arthritis —

***Figure 8-10* Clinical findings in systemic lupus erythematosus (SLE).** This illustration shows SLE's clinical features.

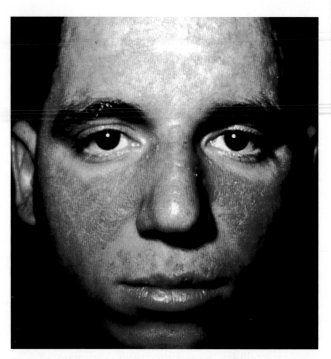

***Figure 8-11* Malar "butterfly" rash of SLE.** The photosensitive butterfly rash is clearly visible in this photograph.

Rheumatoid Arthritis (RA) and Related Diseases

Classic adult **rheumatoid arthritis** (Chapter 22) is an autoimmune disease affecting the tissue (synovium) that lines joints. It often begins slowly with low-grade fever, malaise, and early morning joint pain and stiffness. Joints most commonly affected are the wrists, elbow, shoulder, ankle, and the proximal interphalangeal and metacarpophalangeal joints of the hands. Severe disease of the vertebrae may be especially debilitating.

Two clinical conditions unique to RA are helpful in clinical diagnosis. First is radial deviation of metacarpals with ulnar deviation of the fingers, producing a classic "Z" deformity of the hand. Second are *rheumatoid nodules*, which are painless 1–2 cm subcutaneous granulomatous nodules, not found in other forms of arthritis. The disease usually progresses to a disabling arthritis over a decade or two. Diagnosis is confirmed by laboratory detection in blood of **rheumatoid factor**, an autoimmune antibody in blood that is unique to RA.

Juvenile rheumatoid arthritis is a distinct form of RA that occurs in children. It is a more serious, debilitating disease than is adult RA, and patients lack rheumatoid factor in their blood; that is, they are said to be *seronegative*. Juvenile RA tends to involve a few large joints such as the knees, elbows, and ankles and is closely associated with the HLA-B27 genotype. In about 20% of patients the onset of juvenile RA is explosive, a condition known as **Still disease**, which features high fever, abrupt development of arthritis, and enlarged spleen and lymph nodes, pleuritis or pericarditis, skin rash, and marked increase of the white blood cell count.

The **spondyloarthropathies** are a group of disorders distinct from rheumatoid arthritis in the following ways: 1) vertebral and sacroiliac joints are mainly involved; other joints are less involved or free of disease; 2) inflammation is present in joints but also involves ligaments where they attach to bone; 3) most patients carry the HLA-B27 genotype; and 4) rheumatoid factor is not present in their blood (a fact that causes some to refer to these diseases as the *seronegative spondyloarthropathies*). Among the disorders in this group are **ankylosing spondylitis**, a severe vertebral arthritis; the arthropathies associated with inflammatory bowel disease (Chapter 15) and psoriasis (Chapter 24); and the arthropathy that sometimes follows intestinal infection by *Salmonella, Shigella, Helicobacter,* or *Campylobacter.*

Other Autoimmune Diseases

Sjögren syndrome is an autoimmune inflammatory disease of the lacrimal and salivary glands, which features dry eyes (keratoconjunctivitis sicca) and dry mouth (xerostomia). It mainly affects women over 40 and is often associated with other autoimmune disorders such as SLE or RA.

Systemic sclerosis (Fig. 8-12), historically called **scleroderma**, is a sometimes cripplingly severe disease featuring inflammation and fibrosis of the supporting fibrous intercellular tissue (interstitium) of many organs, especially the dermis. Fibrosis, the hallmark of systemic sclerosis, may affect the GI tract, lungs, kidney, heart, and skeletal muscle. Mainly a disease of young women, it may prove devastatingly disfiguring, disabling, or fatal. Although it may manifest many of the features of systemic lupus or rheumatoid arthritis, it is distinctive because of the striking skin disease and the near uniform presence of **Raynaud phenomenon**, a condition resulting from spasm of small blood vessels that causes coldness, blanching, numbness, and pain in the fingers and toes.

Polyarteritis nodosa is one of several autoimmune diseases dominated by generalized blood vessel inflammation (systemic vasculitis, Chapter 12). One third of the cases are caused by hepatitis B infection (Chapter 16), which is associated with inflammation in the vascular wall owing to deposition of immune complexes (type 3 hypersensitivity reaction). Clinical presentation varies greatly. The disease usually occurs in young adults and may present acutely or subtly, with long intervals of quiet between symptomatic episodes. Malaise, fever of uncertain cause, hypertension, and weight loss are common. Vascular occlusion and infarction may occur in almost any site. Renal involvement is common, and renal failure is often the cause of death.

The **inflammatory myopathies** are a varied group of disorders characterized by autoimmune skeletal muscle injury that occur alone or in conjunction with other autoimmune disease such as SLE or RA. Each disease differs from the others in detail, but all feature widespread muscle weakness, soreness, fatigue, lymphocytic inflammatory cell infiltrates in affected muscle groups, and laboratory evidence of autoimmune disease.

Autoimmunity plays an important role in many other diseases. In some, autoimmune pathogenesis is clear; *type 1 diabetes* is an example. In others, autoimmunity is strongly suspected; for example, *chronic ulcerative colitis* (Chapter 15) and *multiple sclerosis* (Chapter 23).

Immunity in Organ and Tissue Transplantation

Successful tissue transplantation from one person to another requires that donor and recipient be matched antigenically as closely as possible to limit immune reaction and avoid immune rejection of the donated organ. Except for identical twins, every donated organ causes some degree of immune reaction, which can be diminished by careful matching of major histocompatibility complex (MHC, HLA) antigens and major blood group types and carefully administered immunosuppressive therapy. The best donor matches of MHC antigens and blood groups are likely to be found in close relatives of the recipient.

Hyperacute organ rejection is a reaction that occurs in the operating room as the surgeon connects the organ to the recipient's vascular supply. It occurs when *preformed* antibodies in the recipient's blood react immediately with graft endothelial cells, producing instant multivessel thrombosis. Immediate removal of the donated organ is necessary to avoid severe complications.

Acute organ rejection occurs within a few weeks, owing to an immune vasculitis (Chapter 12).

Chronic transplant rejection develops over a period of months to years and is the result of a variety of immune reactions, some of which are not well understood. However, it is clear that an antibody-mediated vasculitis can lead to ischemia and hypoperfusion that slowly starves the donated organ.

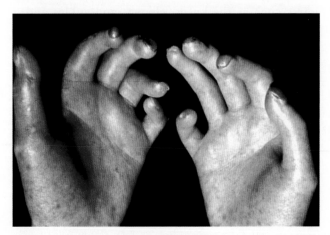

***Figure 8-12* Systemic sclerosis (scleroderma).** This crippling deformity of the hands results from severe skin sclerosis.

An especially devastating complication of bone marrow transplantation is **graft-versus-host (GVH) reaction**. Successful marrow transplantation requires pre-transplant immunosuppression of the recipient. In GVH, the donor's transplanted lymphocytes proliferate to the point that they replace the entire immune system of the recipient. Thus, recipient cells become nonself to the newly transplanted immune system, which attempts to destroy them. Multiple organs are affected, and patients suffer from severe dermatitis, diarrhea, and jaundice. Death from infection is a common result.

Immunity in Blood Transfusion

Blood transfusion is a form of temporary tissue transplantation. Because red blood cells (RBC) are one thousand times more common than white blood cells are and one hundred times more common than platelets are, successful blood transfusion depends primarily on RBC compatibility between donor and recipient.

Transfusion reaction is a complication of blood transfusion in which there is an abnormal response to the transfused blood cells or other components of the transfusion. There are two types of transfusion reactions: *major* reactions of antigenic incompatibility between infused RBCs and patient plasma agglutinins, and *minor* reactions of various types.

To avoid transfusion reactions, donor and potential recipient blood are carefully tested in advance to define the ABO and Rh type of each (**blood typing**). Blood from several potential donors with *presumably* compatible ABO and Rh types is selected from blood bank stores and mixed with recipient blood (a **crossmatch**) to see if agglutination occurs. The **major crossmatch** is a mix of *donor RBCs* with *potential recipient plasma*, and is the key factor in determining compatibility because transfusing incompatible RBCs can be fatal; natural agglutinins in the recipient's plasma immediately agglutinate the infused cells. If a clerical, laboratory, or other error occurs, and the donor and recipient blood would not be compatible, the major crossmatch will reveal the incompatibility, as is shown in Figure 8-13.

A **minor crossmatch** is performed by mixing *donor plasma* with *recipient RBC*. There is little danger in transfusing incompatible *plasma* because it is greatly diluted by the recipient's plasma. *The main function of a minor crossmatch is to confirm that the original ABO typing of both donor and recipient was done correctly.* For example, if through an error type A donor RBCs have been selected for potential transfusion into a patient with type B blood, the minor crossmatch would catch the error, because the anti-B in donor plasma would agglutinate the B antigen on the recipient's RBCs.

Also, tests are conducted to see if antibodies to minor RBC blood groups are attached to the potential recipient's RBCs (usually as a consequence of minor blood group incompatibility at the time of a prior transfusion) or if minor blood group antibodies exist in the potential recipient's plasma. When minor blood group antibodies are detected, donor blood for transfusion is screened to ensure that the donated RBCs do not contain the minor blood group in question, because they can cause a transfusion reaction if antibodies are present in the patient's blood. These antibody-screening tests are known as **Coombs tests**. They are further explained in the accompanying Lab Tools box.

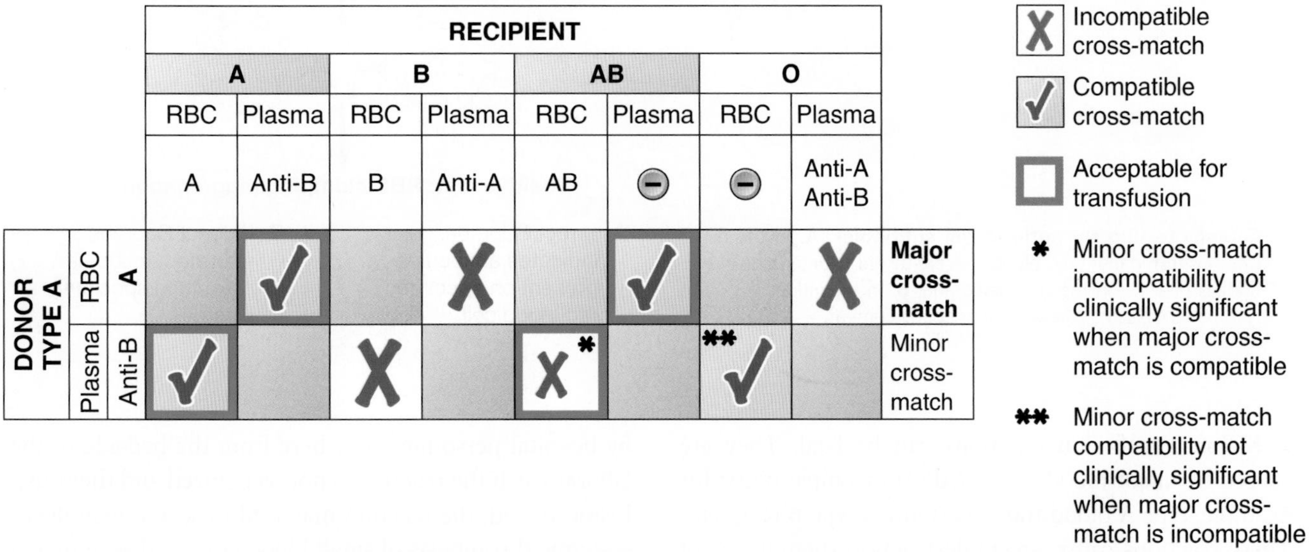

Figure 8-13 **Major and minor crossmatch of blood for transfusion.** The example shows type A blood crossmatched with other blood types. As is shown here, type A can be transfused safely into type A and type AB recipients because the major crossmatches are compatible.

Coombs Tests

Coombs testing is a method used by laboratories and blood banks to detect anti-red cell antibodies attached to red blood cells or free in plasma. The key to understanding Coombs tests is to keep in mind that human *antibodies* (immunoglobulins) are *antigens* to other animals.

The main ingredient in Coombs testing is Coombs reagent, which is prepared by injecting *human* immunoglobulin (antibody protein) into an *animal*, a goat, for example. The goat makes an anti-human antibody that will react with *any* human antibody. The goat anti-human antibody is collected and used as Coombs reagent.

As is depicted in the illustration, the *direct* Coombs test is performed on blood being considered for transfusion or on the blood of patients who have autoimmune hemolytic anemia, in order to determine whether the red cells have any antibody attached to them. The red cells to be tested are washed to remove (elute) any antibody that might be attached. The fluid (the eluant) is mixed with *reagent* (not patient) red cells that contain many different types of antigens. If antibody is present on the *patient* red cells it will be in the eluant and attach to *reagent* red cells. Coombs anti-antibody reagent is added to the mix of red cells and eluant and attaches to any antibody that might be present on the reagent cells, causing them to clump, which is the sign of a positive test.

The *indirect* Coombs test is similar except the specimen is patient plasma that is suspected of having anti-red cell antibodies. The plasma is mixed with the reagent red cells. If antibody is present it will attach to the reagent red cells. Then the Coombs anti-antibody reagent is added, and clumping of reagent red cells signifies a positive test, which indicates that the patient's plasma contains anti-red cell antibody.

COOMBS TEST FOR ANTI-RED CELL ANTIBODIES

Coombs testing for anti-red cell antibodies. A. In the direct Coombs test, patient red blood cells are tested to determine if antibody is present on the cell membrane. **B.** In the indirect Coombs test, patient plasma is tested for antibody content.

Major transfusion reactions can be fatal. They are caused by major blood group (ABO) incompatibility; for example, type A blood transfused into a type B recipient. These reactions cause severe destruction (hemolysis) of the transfused cells and are usually caused by human error by hospital personnel anywhere from the bedside to the laboratory. If the reaction is not recognized and the transfusion halted, the reaction may lead to severe hemolysis, systemic thrombosis of small blood vessels, disseminated intravascular coagulation (DIC), renal failure, and death.

Rh D-related hemolytic reactions occur only if prior sensitization of an Rh D-negative recipient has occurred. For example, if an Rh D-negative woman has an Rh D-positive child, the mother may develop anti-D antibodies. If she is later given Rh D-positive cells by transfusion, a severe hemolytic reaction may occur.

By definition a **minor transfusion reaction** is any reaction that is not potentially life threatening, which usually means any reaction that does not involve major blood group incompatibility or hemolysis of transfused red blood cells. Minor reactions include fever, chills, back pain, hives, or rash. The cause of most reactions is unknown, but one culprit may be an immune reaction to transfused white blood cells (WBC), especially in patients receiving recurring transfusions who have developed antibodies to transfused WBC.

Amyloidosis

Amyloid is an abnormal form of a normal protein, and **amyloidosis** is any dysfunction resulting from the systemic deposition of amyloid protein.

Normal protein molecules are folded in a particular manner. Amyloid is formed when normal protein is folded into abnormal, crystal-like molecules. Deposited between cells (Fig. 8-14) in the interstitial tissues, amyloid appears microscopically as a translucent, smooth, glassy material, which at one time was thought to be like starch, hence "amyloid" from the Latin word, *amylum*, for starch. Diagnosis of amyloidosis requires that a biopsy be performed and the tissue specimen examined microscopically. Amyloidosis can be detected microscopically by its special affinity for Congo red, a dye. Also, the crystalline nature of amyloid refracts light in such a way that it literally glows in the dark when viewed microscopically with polarized light.

The most common causes of amyloidosis are autoimmune diseases, such as rheumatoid arthritis, or chronic infections, such as pulmonary tuberculosis or severe chronic kidney or bone infection, which results in chronic excesses of immunoglobulin that deposit in tissue as amyloid.

Amyloid deposits in the liver and adrenal gland may be associated with liver or adrenal insufficiency; deposits in the glomerulus may cause renal insufficiency; deposits in myocardium may cause heart failure; and deposits in nerves may impair motor and sensory function. Deposits in the brain are associated with Alzheimer disease.

Amyloidosis may be hereditary, but cases are rare and usually found in Middle Eastern ethnic groups. Localized amyloid deposits may occur in some tumors and in the islets of Langerhans in patients with adult-onset (type 2) diabetes.

Amyloidosis cannot be treated effectively; average survival is a few years.

Immunodeficiency Diseases

Immunodeficiency may be caused by a deficiency of T-cell or B-cell origin; it may be either inherited or acquired, and it usually becomes apparent following an unusual or persistent infection. Patients with deficiency in B-cell function do not produce effective antibody response and usually suffer from infections from pyogenic bacteria, such as staphylococcus or streptococcus. Patients with defective T-cell function (cell-mediated immunity) are also prone to infections and to the development of neoplasms as a result of failed immune surveillance (Chapter 6). Infections in immunodeficient patients are usually caused by organisms that ordinarily do not cause infection in people with healthy immune systems. Such infections are called **opportunistic infections**.

> ☞ *Immunodeficiency disease leads to infection and malignancy.*

INHERITED IMMUNODEFICIENCY DISEASES

X-linked agammaglobulinemia (Bruton Disease) results from failed embryonic B-cell development: patients lack the ability to produce antibodies; T cells are unaffected. Inheritance occurs according to Mendelian principles (Chapter 7), and the disorder first comes to attention at about age six months. After age six months, the passive

Epidermis   Dermal deposits of amyloid

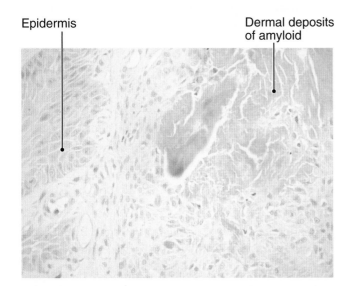

Figure 8-14 **Amyloidosis.** This section of skin has been stained with Congo red to highlight amyloid deposits.

immunity wanes that was conferred on the newborn by maternal antibodies that crossed the placenta from mother to fetus during pregnancy. Patients present with a history of recurrent infections: bronchitis, pneumonia, sinusitis, pharyngitis, and ear and gastrointestinal infections. Some patients develop autoimmune disease, especially arthritis similar to rheumatoid arthritis.

Thymic hypoplasia (DiGeorge syndrome) is the embryonic failure of T-cell development; B-cell immunity is unaffected. These patients suffer from viral, fungal, and protozoan diseases. Because development of the fetal thymus is closely related to nearby anatomic structures, these patients also may lack parathyroid glands (and suffer from hypoparathyroidism, Chapter 18) and may have anomalies of the neck, face, ears, heart, and aorta.

Other than AIDS, the most common immunodeficiency is *isolated deficiency of immunoglobulin A (IgA)*, which is caused by a monogenic (Mendelian) defect that occurs in about 1 in 700 persons of European descent but is rare in people of African or Asian heritage. However, some cases occur as a result of viral infection. As discussed earlier, IgA occurs in high concentration as the mucosal "immune paint" in secretions of the gastrointestinal and respiratory tracts that protects these organs from bacteria in their environment. Deprived of this protection, patients have recurrent gastrointestinal, sinus, and pulmonary infections.

Severe combined immunodeficiency (SCID) is a group of inherited disorders affecting both B-cell and T-cell function. All result from single-gene defects and are inherited in Mendelian fashion; some are X linked and affect males only. In SCID, lymphoid tissues and the thymus are underdeveloped, and blood lymphocyte count is always low. Patients suffer a wide range of infections, many of them caused by *Pneumocystis*, *Candida*, and other opportunistic microbes that do not ordinarily cause infection in patients with normal immune systems.

ACQUIRED IMMUNODEFICIENCY SYNDROME (AIDS)

Most immunodeficiencies are acquired, not hereditary. **AIDS (acquired immunodeficiency syndrome)** is well known, but patients with malnourishment, Hodgkin disease, sarcoidosis, and other acquired (not genetic) conditions also may become immunodeficient, even though they are not infected by the *human immunodeficiency virus* (HIV). The degree of immunodeficiency in non-AIDS cases, however, is usually not serious enough to overshadow the primary clinical condition. Non-AIDS patients develop infections, but they are not as seriously affected as patients with AIDS. AIDS is by far the most common serious acquired immunodeficiency.

AIDS is caused by the **human immunodeficiency virus (HIV)**, which preferentially infects lymphocytes and brain cells; however, it can affect virtually any organ. AIDS is characterized by profound immune deficiency associated with infections, secondary neoplasms, and neurologic disease. HIV infection ranks among the most devastating epidemics in world history. In southern Africa the percent of population infected (prevalence) is about 20%, and in Botswana 36% are infected. In 2003 five million new HIV infections occurred worldwide; there were three million AIDS deaths.

AIDS and HIV infection are not exactly the same. AIDS is a state of severe immune deficiency caused by HIV infection; but many people with HIV infection are not affected severely enough for a diagnosis of AIDS to be made. Criteria for the diagnosis of AIDS include certain laboratory abnormalities and the presence of certain infections, malignancies, or other conditions. In the United States, where laboratory services are plentiful, the diagnosis of AIDS is made according to the following criteria, which are simplified from official United States Centers for Disease Control (CDC) criteria:

- Peripheral blood CD4+ lymphocyte count below 200 cells per microliter

OR

- Other laboratory evidence of HIV infection (detection of HIV antigens or antibodies in blood)

AND

  - Certain types of infections or recurrent infections, usually by organisms that ordinarily do not produce infections in patients with normal immune systems (*opportunistic infections*); for example, avian (bird) tuberculosis

  OR

  - Progressive multifocal leukoencephalopathy, a degenerative disease of brain white matter

  OR

  - Certain kinds of neoplasms (AIDS-defining neoplasms), such as Kaposi sarcoma, B-cell lymphoma of the brain, or invasive cancer of the cervix.

  OR

  - Severe wasting

Among *adolescents and adults*, there are five distinct groups at risk for HIV infection. In descending order of risk, they are:

- homosexual or bisexual males
- intravenous drug abusers

- patients with hemophilia (almost all of whom are male)
- recipients of transfusions of human blood or blood components
- heterosexual contacts of the above

Of HIV-infected patients under age 13, the great majority have been infected by transmission of virus from mother to infant.

The predominant mode of sexual spread varies geographically according to economic conditions. Heterosexual contact is the predominant mode of transmission in underdeveloped areas with inadequate public health education and resources. It is easier for males to infect females than the reverse. As the prevalence of heterosexually transmitted AIDS has increased, so has the number of women affected. In the United States in 1992 14% of patients with AIDS were women; by 2003 that figure had risen to 22%, and worldwide almost 50% of AIDS patients are women. HIV is carried by lymphocytes in semen and enters the body through genital abrasions or sores, lesions that are much more common in the genitalia of persons infected with sexually transmitted disease. However, heterosexual transmission accounts for only about one third of cases in economically privileged nations, where most cases are from contacts with high-risk groups: bisexual males, IV drug abusers, and prostitutes. In developed nations heterosexual transmission of AIDS is very uncommon except in people who have sexual contact with these high-risk groups.

Transmission by needle stick occurs almost solely in association with shared needles and other unsanitary practices by intravenous drug abusers. Transmission by blood or blood products or by medical procedures is rare, although many hemophiliacs and some other transfusion recipients were infected before screening tests for HIV were devised in the early 1980s. The risk to health care workers is real but very small—about 0.3% of workers become infected when accidentally stuck by a needle used in an HIV-infected patient. The overall risk to patients of infection from a health care worker is about 25 infections per 100 million patient encounters. Transmission in utero to the fetus occurs in about 25% of infected mothers. HIV cannot be transmitted by casual contact at home, school, or work by casual contact, nor is HIV transmitted by insect bites.

Etiology and Pathogenesis

As is illustrated in Figure 8-15, the HIV attack on the immune system results from the affinity of the virus for lymphocytes, particularly CD4+ (helper) T lymphocytes. As is depicted in the figure, once inside T lymphocytes, HIV produces abnormal DNA that merges

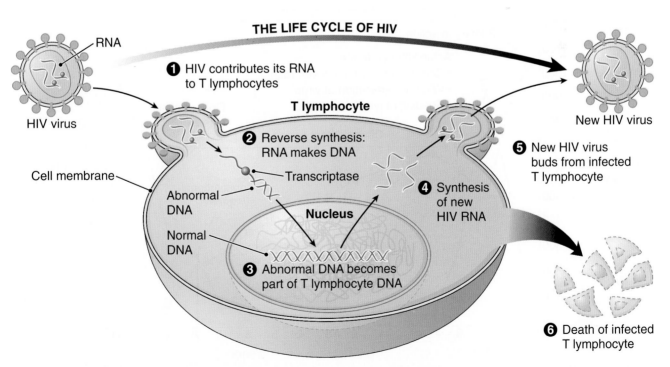

Figure 8-15 **HIV infection of a T lymphocyte.** In the life cycle of HIV, the HIV virus merges with the T lymphocyte's cell membrane and injects its RNA into the cytoplasm, where, in a reverse of the usual process, new DNA is synthesized from RNA. This new HIV DNA is incorporated into the DNA of the T lymphocyte nucleus. The infected T lymphocyte then synthesizes new HIV RNA, which buds from the cell membrane as a new HIV virus, after which the infected T lymphocyte dies.

with normal DNA to become part of a new, corrupted T-cell DNA. Later, the corrupted DNA produces new HIV particles using the patients' infected T lymphocytes as an HIV factory. New HIV viruses exit the dying cell to infect and kill other CD4+ T cells, and the cycle continues until the T-cell population is devastated and the patient dies from AIDS-related opportunistic infection or malignancy.

Some infected CD4+ cells do not die but linger as a population of infected but inactive cells (latently infected cells) that can be stimulated to resume the cycle of T-cell destruction by becoming active again with antigenic stimulation of the immune system. The antigenic stimulation is usually another infection, which stimulates proliferation of latently infected cells and renewed internal proliferation of the virus. In Africa and Asia sexually transmitted disease and HIV infection are closely linked; not only do sexual sores facilitate spread of the HIV virus, they often provide the antigenic stimulation that worsens the infection.

Although the T-cell system is the primary point of HIV attack, the B-cell system is also adversely affected. B cells are stimulated by HIV antigens and the antigens of the *cytomegalovirus (CMV), Epstein-Barr virus (EBV)*,

and other infections that occur in AIDS. The stimulated B cells produce large amounts of antibody (immunoglobulins), but they are ineffective as a defense against infection because they depend on helper T cells, which are impaired by the HIV infection. The net result is that both T-cell and B-cell function is defective.

The Natural Progression of HIV Infection

HIV infection and AIDS develop in distinct phases. Peripheral blood CD4+ T-cell counts are a fairly reliable guide to the progress of the disease—lower counts are usually associated with more advanced disease and a grimmer prognosis. According to current guidelines, HIV-infected patients are defined as having AIDS if the CD4+ T-cell count falls below 200 cells/cu mm (normal CD4+ counts are >500 cells/cu mm).

Immediately after HIV infection, patients are asymptomatic. However, as is illustrated in Figure 8-16, after a few weeks most patients develop an acute "flu syndrome," with sore throat, muscle soreness (myalgia), fever, and rash, which resolves in a few weeks. In this phase HIV is present in blood in high concentration and CD4+ (helper T-cell) cell counts may temporarily fall

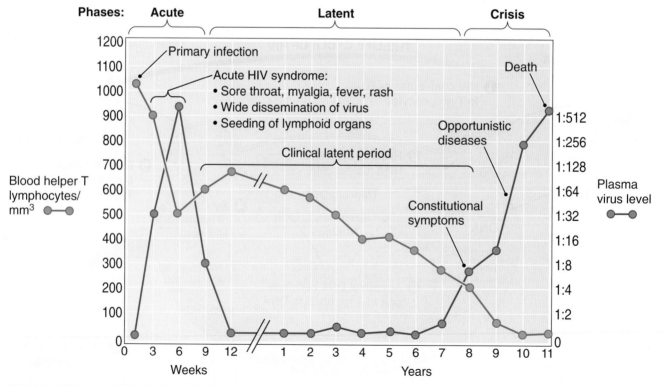

***Figure 8-16* Phases of HIV infection and AIDS.** Shortly after infection with HIV, a flu-like acute HIV syndrome occurs. Blood virus level is high, helper T-cell (CD4+ lymphocytes) count falls, and the virus spreads widely. In the *latent period*, which may last for years, helper T-lymphocyte levels are moderately depressed, and virus levels in blood are low. In the final *crisis phase* the CD4+ T-lymphocyte count falls markedly. Opportunistic infections appear that are usually the cause of death.

markedly. However, CD4+ T cells soon replenish, the number of virus particles in blood falls to low levels, and anti-HIV antibodies appear in blood (seroconversion) as the HIV infection enters a latent phase, during which the virus continues to reproduce, although it is confined to the lymphoid system. During this latent phase, CD4+ T-cell counts in blood remain normal as dying CD4+ T cells are replenished by immune system reserves, and there are few clinical symptoms. Finally, a crisis phase appears as CD4+ T-cell counts fall dramatically and HIV infection evolves into AIDS, and patients become susceptible to organisms that do not infect patients with normal immune systems (*opportunistic infections*, Chapter 9). This pre-death period is characterized by a near-complete breakdown of the immune system as opportunistic infections occur, especially in the lungs and gastrointestinal tract; neurologic symptoms and dementia appear, and secondary neoplasms may develop.

Clinical Features

Figure 8-17 summarizes the clinical and pathologic features of AIDS. The typical patient is a young adult from

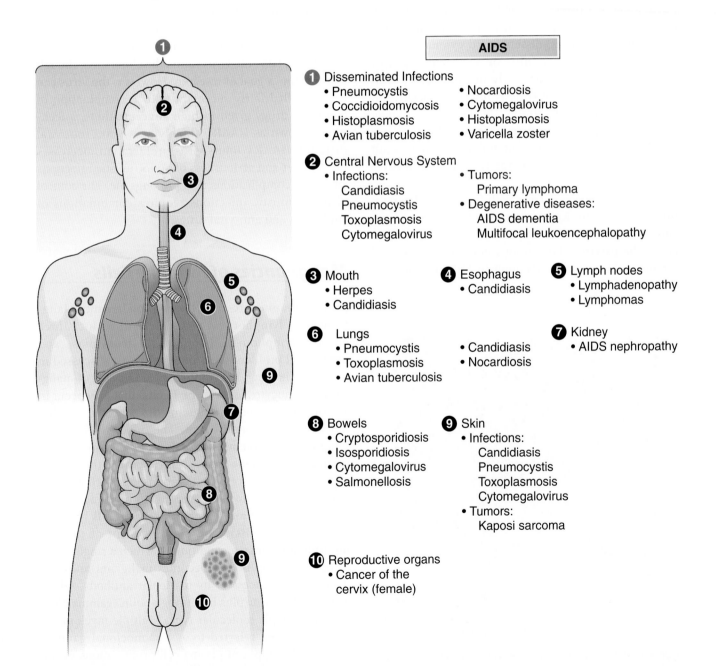

AIDS

1 Disseminated Infections
- Pneumocystis
- Coccidioidomycosis
- Histoplasmosis
- Avian tuberculosis
- Nocardiosis
- Cytomegalovirus
- Histoplasmosis
- Varicella zoster

2 Central Nervous System
- Infections:
  - Candidiasis
  - Pneumocystis
  - Toxoplasmosis
  - Cytomegalovirus
- Tumors:
  - Primary lymphoma
- Degenerative diseases:
  - AIDS dementia
  - Multifocal leukoencephalopathy

3 Mouth
- Herpes
- Candidiasis

4 Esophagus
- Candidiasis

5 Lymph nodes
- Lymphadenopathy
- Lymphomas

6 Lungs
- Pneumocystis
- Toxoplasmosis
- Avian tuberculosis
- Candidiasis
- Nocardiosis

7 Kidney
- AIDS nephropathy

8 Bowels
- Cryptosporidiosis
- Isosporidiosis
- Cytomegalovirus
- Salmonellosis

9 Skin
- Infections:
  - Candidiasis
  - Pneumocystis
  - Toxoplasmosis
  - Cytomegalovirus
- Tumors:
  - Kaposi sarcoma

10 Reproductive organs
- Cancer of the cervix (female)

Figure 8-17 **Clinical and pathologic features of AIDS.**

one of the risk groups discussed earlier, who presents with fever, weight loss, diarrhea, palpable lymph nodes, infection, neurologic symptoms (including psychosis or dementia), and, perhaps, an AIDS-related secondary neoplasm. Two types of AIDS infections occur. First, are those caused by pathogens that also affect patients with healthy immune systems and cause diseases such as pulmonary tuberculosis or diarrhea. A second group includes *opportunistic pathogens* that do not ordinarily cause infection in people with healthy immune systems. Case Study 8-1 at the end of this chapter presents an example.

As is illustrated in Figure 8-18, *Pneumocystis jiroveci* pneumonia is a presenting opportunistic infection in many patients; others present with mucosal candidiasis, ulcerating oral herpes, disseminated cytomegalovirus infection (especially retinitis or gastroenteritis), or disseminated tuberculosis. Early in the disease, ordinary *Mycobacterium tuberculosis* infections occur, but later the avian (bird) strain, *Mycobacterium avium*, predominates. Brain and meningeal infections are common. Diarrhea is a constant problem and may result from a variety of organisms rarely seen in non-AIDS patients.

AIDS patients also have a high incidence of certain tumors, especially Kaposi sarcoma, B-cell lymphoma, and cervical carcinoma. Kaposi sarcoma is caused by type 8 herpesvirus. For reasons not yet clear, Kaposi sarcoma is found more commonly in AIDS patients who are homosexual males. Another virus, the Epstein-Barr virus (EBV), may underlie the highly aggressive B-cell lymphomas that occur in some AIDS patients.

Nervous system involvement is demonstrable at autopsy in the majority of patients. About half have neurologic symptoms, including mental aberrations that may progress to a severe AIDS-related dementia, or multifocal leukoencephalopathy (Chapter 23), a degenerative disease of white matter.

The gross and microscopic changes of HIV infection are neither specific nor diagnostic; rather, the findings are related to the secondary infections, neoplasms, and other consequences of HIV infection.

Treatment of HIV infection and AIDS is a very complex matter and has two main aims: to control the virus and to control infections. Once a patient is infected with HIV, the virus cannot be eliminated, though this remains a goal of research. However, the virus can be controlled fairly successfully by a combination of anti-virus drugs given in high concentrations, a technique known as HAART (highly active anti-retroviral therapy). HAART limits virus proliferation, decreases the number and seriousness of opportunistic infections and other complications, and prolongs life. The control of opportunistic infections requires combinations of antibiotics and anti-viral drugs.

Malignancies of Immune Cells

B or T lymphocytes can become malignant. Malignancies of lymphocytes may be classified into three groups: lymphomas, lymphocytic leukemias, and plasma cell proliferations, all of which are discussed in detail in Chapter 11. **Lymphomas** are masses of malignant lymphocytes (either B or T cells) that may occur in any organ of the body, including the bone marrow, but not in the peripheral blood. The opposite is true of **lymphocytic leukemias**, which are malignancies that originate in the bone marrow and appear in the peripheral blood. Plasma cell proliferations are B-cell growths that have in common the overgrowth of a single clone of stimulated, immunoglobulin-secreting B lymphocytes (plasma cells). The most frequent of these is **multiple myeloma**, a condition in which a single clone of bone-marrow B cells becomes malignant and produces a great excess of its particular antibody, which accumulates as surplus immunoglobulin (gamma globulin) of a single molecular type. Multiple myeloma is, therefore, often referred to as a **monoclonal gammopathy**. Other types of plasma cell proliferations occur, not all of them malignant. ∎

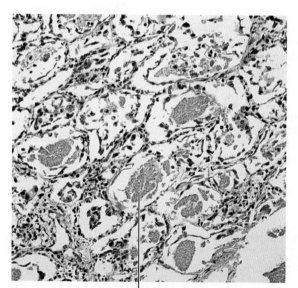

Clouds of tiny *Pneumocystis jiroveci* organisms in pulmonary alveoli

*Figure 8-18 **Pneumocystis jiroveci** pneumonia.* In this microscopic study of lung tissue, clouds of organisms fill the alveoli.

CASE STUDY 8-1 "I'M AFRAID I HAVE AIDS"

TOPICS
AIDS
Opportunistic infections

THE CASE

Setting: You work in the emergency room of a medium-size hospital in the suburbs of a large city. Tonight you are seeing non-urgent, walk-in patients.

Clinical history: MLB is a 38-year-old man who comes right to the point when you ask why he is in the emergency room. "I'm gay," he says, "and I'm afraid I have AIDS." On questioning him, you learn that over the last few months he has lost 25 lb and has a poor appetite, recurrent night sweats, and intermittent fevers. He says he used to use intravenous drugs but quit several years ago, and he adds, "But, I haven't been as careful about sex as I should have been."

Physical examination and other data: Physical examination reveals enlarged lymph nodes in his neck, axillae, and groins. Laboratory studies in the emergency room show him to be anemic and to have low lymphocyte count. Blood tests for HIV and CD4+ lymphocyte count are to be reported later.

Clinical course: After blood tests reveal that he is HIV positive and his CD4+ lymphocyte count is 375 cells/cu mm, he is given a prescription and starter pack of anti-HIV drugs and a clinic appointment, but he fails to fill the prescription or keep his follow-up clinic appointment.

He next appears in the emergency room 14 months later complaining of shortness of breath and severe diarrhea. Chest radiographs showed bilateral pulmonary infiltrates, and study of his stools revealed numerous *Cryptosporidia*. His CD4+ lymphocyte count is 186/cu mm. He is given antibiotics and a clinic appointment but again fails to appear for follow-up care.

His final appearance in the emergency room comes ten months later when he is brought in by friends because his care has become more than they can manage. He is semi-comatose, and his caregivers report that he is suffering from severe memory problems, persistent coughing, diarrhea, and weight loss. Chest radiographs reveal dense bilateral lung infiltrates. He dies the next day, and an autopsy is performed.

At autopsy, MLB's body is found to be very thin. The lungs are meaty, severely congested, and almost airless. Retroperitoneal and mesenteric lymph nodes are enlarged, the spleen is enlarged and congested, and the mucosa of the small bowel and colon are extensively ulcerated and inflamed. The brain shows mild gross atrophy. Microscopic study reveals alveoli filled with *Pneumocystis jiroveci* organisms, and cytomegalovirus nuclear inclusions are identified in intestinal epithelial cells. Microscopic study also reveals widespread, mild chronic inflammation and collections of multinucleated giant cells in brain tissue, suggestive of HIV encephalitis.

DISCUSSION

This patient is representative of the major AIDS risk groups in the United States—male homosexuals and IV drug abusers. Although laboratory studies on his initial appearance documented that he was HIV infected, his CD4+ lymphocyte count was not low enough (<200/cu mm) to warrant a diagnosis of AIDS, nor did he have documented AIDS-related infection or tumor. By the time of his second visit, his HIV infection had progressed to AIDS: his CD4+ count was <200/cu mm and he had diarrhea attributable to an AIDS-related opportunistic infection (*Cryptosporidium*). His final appearance was prompted by dementia and respiratory distress.

Autopsy revealed severe *Pneumocystis jiroveci* pneumonia and severe cytomegalovirus enterocolitis. Infection with opportunistic pathogens like these is a requirement for the diagnosis of AIDS in HIV-infected patients. As the lymphoid system reacts to widespread infections, the spleen and lymph nodes enlarge. The dementia and brain atrophy were the result of HIV encephalitis.

POINTS TO REMEMBER

- The two main AIDS risk groups in the United States are male homosexuals and intravenous drug users.
- The HIV virus attacks the nervous system as well as the lymphoid system.
- Immunodeficiency states are associated with severe infections.

Objectives Recap

1. *Define immunity and autoimmunity*: Immunity is a special function of lymphocytes and macrophages that defends the body against foreign (nonself, alien) threats, mainly microbes, by attacking and destroying the foreign substance. Autoimmune diseases are those in which the immune system attacks the body's own tissues in addition to foreign ones.

2. *Name the two principal nonimmune defense systems*: 1) surface barriers such as skin and mucosa, and 2) cellular and molecular nonimmune systems such as phagocytosis, natural killer cells, lysozymes, and the complement system.

3. *Define antigen and antibody*: An antigen is any substance capable of inciting an immune reaction. An antibody is an anti-antigen protein, an immunoglobulin, made by B cells to attack an antigen.

4. *Describe the two main types of immune cells:* B cells (B lymphocytes) are programmed to produce and secrete circulating antibodies. T cells attack antigen directly by means of programmed receptors on their surface; no antibodies are involved.

5. *Classify antibodies by type of protein, and briefly contrast the differing roles of IgG and IgM in response to antigen challenge:* All antibodies are immunoglobulins and are found in the gamma globulin fraction of blood protein. There are five molecular types: G, A, M, D, and E. IgM antibodies are formed quickly after antigen challenge and constitute the immediate response of the immune system to provide quick, short term protection. IgG antibodies are the most abundant immunoglobulin in blood; they appear after IgM antibodies and confer long-term immunity.

6. *Briefly describe the immune reaction in type 1 hypersensitivity disease:* On first exposure to the antigen, IgE antibodies are produced by B cells and attach to mast cells, coating the mast cell with programmed, specific antibody against the invading antigen. On subsequent exposure the antigen combines with IgE antibody on the surface of mast cells and triggers instant release of inflammatory and vasoactive substances such as histamine from mast cell cytoplasmic granules. The reaction attracts large numbers of eosinophils, causing local and peripheral blood eosinophilia. Typical type I reactions include "hay fever" (allergic rhinitis), hives, and some cases of asthma.

7. *Explain the principal difference between type 4 hypersensitivity reaction and the other three types*: Type 4 hypersensitivity is a T-cell immune reaction; the other three are B-cell system reactions.

8. *Explain the difference between allergic and autoimmune disease:* In allergy the reaction is an exaggerated but otherwise normal immune response against foreign antigen, whereas in autoimmune disease the immune system attacks self antigens. Allergy is an exaggerated immune reactivity (hypersensitivity) to certain environmental substances (allergens) that usually have little effect on most people. The hypersensitivity is established on initial exposure to the allergen (the sensitizing "dose"); subsequent exposure causes the hypersensitivity reaction.

9. *Explain what is meant by "molecular mimicry":* Antigens on microbes or other foreign proteins share common antigenic features with self antigens. Sometimes antibodies made by the immune system against foreign antigens cross-react with self antigens; autoimmune disease is the result.

10. *Briefly discuss the immune mechanism and clinical finding in systemic lupus erythematosus:* Systemic lupus erythematosus is an autoimmune disease resulting from type 3 hypersensitivity: immune complexes deposit in tissues and cause injury and inflammation. The ill effect of SLE is mostly caused by a necrotizing vasculitis that may affect any organ. Heart, kidney, joints, skin, brain, and the serosal surfaces of the lung, pericardium, and peritoneal cavity are most often affected.

11. *Explain why persons with type A blood cannot be safely transfused with type B blood*: People with type A blood have A antigen on their red blood cells and naturally occurring anti-B agglutinin in their plasma. The anti-B agglutinin agglutinates transfused type B red cells. The minor crossmatch incompatibility between type A cells and AB plasma is not clinically significant.

12. *Explain how B and T cells are affected in AIDS*: In AIDS T cells are directly attacked and severely diminished by the effect of HIV infection. B cells are also affected: they react to HIV antigens and opportunistic infections but the activity is ineffective without support by helper T cells, which are diminished in number by HIV infection. The result is increased but ineffective B-cell activity.

13. *Name the most common AIDS risk groups in developed nations*: The most important risk groups are homosexual or bisexual males and intravenous drug users and the heterosexual contacts of the two groups.

14. *Briefly discuss the phases of HIV infection and the appearance of AIDS*: Shortly after infection most patients develop a short "flu syndrome" with sore throat, myalgia, fever and rash, high levels of virus in blood, and low T-cell count. The illness then en-

ters a prolonged clinically quiet latent period in which T-cell count returns to normal, the number of virus particles falls to low levels, and anti-HIV antibodies appear in blood. Finally, a crisis phase appears as T-cell count falls markedly and AIDS-related neoplasms or opportunistic infections appear.

15. *Explain the role of infections and AIDS-defining neoplasms in HIV infection*: Immune impairment in HIV infection makes patients susceptible to infection. Many infections (opportunistic infections) are caused by infective organisms that rarely cause disease in immunologically healthy people. HIV infections also render patients more likely to develop certain neoplasms, such as brain lymphoma and Kaposi sarcoma.

16. *Name the three main types of malignancies of immune cells*: The three types of malignant diseases of immune cells are: lymphoma, lymphocytic leukemia, and plasma cell proliferations such as multiple myeloma.

Typical Test Questions

1. Which one of the following is an immune defense mechanism?
   A. Complement
   B. Phagocytosis
   C. Anaphylaxis
   D. Lysozymes

2. Which one of the following is an antibody?
   A. CD4+ lymphocyte
   B. Macrophage
   C. Complement
   D. Immunoglobulin

3. Which one of the following is a T-cell reaction?
   A. Type 1 hypersensitivity
   B. Type 2 hypersensitivity
   C. Type 3 hypersensitivity
   D. Type 4 hypersensitivity

4. Which one of the following is the hypersensitivity mechanism in lupus erythematosus?
   A. Type 1 hypersensitivity
   B. Type 2 hypersensitivity
   C. Type 3 hypersensitivity
   D. Type 4 hypersensitivity

5. Which one of the following is an incompatible transfusion?
   A. Type O red blood cells transfused into a type A recipient
   B. Type O red blood cells transfused into a type B recipient
   C. Type A red blood cells transfused into a type A recipient
   D. Type A red blood cells transfused into a type B recipient

6. True or false? Natural killer cells require immune programming to be effective.

7. True or false? Only proteins can cause an immune reaction.

8. True or false? Most autoimmune disease is caused by a type 3 hypersensitivity reaction.

9. True or false? Most major transfusion reactions are caused by human error.

10. True or false? Most immune deficiencies are acquired.

This chapter begins with a review of the different varieties of infectious agents, then moves into a discussion of their spread and effects in the body as well as their spread from person to person. It also examines the clinical nature and diagnosis of infection.

BACK TO BASICS
INFECTION
CONTAGION
THE SPREAD OF ORGANISMS IN TISSUE
MECHANISMS OF MICROBIOLOGIC INJURY
THE INFLAMMATORY RESPONSE TO INFECTION
INFECTIONS OF ORGAN SYSTEMS
• Respiratory Infections
• Gastrointestinal Infections
• Genitourinary Infections
• Skin Infections

INFECTIONS BY PYOGENIC BACTERIA
INFECTIONS BY *CLOSTRIDIUM* ORGANISMS AND OTHER
    NECROTIZING AGENTS
OPPORTUNISTIC AND AIDS-RELATED INFECTIONS
TROPICAL, VECTOR-BORNE, AND PARASITE INFECTIONS
• Vector-borne Infections
• Parasite Infections
THE NATURAL COURSE OF AN INFECTION
SIGNS AND SYMPTOMS OF INFECTION
LABORATORY TOOLS

Learning Objectives

After studying this chapter you should be able to:
1. List several of the most common causes worldwide of death resulting from infection
2. Define the following terms: infection, contagion, nosocomial, reservoir, carrier, pathogen, host, vector
3. Name the crucial differences between viruses and bacteria
4. Describe how bacteria vary according to shape, oxygen requirements, and staining characteristics
5. Briefly describe how organisms spread in tissue
6. Describe the cellular inflammatory reaction to bacteria, viruses, mycobacteria and fungi, parasitic worms, and protozoa
7. Name the organ systems most commonly affected by infections and discuss the aspects they share in common
8. Define dysentery
9. Name several types of bacterial enteritis
10. Name several sexually transmitted diseases, the pathogens that cause them, and the genitourinary lesions that are associated with them
11. Name the two types of Gram-positive cocci that cause most pyogenic infections
12. Name several diseases caused by *Streptococcus* organisms.
13. Define the phrase opportunistic pathogen, and offer several examples
14. Name a vector-borne disease, including the pathogen and the vector
15. Discuss the transmission and pathology of amebiasis
16. Name the two parasitic diseases causing the most morbidity and mortality worldwide
17. List the clinical phases of infection that occur after an infective organism invades the body.

Key Terms and Concepts

BACK TO BASICS
- anaerobic
- aerobic
- Gram positive
- Gram negative
- cocci
- bacilli

INFECTION
- infection
- pathogen

CONTAGION
- host
- vector

MECHANISMS OF MICROBIOLOGIC INJURY
- exotoxin
- endotoxin

INFECTIONS BY PYOGENIC BACTERIA
- pyogenic
- *Staphylococcus*
- *Streptococcus*

OPPORTUNISTIC AND AIDS-RELATED INFECTIONS
- opportunistic pathogen

TROPICAL, VECTOR-BORNE, AND PARASITE INFECTIONS
- tropical disease
- parasite
- helminth
- protozoa

THE NATURAL COURSE OF AN INFECTION
- incubation period
- septicemia

LABORATORY TOOLS
- microbial culture
- antimicrobial susceptibility

For each illness that doctors cure with medicine, they provoke ten in healthy people by inoculating them with the virus that is a thousand times more powerful than any microbe: the idea that one is ill.

MARCEL PROUST (1871–1922), FRENCH NOVELIST

BACK TO BASICS

As is illustrated in Figure 9-1, most infections are caused by microscopic organisms (*microorganisms, microbes*), such as bacteria. These organisms vary greatly in size. Most viruses are too small to be seen with an ordinary light microscope, while intestinal worms are visible to the naked eye. Table 9-1 lists some important pathogenic organisms and some of the diseases associated with them.

Bacteria are microscopic organisms with a cell wall and DNA but no chromosomes or nucleus; they have an independent metabolism and can live outside of cells. They populate the intestinal tract and every square millimeter of skin surface. About a billion bacteria are on the skin at any given time, most of them *Staphylococcus epidermidis* and *Propionibacterium acnes*, the pathogen of teenage pimples (acne). The intestines contain about 100 trillion (10^{14}) organisms, almost all of which are **anaerobic** (oxygen is toxic to them). However, most bacteria are **aerobic**; that is, they require oxygen to replicate. Bacteria are larger and more complex than viruses are. Bacteria synthesize their own DNA and proteins and can *reproduce outside of cells*, and they depend on the host only for favorable living conditions. Bacteria have a cell wall and require energy to live, features that make them susceptible to antibiotics (which exert their effect by dissolving the cell wall or interfering with bacterial metabolism).

Bacteria are commonly identified according to their shape and color when stained by dyes. The most common stain is the **Gram stain**, which is performed using a deep purple dye followed by decolorization with an acid wash then restaining with a red dye. As is illustrated in Figure 9-2, thick-walled organisms remain purple and are called **Gram positive**. Thin-walled organisms lose their initial purple in the acid wash and are then stained red by the second stain. They are called **Gram negative**. Bacteria also have two basic *shapes*: round (called **cocci**) and elongated or rod-shaped (called **bacilli** or rods). Several other shapes occur; some have pointed ends (*fusiform*, spindle-shaped) and others are tightly spiraled (**spirochetes**). Table 9-2 lists some common bacteria (and their associated diseases)

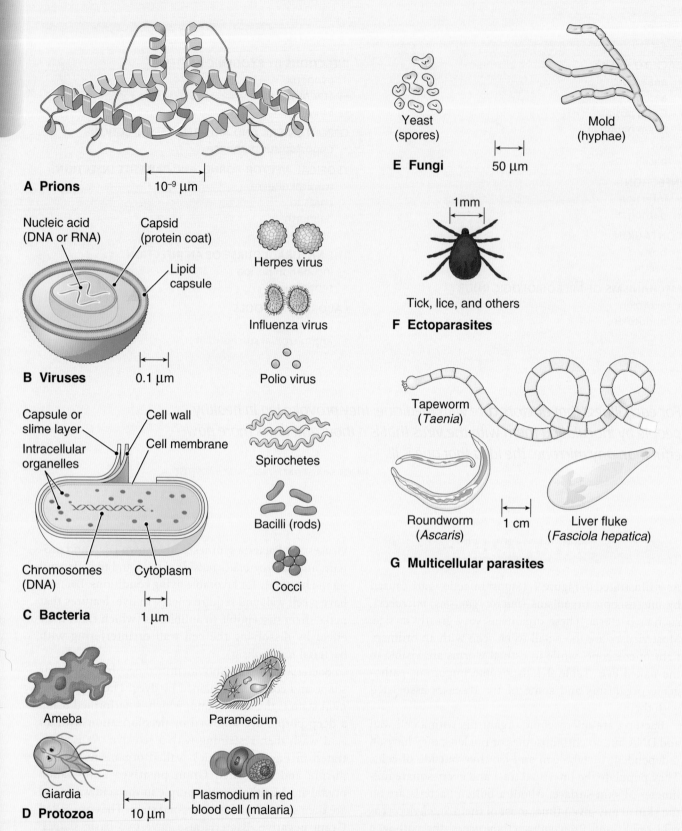

A Prions 10⁻⁹ μm

Nucleic acid (DNA or RNA) Capsid (protein coat) Lipid capsule

B Viruses 0.1 μm

Herpes virus
Influenza virus
Polio virus

Capsule or slime layer Cell wall
Intracellular organelles Cell membrane

Chromosomes (DNA) Cytoplasm

C Bacteria 1 μm

Spirochetes
Bacilli (rods)
Cocci

Ameba Paramecium
Giardia Plasmodium in red blood cell (malaria)

D Protozoa 10 μm

Yeast (spores) Mold (hyphae)

E Fungi 50 μm

1mm
Tick, lice, and others

F Ectoparasites

Tapeworm (*Taenia*)
Roundworm (*Ascaris*) 1 cm Liver fluke (*Fasciola hepatica*)

G Multicellular parasites

Figure 9-1 **Agents of infectious disease.** Arranged from **A.**, the smallest, molecule-size prions to **B.**, **C.**, and **D.**, intermediate-size organisms, to the largest, **F.** ectoparasites and **G.** worms, both of which are visible to the naked eye.

Table 9-1	**Some Important Infectious Diseases**		
Pathogen	**Transmission**	**Incubation Period**	**Symptoms**
VIRUS INFECTIONS			
AIDS Human Immuno-deficiency Virus	Sexual contact, shared needles, mother to child	Variable; usually several years	Fever, weight loss, fatigue, lymphadenopathy, cough, diarrhea
Common cold Rhinovirus, Coronavirus	Airborne droplet; hand-to-hand contact	1–3 days	Sneezing, sore throat, rhinorrhea, aches, cough
Hepatitis A	Fecal contamination of food or water	3–6 weeks	Influenza-like illness and jaundice; many initial infections are asymptomatic
Hepatitis B	Needles, sex	6–8 weeks	Same as hepatitis A
Hepatitis C	Blood and blood products	2–6 weeks	Same as hepatitis A
Influenza Influenza A in adults; influenza B or C in children	Airborne droplets	1–3 days	Fever, malaise, aches, sore throat, photophobia, cough, rhinorrhea
Measles Measles virus	Airborne droplets	7–14 days	Fever, cold symptoms, rash, conjunctivitis
Infectious mononucleosis Epstein-Barr virus	Saliva	1–6 weeks	Lymphadenopathy, fever, sore throat, malaise, fatigue
Rubella Rubella virus	Airborne droplets; mother to child	2–3 weeks	Fever, rash
CHLAMYDIA INFECTION			
Non-gonococcal urethritis and related sexual infections *Chlamydia trachomatis*	Sexual contact	1–4 weeks	Males: urethritis, prostatitis, epididymitis Females: vaginitis, cervicitis, salpingitis
RICKETTSIA INFECTION			
Rocky Mountain spotted fever *Rickettsia rickettsii*	Bite from infected tick	2–7 days	Severe headache, high fever, aches, weakness, rash
BACTERIA INFECTIONS			
Gonorrhea *Neisseria gonorrhoeae*	Sexual contact; mother to child	2–6 days	Males: urethritis, prostatitis, epididymitis Females: vaginitis, cervicitis, salpingitis; conjunctivitis of newborns

(continued)

Table 9-1	Some Important Infectious Diseases (Cont'd)		
Pathogen	**Transmission**	**Incubation Period**	**Symptoms**
BACTERIA INFECTIONS (cont'd)			
Meningitis *Neisseria meningitidis*	Airborne droplets, close contact among youth in closed populations such as dormitories	Variable; occasionally a few hours	High fever, stiff neck, confusion, collapse
Tuberculosis *Mycobacterium tuberculosis*	Airborne droplets	Weeks to years	Malaise, fatigue, weight loss, cough, shortness of breath
Typhoid fever *Salmonella enterica*	Fecal contamination of food or water	1-4 weeks	High, prolonged fever; intestinal upset, lethargy, headache
FUNGUS INFECTIONS			
Athletes' foot *Tinea* species	Direct contact	Weeks, months	Intense itching
Histoplasmosis *Histoplasma capsulatum*	Inhalation of dusty soil, bird droppings, especially in Ohio River valley region	2–3 weeks	Malaise, fever, cough, weight loss, shortness of breath
PROTOZOA INFECTIONS			
Amebiasis *Entamoeba histolytica*	Fecal contamination of food or water	Weeks to years	Severe diarrhea; liver abscess
Giardiasis *Giardia lamblia*	Fecal contamination of food or water	Days to weeks	Severe diarrhea
Malaria *Plasmodium* species	Bite of infected mosquito	10–40 days	Cyclical chills and fever; sweating, fatigue; jaundice

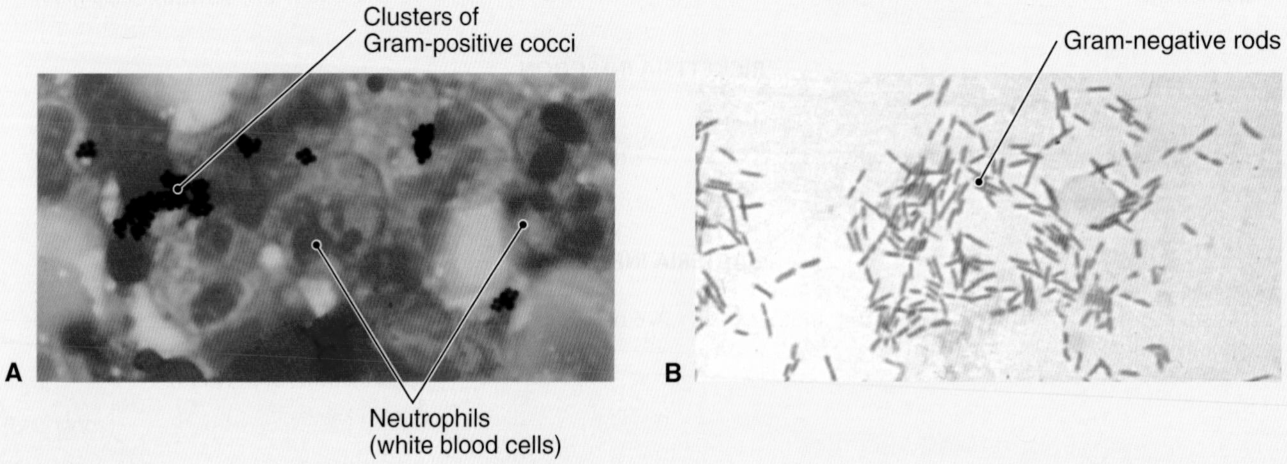

Figure 9-2 Gram stain. A. Gram-positive cocci (*Staphylococcus aureus*) in pus (large, dark-red globules are white cell nuclei). **B.** Gram-negative bacilli, or rods (*Escherichia coli*), from a culture plate.

Table 9-2 Common Pathogenic Bacteria and Associated Diseases

Type of Organism	Examples	Disease
Gram-positive cocci	*Staphylococcus aureus*	Skin abscesses, pneumonia
	Streptococcus	Pharyngitis (strep throat)
	Streptococcus pneumoniae	Lobar pneumonia
Gram-positive bacilli	*Bacillus anthracis*	Anthrax
	Clostridium tetani	Tetanus
Gram-negative cocci	*Neisseria gonorrhoeae*	Gonorrhea
Gram-negative bacilli	*Escherichia coli*	*E. coli* food poisoning
	Salmonella enterica	Typhoid fever
Spirochetes	*Treponema pallidum*	Syphilis
	Borrelia burgdorferi	Lyme disease

sorted according to bacteria shape and staining characteristic.

Mycoplasma are tiny bacteria not much larger than a virus that reproduce outside of cells. Mycoplasma are responsible for some urinary and pulmonary infections. *Chlamydia* and *Rickettsia* are small bacteria that, like viruses, are obligate intracellular parasites, but cannot replicate outside of cells. Like all bacteria they divide by splitting into two parts and are susceptible to antibiotics. Sexually transmitted *Chlamydia trachomatis* (Chapter 20) is the most common *reportable* (to public health authorities) infectious disease in the United States. Ocular infection by *C. trachomatis* (*trachoma*) is the most common cause of blindness in many parts of the world. *Rickettsia* causes infections in rodents and other animals and are incidentally transmitted to humans by insect vectors and cause a family of "spotted fevers," so called because patients have fever, flu-like symptoms, and skin rash.

Compared to bacteria, **fungi** are relatively large organisms. They have a cell wall and complex metabolism, enabling them to grow outside of cells. In disease they have two distinctive forms: those that grow as long, branching, multicellular filaments (*hyphae*), which are known as *molds*, or multicellular clusters of budding round forms called *yeast*. As pathogens, fungi are classified as either mold or yeast according to the form they take at normal body temperature; some can grow in both ways. Some yeasts can produce spores that exist in ice or soil for hundreds of years. Some fungi cause superficial infections of skin or of mucosal membranes. The general term for these infections is *tinea*. Other fungi, such as *Histoplasma capsulatum*, are associated with deep infections in the lungs or other viscera. Still other fungi are normal residents of skin and intestines (*Candida, Aspergillus*) but may cause disease in immunodeficient patients (Chapter 8). *Pneumocystis jiroveci* is a very small fungus that causes serious pneumonia in AIDS patients.

Viruses are very small pathogens that can live only inside of cells and depend on the cell to help them grow; they have no metabolism independent of the infected host and are not ordinarily thought of as living things. Outside of cells, viruses exist in an inert and inactive state. Because they reproduce only inside of cells, viruses are not susceptible to conventional antibiotics, such as penicillin. However, in recent years antiviral drugs have achieved limited success by inhibiting intracellular virus reproduction. Viruses are either RNA or DNA type according to the type of nucleic acid they contain. For example, HIV, the pathogen of AIDS (Chapter 8), is an RNA virus, while the adenovirus, one of the causes of the common cold, is a DNA virus.

Prions are the smallest of all infective agents—they are *molecules* derived from normal brain protein, prion protein (PrP). They are more like a crystal than a life form—prions duplicate themselves much as a snowflake grows by adding to itself. Like viruses, prions grow only within cells, but unlike viruses they have no DNA or RNA. However, once transmitted into a previously uninfected brain, they influence normal brain protein to change into prions, which cause chronic degenerative brain disease in humans (*Creutzfeldt-Jakob disease*) and animals (*mad cow disease*).

Protozoa are motile, single-cell organisms with a nucleus and are responsible for much illness and death in developing countries; *malaria* and *amebic dysentery* are examples. In industrialized nations protozoa cause common, less serious disease such as vaginitis (*Trichomonas vaginalis*) and diarrhea (*Giardia lamblia*). Some, like malaria, are spread by insects; others, like amebic dysentery, are spread by ingestion of fecally contaminated food.

Helminths (worms) are parasitic worms and are the most common of all human pathogens, infecting about one-third of the world population. They are the largest of all pathogens capable of living in the human body, and they have complex life cycles, sometimes living in an intermediate host before infecting humans. For example, in *schistosomiasis*, the most serious of all helminth diseases, the schistosome worm passes through snails before infecting humans. The number of *adult* worms present in the initial infection is important because the severity of the disease is proportional to their number. Once established in humans, adult helminths do not multiply; however, they produce eggs and larvae that account for most of the inflammation and symptoms. For example, a few intestinal helminths are of little consequence, but hundreds may consume enough blood to produce anemia. Most helminths infect the gastrointestinal tract or liver; some infect blood or muscle.

Ectoparasites are small insect-like creatures that attach to or live in the skin. They may transmit organisms—ticks transmit the spirochete *Borrelia burgdorferi*, which causes *Lyme disease*—or, like body lice, they may be an infection themselves.

MAJOR DETERMINANTS OF DISEASE

- Natural barriers and the immune system are critical in preventing infection.
- The body reacts in distinctive ways according to the type of infective pathogen.
- Particular pathogens have a tendency to infect a particular body part.
- Most infections occur in organs that are in direct contact with the environment.
- Inflammation is the primary response to infection.

Infection

Infections are among the oldest and most common afflictions of humankind, as is illustrated in the nearby History of Medicine box, and they remain a very serious problem. Table 9-3 lists the most common causes of fatal infection worldwide. Those dying from infection tend to be underprivileged, elderly, or debilitated or to have AIDS; and infectious diarrhea is an important cause of death in children in developing nations.

The mouth, throat, lungs, intestines, vagina, and skin normally contain or come into contact daily with potentially infectious agents. However, for infection to occur the pathogen must *invade* through the physical barriers (such as skin or gastrointestinal mucosa) and overcome innate and immune defenses (Chapter 8). Thus, **infection** is the *invasion* of the body by an infectious agent (**pathogen**) that causes tissue injury. Most pathogens are microscopic living things (*microbes*), such as bacteria and protozoa, which have their own metabolism apart from the tissues they invade. However, some pathogens

Table 9-3	Deaths from Infectious Disease, Worldwide 2002[1]	
Rank	**Disease**	**Deaths**
1	Pneumonia, influenza, and other respiratory infections	3.8 million
2	HIV/AIDS[2]	2.8 million
3	Diarrheal infections	1.8 million
4	Tuberculosis	1.6 million
5	Malaria	1.3 million
6	Measles	0.6 million
7	Pertussis (whooping cough)	0.3 million
8	Tetanus	0.21 million
9	Meningitis	0.17 million
10	Syphilis	0.16 million
	Total infection deaths[3]	13 million
	World population	6.2 billion
	Total deaths from all causes	57 million

[1]World Health Organization. Excludes deaths from parasitic disease (Table 9-4).
[2]HIV/AIDS deaths in 2002 were quadruple the 700,000 deaths in 1993.
[3]Infection deaths in all categories declined from 1993 except HIV/AIDS and tetanus.

are large enough to be seen by the naked eye; some intestinal worms, for example. What's more, some pathogens are not living things: viruses are packets of DNA and protein that have no metabolism independent of the cells they infect, and prions are infectious proteins

HISTORY OF MEDICINE

MILESTONES IN THE FIGHT AGAINST INFECTIOUS DISEASE

Microbiologic life existed on earth long before humans; we are interlopers in a microbial world, not the other way around. Their staying power is proven; ours is not. That some illnesses are contagious (transferable from one person to another) is among the oldest facts of history, but it took centuries of painstaking experimentation to prove microbes cause infectious disease.

The Greeks did not know of microbes and believed that maggots on decaying animals sprang from spontaneous generation, a theory not disproved until the middle of the 17th century when Francisco Redi, an Italian physician, showed that maggots would not appear if a jar of meat was covered by cloth. About this time Otto von Leeuwenhoek, a Dutch textile merchant, using a combination of lenses designed for inspecting fabric, assembled a powerful microscope that he used to identify the first microscopic living things, which he called animalcules, and we know as protozoa.

The 19th century French scientist Louis Pasteur, as an outgrowth of his studies on yeast and the fermentation of wine and beer, proved in 1865 that microbes could cause disease in humans and began to advocate cleanliness and sterilization as protective measures. Pasteur's cause was taken up by Joseph Lister, an English surgeon after whom Listerine

mouthwash was named. Lister's advocacy of antiseptic surgery achieved dramatic results: the death rate for limb amputation, the most serious surgery of the time, fell from 40% to 3%. In the latter part of the 19th century Robert Koch, a German microbiologist, proved that specific microbes were associated with specific diseases. In 1897, Ronald Ross showed that mosquitoes carry malaria; in 1911 Peyton Rous proved that viruses can cause cancer; and in 1928 Alexander Fleming discovered the antibiotic qualities of penicillin.

A milestone of a different sort occurred in 1796 when Edward Jenner, an English country doctor, observed that milkmaids were resistant to smallpox infection. He correctly concluded that prior infection by cowpox was the reason. Jenner's insight led to the discovery that cowpox pathogen, now known to be a virus related to smallpox, could be used as a vaccine to prevent smallpox.

Although we have known about infectious diseases, such as leprosy, since Biblical times, new infections are discovered regularly—AIDS, hepatitis C, and Lyme disease were discovered in the 1980s and 1990s, and the herpesvirus that causes AIDS-related Kaposi sarcoma in 1995. In 2003 severe acute respiratory syndrome (SARS) was found to be caused by a virus previously known only in animals.

that do not have DNA and "reproduce" somewhat like a crystal grows by adding onto itself.

Not all people and pathogens are equal—some people are more susceptible to infection than others, and some pathogens are more dangerous than others. Impaired immune or non-immune defense mechanisms (Chapter 8) are common causes of infection; for example, severely burned patients lack intact skin to protect them and subsequently acquire skin infections that may invade the rest of the body, and AIDS patients have defective immunity that renders them especially susceptible to infection. Some people are genetically more susceptible or resistant to infection. For example, people of African heritage are resistant to one type of malaria because they lack a red blood cell antigen to which the malaria parasite must attach to enter the red cell, but on the other hand, they are more susceptible to certain fungus infections.

The number of pathogens entering the body is important—a small number may not be enough to establish infection. The characteristics of the pathogen are important, even among pathogens of the same type. For example, the gastrointestinal tract contains *Escherichia coli*, which is part of the normal flora; however, some types of *E. coli* have characteristics that produce epidemic diarrhea and are known as *enteropathogenic E. coli* (Chapter 15).

What's more, despite the near-miraculous cures produced by antibiotics (see the nearby History of Medicine box), the widespread use of antibiotics is producing strains of antibiotic-resistant bacteria because occasional, random mutations of bacterial DNA provide a Darwinian, survival-of-the-fittest, advantage. Because reproduction cycles in bacteria are very short, it does not take long for new, antibiotic-resistant strains to displace older strains that were more susceptible to antibiotics.

Although the ancients used various concoctions to try to cure infections, ancient Peruvians provided the first clear evidence that infection could be treated with medicine. They discovered that the bitter bark of the cinchona tree was effective in treating what we now know as malaria. By the seventeenth century, science had discovered that the active ingredient in the bark was quinine, which remained the only effective antimalarial drug until the 1930s. Because of side effects, however, it is used in modern medicine only for certain types of severe malaria.

In 1928 Alexander Fleming, a Scottish physician working in London, made one of the most important discoveries in the history of medicine when he noted that a strain of the *Penicillium* mold exuded a substance that killed bacteria. Initially, Fleming did not think of the substance as medicine; however, in 1932 a German researcher, Gerhard Domagk, found that prontosil, a synthetic red dye, was effective in treating some bacterial infections. This evidence prompted

Fleming to suggest to colleagues that they try an extract of the mold, which he named penicillin, and in 1940, it was found to be effective in treating patients at London's St. Mary's hospital. By 1942, penicillin was used widely to treat English and American soldiers during World War II.

The widespread use of antibiotics to cure infection has been a boon to humankind. However, success has created a problem: strains of bacteria that are antibiotic-resistant. It is a Darwinian matter: the fittest bacteria survive. Bacteria, like all life forms, constantly mutate. Most mutations are detrimental to the organism, but some produce organisms more fit than others to survive the effects of antibiotics. Because reproduction cycles in bacteria are short, many generations per day, it does not take long for new, antibiotic-resistant strains to displace other forms—a benefit to the microbe but a hazard for the rest of us. The indiscriminate use of antibiotics for viral illnesses, where antibiotics have no effect, has contributed to the emergence of resistant strains of bacteria.

Contagion

Contagion is the spread of infection from one person (host) to another. Contagion can occur in almost any setting: at home or work or even in a hospital. (Infection acquired in a hospital is a **nosocomial** infection.) Infection occurs in a variety of ways: from animal to human or human to human; through skin, blood, lungs, or gastrointestinal tract; by fecal contamination of food or water; by aerosol droplets from sneezes and coughs; and by sexual intercourse, kissing, handshakes, or other contact. The infective organism is the pathogen; the infected person or animal is the **host**. For every pathogen there is a **reservoir**, a place where the pathogen exists and from which it spreads to new hosts. The reservoir may be food, water, soil, equipment, animals or animal products, or humans. The reservoir may be an obviously infected person, or it may be an asymptomatic **carrier**—a person or animal harboring the pathogen but suffering no obvious disease. For example, the hepatitis B virus may infect an intravenous drug addict (the host).

The mode of transmission from reservoir to new host may be by:

- *Direct contact*. Sexual intercourse, for example, transmits certain diseases such as syphilis (a bacterium) or herpes (a virus).

- *Indirect contact*. Contaminated food is sometimes responsible, as in hepatitis A infection. Sometimes **fomites**—inanimate materials such as gloves, bed sheets, or handkerchiefs—carry the pathogen. In each instance, the host contaminates the fomite with feces, nasal secretions, cells, or other material.
- *Droplets*. Respiratory droplets from coughing or sneezing are the mode of transmission for most upper respiratory infections ("colds"), influenza, mumps, and other diseases.
- *Vectors*. Malaria and other parasitic diseases are often transmitted by insect **vectors**, intermediate carriers such as mosquitoes.

Regardless of the mode of transmission, hands often play a role because they are in regular contact with the nose, mouth, genitalia, and other body parts. Frequent hand-washing is effective in controlling the spread of infectious disease. This is especially true in restaurants and hospitals.

The normal or expected rate of infection in a population or geographic area is the **endemic** rate. When cases occur at above normal rates, the infection is termed **epidemic**. For example, in 2003 an epidemic of hepatitis A in a large United States city was traced to a Mexican fast food restaurant. Further investigation revealed the source to be a batch of contaminated green onions. Exactly where between farm and restaurant the contamination occurred was not determined. More than 500 people were infected; three fatally. Most governments require that health care providers report certain infections, including, but not limited to, hepatitis, HIV, measles, sexually transmitted disease, tuberculosis, and enteropathogenic *E. coli*.

The Spread of Organisms in Tissue

It is the normal state of humans and beast that skin, mouth, and gastrointestinal tract teem with trillions of bacteria. This happy state of coexistence largely results from the presence of physical barriers to invasion and the molecular workings of the immune system (Chapter 8).

As is illustrated in Figure 9-3, microorganisms penetrate natural barriers such as skin, gastrointestinal, respiratory, or urogenital epithelium to cause infections such as abscess, diarrhea, pneumonia, or urinary infection, after which they may spread widely by gaining access to blood or the lymphatic system. For example, a skin infection with *Staphylococcus* might invade the lymphatic system to produce *lymphangitis* and spread upward through the thoracic duct and enter the blood stream to cause blood infection (*septicemia*), which in turn might carry organisms to the brain, causing a brain infection (Chapter 23).

In tissues, microorganisms spread along planes of least resistance. For example, bacteria from a ruptured appendix can spread along the smooth surfaces of the

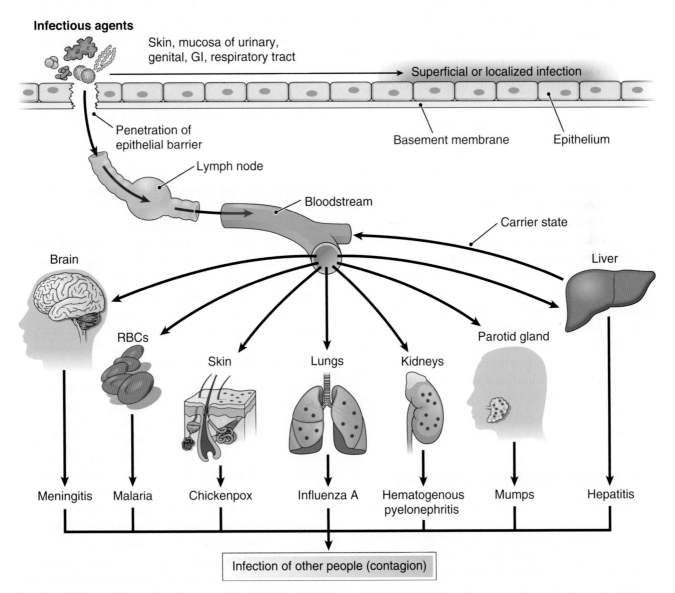

Figure 9-3 **The spread of infectious agents.** To infect and spread, agents (pathogens) must invade the body, usually by penetrating an epithelial barrier. After invading, most pathogens spread first through the lymphatic system before entering the blood and disseminating to distant organs.

peritoneum to cause an infection around the liver. In some infections, spread of organisms is confined to superficial epithelial surfaces. Pharyngitis caused by *Streptococcus* is an example. To the contrary, other organisms produce substances that promote tissue invasion. For example, some bacteria produce enzymes or other substances that enable them to invade tissue.

Mechanisms of Microbiologic Injury

Most viruses have surface protein receptors that attach to specific host cell surface proteins to gain entry into cells. For example, the HIV virus has a specific protein that attaches to the CD4 protein receptor on the surface of helper T cells (Chapter 8), enabling the virus to invade the cell. Some viruses kill cells; the HIV virus is an example. Other viruses stimulate an immune response that kills the infected cell. Still others stimulate cell proliferation; the human papillomavirus (HPV), the cause of cervical cancer (Chapter 21), is an example.

Some pathogens injure cells by producing toxins. Bacterial **endotoxin** consists of substances derived from bacteria that are released upon destruction of the cell wall and death of the bacterium. Most endotoxins come from Gram-negative bacteria and can cause vascular collapse (endotoxic shock), disseminated intravascular coagulation (DIC) (Chapter 5), or severe lung damage (acute respiratory distress syndrome, Chapter 14). In contrast, bacterial **exotoxins** are secreted by living bacteria into the medium in which they grow. Often the medium is outside the patient (food, for example) and the toxin is ingested and produces immediate effect. For example, the most common type of food poisoning features nausea, vomiting, and diarrhea caused by an exotoxin produced by staphylococci growing on unrefrigerated food. *Clostridium botulinum*, a Gram-positive, anaerobic bacillus, grows in contaminated canned or sealed food and synthesizes a neurotoxin that causes muscle paralysis. Botulinum toxin is popularly known as "botox" because of its widespread use to paralyze facial muscles and reduce skin wrinkles.

The Inflammatory Response to Infection

Refer to Chapter 3, Acute and Chronic Inflammation, for a more detailed discussion of the inflammatory response to infection. By way of review, however, recall that:

- Bacteria evoke an acute, pyogenic (pus-forming) inflammation, characterized by neutrophil infiltration

at the site and an increased number of neutrophils in blood (neutrophilia).

- Viruses evoke a less intense (subacute) inflammatory response characterized by lymphocyte and monocyte cellular accumulations in infected tissue and increased blood lymphocyte count (lymphocytosis). Some viruses, herpesvirus, for example, directly damage or kill cells (cytopathic effect), while other viruses may cause cell proliferation (cytoproliferative effect), such as HPV stimulation of cervical epithelium to cause cervical dysplasia or cancer.
- Mycobacteria and fungi typically evoke chronic inflammation, characterized by lymphocyte and monocyte accumulations at the infected site, increased blood lymphocyte count (lymphocytosis), and nodules of macrophages (granulomas, Chapter 3).
- Parasitic worms evoke an eosinophilic inflammatory reaction locally and in blood (eosinophilia).
- Protozoa evoke chronic inflammation and increased blood lymphocyte count (lymphocytosis).

The extent of tissue damage is proportional to the intensity and duration of inflammation. Some inflammation heals with little or no lasting effect, but more intense or long-lasting inflammation produces fibrous repair (scarring).

Infections of Organ Systems

Most infections affect one organ or organ system more than others. Infections of each organ system will be discussed in more detail in the chapter dealing with the organ. However, we will briefly discuss here the most commonly affected systems—those in contact with the environment: the respiratory system, gastrointestinal system, genitourinary system, and skin.

RESPIRATORY INFECTIONS

Respiratory infections are also discussed in Chapter 14. As is illustrated in Figure 9-4, many types of pathogens cause respiratory infections, and it is estimated that each day an average city dweller inhales roughly 10,000 microorganisms, most of which are trapped by nasal and bronchial mucus. Those reaching the bronchi are swept upward to the throat by the bronchial epithelium, which have cilia that move together like wheat in a windswept field and brush bacteria and particulate matter upward so that they can be coughed away or swallowed. However, a few bacteria reach the alveoli, where macrophages ingest and kill them. In addition, the bronchial tract is populated by patches of lymphoid tissue that provide enhanced immune protection by

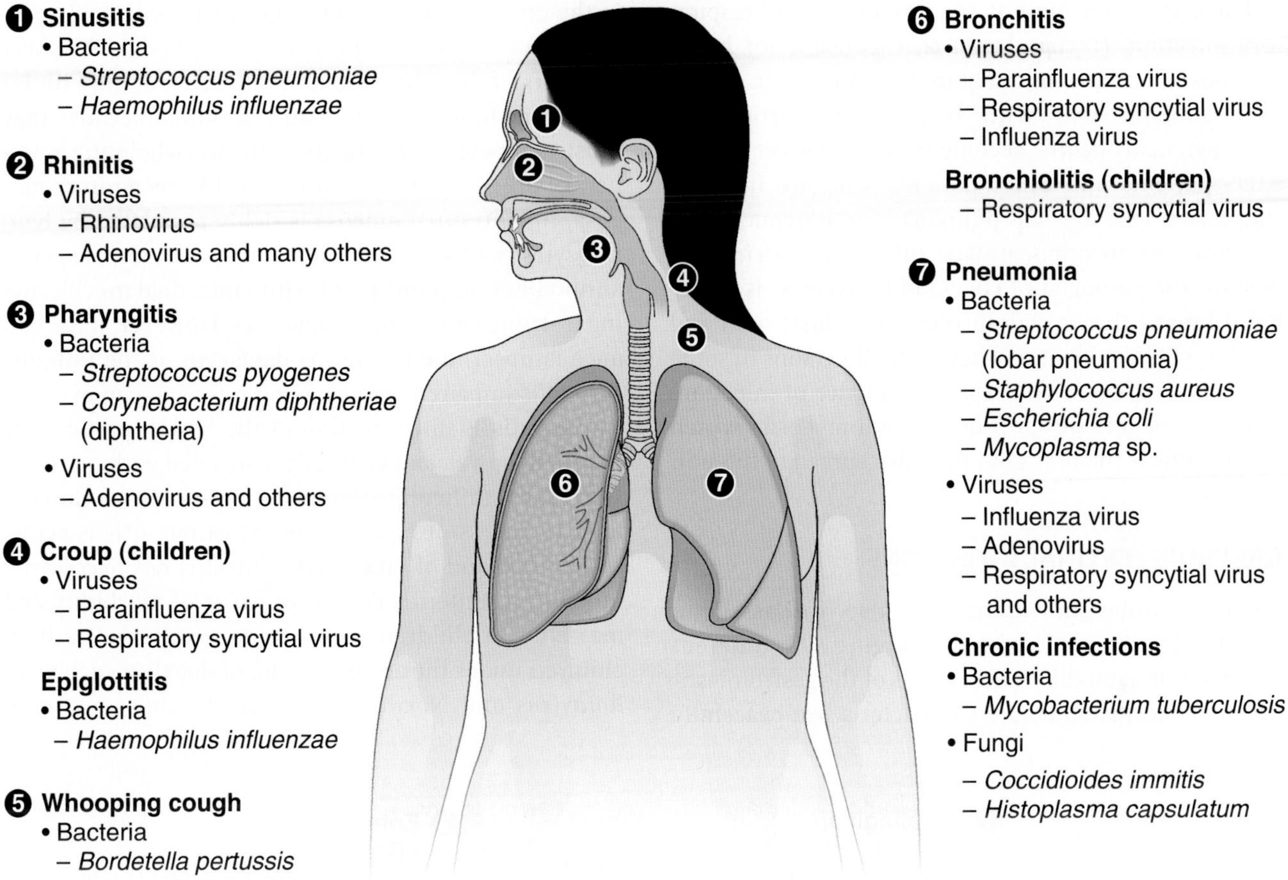

❶ Sinusitis
- Bacteria
  - *Streptococcus pneumoniae*
  - *Haemophilus influenzae*

❷ Rhinitis
- Viruses
  - Rhinovirus
  - Adenovirus and many others

❸ Pharyngitis
- Bacteria
  - *Streptococcus pyogenes*
  - *Corynebacterium diphtheriae* (diphtheria)
- Viruses
  - Adenovirus and others

❹ Croup (children)
- Viruses
  - Parainfluenza virus
  - Respiratory syncytial virus

Epiglottitis
- Bacteria
  - *Haemophilus influenzae*

❺ Whooping cough
- Bacteria
  - *Bordetella pertussis*

❻ Bronchitis
- Viruses
  - Parainfluenza virus
  - Respiratory syncytial virus
  - Influenza virus

Bronchiolitis (children)
  - Respiratory syncytial virus

❼ Pneumonia
- Bacteria
  - *Streptococcus pneumoniae* (lobar pneumonia)
  - *Staphylococcus aureus*
  - *Escherichia coli*
  - *Mycoplasma* sp.
- Viruses
  - Influenza virus
  - Adenovirus
  - Respiratory syncytial virus and others

Chronic infections
- Bacteria
  - *Mycobacterium tuberculosis*
- Fungi
  - *Coccidioides immitis*
  - *Histoplasma capsulatum*

Figure 9-4 **Respiratory infections.**

secreting a special category of antibodies ("immune paint") into bronchial mucus. Anything that interferes with either of these mechanisms promotes infection. For example, alcohol impairs the sweeping motion of the bronchial cilia, at least partially accounting for the fact that chronic alcoholics are prone to bacterial pneumonia.

Infections in children (Chapter 7) differ significantly from those in adults—whooping cough (*Bordetella pertussis*), diphtheria (*Corynebacterium diphtheriae*), and bronchiolitis (viruses) occur almost exclusively in children.

Viruses cause most respiratory infections. For example, the **rhinovirus** accounts for 60% of *common colds*. Infections of nose, pharynx, larynx, and trachea and are known as *upper respiratory infections* (URI). It is common for patients to refer to an upper respiratory infection as "the flu." Health care professionals should avoid this improper use of the term "flu." Real "flu," **influenza**, is caused by the *influenza virus* and is a serious, potentially fatal illness (see the Case Study at the end of this chapter). For example, 20–40 million people died during a 1918 worldwide influenza epidemic.

There are three influenza viruses—A, B, and C. Type A infects humans and animals and is responsible for most human disease; types B and C mainly cause childhood influenza. A few subtypes of influenza A sweep the world each year. Most originate in the bird population in coastal southeast China. Influenza A undergoes mutations each year to become antigenically different with each new flu season ("antigenic drift"), thus escaping immunity created by prior infections; therefore, a new vaccine is required each year. Public health officials note the strain that most successfully circulates in the spring in Asia and design vaccines to ward off infection later in the rest of the world.

Bacteria cause relatively few primary respiratory infections. However, bacterial pneumonia secondary to an underlying illness is the most common immediate cause of death in hospitalized patients, who usually have an array of other problems such as cancer or heart disease. The most serious bacterial respiratory infection is pulmonary **tuberculosis**, discussed in Chapter 14. About one-third of the world's population is infected, and worldwide about 1.5 million people die of tuberculosis each year.

Fungi are an uncommon but serious cause of respiratory infection. *H. capsulatum* is responsible for **histoplasmosis**, an infection acquired by inhalation of soil dust contaminated with bird or bat droppings. Although many people become infected, few become ill. AIDS patients and other patients who are immune suppressed may develop pulmonary or systemic histoplasmosis as an opportunistic infection. *Coccidioides immitis*, the pathogen of **coccidioidomycosis**, is an inhaled fungus that is widespread in the dusty west and southwest United States, where 80% of persons in some areas show positive skin tests as evidence of infection. Very few people develop coccidioidomycosis, which usually affects the lungs but may also spread to the skin or brain.

GASTROINTESTINAL INFECTIONS

Gastrointestinal infections are also discussed in Chapter 15. As is illustrated in Figure 9-5, different pathogens inhabit different sections of the gastrointestinal tract. Normally, trillions of bacteria live peacefully

in the intestines and exist in a mutually beneficial (*symbiotic*) state with one another and the body. The sheer numbers of these bacteria normally make it difficult for pathogens to gain a competitive foothold because they must compete for nutrients with overwhelming numbers of other organisms. Moreover, like respiratory mucosa, the intestinal mucosa is richly populated by lymphocytes, which secrete high concentrations of special antibodies ("immune paint") into intestinal mucus, giving it strong antimicrobial qualities. However, if the balance is upset, the mucosa is damaged, or the immune system is impaired, invasion and infection can occur.

Enteritis is inflammation of the bowel, particularly the small bowel, and is usually associated with diarrhea. **Diarrhea** is difficult to define but most patients think of it as an excess of liquid stools. Most enteritis is acute, self-limited and of viral origin, but it is not necessarily innocuous. Enteritis is a major cause of morbidity and mortality in children—worldwide nearly two million children under the age of five die of diarrhea each year. *Rotavirus* and *Norwalk virus* are the most common

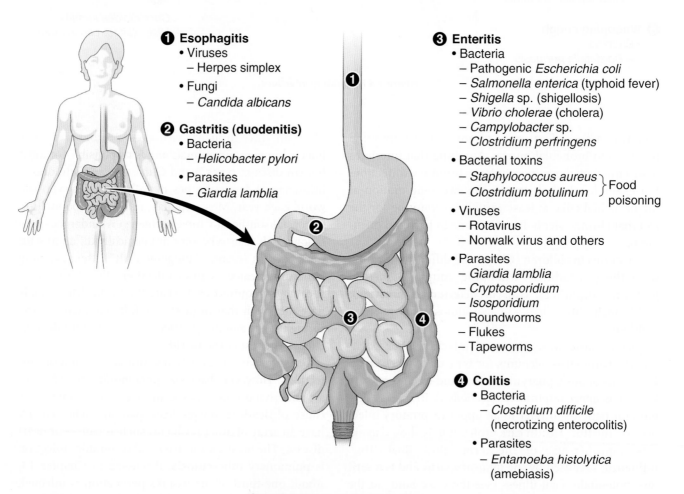

***Figure 9-5* Gastrointestinal infections.**

pathogens and are the culprits for outbreaks of enteritis among people living in close proximity, such as prisons or cruise ships.

Bacterial enteritis is less common but tends to be somewhat more severe. *Shigellosis*, caused by *Shigella* species, is a severe form of enteritis known as **dysentery**, which is a severe diarrhea with cramping and watery stools containing blood, pus, and mucus. *Shigella* is transmitted by oral-fecal contamination and is endemic in underdeveloped nations. *Salmonella* species cause food- and water-borne enteritis. *Salmonella enterica* infection can cause enteritis, septicemia, and shaking chills, a syndrome known as **typhoid fever**. *Campylobacter* species, responsible for many times more cases of enteritis than *Salmonella* or *Shigella*, causes sporadic, acute enteritis, usually from ingestion of improperly cooked chicken. ***Helicobacter pylori*** causes *chronic gastritis* and *peptic ulcers* (Chapter 16). **Cholera**, epidemic enteritis owing to *Vibrio cholerae*, is especially common on the Indian subcontinent. Although fatal in 50% of untreated cases, simple hydration and electrolyte replacement can reduce the mortality to less than 1%.

Parasitic intestinal infections are a severe problem in developing nations, but they also occur from time to time in the United States They are discussed in detail later in this chapter.

GENITOURINARY INFECTIONS

Urinary tract infections are also discussed in detail in Chapters 19 and 20. Infections of the genitals and urinary tract are closely related because of their intimate anatomic relationships and functions. The genitals are directly exposed to infection from the environment; the urinary system is indirectly exposed because organisms can spread up the urethra or vagina. For example, infection of the bladder (cystitis) is common in women because their urethra is short and opens onto the vaginal mucosa, which is warm and moist and supports bacterial growth. Moreover, most bacterial infections of the kidney (pyelonephritis) arise from infections of the bladder that ascend the ureter. Figure 9-6 illustrates the most common genitourinary infections.

Most genital infections are **sexually transmitted diseases (STD)**, which are reviewed in more detail in Chapters 20 (Male Genital System) and 21 (Female Genital System). The risk of STD is influenced by the number and variety of sexual contacts and lack of condom use or other protection. However, some diseases that are transmitted primarily by non-sexual means also can be transmitted sexually; for example, hepatitis B virus infection (Chapter 16).

Most STDs affect the genitalia, but some infections spread widely from the genitalia. For example, *syphilis* usually appears first as a genital ulcer (the *chancre*), but also invades the blood and spreads widely, causing widespread vasculitis that can affect almost any organ (for example, untreated syphilis can cause aortic aneurysm or dementia).

The most common sexually transmitted disease is **human papillomavirus (HPV)** infection (Chapters 20 and 21). HPV is a family of viruses, about two thirds of which are passed by casual skin-to-skin contact, especially among children, and are the cause of common skin warts. The remaining one-third of HPV viruses are genitally transmitted and are the cause of genital warts and dysplasia and cancer of the cervix. The most common genital disease caused by HPV is genital warts (**condyloma acuminatum**), a wart-like growth on the cervical or vulvar mucosa in females, or on the glans or prepuce in uncircumcised males. Cervical dysplasia and carcinoma are caused by genital HPV infections acquired from an infected partner or from several infected partners. Repeated infections are necessary to produce cervical dysplasia or carcinoma. Many women are infected but few develop dysplasia, and very few develop carcinoma.

Gonorrhea is a sexually transmitted bacterial disease caused by the Gram-negative diplococcus (cocci in pairs) *Neisseria gonorrhoeae*, also known as *the gonococcus*. It provokes an intense acute, purulent inflammatory reaction, which in males is a urethral exudate; however, infection may spread to cause acute infection of the prostate or the testicular epididymis. Repeated infection may cause urethral strictures and obstructed urine flow (Chapter 20). In females, infection produces clinically less noticeable inflammation of the urethra, vagina, and cervix; however, infection of the fallopian tubes produces intense acute inflammation (salpingitis). Repeated salpingitis (chronic pelvic inflammatory disease) may produce tubal obstruction with infertility or ectopic pregnancy (Chapter 21).

Nongonococcal urethritis (any acute urethritis that is not of gonorrheal origin) is the most common acute genital infection in males. Most cases are associated with *C. trachomatis*, but identifying the organism is difficult and often not worth the effort, because antibiotic treatment usually kills whatever organism is present. About 10% of college-age youths are infected, and about 90% of these infections are asymptomatic. *Chlamydia* infections occur in the same tissues that gonorrhea does: in men the urethra, prostate, and epididymis; in women, the vagina, cervix, and fallopian tubes.

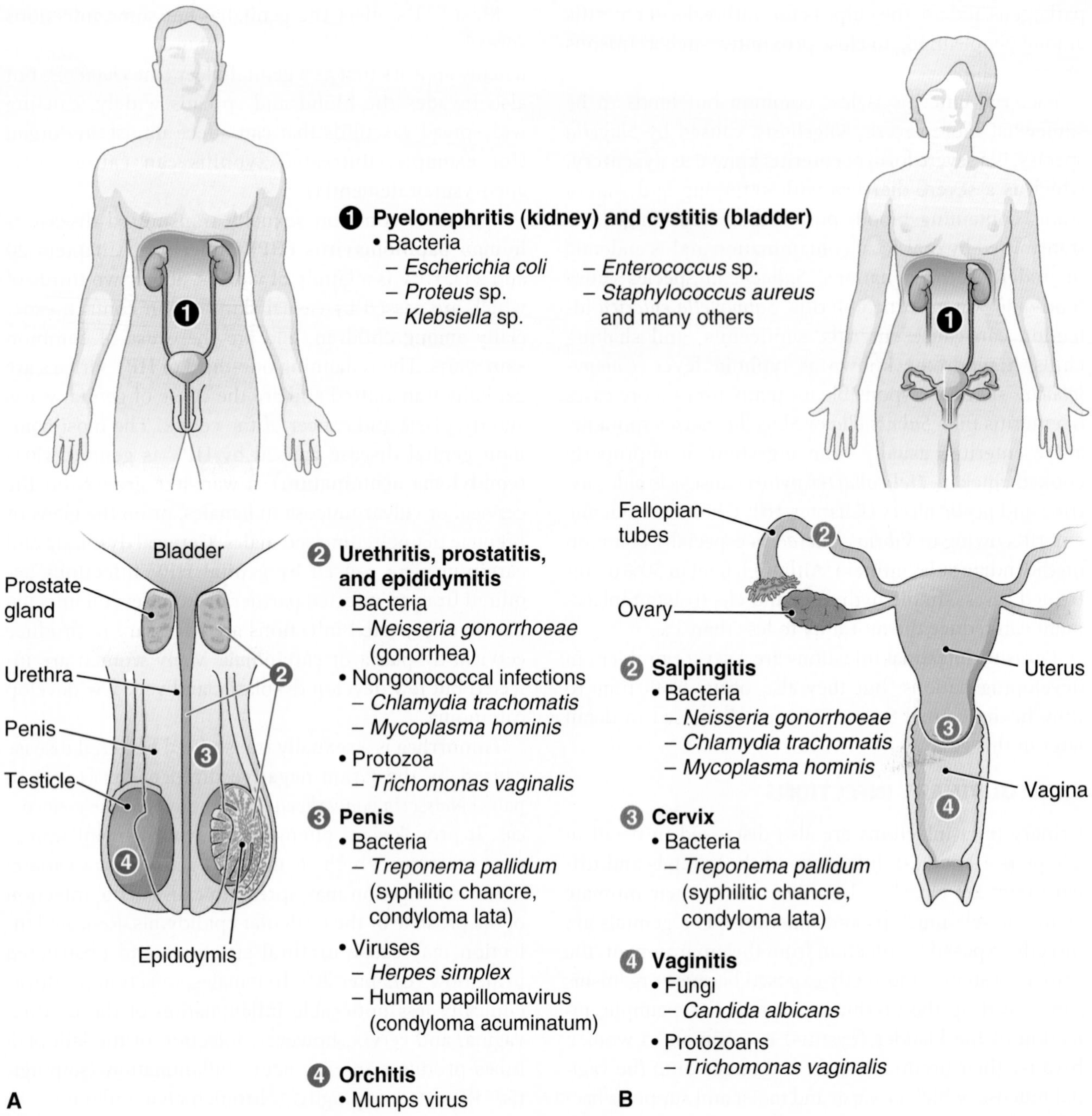

❶ **Pyelonephritis (kidney) and cystitis (bladder)**
- Bacteria
  - *Escherichia coli*
  - *Proteus* sp.
  - *Klebsiella* sp.
  - *Enterococcus* sp.
  - *Staphylococcus aureus* and many others

Bladder

Prostate gland

Urethra

Penis

Testicle

Epididymis

❷ **Urethritis, prostatitis, and epididymitis**
- Bacteria
  - *Neisseria gonorrhoeae* (gonorrhea)
- Nongonococcal infections
  - *Chlamydia trachomatis*
  - *Mycoplasma hominis*
- Protozoa
  - *Trichomonas vaginalis*

❸ **Penis**
- Bacteria
  - *Treponema pallidum* (syphilitic chancre, condyloma lata)
- Viruses
  - *Herpes simplex*
  - Human papillomavirus (condyloma acuminatum)

❹ **Orchitis**
- Mumps virus

A

Fallopian tubes

Ovary

Uterus

Vagina

❷ **Salpingitis**
- Bacteria
  - *Neisseria gonorrhoeae*
  - *Chlamydia trachomatis*
  - *Mycoplasma hominis*

❸ **Cervix**
- Bacteria
  - *Treponema pallidum* (syphilitic chancre, condyloma lata)

❹ **Vaginitis**
- Fungi
  - *Candida albicans*
- Protozoans
  - *Trichomonas vaginalis*

B

Figure 9-6 **Genitourinary infections. A.** Infections of men. **B.** Infections of women.

Chlamydia infection also causes **lymphogranuloma venereum (LGV)**, a recurring, suppurative infection of lymph nodes in the groin and rectal area. It is rare in the United States but common in developing nations. *Chlamydia* also may be associated with **Reiter syndrome**, a systemic condition characterized by urethritis, arthritis, conjunctivitis, iritis, and mucocutaneous lesions.

Genital **herpes** infection is caused by herpesvirus (*herpes simplex*), the virus that also causes cold sores. Most genital lesions are caused by herpesvirus type 2; most oral lesions are caused by type 1. Type 2 spreads mainly by direct contact with genital lesions, type 1 via oral secretions. The signs and symptoms are similar: clusters of small, painful blisters on the lips or genitals, which disappear in about 7–10 days.

T. vaginalis is a protozoan parasite and the pathogen responsible for a common form of mild vaginitis (**trichomoniasis**). The organism is often seen on routine pap smears in asymptomatic women. In men, *T. vaginalis* is one of the causes of mild, non-gonococcal urethritis.

Most cases of **human immunodeficiency virus (HIV)** infection are transmitted sexually. According to the United States Center for Disease Control and Prevention, in 2003 about 60% of cases in the United States occurred in male homosexuals and 20% in intravenous drug users, 10% were acquired by heterosexual contact, and 10% occurred in male homosexuals who were also intravenous drug abusers. However, in developing nations 75% of cases are transmitted by *heterosexual* contact, because the HIV virus finds easy entry through the genital sores created by other sexually transmitted diseases such as gonorrhea and syphilis, which are much more prevalent in developing nations.

SKIN INFECTIONS

The skin (Chapter 24) is more exposed to the environment than is any other organ, but it suffers relatively few, minor infections because it is covered by a surface layer of tough, dry keratin that contains few nutrients to support microbial growth.

Streptococci and staphylococci can cause small abscesses. *Impetigo* and *erysipelas* are superficial staphylococcus or streptococcus infections that often disappear without treatment (that is, they are self-limiting). *Dermatophytes*, a type of fungus that can digest keratin, can cause chronic superficial skin infections such as "ringworm" and "athletes foot." Herpesvirus infection causes common *cold sores*, and certain varieties of HPV cause *common warts* (verrucae).

Infections by Pyogenic Bacteria

Most bacteria that cause acute, **pyogenic** (pus-forming) infection require oxygen to live; that is, they are *aerobic*. However, many bacteria, especially those of the mouth, intestines, and vagina, and some on skin, are *anaerobic*; that is, oxygen kills them. Anaerobes cause diseases as varied as acne, septic abortion, periodontal abscess, and intra-abdominal abscess following intestinal perforation. Unless otherwise noted, the bacteria discussed below are aerobic.

Most pyogenic infections are the result of Gram-positive cocci. **Staphylococci**, usually *Staphylococcus aureus* (to be distinguished from *S. epidermidis*, a much less potent troublemaker), cause boils, impetigo, pha-

ryngitis, pneumonia, and endocarditis. Some varieties secrete toxins, which on ingestion cause severe diarrhea and vomiting (food poisoning). While staphylococcal infections tend to localize as abscesses, streptococcal infections tend to spread superficially. *S. aureus* is the major cause of skin infection in burns and is second only to *E. coli* as a cause of hospital-acquired (nosocomial) infections. *S. epidermidis* is a normal resident of skin and an opportunistic pathogen that infects vascular and urinary catheters, artificial heart valves, and other medical devices and is a common cause of endocarditis in intravenous drug users.

Streptococci (Fig. 9-7) also cause a wide variety of infections of skin, pharynx, lungs, and heart valves. In contrast to staphylococcus infections, those caused by streptococci tend to spread along surfaces and tissue planes because streptococci secrete a digestive enzyme that dissolves tissue barriers. Streptococci are classified into several groups according to surface antigens—A, B, and D are clinically important.

- *Group A* streptococci typically cause infection of superficial surfaces such as skin or pharynx.
  - *Acute streptococcal pharyngitis* (Chapters 8 and 14) is a painful, superficial throat infection commonly called "strep throat."
  - Two types of skin infection occur (Chapter 24): *Erysipelas* (Chapter 3, Figure 3-6) is a superficial, edematous, erythematous infection of skin and lymphatics.
    Impetigo (Chapter 24, Figure 24-21) is a superficial skin infection of young children that appears first as transient, small blisters, which break to form patches of red, "honey-crusted" lesions covered with dried exudate.
- *Group B* streptococci cause neonatal and urinary tract infections (Chapter 19).
- *Group D* streptococci cause infections of heart valves (bacterial endocarditis) and the urinary tract.
- *Streptococcus pneumoniae* (pneumococcus) is a major cause of pneumonia (lobar pneumonia, Chapter 14) and meningitis (Chapter 23) in adults.
- *Streptococcus mutans* is a major cause of dental caries.

In addition to direct infection, streptococci invade the bloodstream to cause serious blood infections (*septicemia*) or infection of the meninges (meningitis) or heart valves (bacterial endocarditis, Chapter 13). Moreover, streptococci can stimulate an autoimmune reaction (Chapter 8) in the kidney (glomerulonephritis, Chapter 19) or the heart (myocarditis and valvulitis in rheumatic fever, Chapter 13). Finally, *scarlet fever* (*scarlatina*), an intensely red skin reaction caused by an

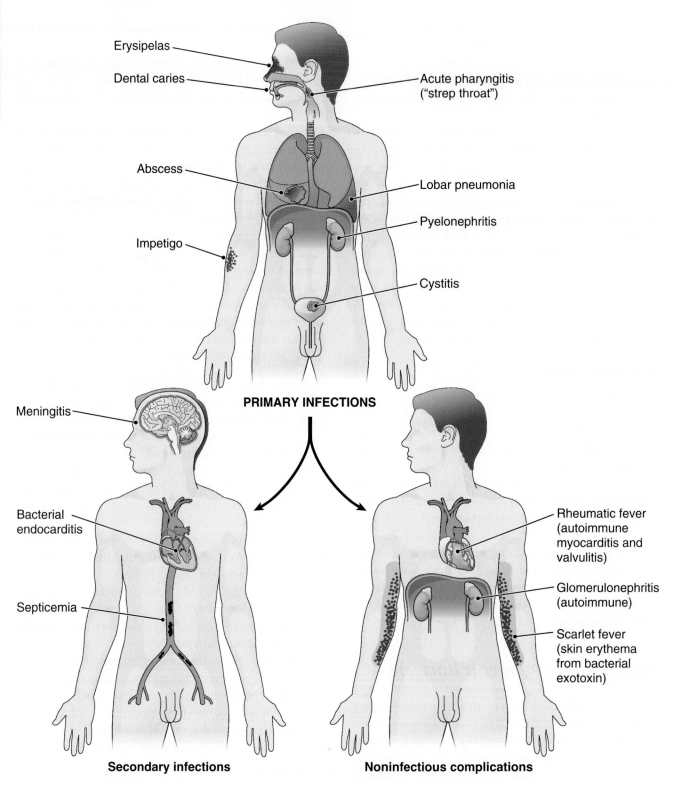

Erysipelas

Dental caries

Acute pharyngitis ("strep throat")

Abscess

Lobar pneumonia

Pyelonephritis

Impetigo

Cystitis

PRIMARY INFECTIONS

Meningitis

Bacterial endocarditis

Septicemia

Rheumatic fever (autoimmune myocarditis and valvulitis)

Glomerulonephritis (autoimmune)

Scarlet fever (skin erythema from bacterial exotoxin)

Secondary infections

Noninfectious complications

Figure 9-7 Streptococcal diseases.

exotoxin produced by some streptococci, is seen as an added feature in conjunction with a primary infection.

Infections by *Clostridium* Organisms and Other Necrotizing Agents

Clostridium species are large, Gram-positive, anaerobic bacilli frequently found in soil. They cause four infection syndromes in humans:

- *Clostridium difficile* is a normal inhabitant of the colon. It can proliferate and cause disease if the more populous, normal flora becomes suppressed by antibiotic therapy. Proliferation of *C. difficile* is associated with production of a toxin that causes **pseudomembranous colitis** (Chapter 15), a severe, necrotizing inflammation of the colon.
- *C. tetani* infects deep skin puncture wounds and releases a neurotoxin that causes severe muscle spasms and convulsions, a syndrome known as *tetanus*, or lockjaw.
- *C. perfringens* and related species ferment tissue to produce gas; they infect wounds and amateur abortions to cause anaerobic infection of deep soft tissues and muscles (*gas gangrene*).
- *C. botulinum* grows in incompletely sterilized food and synthesizes a neurotoxin that causes *botulism*, a syndrome of muscle and respiratory paralysis caused by neurotoxin blockage of acetylcholine release at the neuromuscular synapse.

Uncommonly, other organisms may cause severe tissue necrosis (gangrene); sometimes more than one organism is involved. Patients often are elderly and suffer from diabetes and vascular or immune disease. These infections often spread along fascia and tissue planes (*necrotizing fasciitis*), and they may be fatal or cause devastating local damage. For example, *Fournier gangrene* involves the penis, scrotum, and abdominal wall, usually in diabetics. *Meleney synergistic bacterial gangrene*, a progressive soft tissue necrosis usually resulting from a mixture of streptococcus and staphylococcus infections, is seen most often in an abdominal surgical wound or on an extremity.

Opportunistic and AIDS-Related Infections

Patients with impaired immunity (AIDS patients, for example) may be infected by any pathogen; however, many infections in these patients are caused by **opportunistic pathogens** (Chapter 8), agents that are not ordinarily pathogenic, or that rarely cause infection in people with healthy immune systems. Figure 9-8 illustrates that these ordinarily non-pathogenic organisms can infect almost any site.

Cytomegalic inclusion disease is caused by the *cytomegalovirus*. In healthy people, infection produces a mild febrile illness; however, in patients with impaired immunity it can produce hepatitis, gastroenteritis, esophagitis, chorioretinitis (inflammation of the retina and iris), and encephalitis (Chapter 23). Cytomegalovirus infection is one of the TORCH syndrome infections discussed in Chapter 7 as a cause of severe fetal deformities. Neonatal infection with cytomegalovirus is usually not fatal, but it can be associated with destruction of red blood cells (hemolytic anemia), enlarged liver and spleen, skin hemorrhages (purpura), pneumonia, and inflammation of the brain and meninges.

Pneumocystis jiroveci is a small fungus that causes no disease in people with normal immune function; however, *Pneumocystis* pneumonia is the foremost cause of AIDS death.

Cryptosporidium parvum and related protozoa cause chronic watery diarrhea in AIDS patients. Another protozoan, *Toxoplasma gondii*, causes **toxoplasmosis**, which may produce abortion or TORCH syndrome deformities (Chapter 7) in an infected fetus, or encephalitis in AIDS patients.

Cryptococcosis is a fungal infection caused by *Cryptococcus neoformans*. It causes infection of the brain and meninges in patients with deficient defense mechanisms, such as patients with AIDS, leukemia, Hodgkin disease, or sarcoidosis or in organ transplant patients being treated with immunosuppressive therapy.

Candidiasis (also called *moniliasis*) is an infection with *Candida* species fungi, which are normal inhabitants of skin, mouth, and gastrointestinal tract. *Candida* favors warm moist environments, such as the mouth or vagina. In infants it is a common cause of mild stomatitis (inflammation of the mouth) and diaper rash, and it is a common cause of vaginitis at any age. Chronic candidiasis of the mouth, nose, lips, and anus (*proctitis*) is a problem in AIDS. Severe, disseminated candidiasis may occur with leukemia, cancer chemotherapy, or immunosuppression associated with organ transplantation.

Pseudomonas infection is caused by *Pseudomonas aeruginosa*, an opportunistic and often deadly Gram-negative bacillus that is the third most common hospital-acquired infection (after *S. aureus* and *E. coli*). It is often a pathogen in cystic fibrosis, where *Pseudomonas*

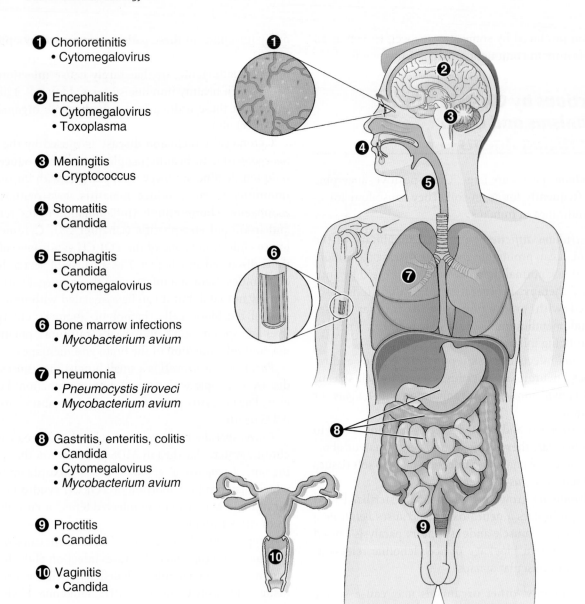

❶ Chorioretinitis
  • Cytomegalovirus

❷ Encephalitis
  • Cytomegalovirus
  • Toxoplasma

❸ Meningitis
  • Cryptococcus

❹ Stomatitis
  • Candida

❺ Esophagitis
  • Candida
  • Cytomegalovirus

❻ Bone marrow infections
  • *Mycobacterium avium*

❼ Pneumonia
  • *Pneumocystis jiroveci*
  • *Mycobacterium avium*

❽ Gastritis, enteritis, colitis
  • Candida
  • Cytomegalovirus
  • *Mycobacterium avium*

❾ Proctitis
  • Candida

❿ Vaginitis
  • Candida

Figure 9-8 Opportunistic and AIDS-related infections.

pneumonia is the most common cause of death. It frequently infects the skin of burn patients and may invade the bloodstream (septicemia). Patients with extremely low white blood cell counts (leukopenia) are susceptible to *Pseudomonas* infection.

Atypical tuberculosis is tuberculosis caused by any *Mycobacterium* other than *Mycobacterium tuberculosis*. A common opportunistic pathogen in AIDS patients, *Mycobacterium avium* (the pathogen of bird tuberculosis) causes infection of the lungs and spreads widely to the bone marrow and other organs.

Tropical, Vector-borne, and Parasite Infections

Tropical diseases, by definition, occur in tropical climates, and most are caused by parasites or are borne by *vectors*, such as insects. Tropical diseases are numerous and widespread, accounting worldwide for billions of illnesses and millions of deaths annually. With increased worldwide air travel, tropical infections (especially malaria, Chapter 11) are becoming more common in the United States.

Two important tropical diseases *not* associated with vectors include leprosy and trachoma. **Leprosy** (Hansen disease) is caused by *Mycobacterium leprae*, a mycobacterium related to tuberculosis. It affects skin and peripheral nerves in the cool parts of the body, especially extremities and scrotum. Leprosy's fearsome reputation derives from the terrible disfigurement of a few of its victims and the erroneous belief that it is highly contagious. To the contrary, leprosy is probably transmitted by aerosol inhalation, not by skin-to-skin contact, and it is very difficult to transmit. The accompanying History of Medicine box relates an interesting aspect of leprosy research.

Trachoma is an eye disease caused by *C. trachomatis*, the same organism mentioned in Chapter 21 as the principal cause of urethritis in men and chronic fallopian tube infection in women. When *C. trachomatis* infects the underside of the eyelid (the conjunctiva), it is known as *trachoma*, a disease principally found in nomads in dry, sandy, developing nations. It blinds millions annually by scarring the mucosal surface of the eyelid—contraction of the scars turns the eyelashes inward (entropion) so that they scratch the cornea with each blink. Corneal scarring is the result. Infection is usually acquired in childhood from fomites (foreign objects) and possibly from flies.

VECTOR-BORNE INFECTIONS

A **vector** is an invertebrate animal that transmits disease to vertebrates. Most vectors of human disease are insects, such as mosquitoes, or arachnids, such as ticks.

HISTORY OF MEDICINE

ARMADILLOS TO THE RESCUE

For many years leprosy research was hampered by the lack of an animal model because the bacterium can live only at relatively low temperatures, and the body temperature of laboratory animals was too high. This also accounts for the fact that in humans leprosy mainly infects the cooler parts of the human body: the ears, nose, and fingers and toes. However, in 1971 it was discovered that the humble armadillo, which has a low body temperature, could propagate the bacillus. About 10% of wild armadillos in Texas are infected. Whether armadillo leprosy is contagious remains a matter of debate, especially around campfires in Texas, where the armadillo's status as the "national" mascot is undisputed—as is its favored status in roadkill recipes.

For example, *Plasmodium,* the pathogen of **malaria,** infects red blood cells and is transmitted by mosquitoes from an infected patient to the new host.

Rickettsia is a family of obligate intracellular bacteria (they cannot live outside of cells) transmitted by ticks, lice, or chiggers. After a variable incubation period of up to several weeks, the typical case erupts with a prominent hemorrhagic rash (petechiae), fever, enlarged lymph nodes, and a hemorrhagic, crusted sore (the eschar) at the site of the bite. Diseases vary and are named according to the causative organism: for example, *Rocky Mountain spotted fever* is caused by *Rickettsia rickettsii,* and *epidemic typhus* (not to be confused with typhoid fever) is caused by *Rickettsia prowazekii.*

Lyme disease is discussed in detail in Chapter 22 and is caused by a corkscrew-shaped bacterium (spirochete), *Borrelia burgdorferi.* It is transmitted to humans by deer ticks.

Plague, which killed about one-fourth of the population of 14th century Europe, is still with us—it infects wild rodents in the southwest United States, prairie dogs especially. A few human cases are reported annually. The pathogen is *Yersinia pestis,* a Gram-negative bacterium transmitted by rodent fleabites and by aerosol droplets from patients with plague pneumonia.

PARASITE INFECTIONS

Infestation by parasites is the most widespread of all human disease. A **parasite** is an organism that draws nourishment from another organism, the host, and coexists with the host while contributing nothing to the survival of the host. The word is derived from the Greek *parasitos,* for one who lives at the expense of another and offers nothing in return. Table 9-4 presents broad-brush estimates of the prevalence of parasitic disease (the number affected at any given time) and the death incidence (the number of deaths per annum), but such statistics can vary, sometimes greatly, from one expert analysis to another. Most parasitic disease occurs in developing nations with poor public health capabilities.

Worm Infections

Worm (**helminth**) infections deserve special attention because worldwide they infect about 3 *billion* people, nearly half of people on the planet. Most parasite infections are little more than a nuisance, but many patients are severely affected: helminth infection is a leading cause of global morbidity and mortality. Worms vary from a few millimeters to over a meter long, and most migrate from the point of entry through various organs as they grow and mature. Many have very complex life

Table 9-4	Human Parasitic Infections	
Disease Category	People Infected (approximate)	Deaths per Year (approximate)
Helminths (worms) Intestinal nematodes	4.5 billion	1,000,000+
Ascariasis	1 billion	20,000
Trichuriasis (whipworm)	500 million	Rarely fatal
Hookworms	1.3 billion	Rarely fatal
Enterobiasis (pinworm)	300 million	Not fatal
Other nematodes: Filariasis	140 million	35,000
Trematodes: Schistosomiasis	200 million	1,000,000+
Cestodes: Tapeworms	50 million	50,000, all caused by cysticercosis or echinococcosis
Malaria	500 million	1,500,000+
Amebiasis	500 million	100,000

cycles that require passage through other hosts before reinfecting humans.

Roundworm Infections

Roundworms (nematodes) infect either the intestines or subcutaneous tissues. The clinical presentation of worm infections varies greatly; however, most are accompanied by increased numbers of blood eosinophils (eosinophilia).

Filariasis (from Latin, filum, for thread) is an infection by small (1–3 cm) roundworms transmitted by mosquitoes and found most commonly in Asia and Africa. The most common variety infests lymphatics and subcutaneous tissue and can cause massive lymphedema of the scrotum and legs (elephantiasis).

Intestinal roundworms are common in tropical climates but rarely cause problems. They live in the intestine and spread by oral-fecal contamination. Affecting over one billion people worldwide, ascariasis is caused by intestinal infestation with the Ascaris species of large roundworms. Transmission is by oral-fecal contamination, and the life cycle is fascinating—ingested eggs hatch and larvae invade the intestinal mucosa to enter the blood, where they migrate to the lungs, crawl up the trachea and are swallowed. They reenter the intestine, where they attach to the mucosa and suck blood for

nourishment. Most infections are asymptomatic but can be suspected by blood eosinophilia. Severe infections may cause intestinal bleeding, anemia, or intestinal obstruction.

Hookworms are intestinal roundworms that infect over one billion persons, mostly in tropical climates. There are several varieties and their life cycle is similar to ascariasis but they initially enter through skin and then into blood. Most infections are asymptomatic, but severe infestation may cause intestinal bleeding and anemia.

Pinworm infection, caused by Enterobius vermicularis, a small (1 cm long) roundworm, is a common pediatric infection in the United States. Transmitted by the oral-fecal route, pinworms live in the intestine and usually cause no symptoms; however, in some patients the worm crawls onto perianal skin and causes intense itching. Diagnosis is made by pressing clear acetate tape to the perianal region and examining it microscopically for eggs.

Trichinosis is infection by the Trichina roundworm, which is transmitted by eating infected pork (pig muscle containing Trichina larvae) that is inadequately cooked. The ingested larvae mature in the intestine, invade blood, and spread to muscle, where they remain and cause myositis.

Flatworm Infections

Flatworms (flukes) are also called trematodes, from Greek, meaning pierced with holes, because they attach by suckers that pierce the mucosal lining of hollow tissues such as blood vessels and bile ducts.

Schistosomiasis, caused by one of several types of flukes from the Schistosoma family, is by far the most important of all worm infections, affecting about 10% of world population and ranking near malaria in terms of the death and disability it causes. Most common in central Africa and other tropical climates, eggs are passed in urine and stool into water, from whence larvae infect snails and mature before reentering water to invade the skin of humans and disseminate widely via blood. Severe infections are characterized by intense liver, intestinal, and bladder inflammation.

Tapeworms

Tapeworms (cestodes) are segmented, ribbon-shaped worms that infect about 50 million people worldwide, most commonly in developing nations. Infection occurs with consumption of inadequately cooked beef or pork that contains larvae. Though infection is common, infected people are often not ill, although they may suffer weight loss and minor abdominal discomfort and may become alarmed upon finding pieces of worm in their stool.

The *pork* tapeworm can cause severe illness if *eggs* (as opposed to larvae in muscle) are ingested from fecally contaminated food or drink. The eggs release a form of the worm that invades blood vessels and disseminates to deposit widely in many tissues as small (1 cm) cysts, *cysticerci* (**cysticercosis**). Cysticerci do not cause inflammation, but remain alive and create problems by mass effect. Severe infestation of the brain can cause seizures or death.

Echinococcosis (*hydatid disease*) is a tapeworm infection caused by larvae of several varieties of tapeworm passed back and forth between dogs and cows: cattle eat grass contaminated by dog feces; dogs eat cow flesh. Human infection occurs by ingestion of food contaminated by infected dog feces. Larvae invade blood vessels and lodge in deep organs, especially liver and lungs, where they may mature into large cysts (*hydatids*) several centimeters in diameter. Most infections are acquired in childhood but do not become symptomatic for many years.

Protozoal Infections

Protozoa are unicellular, motile, microscopic pathogens with a nucleus. They are larger and more complex than are bacteria, which, for example, do not have a nucleus.

Malaria, discussed in detail in Chapter 11, a protozoal infection spread by mosquitoes, infects 200 million people worldwide, mostly in tropical climates, and kills more than a million people annually. Malaria parasites invade red blood cells and destroy them in febrile, hemolytic cycles as immature new organisms burst from infected red cells.

Amebiasis (Fig. 9-9) refers to infection by *Entamoeba histolytica*, a protozoan that infects hundreds of millions of persons annually on the Indian subcontinent, Mexico, and South America. Most cases (90%) are asymptomatic; however, amebiasis is the third most common fatal parasitic disease after malaria and schistosomiasis. Infection is acquired through consumption of food contaminated by human feces that contains amebic cysts, which are capsules of amebae designed to survive in the environment. After ingestion the amebae break out of the cyst in the intestine; some invade the colon mucosa and others form new cysts that are passed in feces. Invasion of bowel mucosa produces abdominal pain and diarrhea. Invasion into the portal blood often produces amebic liver abscesses, but brain, lung, and other organs may be involved.

Leishmaniasis is a chronic inflammatory disease of skin, mucous membranes, and viscera. Most common in underdeveloped nations, it is caused by microscopic, intracellular protozoa that infect white blood cells, and it is transmitted from infected animals by sandflies. **Trypanosomiasis** is a disease caused by several varieties of microscopic protozoa that infect blood and are transmitted from human to human by insects. One variety, *African trypanosomiasis*, or sleeping sickness, causes intermittent fevers, enlarged lymph nodes and spleen, and progressive brain dysfunction. *Chagas disease* occurs mainly in South America. Many Chagas infections are asymptomatic, but severe infection can cause myocardial damage; Chagas disease is the most common cause of heart disease in South America.

Giardiasis, caused by the protozoan *Giardia lamblia*, arguably the world's most common intestinal parasite infection, is acquired by ingesting fecally contaminated water or unwashed vegetables or fruits. Most infections are asymptomatic, but some cause acute or chronic diarrhea. *G. lamblia* is not killed by water chlorination; it must be filtered out. Giardiasis is a common infection in campers drinking stream water, especially near cattle or human habitation.

Cryptosporidiosis and **isosporidiosis** are infections caused by small protozoa, which may cause diarrhea in otherwise healthy people but are most notable as opportunistic intestinal pathogens in AIDS and other immunodeficiency states.

T. vaginalis is a protozoan and the pathogen of vaginal **trichomoniasis** and is discussed in greater detail in Chapter 21.

The Natural Course of an Infection

The natural course of infection is depicted graphically in Figure 9-10. The initial event in every infection is the invasion of the organism into the body. The time between invasion and appearance of signs or symptoms is the **incubation period**, during which the organism attempts to proliferate. If the body's defenses are effective, no illness occurs. Otherwise, the organism multiplies to the point that it produces damage sufficient to cause signs and symptoms. After the incubation period, a **prodromal period** may occur in which the patient suffers from mild, non-specific symptoms. Headache, loss of appetite, and fatigue are common prodromal symptoms. The prodrome is followed by the **acute phase** of the illness, a time of maximum acute, typical clinical signs and symptoms. There follows a period of **convalescence**, during which symptoms fade. Finally is the **recovery**

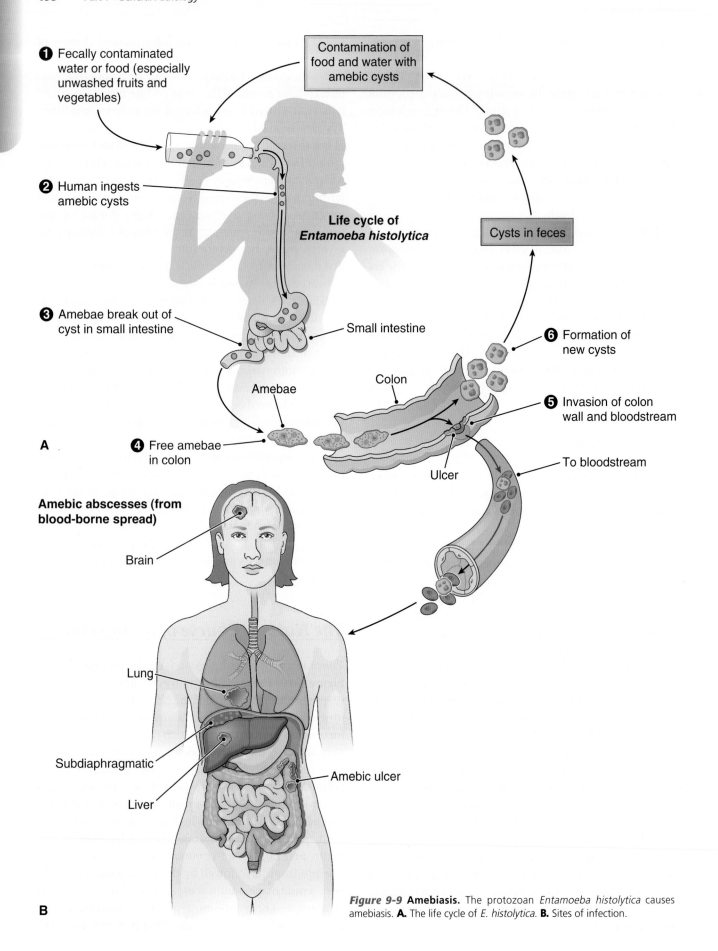

A

① Fecally contaminated water or food (especially unwashed fruits and vegetables)

Contamination of food and water with amebic cysts

② Human ingests amebic cysts

Life cycle of *Entamoeba histolytica*

Cysts in feces

③ Amebae break out of cyst in small intestine

Small intestine

⑥ Formation of new cysts

Colon

Amebae

⑤ Invasion of colon wall and bloodstream

④ Free amebae in colon

Ulcer

To bloodstream

B

Amebic abscesses (from blood-borne spread)

Brain

Lung

Subdiaphragmatic

Liver

Amebic ulcer

***Figure 9-9* Amebiasis.** The protozoan *Entamoeba histolytica* causes amebiasis. **A.** The life cycle of *E. histolytica*. **B.** Sites of infection.

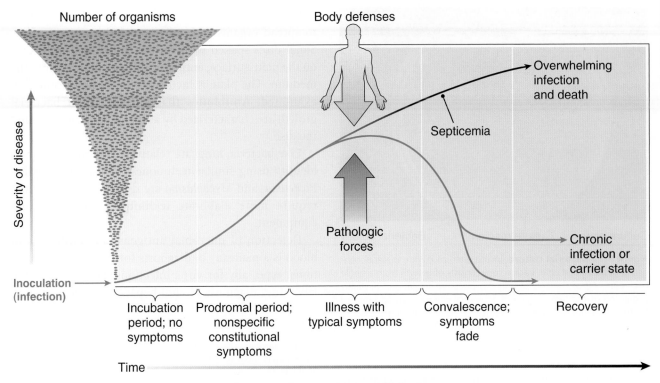

Figure 9-10 **The natural course of infection.**

period, during which no symptoms are present, but the patient may feel fatigued.

However, the picture is not always so simple. If the patient's defenses are inadequate, the organism may continue to proliferate and invade the bloodstream, colonizing various organs. For example, if the brain coverings (meninges) are colonized, meningitis may occur. Severe infection of blood by bacteria, called **septicemia**, can cause shock, DIC, or other calamity.

Most infections are cleared completely by body defenses or medical therapy. However, some patients may regain good health but harbor the organism. They are **carriers**, a potential source of infection for others.

Signs and Symptoms of Infection

Local signs of infection are those of local tissue damage as discussed in Chapter 2—swelling, redness, warmth, and pain. *Systemic symptoms* of infection include fever, malaise, myalgia, loss of appetite, and fatigue. Of course, there are symptoms specific to the organ or system involved: headache with brain or meningeal infections, jaundice with viral hepatitis, and cough with influenza. *Laboratory findings* include elevated white blood cell count (neutrophilia in bacterial infections; lymphocyto-

sis in viral infections; eosinophilia in parasitic infections) and elevated erythrocyte sedimentation rate and levels of C-reactive protein (Chapter 3) because of increased liver synthesis of defensive proteins.

Laboratory Tools

Laboratory tools are important in investigating the cause of infection, choosing appropriate therapy, and monitoring patient progress. The simplest, most widely available and reliable tool is the **Gram stain**, explained earlier. Merely identifying the shape (bacillus or coccus) and the Gram stain properties (Gram positive or Gram negative) can be invaluable and, when combined with clinical findings, may be enough to make a provisional diagnosis and begin therapy. Occasionally other organisms, fungi, for example, may be visible on a Gram stain. Viruses and other small non-bacterial pathogens are usually not visible by Gram stain study but may be detected by other stains and techniques in particular circumstances.

Of perhaps greater importance is **microbial culture**, as is illustrated in Figure 9-11. Obtaining a specimen for culture may be as simple as swabbing pus from a wound or collecting a urine specimen. On the other hand, ob-

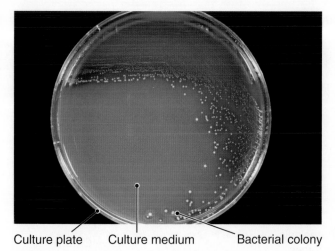

Culture plate   Culture medium   Bacterial colony

Figure 9-11 Bacterial culture. In this plate of culture material consisting of blood and agar, each colony consists of growth from a single bacterium. All of the colonies on this plate are similar and probably composed of the same organism. Individual colonies can be sampled for further identification and antimicrobial sensitivity testing.

taining a specimen may require an invasive technique such as a spinal tap to obtain cerebrospinal fluid in cases of suspected meningitis.

Cultures are performed by smearing the specimen on one or more types of special nutrient *media*, which are incubated at body temperature to encourage the growth of organisms. Typically, the specimen is smeared in a way that spreads the specimen thinly, so that it is likely that a single bacterium will be isolated and reproduce itself to form a **colony** apart from others. Colonies are pure cultures of a single bacterium, and can be re-sampled and re-cultured to determine other bacterial characteristics.

The type of media varies according to the type of specimen and the organism suspected. For example, stool specimens are usually cultured on media that inhibit the growth of normal intestinal bacteria and encourage the growth of intestinal pathogens such as *Shigella* or *Salmonella*. Throat swabs of suspected streptococcus infection, an important cause of pharyngitis, are inoculated onto media especially conducive to the growth of streptococci but not to other bacteria. If a suspected pathogenic organism grows, it is subjected to other identifying tests and re-cultured (regrown) in the presence of different antibiotics, a technique known as **antimicrobial susceptibility** testing (Fig. 9-12) to determine which antibiotics inhibit growth or kill the organism and which have no effect. Modern antimicrobial susceptibility testing is automated, but the underlying principle is illustrated by the following simple manual technique. Bacteria from a single colony are suspended

in fluid and poured onto a culture plate in such a way as to spread organisms evenly across the entire surface. Small discs soaked with various antibiotics are placed on the plate surface; antibiotic diffuses outward into the medium. The plate is incubated for 24 hours and then examined. Antibiotics that kill or inhibit bacterial growth are characterized by a ring of no growth around the disc.

Like bacteria, fungi are relatively easy to culture and identify using similar techniques. Viruses, *Chlamydia*, *Rickettsia*, and *Mycoplasma* are difficult to culture and require more elaborate techniques, expertise, and equipment.

Detection of microbial antigens and antibodies in blood is a mainstay of diagnosis for nonbacterial infections, especially for virus infections. For example, the laboratory diagnosis of viral hepatitis (Chapter 16) de-

Large area of growth inhibition – bacterium is <u>most sensitive</u> to antibiotic C

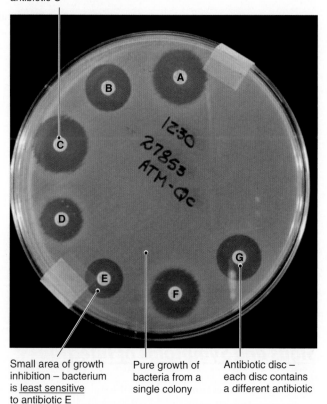

Small area of growth inhibition – bacterium is <u>least sensitive</u> to antibiotic E

Pure growth of bacteria from a single colony

Antibiotic disc – each disc contains a different antibiotic

Figure 9-12 Antibiotic sensitivity testing. The surface of the culture plate is overgrown by bacteria that were collected from a *single colony* of the culture plate in Figure 9-11 and evenly spread across the surface. White paper discs soaked with different antibiotics are placed on the plate, and the plate is incubated 24 hours. Clear areas around discs are where bacterial growth has been inhibited. Bacterial sensitivity to a particular antibiotic is related to the size of the zone of inhibited: a large zone suggests the antibiotic may be effective in treating the patient's infection.

pends exclusively on detection of viral antigens and antibodies in blood.

Finally, direct detection of organisms in tissue, fluids, or smears may be accomplished by a variety of immune and genetic techniques or by direct microscopic exami-

nation. For example, the *Plasmodium* parasite of malaria can be seen in red blood cells on ordinary smears of peripheral blood, or in the case of intestinal parasitism, the eggs or the worms themselves can be detected by direct microscopic examination of stool smears. ■

CASE STUDY 9-1 *"I KNEW SHE WAS SICK WHEN SHE DIDN'T WANT A CIGARETTE"*

TOPICS
The effects of cigarette smoking
Influenza
Bronchopneumonia

THE CASE

Setting: Your job is to see patients in the campus walk-in clinic at a large university.

Clinical history: Ruth R. is a 63-year-old retired bookkeeper who comes to the exam room when you call her name to the crowded waiting room. Making small talk on the way to the exam room, you learn that she and her husband, a university administrative official, attended a volleyball game earlier in the day, and when you inquire about the problem her husband interrupts to say, "I knew she was sick when she didn't want a cigarette in the car after the game." She complains of cough, scratchy throat, and fever, which she has had for several days. The last few days she has been feeling "bum," and she spent most of the previous day in bed.

Her past medical history is unremarkable except for minor surgery and the usual childhood illnesses. She has smoked a pack of cigarettes a day for more than 40 years. She says she "doesn't believe in vaccinations" and has not had a flu shot.

Physical examination and other data: She is a small, thin woman in moderate distress. Vital signs are: temperature 100.8 °F, heart rate 82, respiratory rate 20, and blood pressure 142/88. Physical exam is remarkable only for distant breath sounds, mild barrel-chest deformity, and a few wheezes. Lab studies were unremarkable except for mild lymphocytosis in the peripheral blood. Chest radiograph reveals signs of moderate emphysema. No infiltrates are present.

Clinical course: You make a diagnosis of viral upper respiratory infection and resist the patient's demand for a shot of penicillin. You prescribe aspirin, aerosol inhalations, and supportive care.

You next see the patient three days later when she returns before her scheduled follow-up visit. She is so weak she is brought into your office in a wheelchair. She complains of severe aching with high fever and chills. She is short of breath and complains that her eyes hurt "as if they are going to pop out of my head." She also asks that you close

the blinds to darken the room, saying the light hurts her eyes. She is hot and flushed, her eyes are red and watery, and her chest if full of crackling rales. Chest radiograph reveals patchy infiltrates throughout both lungs. Laboratory studies are unremarkable except for a white blood count of 17,200/cu mm, mostly neutrophils.

You consult a pulmonary specialist who agrees with your diagnosis of influenza but also concludes that she has a superinfection with bacterial pneumonia. The consultant decides to hospitalize her for ventilatory assistance, intravenous rehydration, and antibiotic therapy. You learn later that she was hospitalized for ten days with severe pneumonia and nearly died of it.

DISCUSSION

This case illustrates that influenza can be extremely serious, even fatal, in elderly or debilitated persons. The most significant facts in this case were the history of cigarette smoking and failure to obtain an influenza vaccination. When the patient first appeared in your office, she was in the prodromal phase of influenza. Mild lymphocytosis confirmed the viral nature of her illness. Her second appearance was at the height of the acute phase of the influenza syndrome, but the marked granulocytosis (neutrophilia) and widespread pulmonary infiltrates suggested a secondary bacterial infection. Bacterial pneumonia can be a nosocomial (hospital or clinic-acquired) infection, and she might have picked it up on her initial visit to your office. An important question is whether or not you should have prescribed antibiotics on her initial visit. In light of the near-fatal course of this case of influenza, it is tempting to believe that doing so might have prevented the bacterial pneumonia. However, there is no guarantee that the bacterium that infected her would have been susceptible to the antibiotic you chose, and there remains the possibility that killing off her normal flora might have encouraged infection by an even more dangerous bacterium.

POINTS TO REMEMBER
- Cigarette smoking causes lung disease and increases risks associated with other lung disease.
- Influenza vaccination is important in elderly or debilitated people, especially those with lung disease.
- Bacterial pneumonia is a common complicating illness in patients with chronic lung disease. ▶

CASE STUDY 9-1 *THE ROAD NOT TAKEN—AN ALTERNATIVE SCENARIO*

For all sad words of tongue or pen,
The saddest are these: "It might have been."
JOHN GREENLEAF WHITTIER (1807–1892),
AMERICAN QUAKER POET AND REFORMER, *MAUD MULLER*

THE CASE

With a bit of imagination, we can speculate how Ruth R's case might have had a happier ending.

Setting: Your job is in a private medical office near a large university, where many of the faculty and administrative personnel are patients of the internist for whom you work. Your job is to do histories and physicals on new patients before they see the physician.

Clinical history: Ruth R. is a 48-year-old bookkeeper who recently moved to town with her husband, who has just taken an administrative job in the Dean's office.

You ask why she is in need of care, and she replies, "It's kind of embarrassing, but I'm here because of a television ad I saw last month."

"Tell me about it," you say.

"Well," she says, "it was horribly graphic and scared the wits out of me. It showed this man, not much older than me, speaking directly into the camera. He was gasping for breath and told how he'd smoked since he was a teenager and now he was dying of lung cancer. 'Don't smoke,' he said. 'It's killing me and it'll kill you.' The screen faded to black and this voice came on saying he'd died right after making the ad."

You ask, "Are you a smoker?"

"Yes," she replies. "I've been smoking since I was in college—about a pack a day for 25 years."

You continue to question her and learn she is worried because in the last year or so she has begun to cough and wheeze, and she finds she becomes short of breath while doing routine tasks. She worries that she might have lung cancer or emphysema.

Physical examination and other data: She is a small, trim woman in no distress. Vital signs are unremarkable. Physical exam is normal except for occasional expiratory wheezes. Laboratory blood tests are within normal limits. A chest radiograph is reported as "essentially normal" but with a comment by the radiologist that describes certain findings that in light of the clinical history could be interpreted as early emphysema and chronic bronchitis.

Clinical course: When the patient returns for a follow-up visit, you join the internist in her office.

After a brief exchange of pleasantries, the internist says, "Mrs. R. I have good news and bad news. The good news is that the radiographs don't show any lesions to suggest lung cancer, and the radiologist says your lungs are in relatively good shape for someone who has smoked so long. The bad news is that your lungs may show early changes of emphysema and chronic bronchitis. Knowing your smoking history, I think the radiologist is right, and I feel confident in predicting that if you continue to smoke you're going to get emphysema or even a lung cancer."

Mrs. R. says, "I was afraid of that. But quitting smoking is so hard; I've tried several times and just never could manage to quit."

The internist says, "That's not so bad; in fact, that's a good sign. At least you recognize you have a problem. I work with another physician who operates an anti-smoking program. He has been successful with many of my patients. Would you care to give it a try?"

Mrs. R. nods, "Yes; I know I've got to do something. I just can't go on this way."

"Good," the internist says. "There is one other important thing you need to do. I see from your chart that you haven't been taking flu shots each year. I strongly recommend you do so. Long-time smokers are especially vulnerable to pneumonia and other lung complications if they get influenza. The front office will set you up for a vaccination."

You continue to see Mrs. R. on an annual basis when she comes in for her physical examination and flu shot. She quit smoking in the first year, and the wheezing and coughing have stopped. She gained a few pounds after quitting smoking but managed to control her weight by watching her diet and by taking a daily walk during her lunch hour. Fifteen years later she is healthy and remains a non-smoker.

DISCUSSION

The best medical outcomes are achieved by a motivated patient and conscientious care by an experienced practitioner. Mrs. R. had enough self-awareness to take the TV anti-smoking ad seriously and acted on her concern. She also had the good sense to seek professional help and the will to change her habits. The internist's prescription of an annual flu shot is a very important part of the overall treatment plan, which produced a desirable outcome.

Objectives Recap

1. *List several of the most common causes worldwide of death associated with infection:* The most common cause of infection-associated death is respiratory infection, followed by HIV/AIDS, diarrheal disease caused by infection, tuberculosis, and malaria.

2. *Define the following terms: infection, contagion, nosocomial, reservoir, carrier, pathogen, host, vector:* Infection is the invasion of the body by a pathogen that results in tissue injury and inflammation. The infective organism is the pathogen. Contagion is the spread of infections from one person to another. Infection acquired in a hospital is a nosocomial infection. A reservoir is a place where the pathogen exists and from which it spreads to new hosts. A carrier is a person or animal harboring the pathogen but suffering no obvious disease. The infected person or animal is the host. A vector is intermediate carriers, such as a mosquito, that carries the pathogen from reservoir to patient.

3. *Name the crucial differences between viruses and bacteria:* Viruses are obligate intracellular parasites. Bacteria can live outside of cells. Viruses are packets of protein without a cell wall; bacteria are more complex structures with a cell wall.

4. *Describe how bacteria vary according to shape, oxygen requirements, and staining characteristics:* Most bacteria are either round (cocci) or rod-shaped (bacilli), they are either Gram positive (black-purple) or Gram negative (red-pink) when stained according to standard technique, and they are aerobic, requiring oxygen, or anaerobic, if oxygen is toxic to them.

5. *Briefly describe how organisms spread in tissue:* Microorganisms penetrate natural barriers such as skin, gastrointestinal, respiratory, or urogenital epithelium to cause infections such as abscess, diarrhea, pneumonia, or urinary infection, after which they may spread widely by gaining access to blood or the lymphatic system.

6. *Describe the cellular inflammatory reaction to bacteria, viruses, mycobacteria and fungi, parasitic worms, and protozoa:* Bacteria usually evoke neutrophil infiltration at the site and an increased number of neutrophils in the peripheral blood (neutrophilia). Viruses evoke a lymphocyte and monocyte reaction with a few neutrophils. Mycobacteria and fungi evoke lymphocyte and monocyte reaction and formation of giant cell granulomas at the site of infection. Parasitic worms usually cause an eosinophilic inflammatory reaction. Protozoa usually cause lymphocyte and monocyte inflammation.

7. *Name the organ systems most commonly affected by infections. What do they share in common?* The organ systems most commonly infected are the gastrointestinal tract, the respiratory tract, the genital tract, and the skin. They are alike in that all are in direct contact with the environment.

8. *Define dysentery:* Dysentery is severe, watery diarrhea with abdominal cramping and watery stools containing blood, pus, and mucus.

9. *Name several types of bacterial enteritis:* Salmonellosis, shigellosis, cholera.

10. *Name several sexually transmitted diseases, the pathogens that cause them, and the genitourinary lesions that are associated with them:* Syphilis is caused by *Treponema pallidum* and is associated with an ulcer (the chancre); gonorrhea is caused by *Neisseria gonorrhoeae* and is associated with urethritis, prostatitis, and epididymitis in men, and salpingitis in women; *Chlamydia trachomatis* causes chlamydia infections, associated with gonorrhea-like manifestations in both sexes; and human papillomavirus causes condyloma acuminatum or dysplasia and cancer of the cervix.

11. *Name the two types of Gram-positive cocci that cause most pyogenic infections:* Staphylococci and streptococci.

12. *Name several diseases caused by Streptococcus organisms:* Acute streptococcal pharyngitis, erysipelas, impetigo, urinary tract infections, bacterial endocarditis, pneumonia, meningitis, dental caries, scarlet fever, and acute rheumatic fever.

13. *Define the phrase opportunistic pathogen, and offer several examples:* An opportunistic pathogen is one that does not cause disease in people with healthy immune systems but can become an infectious pathogen in patients with impaired immunity. Examples include *Pneumocystic jiroveci* pneumonia, cryptosporidial gastroenteritis, atypical tuberculosis, cytomegalic inclusion disease, cryptococcosis, toxoplasmosis, candidiasis, *Pseudomonas aeruginosa* infection.

14. *Name a vector-borne disease, including the pathogen and the vector:* Malaria is caused by *Plasmodium* protozoa and transmitted by mosquitoes. Rocky Mountain spotted fever is caused by one of the *Rickettsia* and transmitted by ticks. Lyme disease is caused by the spirochete *Borrelia* and transmitted by ticks. Plague is cause by *Yersinia pestis* and transmitted by rodent fleas.

15. *Discuss the transmission and pathology of amebiasis:* Amebiasis is an infection by *Entamoeba histolytica*, which infects hundreds of millions of persons annually in tropical nations. Most cases are asymptomatic; however amebiasis is the third most common fatal parasitic disease after malaria and

schistosomiasis. Infection is acquired by eating food contaminated by human feces containing amebic cysts, a capsule of amebae designed to survive in the environment. After ingestion the amebae break out of the cyst and invade the colon, producing abdominal pain and diarrhea. Invasion into the portal blood often produces amebic liver abscesses, but brain, lung, and other organs may also be involved.

16. *Name the two parasitic diseases causing the most morbidity and mortality worldwide:* Malaria and schistosomiasis.

17. *List the clinical phases of infection that occur after an infective organism invades the body:* After inoculation the organism enters an incubation period during which it proliferates quietly or is destroyed by the body's defenses. Next comes a prodromal period, during which the patient suffers from mild, non-specific symptoms. The prodromal period gives way to the acute phase of the illness, during which typical symptoms are present. During the convalescent phase symptoms fade and give way to the final phase, the recover phase during which no symptoms are present.

Typical Test Questions

1. Which one of the following have a cell wall and DNA but have no nucleus?
   A. Prions
   B. Bacteria
   C. Viruses
   D. Helminths

2. Which one of the following means "hospital acquired?"
   A. Contagious
   B. Nosocomial
   C. Endemic
   D. Fomite

3. Which one of the following is a deep mycosis?
   A. Tuberculosis
   B. Reiter syndrome
   C. Schistosomiasis
   D. Histoplasmosis

4. Which one of the following is transmitted sexually?
   A. Condyloma acuminatum
   B. Malaria
   C. Leprosy
   D. Cytomegalic inclusion disease

5. Which one of the following is the cause of most non-gonococcal urethritis in males?
   A. *Salmonella enterica*
   B. *Chlamydia trachomatis*
   C. *Mycobacterium avium*
   D. Herpes simplex

6. True or false? The number of pathogens entering the body has little to do with whether or not infection develops.

7. True or false? *Clostridium difficile*, the pathogen of pseudomembranous colitis, is a normal inhabitant of the colon.

8. True or false? A "carrier" is a reservoir of infectious pathogens.

9. True or false? "Pyogenic" inflammation is characterized by marked numbers of lymphocytes in the inflamed tissue.

CHAPTER

10 *Disorders of Daily Life and Diet*

This chapter discusses the adverse health effects of our personal habits, workplace conditions, and activities. It also examines the effects of environment and improper nutrition on health.

INJURY RESULTING FROM TRAUMA
INJURY RESULTING FROM EXTREMES OF TEMPERATURE
- Thermal Burns
- Cold Injury
- Heat Cramps, Heat Exhaustion, and Heat Stroke
POLLUTION AND OCCUPATIONAL DISEASE
EXPOSURE TO TOXIC MATERIALS
- Chemicals
- Adverse Reactions to Therapeutic Drugs
- Radiation
- Inhalant Lung Disease

TOBACCO, ALCOHOL, AND DRUGS
- Cigarette Smoking
- Alcohol Abuse
- Drug Abuse
NUTRITIONAL DISEASE
- Malnutrition
- Obesity
- Morbid Obesity
- The Metabolic Syndrome

Learning Objectives

After studying this chapter you should be able to:
1. Name several of the most common causes of death in the United States, and discuss the environmental aspects
2. Name several of the most common causes of accidental death in the United States
3. Define first-degree, second-degree, and third-degree burns
4. Define toxin, and briefly discuss some examples
5. Briefly discuss several types of drugs and their associated adverse reactions
6. Name several diseases other than lung cancer that are related to cigarette smoking
7. Name several conditions associated with alcohol abuse
8. List some of the complications of drug abuse, and explain why intravenous drug abuse is especially risky
9. Name and differentiate the two stages of protein-energy malnutrition
10. Define obesity, and discuss Body Mass Index
11. Give a brief description of the metabolic syndrome and the associated risks

Key Terms and Concepts

INJURY OWING TO TRAUMA
- trauma

INJURY OWING TO EXTREMES OF TEMPERATURE
- thermal burns
- frostbite
- hypothermia
- heat stroke

POLLUTION AND OCCUPATIONAL DISEASE
- pollutant
- occupational disease

EXPOSURE TO TOXIC MATERIALS
- toxin
- dose
- radiation sickness
- pneumoconiosis

TOBACCO, ALCOHOL, AND DRUGS
- nicotine
- ethanol
- Wernicke encephalopathy
- Korsakoff psychosis
- fetal alcohol syndrome
- depressant
- stimulant
- narcotic
- hallucinogen

NUTRITIONAL DISEASE
- malnutrition
- protein-energy malnutrition
- obesity
- body mass index
- leptin
- morbid obesity
- metabolic syndrome

For thy sake, Tobacco, I
Would do anything but die.

CHARLES LAMB (1775–1834), ENGLISH ESSAYIST, A FAREWELL TO TOBACCO

MAJOR DETERMINANTS OF DISEASE

- Accidents and workplace activities are an important cause of death and disease
- Personal habits are important factors in the cause of most deaths in the United States:
  - Smoking has a devastating effect on health
  - Diet is an important factor in cancer and vascular disease
  - Obesity is an important factor in vascular disease and diabetes
  - Drug and alcohol abuse are associated with predictable health problems

This chapter focuses on disorders that arise from the more or less regular routines and exposures of daily life: our air and water, our work, our recreation, our personal habits, and our food and drink.

An important part of how we live is the *environment*. In our study of genetic disease (Chapter 7), we used the term *environment* in the broadest possible sense; that is, to refer to any non-genetic influence. However, in this chapter "environment" has a much narrower definition, referring to the effects of 1) physical forces and extremes of temperature; 2) air and water pollution; 3) occupational exposures; 4) personal exposures to chemicals and drugs, legal and illegal, including alcohol; 5) radiation; 6) personal exposure to tobacco; and 7) too much or too little food.

Most environmental disease is the result of personal habits—cigarette smoking, alcohol or drug use, and dietary practices. Environmental disease is an important factor in most deaths in the United States. Figure 10-1 illustrates the major causes of death in the United States for 2003. Smoking and diet are very important in death associated with heart disease; smoking directly accounts for most chronic lung disease and lung cancer and contributes to the development of cancers in other organs.

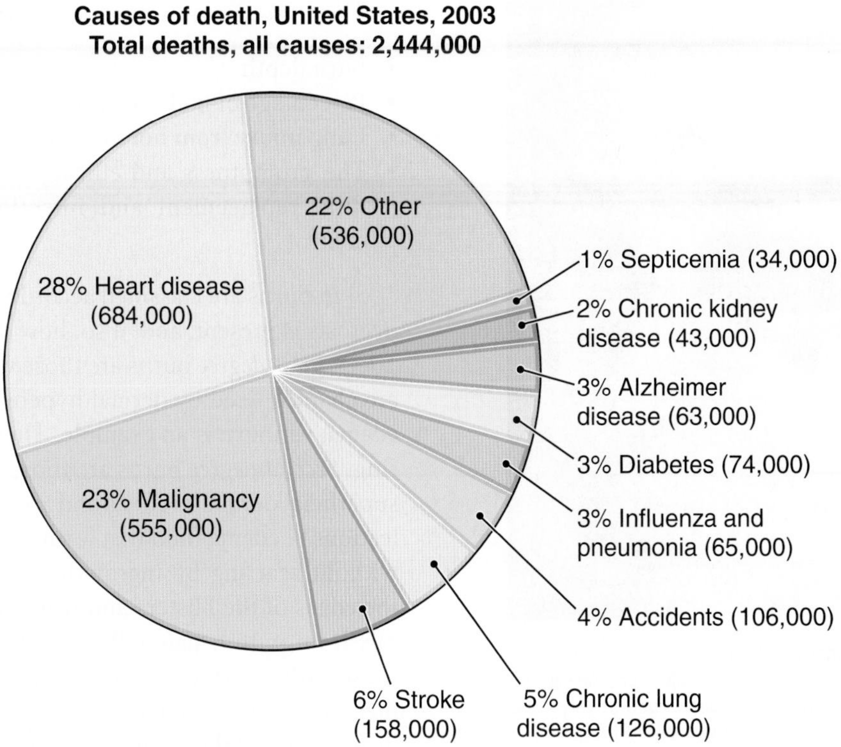

Causes of death, United States, 2003
Total deaths, all causes: 2,444,000

22% Other (536,000)

1% Septicemia (34,000)

2% Chronic kidney disease (43,000)

3% Alzheimer disease (63,000)

3% Diabetes (74,000)

3% Influenza and pneumonia (65,000)

4% Accidents (106,000)

28% Heart disease (684,000)

23% Malignancy (555,000)

6% Stroke (158,000)

5% Chronic lung disease (126,000)

Figure 10-1 **Causes of death in the United States, 2003.** Environmental factors are important in many categories but are not listed separately. For example, cigarette smoking is an important cause of heart disease, malignancy, stroke, and chronic lung disease. Lack of exercise is important in heart disease and stroke. Alcohol abuse plays an important role in accidents. (Adapted from Centers for Disease Control, National Vital Statistics Report, 2003.)

Accidents are the only purely environmental category, and they claim in excess of 100,000 lives per year.

Injury Resulting from Trauma

Trauma is any injury to the body caused by violence or accident, usually physical force associated with accidents, suicide, or homicide. In this discussion, we include acute fatal toxic exposures (poisonings) as acute injuries in order to separate them from chronic toxic exposures.

Physical force injuries are an important cause of skeletal (Chapter 22) and neurologic (Chapter 23) problems. Skin is the most common site of physical force injury. An **abrasion** is an injury to skin that scrapes away epidermis. A **laceration** is a tearing of tissue. Internal tissues or organs such as liver or spleen may be lacerated without apparent skin injury. A **contusion** is a blunt force injury that results in local hemorrhage in any tissue or organ.

Figure 10-2 illustrates the causes of traumatic death in the United States for 2002. According to the United States Centers for Disease Control, trauma accounts for about 160,000 deaths each year.

Deaths from traumatic injury, United States, 2002
Total traumatic deaths: 161,000

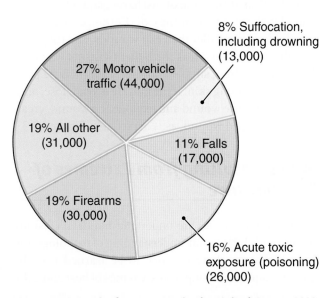

8% Suffocation, including drowning (13,000)

27% Motor vehicle traffic (44,000)

19% All other (31,000)

11% Falls (17,000)

19% Firearms (30,000)

16% Acute toxic exposure (poisoning) (26,000)

Figure 10-2 **Deaths from trauma in the United States, 2002.** Deaths from the direct effect of alcohol are not included, though alcohol plays a role in many categories. For example, alcohol is implicated in 40% of motor vehicle traffic deaths. Most gunshot deaths are suicide or homicide. (Adapted from Centers for Disease Control, National Data on Injuries, 2002.)

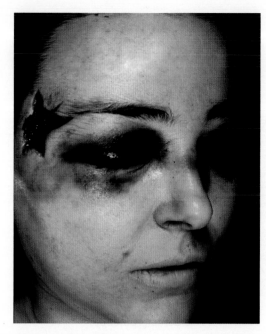

***Figure 10-3* Contact gunshot wound.** Gunshot wounds tell a story. Note the star shape of the defect, which results from the explosive force of muzzle blast gas (the weapon was discharged at very close range, perhaps in contact with the skin). Orbital hemorrhage indicates the wound was not immediately fatal. The patient lived long enough to bleed.

About 30,000 people die of gunshot wounds each year in the United States. Of these deaths about 55% are suicide, 40% are homicide, and 5% are accidents or related to law enforcement. Gunshot wounds tell a story. Important in the assessment of a gunshot wound are the size and velocity of the bullet, the distance of the muzzle from the skin at the time of discharge, and whether the wound is the entrance or the exit. Entrance wounds are usually slightly smaller than exit wounds, and they have a small rim of abrasion as the bullet twists its way in. If the muzzle is close, stippled powder burns may be present on surrounding skin. If the muzzle is very close, blast gas may enter the wound and explode the wound, creating a star-shaped wound, as is depicted in Figure 10-3.

Injury Resulting from Extremes of Temperature

Physical force injuries are important, but detailed study of them adds little to our understanding of pathology. On the other hand, there is much to be learned from by studying injury resulting from extremes of heat and cold.

THERMAL BURNS

Thermal burns are a serious medical and social problem, causing 5,000 deaths and 50,000 hospitalizations each year in the United States.

The clinical significance of a burn depends on:

- Burn depth
- Percentage of body surface affected
- Lung injury from hot or toxic gas
- The promptness and efficacy of therapy, especially fluid replacement and infection prevention and control

Skin burns are classified according to whether or not necrosis is present, and, if so, how deep it extends (Fig. 10-4). *First-degree* burns are those without necrosis and are characterized by dermal hyperemia (erythema) and edema; sunburn is an example. They heal without scarring. *Second-degree* burns are those with epidermal and superficial dermal necrosis and are characterized by collections of edema fluid that form into blisters. They heal without scarring by ingrowth of new epidermis from the edges of the blisters and from outgrowth of epidermis from within hair follicles. *Third-degree* burns are those with full-thickness necrosis of epidermis and dermis; only deep skin appendages may be spared. Third-degree burns take a long time to heal, produce scars, and usually require extensive, specialized treatment and skin grafting.

The *rule of nines* is a convenient way to estimate percent of body surface burned. The front and the back of the legs are 9% each (total 36%), the front and back of the torso are 18% each (total 36%), the front and the back of the arms are 4½ % each (total 18%), the head, neck and face are 9%. The genitalia account for 1%.

Burns exceeding 50% of body surface area are potentially fatal, no matter how deep. Any burn of 20% of body surface results in rapid fluid shifts: fluid seeps from the wound and is absorbed into damaged skin as edema. Fluid can be lost in such large quantities that the vascular space becomes depleted, and hypovolemic shock may develop. Intense intravenous electrolyte fluid support is a critical aspect of burn care. An additional, important aspect of burn injury is heat loss (one of the first complaints of a burn victim is that they feel cold) and the onset of a hypermetabolic state that consumes huge numbers of calories and requires intense nutritional support.

Smoke or hot air injury to the airways and lungs can injure alveoli and cause pulmonary edema, which may not develop until 24–48 hours after the injury. Burn infections are a constant threat in burn victims because the natural barrier of skin is breached; pathogens easily invade blood vessels and spread widely. Pneumonia, septic shock, renal failure, and acute respiratory distress syndrome (Chapter 14) are common consequences of blood infection (septicemia) associated with burns.

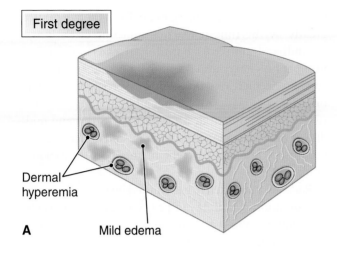

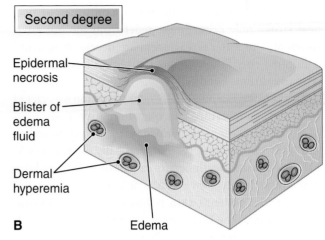

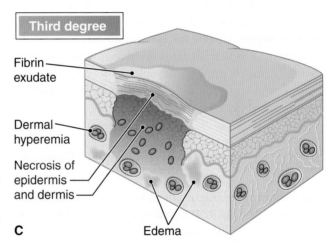

Figure 10-4 **The pathology of skin burns. A.** First-degree burn shows only dermal hyperemia and mild edema. No blistering or necrosis is present. **B.** Second-degree burn shows epidermal necrosis, blister formation, and dermal hyperemia and edema. **C.** Third-degree burn shows necrosis of the full thickness of the epidermis and dermis.

COLD INJURY

Susceptibility to cold injury is increased by substance abuse, hunger, dehydration, and impaired cardiovascular function.

Frostnip is a recoverable injury of skin occurring in cold but not freezing conditions. It is characterized by firm, white patches on the face, ears, fingers, or toes and results in peeling and blistering on rewarming.

Frostbite is cold injury to skin that occurs in subfreezing temperatures: ice crystals within cells rupture cell membranes and cause tissue necrosis. Affected areas are hard and white and lack feeling. When warmed, the lesion becomes swollen, red, blistered, and painful as blood flow returns, and inflammation occurs in response to tissue necrosis. Superficial frostbite may heal without residual tissue loss, but deep frostbite always results in necrosis, referred to as gangrene.

Hypothermia, exceptionally low body temperature, results in a slowing of all physiologic functions. It is favored by low temperatures, high humidity, wet clothing, and the peripheral vasodilation caused by ingestion of alcohol—a combination common in homeless people. Hypothermia causes lethargy, clumsiness, confusion, hallucinations, and slow respirations and heart rate. At body core temperature of about 90° F, loss of consciousness occurs and death may follow, owing to cardiac arrhythmia or cardiac arrest.

HEAT CRAMPS, HEAT EXHAUSTION, AND HEAT STROKE

Heat cramps are spasms of voluntary muscle caused by electrolyte loss, most often following vigorous exercise. **Heat exhaustion**, a more serious condition, is characterized by profuse sweating and sudden weakness and disorientation or fainting owing to the inability of the cardiovascular system to compensate for water loss. Body temperature may rise to near 102° F, but after a brief period of instability, homeostasis (equilibrium) is reestablished. If body temperature continues to rise, heat stroke may occur. Rest, relief from the hot environment, and water replacement are necessary to avoid continued rise of body temperature and heat stroke, a far more serious condition.

Heat stroke is a potentially fatal condition associated with high temperature and high humidity. Body temperature regulation mechanisms fail, sweating stops, and body temperature rises dramatically, sometimes to 110° F or more. Death occurs in half of patients whose temperature rises above 106°F. Because sweating has stopped, the patient's skin is flushed from peripheral vasodilation as the body attempts to shed heat through the skin. Hypotension and shock follow. Other problems include cardiac arrhythmias or cardiac arrest, seizures, coma, disseminated intravascular coagulation (DIC; Chapter 5), and skeletal muscle necrosis (rhabdomyolysis), which liberates massive amounts of myoglobin (a muscle protein). Myoglobin is excreted by the kidney, and large amounts can obstruct renal tubules, causing renal failure.

Pollution and Occupational Disease

A **pollutant** is a substance in air or water that can injure those exposed to it. Pollutants may have short-term effects, such as the acute toxicity of carbon monoxide poisoning from incomplete burning of fuel in a faulty room heater or water heater, or long-term effects, such as the lung cancers and vascular diseases that plague cigarette smokers. Outdoor air pollutants are produced by combustion of fossil fuels, non-nuclear power plant emissions, waste incinerators, and industrial plants. Some air pollutants undergo photochemical reactions to produce ozone (O_3, a powerful oxidant), which can damage lungs directly or aggravate pre-existing chronic lung disease.

Air pollution is a problem in industrial societies. For example, average pulmonary function is permanently impaired in people who live downwind of factories that put pollutants into the air; people living upwind are unaffected.

Indoor pollutants accumulate in poorly ventilated spaces. For nonsmokers, cigarette smoke is an important hazard. **Secondhand smoke**, also known as passive smoke, is a mixture of two forms of smoke from burning tobacco products. Smoke flowing into the air from the tip of a burning cigarette is called *sidestream smoke*. Smoke inhaled and exhaled by a smoker is *mainstream smoke*. Sidestream smoke contains twice the tar of mainstream because sidestream has not been filtered by

being drawn through the cigarette. Even though diluted greatly by the time it reaches someone else's lungs, secondhand smoke is harmful. It causes increased numbers of heart attacks and lung cancers in nonsmokers, it increases the number of respiratory infections and asthmatic attacks in children, it increases the risk of sudden infant death syndrome (SIDS) and middle ear infections in young children, and it increases the number of low birth weight infants born to exposed mothers.

Radon is a radioactive gas emitted by naturally occurring uranium in soil. It can be trapped in poorly ventilated homes, and it may be responsible for some lung cancers. Inhalation of *asbestos* particles is a well-known hazard of asbestos miners (Chapter 14). At one time asbestos was a significant indoor air hazard because of its use in spray-on insulation in United States office buildings and industry. It is no longer used for this purpose, and insulation of this type presents no hazard if it remains undisturbed.

Carbon monoxide (CO) is the leading cause of accidental poisoning death in the United States. It is an odorless gas product of incompletely burned fuels. For example, 5% of auto exhaust is CO, and gas from burning charcoal has high CO content. Carbon monoxide has a great affinity for hemoglobin, combining with it to form carboxyhemoglobin, a bright red form of hemoglobin to which oxygen cannot attach. The result is anoxia despite adequate pulmonary ventilation. Carbon monoxide poisoning can prove rapidly fatal. The bright red color of carboxyhemoglobin provides an important clinical or postmortem clue to the problem: the patient's skin is cherry red, even in death, as is depicted in Figure 10-5. Chronic poisoning may induce hypoxic brain injury and permanent brain dysfunction.

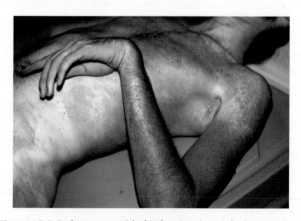

Figure 10-5 **Carbon monoxide (CO) poisoning.** A faulty natural gas room heater caused this fatal poisoning. The characteristic cherry-red coloration of skin persists in death. CO binds irreversibly with hemoglobin to produce bright red hemoglobin, which retains its color even though no oxygen is present.

HISTORY OF MEDICINE

CHIMNEY SWEEPS' CANCER

The first physician to recognize and treat an occupational illness was Sir Percival Pott, who is famous in medical history for his observation regarding scrotal cancers in chimney sweeps. Pott, an English physician advising Dutch tradesmen, observed in 1775 that the chimney sweeps, all of whom were male, had an exceptionally high incidence of cancer of the scrotal skin. In his report he wrote, "The disease in these people seems to derive its origin from the lodgment of soot in the rugae of the scrotum . . . . " He advised the workers to bathe regularly, which solved the problem.

Occupational disease in the form of work-related disorders claims about 5,000 lives per year. Other occupational disease and death include chronic occupational exposures that cause cancer or other illness, such as lung cancer that is associated with asbestos inhalation in asbestos miners, and bladder cancer in aniline dye workers, caused by urinary excretion of chemicals inhaled or absorbed through the skin. See the above History of Medicine box for the story of the first recognized occupational disease.

The most common workplace disorders are associated with repeated trauma; for example, arthritis in the hands of persons operating vibrating equipment. Second most common are skin diseases (Chapter 24), often owing to contact allergy or direct irritation resulting from contact with solvents, acids, or alkalis. Table 10-1 offers a brief list of some of the more important occupational toxic exposures.

Exposure to Toxic Materials

A **toxin** is any substance that is injurious to health or dangerous to life. "Toxin" and "poison" mean much the same thing; however, "poison" is often used to connote deliberate acts, so in this discussion "toxin" will be used because it carries a broader meaning.

Almost any substance is capable of being toxic in the right set of circumstances. Even the most innocuous substances can be injurious if taken in large quantity over a short period of time. For example, forced ingestion of very large amounts of water, as in a college hazing prank, can produce fatal brain edema. Moreover, prolonged therapeutic use of inhaled oxygen can cause direct damage to the lungs.

CHEMICALS

About 10,000,000 natural and synthetic chemicals are known to exist. Almost any substance delivered at the right dose can be toxic, and the workings of toxins can be slow and not necessarily fatal, but most toxic exposures derive from a group of about 2,500 compounds.

Toxicity is dependent on the properties of the chemical and the amount (*dose*). A few milligrams of some substances can be fatal; on the other hand, it requires upwards of 100 grams of *ethanol*, the active ingredient in alcoholic drinks, to cause fatal respiratory arrest. A convenient way of discussing the harmful effect of a toxin is to determine the dose at which half of the recipients (humans or lab animals) die—the "lethal dose to kill fifty percent" or LD_{50} *dose*.

About 26,000 people in the United States die each year of acute toxic exposure (Fig. 10-2). Eighty-percent (80%) are attributed to drug overdose, primarily over-

Table 10-1	**Occupational Toxic Exposures and Disease**	
System	**Effect**	**Toxins**
Respiratory	Lung cancer Chronic pulmonary disease	Asbestos, rock dust (silica), arsenic, chromium, nickel Grain dust, coal dust, rock dust (silica), asbestos, cobalt, beryllium, cadmium
Nervous	Peripheral neuropathy CNS toxicity	Mercury, lead, arsenic, solvents Mercury, toluene, solvents, aldehydes, ketones
Urinary	Bladder cancer	Benzidine, naphthylamines, aniline dyes, rubber products
Reproductive	Infertility, teratogenesis	Lead, cadmium, mercury, polychlorinated biphenyls (PCB)
Hematopoietic	Leukemia	Benzene, uranium

dose of illegal drugs; a few are the result of acute alcohol toxicity. Poison center data show that accidental interaction with toxic substances is common but rarely fatal. The most serious incidents are usually in the home, and young children are the victims most of the time. One of the most common sources of fatal accidental poisoning is furniture polish. It has a pleasant smell, and attempted ingestion by children often causes aspiration and severe lung damage. Vitamins, minerals, and other dietary supplements, such as iron, are not toxic in recommended doses; however, overdose can be very serious. Iron overdose is especially harmful to children. By law in the United States, no dietary supplement tablet may contain more than 30 mg of iron per tablet; nevertheless, 20 such tablets can contain enough iron (600 mg) to cause fatal iron poisoning in a child.

Occupational exposure to a substance is usually more intense than is casual, everyday exposure, because in the workplace, potentially toxic substances are in active use in high concentration. There are large numbers of workplace hazardous materials, some of which are listed in Table 10-1.

Volatile organic compounds and *petroleum products* are used in industry and at home. They are an important ingredient in solvents, glue, paint remover, and charcoal lighter fluid, and they may be abused (glue sniffing, for example). Acute exposure can be associated with dizziness, unsteady gait, confusion, and nausea. In severe cases coma and death may occur. Bone marrow suppression (aplastic anemia, Chapter 11) and leukemia are long term risks for misuse of some compounds.

Agricultural chemicals may prove acutely toxic or fatal to farm workers. Because these chemicals tend to accumulate in water and soil, they pose a long-term threat to wildlife and humans. The pesticide DDT is a classic example. It has low acute toxicity in humans and was effective in controlling mosquitoes and insect damage to crops, but it accumulated in birds and other animals, most famously the American bald eagle, causing thinned eggshells and otherwise impairing reproduction. DDT was banned by the United States government in 1972, and today the bald eagle population has rebounded to the point that the bald eagle soon may no longer be considered an endangered species. DDT remains in use in some tropical countries that have severe problems with mosquito-borne diseases, especially malaria.

Organophosphates (such as parathion) are insecticides that are easily absorbed through skin or lungs and have their effect at the neuromuscular synapse, causing paralysis by blocking nerve signal transmission. Acute toxicity causes sweating, blurred vision, constricted pupils, salivation, bronchospasm, muscle twitching (fasciculation), paralysis, and respiratory arrest.

Dioxin is an herbicide that first came to worldwide attention because of the toxicity associated with its use as a defoliant in the Vietnam War (1969–1975). It continues to receive attention, most recently in the 2004 Ukrainian presidential campaign, when a leading politician was deliberately poisoned with it by the political opposition.

Exposure to *metals* poses acute toxic hazards; long-term risk includes increased cancer risk. Table 10-2 summarizes some of these hazards.

Lead poisoning warrants special mention because lead is widespread in urban air, soil, water, and food, and

Table 10-2 Hazardous Metals

Metal	Hazard	Occupation
Lead	Renal toxicity, anemia, peripheral neuropathy, cognitive defects	Battery plants, metal casting, spray painting, auto repair
Mercury	Renal toxicity, CNS damage	Various
Arsenic	Cancer of skin, lung, liver	Mining, smelting, oil refining, agriculture
Cobalt and tungsten carbide	Pulmonary fibrosis	Toolmakers, grinders
Cadmium	Renal toxicity	Battery plants, smelters, welders, soldering
Chromium	Cancer of lung and nasopharynx	Pigment production, smelting, steel production
Nickel	Cancer of lung and paranasal sinuses	Electroplating, smelting, steel production

because chronic exposure can be damaging, especially to children. Lead poisoning, which is now uncommon in the United States, has been a problem for a very long time, as the nearby History of Medicine box indicates. Despite elimination of lead from gasoline and paint, older urban homes and factories often contain large amounts of flaking lead-based paint and contaminated soil. In some developing nations lead is present in earthen cookware and can contaminate food and drink. Another hazard is lead-based paint used to decorate souvenir plates and cups bought by tourists.

As is illustrated in Figure 10-6, lead primarily affects the nervous system, the bone marrow, and the kidney. Children absorb a much higher percentage of ingested lead than adults do, and children are more susceptible than adults are to its toxic effects. In children lead causes brain edema and encephalopathy (unsteady gait, sleepiness or irritability, seizures, or coma), whereas in adults peripheral motor nerves are most affected (foot- or wrist-drop). Anemia is a prime sign of lead toxicity in both adults and children; it impairs bone marrow production of red cells and shortens their life span, causing microcytic, hypochromic anemia that mimics iron deficiency anemia (Chapter 11). However, lead toxicity causes a bluish-gray ("basophilic") stippling of red cells that is not present in iron deficiency anemia. Lead also damages the kidney and may cause chronic

renal failure. Lead toxicity may also produce very painful intestinal spasms that mimic an acute surgical emergency such as intestinal obstruction or perforation. In children lead deposits in the growing ends of long bones can leave a characteristic and diagnostic "lead line" visible on radiograph examination.

Long-term exposure to low levels of lead may not cause clinically detectable effects; however, exposed children suffer subtle neurologic problems and lower intelligence, which persist into adult life.

ADVERSE REACTIONS TO THERAPEUTIC DRUGS

Apothecary, n. The physician's accomplice, the undertaker's benefactor, and the grave worm's provider.
AMBROSE BIERCE (1842–1914?), AMERICAN SATIRIST, JOURNALIST, AND SHORT-STORY WRITER, *THE DEVIL'S DICTIONARY*

Adverse reaction to therapeutic drugs is common. Acute reactions, such as allergy or accidental overdose, are uncommon; the most frequent problems occur in patients on long-term therapy, such as extended steroid treatment of rheumatoid arthritis. For example, prolonged steroid therapy induces Cushing syndrome (Chapter 18), which is characterized by obesity, excess facial hair in females, diabetes, high blood pressure, fragile bones, and susceptibility to infections. Supplemental estrogen was until recently very widely prescribed to prevent

HISTORY OF MEDICINE

BENJAMIN FRANKLIN AND LEAD TOXICITY

Before the American Revolution, Founding Father Benjamin Franklin was the most famous American and, perhaps, the most famous scientist in the world. Long known for his kite-flying experiment that proved lightning was an electrical phenomenon, Franklin was a not a mere tinkerer: he was a meticulous scientist who conducted elegant experiments that brought him worldwide acclaim for his inquiring mind and scientific accomplishments long before the world knew of George Washington, Thomas Jefferson, Alexander Hamilton, and John Adams.

Franklin began his career as a printer, which necessitated melting lead to make typeface. In 1724, he wrote about two of his coworkers who had lost the use of their hands after years of handling hot lead. He described how they had "a kind of obscure Pain that I had sometimes felt . . . in the Bones of my Hand . . . (which) induc'd me to omit the Practice."

Nevertheless, many workers melted lead over the fires and, their hands blackened with lead fumes, went home to eat without washing. Additionally, workers inhaled lead fumes and drank rainwater collected from lead roofs. Lead was somewhat of a miracle metal in the 18th century: in addition to its use in printing, it was used in paint for buildings and to decorate ceramics, to make musket balls and cannon shot, in pewter for buttons and tableware, as roofing material, in glass to make windows, to make plumbing pipes (*plumbum* is Latin for lead), and dozens of other uses. Franklin lamented that people were reluctant to accept what was, to him, obvious: lead was toxic. He wrote, "You will observe with Concern how long a useful Truth may be known, and exist, before it is generally receiv'd and practis'd on." It took nearly two centuries for medicine to pay attention.

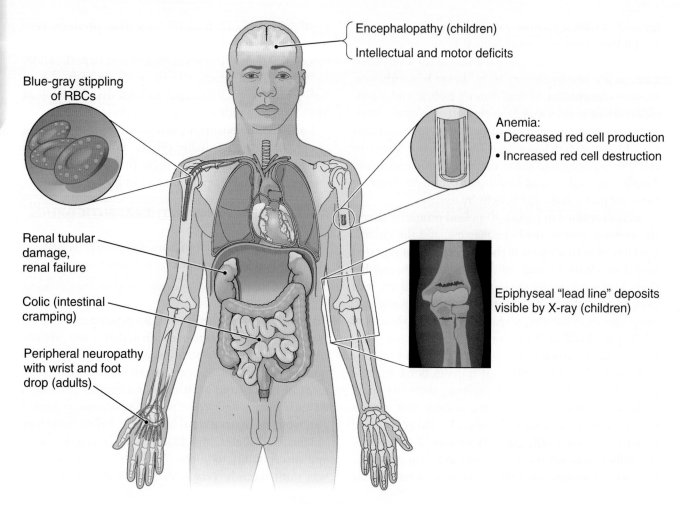

Encephalopathy (children)

Intellectual and motor deficits

Blue-gray stippling of RBCs

Anemia:
• Decreased red cell production
• Increased red cell destruction

Renal tubular damage, renal failure

Colic (intestinal cramping)

Epiphyseal "lead line" deposits visible by X-ray (children)

Peripheral neuropathy with wrist and foot drop (adults)

Figure 10-6 **The effects of lead toxicity.**

brittle bones in post-menopausal women (Chapter 21). Evidence suggests that estrogen replacement therapy carries risks that are unacceptable for many women because it is associated with a slightly increased risk for breast cancer, thrombophlebitis, heart attack, and stroke. However, estrogen is very effective at relieving disabling post-menopausal hot flushes, and it continues to be prescribed in selected circumstances.

After many years of uncertainty, it is now clear that *oral contraceptives* are safe, but they are not entirely risk free. Data show that women taking oral contraceptives probably have below normal risk for heart disease and stroke, and they also have decreased risk for ovarian and uterine (endometrial) cancer. Oral contraceptives appear to have no effect on a woman's chance of developing breast cancer. The most significant risk is for women over age 35 who take contraceptives and smoke; they have a very high (3–10 times normal) risk of heart attack (myocardial infarction). And all women who use oral contraceptives have a slight increased risk of ve-

nous thrombosis (Chapter 5) and pulmonary thromboembolism (Chapter 13).

Aspirin is the most widely used medicine in the world because it is cheap and effective as a pain-reliever and fever-reducer. Ingestion by a child of 10–20 standard adult doses (one 325 mg tablet) can be toxic; in adults acute aspirin toxicity, causing severe acidosis, requires 30–100 standard tablets. Childproof containers have almost completely eliminated accidental overdose among children, which at one time was common. Furthermore, aspirin use in children is now not recommended because of its possible association with *Reye syndrome* (Chapter 15), a combination of fatty liver and acute brain disease (encephalopathy) in children, which most often develops a few days after an acute viral illness treated with aspirin.

Chronic aspirin toxicity (**salicylism**) may occur in patients taking more than 10–12 tablets per day, usually for pain control associated with chronic disease, such as rheumatoid arthritis. Doses in this range can cause gastrointestinal problems (including irritation and ulceration of the stomach), dizziness, ringing in the ears (tinnitus), deafness, and mental problems. Bleeding tendencies may occur, because aspirin inhibits platelet "stickiness" (Chapter 10), an effect that can be achieved by a single daily tablet. This effect has therapeutic value in preventing heart attack and stroke, both of which are often initiated by aggregations of platelets in arteries. When administered quickly after onset of acute myocardial infarction, aspirin can limit the size and severity of myocardial damage.

Acetaminophen, the active ingredient in Tylenol®, has fewer side effects than aspirin does and has replaced aspirin as a pain reliever and fever reducer. However, accidental or suicidal doses (30–50 tablets) of acetaminophen can cause fatal liver necrosis.

RADIATION

The word "radiation" usually calls to mind the rays emitted from nuclear power plant fuel, atomic weapons, and x-ray machines. However, as indicated in Table 10-3, radiant energy encompasses much more, including sunlight and radio waves. Low energy waves (such as radio waves and radar) carry little risk, whereas high energy waves can cause very serious tissue damage.

Radiant energy does its damage by ionizing molecules; that is to say, the molecules gain or lose an electron and become unstable and liable to react with other molecules in an abnormal way. For example, DNA is vulnerable to ionization, especially during cell division when it is unwinding to combine with nucleotide bases in the formation of new DNA. Tissues with rapid cell division—bone marrow, lymphoid tissues, GI mucosa, and skin—are most susceptible to radiation damage.

The most common form of radiation exposure is sunlight. The ultraviolet bands (short, high-frequency waves) carry the most energy and therefore have the most ionizing potential. They damage skin cell DNA, and can induce malignancy or excess wrinkling (photoaging) in chronically over-exposed skin

Apart from sunlight, radiation therapy causes most radiation damage. Some exposure to the more powerful energy of x-rays is a necessary hazard for medical professionals and patients. However, modern diagnostic radiographic techniques have reduced the dosage to very low levels, so that the exposure for most diagnostic tests is less than that obtained from a day at the beach. Nevertheless, other body parts, the gonads in particular, should be shielded during x-ray studies.

Patients receiving high doses of radiation over a short period of time suffer short- and long-term effects. Acute **radiation sickness** follows intense exposure and is characterized by severe infections, owing to bone marrow and lymphoid (immune) system failure, and by severe diarrhea and intestinal infections owing to damage to intestinal mucosa. Long-term radiation injury is associated with scarring (bone marrow fibrosis, for example) and increased cancer risk (leukemia, for example) in affected organs. Examples include survivors of the atomic bomb blasts at Hiroshima and Nagasaki in 1945, and the Chernobyl nuclear plant accident in 1986 in Ukraine.

INHALANT LUNG DISEASE

The **pneumoconioses** (Chapter 14) are lung diseases caused by inhaled substances (inhalants). Long-term exposure, typically in the workplace, is usually necessary to produce ill effect. Common offenders are mineral dusts, such as rock dust (silica), coal dust, asbestos, and beryllium, and organic materials, such as cotton lint or grain dust. The most common reaction is lung scarring, which may be debilitating, even fatal. Moreover, some inhalant exposures are associated with increased prevalence of malignancy; for example, pulmonary asbestosis

Table 10-3	*The Radiant Energy Spectrum*	
Energy	**Type of Radiation**	**Effect**
Highest energy, highest frequency, shortest wavelength	Cosmic rays	Unknown
	X-rays; gamma rays	Cancer; acute and chronic radiation sickness
	UV light	Sunburn, skin cancers
	Visible light	Laser burns
	Infrared light	Cataracts
	Microwaves	Cataracts
	Radio and radar	Cataracts
Lowest energy, lowest frequency, longest wavelength	Electric power radiation	Probably none

is associated with increased risk for malignant mesothelioma, a malignant tumor of the pleura.

Tobacco, Alcohol, and Drugs

In the United States, tobacco use, mainly cigarette smoking, causes about 400,000 deaths per year, most of which can be attributed to lung cancer or cardiovascular disease. Each year alcohol abuse accounts for about 100,000 deaths; drug abuse accounts for about 20,000.

CIGARETTE SMOKING

It is not much of a stretch to say that, for any given disease, cigarette smokers have more of it than those who do not smoke. Cigarette smoking is arguably the most corrosive, health-destroying habit ever adopted by humankind. Smoking kills more than 400,000 Americans annually, about ten times as many as auto accidents do. Smoking is widespread in every society; about 50% of smokers die from the habit. Figure 10-7 offers a summary of the ill effects of smoking.

Cigarette smoke contains over 40 known carcinogens, plus toxic metals and formaldehyde. Adding to the damage is the effect of carbon monoxide, which has $200\times$ greater affinity for hemoglobin than oxygen does and deprives tissue of oxygen by occupying red blood cell space where oxygen belongs. All of these effects are dose related; that is, they are directly proportional to the number of cigarettes smoked in a lifetime. Figure 10-8 illustrates the close relationship between the num-

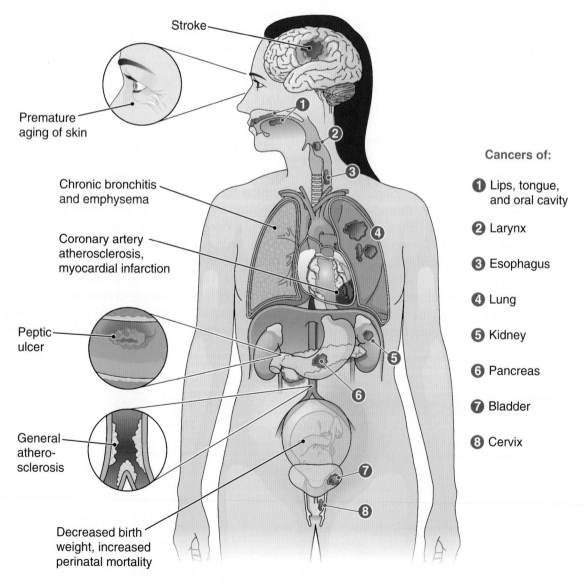

Figure 10-7 **The effects of smoking.**

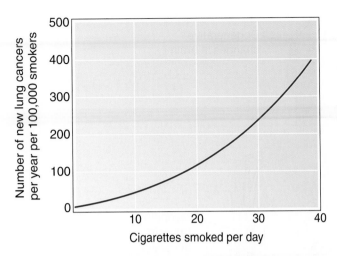

Figure 10-8 The relationship between smoking and lung cancer. The number of new lung cancers increases directly with the number of cigarettes smoked per day. A similar relationship exists between the number of new lung cancers and the number of years smoking.

ber of new lung cancers diagnosed per year in smokers and the number of cigarettes smoked per day.

Cigarette smokers not only have higher rates of lung cancer than nonsmokers do, but cigarette smokers also have a higher prevalence of other kinds of cancer than do nonsmokers. Cigarette smoke accelerates disease in almost every organ system—cigarettes smokers have higher rates of emphysema, chronic bronchitis, heart attack, stroke, atherosclerosis, gastric ulcers, hypertension, and other diseases than nonsmokers do.

The ill effect of passive inhalation of cigarette smoke by nonsmokers is real. Passive smoke inhalation increases the risk of lung cancer, stroke, heart attack, asthma, and sudden infant death syndrome (SIDS, Chapter 7).

> *Half of smokers die of the habit.*

Most of the ill effects of cigarette smoke are *not* associated with **nicotine**. Nicotine is a stimulant that is responsible for *addiction* to tobacco—it is, perhaps, the most addictive of all substances—but it has little pathologic effect compared to the tars, phenol, benzopyrene, formaldehyde, and hydrocarbons also found in smoke. Some of these compounds cause cancer by damaging bronchial DNA. Others irritate the bronchial mucosa, causing chronic inflammation, excess mucus production, and paralysis of bronchial cilia, which inhibits their cleansing sweep.

Fetuses are vulnerable to the effects of maternal smoking. Smoking half a pack a day causes fetal hypoxia, low birth weight, and prematurity. There is increased risk of abnormal implantation of the placenta, placental

bleeding, abortion, and early rupture of amniotic membranes.

It helps to quit smoking—the life expectancy of smokers who quit before age 30 is equal to that of people who have never smoked. Older smokers benefit, too. After one year, smoking-related cardiovascular risk decreases 50%. Cancer risk fades more slowly than cardiovascular risk does, falling to near nonsmoker risk after 15–20 years. For those who find it impossible to quit, smoking fewer cigarettes helps: recent evidence indicates that, for heavy smokers, smoking half as many cigarettes significantly reduces lung cancer risk.

ALCOHOL ABUSE

In discussing alcohol consumption, it is important to distinguish between *use* and *abuse*. Each year the *use* of alcohol accounts for about 80,000 deaths, which include accidents and medical conditions caused by alcohol *abuse*. Moderate use appears to be beneficial, but the balance of benefit versus harm depends on age, sex, weight, and genetic and other factors.

Moderate *use* is considered to be about two 150 ml glasses of wine, two beers, or two cocktails per day. Many studies document the benefit of moderate consumption of alcohol—it clearly decreases risk of developing cardiovascular disease and type II diabetes. The positive cardiovascular effect is attributed to increases in HDL cholesterol and decreases of fibrinogen levels and platelet agglutination. The latter two are important in thrombus formation, which is important in the pathogenesis of heart attack and stroke. However, *any* amount of ethanol can impair physical and mental performance for a short time, and few, if any, health care professionals would encourage non-drinkers to start drinking for the cardiovascular or anti-diabetic benefits.

Alcohol *abuse* is a chronic disease in which people refuse to stop drinking even though it causes neglect of important family and work obligations. Figure 10-9 illustrates the medical conditions associated with abuse of alcohol. The social characteristics of chronic alcohol abuse are:

- Drinking when it is dangerous (e.g., while driving)
- Difficulties with family, friends, or coworkers caused by alcohol
- Legal problems related to drinking

A common legal definition of drunkenness is blood alcohol (**ethanol**) of 80 mg/dL (0.08%). In a 140-lb woman, it takes about three 12-ounce bottles of beer, or one-ounce shots of 100 proof whiskey, or half a bottle of wine in a short period of time to produce legal intoxication. A blood alcohol level of 200 mg/dL is associated

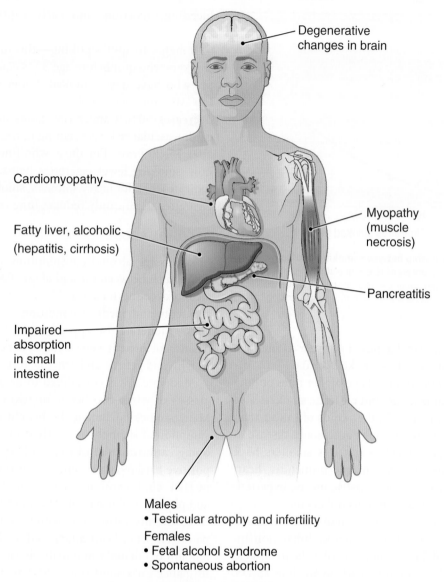

- Degenerative changes in brain
- Cardiomyopathy
- Myopathy (muscle necrosis)
- Fatty liver, alcoholic (hepatitis, cirrhosis)
- Pancreatitis
- Impaired absorption in small intestine

Males
- Testicular atrophy and infertility

Females
- Fetal alcohol syndrome
- Spontaneous abortion

Figure 10-9 The effects of chronic alcohol abuse.

with severe drunkenness; coma and death may occur at levels of 300–400 mg/dL. However, heavy drinkers can tolerate higher levels.

About 5% of drinkers are abusers. As is illustrated in Figure 10-9, chronic alcoholism may cause disease in almost any organ, but it primarily affects the brain, liver, and stomach. Alcohol may ulcerate the gastric mucosa, and its adverse effect on the liver is clear and devastating: all chronic alcoholics have fatty livers (Fig. 10-10), and about 15% develop cirrhosis (severe scarring) of the liver, which is discussed in detail in Chapter 16.

Chronic alcohol abuse severely affects the brain (Chapter 23) and may lead to cerebellar degeneration (Fig. 10-11), which leaves sober patients with severe motor incoordination and stumbling gait. Other effects on the brain are attributable to alcoholic nutritional

deficiencies—alcohol supplies calories but no vitamins or other nutrients. One of the most noteworthy deficiencies is thiamine (vitamin B_1) deficiency (**beriberi**), which is characterized by peripheral neuropathy, cardiac failure, and central nervous system (CNS) symptoms. CNS symptoms take either or both of two syndromes: Wernicke encephalopathy and Korsakoff psychosis. **Wernicke encephalopathy** consists of impaired eye motility, pupillary alterations, nystagmus (a rapid, jerky oscillation of the globe), tremors of the extremities, and ataxia (a staggering gait). **Korsakoff psychosis** is characterized by amnesia for recent events and an attempt to disguise the memory loss by *confabulation*—a tactic adopted by alcoholics trying to disguise short-term memory loss. They make fluent but rambling statements full of fabrications, which go nowhere be-

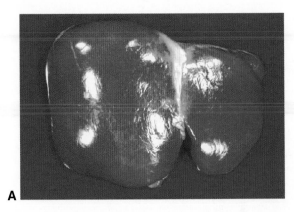
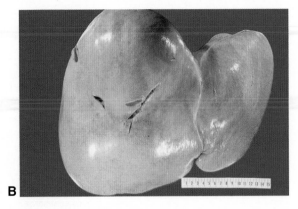

Figure 10-10 **Fatty liver of chronic alcoholism. A.** Normal liver. **B.** Fatty liver in a chronic alcoholic. The cuts are postmortem artifacts.

cause they can't remember where the conversation is supposed to go.

Alcohol abuse is also associated with increased incidence of cancers of the mouth, throat, larynx, esophagus, pancreas, kidney, and bladder. Other adverse effects include testicular atrophy and infertility, spontaneous abortion (Chapter 7), hypertension (Chapter 12), cardiomyopathy (Chapter 13), and acute and chronic pancreatitis (Chapter 17). Alcohol consumption is a contributing or direct factor in other conditions. **Fetal alcohol syndrome** (Chapter 7) is the most common form of preventable mental retardation in the United States. In addition, alcohol is a contributing factor in 40% of motor vehicle deaths and is a contributing factor in other types of accidents.

DRUG ABUSE

In this discussion, "drug" refers to any substance other than alcohol and nicotine that is used to excess to

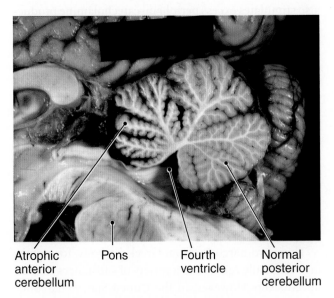

Figure 10-11 **Cerebellar atrophy of chronic alcoholism.**

Atrophic anterior cerebellum   Pons   Fourth ventricle   Normal posterior cerebellum

achieve an altered mood. Most types of abused drugs are legally manufactured and are available in limited quantity by prescription to be used only for medical treatment (morphine is an example). However, abuse depends on illegal production, possession, and distribution. In 2001 when questioned about illegal drug use, 7% of persons in the United States age 12 and older admitted illegal use in the prior month. Drug abuse is associated with suicide, homicide, and violence, motor-vehicle injury, HIV infection, pneumonia, mental illness, hepatitis, and sudden death from cardiac disease or coma. Drug abuse accounts for about 20,000 deaths each year in the United States (for comparison, traffic accidents account for about 40,000).

Drugs can be ingested, sniffed or inhaled, or injected. Intestinal absorption is slow and produces less of the desired effect. Greater effect is produced by injection, or by sniffing or inhaling (including smoking) for quick absorption into the bloodstream via the nasal or bronchial mucosa. Intravenous injection is particularly risky (Fig. 10-12). Shared needles and other unsanitary practices lead to injection of microbes and foreign material. The most common infections obtained by injection are HIV/AIDS, hepatitis virus, and bacteria infections, including bacterial endocarditis (Chapter 13). Injected foreign material can also stimulate formation of antigen-antibody complexes (circulating immune complexes, Chapter 8) that lodge in the glomeruli to produce chronic kidney disease. Some foreign substances, such as talc (used to dilute the drug dose), lodge in the lungs to produce "narcotic lung," characterized by inflammatory nodules and scarring. Finally, there is the risk of coma with brain damage or death if the user miscalculates.

Illegal drugs fall into four main categories:

1. Depressants: ethanol, barbiturates, benzodiazepines
2. Stimulants: cocaine, amphetamines

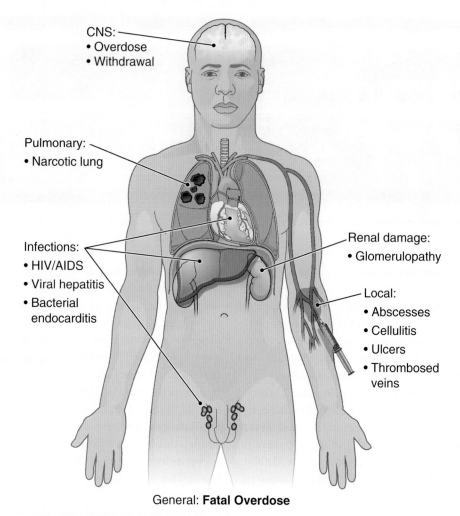

CNS:
• Overdose
• Withdrawal

Pulmonary:
• Narcotic lung

Infections:
• HIV/AIDS
• Viral hepatitis
• Bacterial endocarditis

Renal damage:
• Glomerulopathy

Local:
• Abscesses
• Cellulitis
• Ulcers
• Thrombosed veins

General: **Fatal Overdose**

Figure 10-12 **The effects of intravenously injected illegal drugs.** Illegal drugs affect the lungs, kidneys, and brain cause a variety of infections and produce local effects such as vein thrombosis and abscess.

3. Narcotics: morphine, heroin, meperidine (Demerol®)
4. Hallucinogens: marijuana, LSD, mescaline

The list is partial; new compounds appear regularly.

Depressants have a sedative or calming effect. At low doses they loosen inhibition, but at high doses they can produce coma and death. *Ethanol* is the most commonly abused depressant. *Barbiturates* are sedatives that relieve anxiety. Barbiturate tolerance develops quickly, and abrupt withdrawal may be accompanied by seizures and death. Safer alternatives such as *benzodiazepines* are infrequently abused.

Stimulants enhance the sense of awareness and awakeness and produce euphoria. The most popular illegal stimulant drug is *cocaine*. Among drug users cocaine abuse is second only to marijuana abuse—about 1% of all persons age 12 and over in the United States report recent cocaine use. The stimulating effects of cocaine are so seductive that it is one of the most addictive and destructive of all illegal drugs. Cocaine produces its euphoria by causing repeated firing of neurons in brain centers responsible for feelings of pleasure. Cocaine use also stimulates excess peripheral catecholamine production, which causes hypertension, cardiac arrhythmias, and sudden cardiac death. Acute overdose of cocaine can produce seizures and cardiorespiratory arrest. Chronic abuse is also associated with nasal septal perforation (in chronic snorters), premature atherosclerosis, coronary spasm, heart attack, and stroke. Cocaine use during pregnancy can cause placental hypoperfusion, which leads to spontaneous abortion, fetal growth retardation, and congenital anomalies, and fetal hypoxia with permanent fetal brain damage.

Amphetamines are widely abused stimulants as well. Overdose produces delirium, convulsions, cardiac arrhythmias, coma, and death.

The word **narcotic** (from Greek *narkosis*, for numbing) originally referred to a variety of substances that induced sleep. However, in the United States "narcotic" has a strict legal definition: it refers to 1) drugs derived from the opium poppy plant; 2) cocaine and other derivatives of the cocoa plant; and 3) synthetic substitutes that have similar pharmacologic action. *Heroin* is the most widely abused narcotic—0.1% of people 12 and over in the United States report recent use. Heroin is an opium derivative originally touted as a non-addictive pain reliever. However, it is more powerfully addictive than cocaine is and has a sedative, rather than stimulatory, effect. It creates a mental and *physical* addiction associated with an agonizingly painful withdrawal syndrome that can prove fatal. On a case-by-case basis heroin is more dangerous than cocaine is, because heroin is often taken intravenously, and accidental overdose can prove fatal, usually owing to respiratory depression or cardiac arrhythmias. Intravenous use is associated with the constant threat of hepatitis, AIDS, staphylococcal abscesses, bacterial endocarditis, and other infections. Pulmonary edema and renal disease occur regularly. The ready availability of medical narcotics—morphine, meperidine (Demerol®), and others—make them a particular problem among health care workers.

A **hallucinogen** is a drug that distorts reality or produces altered sensory experiences. Hallucinogens such as mescaline, LSD, and phencyclidine (PCP) are in general less physically dangerous than the drugs mentioned above, but their power to distort reality may lead to lethal behavior. *Marijuana* is the most widely abused of all illegal drugs—75% of drug users abuse marijuana alone or with other drugs. The physical effects of chronic marijuana use are well known. On the negative side, chronic use is associated with gynecomastia (enlarged male breasts) and testicular atrophy. On the positive side it lowers intraocular pressure in chronic ocular hypertension (glaucoma, Chapter 25) and relieves the nausea associated with cancer chemotherapy.

Nutritional Disease

Diet has been alleged to have a role in, or be the salvation for, almost every condition known to humankind. While many "diet cure" regimens are more imaginary than real, there is no doubt that diet plays an important role in some diseases. The diet of industrialized nations is high in fat and processed foods and low in fiber. Diet is clearly associated with increased death and illness from cardiovascular disease and cancer when compared to the diet of people in developing nations, who eat a diet containing less meat and processed food but more fish and fresh vegetables, and have less cardiovascular disease and cancer. The Western diet is also high in salt

(sodium), a fact linked to high prevalence of hypertension. Nevertheless, it is difficult to prove a *causative* relationship between diet and many of these conditions. For example, people living in Africa eat a diet with high fiber content, and they have low rates of colon cancer, whereas people living in the United States eat a diet containing relatively little fiber and have a high rate of colon cancer. Even so, studies prove conclusively that low dietary fiber does not *cause* colon cancer.

MALNUTRITION

Malnutrition may be a deficiency either of calories or of dietary essentials, such as vitamin D or iron. Malnutrition can be:

- self-induced, as in *anorexia nervosa* (self-starvation caused by fear of becoming obese) and *bulimia* (avoidance of weight gain by self-induced vomiting after a meal)
- the result of poverty and ignorance
- the result of a disease process, such as chronic alcoholism, gastrointestinal malabsorption syndrome, or the cachexia of malignancy (Chapter 6)

Children are particularly susceptible to nutritional deficiencies because their growing bodies need an ample supply of calories and nutrients. Both caloric deficiency and deficiency of specific nutrients are widespread public health problems in poor nations, but they are not absent in wealthy ones. In any particular individual, the effect may be as devastating as death or as subtle as mildly impaired intelligence.

Vitamin deficiency is an important aspect of malnutrition. Vitamins are organic substances essential in minute amounts for normal growth and activity of the body and are obtained naturally from plant and animal foods. Vitamins are involved in virtually every aspect of human physiology, and their deficiency syndromes offer a complex array of signs, symptoms, and pathophysiological relationships, far too varied for discussion here. It is important to know that four vitamins (A, D, E, and K) are *fat soluble*; the remainder are water soluble. This distinction is important because fat-soluble vitamins are stored in body fat and are, therefore, more difficult to deplete by dietary deficiency. On the other hand, fat-soluble vitamins are subject to rapid depletion in diseases associated with poor intestinal fat absorption (malabsorption syndromes, Chapter 15). Vitamin toxicity (overdose) is usually of one of the fat-soluble vitamins, which are efficiently stored in body fat, facilitating accumulation of a toxic dose.

Vitamin deficiency, although rare in the United States, occurs in conjunction with malnutrition in developing nations. Among the more important syndromes are the anemia of B_{12} or folic acid deficiency (Chapter 11), the bleeding tendency of vitamin K deficiency (Chapter 11), and the bony deformities of *rickets* (a syndrome of vitamin D deficiency in children).

Historically important but uncommon now are *scurvy* (vitamin C deficiency) and *beriberi* (thiamine, also known as B_1, deficiency). Thiamine deficiency rarely occurs except in chronic alcoholics—about one-fourth of chronic alcoholics admitted to hospitals are thiamine deficient and may suffer from peripheral neuropathy, cardiac failure, or Wernicke-Korsakoff syndrome (discussed above).

Vitamin toxicity is uncommon and usually occurs in association with food or dietary supplement faddism (dietary practice based upon an exaggerated belief in the beneficial effects of food or nutrition on health and disease). The fat-soluble vitamins A, D, E, and K are most often the culprit.

In addition to the need for calories, the body has a requirement for *protein* to maintain the body's two protein compartments: the somatic compartment, mainly skeletal muscle, and the visceral compartment, mainly the liver. Diets deficient in protein are almost always deficient in calories, and vice versa, so that protein and energy deficiencies usually go hand-in-hand as **protein-energy malnutrition**. Deprivation of *both* protein and calories leads to **marasmus**, a widespread condition in some developing nations, particularly after children are weaned from the breast. Marasmus is characterized by skeletal thinness, particularly in the limbs. Muscles waste away, but the liver and other viscera are initially spared, and the abdomen bulges. These children also have an aged, wrinkled appearance because their bodies shrivel to the point that their skin no longer "fits."

If the diet contains some calories from carbohydrate but remains very low in protein, the child develops **kwashiorkor** (from the Niger-Congo language of Ghana, in West Africa), a state of malnutrition in which the liver and other viscera are also affected (Fig. 10-13). Intestinal villi atrophy and cannot absorb food properly; diarrhea is the result. Blood levels of albumin and other proteins made by the liver fall dramatically. Low plasma albumin causes decreased intravascular osmotic pressure (Chapter 5), resulting in extravascular accumulations of fluid as tissue edema and ascites. This accumulation of fluid gives the patient a puffy appearance that can mask underlying skeletal thinness. Hair, composed of keratin, a protein, loses its color and becomes sandy or reddish, and epidermis, also composed partially of keratin, develops splotches of white depigmentation and other skin disease. The typical clinical picture of

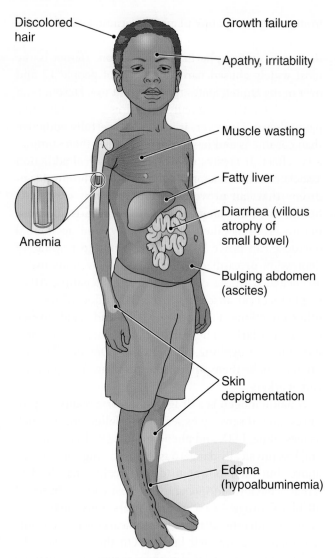

Figure 10-13 Kwashiorkor.

kwashiorkor is an infant near death with a potbelly, puffy face, red or sandy discolored hair, skin lesions, thin arms and legs, and swollen feet.

OBESITY

Thou seest I have more flesh than another man, and therefore more frailty.

WILLIAM SHAKESPEARE (1564–1616),
ENGLISH PLAYWRIGHT, *HENRY IV, PART 1* (III.ii)

The standard dictionary definition of **obesity** is an excess of body fat, and, as the accompanying History of Medicine box relates, it was rare anywhere in the world until about 200 years ago. Just as smoking plays a key role in the development of lung and other cancers and cardiovascular disease, diet and obesity contribute to the development of many diseases, especially cardiovascular disease.

So, who is fat and who is not? To separate accurately those who are obese from those who are not requires body fat measurement, which is cumbersome and expensive. However, because excess fat is responsible for weight gain in most people, a very good substitute for body fat measurements is **Body Mass Index** (BMI), a ratio of body weight and height, which is discussed in Basics in Brief 10.1. BMI is used to define underweight, normal, overweight, obese, and morbidly obese.

> ☞ *Among adult Americans nearly 60% are overweight or obese.*

Body weight is related to body height. All other things being equal, body weight varies with the square of height; in mathematical terms, the ratio of weight to the square of height is constant ($w/h^2 =$ constant).

Stated another way, a person six feet tall ($6^2 = 36$) should weigh four times as much as someone three feet tall ($3^2 = 9$). Normal and abnormal body weight and various stages of excess weight are defined by BMI, which is the body weight in kilograms divided by the square of the height in meters. BMI is not perfect, however. Some athletes, especially those with high muscle mass, have abnormally high BMI but are not actually obese because they have a low percentage of body fat. Basics in Brief 10.1 offers more detail.

It is incontestable that being obese is bad for health; however, the number of annual deaths that can be attributed to obesity is difficult to calculate and is the subject of some controversy. Table 10-4 quantifies the relationship between obesity and ill health.

Obesity is strongly related to increased odds of developing cancer, cardiovascular disease, and diabetes.

HISTORY OF MEDICINE

FRENCH FOOD, FAST FOOD, FAT FOOD

For most of human history, the average person ate to satisfy hunger; eating for pleasure was unknown except to kings, queens, and tyrants, among whom obesity occurred because only they could afford cooks and inventories of food. The average person's meal was simple and was determined more by availability than choice. Travelers staying overnight at an inn could obtain drink, but food was only what the innkeeper was having for supper—if there was some to spare. There was no such thing as a restaurant as we know it until 1765 in Paris when Monsieur A. Boulanger opened a business that was not an inn and that specialized in prepared food. Thinking to trade on the idea of food as a cure (like chicken soup for a cold) the sign above the door said, "Restaurants," French for "restoratives." However, politics made his experiment short lived and this, the first-ever restaurant, was closed.

In 1782 the first truly luxury restaurant was opened in Paris, but the idea of restaurants did not really catch on until 1789, when the French Revolution destroyed French royalty and nobility and emptied kitchens of hundreds of chefs, many of whom opened places to eat, which they also called "restaurants." Monsieur Boulanger was among them, and his restaurant became the first to offer a menu with a choice of dishes. By 1804, Paris had more than 500 restaurants, and the concept swept around the world.

Restaurants were slow to come to America. The first true American luxury restaurant was Delmonicos, which opened in 1827 in New York City. However, Americans, always

wanting more of everything faster and cheaper, soon invented fast food. Some food historians consider that the first fast food restaurant was established 1891 when the YWCA of Kansas City, Mo., established a cafeteria—a place where prepared food is set on display and sold by the dish. Others suggest that fast food had its origins in San Francisco in 1849 during the California gold rush when prepared food was set out on open-air tables and sold by the dish to the "forty-niners" who flocked to California to make their fortune.

With the coming of the automobile in the early 1900s, restaurants began to serve patrons in their cars. After World War II (1939–1945), with the development of the American interstate highway system and the idea of franchising pioneered by Holiday Inn motel chain, "fast food" restaurants spread across America. McDonald's restaurant chain began in 1955, Kentucky Fried Chicken in 1956, and Pizza Hut in 1958, and each followed the burgeoning interstate highway system.

About the same time, the United States government began to subsidize corn production, which brought down the cost of processed food. All of these developments—cheap corn sugar, standard quality, and easy access—made "fast food" calories cheap and readily available.

In 1950, there was no state in the United States with *more* than 10% of the population overweight. In 2004 there was no state with *less* than 60% of the population overweight: an entire nation became fat in 50 years.

▶ **BASICS IN BRIEF 10-1**

BODY MASS INDEX (BMI) AND OBESITY

By widely accepted agreement, people are classified as underweight, normal, overweight, or obese according to their body mass index (BMI), a calculation that relates body weight and height.

The kilograms and meters formula for BMI is:

$$[\text{weight in kilograms}] \div [\text{height in meters}]^2$$

The pounds and inches formula is:

$$[\text{weight in pounds} \times 704.5] \div [\text{height in inches}]^2$$

For example: the BMI for a person 6 feet tall (72 inches), weighing 200 lb is calculated thus:

$$200 \text{ (weight in lb)} \times 704.5 = 140{,}900$$

$$72 \text{ (height in inches)} \times 72 = 5{,}184$$

$$140{,}900 \div 5{,}184 = 27.18, \text{ which rounds to BMI of 27}$$

The table in this box displays the prevalence of various BMI categories in the United States according to the most recent United States National Health and Nutrition Examination Survey (NHANES III).

Prevalence (%) of Various BMI Groups in the United States, 1988-1994

Category	BMI	Prevalence (%)
Underweight	<18.5	2%
Normal	18.5–<25	41%
Overweight	25–<30	34%
Obese*	>30	23%

*People with BMI >40 are defined as morbidly obese

For example, for a person 5'8" tall:

- 165 lb is overweight
- 198 lb is obese
- 263 lb is morbidly obese

Some athletes are heavy because of large muscle mass, and they have lower body fat than most others with the same BMI.

The obese are also at increased risk for wear-and-tear joint disease (osteoarthritis, Chapter 22), stroke (Chapter 23), gallstones (Chapter 16), and pulmonary disease (Chapter 14).

Obesity is a very complex matter physiologically, psychologically, and socially. On one hand it is a simple matter of energy balance—take in more calories than you burn, and the excess is stored as fat. On the other hand, it is maddeningly difficult to treat with sustained success—diet regimens work wonders for a while, but only about 5% of dieters maintain their weight loss.

It is becoming clear that *obesity is an inflammatory state*. That is, a smoldering inflammation occurs in tissue with excess fat, which causes production of certain inflammatory products (including C-reactive protein, Chapter 12) that damage endothelial cells. Damage to

Table 10-4	Relative Risk for Cancer, Cardiovascular Disease, and Diabetes in People with Various Body Mass Indices (BMI)		
Classification (defined by BMI, with examples)	**Relative Cancer Risk***	**Relative Cardiovascular Risk***	**Relative Type II Diabetes Risk***
Normal (BMI 18.5–25) 5′8″, <165 lb	1.0	1.0	1.0
Overweight (BMI 25–30) 5′8″, 165–197 lb	1.1	1.2	2.0
Obese (BMI 30–40) 5′8″, 198–263 lb	1.3	1.9	3.5
Morbidly Obese (BMI >40) 5′8″, >263 lb	1.7	2.4	6.5

*The risk of cancer, cardiovascular disease, and type II diabetes in people with normal BMI is 1.0. The relative risk of disease among the overweight or obese is their risk compared to normal. For example, people with BMI 25–30 are 1.1 times (ten percent) more likely to develop cancer than people with BMI <25.

endothelial cells is the first step in atherosclerosis (Chapter 12). What's more, obesity induces in non-fat cells a resistance to the effect of insulin, which is the primary cause of type II diabetes mellitus (Chapter 17).

Manifold hormonal factors have been identified in the biologic regulation of body weight and fat deposition. Figure 10-14 demonstrates a simplified scheme showing the normal function of this regulatory system, which operates in a typical negative feedback loop (Chapter 18) designed to maintain physiologic balance (homeostasis, Chapter 2). Accumulation of fat signals the brain to decrease hunger pangs, to increase energy burn and heat production, and to metabolize fatty acids. An important regulator of these reactions is **leptin** (*ob protein*), an anti-obesity hormone produced under the influence of *ob gene*. Leptin is secreted by fat cells and appears to have three functions: 1) to decrease food intake by lowering appetite; 2) to increase energy burn; and 3) to prevent fat from accumulating in cells that are not lipocytes—the accumulation of fat in non-fat cells, such as heart muscle, is toxic. In normal people as fat accumulates, additional leptin is produced, which is carried to the hypothalamus where it binds to leptin receptors, causing a signal to the cerebral cortex that says, in effect, "I'm full." As fat accumulates, the hypothalamus also increases energy burn by stimulating the sym-

pathetic (adrenergic) nervous system and adrenal medulla to produce norepinephrine, which increases heat production and the breakdown of fatty acids that otherwise would be converted into fat. In addition, accumulation of fat causes the hypothalamus to stimulate the thyroid to release its hormones, which increase the metabolic rate.

It now seems likely that dysfunction of the leptin system is important in obesity. Obese people have high leptin but remain hungry, which suggests the brain may be resistant to the "I'm full" signal. Moreover, obese people tend to accumulate fat in other organs, also suggesting that leptin is unable to prevent fat from accumulating in them. Together these facts suggest that the peripheral tissue of obese people is resistant to the effect of leptin.

Abdominal obesity, a "beer gut" in American slang, is especially perilous, as is indicated in the discussion below of the *metabolic syndrome*. Abdominal obesity is very important; it is not merely a convenient measure. Large abdominal girth caused by abdominal fat is much more of a health hazard than is the same amount of extra fat stored elsewhere. Waist size is an independent risk factor for type II diabetes, hypertension, coronary artery disease, gallstones, stroke, cancer (especially of the endometrium and breast), pulmonary disease, and osteoarthritis. That is to say, if fat is distributed widely, not concentrated in the abdomen, it is less risky.

Abdominal obesity is defined as a man with a 40″ waist or a woman with a 35″ waist. Waist size is properly measured horizontally, across the fat part of the belly, not below it. In 2003 the average American man and woman over age 55, regardless of race, exceeded these measurements; that is to say, the average American over age 55 is centrally obese.

The ill effect of obesity is pervasive and appears in unexpected ways. Obese people are more prone to home accidents because they are less fit and unable to manage their bulk; and on average they are twice as likely to suffer from hearing loss, poor eyesight, mental illness, and mobility disorders of the arms or legs. Obesity also is linked to increased prevalence of cancers of the colon, stomach, pancreas, lung, prostate, breast, and brain, as well as leukemia and lymphoma. Morbidly obese people (BMI >40, for example a person 5′8″, weighing 263 lb) experience about 70% more cancers than do people who are not obese.

Genes play a role in obesity. For example, studies of identical twins reared separately show that if one is obese the other very likely is, too. An *OB* gene has been discovered, which codes for *leptin*, a hormone that influences appetite and fat accumulation.

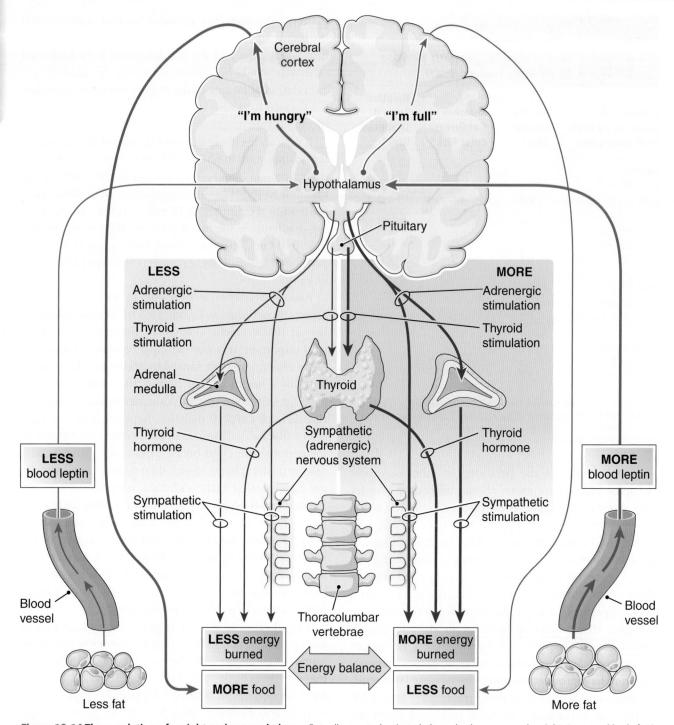

Figure 10-14 The regulation of weight and energy balance. Fat cells secrete leptin to balance body energy and weight. Increased body fat is associated with increased leptin secretion. Leptin travels to the hypothalamus, where it performs three functions. 1) It stimulates an "I'm full" signal to the cerebral cortex, which suppresses appetite. 2) It stimulates the pituitary to stimulate the thyroid gland, which secretes thyroid hormones to increase the metabolic rate and burn more energy. 3) It stimulates the adrenal medulla and the sympathetic (adrenergic) nervous system, which further increases energy metabolism.

Morbid Obesity

Morbid obesity is defined as BMI >40. The degree of obesity is important: morbidly obese patients are even more vulnerable than are those who are merely obese (BMI >30). Morbidly obese patients are especially

likely to develop diabetes, cancer, and cardiovascular disease. They also are at increased risk for:

- Obstructive sleep apnea and chronic hypoventilation, which is associated with hypoxia and CO_2 retention (see Pickwickian syndrome, on the next page)

- Pulmonary hypertension and right heart failure (cor pulmonale)
- Esophageal reflux
- Urinary incontinence
- Irregular menses and infertility
- Osteoarthritis

There is evidence that very obese people can suffer from **fatty heart syndrome**, a condition in which heart muscle accumulates fat and loses contractile power. Congestive heart failure and other problems may result.

Morbid obesity may be associated with the **Pickwickian syndrome**, a combination of morbid obesity, hypoventilation, chronic hypoxia, and CO_2 retention, which takes its name from Charles Dickens' The *Pickwick Papers*, as is described in the nearby History of Medicine box. The enormous amount of fat in the belly and the pelt of fat on the chest wall press down on the ribs and up on the diaphragm and mechanically limit each breath. Chronic hypoxia causes vasoconstriction in the systemic and pulmonary circulation, causing high blood pressure, pulmonary hypertension, and right heart failure (Chapter 13). Chronic hypoxia also produces increased peripheral red blood cell count (*erythrocytosis*, Chapter 11) as the bone marrow makes extra red cells to carry more oxygen to tissues.

Patients with Pickwickian syndrome typically have *Cheyne-Stokes respirations*, a pattern of breathing with alternating periods of very shallow breaths or apnea followed by periods of deeper breathing. During apnea, CO_2 builds up until it reaches levels high enough to stimulate deeper breathing; deep breathing then blows

THE CLINICAL SIDE

METABOLIC RATE AND AGING

One of the best ounces of prevention is the ounce of fat you do not gain. Obesity is a killer—heart disease, cancer, stroke, diabetes, accidents, and other causes of death and disease are much more common in the obese than in the non-obese. To move and maintain their bulk, obese people must burn more calories than the non-obese. That is right: the obese burn more calories; their metabolic rate is higher. Of course, they take in a lot more to make up for it.

A high metabolic rate is associated with more rapid aging and earlier death than occur with a low metabolic rate. It has been documented in numerous studies that animals fed near-starvation diets live much longer and healthier lives than do those given normal diets. Obese animals fattened on excessive diets are less healthy and live the shortest time. The near-starving animals use less energy and oxygen and age less rapidly than the others do.

off CO_2, the stimulus to breathe disappears, and the patient becomes apneic again. During apneic periods these patients may fall asleep, even in mid-sentence, owing to the sedative effect of retained CO_2 (CO_2 narcosis), and reawaken during the next phase of the cycle and take up conversation where they left off. However, they become most apneic and hypoxic at night—90% of Pickwickian syndrome patients suffer from sleep apnea.

THE METABOLIC SYNDROME

Obesity is a key aspect of the **metabolic syndrome**, illustrated in Figure 10-15. It is important to note that, while most patients with the metabolic syndrome are obese, obesity is not a necessary requirement for the diagnosis. Nevertheless, one fourth of obese people have the metabolic syndrome.

Precise definitions of the metabolic syndrome vary, but patients typically have a lifestyle characterized by a high carbohydrate diet and lack of exercise. People with metabolic syndrome usually have several of the following metabolic abnormalities:

- *Abdominal obesity*: waist measurement 40″ or more in men, 35″ or more in women
- *Abnormal glucose metabolism*: fasting blood glucose levels >110 mg/dL
- *Abnormal plasma lipids (dyslipidemia)*: triglyceride levels >150 mg/dL; or HDL cholesterol <40 mg/dL in men, or <50 mg/dL in women
- *Hypertension*: blood pressure >140/90 mm Hg

HISTORY OF MEDICINE

THE PICKWICKIAN SYNDROME

Most syndromes are named after the first patient or the first physician to describe them. The Pickwickian syndrome is unusual because the name is traceable to a memorable character in Charles Dickens' first novel, *The Pickwick Papers*, published in 1837. At the end of Chapter 53 Dickens introduces a scene involving the fat boy Joe:

> *A most violent and startling knocking was heard at the door . . . . The object that presented itself to the eyes of the astonished clerk was a boy—a wonderfully fat boy—habited as a serving lad, standing upright on the mat, with his eyes closed as if in sleep. He had never seen such a fat boy, in or out of a traveling caravan . . . .*

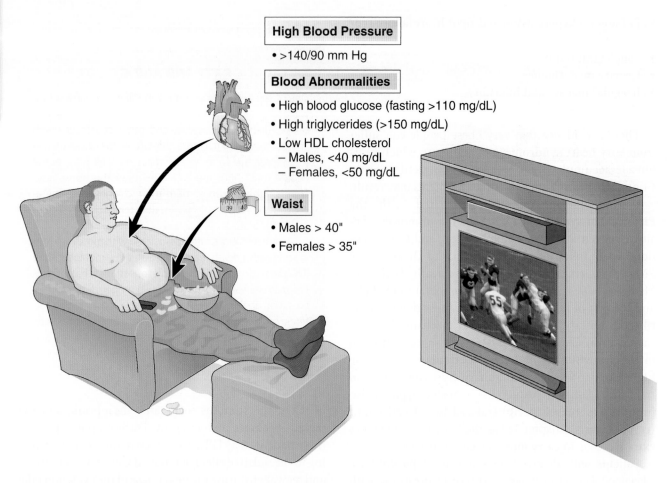

High Blood Pressure

• >140/90 mm Hg

Blood Abnormalities

• High blood glucose (fasting >110 mg/dL)
• High triglycerides (>150 mg/dL)
• Low HDL cholesterol
  – Males, <40 mg/dL
  – Females, <50 mg/dL

Waist

• Males > 40"
• Females > 35"

Figure 10-15 **The metabolic syndrome.** As the figure illustrates, people with this syndrome typically have central obesity, do not get enough exercise, and eat a high carbohydrate diet. They are at grave risk for cardiovascular disease.

Depending on precise diagnostic criteria, which vary from institution to institution, diagnosis typically depends on the presence of any three of the above factors. A characteristic example is reported in the case study at the end of this chapter.

No matter the particular criteria, about 70% of patients with type II diabetes and 40% of patients with abnormal glucose metabolism (but not frank diabetes) have the metabolic syndrome.

There is a distinct genetic tendency to develop the metabolic syndrome. In the United States, Hispanics and Native Americans are especially vulnerable.

The metabolic syndrome is associated with grave cardiovascular risk. For example, compared to people with no metabolic syndrome factors, patients with two of the required diagnostic factors in the list above are twice (2×) as likely to die of coronary artery disease (Chapter 13); patients with three factors are three-and-a-half times (3.5×) more likely to die of coronary artery disease.

Weight loss and exercise reduce the risk dramatically. Exercise alone (without weight loss) reduces risk significantly, but not to the level of non-obese patients. ■

CASE STUDY 10-1 *"MY CHEST FEELS FUNNY"*

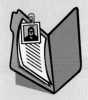

TOPICS
Angina pectoris
Obesity
The metabolic syndrome

THE CASE

Setting: You are one of several professionals staffing an urgent care clinic.

History: MB is a 48-year-old very obese man whose main complaint is "my chest feels funny."

You question him about the chest sensation, and he has a hard time finding words to describe it, saying that sometimes it is "almost a pain," and at other times it just "feels funny," and that it has been occurring for over a year. When you ask why he chose this particular time to seek medical care rather than some earlier time, he says the sensation is more severe and occurs more often now, and it is accompanied by shortness of breath. He says "it comes and goes" and is "sometimes" related to walking and "sometimes" related to meals. He says it occurs in the middle of his chest some of the time and in his upper abdomen other times. It does not radiate into his neck or jaw or left shoulder or arm. Further questions reveal that his mother is diabetic and his father died of a "heart stroke" in his fifties. He works from his home in the real estate business and "doesn't have time for exercise." He drinks "a few beers" every night.

Physical examination and other data: He is markedly obese, refuses to be weighed or measured, and answers "about 250" when asked about his weight. His blood pressure is 158/92. He appears to be about 5' 8" and wears size 44 pants. His lungs are clear, and his heart sounds are normal but distant. His peripheral pulses are good, and there is no edema in his feet. An electrocardiogram shows low voltage but no other abnormality.

You order a chest radiograph, urinalysis, and blood work and advise him that the pain could be from his heart or his stomach. You ask him to return in a week. In the interim you calculate that his BMI is about 38, perhaps more if he was not truthful about his weight. The chest radiograph shows slightly enlarged pulmonary vessels. Urinalysis is normal. Fasting blood glucose level is high: 112 mg/dL (normal <110; diabetes >126 mg/dL); total cholesterol is high: 265 mg/dL (desirable <200 mg/dL); HDL cholesterol is 43 mg/dL, much less than optimal for a man (male desirable >60 mg/dL), and triglyceride level is 307 mg/dL, markedly elevated (desirable <150 mg/dL). A complete blood count is unremarkable, but you notice that his hemoglobin level is near the upper end of the normal for a man, 17.1 gm/dL (normal 13.5 mg/dL–17.5 gm/dL).

Clinical course: When he returns for follow-up, you tell him you would like to refer him to a gastroenterologist to rule out esophageal reflux and to a cardiologist to rule out heart disease. You show him the laboratory results and tell him he appears to be pre-diabetic and has serious plasma lipid abnormalities and high blood pressure, all of which need attention if he is to avoid stroke or heart attack. You emphasize that his weight is a factor in all of these problems and give him the name of a clinic that specializes in weight control. He agrees to a referral, and you schedule him to return in a month, after the consultants' reports have been received.

The consultants' reports are not completely conclusive, but both believe he probably has angina pectoris (cardiac pain); the cardiologist recommends a coronary angiogram to study coronary blood flow.

On his follow-up visit, you explain the consultants' reports and urge him to have the angiogram and to enroll is a weight loss program. He says, "I'll think about it, Doc; but right now I feel pretty good."

DISCUSSION

This man was a cardiovascular time bomb waiting to explode, probably as a heart attack (coronary artery occlusion with myocardial infarct). He was very obese, and he fit the diagnostic criteria for metabolic syndrome: obesity, abnormal glucose metabolism, hypertension, and dyslipidemia (high triglyceride levels). Given that his fasting blood glucose level was abnormally high, but not high enough to diagnose diabetes, and given that 90% of diabetics are obese, it was likely that he would soon become frankly diabetic. He was hypertensive, too, a condition that will, with diabetes, accelerate atherosclerosis. The high hemoglobin level suggested he suffered from chronic hypoventilation, which may in turn have caused chronic pulmonary hypertension, which his prominent pulmonary vessels suggested may have already been present.

The cause of his chest pain was unexplained when you saw him. It could have been cardiac pain (angina)—he had plenty of reason to have coronary atherosclerosis. His shortness of breath added to the suspicion, but he could have been short of breath for no reason other than he was extremely obese and got little exercise. The chest pain could also have been from pulmonary hypertension—patients with severe pulmonary hypertension may develop atypical chest pain. Alternatively, the chest pain could have been from esophageal reflux—extremely obese patients may have so much abdominal fat that intra-abdominal pressure forces gastric juice up the esophagus, where it causes spasm, ulcers, and pain.

POINTS TO REMEMBER
- Chest pain can by a difficult diagnostic problem.
- Obesity is bad for your health.

CASE STUDY 10-1 *THE ROAD NOT TAKEN—AN ALTERNATIVE SCENARIO*

For all sad words of tongue or pen,
The saddest are these: "It might have been."
JOHN GREENLEAF WHITTIER (1807–1892),
AMERICAN QUAKER POET AND REFORMER, *MAUD MULLER*

THE CASE

With a bit of imagination, we can speculate how MB's case might have had a happier ending.

Setting: You are employed in the office of a physician who specializes in weight reduction, with an emphasis on changing dietary, exercise, and other habits to create a healthy lifestyle. While enrolled in the program, patients are required to come for an office visit once per week. Your job is to interview patients, monitor progress, authorize prescription refills and other tasks, and offer emotional support.

History: MB is a 38-year-old very obese man who is 5' 8" tall. You have come to know MB fairly well in the six weeks he has been in the program. Initially, you were not optimistic about his prospects because he was a reluctant patient. You recall his opening remark in the initial interview: "Look, Doc," he said, "I'm in this thing because my wife is driving me crazy about my weight. Yeah, I guess I'm a bit tubby, but I'm in the real estate business; I don't sell houses with my stomach; I sell them with my head."

Knowing that he will not be successful until he can participate for his own benefit, not his wife's, and sensing a challenge, you try very hard to win his confidence and to scare him a bit, too, hoping it will improve his chances of sticking to the task. You give him your well-rehearsed mini-lecture on the concept of Body Mass Index, the many ill effects of obesity, and the value of exercise. After you finish, he remarks with a laugh, "I guess the only thing I'm doing right is that I'm not a smoker. My wife made me quit when we got married." You agree and fill out his "contract," which lists his initial weight at 245 lb (BMI 37), his "optimal weight goal" of 164 lb or less (BMI <25), and his "acceptable weight goal" of 196 lb or less (BMI <30). The contract further specifies that he follow the agreed-upon dietary plan

to begin walking daily for exercise—10 minutes each day for the first month, then an additional 5 minutes per day until he reaches 30 minutes per day.

Physical examination and other data: Today, after six weeks in the program, he tips the scales at 224 lb—a loss of 21 lb. Blood tests collected the previous week are now in his record, and you see that there is important progress: his cholesterol level has fallen from 248 mg/dL to 227 mg/dL, and his triglyceride level has come down from 385 mg/dL to 225 mg/dL.

Clinical course: You congratulate him on his progress. "Thanks, Doc," he says, "You know, I can't believe how much better I feel. I'm glad the numbers show it. I don't even get short of breath anymore walking from the car to soccer practice with my girls, and my knees don't bother me as much as they used to."

You encourage him further: "You're about half way to 196 lb. When you get there you'll feel even better."

Eventually he completes the course, and his weight stabilizes near 205 lb (BMI 31), still in the obese range but much better than before. He walks regularly for exercise, but his total cholesterol remains over 200 mg/dL; however, it falls to 188 mg/dL when you add a statin drug to the program.

For the next ten years you see him periodically for prescription refills and minor ailments and are very pleased to see that he does not regain the weight, his cholesterol remains under control, and he appears in general good health.

DISCUSSION

Although MB fell short of his ambitious goals, this case was a resounding success even though he remained obese by BMI calculation. First, he was less likely to become diabetic at 205 lb than at 245 lb. Second, he improved symptomatically: his mental outlook improved, he did not get short of breath as easily as before, and the osteoarthritis in his knees did not bother him so much. In addition, his levels of blood lipids were markedly improved, which materially lessened his risk for cardiovascular disease.

Objectives Recap

1. *Name several of the most common causes of death in the United States, and discuss the environmental aspects*: Cardiovascular disease, stroke, and malignancies account for more than half of all deaths. Diet, smoking, and lack of exercise are important in each of the three. Alcohol use plays an important role in many fatal accidents.

2. *Name several of the most common causes of accidental death in the United States*: The four most common are motor vehicle traffic accidents, firearms, acute toxic exposure (poisoning)s, and falls. Alcohol use plays a part in many of these deaths.

3. *Define first-degree, second-degree, and third-degree burns*: First-degree burns are those without significant skin cell necrosis and are characterized by erythema and edema only. Second-degree burns are those with epidermal and superficial dermal necrosis and are characterized by blisters. Third-degree burns are those with full-thickness necrosis of epidermis and dermis; only deep skin appendages may be spared.

4. *Define toxin, and briefly discuss some examples*: A toxin (poison) is any substance that is injurious to health or a threat to life. Carbon monoxide and lead poisoning are examples. Carbon monoxide (CO) is the leading cause of accidental poisoning death in the United States. CO is an odorless gas product of imperfectly burned fuels. It is the normal product of combustion of gasoline and other engines (5% of auto exhaust is CO). It has a great affinity for hemoglobin, combining to form carboxyhemoglobin, a bright red chemical form of hemoglobin to which oxygen cannot attach, and resulting in acute anoxia despite adequate cardiopulmonary function. Lead is found in older urban homes and factories in the United State in flaking lead-based paint and contaminated soil. In some poor nations lead is present in earthen cookware and can contaminate food and drink. Lead has a toxic effect on the brain (impaired intellect, seizures), bone marrow (anemia), and kidney (renal failure).

5. *Briefly discuss several types of drugs and their associated adverse reactions*: Adverse reaction to therapeutic drugs is common. Acute reactions, such as allergy or accidental overdose, are uncommon. The most frequent problems occur in patients on long-term therapy, such as extended steroid treatment of rheumatoid arthritis, or estrogen replacement therapy. Prolonged steroid therapy induces Cushing syndrome, which is characterized by obesity, excess facial hair in females, diabetes, high blood pressure, fragile bones, and susceptibility to infections. Supplemental estrogen therapy for postmenopausal osteoporosis or hot flushes carries a slightly increased risk for breast cancer, thrombophlebitis, heart attack, and stroke. Oral contraceptives are safe, but they are not entirely risk free. Women taking oral contraceptives probably have below normal risk for heart disease and stroke, and they also have decreased risk for ovarian and uterine (endometrial) cancer. However, women who smoke and take oral contraceptives have a very high (3–10 times normal) risk of heart attack (myocardial infarction). All women who use oral contraceptives have a slight increased risk for venous thrombosis and pulmonary thromboembolism.

6. *Name several diseases other than lung cancer that are related to cigarette smoking*: Emphysema, generalized atherosclerosis, myocardial infarct, peptic ulcers, and cancers of the larynx, oral cavity, bladder, and esophagus.

7. *Name several conditions associated with alcohol abuse*: Fatty liver is a common finding in both acute and chronic alcohol abuse. Chronic alcohol abuse is associated with cirrhosis, gastric ulcers, accidents, thiamine deficiency, cardiomyopathy, pancreatitis, hypertension, spontaneous abortion, and fetal alcohol syndrome. It is also associated with cancers of the mouth, throat, larynx, esophagus, pancreas, and bladder.

8. *List some of the complications of drug abuse, and explain why intravenous drug abuse is especially risky*: Drug abuse is associated with suicide, homicide, motor-vehicle injury, HIV infection, pneumonia, violence, mental illness, hepatitis, and sudden death from cardiac disease or coma. Intravenous drug use can cause coma and death if the user miscalculates the dose. IV drug use is also associated with 1) pulmonary disease caused by injected foreign materials that lodge in the lungs; 2) kidney disease caused by immune complexes that lodge in the glomeruli; and 3) bacterial endocarditis from injected bacteria that attach to cardiac valves.

9. *Name and differentiate the two stages of protein-energy malnutrition*: Marasmus is the first stage, characterized by skeletal thinness owing to loss of muscle mass. Kwashiorkor is the second, more severe stage, characterized by loss of visceral protein that results in poor liver and immune function and is characterized by generalized edema because of low plasma albumin and because of infections resulting from low levels of immune protein.

10. *Define obesity, and discuss Body Mass Index*: Body weight is related to body height. All other things being equal, body weight varies with the square of height; in mathematical terms, the ratio of weight to the square of height is constant (w/h^2 = constant). Normal and abnormal body weight and various stages of excess weight are defined by Body Mass Index (BMI), which is the body weight in kilograms divided by the square of the height in meters. Obesity is defined as Body Mass Index of 30 or more.

11. *Give a brief description of the metabolic syndrome and the associated risks*: Patients typically have a lifestyle characterized by high carbohydrate diet and lack of exercise and have several of the following abnormalities: abdominal obesity, abnormal glucose metabolism, abnormal plasma lipid levels, and hypertension. The metabolic syndrome is associated with very high risk for diabetes and cardiovascular disease.

Typical Test Questions

1. Which one of the following causes the most deaths annually in the United States?
    A. Pollution
    B. Heart disease
    C. Cancer
    D. Trauma

2. Which one of the following is a third-degree burn?
    A. Deep necrosis of skin
    B. No necrosis of skin
    C. Erythema only
    D. Lung damage from inhaled gases

3. Which one of the following is a risk associated with oral contraceptive use?
    A. Ovarian or uterine (endometrial) cancer
    B. Breast cancer
    C. Venous thrombosis
    D. None of the above

4. Which one of the following is the cause of the most acute toxic deaths per annum?
    A. Drug overdose
    B. Childhood accidental ingestions
    C. Work-related toxin exposures
    D. Carbon monoxide poisoning

5. Which one of the following suffers most in acute radiation sickness?
    A. The brain and spinal cord
    B. Bronchial epithelium and skin
    C. Bone marrow and intestinal epithelium
    D. Liver and kidneys

6. True or false? Cigarette smokers have an increased risk for gastric ulcers and high blood pressure.

7. True or false? Heavy drinkers can tolerate higher blood alcohol levels than non-drinkers can.

8. True or false? Regarding malnutrition: most diets that are low in calories are also low in protein.

9. True or false? Abdominal girth is a health risk factor independent of weight.

10. True or false? Most patients with the metabolic syndrome are obese or have abnormal glucose metabolism.

Diseases of Organ Systems

The chapters in Part 2 focus on the pathologic anatomy and pathophysiology of diseases that originate in, or exert their primary effects on, particular organ systems.

Chapter 11 Diseases of Blood Cells and Blood Coagulation

Reviews the composition of normal blood and normal blood cell formation. Discusses anemia, leukemia, lymphoma, and coagulation dysfunction, as well as other disorders.

Chapter 12 Diseases of Blood Vessels

Reviews normal vascular anatomy and blood flow and discusses atherosclerosis, hypertension, and other vascular diseases.

Chapter 13 Diseases of the Heart

Reviews normal cardiac anatomy and cardiopulmonary blood flow, and discusses coronary artery disease, valvular disease, congestive heart failure, congenital heart disease, and other disorders.

Chapter 14 Diseases of the Respiratory System

Reviews normal pulmonary anatomy, ventilation, and gas exchange, and discusses asthma, cigarette smoking, chronic bronchitis, and emphysema. Also covers pulmonary edema and thromboembolism, pneumonia, tuberculosis, lung cancer, and other disorders.

Chapter 15 Diseases of the Gastrointestinal Tract

Reviews normal gastrointestinal anatomy and digestion. Discusses intestinal bleeding and obstruction; gastritis and peptic ulcers; diarrhea, parasitic disease, and malabsorption syndromes; ulcerative colitis and Crohn disease; benign and malignant gastrointestinal tumors; and other disorders.

Chapter 16 Diseases of the Liver and Biliary Tract

Reviews the normal anatomy and physiology of the liver and biliary tract. Discusses cirrhosis, hepatitis, and alcoholic and metabolic liver disease; gallstones and other gallbladder disease; cancers of the liver and biliary tract; and other disorders.

Chapter 17 Diseases of the Pancreas

Reviews the normal anatomy and physiology of the digestive and endocrine functions of the pancreas. Discusses diabetes, pancreatitis, pancreatic cancer, and other disorders.

Chapter 18 Diseases of Endocrine Glands

Reviews the normal anatomy and physiology of the pituitary, thyroid, parathyroid, and adrenal glands, their interrelationships, and their role in homeostasis, as well as the importance of negative feedback loops. Discusses overactivity and underactivity of the endocrine glands, as well as tumors and other disorders of each.

Chapter 19 Diseases of the Kidney

Reviews the normal gross anatomy of the urinary tract, the microscopic anatomy of the glomerulus and renal tubules, the formation and flow of urine, the regulation salt and water balance, and normal urinalysis. Discusses glomerulonephritis and other inflammatory disease, the role of the kidney in hypertension, cancers of the kidney, and other disorders.

Chapter 20 Diseases of the Lower Urinary Tract and Male Genitalia

Reviews the normal anatomy and physiology of the lower urinary tract and male genitalia. Discusses cystitis, urethritis, epididymitis, and other inflammations; erectile dysfunction and infertility; syphilis and other sexually transmitted diseases; prostate enlargement; cancers of the penis, prostate, and bladder; and other disorders.

Chapter 21 Diseases of the Female Genital Tract and Breast

Reviews the normal anatomy and physiology of the female genitalia and breast, including ovulation, fertilization, menstruation, pregnancy, lactation, and menopause. Discusses sexually transmitted disease, ectopic pregnancy, abortion, infertility, endometriosis, placental disease, dysplasia and cancer of the cervix, cancers and other tumors of the ovary, and other disorders.

Chapter 22 Diseases of Bones, Joints, and Skeletal Muscle

Reviews the normal anatomy and physiology of bone and bone types, muscle and muscle types, and ligaments and tendons. Discusses bone infection and infarction, osteoporosis and fractures, arthritis and joint injury, tumors and tumor-like conditions of bone and muscle, and other disorders.

Chapter 23 Diseases of the Nervous System

Reviews the normal anatomy and physiology of the brain, spinal cord, peripheral nerves, and autonomic nervous system, their interconnections, and their connections to other cells. Discusses increased intracranial pressure, stroke, brain trauma, and brain hemorrhage; encephalitis and meningitis; degenerative diseases and brain toxins; benign and malignant tumors of nerve cells; and other disorders.

Chapter 24 Diseases of the Skin

Reviews the peculiar language of skin disease, the normal physiology and microscopic anatomy of skin, and the role of skin in body defense against the environment. Discusses selected skin conditions, including the effects of systemic disease, sunlight, and pregnancy. Also covers hair loss, eczema, acne, allergies, autoimmune disease, infections and other inflammations, premalignant and malignant lesions including malignant melanoma, and other diseases.

Chapter 25 Diseases of the Eye and Ear

Reviews the normal anatomy of the eye and the optics and physiology of vision. Discusses refractive disorders, infections, cataract, glaucoma, chorioretinitis, and other inflammations; neoplasms of the eye; and other disorders. Also reviews the normal anatomy of the ear and the physiology of hearing and balance. Discusses acute otitis media, deafness, vertigo, and other disorders.

Diseases of Blood Cells and Blood Coagulation

This chapter begins with a review of the composition of normal blood and normal blood cell formation. Later sections discuss anemia, leukemia, lymphoma, coagulation dysfunction, and other disorders.

Section 1: Diseases of Blood Cells

BACK TO BASICS
- Normal Blood Production (Hematopoiesis)
- Cell Compartments and Life Span
- Laboratory Assessment of Blood Cells

TOO LITTLE HEMOGLOBIN (ANEMIA)
- The Anemia of Hemorrhage
- Anemia of Red Cell Destruction (Hemolytic Anemia)
- Anemia of Insufficient Red Cell Production

TOO MANY RED CELLS—POLYCYTHEMIA

TOO FEW WHITE CELLS—LEUKOPENIA AND AGRANULOCYTOSIS

TOO MANY WHITE CELLS—BENIGN AND MALIGNANT DISORDERS OF LEUKOCYTES
- Peripheral Leukocyte Responses to Infection or Injury
- Lymph Node Response to Injury or Infection
- Lymphoid Neoplasms
- Myeloid Neoplasms

DISORDERS OF THE SPLEEN AND THYMUS

Section 2: Bleeding Disorders

BACK TO BASICS

BLEEDING DISORDERS
- Vascular or Platelet Deficiency
- Coagulation Factor Deficiency
- Disseminated Intravascular Coagulation (DIC)

THROMBOTIC DISORDERS

Learning Objectives

After studying this chapter you should be able to:

1. Give a reasonable estimate of the life span of blood cells and platelets
2. Explain what is meant by red cell indices, and understand how to calculate them
3. Define anemia, and list the major types of anemia
4. Regarding sickle cell anemia, explain the cause and discuss what happens to red cells
5. Explain blood and bone marrow ferritin, iron, transferrin, and iron binding capacity in iron deficiency anemia
6. Explain the difference between relative and absolute erythrocytosis
7. Explain the significance of a left shift in the white cell differential count in peripheral blood
8. Name the two major groups of bone marrow malignancies, and list some of the diseases associated with each
9. Distinguish between leukemia and lymphoma
10. Explain why patients with plasma cell proliferation have abnormal blood proteins
11. Name the two major types of lymphoma
12. Name the two types of non-Hodgkin lymphoma according to microscopic patterns, and explain why this distinction is important
13. Define hypersplenism
14. Name the elements of normal hemostasis
15. Characterize bleeding due to platelet disease
16. Briefly characterize classic hemophilia (hemophilia A)
17. Explain why patients with disseminated intravascular coagulation have bleeding problems

Key Terms and Concepts

BACK TO BASICS
- myeloid
- lymphoid
- hemoglobin
- hematocrit
- red cell indices
- mean cell volume
- macrocytic
- normocytic
- microcytic
- normochromic
- hypochromic
- reticulocyte

TOO LITTLE HEMOGLOBIN (ANEMIA)
- anemia
- hemolysis
- hemoglobinopathy
- megaloblastic anemia

TOO MANY RED CELLS—POLYCYTHEMIA
- polycythemia vera

TOO FEW WHITE CELLS—LEUKOPENIA AND AGRANULOCYTOSIS
- leukopenia

TOO MANY WHITE CELLS—BENIGN AND MALIGNANT DISORDERS OF LEUKOCYTES
- leukemia
- lymphoma
- multiple myeloma
- Hodgkin lymphoma
- non-Hodgkin lymphomas (NHL)
- follicular lymphoma
- diffuse lymphoma
- chronic myeloproliferative disorders

NORMAL HEMOSTASIS, COAGULATION, AND LABORATORY TESTING
- hemostasis
- coagulation
- extrinsic coagulation pathway
- intrinsic coagulation pathway

BLEEDING DISORDERS
- hemorrhagic diathesis
- disseminated intravascular coagulation (DIC)

Blood is thicker than water.

THE SENTIMENT OF THIS PROVERB—THAT FAMILY TIES ARE THE CLOSEST OF ALL RELATIONSHIPS—

IS AS OLD AS WRITING. IN ABOUT 1800 BC, THE SUMERIANS, INVENTORS OF WRITING WHO LIVED IN

WHAT IS MODERN-DAY IRAQ, WROTE IT THIS WAY: "FRIENDSHIP LASTS A DAY; KINSHIP IS FOREVER."

Section 1: Diseases of Blood Cells

BACK TO BASICS

Blood is liquid tissue; a mixture of cells and water. The water contains protein, glucose, cholesterol, calcium, hormones, metabolic waste, and hundreds of other substances. **Plasma** is the liquid part of blood; the term refers to blood circulating *in vivo* and to *anticoagulated* blood *in vitro* (in a laboratory tube, for example). **Serum**, the fluid remaining after blood clots, differs from plasma in that serum contains no fibrinogen, which was consumed in formation of the clot. When blood clots it forms a gelatinous mass that traps cells in a mesh of fibrin (Chapter 5). The clot shrinks and after an hour is about half its original size. Serum is the remaining fluid, which was squeezed from the clot. Serum contains no fibrinogen and cannot clot again, and for this reason is widely used for laboratory analyses because clots can interfere with the operation of delicate laboratory equipment. However, sometimes tests are done on *anticoagulated* whole blood or plasma. When referring to concentrations of substances, the words "blood," "serum," and "plasma" are often used interchangeably; as for example, when referring to blood or serum or plasma glucose. The composition of normal blood is detailed in Table 11-1 and Figure 11-1.

Value	Units	Men	Women
Table 11-1		*Normal (Reference) Ranges for Blood Cells**	
		RED CELLS	
Hemoglobin (HGB)	mg/dL	13.5–17.1	12.1–15.1
Hematocrit (HCT)	%	39–49	33–43
Red cell count (RBC)	10^6 cells/cu mm	4.3–5.9	3.5–5.0
Red cell MCV	fL	76–100	Same
Red cell MCHC	g/dL	33–37	"
Red cell MCH	pg	27–33	"
Reticulocyte count	%	0.5–2.0	"
		WHITE CELLS	
Total WBC	10^3 cells/cu mm	4.5–10.5	Same
Neutrophils	%	60–70	"
Bands	%	<5	"
Eosinophils	%	2–4	"
Basophils	%	0–1	"
Lymphocytes	%	20–25	"
Monocytes	%	3–8	"
		PLATELETS	
Platelet count	10^3 cells/cu mm	150–350	Same

*Ranges vary slightly from laboratory to laboratory. Most normal ranges are established by statistical technique to include 95% of healthy persons; therefore 5% of healthy persons have abnormally high or low values.

NORMAL BLOOD PRODUCTION (HEMATOPOIESIS)

The cells in blood are red cells (**erythrocytes**), white cells (**leukocytes**), and **platelets** (cytoplasmic fragments of bone marrow platelet-producing cells, **megakaryocytes**). In the fetus, production of blood cells takes place in the liver, but by birth most blood cell production has shifted to the bone marrow.

As is depicted in Figure 11-2, all blood cells arise from a common ancestor, the totipotent stem cell. This primitive stem cell gives rise to two other stem cells: a

myeloid stem cell that in turn gives rise to red cells, megakaryocytes, monocytes and macrophages, and granulocytes (neutrophils, basophils, eosinophils), and a **lymphoid** stem cell that give rise to lymphocytes.

Bone marrow *red cell* production is stimulated by **erythropoietin**, a hormone synthesized by the kidney. Erythropoietin production is stimulated by low delivery of oxygen to the kidney. Mild general hypoxia occurs in people living at high altitude. Their bone marrow makes extra red cells to compensate, and they have higher red blood cell counts than do people living at lower altitudes. General hypoxia also occurs in patients with chronic lung disease; they, too, have high red cell counts. Local kidney hypoxia can also stimulate erythropoietin production; for example, impaired renal blood flow (ischemia) owing to renal vascular disease can cause increased erythropoietin and very high red cell counts.

Production of *white blood cells* and *platelets* is controlled by other hormones and factors.

Red cells have no nucleus and no need for one. Their role is to carry oxygen, and a nucleus would take up unnecessary room. *Leukocytes* have a nucleus. There are three kinds of leukocytes: granulocytes, lymphocytes, and monocytes. *Monocytes* are phagocytic: they ingest and digest foreign antigen and present it for action to immune cells for immune response. *Lymphocytes* are the main cells of the immune system: their task is to react to foreign antigen. *Granulocytes* have cytoplasmic granules of digestive enzymes and other substances that play an important role in inflammation (Chapter 3). The three granulocytes are: neutrophils, eosinophils, and basophils. *Neutrophils* are the most abundant granulocyte. Their task is to react to acute injury and infection by ingesting (phagocytosis) and digesting foreign agents, especially bacteria, and by cleaning up inflammatory debris. *Basophils* and *eosinophils* are the inflammatory cells of allergic reactions (Chapter 8) and reactions to parasites. *Platelets* are small fragments of megakaryocyte cytoplasm and have no nucleus. Their task is to stop bleeding by sticking together at points of vascular injury to obstruct hemorrhage, and to initiate the clotting process at the site of bleeding.

CELL COMPARTMENTS AND LIFE SPAN

Blood cells exist in several body compartments (blood, bone marrow, spleen, lymph nodes, and, to a great extent in the fetus and a lesser extent in adults, the thymus), and there is constant cell trafficking among them.

How long cells live (and circulate) is critical. Compared to cells in most other tissues, the life span of

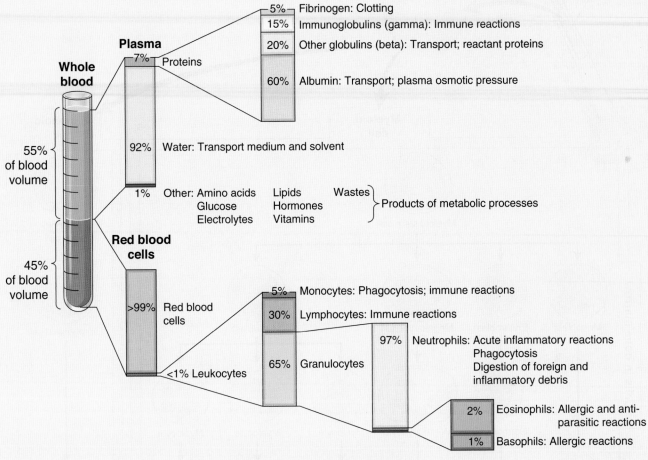

Figure 11-1 **The composition of blood.**

blood cells is short; therefore, cell turnover is rapid. Red cells have the longest life span of blood cells: about 120 days. Neutrophils, basophils, and eosinophils live about 4 days; lymphocytes and monocytes, a week or two; platelets, a day or two. Old (senescent) blood cells and platelets are removed from circulation by the spleen. This rapid turnover means that it is critical that new cells be produced at a rate that equals the rate at which cells are dying. Many diseases of blood cells are caused by production failure or early cell death or destruction; that is to say, by shortened cell life span. Anemia (too little hemoglobin) is usually attributable to too few red blood cells (anemia can also occur with normal numbers of red cells that do not contain enough hemoglobin). Some patients have low red blood cell count because bone marrow fails to produce enough red blood cells (RBCs); in other cases of anemia, RBC life span is short because RBCs are destroyed (*hemolysis*). The same holds true for platelets and white blood cells—some conditions are attributable to failed cell or platelet production, others to early destruction or death.

Hemoglobin is the compound in RBCs to which oxygen attaches for transport from lungs to tissues, there-

fore the amount of hemoglobin in blood is critical. Hemoglobin cannot be synthesized without iron, vitamin B_{12}, vitamin B_6, and folic acid. The character of hemoglobin is important. There are many types of abnormal hemoglobin, most of them stemming from genetic defects of hemoglobin synthesis.

LABORATORY ASSESSMENT OF BLOOD CELLS

Laboratory assessment of blood cells is usually performed on a sample of blood collected from an arm vein. Such a blood sample is typically referred to as "peripheral blood" to distinguish it from the pool of blood in large vessels and the viscera, which is slightly more dilute than peripheral blood. Cellular elements typically are measured in anticoagulated whole blood. Conversely, chemical elements, such as glucose, are typically measured in the liquid part of blood, usually serum obtained from a tube containing clotted blood.

The most common standard laboratory study of blood is referred to as a **complete blood count (CBC)**. In modern laboratories the process is automated and consists of a determination of white blood cells (**white**

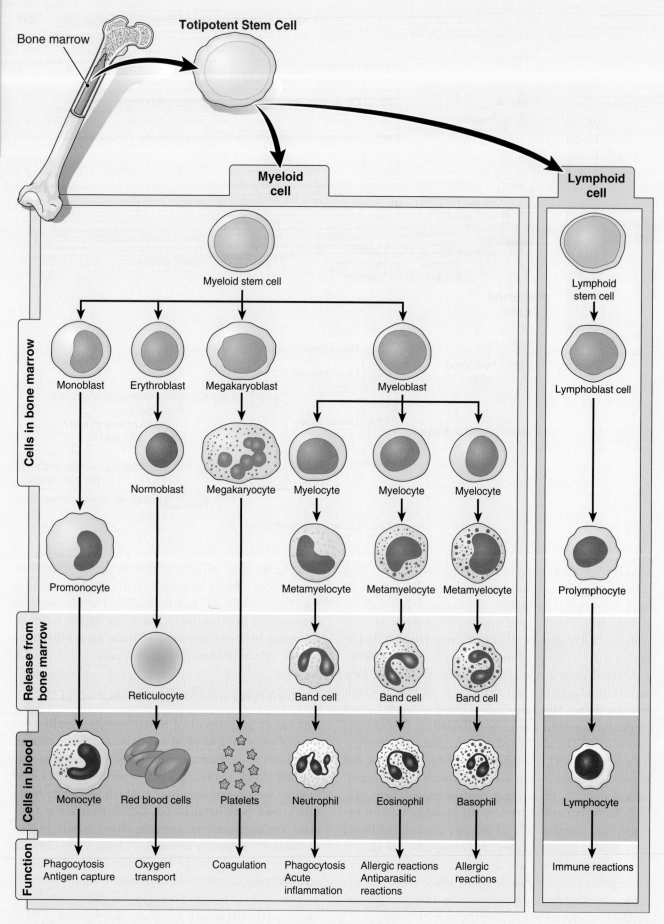

Figure 11-2 Hematopoiesis. There are two main groups of blood cells: myeloid and lymphoid, each derived from a primitive stem cell.

blood cell [WBC] count), red blood cells (**red blood cell count**), the percentage of white cells that are neutrophils, eosinophils, or basophils (the **white cell differential count**), the amount of **hemoglobin**, and the hematocrit. The **hematocrit** is the percent of blood volume occupied by red blood cells (RBCs). It is measured by centrifuging whole blood to compact red blood cells and observing the percentage of whole blood volume occupied by red blood cells. The number of white cells and platelets is so small that their volume is negligible.

Also important in a complete blood count is determination of the **red cell indices**, which are measures of the size and hemoglobin content of the *average* RBC. The average *size* of an RBC is the **mean cell volume (MCV)**; the average *amount* of hemoglobin in an average RBC is the **mean cell hemoglobin (MCH)**; and the average *concentration* of hemoglobin per unit of volume in an average RBC is the **mean cell hemoglobin concentration (MCHC)**. As is indicated in Figure 11-3, each of the indices can be calculated using hemoglobin, hematocrit, and red blood cell count. Red cell indices are important in the diagnosis of diseases of red blood cells—in anemia red blood cells may be too large (**macrocytic**), normal size (**normocytic**) or too small (**microcytic**). Additionally, diseased RBCs may have a normal amount of hemoglobin per cell (**normochromic**) or too little hemoglobin (**hypochromic**). There is no such thing as a red cell with too much hemoglobin.

Visual examination of blood cells is an important tool, but it is ordinarily not necessary unless there are significant abnormalities in the measurements obtained on a complete blood count. Every laboratory has criteria defining when visual examination is necessary. For example, visual examination may be required if the hemoglobin is below 10 gm/dL, or the WBC count is above 15,000 cells/cu mm. Additionally, the clinician may know of signs and symptoms that indicate need for visual examination of blood cells and can request visual examination. Among the important things detectable by visual examination are the presence of malignant white cells in leukemia, abnormally shaped RBCs, malaria parasites in RBC, RBCs with nuclei, and giant platelets.

Laboratories also seek to identify normal red cell blood antigens for blood group typing, as discussed in Chapter 8, or antibodies attached to the red cell membrane that might account for red cell destruction (hemolysis). Additionally, tests are performed to determine the percentage of new (young) red cells (**reticulocytes**), which are elevated when red cell production increases as the bone marrow compensates for anemia, red cell destruction, or short red cell life span. Additionally, laboratories can determine the type of hemoglobin in red cells. Normal hemoglobin is *hemoglobin A*. Hundreds of types of abnormal hemoglobin have been described. Among the most common abnormal hemoglobin is *hemoglobin S*, the hemoglobin of sickle cell disease.

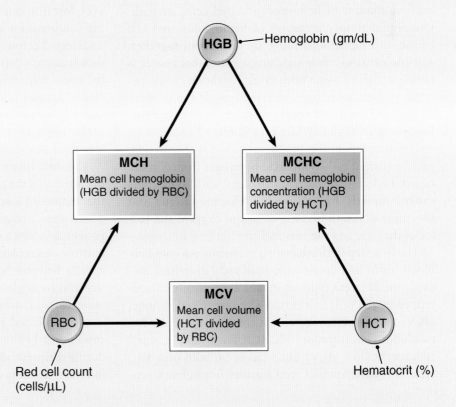

Figure 11-3 **Red blood cell indices.** Measurement of red cell size (MCV) as well as hemoglobin content (MCH) and concentration (MCHC) are calculated from blood hemoglobin (HGB), red cell count (RBC), and hematocrit (HCT).

Too Little Hemoglobin (Anemia)

Anemia is abnormally low hemoglobin in blood and is caused by decreased numbers of red blood cells, decreased amount of hemoglobin in red cells, or both. Usually laboratory measures of hemoglobin, red cell count, and hematocrit move up and down together. Anemia demands thorough investigation because it is always a sign of some underlying condition. Some patients present with signs or symptoms of the primary disease and are found upon investigation to be anemic. For example, a slowly bleeding intestinal cancer may not be detected until it produces intestinal obstruction; and the patient is then found to be anemic from chronic blood loss. Other patients present with symptoms caused directly by the anemia: chronic fatigue and shortness of breath because of lack of oxygen; and pallor of the skin and the oral and conjunctival mucosae.

The first step in the diagnosis of anemia is a complete blood count and determination of red cell indices, because the different types of anemia are typically characterized by red cells of a certain size (mean cell volume, MCV) and hemoglobin content (mean corpuscular hemoglobin concentration, MCHC). For example, small (microcytic, low MCV) RBCs can occur with iron deficiency. A deficiency of iron impairs hemoglobin syn-thesis, so iron-deficient RBCs contain less hemoglobin than normal and are pale (hypochromic, low MCHC). Few diseases other than iron deficiency produce small, pale RBCs. Knowing the red cell indices dramatically narrows the number of diseases to be considered in the differential diagnosis.

The second step in the diagnostic routine for anemia is to determine if the anemia is associated with blood loss, red cell destruction, or failed bone marrow production of red cells. In this regard it helps to think of the intravascular space (blood) as a tank into which red blood cells are pumped from the bone marrow. They enter the intravascular space and survive an average of 120 days before they die a natural death (apoptosis) and are filtered out by the spleen. Figure 11-4 illustrates the production, circulation, and destruction of RBCs. Anemia occurs 1) if *production fails* (either not enough cells are added to the circulation to replace the daily natural loss, or red cells do not contain enough hemoglobin); 2) if blood *leaks* (hemorrhages) from the circulation tank; or 3) if cell *life span is shortened* (hemolysis), and cells die quicker than they can be replaced by the bone marrow.

THE ANEMIA OF HEMORRHAGE

Hemorrhagic blood loss creates two problems: 1) loss of oxygen-carrying capacity when red cells are lost; and 2) loss of iron (80% of body iron is in hemoglobin). If bleeding is limited, lost red cells can be replaced in a few weeks or months by normal bone marrow; however, lost iron is not easily or quickly replaced. If bleeding continues for a long time (as from, for example, an undetected colon cancer), the patient may become iron deficient. Iron deficiency, in turn, hinders the ability of the bone marrow to make hemoglobin, and iron deficiency anemia is the result. By far the most common cause of iron deficiency anemia is chronic blood loss; other causes, such as dietary iron deficiency or defective intestinal absorption of iron, are uncommon.

The main threat of acute blood loss is shock or death, not anemia. If the patient survives an acute hemorrhage, the volume of lost red cells is initially replaced by ingested water and albumin synthesis by the liver, and the patient develops a temporary *dilutional anemia* until the marrow can replace the lost red blood cells. Dilutional anemia features healthy red cells, which have normal size and hemoglobin content; that is, the red cells are *normochromic, normocytic* (normal MCV and MCHC).

Chronic blood loss usually occurs with one of two conditions: 1) abnormal menstrual bleeding in women during their reproductive years; or 2) intestinal bleeding in either sex, especially from undetected colon cancer

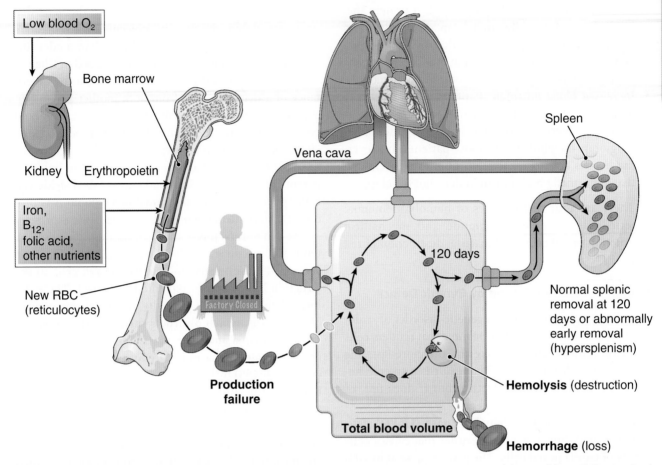

Figure 11-4 Production, circulation, and death of red blood cells. Every anemia is caused by at least one of three problems: 1) decreased red cell production, 2) loss of red cells by hemorrhage, or 3) early death (destruction) of red blood cells.

(see Case Study 11.1 at the end of this chapter). If bleeding is very slow, lost red cells are replaced by new cells from the bone marrow, and the patient does not develop a dilutional anemia. If, however, the rate of red cell loss is greater than the marrow can produce, the lack of red cells in the vascular space is made up by fluid and the patient *initially* develops a dilutional anemia until the bleeding stops. However, in chronic bleeding the intestinal absorption of dietary iron usually cannot make up for iron lost by hemorrhage, and the patient eventually becomes *iron deficient*. In iron deficiency the bone marrow has the capacity to produce red *cells*, but it cannot produce enough *hemoglobin* for each new cell, and the patient develops *iron deficiency anemia*, in which red blood cells are small (low MCV) and pale (low MCHC). Therefore, *iron deficiency anemia in a man or in a postmenopausal woman is to be considered bleeding from gastrointestinal cancer until proven otherwise.* This does not mean that cancer is the most common cause of iron deficiency anemia. It is not. Other gastrointestinal diseases are often the cause, but cancer cure depends so heavily

on early detection that a search for intestinal malignancy is always the first priority.

ANEMIA OF RED CELL DESTRUCTION (HEMOLYTIC ANEMIA)

Premature destruction of red blood cells is called **hemolysis**, which shortens red cell life span. Hemolytic anemia is associated with:

- *An active, hypercellular, bone marrow,* which must work overtime to replace dying cells.
- *Blood that contains a high count of new red blood cells (reticulocytes).* These new red cells are easy for laboratory technicians to identify on conventional microscopic examination because they have a bluish cast; they can be revealed even more clearly by special stains.
- *Increased blood lactic dehydrogenase (LDH).* Red blood cells are packed with LDH, an enzyme that is released from dying red cells and rises to high levels in hemolysis.

- *Low blood haptoglobin.* Haptoglobin is a protein that binds hemoglobin liberated from dead RBCs and carries it away for disposal, which destroys haptoglobin and decreases its concentration in blood. Low plasma haptoglobin is a key diagnostic indicator of hemolysis.
- *Increased blood bilirubin.* Patients with especially high rates of red cell destruction may have abnormally high levels of blood bilirubin, a product of hemoglobin metabolism. In most patients, however, the liver is able to excrete bilirubin rapidly enough that abnormally high bilirubin does not develop.

There are four main causes of hemolytic anemia: genetic red cell defects, immune and mechanical destruction of red cells, and malarial destruction of red cells.

Hemolytic Diseases Caused by Genetic Defect

Hereditary spherocytosis is a genetic disorder of structural protein in the red cell *membrane* that renders cells spherical rather than biconcave and therefore less able to pass through the spleen. The result is a splenic hemolysis. Splenectomy is effective, but it does not, of course, remedy the genetic defect.

Glucose-6-phosphate dehydrogenase (G6PD) deficiency is an X-linked genetic disorder that causes deficiency of G6PD in red cells. The gene is present in 10% of African American men, rendering them subject to acute hemolytic episodes upon exposure to certain oxidizing drugs, toxins, or infections.

The **hemoglobinopathies** are genetic disorders of hemoglobin synthesis. More than 300 genetically flawed hemoglobins have been identified. They are *molecularly defective* and are unstable, causing early red cell death (hemolysis). Normal, molecularly correct hemoglobin is **hemoglobin A**; abnormal hemoglobins have other names. Most notable among these is **hemoglobin S**, the cause of **sickle cell anemia**. Additionally, there are hemoglobins C, E, and many others, most very rare. The **thalassemias** are an important group of hemoglobinopathies that differ from the molecularly imperfect hemoglobins—the hemoglobin of thalassemia is molecularly correct but is not produced in sufficient volume because the production mechanism is genetically faulty.

Sickle Cell Anemia (Hemoglobin S Disease)

About 8% of African Americans and 30% of African blacks are carriers of the **hemoglobin S** genetic mutation. The higher rate in Africa is Darwinian: hemoglobin S gene conveys resistance to *P. falciparum* malaria, the most severe form of malaria, and provides an advantage in the battle to survive.

The sickle cell defect is a mutation in the gene that codes for globin, the protein molecule of hemoglobin, and is inherited according to the Mendelian model (the genetic defect and its inheritance is discussed in Chapter 7). The gene defect is a recessive trait, requiring inheritance of a defective gene from both mother and father. When the patient inherits the defective gene from both parents (genotype: SS), hemoglobin S is produced, and **sickle cell disease** (phenotype: *sickle cell anemia*) is the result. If the patient has a defective gene from only one parent (genotype: SA), the condition is called **sickle cell trait** (phenotype: normal; normal hemoglobin A is produced). The patient is a *carrier,* and no disease is present.

Even in normal physiologic conditions hemoglobin S tends to crystallize (sickle), deforming red cells into a crescent (sickle) shape and subjecting red cells to destruction by the spleen (splenic hemolysis). These deformed cells also have difficulty passing through small blood vessels, which obstructs small blood vessels and causes ischemia and infarcts (Chapter 5). Sickling can be precipitated in carriers (SA) or patients with sickle cell disease (SS) by low oxygen tension (local or general hypoxia), infections, dehydration, and acidosis. For example, the low oxygen tension at high altitudes can induce sickling. A simple laboratory test for the presence of sickle hemoglobin (SA or SS) consists of adding a chemical to bind all oxygen in a drop of blood and then inspecting the specimen for sickled cells. The microscopic appearance of sickled red cells in smears of untreated patient blood is also diagnostic (Fig. 11-5).

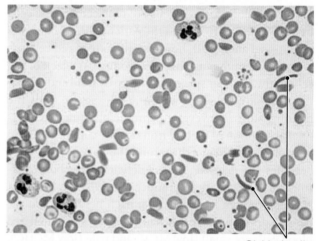

Sickled cells

Figure 11-5 Blood in sickle cell disease. Sickled red cells appear in peripheral blood specimens only in patients with sickle cell *disease* because all of their hemoglobin is hemoglobin S. Sickled cells do not normally appear in the blood of patients with sickle cell *trait* because their red cells contain roughly equal amounts of hemoglobin S and normal hemoglobin. However, red cells with any amount of hemoglobin S can be induced to sickle as part of a laboratory test for the presence of hemoglobin S.

Sickle cell disease usually becomes evident shortly after birth, presenting as a severe anemia with chronic hemolysis. The clinical and pathologic findings in sickle cell disease are depicted in Figure 11-6. These findings result from:

- *Obstruction of small blood vessels*, which causes is-chemia and infarction of various organs, or gangrene of fingers and toes
- *Anemia*, which causes high-output heart failure and cardiomegaly, bone marrow hyperplasia, and bone deformities induced by the overactive bone marrow
- *Hemolysis*, which produces pigment gallstones (Chapter 16) caused by bilirubin overload on the liver and biliary system
- *Infections*, caused by infarct-associated loss of splenic immune function; or by pathogens that find their way into necrotic bone, lung, and other tissues

About half of patients with sickle cell disease (SS) reach mid-life, but others succumb to a variety of infections—such as *Salmonella* bone infections or pneumococcal sepsis—or to bone marrow failure (aplastic crisis), which is triggered by parvovirus infection of red cell precursors in the bone marrow.

On the other hand, patients who are carriers (sickle cell trait, SA) remain asymptomatic unless the patient's blood oxygen content falls, as happens in ascent to high altitude, severe lung disease, or other conditions.

Thalassemia

The **thalassemias** are a group of recessive genetic disorders inherited in Mendelian fashion (Chapter 7) in which hemoglobin is molecularly perfect, but the defect causes a decreased *amount* of hemoglobin production. There are several varieties of thalassemia, which vary from mild to severe depending on the particular genetic defect.

Detailed discussion of the classification of the many types of thalassemia is beyond the scope of this textbook. The most severe form of thalassemia (*thalassemia major*) appears in childhood; many patients die before age 20. Less severe forms of thalassemia (*thalassemia minor*) cause anemia but are not associated with decreased life expectancy.

The most common type of thalassemia presents as a severe *microcytic hypochromic* anemia with small, pale red cells similar to the red cells seen in iron deficiency anemia. In addition to anemia from inadequate *production* of hemoglobin, the anemia is compounded by a *hemolytic* component, some of which takes place in the bone marrow before the red cells mature (intramedullary hemolysis). This ineffective red cell production stimulates increased iron absorption from the gastrointestinal tract. This often leads to iron overload (*hemochromatosis*, Chapter 16) because the body cannot easily excrete iron. Excess amounts of iron are present in blood and bone marrow, which offers an easy way to distinguish thalassemia from iron deficiency: both thalassemia and iron deficiency are characterized by small, pale (low MCV and MCHC) red cells; however, patients with iron deficiency have no iron stores and patients with thalassemia are flooded with iron. As with sickle cell anemia (SS), patients with thalassemia can have skeletal abnormalities because chronically hyperactive bone marrow has a deforming effect. Additionally, the liver and spleen may enlarge markedly as some of their cells transform into bone marrow cells (*myeloid metaplasia*) in an effort to make up for bone marrow deficiency. The liver is naturally inclined to undergo myeloid metaplasia: recall that in the fetus the liver, not the bone marrow, produces most blood cells. The cause of splenic myeloid metaplasia is not clear.

Patients with mild disease are mildly anemic for life and need no treatment. Patients with severe disease need regular transfusions; and bone marrow transplant may be effective.

Non-genetic Hemolytic Anemia

Immune hemolytic anemia is caused by antibodies directed against antigens on the red cell membrane. Red cells become coated by antibody, which renders them susceptible to premature removal by the spleen. These antibodies may be detected on red cells or in plasma by a laboratory test (Coombs test, Chapter 8). Immune hemolytic disease often occurs in association with autoimmune disease (especially systemic lupus erythematosus), malignancies of white blood cells (lymphoma and leukemia), infectious mononucleosis, and *Mycoplasma pneumoniae* pneumonia (Chapter 14), and as a reaction to certain drugs.

Mechanical hemolytic anemia is caused by physical shredding of red cells as they pass through mechanical devices, such as artificial heart valves. A similar mechanical effect may occur as red cells squeeze through swollen, inflamed small blood vessels affected by autoimmune disease (*autoimmune vasculitis*, Chapter 12), or as red cells pass through blood vessels partially blocked by intravascular blood clotting (*disseminated intravascular coagulation*).

Hemolytic disease is also associated with **malaria**, a parasitic disease that infects red cells. Malaria is one of the most widespread diseases in the world and is very common in the tropical areas of Africa and Asia. The word "malaria" is derived from Italian, *mala aria*, for "bad air." Before science understood that malaria is

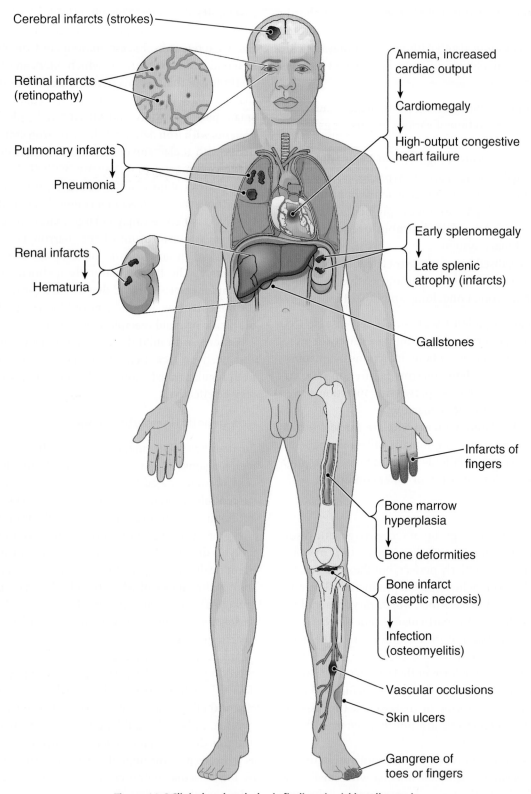

Figure 11-6 Clinical and pathologic findings in sickle cell anemia.

caused by a that parasite transmitted by mosquito bites, it was believed the disease was a product of the "bad air" in swampy, tropical zones.

As is illustrated in Figure 11-7, malaria is caused by four varieties of tiny amoebae smaller than a red blood cell, the *Plasmodium* species, which are transmitted by mosquitoes from infected to non-infected persons. No immunity develops and reinfection may occur.

Clinically, malaria parasites infect and destroy red cells, causing episodes of hemolysis, fever, and jaundice that occur every 48–72 hours as new generations of parasite are reproduced. *Plasmodium falciparum* malaria is especially dangerous because it has a high fatality rate caused by its effect on the brain. Antimalaria drug prophylaxis is effective for all types, but some drug-resistant strains now exist.

ANEMIA OF INSUFFICIENT RED CELL PRODUCTION

Inadequate bone marrow red cell production is another cause of anemia. Inadequate supply of some essential substance necessary for red cell production, such as iron, folic acid, or vitamin B_{12}, can cause anemia. Marrow cell output may fail, associated with adverse effect of drugs, toxin, or radiation or some other, unknown, cause. Destruction or replacement of the marrow by scar tissue or tumor can also result in a decrease in the production of red cells, with consequent anemia.

Iron Deficiency Anemia

The body is stingy with iron—natural losses from shedding skin and cells of the GI tract are on the order of

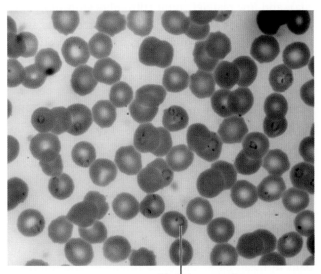

Malaria parasite

Figure 11-7 **The blood in malaria.** Red cells contain *Plasmodium* organisms.

0.1% of total body iron per day. The average diet contains more than enough iron for men, but barely enough for menstruating women, who normally have low iron reserves. Iron balance is maintained largely by intestinal absorption of dietary iron. About 80% of total body iron is in the hemoglobin of red cells; the remaining 20% is stored as ferritin and hemosiderin. **Ferritin** is an iron-protein complex found in the bone marrow, liver, spleen, and skeletal muscle. Plasma ferritin levels vary directly with the amount of ferritin stored in bone marrow; therefore, the level of plasma ferritin is a good indicator of the amount of body iron stores.

Iron is transported from one place to another bound to a special blood protein, **transferrin**, made by the liver. Total transferrin is measured by testing the ability of plasma protein to bind to iron and is expressed as **total iron binding capacity (TIBC)**. The degree to which this *potential* transporting capacity is occupied by *actual* plasma iron is referred to as the percent *saturation* of TIBC and is calculated by dividing plasma iron by TIBC. When patients are iron deficient, the liver increases plasma transferrin in an effort to deliver more iron to the bone marrow. Therefore, in *iron deficiency*:

- plasma transferrin (total iron binding capacity) is high
- plasma iron is low
- the percent saturation of transferrin by iron is low

Most iron deficiency can be attributed to blood loss. Other, less common causes include intestinal absorption, owing to intestinal disease, or increased need for iron. For example, infants are at risk of iron deficiency because milk contains little iron, and the rapid growth of children demands iron for expansion of blood volume and other tissues.

> 🔑 *Iron deficiency is the most common of all nutritional deficiencies, affecting perhaps 5% of the population of developed nations and many times more in developing ones.*

When patients lose more iron than they absorb intestinally, iron stores gradually become depleted. Iron stores must be completely exhausted before red cell production is affected, and, therefore, patients become *iron deficient before they become anemic*, and they become anemic only if iron deficiency persists. This pre-anemic stage is characterized by normal levels of plasma iron and transferrin (expressed as total iron binding capacity, TIBC), but levels of plasma ferritin are low, reflecting low marrow iron stores. As negative iron balance persists, plasma iron levels fall and ferritin (TIBC) levels rise. Finally, **iron deficiency anemia** develops as red cell production becomes impaired owing to lack of iron. The bone marrow, lacking sufficient iron to make hemoglobin, produces red blood cells that are small (microcytic, low MCV) and pale (hypochromic, low MCHC), illustrated in Figure 11-8.

Iron deficiency anemia is common but rarely fatal. By far the most common cause is chronic blood loss; low dietary intake of iron is rarely the case. The most common causes of chronic blood loss are menstrual abnormalities and gastrointestinal bleeding. The diagnosis of menstrual loss is usually easy to establish; however, loss from gastrointestinal bleeding is much more sinister—it is difficult to document and is often associated with intestinal malignancy, especially carcinoma of the colon. Therefore, it is a good rule to assume that, *until proven otherwise, the source of iron deficiency anemia in adult men or postmenopausal women is occult (undetected) bleeding from a gastrointestinal carcinoma.*

Think of iron deficiency anemia as a *symptom*, not a disease; there is always some other, underlying, condition. Oral iron supplementation can rebuild iron stores, but the underlying condition must also be found and treated.

> ☞ *Iron deficiency anemia in an adult man or postmenopausal woman is to be considered to be caused by bleeding from a gastrointestinal cancer until proven otherwise.*

Vitamin B$_{12}$ and Folic Acid Deficiency

Anemia associated with deficiency of either vitamin B$_{12}$ (cobalamin) or folic acid is characterized by enlarged (macrocytic) red cells, depicted in Figure 11-9. Together

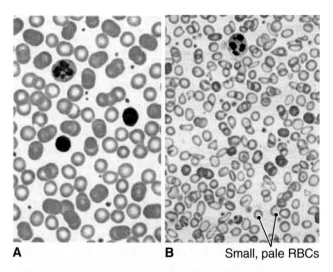

A   B   Small, pale RBCs

Figure 11-8 **The blood in iron deficiency anemia. A.** Normal blood smear. **B.** Blood smear in iron deficiency anemia. The red cells are small (microcytic) and pale (hypochromic).

Abnormally large (macrocytic) red blood cells

A   B

Figure 11-9 **The blood in vitamin B$_{12}$ (folic acid) deficiency. A.** Normal blood smear. **B.** Macrocytic anemia. Deficiency of vitamin B$_{12}$ (folic acid) causes red cells to be much larger than normal.

these are known as the **megaloblastic** or **macrocytic anemia.** "Megalo" and "macro" mean large, and in these anemias the red cells and their bone marrow precursors (blasts) are unusually large.

Vitamin B$_{12}$ and folic acid are necessary for DNA synthesis. If nuclear DNA cannot be produced, cells cannot be made, hence a deficiency of either B$_{12}$ or folic acid results in decreased production of red cells, white cells, and platelets (because megakaryocytes are affected as well). Both of these deficiencies result in *macrocytic* red cells (high MCV), low white blood cell count (leukopenia), and low platelet count (thrombocytopenia). Bone marrow studies in each reveal a hypercellular, active bone marrow filled with enlarged (megaloblastic) red and white cell precursors. The marrow is overly cellular because it is striving ineffectively to produce red and white cells.

Inadequate diet or deficient intestinal absorption may cause deficiency of either B$_{12}$ or folic acid. Megaloblastic anemia associated with **folic acid (folate)** deficiency is uncommon because folate is abundant in raw vegetables (however, it is largely destroyed by cooking). Nevertheless, depressed folic acid levels may be found in anyone with a poor diet; chronic alcoholics are especially prone to folic acid deficiency.

Dietary **vitamin B$_{12}$** deficiency is rare—B$_{12}$ is abundant in meat, eggs, and dairy products, and multiyear reserves are stored in the liver. It is almost impossible to devise a diet deficient in B$_{12}$ except by observing an unusually strict vegetarian diet over a decade. The most common cause of B_{12} deficiency is defective intestinal absorption. B_{12} absorption requires **intrinsic factor** (IF), a protein secreted by the gastric mucosa. IF binds to B_{12} and travels to the lower end of the small bowel (ileum), where absorption takes place. B_{12} cannot be absorbed by the ileum unless it is bound to IF. Causes of insufficient B_{12} absorption include gastrectomy (which limits IF production), surgical resection of the ileum (which removes the absorbing site), inflammatory bowel disease (Chapter 15), and other diseases affecting the distal ileum, all of which interfere with absorption of the B_{12}-IF complex.

An additional cause of B_{12} deficiency that deserves special mention is **pernicious anemia**, an autoimmune disease featuring autoantibodies against gastric mucosal cells and IF. Without treatment, the disease can cause a destructive disease of the spinal cord and is usually fatal, thus the name "pernicious," meaning deadly, evil, or destructive.

The primary pathologic abnormality in pernicious anemia is *chronic atrophic gastritis*, discussed in detail in Chapter 15. In pernicious anemia atrophic gastric mucosa does not secrete enough intrinsic factor to allow normal B_{12} absorption in the intestine.

Anemia of Chronic Disease

Patients with chronic disease develop anemia due to low output of RBC by the bone marrow. The reasons are not clear. The chronic diseases usually involved are malignant neoplasms, chronic infections, and chronic autoimmune disorders. Red cells are normal size (normocytic, normal MCV) and have a normal amount of hemoglobin (normochromic, normal MCHC).

The anemia of chronic disease may look somewhat like iron deficiency because plasma iron is often low and patients are anemic. Plasma iron is usually low because plasma proteins, including transferrin, are reduced secondary to the wasting usually associated with chronic diseases, not because the patient is iron deficient. The distinguishing point between the two is that patients with iron deficiency have small, pale (microcytic, hypochromic) red cells. Furthermore, patients with anemia of chronic disease have normal or high plasma ferritin because iron stores are plentiful and abundant iron is found on bone marrow exam.

Primary Bone Marrow Failure (Aplastic Anemia)

Primary bone marrow failure is called **aplastic anemia**. The name, however, is a misnomer: the disease is not just a failure to produce red blood cells, it is a primary failure of *all* marrow elements—red cells, white cells, and megakaryocytes. However, anemia is usually the

presenting problem. In fatal cases the cause of death is usually *hemorrhage*, because of low platelet count, or *infection*, secondary to low WBC count. The cause of aplastic anemia is unknown (idiopathic) in most cases. When the cause is known, drugs and chemicals are usually responsible because they exert a toxic effect on bone marrow cells. In some cases the toxic effect is dose-related, as is the case with chemotherapy drugs given to patients with a malignancy. In others, the reaction is termed *idiosyncratic*; that is, the toxic effect is far out of proportion to the dose.

In addition to the fatigue and pallor of anemia, patients with aplastic anemia have low platelet count (thrombocytopenia), resulting in hemorrhages (skin petechiae and ecchymoses, or internal bleeding), and low white blood cell counts (granulocytopenia), resulting in bacterial infections. Bone marrow biopsy reveals a hypocellular (mostly fat, few hematopoietic cells) bone marrow, as is depicted in Figure 11-10.

Anemia Caused by Bone Marrow Replacement or Destruction (Myelophthisis)

In some situations the bone marrow is replaced by malignancy or fibrosis (**myelophthisis**). Some cancers—notably prostate, lung, breast, and thyroid—metastasize to bone and occupy so much marrow space that there is no room for hematopoietic elements. Radiation, lymphoma, leukemia, and multiple myeloma may have a similar effect. Bone marrow fibrosis warrants special mention. In the absence of known cause, such as radia-

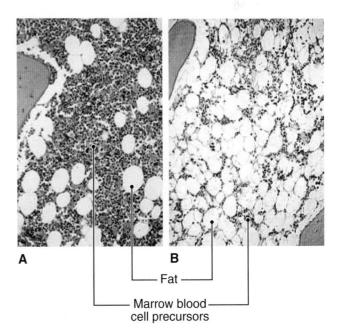

Figure 11-10 **Bone marrow in aplastic anemia. A.** Normal bone marrow. **B.** Bone marrow in aplastic anemia. Few bone marrow cells are present. Most of the tissue shown is fat.

tion damage, marrow fibrosis is usually a manifestation of one of several primary malignant disorders of the bone marrow, the *chronic myeloproliferative syndromes*, discussed later in this chapter.

Too Many Red Cells—Polycythemia

Polycythemia (**erythrocytosis**) is an excess number of red cells in blood. The most common cause of *apparent* polycythemia is low plasma volume (*relative* polycythemia). For example, in dehydration, loss of fluid causes blood to become concentrated, but the *absolute* number of red cells is unaffected. Dehydrated patients, therefore, have *relative* polycythemia; the *absolute* number of RBC is not increased. Among the most common causes of relative polycythemia is a poorly understood condition called "stress polycythemia," which is usually seen in obese, anxious (stressed), hypertensive patients. For reasons that are not well understood, these patients have low plasma volume. Although the total number of red cells in the body does not change, the decreased plasma volume produces a relatively higher than normal number of red cells per unit of blood volume, which increases hematocrit and red cell count.

Other patients have an increased red cell count because there is an *actual* increase in the total number of RBCs in the body; these patients have *absolute* polycythemia. Absolute polycythemia can be primary or secondary. *Secondary* absolute polycythemia is caused by conditions outside the bone marrow that stimulate the marrow to produce red cells. For example, hypoxia, as in a patient with chronic lung disease, stimulates the kidney to produce **erythropoietin**, a hormone whose release is stimulated by low oxygen levels and whose function is to increase marrow production of red blood cells. For the same reason, people living at high altitudes have secondary polycythemia as compared to those living at lower altitudes. Secondary polycythemia can also be caused by renal tumors (Chapter 19) that secrete erythropoietin.

Primary absolute polycythemia occurs with a bone marrow malignancy called **polycythemia vera** (literally, true polycythemia), a proliferation of primitive bone marrow red cell precursors that is related to myeloid leukemia and other myeloid neoplasms, discussed later in this chapter.

Most of the time an abnormally high red cell count is accompanied by increased hematocrit and hemoglobin and can be explained by conditions other than polycythemia vera. For example, patients who smoke more than just an occasional cigarette damage their lungs enough to reduce oxygen uptake, which stimulates red cell production and a secondary increase of red blood cells. Determining whether or not patients have an absolute or relative increase of red cells can be very difficult because red cell count in *peripheral* blood is significantly higher than the relatively dilute *central* pool of blood in viscera and large blood vessels. The accompanying Lab Tools box explains how to distinguish

LAB TOOLS

Measurement of Total Red Cell Mass

Determining red cell mass requires a special procedure because the concentration of red cells in blood is higher in peripheral blood than it is in the central pool in the viscera, heart, and lungs, where it is more dilute. For example, a male patient might have a peripheral blood hematocrit of 53% (normal: 39–49), but blood from his heart might have a hematocrit of 44%. Hematocrit levels in the peripheral blood are always higher than hematocrit levels in the central pool because *peripheral blood is a bit "sludgy" and concentrated.*

Determining the total amount of red cells in the body is relatively easy. The test is simple and is much like measuring the amount of water in a large tank by dumping into it a known volume, say one gallon, of red dye of known concentration, say 100% pure. After mixing tank water and dye, remove some water and measure the concentration a second time. If the concentration is 1% dye and 99% water, it is easy to see that the tank holds 100 gallons of water because the original one gallon of pure dye has been diluted 100 times.

To measure total red cell mass the method is similar. A known volume, say 10 ml, of patient red cells is tagged with radioactive chromium-51, and a radioactive count of the specimen is taken. Let's say it is 10,000 counts per minute. The tagged cells are injected back into the patient and circulate to become diluted in the patient's untagged red cell mass. A second 10 ml specimen is collected and counted. Let's say the count is 40 counts per minute, or 1/250th of the original. It is easy to see that the patient's red cell mass is 250 x 10 ml (2500 ml). This result is compared to tables of normal ranges for men and women of various weights to determine if it is normal or high.

between absolute and relative polycythemia by determining total body red cell mass.

Too Few White Cells—Leukopenia and Agranulocytosis

Leukopenia is low blood white cell count. It is usually caused by a decrease of granulocyte numbers, especially neutrophils, a condition called **neutropenia**. Low numbers of lymphocytes (**lymphopenia**) is uncommon and is usually associated with immune deficiency diseases (Chapter 8), AIDS most notably, or steroid therapy.

Neutropenia may result from accelerated destruction of neutrophils or from a failure of production. Among the causes of increased destruction are increased filtering of neutrophils from blood by the spleen (hypersplenism), autoimmune disease, and overwhelming sepsis. Leukopenia also can be caused by failing bone marrow white cell production, which can be caused by drugs or toxins or when bone marrow is replaced by neoplasm.

When neutropenia is severe it is called **agranulocytosis**. Most agranulocytosis is caused by drugs. In most instances the degree of white cell decline is dose related, and the drugs are those administered as cancer chemotherapy. However, many drugs are known to cause a rare, idiosyncratic (not dose-related) agranulocytosis. The major clinical problem resulting from agranulocytosis is bacterial or fungal infection, either of which may prove fatal, but white cell counts must be profoundly depressed for severe infection to occur.

Too Many White Cells—Benign and Malignant Disorders of Leukocytes

Leukocytosis is an increase of white blood cells in the peripheral blood. It may be benign (reactive) or malignant (leukemia). **Leukemia** is a malignant proliferation of white cells, either *lymphoid cells* (lymphocytes) or *myeloid cells* (granulocytes or monocytes), in which the malignant cells appear in the peripheral blood. Leukemia is related to **lymphoma**, which is a malignant neoplasm of lymphocytes in lymph nodes and organs that grows as nodular masses, However, in lymphoma *no malignant cells are detectable in blood*.

Review of normal blood cell production helps understand the relationship of lymphoma to leukemia and to leukemia-related bone marrow neoplasms. As is illustrated in Figure 11-11, all blood cells, and all blood cell malignancies, originate from primitive stem cells:

lymphoid stem cells differentiate into lymphocytes, which in turn may develop into lymphocytic leukemia, lymphoma, or plasma cell disorders; and *myeloid* stem cells differentiate into red blood cells, granulocytes, monocytes, and megakaryocytes, which in turn develop into myeloid malignancies.

Modern laboratory tools allow precise classification of malignant diseases of white cells into dozens of types according to the type of DNA defect present and the precise type of white cell involved, a topic far beyond the scope of this discussion. Our approach is simpler: we will discuss malignancies of white blood cells according to the basic cell type involved, lymphoid or myeloid, and their clinical behavior, either acute or chronic leukemia.

Leukemia of cells in the lymphoid line is called **lymphocytic leukemia**. Leukemia of cells in the myeloid line is called **myelocytic leukemia**. *Clinically* leukemias are called acute or chronic, according to the maturity of the malignant cells seen in the peripheral blood. When the malignant cells are immature (blasts) the disease is **acute leukemia**, which is aggressive and runs a short course. When the malignant cells are mature the disease is **chronic leukemia**, which is less aggressive and runs a longer course. In everyday practice leukemias are usually designated as a combination of these terms; for example, acute myelocytic or chronic lymphocytic.

Acute leukemia is characterized by:

- Abrupt onset, which often presents as acute infection or hemorrhage
- Symptoms related to a decrease in the numbers of normal marrow cells, such as might be seen in anemia, infection, or bleeding from thrombocytopenia
- Bone pain and tenderness when bone marrow becomes packed with cells
- Enlarged lymph nodes, spleen, and liver because of accumulations of malignant cells
- Nervous system symptoms such as headache, vomiting, or nerve palsies from malignant cells infiltrating the meninges

In acute leukemia, peripheral blood WBC counts often are very high; sometimes >100,000 cells/cu mm, but about half the cases have total WBC counts near normal. It is the microscopic appearance of the cells in bone marrow and peripheral blood that is diagnostic—both contain many immature WBCs (blasts).

By contrast, the onset of *chronic leukemia* is insidious—patients present with fatigue or pallor from anemia, night sweats, low-grade fever, secondary infection, or enlarged spleen or liver. The clinical course is less rocky and the prognosis is better than for acute

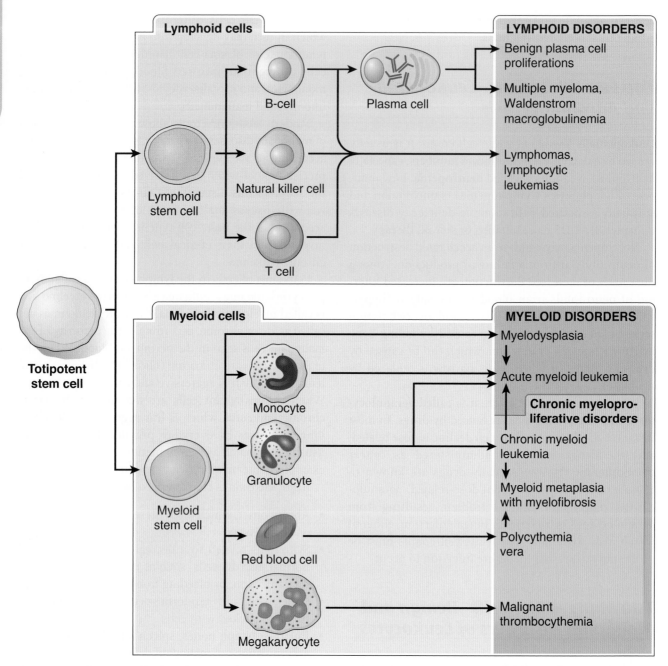

Figure 11-11 **The origin of bone marrow malignancies.** Arrows indicate the ways in which an initial malignancy may evolve into a related, but different, malignancy.

leukemia, although ultimately the cause of death is similar in both acute and chronic leukemia: hemorrhage as a result of low platelet count, or infection because leukemic white blood cells are not effective at fighting infection.

An important shortcoming of this simple classification is that it does not account for the very important fact that leukemias, whether of lymphoid or myeloid origin, can be understood in greater detail and treated more effectively by identifying other characteristics, such as whether malignant lymphocytes are B cells or T cells. However, we will avoid a more precise description of leukemias because these classifications are complex and beyond the scope of this discussion.

PERIPHERAL LEUKOCYTE RESPONSES TO INFECTION OR INJURY

Most leukocytosis is secondary (reactive), resulting from *bacterial* infection or inflammation associated with tissue necrosis. Most leukocytosis occurs owing to increased numbers of granulocytes (**granulocytosis**), most of which are neutrophils (**neutrophilia**). The normal WBC count is usually <10,000 cells per microliter (10,000/cu mm). In most instances of infection the WBC count does not rise above 20,000/cu mm. However, sometimes very high reactive white counts occur that may appear alarming, especially in uncommon cases when it rises to over 50,000/cu mm. Such a high reactive WBC count is termed **leukemoid reaction** (literally, "like leukemia").

Viral infection usually causes **lymphocytosis**, an increase in the number of lymphocytes in blood. *Eosinophilic* leukocytosis is uncommon and when present is almost always associated with *allergic* reactions or *parasitic* infection.

Parasitic infections, such as intestinal worms, cause **eosinophilia**, an increase in the number of blood eosinophils. Allergic reactions (Chapter 8), such as hay fever or allergic asthma, also produce eosinophilia.

Sometimes bacterial infection or other injury causes such demand for neutrophils from the bone marrow that an excess number of immature granulocytes is released into blood. The least mature WBC normally found in the peripheral blood is the **band neutrophil** (normally <5% of WBC count), which has a banana-shaped nucleus. Release of immature cells is commonly referred to clinically as a "left shift" because the point of release is further to the left if neutrophils are visualized as maturing from immature on the left to mature on the right. *Immature* lymphocyte cells do not normally appear in the peripheral blood unless leukemia is present.

Infectious mononucleosis is an acute, self-limited (self-curing) infectious disease associated with lymphocytosis, occurring most often in adolescents and young adults. It is caused by the **Epstein-Barr virus (EBV)**, which infects B lymphocytes and in typical cases causes fever, sore throat, enlarged neck and jaw lymph nodes, and increased lymphocytes in the peripheral blood, many of which are large "atypical" lymphocytes, depicted in Figure 11-12. Hepatitis and skin rash sometimes occur. The typical acute syndrome usually resolves in 4–6 weeks. The virus is shed into saliva and passed almost solely by kissing. The risk of transmission for any single kissing exposure is about 10%.

Diagnosis depends on observation of typical clinical signs and symptoms and on laboratory confirmation by finding characteristic atypical lymphocytes in blood or by detecting anti-EBV antibodies. The blood of patients with infectious mononucleosis typically contains characteristic **heterophil antibodies**, so named for their ability to agglutinate red cells from non-human species. A simple office test for heterophil antibodies, usually

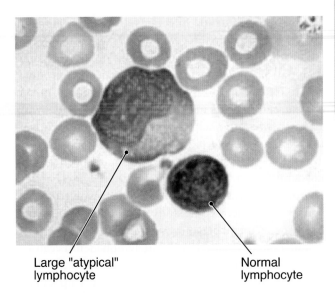

Large "atypical" lymphocyte   Normal lymphocyte

Figure 11-12 The blood in infectious mononucleosis. The large "atypical" lymphocyte is characteristic.

called the "monospot" test, is positive in over 90% of patients with infectious mononucleosis.

EBV infection may be severe or fatal in immunocompromised patients, such as those with AIDS. EBV infection is also the cause of some lymphomas.

LYMPH NODE RESPONSE TO INJURY OR INFECTION

Lymph nodes are involved in the most common diseases: infection, malignancy, immune reactions, and autoimmune disease. The lymphatic system filters bacteria, cancer cells and other alien substances from tissues. Lymph node lymphocytes are involved in immune reactions, and most lymphomas arise in lymph nodes. Therefore, most lymph nodes involved in a disease process are enlarged (**lymphadenopathy**).

In the absence of apparent infection or injury enlarged lymph nodes are worrisome and deserve investigation, primarily because they may contain malignant cells, either metastatic from a nearby cancer or a lymphoma that may involve the node. Enlarged, *tender* nodes are not so worrisome because the cause is almost always infectious even if the specific cause cannot be demonstrated. However, enlarged *nontender* nodes raise the possibility of malignancy.

Lymphadenitis is infection of a lymph node, usually resulting from the spread of organisms into nodes draining an infected site. If the node is reacting to the infection but is not actually infected, the condition often called **reactive hyperplasia** or **reactive lymphadenitis**. *Acute lymphadenitis* is characterized by enlarged, *tender* nodes. It is usually seen in cervical (neck) nodes in association with dental infections or sore throat, or in the axillae or inguinal regions in association with genital infections or infections of the arms or legs. Systemic bacterial or viral infections in children may produce generalized acute nonspecific lymphadenitis. *Chronic lymphadenitis* occurs in two varieties: 1) associated with a specific disease such as tuberculosis and 2) *chronic non-specific lymphadenitis* for which no etiology can be discovered. Patients with chronic, non-specific lymphadenitis usually have large, *non-tender* lymph nodes, a clinical finding similar to lymph nodes involved by malignancy. On microscopic study pathologic findings vary but evidence of malignancy is absent.

Catscratch disease is an acute lymphadenitis caused by a rickettsia-like microorganism, *Bartonella henselae*. It is an acute syndrome of axillary or neck lymphadenitis in children and adolescents that arises about two weeks after a cat scratch (or, rarely, thorn or splinter injury). Lymph node biopsy demonstrates a characteristic granulomatous inflammatory reaction.

LYMPHOID NEOPLASMS

Figure 11-11 illustrates the important point that there are two major categories of white blood cells: lymphoid cells and myeloid cells. Lymphoid neoplasms are lymphocytic leukemia, lymphoma, and plasma cell proliferations.

Lymphocytic Leukemia

Acute lymphocytic leukemia (ALL) is an uncommon malignant proliferation of immature lymphocytes, usually B cells, that most often occurs in children and young adults. Onset is typically abrupt and accompanied by widespread malignant cell infiltration of bones, lymph nodes, liver and spleen, which cause bone pain, lymphadenopathy, and hepatosplenomegaly. Infiltration of the meninges often occurs, producing headaches, nerve paralysis, and pain. Blood and bone marrow (Fig. 11-13) are overrun by malignant cells; red cell, granulocyte, and platelet counts fall; and anemia, infection, and hemorrhage follow. Chemotherapy induces remission in most patients, and about half of patients are ultimately cured.

Chronic lymphocytic leukemia is a malignant proliferation of B cells that accounts for about a third of all leukemias and is indistinguishable from **small cell lymphocytic lymphoma**, discussed below, except that small cell lymphocytic lymphoma has few malignant cells in the peripheral blood. The malignant cells in both conditions have a gene defect that stops lymphocyte apoptosis (normal cell death), so that "immortal" lymphocytes overpopulate the blood, lymph nodes, and

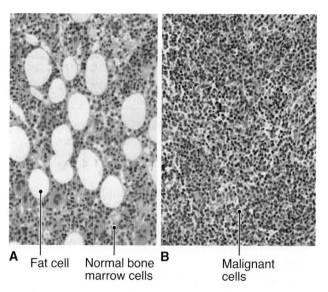

Figure 11-13 **The bone marrow in leukemia. A.** Normal bone marrow. **B.** The marrow in leukemia. The marrow is packed with cells of a single type. No fat remains.

bone marrow. As malignant B cells proliferate, normal B cells are in short supply. Because B cells produce immunoglobulins (antibodies) to fight infection, little immunoglobulin is made, and patients are predisposed to developing infections.

Chronic lymphocytic leukemia, the most sluggish of all leukemias, occurs primarily in mature adults, as a slowly developing disease that may initially cause only fatigue, weight loss, and poor appetite. Malignant cells multiply in blood, lymph nodes, and spleen, causing lymphocytosis, lymphadenopathy (Fig. 11-14), and splenomegaly. In all cases, however, there is moderate blood lymphocytosis, which sometimes is discovered incidentally in patients under care for other reasons. Chemotherapy is the main form of therapy. Some early, indolent cases require no therapy. Average survival is nearly ten years, and some cases extend for much longer.

Plasma Cell Proliferations

Plasma cells are B lymphocytes that are actively making antibodies (immunoglobulins, Chapter 8). In some circumstances, a *clone* of plasma cells (a group of identical cells derived from a single ancestor cell) proliferates abnormally. These proliferations are referred to as **plasma cell dyscrasia**. *Dyscrasia* is an old but useful term that essentially means *disease*. Most plasma cell dyscrasias are malignant, but some are benign. The proliferating clone of plasma cells makes too much of its particular antibody (immunoglobulin), and the result is a very large amount of homogeneous (uniform) immune pro-

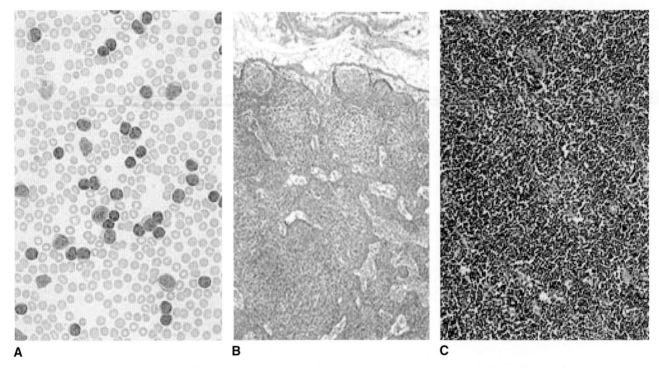

A   B   C

Figure 11-14 **Chronic lymphocytic leukemia. A.** All of the white cells are lymphocytes. No granulocytes are present. **B.** Normal lymph node. **C.** Lymph node in chronic lymphocytic leukemia. Malignant lymphocytes have displaced normal lymph node structure.

tein circulating in blood. This protein appears as a dense band in the gamma globulin region when plasma protein components are separated by **protein electrophoresis**, illustrated in Figure 11-15. The abnormal protein is called a **monoclonal spike, M-spike, M-protein,** or **monoclonal gammopathy**. About 1% of people over 50 have an M-protein in their plasma. Most are not associated with an identifiable abnormal proliferation of plasma cells and are considered benign, but some later prove to have a plasma cell malignancy or develop plasma cell malignancy over the years. Because of this uncertainty, these patients are said to have a *monoclonal gammopathy of uncertain significance*.

Normal immunoglobulins and abnormal M-proteins are made of two components, *heavy chain* proteins and *light chain* proteins (Chapter 8). Sometimes the plasma cell proliferation makes only heavy chains or light chains, in which case the diseases are called *heavy chain disease* and *light chain disease*. Light chains are also liberated by the metabolic breakdown of M-proteins. Whatever the cause, light chains are small enough to pass through the glomerulus and into urine, where they are known as **Bence-Jones protein**.

Multiple Myeloma

Multiple myeloma is a malignant proliferation of plasma cells. The malignant plasma cells do not circulate in

blood but appear as nodular masses in bone marrow (Fig. 11-16). These nodules destroy bone and produce solitary, "punched out" bone defects, especially in the spine and skull (Fig. 11-17), which are so distinctive radiographically that the appearance is diagnostic.

As the clone of malignant plasma cells grows, it replaces normal plasma cells, causing a decline in the production of normal immunoglobulin and normal antibodies. The result is low levels of gamma globulin (*hypogammaglobulinemia*) and subsequent susceptibility to infections.

Multiple myeloma occurs most frequently in elderly adults. Bone pain, hypercalcemia (as a result of bone destruction), and anemia (because of bone marrow replacement) are common complaints. Low gamma globulin levels cause recurrent infections, and about half of patients develop renal failure because of the toxic effect of *Bence Jones protein* on the renal tubules.

The diagnosis of multiple myeloma can be made by finding characteristic "punched out" bone lesions on radiographs or by finding monoclonal proteins in plasma or urine. Chemotherapy is usually not effective. Average survival is short, about three years.

Waldenström Macroglobulinemia

Waldenström macroglobulinemia can be conceived of as a cross between multiple myeloma and small cell

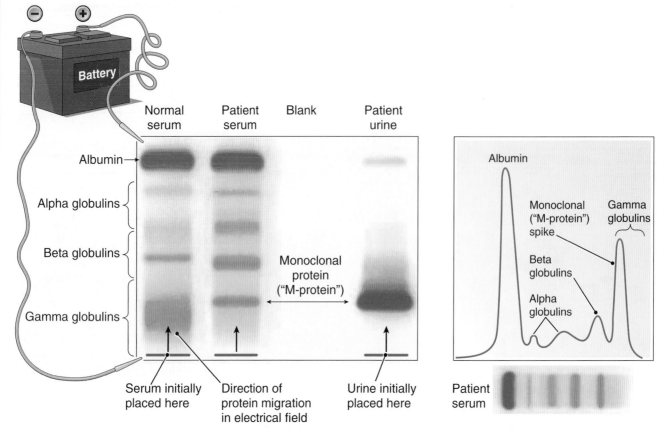

Figure 11-15 **Protein electrophoresis in plasma cell disease.** Serum or urine is placed at one end of a strip of gel, across which an electrical current is applied. Most proteins have a negative charge and migrate toward the positive pole at various speeds according to their molecular weight and charge. The serum on the left shows a narrow band in the gamma globulin region. Serum protein has spilled into urine, which demonstrates a matching band. In the scan of patient serum on the right, the height of the tracing is proportional to the amount of protein stained in each band. Monoclonal protein appears as a tall, narrow (monoclonal) "M-protein."

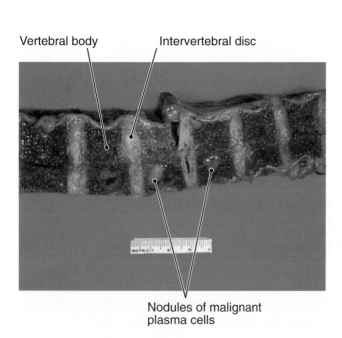

Figure 11-16 **Multiple myeloma.** In this autopsy study of vertebrae, nodules of malignant plasma cells are visible.

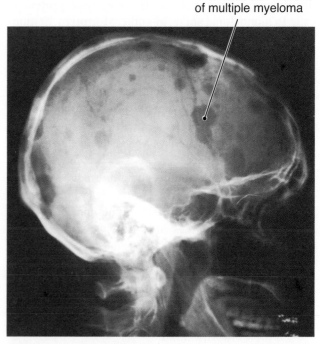

Figure 11-17 **Multiple myeloma.** In this radiograph of the skull in multiple myeloma, the "punched out" radiolucent lesions are the result of destruction by nodules of plasma cells. (Reprinted with permission from Rubin E. Pathology. 4th ed. Philadelphia. Lippincott Williams and Wilkins, 2005.)

lymphocytic lymphoma. The malignant cells look like lymphocytes, but they produce a particular type of M-protein—IgM, the largest and heaviest of the immunoglobulin molecules, hence the name *macro*globulinemia.

Waldenström macroglobulinemia mainly affects adults over 60. In most patients the symptoms are similar to multiple myeloma: anemia, weight loss, fatigue, weakness, lymphadenopathy, and splenomegaly. Waldenström macroglobulinemia differs from multiple myeloma in that the IgM is thick and syrupy (highly viscous) and causes sluggish blood flow. Impaired blood flow to the brain causes dizziness, headache, confusion, and stroke, and poor flow to the eyes causes visual symptoms. Patients may also suffer from hemorrhages because increased levels of IgM interfere with the clotting process. Average survival is a few years, similar to multiple myeloma.

Lymphoma

Lymphomas are malignant neoplasms of lymphocytes or lymphoblasts that grow as nodular masses, usually in lymph nodes (Fig. 11-18) but sometimes in organs. In contrast to leukemic cells, lymphoma cells are not detectable in peripheral blood.

There are two broad types of lymphoma: *Hodgkin lymphoma*, and all the rest, which are designated *non-Hodgkin lymphomas (NHL)*.

Hodgkin Lymphoma

The malignant cell of **Hodgkin lymphoma** is a lymphoid cell known as the **Reed-Sternberg (RS) cell**, but the exact nature of the cell remains a mystery. However, there is substantial evidence that it becomes malignant because of infection by the *Epstein-Barr virus (EBV)*.

Hodgkin lymphoma is the most common malignant neoplasm of Americans between ages 10–30 years. Among Americans it is a bit more common in men than women and occurs almost twice as frequently in Caucasians as in African-Americans.

Immunity is important in Hodgkin lymphoma. Immunocompromised patients have a tendency to develop Hodgkin lymphoma; and patients with Hodgkin lymphoma often have poor T-cell (cellular, delayed) immunity and develop infections as a result.

Hodgkin lymphoma differs from NHL in three important respects:

- Hodgkin lymphoma arises in a single lymph node or chain of nodes and spreads in an orderly, predictable manner to adjacent nodes, rather than spreading widely, like non-Hodgkin lymphoma does
- Hodgkin lymphoma rarely involves structures other than lymph nodes
- All types of Hodgkin lymphoma are associated with defective cell-mediated (T-cell) immunity that is manifest by infections.

Based on microscopic characteristics, several types of Hodgkin disease are recognized. The most important of these is **nodular sclerosis Hodgkin lymphoma**, which accounts for about 70% of cases. Nodular sclerosis Hodgkin lymphoma differs from other types of Hodgkin lymphoma on several counts:

- It is the only variety of Hodgkin lymphoma that is more common in women than men
- It has a conspicuous tendency to involve neck, upper chest, and mediastinal lymph nodes (Fig. 11-19)
- It is the least aggressive

The first manifestation of Hodgkin lymphoma usually is painless, non-tender enlargement of lymph nodes, often in the neck. As tumor mass grows, however, patients may lose weight and develop night sweats, fever, and fatigue. If T-cell function becomes impaired, infections may occur. For reasons unknown, in about 10% of patients with Hodgkin lymphoma the consumption of alcohol causes pain in affected areas.

Radiotherapy and chemotherapy secure permanent remission in most patients with Hodgkin lymphoma, but survival rates vary inversely with the extent of disease at the time of original diagnosis and to a lesser extent with the histologic subtype. Five-year survival for early stage patients is about 90%, and about three fourths can be considered cured. Survival with modern

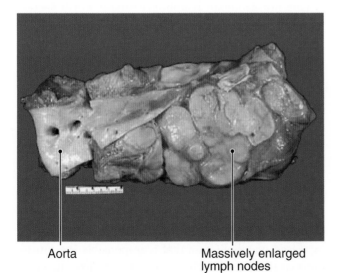

Aorta   Massively enlarged lymph nodes

Figure 11-18 **Malignant lymphoma in lymph nodes.** Shown here is a gross autopsy study of paraaortic, retroperitoneal lymph nodes.

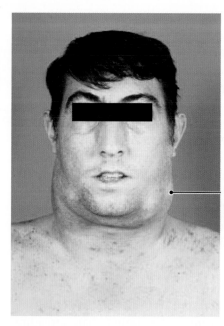

Marked
cervical
lymphadenopathy

Figure 11-19 **Hodgkin disease.** This clinical study shows a patient with nodular sclerosis type and marked enlargement of the cervical lymph nodes.

chemotherapy and radiation is in the 60–70% range for those with one of the more aggressive subtypes or with clinically advanced disease.

Therapeutic success, however, presents other problems—long-term survivors are at increased risk for other malignancies, especially myeloid bone marrow neoplasms and lung cancer, which can be attributed to failure of immune surveillance (Chapter 8) by the immune system. Risk for breast cancer is also high in young women treated with chest irradiation for mediastinal nodular sclerosis Hodgkin lymphoma.

Non-Hodgkin Lymphomas

Most **non-Hodgkin lymphomas** are malignant tumors of B lymphocytes. These lymphomas are similar to Hodgkin lymphoma in that both are tumors of lymphocytes, both usually present as a painless enlargement of lymph nodes, and both are associated with immune deficiency and infections.

However, non-Hodgkin lymphomas differ from Hodgkin lymphomas in important ways. On average they are more aggressive and are in a more advanced clinical stage at time of diagnosis, and their microscopic appearance and behavior vary greatly from one type to the next and from one case to the next. One third of non-Hodgkin lymphomas arise not in lymph nodes but in other organs, such as brain, bone, or bowel, whereas Hodgkin lymphoma rarely arises in tissues other than lymph node. Non-Hodgkin lymphomas tend to spread widely from the original site into other lymph nodes, spleen, liver, and bone marrow, and at time of diagnosis most patients are presumed to have widespread disease; therefore, clinical staging is not as important as in Hodgkin disease

The pathologic classification of non-Hodgkin lymphomas is complex—the World Health Organization classification lists dozens of types. A simpler but useful method classifies non-Hodgkin lymphomas into two main groups: those with a follicular microscopic appearance are called **follicular lymphoma**, and the rest are called **diffuse lymphoma**. Follicular lymphoma, depicted in Figure 11-20B, is so-named because its growth pattern is similar to the lymphoid follicles of normal lymph nodes (Fig. 11-20A). Of all non-Hodgkin lymphomas, about half have a follicular microscopic appearance and half diffuse.

Follicular lymphomas are less aggressive and have a better prognosis than do diffuse lymphomas. Follicular lymphomas arise, mainly in adults, as painless, enlarged lymph nodes. Median survival is nearly ten years. Despite this sluggish behavior they do not respond well to chemotherapy.

About half of non-Hodgkin lymphomas are **diffuse lymphoma**, which grow in a uniform microscopic pattern without follicles. They occur mainly in people over 60 years old, but there are two notable age exceptions: childhood lymphomas and the lymphomas associated with AIDS. Most appear quickly, grow rapidly, and are lethal unless treated. After chemotherapy about 30% of patients experience a permanent remission and can be considered cured. Most of the others undergo temporary complete remissions, but the disease recurs in a few years.

One non-Hodgkin lymphoma variant worth special mention is *small cell lymphocytic lymphoma*, an especially low-grade diffuse lymphoma discussed above in connection with *chronic lymphocytic leukemia*. These are essentially the same disease except that in chronic lymphocytic leukemia the peripheral blood lymphocyte count is high, and in small cell lymphocytic lymphoma it is not.

Prognosis and therapy are guided by the microscopic type (follicular pattern or not, nuclear size), immunotype (B cell or T cell), and clinical stage (extranodal or organ involvement).

The clinical features of non-Hodgkin lymphoma include 1) enlarged, non-tender lymph nodes; 2) an increased metabolic rate that is responsible for constitutional symptoms such as fever, weight loss, malaise, and sweating; and 3) autoimmune phenomena or immunodeficiency problems such as infection.

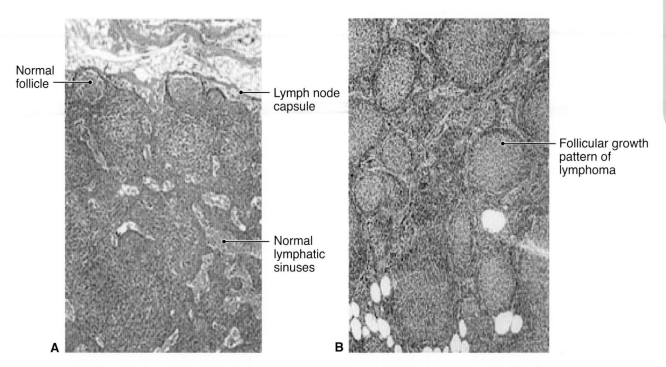

Figure 11-20 **Nodular lymphoma, microscopic study. A.** Normal lymph node demonstrating follicular pattern. **B.** Malignant lymphoma with nodular pattern.

MYELOID NEOPLASMS

Figure 11-2 illustrates that there are two groups of white blood cells: lymphoid cells and myeloid cells. Lymphoid stem cells give rise to B and T lymphocytes. Myeloid stem cells give rise to granulocytes, monocytes, red blood cells, and megakaryocytes. Under this heading we will discuss neoplasms of each of these types of myeloid cells.

Acute Myeloid Leukemia

Figure 11-11 illustrates that malignancies arising from myeloid stem cells can differentiate into malignant granulocytes, red cells, monocytes, or megakaryocytes. If the malignant proliferation is of immature *granulocyte* precursor cells, the disease is called **acute myelocytic leukemia.**

Acute myelocytic leukemia is a malignant proliferation of *immature* granulocyte precursor cells (myeloblasts) that do not mature enough to develop neutrophilic, eosinophilic, or basophilic granules. All leukemic cells in acute myelocytic leukemia have gene mutations that prevent cells from maturing, and as a result immature myeloid cells overrun blood (Fig. 11-21) and bone marrow.

Acute myelocytic leukemia is a disease primarily of middle-aged and older adults. As malignant cells crowd out normal bone marrow, granulocytes, red cells, and

megakaryocytes fail to develop. Onset is typically sudden, and symptoms of marrow failure appear rapidly as the bone marrow becomes packed with malignant cells. Red cell, granulocyte, and platelet counts fall, and anemia, infection, and hemorrhage occur. Symptoms in include bone pain, lymphadenopathy, enlarged spleen and liver, and neurologic defects from leukemic infiltrates in brain and peripheral nerves.

Chemotherapy causes remission in about two thirds of younger patients, but only half of those survive five years. In older patients only about 10% survive five years.

Chronic Myeloproliferative Disorders

As is illustrated in Figure 11-11, the **chronic myeloproliferative disorders** are related neoplastic diseases, all of which arise from myeloid stem cells and can be considered one condition with various expressions. Each has a tendency to evolve toward acute myelocytic leukemia.

Four disorders are recognized, according to the manner in which the stem cells differentiate, but there is considerable overlap among them.

• *Polycythemia vera,* malignant red cells predominate
• *Chronic myelogenous leukemia,* malignant granulocytes predominate

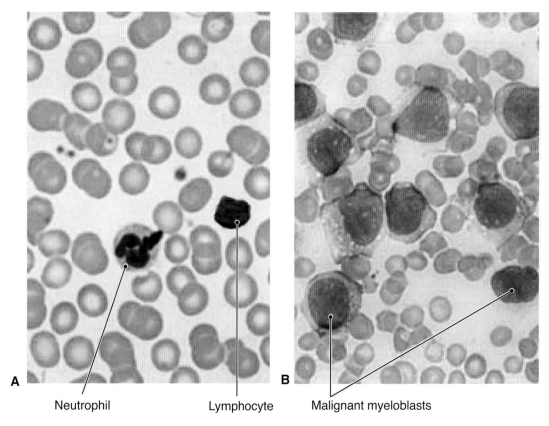

A — Neutrophil   Lymphocyte   B — Malignant myeloblasts

Figure 11-21 **Acute myelocytic (myeloid) leukemia. A.** Normal blood showing normal neutrophil and lymphocyte. **B.** Acute myelocytic (myeloid) leukemia showing immature myeloid cells (malignant myeloblasts).

- *Malignant* (essential) *thrombocythemia,* malignant megakaryocytes predominate
- *Myeloid metaplasia with myelofibrosis,* malignant cells differentiate toward fibrous tissue

Two features occur to some degree in each of these disorders: myelofibrosis and extramedullary hematopoiesis.

Myelofibrosis is replacement of normal bone marrow by fibrous tissue that grows as a result of fibrogenic factors released by neoplastic megakaryocytes. Marrow fibrosis tends to appear as a final, fatal phase in many of the chronic myeloproliferative syndromes. As is illustrated in Figure 11-22, bone marrow biopsy reveals fibrosis and varying numbers of megakaryocytes but few WBCs or RBCs. Severe anemia, thrombocytopenia, and leukopenia result in hypoxia, bleeding, and infection.

Extramedullary hematopoiesis is the production of blood cells (hematopoiesis) in organs other than the bone marrow. Most occurs in the spleen and liver. Red cells made outside the bone marrow tend to be deformed and are released into the circulation before los-

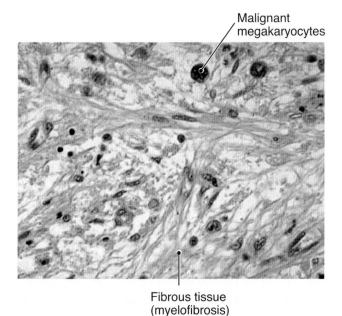

Malignant megakaryocytes

Fibrous tissue (myelofibrosis)

Figure 11-22 **Myeloid metaplasia with myelofibrosis.** This high-power microscopic view reveals that the marrow is completely replaced by malignant fibrous tissue. No normal marrow elements remain.

ing their nucleus. Clinical features of extramedullary hematopoiesis include deformed, nucleated red cells in peripheral blood and hepatosplenomegaly. The spleen is sometimes gigantic.

Chronic Myelocytic Leukemia

In chronic myeloproliferative disorders the malignant myeloid stem cells can differentiate in various ways; if they differentiate toward mature granulocytes with visible neutrophilic, eosinophilic, or basophilic granules, the condition is called **chronic myelocytic leukemia (CML)**.

CML usually affects middle-aged adults and accounts for about 15% of adult leukemias. Median survival is about three years. The onset and progress of CML is slow but worsens progressively. Clinical features include fever, malaise, weight loss, weakness, and anorexia. The spleen can grow so large that patients may see or feel it and seek care. In contrast to acute myelocytic leukemia, most of the malignant cells are mature neutrophils, but some eosinophils and basophils are usually present. White blood cell counts tend to be very high, sometimes >100,000 cells/cu mm. Red blood cell precursors and megakaryocytes proliferate to a lesser degree—*nucleated* RBC may be found in the peripheral blood, and platelet counts may be high (*thrombocytosis*).

Prior to modern chemotherapy, average survival was about three years, and chronic myelocytic leukemia was rapidly fatal, often ending in a "blast crisis" of acute myeloid leukemia as immature myeloblasts proliferated. However, modern chemotherapy has improved survival figures dramatically: over 90% of patients survive three years, and half of those can be considered cured.

Polycythemia Vera

Polycythemia vera is a chronic myeloproliferative disorder in which malignant proliferation of primitive bone marrow *red cell* precursors predominates. It is usually accompanied by a limited overgrowth of granulocytes and megakaryocytes. In polycythemia vera red cell elements predominate, and there is an absolute increase of total red cell mass, a condition uniformly accompanied by high red cell counts and elevated levels of hemoglobin and hematocrit.

Polycythemia vera usually appears slowly in middle-aged adults as vague constitutional symptoms. Other manifestations include intestinal bleeding, gout (Chapter 22) caused by joint deposits of uric acid crystals metabolized from the DNA of bone marrow RBC

precursors, hypertension because of expanded intravascular volume, intense pruritus (itching) of unknown cause, and a flushed complexion. Hematocrit is usually above 60%, and red cell count and hemoglobin levels are increased correspondingly. The white cell count may be as high as 50,000/cu mm; the platelet count is also high, with counts often near 500,000/cu mm. Giant platelets and nucleated red cells are seen on microscopic study of blood cells. Some patients have tendency toward deep vein thrombophlebitis; others have problems with hemorrhages. The natural history of polycythemia vera is to evolve over about a decade to a burned-out state with most of the features of *myelofibrosis with myeloid metaplasia*.

Conclusive diagnosis usually requires determination of total red cell mass, as is discussed in the Lab Tools box earlier in this chapter.

Malignant Thrombocythemia

Malignant thrombocythemia (*essential thrombocythemia*) is a rare, chronic myeloproliferative disorder in which the predominant malignant cell is the megakaryocyte. Platelet counts can be 500,000/cu mm or higher, but high platelet counts are common in all chronic myeloproliferative syndromes, so the diagnosis is one of exclusion. Circulating giant platelets are common. Bone marrow exam reveals an increase of megakaryocytes, some of them quite large. Myelofibrosis is absent. Thrombosis and hemorrhage are the most common clinical problems. It is a sluggish disorder with periods of quiet; average survival is about 10–15 years.

Myeloid Metaplasia with Myelofibrosis

Myeloid metaplasia with myelofibrosis is a myeloproliferative disorder in which marrow fibrosis predominates. It is caused by a release of fibrogenic factors from neoplastic megakaryocytes. It usually occurs in older adults, most of whom have very large spleens because there is splenic growth of bone marrow cells (extramedullary hematopoiesis, myeloid metaplasia). Red cells made outside the marrow tend to be deformed and retain their nuclei, so the peripheral blood contains many odd-shaped and nucleated red cells. Other blood findings include giant platelets, increased basophil count, and increased uric acid owing to metabolism of malignant cell DNA. Patients also suffer hemorrhagic or thrombotic problems associated with platelet defects. Typically the bone marrow is hypocellular or fibrotic, as is depicted in Figure 11-22. The final phase in some cases is a "blast crisis" that occurs as the case evolves rapidly into acute myeloid leukemia. Chronic myeloid leukemia and polycythemia vera may evolve ("burn out") into myeloid metaplasia with myelofibrosis. Average survival is a few years.

Myelodysplasia

Myelodysplasia is a group of bone marrow stem cell proliferations characterized by *ineffective RBC production* and a tendency to evolve into acute myelocytic leukemia. Cases occur spontaneously in older adults or as a result of prior chemotherapy or radiation, usually a few years after treatment. Myelodysplasia is also referred to as *preleukemia* or *smoldering leukemia*; both terms conveying a correct sense of the disease. The marrow typically is hypercellular and contains many dysplastic red and white cells. Because hematopoiesis is ineffective, patients may come to attention initially because of fatigue (low red cell count), bleeding (thrombocytopenia), or infection (leukopenia). Sometimes one cell type is more affected than others are. For example, red cell production may be especially impaired, giving rise to a syndrome called *refractory anemia*. Average survival is a few years.

Disorders of the Spleen and Thymus

The *spleen* filters unwanted microbes and substances from blood, the same as lymph nodes do from lymphatic fluid—splenic macrophages trap bacteria, foreign material, and antigens for elimination or presentation to the immune system. The spleen also removes from the circulation old blood cells and platelets, or blood cells to which antibody is attached. For example, in immune hemolytic anemia red cells coated with antibody are trapped and hemolyzed by the spleen. Overactivity of splenic function (**hypersplenism**) can cause decreased numbers of red cells, white cells, or platelets.

The catalog of conditions that affect the spleen is too long to list in its entirety, but among the most common are viral infections, chronic autoimmune disease, malaria, lymphoma and leukemia, chronic passive congestion owing to right heart failure, and portal hypertension (usually associated with cirrhosis). In almost every instance the result is an enlarged spleen (*splenomegaly*). Regardless of cause, an enlarged spleen may become overactive and remove more cells from blood than it normally should, destroying normal blood cells and platelets.

The *thymus* sits behind the upper end of the sternum and is critical to the development of the T lymphocytes of the immune system. It features a cortex of lymphocytes and a medulla of thymocytes (thymic epithelial cells). Relative to body size, it is largest at birth, but in absolute terms it becomes largest at puberty and shrinks to a few grams in adults.

Underdevelopment of the thymus causes serious immune deficiency, discussed in Chapter 8.

Hyperplasia of thymic lymphocytes or epithelial cells is associated with a variety of endocrine and autoimmune disease but is most commonly found in association with **myasthenia gravis** (Chapter 22), a rare, acquired autoimmune disease in which antibodies block transmission of nerve signals across the neuromuscular synapse—about half of cases have thymic hyperplasia or thymoma.

Thymoma is a tumor of thymic epithelial cells. It is very rare and may be either benign or malignant. Most are discovered in association with myasthenia gravis.

Section 2: Bleeding Disorders

Don't worry; the bleeding always stops.
ADVICE FROM OLDER SURGEONS TO WORRIED YOUNGER ONES.

▶ BACK TO BASICS

Hemostasis (Fig. 11-23) is a natural reaction, the purpose of which is to stop bleeding. It depends upon the interplay of blood vessels, platelets, and coagulation (clotting). After injury, damaged vessels undergo temporary constriction (vasospasm), and platelets begin to accumulate at the edges of the vascular defect to obstruct blood flow and to release factors to stimulate coagulation. At the same time, escaping blood is exposed to extravascular tissue factors that also stimulate coagulation, resulting ultimately in the weaving of a web of fibrin (a **clot**) to trap red cells and obstruct further escape of red cells from the vascular defect.

Coagulation begins when blood or platelets contact something they should not: extravascular tissue or a foreign surface. Coagulation is the result of interactions

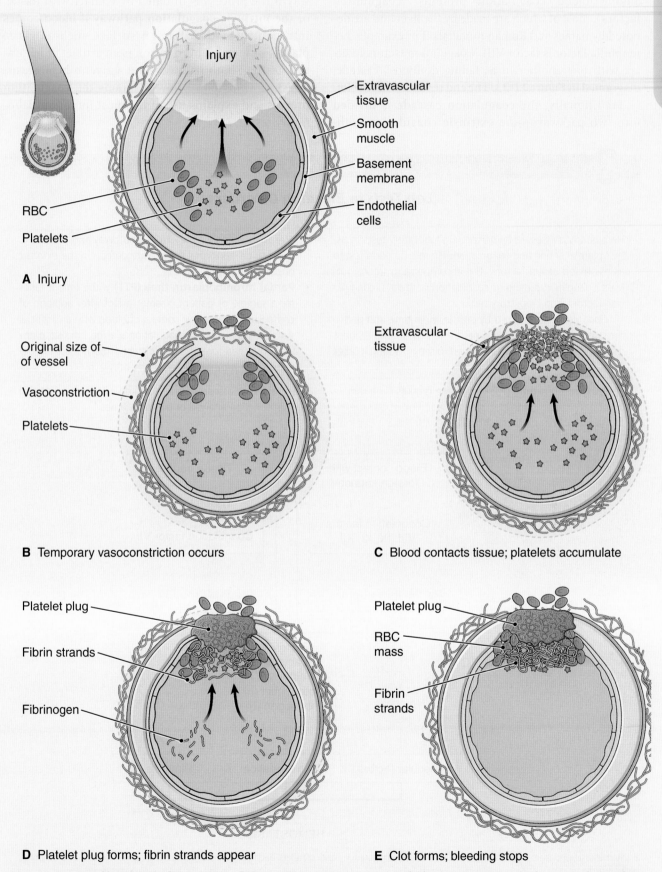

A Injury

B Temporary vasoconstriction occurs

C Blood contacts tissue; platelets accumulate

D Platelet plug forms; fibrin strands appear

E Clot forms; bleeding stops

Figure 11-23 **Normal hemostasis. A.** Injury occurs. **B.** Temporary vasoconstriction occurs. **C.** Blood contacts tissue, platelets accumulate, and co-agulation begins. **D.** Further platelet aggregation occurs, and coagulation produces a web of fibrin in the wound. **E.** Hemorrhage stops as fibrin traps red cells and blocks further bleeding.

among blood coagulation proteins (**coagulation factors**), most of which are made by the liver and are denoted by names and Roman numerals. For example, hemophilia factor is factor VIII. Coagulation factors interact with one another in a "falling dominos" cascade, diagramed in Figure 11-23. The end result is a fibrin clot.

Traditionally, the coagulation cascade is divided into two pathways—the **extrinsic coagulation path-**way if the process is initiated by contact with tissue, or the **intrinsic coagulation pathway** if blood comes into contact with a foreign surface such as glass, plastic, or metal. This division is an artifact of laboratory testing; both pathways are active in hemostasis. The Lab Tools box below diagrams the coagulation process and explains use of the most important laboratory tests.

LAB TOOLS

Lab Tests in Bleeding Disorders

Hemostasis is assessed by performing laboratory tests to assess platelet action and coagulation. There is no good test to assess blood vessel factors. The accompanying figure outlines a simplified outline of coagulation pathways, coagulation factors, and laboratory tests.

Coagulation is assessed by prothrombin time and partial thromboplastin time. Each is performed by adding reagent to anticoagulated plasma and timed to see how long it takes for a clot to form.

- **Prothrombin time (PT)** is the time it takes for a sample of patient plasma to clot after the addition of a tissue extract that mimics contact of blood with tissue. This initi-

ates coagulation via the *extrinsic* pathway and, therefore, the result is abnormal if there are defects in the *extrinsic* or *common* pathways.

- **Partial thromboplastin time (PTT)** is the time it takes for a sample of patient plasma to clot after addition of compounds that mimic contact of blood with an artificial surface. This initiates coagulation via the intrinsic pathway and, therefore, the result is abnormal if there are defects in the *intrinsic* or *common* pathways.

Platelets are assessed by performing a platelet count and platelet function analysis or bleeding time:

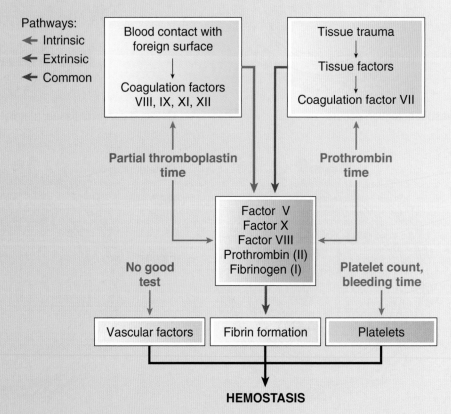

Hemostasis and hemostasis tests. Vascular factors, coagulation, and platelets each play a role in maintaining hemostasis and stopping hemorrhage.

- **Platelet count**: measures platelet *numbers* only; it does not account for platelets that do not *function* properly.
- **Platelet function analysis** detects defective platelet function and can be performed by specialized analyzers in large laboratories. In the absence of these devices, a **bleeding time** can be performed, which measures the length of time required for a patient to stop bleeding after skin prick with a standardized lancet. An abnormally long bleeding time is the result either of a low platelet count or of defective platelet function.

There is no test to assess vascular factors that contribute to abnormal bleeding.

The accompanying table shows how to interpret the results.

With results in hand from the four tests above and by process of elimination, the problem usually can be identified. For example, patients with liver failure may have a prothrombin deficiency because prothrombin is made by the liver. Patients with prothrombin deficiency have a normal platelet count and bleeding time. However, both PT and PTT are prolonged because prothrombin acts in the common pathway.

Interpretation of Tests of Hemostasis Function

Platelet Count	Bleeding Time	Conclusion
	Test and Result	
Normal	Normal	Platelets not part of the bleeding problem; suspect coagulation factor defect
Low	Prolonged	Bleeding because of low platelet count
Normal	Prolonged	Bleeding because of abnormal platelet function

Prothrombin Time	Partial Thromboplastin Time	
Normal	Normal	NORMAL coagulation function; suspect vascular or platelet factors
Abnormal	Abnormal	Coagulation defect in the COMMON pathway
Normal	Abnormal	Coagulation defect in the INTRINSIC pathway
Abnormal	Normal	Coagulation defect in the EXTRINSIC pathway

Bleeding Disorders

MAJOR DETERMINANTS OF DISEASE

- Excessive bleeding is always associated with at least one of three factors:
  - fragile blood vessels
  - low platelet count or defective platelet function
  - decreased coagulation factor activity
- Bleeding related to platelet disorders usually occurs from capillary-sized blood vessels.
- Bleeding related to coagulation factors usually occurs from larger vessels.
- Most coagulation factors are proteins made by the liver, and severe liver disease is often accompanied by excessive bleeding.
- Intravascular clotting is always abnormal and secondary to another disease.

Bleeding is usually the result of vascular injury. *Excessive* bleeding (**hemorrhagic diathesis**) is bleeding beyond the expected amount for a certain injury, or bleeding without obvious injury. Excessive bleeding is caused by one of three factors:

1. Fragile small blood vessels
2. Decreased platelet count or ineffective platelet function
3. Decreased coagulation factor activity

Hemorrhage occurs either from capillaries or from larger blood vessels. Patients with platelet problems or fragile small blood vessels usually bleed from capillary-size blood vessels, and the bleeding usually presents as tiny skin or mucosal hemorrhages (petechiae), nosebleed, hematuria, or excessive menses. On the other hand, patients with *coagulation factor deficiency* bleed from larger vessels and usually bleed into deep tissues, joints, and body spaces.

VASCULAR OR PLATELET DEFICIENCY

Other than trauma, few bleeding problems result solely from fragile small blood vessels. Some people, especially the elderly, do bruise easily, but the reasons are not clear and may relate to weakening of supporting connective tissue. Other causes include autoimmune vasculitis and vitamin C deficiency (scurvy), which weakens the intercellular cement that holds together small blood vessels.

Low platelet count (**thrombocytopenia**) occurs in a great variety of disorders and is usually characterized by tiny hemorrhages (petechiae, Chapter 5) in skin or mucosa. The normal range for platelet counts in most laboratories is about 130,000–400,000/cu mm. Because of this wide range, most practitioners do not grow concerned unless the platelet count falls below 100,000/cu mm. Even so, excessive bleeding after trauma rarely occurs until the count falls below 50,000/cu mm, and spontaneous hemorrhage usually does not occur until counts fall to about 20,000/cu mm. However, with severe thrombocytopenia, hemorrhage may occur at any site. CNS hemorrhage is a particular hazard for patients with very low platelet counts. In addition to a low platelet count, patients with thrombocytopenia have an abnormal bleeding time (see the related Lab Tools box).

Thrombocytopenia also may also occur when platelet production is low because of a primary bone marrow disorder, toxic effect of drugs or chemicals such as thiazide diuretics, or with ineffective platelet production, as in the case of folate or B_{12} deficiency. Decreased platelet survival may also lead to low counts. The spleen normally filters old platelets out of the blood after about 12 days, so an overactive spleen (hypersplenism) may cause thrombocytopenia.

A much more common cause of low platelet count is **immune thrombocytopenic purpura (ITP)**, in which the body's immune system destroys its own platelets. ITP usually occurs as an isolated disease, but can be seen in association with other autoimmune disorders, or it rarely may occur as a complication of acute pediatric viral illnesses. Platelets become coated with anti-platelet autoantibodies and are quickly removed by the spleen. Onset of ITP is insidious and may be first noticed by an astute clinician who detects subungual (beneath a fingernail) or conjunctival petechiae. More commonly, however, thrombocytopenia first shows itself as easy bruisability, epistaxis (nosebleed), bleeding gums, or unusual bleeding after minor trauma. Treatment with steroids is effective, and splenectomy is curative in most cases.

COAGULATION FACTOR DEFICIENCY

The liver produces most coagulation factors, and liver disease is an important cause of coagulation disorders. For example, patients with cirrhosis (Chapter 16) usually have bleeding tendencies because of coagulation defects.

On the other hand, many coagulation defects are inherited and involve single coagulation protein deficiencies, which are inherited in Mendelian fashion (Chapter 7). For example, classic hemophilia is a factor VIII deficiency. Vitamin K is essential for the production of factors VII, IX, and X and prothrombin. Coagulation defects resulting from vitamin K deficiency are most often seen with lengthy antibiotic therapy that eliminates vitamin K-producing bacteria from the intestine.

von Willebrand disease stems from a deficiency of von Willebrand factor (vWF), a coagulation factor made in endothelial cells and megakaryocytes. von Willebrand disease is one of the most common inherited coagulation disorders and is characterized by spontaneous bleeding from mouth, nose, and other mucous membranes and by excessive wound bleeding, and excessive menstrual bleeding. Bleeding time is prolonged despite normal platelet count because lack of vWF interferes with platelet adhesion to endothelium.

Classic **hemophilia** (hemophilia A or factor VIII deficiency) is the most common serious inherited coagulation disorder. An X-linked gene defect impairs factor VIII production and therefore this disorder occurs almost exclusively in males; however, about one third of cases are new mutations without positive family history. Spontaneous hemorrhage occurs only in severe deficiency (factor VIII levels about 1% of normal). Lesser deficiencies show varying amounts of post-traumatic bleeding. Intracapsular joint hemorrhage (**hemarthrosis**, especially in the knee) is a particular problem in patients with severe deficiencies. Repeated episodes may produce crippling joint strictures and immobility (ankylosis). Patients with hemophilia characteristically have a normal bleeding time and platelet count because neither platelets nor vascular factors are at fault. Patients with hemophilia have a normal prothrombin time because the extrinsic and common pathways do not require factor VIII; however, PTT is prolonged because factor VIII is in the intrinsic pathway (see the related Lab Tools box). For those with severe deficiency, periodic transfusion with factor VIII is effective. The accompanying History of Medicine box offers a glimpse into the interesting story of hemophilia.

Severe **Christmas disease** (hemophilia B, factor IX deficiency) is clinically similar to classic hemophilia but is much less common. (It is named for the first patient in whom the disease was identified, not for the annual holiday season.) Like classic hemophilia it is caused by an X-linked recessive gene defect, and it has test abnormalities similar to classic hemophilia (see the related Lab Tools box). Christmas disease may or may not be associated with significant bleeding problems. Diagnosis requires highly specialized testing specifically for factor IX deficiency.

DISSEMINATED INTRAVASCULAR COAGULATION (DIC)

Blood is not intended to clot *inside* the vascular space; blood normally clots only when it comes into contact with tissues outside the vascular space. A major function of the vascular endothelium is to prevent blood from contacting extravascular tissue, thereby preventing coagulation. If the vascular wall is disrupted, clotting occurs.

DIC is a condition in which clotting occurs inside the vascular space. One consequence is obstruction of small vessels by clots. However, a somewhat surprising aspect of DIC is that patients eventually have a bleeding tendency because clotting factors consumed by the clotting process no longer exist in high enough concentra-

tion to prevent abnormal bleeding. Therefore, DIC is said to be a **consumptive coagulopathy**.

DIC is never a primary disease; it is a complication of other diseases. For example, it may occur in bacterial septicemia when coagulogenic products released by bacteria activate the coagulation cascade.

DIC may be initiated by a variety of conditions, which can be grouped into several major categories:

- *Obstetrical complications*: toxemia, premature separation of the placenta (abruptio placentae), amniotic fluid embolism, retained dead fetus
- *Infections*: Gram-negative sepsis, meningococcal meningitis, malaria
- *Neoplasms*: carcinoma of stomach, pancreas, lung, and prostate and acute promyelocytic leukemia
- *Massive tissue trauma*: crush injury, burns
- *Others*: snakebite, heat stroke, acute hemolysis, and vasculitis

Regardless of cause, DIC is usually characterized by *hemolytic anemia* (as RBCs are shredded by passing through intravascular fibrin webs), *thromboses*, and *hemorrhage* as coagulation components are consumed by the clotting process.

HISTORY OF MEDICINE

"THE ROYAL DISEASE"

The oldest recognition of hemophilia (deficiency of coagulation factor VIII) is an indirect reference in the Talmud, a collection of Jewish religious writings from the 2nd century AD, which notes that male infants did not have to be circumcised if two brothers had died from the procedure.

In the 12th century AD an Arab physician, Albucasis, wrote of a family whose males died of bleeding after minor injuries.

In 1803, the year Lewis and Clark began their epic voyage up the Missouri River, John Otto, a Philadelphia physician, wrote an account of "a hemorrhagic disposition affecting certain families" and recognized that it was hereditary and affected males only.

Hemophilia has been called "The Royal Disease" because it afflicted the royal families of Europe during the reign of Queen Victoria, who ruled England from 1837 to 1901. Hemophilia is a sex-linked, autosomal recessive gene defect (Chapter 7), and the Queen was a carrier who passed the

trait on to her daughters, who in turn passed it on to German, Spanish, and Russian royalty in the nineteenth century.

A case can be made that hemophilia dramatically altered the course of history. In 1894, Queen Victoria's granddaughter, Alexandra, a carrier of the gene for hemophilia, married Nicholas, Tsar of Russia. Their son, Alexei, heir to the throne, was born in 1904 and suffered from severe hemophilia. During the crisis years leading up to the Bolshevik (communist) revolution in 1917, Nicholas and Alexandra's preoccupation with Alexei's health led them to an unusual, and eventually fatal, reliance on the advice of the mad monk Gregory Rasputin, the only person who seemed to be able to help the suffering boy. The illness of the heir to the Russian throne, the strain it placed on the Royal family, and the influence of the crazed monk were important factors that led to the bloody overthrow of the Tsar and the installation of a communist state in Russia.

Thrombotic Disorders

In most instances, venous thrombosis is caused by local factors such as turbulent blood flow or local endothelial injury (Chapter 5). However, two conditions exist in which *venous* thrombosis is promoted by abnormalities of blood coagulation proteins. These disorders do not promote *arterial* thrombosis (stroke or myocardial infarction), however.

Lupus anticoagulant (also called *anti-phospholipid antibody*) is an autoantibody that occurs in about 10% of patients with systemic lupus erythematosus (Chapter 8) and gets its name from the fact that it interferes with laboratory tests of blood coagulation, causing the tests to suggest that coagulation is deficient when, in fact, the opposite is true: lupus anticoagulant promotes venous thrombosis.

Patients with lupus anticoagulant are at increased risk for recurrent venous thrombosis, pulmonary thromboembolism, and recurrent spontaneous abortions. However, *most patients with lupus anticoagulant do not have systemic lupus erythematosus* or other clinical disease. Lupus anticoagulant also should also be suspected in patients who have abnormal laboratory tests of blood coagulation (prolonged prothrombin or partial thromboplastin time; see the related Lab Tools box) but who do not have clinical evidence of a bleeding disorder.

Factor V Leiden is an abnormal form of coagulation factor V produced by a defective gene. Factor V Leiden promotes a generalized tendency to form venous thrombi. The abnormal gene is an autosomal recessive defect (Chapter 7) that is surprisingly common—it is present in about 5% of Caucasians and 1% of African-Americans. The heterozygous state is associated with an approximate five-fold increased risk for venous thrombosis; the risk for the homozygous state is much higher. Oral contraceptive use further increases the risk. Factor V Leiden should be suspected in patients with venous thrombosis of any type, pulmonary thromboembolism, or recurrent spontaneous abortions. Laboratory tests are necessary to confirm the diagnosis. ■

CASE STUDY 11-1 "I'M TIRED AND SHORT OF BREATH ALL THE TIME"

TOPICS
Intestinal bleeding
Iron deficiency anemia
Colon cancer

THE CASE

Setting: You practice with a primary care physician in an office in a large city. Your principal duty is to see new patients before they see the physician.

Clinical history: Janice K. is a 52-year-old female new patient. When you ask about her main complaint she says, "I'm tired and short of breath all the time." In the last year she has given up walking for exercise and has to stop to catch her breath when climbing the stairs at home. She has never smoked and has never been hospitalized except for pregnancy. Her only physician visits over the last 10 years have been for occasional gynecologic exams and pap smears, the most recent one 3 years ago. Routine questions about diseases in various organ systems reveal no significant problems.

Physical examination and other data: Vital signs are unremarkable except that her resting heart rate is 82/min. She is pale, with fair skin and graying red hair. She is of medium height and average weight. Her conjunctivae are pale. Her chest is clear, and her abdomen is soft and without palpable masses. There are no palpable lymph nodes. Vaginal exam is unremarkable. Digital rectal exam reveals no masses. Stool on the exam glove tests positive for blood. Laboratory studies reveal: ▶

[Case 11-1, continued]

Initial Lab Data on Patient Janice K.

Value	Units	Patient Hi/Lo	Normal (Reference) Women
COMPLETE BLOOD COUNT			
HGB	mg/dL	9.4 Lo	12.1–15.1
HCT	%	29 Lo	33–43
RBC	10^6 cells/ cu mm	4.3	3.5–5.0
MCV	fL	67 Lo	76–100
MCHC	g/dL	32 Lo	33–37
MCH	pg	22 Lo	27–33
Total WBC	10^3 cells/ cu mm	6.6	4.5–10.5
Neutrophils	%	70	60–70
Bands	%	1	<5
Eosinophils	%	2	2–4
Basophils	%	0	0–1
Lymphocytes	%	22	20–25
Monocytes	%	5	3–8
Platelets	10^3 cells/ cu mm	202	150–350
OTHER PRE-SURGICAL LABORATORY DATA			
Reticulocyte count	As % of RBC	0.3 Lo	0.5–2.0
Iron, plasma	μg/dL	14 Lo	60–170

Clinical course: You review her CBC results and conclude that she almost certainly has iron deficiency anemia, probably because of chronic intestinal bleeding. After consulting with the physician, you order a reticulocyte count, plasma iron level, and a barium enema radiograph of her colon. The radiographs reveal a mass in the transverse colon, which the radiologist says is "suspicious for malignancy." The patient is referred to a colon and rectal surgeon, who performs a colonoscopy and biopsy, which reveals that the suspicious mass is a carcinoma of the colon. A few days later a partial colectomy is performed. The tumor is found to deeply invade the colon wall, and evidence of spread is found in nearby lymph nodes; no liver metastases are found.

Six weeks later she is discharged from the surgeon's care and returns to your office. The surgeon has instructed her to take oral iron tablets, and you advise her to follow his instructions and come back in 6 weeks to for follow-up laboratory studies, at which time her reticulocyte count is 6%, indicating a brisk outpouring of new RBCs. Plasma iron levels have risen into the normal ranges, and hemoglobin, hematocrit, and red cell count have improved substantially.

DISCUSSION

This patient presented with fatigue and shortness of breath. Coupled with rapid resting heart rate and pallor, the findings strongly suggested anemia. Lab studies confirmed your conclusion and revealed that the anemia was microcytic (low MCV) and hypochromic (low MCHC). Follow-up reticulocyte count and plasma iron confirmed the diagnosis of iron deficiency anemia: plasma iron was low, as it is in iron deficiency anemia, and the reticulocyte count was low, indicating that few new RBCs were being made by the bone marrow because there was not enough iron to form the necessary hemoglobin.

By far the most common cause of iron deficiency anemia in patients older than 50 is intestinal bleeding, which is strongly suggested in this case by the fact that the patient's stool is positive for blood. The most serious common cause of intestinal bleeding in men and women older than 50 is colon cancer, which was found by barium enema radiograph and proved by biopsy.

After the tumor was removed and the patient was put on oral iron, a brisk reticulocytosis was exhibited. Removal of the tumor stopped the bleeding, and the supplemental iron allowed new red cells to be produced.

Almost every colon cancer arises from pre-existing benign polyps, which take many years to become fully malignant. Regular stool tests for occult blood and periodic colon exams for all patients older than 50 detect almost all colon cancers before they metastasize.

This patient had not had a test for stool blood in at least 10 years, perhaps longer. With regular physical exams, lab studies, and stool exams, her cancer probably could have been detected years earlier, and her prognosis would be better.

Colon cancer is the third leading cause of cancer death in women, behind lung cancer and breast cancer, and it is third behind lung and prostate cancer in men. When statistics for men and women are lumped together, colon cancer is the number two cancer killer after lung cancer.

POINTS TO REMEMBER

- Cancer of the colon is almost entirely preventable with regular stool blood tests and periodic colon examinations.
- Iron deficiency anemia in an adult man or postmenopausal woman should be considered to be caused by an intestinal malignancy until proven otherwise.

Objectives Recap

1. *Give a reasonable estimate of the life span of blood cells and platelets*: Blood cells are produced in the bone marrow, circulate for a number of days, and are removed, mainly by the spleen. Red cells have a life span of about 120 days; neutrophils, basophils, and eosinophils about 4 days; lymphocytes and monocytes, a week or two; platelets, a day or two.

2. *Explain what is meant by red cell indices, and understand how to calculate them*: Red cell indices are measures of red cell size and hemoglobin content. They are calculated ratios among red cell count, hemoglobin, and hematocrit.

3. *Define anemia, and list the major types of anemia*: Anemia is lower than normal blood hemoglobin or hematocrit levels or red cell counts. Anemia can be caused by 1) decreased production of red cells; 2) increased destruction of red cell; or 3) loss of red cells (hemorrhage).

4. *Regarding sickle cell anemia, explain the cause and discuss what happens to red cells*: Sickle cell anemia occurs when there is a genetic defect in hemoglobin formation. The altered hemoglobin causes red cells to be deformed into a sickle (crescent) shape. Malformed (sickled) RBCs clog capillaries and impair blood flow. They are prematurely destroyed or removed from circulation after circulating for less than the normal 120 days.

5. *Explain blood and bone marrow ferritin, iron, transferrin, and iron binding capacity in iron deficiency anemia*: Blood iron and ferritin and marrow ferritin are low because body iron stores are depleted. Blood iron binding capacity is increased as a reflection of increased blood transferrin, a protein made by the liver, which is increased in order to attempt to transport more iron to tissues.

6. *Explain the difference between relative and absolute erythrocytosis*: Relative erythrocytosis is increased peripheral red cell count that is not associated with increased total body red cell mass. Absolute erythrocytosis is associated with increased total body red cell mass.

7. *Explain the significance of a left shift in the white cell differential count in peripheral blood*: A "left shift" is caused by release of immature granulocytes from bone marrow into peripheral blood. It occurs most often when the marrow is under stress, as when responding to acute infection.

8. *Name the two major groups of bone marrow malignancies, and list some of the diseases associated with each*: There are two major groups of bone marrow malignancies: myeloid and lymphoid. Myeloid neoplasms are a very varied group and consist of acute and chronic myeloid leukemia, and a family of related malignancies known as the chronic myeloproliferative syndromes. Lymphoid neoplasms consist of acute and chronic lymphocytic leukemia, lymphomas, and plasma cell proliferations.

9. *Distinguish between leukemia and lymphoma*: Both are malignancies of leukocytes. In leukemia malignant cells are present throughout the bone marrow and are found in high numbers in peripheral blood. In lymphoma malignant cells occur as nodular masses in lymph nodes and other organs; the bone marrow and blood are not much involved.

10. *Explain why patients with plasma cell proliferation have abnormal blood proteins*: Plasma cell proliferations include benign and malignant growths of plasma cells that produce an excess of immunoglobulin.

11. *Name the two major types of lymphoma*: Hodgkin lymphoma and non-Hodgkin lymphoma.

12. *Name the two types of non-Hodgkin lymphomas according to microscopic patterns, and explain why this distinction is important*: The two types are follicular and diffuse. The distinction is important because they behave much differently: follicular lymphomas are less aggressive and have a better prognosis than diffuse ones.

13. *Define hypersplenism*: Overactivity of the spleen that consumes more than the normal amount of WBC, RBC, or platelets. Hypersplenism is associated with enlarged spleen.

14. *Name the elements of normal hemostasis*: Hemostasis depends upon the interplay of 1) coagulation, 2) blood vessel factors, and 3) platelets.

15. *Characterize bleeding caused by platelet disease*: Bleeding is usually the result of low platelet count; bleeding because of platelet malfunction is uncommon. The bleeding is usually from small, capillary-size blood vessels and appears as petechiae or other small hemorrhages.

16. *Briefly characterize classic hemophilia (hemophilia A)*: It is an X-linked genetic deficiency of coagulation factor VIII that occurs in males; mild deficiencies may cause excess post-traumatic bleeding; severe deficiency may cause spontaneous bleeding, especially in joints.

17. *Explain why patients with disseminated intravascular coagulation have bleeding problems*: Disseminated intravascular coagulation consumes clotting proteins (factors), leaving insufficient clotting proteins to support normal clotting. The result is a tendency toward hemorrhage.

Typical Test Questions

1. Mean cell volume (MCV) is calculated using which of the following:
   A. Hemoglobin and hematocrit
   B. Red cell count and hemoglobin
   C. Red cell count and hematocrit

2. Red cells, granulocytes, and platelets arise from which one of the following?
   A. Monocyte stem cells
   B. Myeloid stem cells
   C. Lymphoid stem cells

3. Hemoglobinopathies are characterized by which one of the following?
   A. Bone marrow red cell aplasia
   B. Autoimmune hemoglobin precipitation
   C. Defective hemoglobin synthesis
   D. Excess hemoglobin

4. Follicular lymphoma is characterized by which one of the following?
   A. Growth in large, nodular masses in the chest and neck
   B. Myelofibrosis with myeloid metaplasia
   C. Very aggressive growth
   D. Microscopic pattern resembling normal lymphoid follicles

5. Which of the following statements is true?
   A. Blood normally clots only in the extravascular space
   B. Most coagulation factors are made in the spleen
   C. Platelet-related bleeding usually occurs from large blood vessels
   D. Most coagulation factors are immunoproteins

6. True or false? Most of plasma volume is protein.

7. True or false? Intrinsic factor is secreted by the gastric mucosa.

8. True or false? Small cell lymphocytic lymphoma is very aggressive.

9. True or false? Nodular sclerosis type is the most common type of Hodgkin lymphoma.

10. True or false? Chronic leukemia is characterized by mature white cells in the blood.

12

Diseases of Blood Vessels

This chapter begins with a review of normal vascular anatomy and blood flow. Following the review are discussions of atherosclerosis, hypertension, and other vascular diseases.

BACK TO BASICS
- The Normal Vascular System
- Regulation of Blood Pressure
- Lipid Classification and Metabolism
- Desirable Plasma Lipid Concentrations

NOMENCLATURE OF BLOOD VESSEL DISEASE

ATHEROSCLEROSIS
- The Causes and Consequences of Atherosclerosis
- The Pathogenesis of Atherosclerosis
- Risk Factors for Atherosclerosis
- The Pathologic Anatomy of Atherosclerosis
- Clinical Manifestations of Atherosclerosis

HYPERTENSION
- Types of Hypertension
- Pathogenesis of Hypertension
- The Pathology of Hypertension
- Clinical Aspects of Hypertension

ANEURYSMS AND DISSECTIONS

VASCULITIS

RAYNAUD PHENOMENON

DISEASES OF VEINS

TUMORS OF BLOOD AND LYMPHATIC VESSELS

Learning Objectives

After studying this chapter you should be able to:

1. Describe the normal functions of endothelial cells
2. Classify plasma lipids
3. Explain why "normal" is not a useful concept in study of plasma lipids
4. Explain the difference between atherosclerosis and arteriolosclerosis
5. Name the pathologic processes important in the formation of an atheroma
6. List the factors that predispose to atherosclerosis and name some indicators of risk
7. Name the most important clinical complications of atherosclerosis
8. Discuss the pathologic differences between young and old atheromas
9. Name the two main components that determine blood pressure
10. Name and define the two major types of hypertension
11. Name the characteristic kidney findings in hypertension
12. Give a clinical definition of hypertension
13. Name the cause of most aneurysms
14. Name the most common basic mechanism of vasculitis
15. Briefly explain Raynaud phenomenon
16. Explain the clinical importance of thrombophlebitis

Key Terms and Concepts

BACK TO BASICS
- endothelial cells
- lipoprotein
- cholesterol
- triglyceride
- HDL cholesterol
- LDL cholesterol

NOMENCLATURE OF BLOOD VESSEL DISEASE
- atherosclerosis
- arteriolosclerosis

ATHEROSCLEROSIS
- atheroma
- C-reactive protein
- aneurysm
- peripheral vascular insufficiency
- statin

HYPERTENSION
- hypertension
- cardiac output

- vascular resistance
- renin
- malignant hypertension
- essential hypertension
- secondary hypertension
- nephrosclerosis

VASCULITIS
- vasculitis

RAYNAUD PHENOMENON
- Raynaud phenomenon

DISEASES OF VEINS
- varicose veins
- thrombophlebitis

TUMORS OF BLOOD AND LYMPHATIC VESSELS
- hemangioma

Humorous health definitions:
Artery: the study of fine paintings
Varicose: nearby
Vein: conceited
Capillary: a boy's hat

ANONYMOUS, 2005

BACK TO BASICS

Unlike an ameba, which can wander about to find life's necessities, the cells of our body are fixed in place and must have oxygen, food, and other requirements brought to them by a transport vehicle—blood. Blood travels to and from tissues through a vast network of 50,000+ miles of arteries and veins (Fig. 12-1), which are large near the heart and grow progressively smaller as they branch, finally becoming microscopic. Oxygen (O_2) is absorbed from inhaled air by blood as it passes through the lungs and is delivered to the body by arteries. Blood then circulates back to the lungs through veins. In the lungs carbon dioxide (CO_2) diffuses into inhaled air and is expelled with each breath.

THE NORMAL VASCULAR SYSTEM

Arteries are thick-walled and tense, much like the wall of a basketball; because they contain blood under much higher pressure than that in veins, arteries are subject to a great deal more disease than veins are. With each left ventricular contraction (*systole*), arterial pressure rises as blood is forced into and expands the aorta and large branches, which contain stretchable elastic fibers in the muscular wall. As the left ventricle relaxes and refills (*diastole*), blood pressure and flow are maintained by the elastic squeeze of the wall aorta and large arteries until the next systole.

Veins are a low-pressure system and much less subject to disease than arteries are. They are pliable and relatively underfilled, much like a rubber balloon partially

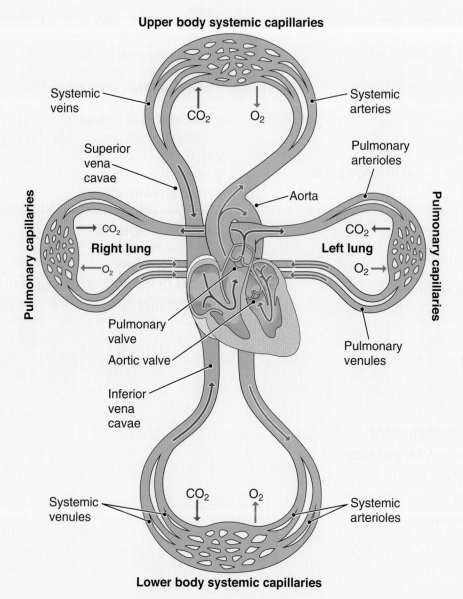

Upper body systemic capillaries

Systemic veins

CO_2 O_2

Systemic arteries

Superior vena cavae

Pulmonary arterioles

Pulmonary capillaries

CO_2 **Right lung** O_2

Aorta

CO_2 **Left lung** O_2

Pulmonary capillaries

Pulmonary valve

Aortic valve

Pulmonary venules

Inferior vena cavae

Systemic venules

CO_2 O_2

Systemic arterioles

Lower body systemic capillaries

Figure 12-1 The circulation of blood.

filled with water, which can expand and contract easily to accommodate more or less blood volume with little pressure change. Venous blood flow back to the heart is facilitated by one-way valves and the massaging action of skeletal muscle activity.

As Figure 12-2 illustrates, the anatomy of arteries and veins varies as the vessels branch into smaller diameter tubes. Large arteries and veins are thick walled and contain several layers. As vessels become smaller they have fewer layers and thinner walls, until the tiniest vessels, capillaries, have a very thin wall, which promotes free exchange of gases and fluids.

Both arteries and veins have a central, hollow core (the *lumen*) and are formed of concentric layers of tissue.

Innermost are **endothelial cells**, which form the *endothelium* (Fig. 12-3), the internal lining of all blood vessels. Endothelial cells serve two important functions: 1) they control diffusion of substances across the wall into adjacent tissues and 2) they are in constant contact with blood and keep it in a smooth, unclotted state by preventing coagulation (Chapter 11). The next layer outward is the **basement membrane**. Surrounding the endothelium and basement membrane are layers of elastic fibers and smooth muscle cells (the **media**) and an outer layer of fibrous tissue (the **adventitia**), which occur in varying proportions according to the size and type of vessel; arteries have thicker walls with more muscle and elastic tissue than veins and smaller arteries (arterioles).

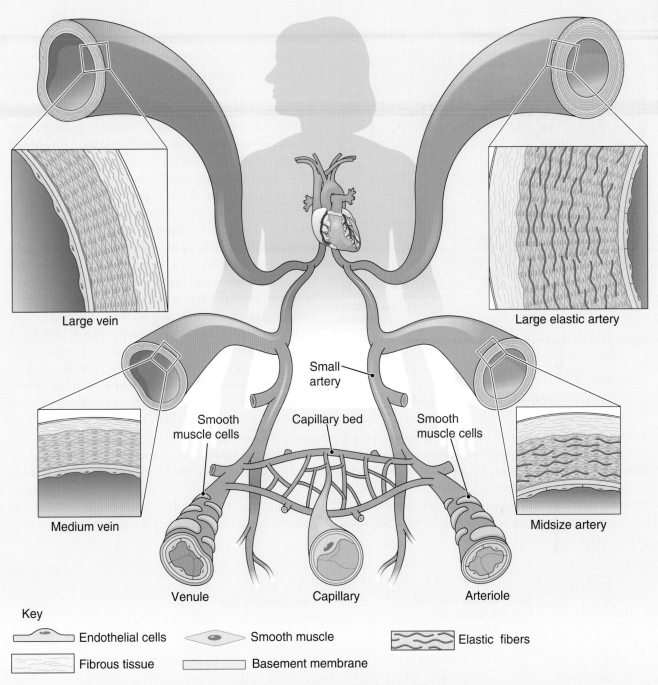

Large vein

Large elastic artery

Small artery

Smooth muscle cells

Capillary bed

Smooth muscle cells

Medium vein

Midsize artery

Venule

Capillary

Arteriole

Key

Endothelial cells

Smooth muscle

Elastic fibers

Fibrous tissue

Basement membrane

Figure 12-2 **The anatomy of blood vessels.**

Smooth muscle cells in the vascular wall influence lumen size by contracting (*vasoconstriction*) or relaxing (*vasodilation*), properties that act to control blood pressure by enlarging or narrowing vessel diameter to increase or decrease resistance to blood flow. Increased arterial resistance results in higher blood pressure; decreased arterial resistance results in lower blood pressure. In the venous system, constriction and dilation act mainly to accommodate changes in blood volume and have little effect on venous pressure.

REGULATION OF BLOOD PRESSURE

Blood pressure is a necessity of life: it is required in order to move blood through the body. Blood pressure is the product of *cardiac output* and *vascular resistance,* depicted in Figure 12-4. Because tissues *must* have oxygen, **cardiac output** (the volume of blood pumped by the heart over a given period of time) *must* keep up with demand, whether the patient is resting or exercising. **Vascular resistance** is the resistance to flow that must be

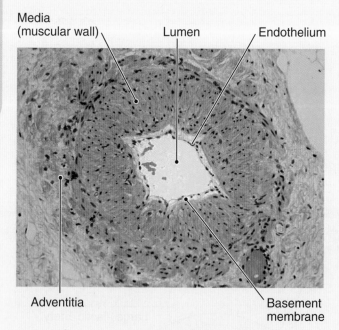

Media
(muscular wall)   Lumen   Endothelium

Adventitia   Basement
membrane

Figure 12-3 **Normal small muscular artery (arteriole).**

overcome to push blood through the circulatory system. If peripheral vascular resistance increases and if cardiac output *must* be maintained to ensure adequate oxygen delivery, it follows that blood pressure *must* rise to maintain blood supply to tissues. The opposite is also true: if blood volume or peripheral resistance fall, blood pressure falls also. It is important to keep in mind when considering cardiac output the simple fact that *increased*

blood volume causes increased cardiac output; *decreased* blood volume causes decreased cardiac output.

The kidneys play a major role in blood pressure regulation by modulating blood volume and peripheral vascular resistance. The kidney senses blood pressure and acts to increase or decrease peripheral resistance and increase or decrease blood volume as pressure rises or falls. For example, if blood pressure falls, blood vessels constrict, including those to the kidney. Renal vasoconstriction has two effects. First, constriction decreases the amount of blood passing through the kidney, which limits urine output and preserves water, making it available for blood volume. Second, as blood pressure falls the kidney receives less blood and is stimulated to secrete **renin**, a hormone that increases peripheral resistance and increases vascular volume, both of which increase blood pressure. Renin acts in concert with **angiotensin-converting enzyme**, to produce **angiotensin**, which in turn causes peripheral and renal vasoconstriction. The actions of renin and angiotensin-converting enzyme also stimulate the adrenal cortex to release **aldosterone**, a hormone that acts on the kidney to cause retention of sodium, thereby attracting water to expand blood volume, which increases cardiac output and blood pressure.

Peripheral vascular resistance is also influenced by local factors such as blood pH, anoxia, certain hormones, and the autonomic nervous system (Chapter 23). The adrenal cortex secretes epinephrine and norepinephrine (collectively called *catecholamines*), which

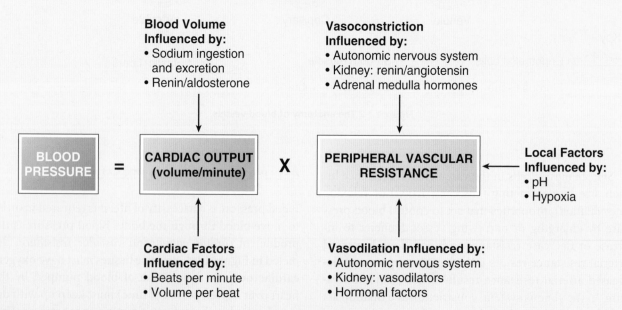

**Blood Volume
Influenced by:**
• Sodium ingestion
and excretion
• Renin/aldosterone

**Vasoconstriction
Influenced by:**
• Autonomic nervous system
• Kidney: renin/angiotensin
• Adrenal medulla hormones

BLOOD PRESSURE = **CARDIAC OUTPUT (volume/minute)** X **PERIPHERAL VASCULAR RESISTANCE**

**Local Factors
Influenced by:**
• pH
• Hypoxia

**Cardiac Factors
Influenced by:**
• Beats per minute
• Volume per beat

Vasodilation Influenced by:
• Autonomic nervous system
• Kidney: vasodilators
• Hormonal factors

Figure 12-4 **The regulation of blood pressure.** Blood pressure is a product of cardiac output (volume of blood flow) and peripheral vascular resistance.

are vasoconstrictors. Other substances, especially *nitric oxide*, act as vasodilators. Moreover, the autonomic nervous system is directly attached to small arterioles and stimulates smooth muscle contraction to maintain a normal level of tension (muscular tone) in the vascular wall. Increased or decreased autonomic activity can either increase or decrease peripheral vascular resistance, which increases or decreases blood pressure.

LIPID CLASSIFICATION AND METABOLISM

Lipids (fats) are very important in human physiology and disease. Blood lipids circulate in blood attached to specialized plasma proteins (**apoproteins**). The combination of an apoprotein and a lipid is a **lipoprotein**. Lipoproteins are classified according to their *molecular density*—high density lipoprotein (**HDL**), low density (**LDL**) and very low density (**VLDL**). On the other hand, the purely lipid part of lipoprotein is classified according to its *chemical* composition, either **cholesterol** or **triglyceride**. The lipid portion of HDL and LDL is mostly cholesterol, referred to as **HDL cholesterol** and **LDL cholesterol**. On the other hand, VLDL lipid is about 80% triglyceride and only 20% cholesterol. **Total cholesterol** is the sum of LDL, HDL, and VLDL cholesterol. For example, a patient with total blood cholesterol 240 mg/dL and triglyceride 150 mg/dL might be composed of the following: LDL cholesterol 160 mg/dL, HDL cholesterol 50 mg/dL, and VLDL cholesterol 30 mg/dL.

After ingesting a meal containing fat, lipid first appears in the plasma as chylomicrons, microscopic droplets of oily fat that do not mix well with plasma. Laboratory blood collection tubes that contain blood with a large amount of chylomicrons will, if left standing for an hour or so, develop a superficial milky layer as the "cream" rises to the top. Chylomicrons are about 90% triglyceride and 10% cholesterol and are cleared from plasma by the liver and attached to apoproteins to form HDL, LDL, and VLDL lipoproteins, which are soluble in plasma. *LDL cholesterol promotes atherosclerosis* and is often called "bad cholesterol" because most of the cholesterol in atheromas is derived from LDL cholesterol. *HDL cholesterol, on the other hand, is protective against atherosclerosis* and is called "good cholesterol," because it represents cholesterol that is on its way to be excreted from the body by the liver. Therefore, *high levels of HDL cholesterol are protective against atherosclerosis*. VLDL is nearly all triglyceride. High triglyceride *alone* may not promote atherosclerosis; however, *high triglyceride amplifies the atherosclerosis risk of high LDL cholesterol or low HDL cholesterol*.

DESIRABLE PLASMA LIPID CONCENTRATIONS

In regard to plasma lipids, the concept of *normal* (Chapter 1) is misleading because it relies on calculations to determine the *average* cholesterol of presumably healthy people, and the *average* cholesterol of presumably healthy Americans is unhealthily high. *Desirable* is a better concept. (The nearby Lab Tools box contains more information about plasma lipids.)

In the United States prior to around 1970 total plasma cholesterol less than 260 mg/dL was considered

---

LAB TOOLS

Plasma Lipids

Patient plasma lipids can be assessed by direct measurement of total plasma cholesterol, HDL cholesterol, and triglyceride. LDL cholesterol is more difficult and expensive to measure than are the others and is usually calculated according to the following formula:

LDL cholesterol = total cholesterol − (HDL cholesterol + [triglyceride/5])

However, calculated LDL is not valid for triglyceride levels >400 mg/dL, and a direct LDL assay must be performed.

After a 12-hour fast, generally accepted ranges for plasma lipids are:

Component*	Desirable (mg/dL)	Increased Risk (mg/dL)	High Risk (mg/dL)
Total cholesterol	<200	200–240	>240
HDL cholesterol	>60	40–60	<40
LDL cholesterol	<100	100–160	>160
Triglyceride	<150	High levels increase risks of high LDL or low HDL	

*Results obtained with less than a 12-hour fast are not reliable.

normal; now total cholesterol below 200 mg/dL is considered desirable for good health. When it comes to total plasma cholesterol, lower is better—lowering total cholesterol has benefits at almost any initial cholesterol level (any starting point). That is to say, people benefit by lowering their total cholesterol, whether they start with total cholesterol of 260 mg/dL or 200 mg/dL. As is shown in Figure 12-5, *decreasing total cholesterol by 40 mg/dL cuts the prevalence atherosclerosis complications in half,* whether it's a drop from 260 mg/dL to 220 mg/dL or from 200 mg/dL to 160 mg/dL. Lowering it by another 40 mg/dL cuts the risk by half again. Evidence suggests that atherosclerosis may not develop with total cholesterol levels below 150 mg/dL, a level unreachable without a strict, low fat vegetarian diet, something few people in industrialized nations are willing to do.

> *Lowering total plasma cholesterol by 40 mg/dL reduces cardiovascular risk by half; each additional 40 mg/dL decrease cuts the rate in half again.*

A desirable *LDL cholesterol* (LDL-C) level is considered to be <100 mg/dL, but as with total cholesterol, lower is better: evidence suggests that people are likely to benefit further by lowering LDL cholesterol below 80 mg/dL, and studies suggest that atherosclerosis does not occur in people with LDL cholesterol of about 50-60 mg/dL. The desirable *HDL cholesterol* (HDL-C) level appears to be above 60 mg/dL, a level that is not associated with cardiovascular risk. Values less than 40 mg/dL are associated with very high atherosclerosis risk. HDL-C levels are strongly influenced by genetics and improving a low HDL-C level is more difficult to change than is total cholesterol or level of LDL cholesterol, both of which are more influenced by diet than is HDL-C. However, low HDL-C can be treated, and the effort is worthwhile—for every 1 mg/dL HDL-C is increased, coronary risk declines by 2–3%. Smoking lowers HDL-C 5–10 mg/dL, and is one of the reasons cessation of smoking is a very effective cardiovascular risk-reduction strategy. Exercise and consumption of moderate amounts of alcohol are also effective in raising HDL-C.

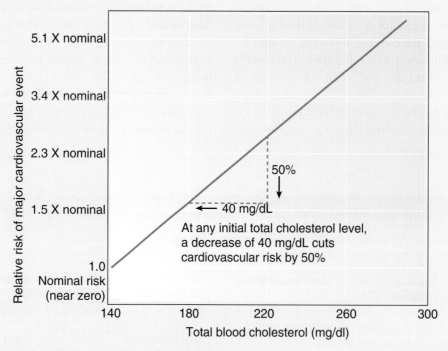

Figure 12-5 **Total plasma cholesterol and relative cardiovascular risk.** Reducing total plasma cholesterol 40 mg/dL from any given initial point cuts relative cardiovascular risk in half.

- Atherosclerosis begins in the crib and progresses with age.
- Atherosclerosis begins with vascular endothelial cell damage and associated inflammation.
- Atherosclerosis is accelerated by lifestyle: diet, obesity, smoking, and lack of exercise are key factors.
- Plasma lipid abnormalities are of paramount importance in the pathogenesis of atherosclerosis.
- High blood pressure and diabetes accelerate atherosclerosis.
- Vascular disease is strongly associated with:
  - Smoking
  - High blood pressure
  - Familial genetic influence

Nomenclature of Blood Vessel Disease

Atherosclerosis is a lifestyle disease related to *smoking, lack of exercise, obesity, and a high-fat diet.* Atherosclerosis is characterized by chronic inflammation, scarring, and cholesterol deposits in large and medium-size arteries. **Arteriolosclerosis** is a disease of small blood vessels that occurs mainly in patients with hypertension and diabetes; inflammation, scarring, and cholesterol are not significant factors. The kidneys (Chapter 19), retina (Chapter 25), and small vessels in the legs and feet are most often affected by arteriolosclerosis.

There are two varieties of arteriolosclerosis:

1. **Hyaline arteriolosclerosis**, a homogeneous thickening of arteriolar walls, is an inevitable part of the ageing process; it is accentuated by *hypertension* and *diabetes*. It is most easily detected in the afferent arterioles of renal glomeruli.
2. **Hyperplastic arteriolosclerosis** is onionskin hyperplasia of cells in arteriolar walls, mainly seen in the kidneys in *very severe (malignant) hypertension.*

> *Three of the most common diseases of humankind—atherosclerosis, hypertension, and diabetes—primarily affect arteries.*

Atherosclerosis

Atherosclerosis accounts for about one third of deaths in the industrialized world. The basic lesion of atherosclerosis is the **atheroma**, a thickening of the arterial wall that occurs with accumulation of scar tissue and cholesterol deposits. Atheromas tend to obstruct arterial blood flow and cause hypoxia of downstream tissue (ischemia, Chapter 5) by hampering the swift, smooth flow of blood. Atheromas also weaken the arterial wall, causing dilation (*aneurysm*) and increasing the risk of arterial rupture and hemorrhage.

The term *atherosclerosis* derives from Greek *athero*, meaning gruel or thick soup, and *scleros*, meaning hard, terms that describe the fibrous (hard) scar portion an atheroma and the fatty (soft) nature of atheroma cholesterol deposits. The character of atheromas changes with time. Young atheromas are soft and have a mealy, semisolid consistency and are the most dangerous because they are prone to sudden thrombosis and occlusion, with infarction (Chapter 5) of downstream tissue. For example, sudden occlusion of a coronary artery usually produces infarction of the heart muscle supplied by the artery (myocardial infarct). On the other hand, old lesions contain much less fat and have an abundance of hard scar tissue and calcium, hence the common practice of calling atherosclerosis "hardening of the arteries."

THE CAUSES AND CONSEQUENCES OF ATHEROSCLEROSIS

Atherosclerosis begins in the crib. Autopsy evidence of people in their twenties who die of violence and accidents demonstrate that the majority have atherosclerosis, which, of course, began many years earlier. Some of these young people have serious disease: about one in five has more than 50% narrowing of one coronary artery. Risk of heart attack, stroke, and other consequences increases with age. Most patients with symptomatic atherosclerosis are in their sixties or seventies, although most practitioners have seen strokes and heart attacks in patients in their thirties or forties. Before age 50, men are more affected than women, who are somewhat protected by estrogen, but after menopause the prevalence of atherosclerosis in women rises dramatically—after age 50 more women than men die each year of vascular disease.

Family history is important in the pathogenesis of atherosclerosis—genetic makeup provides fertile soil for the seeds of unhealthy lifestyle habits that promote atherosclerosis, some of which are:

- high-fat diet
- obesity
- high-sodium (salt) diet
- cigarette smoking
- lack of exercise

Each of these factors promotes atherosclerosis in a somewhat different fashion. How exercise protects against atherosclerosis is beyond the scope of this review, but the positive effect of exercise is clear.

The most important consequence of atherosclerosis is decreased or completely obstructed blood arterial flow, which causes ischemia and necrosis of downstream tissue (Chapter 5). Atherosclerosis accounts for most deaths from heart disease (Chapter 13) and stroke (Chapter 23).

THE PATHOGENESIS OF ATHEROSCLEROSIS

Endothelial cell damage is the initial and most crucial lesion in the pathogenesis of atherosclerosis. As is depicted in Figure 12-6, atherosclerosis begins with subtle, nonlethal damage to endothelial cells. The cause of this endothelial damage is not clear in most patients, but it is serious enough to produce laboratory evidence of inflammation (increased blood C-reactive protein, Chapter 3). Abnormally high concentration of blood uric acid or blood homocysteine (an amino acid) is known to injure endothelium and induce atherosclerosis. High blood pressure and high blood glucose levels also cause vascular damage that induces atherosclerosis or accelerates its development.

The earliest visible change of atherosclerosis is accumulation of lipid (mainly cholesterol) deposits in the arterial wall immediately beneath endothelial cells. These flat, yellow fatty streaks are evidence that damaged endothelium has become "leaky" and has lost its ability to prevent passage of cholesterol into the arterial wall. Cholesterol, cigarette smoke, infectious agents,

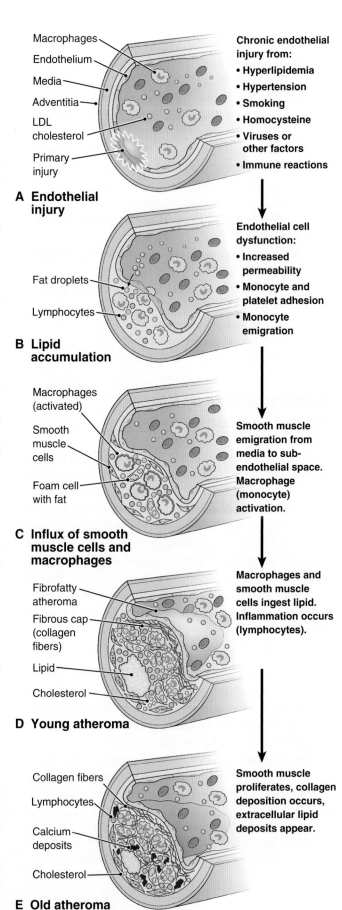

Figure 12-6 **Formation of an atheroma. A.** Subtle injury to intact endothelium. **B.** LDL cholesterol and other lipids "leak" into the site across damaged endothelium. Macrophages invade and phagocytize the lipids. **C.** The atheroma grows as smooth muscle cells invade and evolve into fibroblasts and phagocytes. Lymphocytes and other inflammatory cells appear. Cells with phagocytized fat appear as foam cells. **D.** Further accumulation of fat, foam cells, inflammatory cells, and migrating, evolving smooth muscle cells form an unstable, soft, young atheroma prone to ulceration, hemorrhage, thrombosis, and sudden vascular occlusion. **E.** Fibrosis (scarring) and chronic inflammation produce a hard, sometimes calcified, old, stable atheroma.

and homocysteine are suspected as causes of this early endothelial damage.

Vascular *inflammation* is important in the progress of atherosclerosis. Damaged endothelial cells become "sticky," and neutrophils and lymphocytes attach to them and invade the wall of the vessel. Macrophages invade the site and engulf (phagocytize) the lipid. Finally, as the atheroma ages, scar tissue matures and calcification may occur.

Cholesterol is also a very important element in the development of atherosclerosis: abnormally high levels of LDL cholesterol damage endothelium, allowing cholesterol to cross into the arterial wall, where it accumulates in atheromas. High levels cause more damage and more rapid formation of atheromas.

Arterial *smooth muscle cells* are also important in the development of atherosclerosis: they react to the presence of lipids and inflammation and migrate into the developing atheroma where they change into fibrocytes that produce scar tissue, and into macrophage-like cells that engulf and store cholesterol.

In summary, atherosclerosis is a complex process that is the result of multiple related events. As a result of endothelial injury, cholesterol seeps across the damaged endothelium and accumulates in the arterial wall, where it is ingested by macrophages and other cells, which take on a foamy appearance (*foam cells*). Inflammatory cells, smooth muscle cells, and macrophages migrate into the area, where they accumulate cholesterol and assemble as a soft, fatty mass. These early, soft atheromas obstruct flow. They are unstable and especially dangerous because they may break open or hemorrhage, stimulating thrombosis, acute occlusion, and downstream tissue infarction. By contrast old atherosclerosis lesions tend to be scarred, hard, and calcified. They may impede blood flow gradually, producing downstream ischemia, but they are stable and not commonly the cause of acute thrombosis and infarction because they are not as likely to occlude suddenly.

RISK FACTORS FOR ATHEROSCLEROSIS

Age is a major risk factor: atherosclerosis worsens steadily with age. From age 40 to age 60 the number of heart attacks increases fivefold. By age 60–70, age accounts for 80–90% of the risk in men, but only about 60–70% of the risk in women, in whom other risk factors at this age are relatively more important. This is to say, the risk from hypertension, smoking, and high cholesterol are relatively less important as age-related risk increases. Nevertheless, it remains important to pay attention to smoking, cholesterol, blood pressure, and other risk factors regardless of patient age.

Gender is also influential: before age 60–70, men are much more prone than women are to develop atherosclerosis and its complications. Women have higher estrogen levels, which are protective until menopause, after which atherosclerosis appears in women with increasing regularity, until rates for men and women become nearly equal by age 60–70.

Genetics are important, too: a family history of cardiovascular disease or stroke increases risk.

A high level of blood cholesterol, especially a high level of LDL cholesterol, is the single most important risk factor. The risk for heart attack, stroke, and other complications of atherosclerosis doubles with every 40 mg/dL rise of total cholesterol. In most patients, high cholesterol is attributable to a diet high in cholesterol and animal fats, which are easily converted into cholesterol.

Hypertension (high blood pressure) damages endothelium and initiates atherosclerosis or accelerates established atherosclerosis. For example, patients with diastolic blood pressure >95 mm Hg have five times as much atherosclerosis risk as do those with normal blood pressure. Hypertension is encouraged by a high-salt diet.

Smoking accelerates atherosclerosis. Smoking promotes atherosclerosis by lowering HDL cholesterol levels, by increasing blood pressure, by impairing fitness owing to decreased pulmonary function, and by directly damaging endothelium. Smokers have a 70% greater risk of death from coronary artery disease than do nonsmokers. The younger the person the more dangerous smoking is—smoking accounts for about 50% of coronary risk in people under 65, but only 15% of the coronary risk for people over 65. Cessation of smoking cuts smoking-related cardiovascular risk by 50% in one year.

Patients with *diabetes* are predisposed to developing vascular disease for two reasons: 1) they have abnormally high plasma lipids; and 2) they are predisposed to develop diabetic microangiopathy, a non-atherosclerotic disease of small blood vessels caused by high blood glucose levels (Chapter 17).

Homocysteine, a blood amino acid, is toxic to endothelial cells. Patients with congenital homocysteinemia, an autosomal recessive genetic disease, have severe atherosclerosis with heart attacks and strokes before age 20. Increased levels of plasma homocysteine are fairly common in the general population. It is an independent risk factor for atherosclerosis, but it is relatively less important than other risk factors.

Inflammation is a key element in the pathogenesis of atherosclerosis. In the absence of known inflammation anywhere else—an infection or arthritis, for example—

it can be safely assumed that laboratory evidence of inflammation is due to vascular inflammation or the inflammatory effect of obesity (Chapter 10). The presence of inflammation can be assessed by measurement of levels of plasma **C-reactive protein** (CRP), a reactive protein made by the liver in response to inflammation anywhere in the body. There is a striking relationship between the development of atherosclerosis and increased levels of plasma CRP. However, it is important to keep in mind that increased levels of CRP are like smoke from a fire: it is a *response* not a *cause. In the absence of any other known inflammatory condition,* elevated CRP can be attributed to one of two things: the inflammatory component of atherosclerosis, or the inflammatory component of obesity. Studies show that an increased level of CRP is an independent risk factor for atherosclerosis; that is to say, patients with an increased CRP level have an increased risk for heart attack, stroke, and other atherosclerosis complications even if all other risk factors (e.g., blood pressure, cholesterol) are normal.

Many other factors have been linked with increased risk for atherosclerosis. They include, but are not limited to: psychologic stress, obesity, increased levels of blood uric acid, and a high-carbohydrate diet.

THE PATHOLOGIC ANATOMY OF ATHEROSCLEROSIS

Figure 12-7 illustrates that the normal aortic endothelium is smooth and pink. The earliest lesions in the pathologic anatomy of atherosclerosis are yellow, slightly raised fatty streaks. As is depicted in Figure 12-8, these initial lesions evolve into large fibrofatty atheromas that microscopically are a mixture of fat, fibrous tissue, macrophages, and a sprinkling of lymphocytes, imparting a rough, stiff, caked appearance to the endothelial lining. Atheromas may occur anywhere, but they are most common in (in descending order): the lower abdominal aorta, coronary arteries, popliteal arteries in the back of the knee, descending thoracic aorta, internal carotid arteries in the neck, and the circle of Willis, at the base of the brain. Atheromas can grow slowly, gradually choking blood flow; or they can crack or ulcerate, initiating instant thrombosis or intra-atheroma hemorrhage, either of which can produce sudden vascular occlusion and infarction.

Weakening of the arterial wall can allow bulges (**aneurysms**), which are less common than are complications from blocked blood flow. Aneurysms occur most commonly in the abdominal aorta and may become caked with thick layers of old thrombus material, as is shown in Figure 12-9.

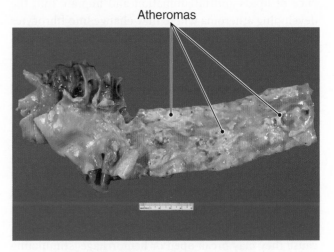

Figure 12-8 **Atherosclerotic aorta.**

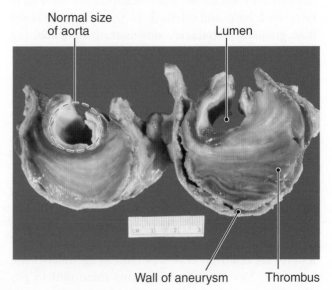

Figure 12-9 **Thrombus in an aortic aneurysm.** Layers of thrombus material fill most of the aneurysm.

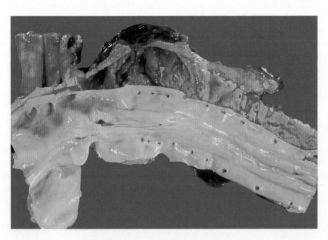

Figure 12-7 **The normal aorta.**

CLINICAL MANIFESTATIONS OF ATHEROSCLEROSIS

For most of their existence, atheromas are silent and subclinical. Figure 12-10 illustrates that atheromas enlarge over the decades until they become symptomatic, usually by obstruction of blood flow, which causes ischemia or infarction of downstream tissue. Less commonly the weakened wall of a diseased vessel balloons into an aneurysm. Coronary artery atheromas cause ischemia and chest pain (*angina*) owing to the "cramps" of oxygen-starved heart muscle. If **coronary occlusion** occurs, a **myocardial infarct** ("heart attack") follows. Common consequences of myocardial infarct include heart failure, arrhythmia, and sudden death (Chapter 13). The abdominal aorta is often the site of aneurysms, which can rupture with fatal results. Atherosclerosis of carotid or intracranial arteries may cause brain infarction (**stroke**, Chapter 23) or other brain disease. Atherosclerosis of the aorta or its major branches may impair blood flow to the extremities (**peripheral vascular insufficiency**). The legs are most often affected, and a syndrome of leg pain or cramps with exercise (*intermittent claudication*) may develop. Flow to internal organs also may be impaired. For example, decreased blood flow to the kidney (*renovascular insufficiency*, Chapter 19) is one cause of high blood pressure, and atherosclerotic obstruction of blood flow in the superior mesenteric artery can cause infarction of the bowel.

Atherosclerosis is epidemic in the United States and other developed nations. Prevention is a laudable goal, but few people can afford the cost of drugs or are willing to stop smoking, lose weight, eat less animal or saturated fat, increase their intake of healthy fish or vegetable oils, reduce dietary salt, and exercise regularly. By whatever means it is achieved, lowering plasma cholesterol levels (especially those of LDL cholesterol) reduces the incidence of atherosclerosis and its complications. The effect is incremental—a 10% reduction is not as effective as 20%, and so on. Until now most treatment efforts have been reparative—surgery to bypass or reopen clogged arteries, and drugs to aid failing hearts. However, emphasis on maintaining desirable plasma lipid levels shows promise of preventing atherosclerosis.

Statin drugs have proven very effective at lowering levels of LDL-C and total cholesterol by inhibiting liver synthesis of cholesterol. In 2001, the United States National Heart, Lung, and Blood Institute issued

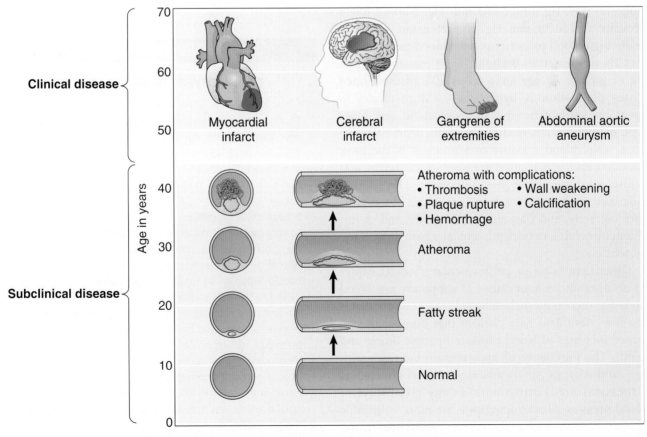

Figure 12-10 **The evolution of atherosclerosis.**

new guidelines for desirable (optimal) cholesterol, calling for more aggressive treatment of high cholesterol than had been exerted previously. The number of people in the United States falling within the guidelines of recommendation for statin therapy was tripled—to about one in every six adults. Good as they are, statins cannot lower cholesterol to optimal levels in all treated people. New drugs are proving effective that inhibit cholesterol absorption by the bowel. However, most plasma cholesterol is made by the body from dietary animal fat; cholesterol in food is a less important source of cholesterol. A large portion of blood cholesterol is cholesterol reabsorbed by the intestine after being excreted in the bile, an excretion-reabsorption circle known as the *enterohepatic circulation* (Chapter 16). The result is that intestinal reabsorption of cholesterol excreted by the liver has much more effect on plasma cholesterol than does cholesterol obtained in the diet. In recognition of this fact, new oral drugs are now available that block intestinal cholesterol absorption.

Hypertension

Optimal blood pressure is systolic 120 mm Hg, diastolic 80 mm Hg, or 120/80 mm Hg. *Normal* blood pressure is 130/85 mm Hg. **Hypertension** is abnormally high blood pressure: systolic blood pressure 140 mm Hg or greater; *or* diastolic blood pressure 90 mm Hg or greater. By age sixty about 60% of the United States population is hypertensive. More money is spent on antihypertensive drugs than on any other type of prescription medication. Aside from stepping on a scale, blood pressure measurement is the most common and widely used measure of cardiovascular health, and one of the most important. The Clinical Side box nearby explains how to measure blood pressure correctly, and Case Study 12.1 at the end of this chapter provides an in-depth look at a patient with hypertension.

Other than being in cardiovascular shock (Chapter 5) or other uncommon causes of temporary low blood pressure, there is no such thing as blood pressure that is too low. Abundant data confirm that even small sustained increases of blood pressure increase illness and death. The prevalence of hypertension increases with age, and African Americans are twice as affected as Caucasians are. Furthermore, at any given level of blood pressure African Americans are more vulnerable to complications such as stroke, myocardial infarct, and renal failure.

THE CLINICAL SIDE

MEASURING BLOOD PRESSURE

Blood pressure is often measured incorrectly. Blood pressure varies with body position: it is lower when a person is lying down than when the person is sitting or standing. Blood pressure also varies with physical activity and emotion: it is higher with physical activity or emotional stress. Blood pressure is also increased by other activities such as smoking and caffeinated beverages.

For a correct measurement the patient should be rested, not recovering from climbing a flight of stairs or walking a long way to get to an appointment. For several hours before the measurement, the patient should not smoke and should ingest nothing but water. Seat the patient in a chair with back and armrests, the absence of which increases blood pressure. The arm to be used for the measurement should be supported by an armrest; an unsupported arm causes higher readings. If the patient is wearing long-sleeved clothing, ask for it to be removed rather than rolling up the sleeve, which interferes with the measurement. Wrap the cuff around the arm at heart level. Use special large or small size cuffs for obese or pediatric patients. Cuffs too large for the patient produce erroneously low readings; cuffs too small produce erroneously high readings.

HISTORY OF MEDICINE

THE DISCOVERY OF BLOOD PRESSURE

That blood moves and has pressure is a fairly recent discovery in medicine. Greek physician Hippocrates (~400 BC) knew of blood vessels but believed they contained air and foodstuffs. About 600 years later Roman physician Galen (131–201 AD) theorized that blood surged and ebbed like the ocean's tide. Galen's idea persisted until English physician William Harvey (1578–1657), in a series of very careful animal experiments and human observations, concluded that blood flowed circularly in a closed system and inferred that arteries and veins were connected, although he never observed them.

In 1733 an English clergyman, Stephen Hales, became the first person to demonstrate blood pressure. His subject was a horse, and his equipment consisted of a small brass pipe, which he connected to a 12-foot long glass tube using the long, thin, flexible windpipe removed from a goose. The intrepid cleric bound the struggling horse and, stabbing the sharpened brass pipe into a carotid artery, was astonished to see blood rise 9 feet in the glass tube.

TYPES OF HYPERTENSION

As is illustrated in Table 12-1, blood pressure varies from optimal to severely hypertensive. The cause of 90% of hypertension is unknown and is referred to as **essential hypertension** (primary hypertension). The remaining 10% have **secondary hypertension**, for which a specific underlying cause can be identified, such as kidney disease that causes plasma renin to rise or tumors of endocrine glands that secrete hormones that raise blood pressure.

PATHOGENESIS OF HYPERTENSION

All hypertension is caused by an imbalance in the relationship between cardiac output and peripheral vascular resistance.

The cause of *essential* hypertension is not known with certainty, but the kidney is the prime suspect. For example, animal renal transplant experiments show "hypertension travels with the kidney." Studies demon-

Table 12-1	Classification of Blood Pressure in Adults*			
Category	**Systolic Pressure mm Hg**	**Diastolic Pressure mm Hg**	**Action**	
Optimal	<120	<80	Recheck in 2 years	
Normal	<130	<85	Recheck in 2 years	
High-normal	130–139	85–90	Recheck in 1 year Lifestyle counseling	
Hypertension,** Stage 1 (mild)	140–159	90–99	Confirm within 2 months	
Hypertension,** Stage 2 (moderate)	160–179	100–109	Evaluate or refer within 1 month	
Hypertension,** Stage 3 (severe)	>180	110	Evaluate or refer within 1 week	

*When systolic and diastolic pressures fall into different categories, choose the higher category for classification.
**All patients with confirmed hypertension deserve treatment.

strate that patients with hypertension have about half the number of renal glomeruli as do people with normal blood pressure. However, a single cause is unlikely; rather, hypertension derives from a combination of forces that vary from patient to patient. Genetic factors (familial tendencies) are important. For example, the concordance rate in identical twins is high. That is to say, if one identical twin has hypertension, the other is very likely to be hypertensive as well. Environmental factors, such as a high-salt (high-sodium) diet, lack of exercise, smoking, obesity, and psychological stress, also play a role.

The most important environmental influence on blood pressure is *dietary sodium*. Increased sodium intake expands blood volume, which increases cardiac output and blood pressure. However, apparently some patients are better endowed genetically than others to excrete the increased dietary sodium load. Those who cannot excrete it are more likely to develop hypertension than others are.

A significant factor in some patients with hypertension is **obstructive sleep apnea**. *Apnea* (from Greek, *a-*, without, and *pnein*, breathing) is temporary cessation of breathing. Obstructive sleep apnea is a syndrome of repeated nighttime apnea—sometimes 100 or more episodes per night. It usually occurs in obese patients who have accumulations of fat in the throat and a receding chin that forces the tongue backward. Apnea is most severe when the patient is sleeping on his or her back: the relaxed tongue falls backward and obstructs the air passage. The result is strangling-like snoring that affects about 5% of adults, especially men. Patients become hypoxic during the apneic period, and hypoxia causes compensatory increase of cardiac output and increased sympathetic activity of the autonomic nervous system, which combine to increase blood pressure.

THE PATHOLOGY OF HYPERTENSION

Hypertension can initiate atherosclerosis or accelerate existing atherosclerosis. Patients with hypertension usually have severe generalized atherosclerosis, coronary artery disease, and muscular enlargement of the left ventricle (ventricular hypertrophy), making them vulnerable to heart attack, stroke, and heart failure.

In addition to systemic atherosclerosis, kidney blood vessels are particularly affected by hypertension. A lifetime of *normal* blood pressure causes distinctive changes in renal arterioles collectively called **nephrosclerosis**, a wear-and-tear change that gradually increases with age. Recall that the glomerulus is supplied with blood from the systemic circulation via the afferent arteriole, which is directly affected by systemic blood pressure. Hypertension accelerates nephrosclerosis and consequently nephrosclerosis is found more often and in a more advanced state in patients with hypertension. In mild and moderate hypertension the pathologic lesion is **benign nephrosclerosis**, an exaggeration of the wear and tear of age-related nephrosclerosis. The distinctive lesion of benign nephrosclerosis is **hyaline arteriolosclerosis** (Fig. 12-11), a thickening and smudging of the fine structure of arteriolar walls, especially the afferent arteriole. As these changes progress, the affected glomerulus and associated tubules (which together form a *nephron unit*) atrophy into a small scar. As a result, on gross inspection the kidney is shrunken and has a granular cortex pitted by small scars.

In severe hypertension, damage is more serious and is known as **malignant nephrosclerosis**. The afferent arterioles are assaulted by much higher pressure and undergo two distinctive changes: **necrotizing arteriolitis**, inflammatory death of the afferent arteriole, or **hyperplastic arteriolitis**, an onionskin layering and thickening of the vascular wall. On gross inspection the kidneys may have some of the granular cortex associated with pre-existing benign nephrosclerosis, but the cortex also contains innumerable tiny hemorrhages from bleeding glomeruli, giving it a "flea-bitten" appearance.

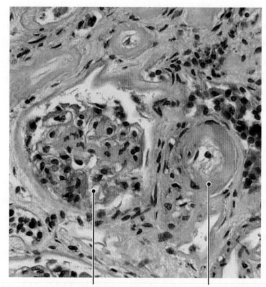

Atrophic glomerulus   Afferent arteriole with hyaline arteriolosclerosis

Figure 12-11 **Hyaline arteriolosclerosis.** In this lesion of benign nephrosclerosis, the waxy, red change in the afferent arteriole (hyaline arteriolosclerosis) and atrophy of the nearby glomerulus are characteristic.

CLINICAL ASPECTS OF HYPERTENSION

Definitions of hypertension vary somewhat, but for this discussion hypertension will be defined as systolic blood pressure 140 mm Hg or greater, or diastolic blood pressure 90 mm Hg or greater (Table 12-1). At least one fourth of Americans are hypertensive; some estimates put the figure closer to half. African Americans are affected much more frequently than are Caucasians. Because of their blood estrogen levels, women are less frequently affected than men are, but after menopause vascular disease increases as blood estrogen levels fall. In addition to race and gender, other factors that accentuate the ill effect of hypertension are smoking, diabetes, and obesity. However, these epidemiologic characteristics offer little help in an individual patient: the cause of hypertension in most patients is unknown (essential hypertension). Even if a patient does not fit the 140/90 mm Hg criteria, every patient with blood pressure higher than normal (130/85) deserves attention because even small, sustained increases in blood pressure are associated with increased incidence of hypertension-related disease.

The diagnosis of essential (primary) hypertension is a diagnosis of exclusion made after causes of secondary hypertension have been eliminated. Secondary hypertension may be caused by:

- *Pheochromocytoma of the adrenal medulla* (Chapter 18): Pheochromocytoma is a tumor of the adrenal medulla that increases peripheral resistance by secreting vasoconstrictive hormones such as epinephrine.
- *Tumor or hyperplasia of the adrenal cortex* (Chapter 18): Either tumor or hyperplasia may produce an excess of steroid hormones such as cortisol or aldosterone, which increase blood volume.
- *Renal disease*: Hypertension may result from almost any kind of kidney disease (Chapter 19). Of special interest is disease of renal arteries that impairs renal blood flow, because most of these lesions can be corrected surgically to cure the hypertension.

It is important to realize that *hypertension per se has no symptoms*—only the complications are symptomatic. Patients with hypertension die prematurely, usually from heart disease, but stroke and renal failure are also frequent. Severe hypertension may cause impaired vision subsequent to retinal disease (*hypertensive retinopathy*, Chapter 25) or may cause seizure when intracranial blood pressure (*hypertensive encephalopathy*, Chapter 23) is increased.

Accelerated hypertension (**malignant hypertension**) is a state of relentlessly progressive increase of blood pressure, which evolves from less severe hypertension.

The presence of hypertension year after year tends to damage blood vessels in the kidney and elsewhere. As kidney vessels are damaged, renal blood flow diminishes, and the kidney secretes additional renin to increase blood pressure in order to force more blood through the kidney. Finally, this feedback mechanism becomes a vicious circle, and blood pressure rises dramatically. Malignant hypertension cannot be defined solely by blood pressure measurements, but it is seldom evident at pressures below 160/110 mm Hg.

Malignant hypertension is not simply severe hypertension. It is an especially aggressive form that feeds on itself and is uniformly and quickly fatal unless treated very aggressively. Malignant hypertension puts great strain on the heart—marked cardiac hypertrophy, accelerated coronary artery disease, and congestive heart failure are common consequences. Untreated malignant hypertension is characterized by brain edema, seizures, renal failure, and cardiac failure. Often massive intracranial hemorrhage is the terminal event. Modern hypertensive drugs control lesser degrees of hypertension so successfully that nowadays malignant hypertension is rare.

Laboratory findings in hypertension vary according to the cause and degree of renal involvement. Patients with essential hypertension may have no laboratory abnormalities. Study of blood renin levels is not helpful in most cases because levels may be normal, low, or high depending on the cause; however, measurement of blood renin levels can be useful in differential diagnosis of certain causes of secondary hypertension. Patients with significant nephrosclerosis may have blood or protein in the urine and increased blood urea nitrogen (BUN) and creatinine. Patients with adrenal tumors that secrete steroid hormones may have low blood potassium levels or increased levels of breakdown products of hormone metabolism that can be detected by analysis of urine collected over a 24-hour period.

Treatment of essential hypertension relies on dietary salt restriction and drug therapy. Treatment of secondary hypertension is specific to the cause—most cases can be corrected surgically if discovered and treated before hypertension has irreversibly damaged the kidneys.

Aneurysms and Dissections

An **aneurysm** is a localized dilation of an artery or heart chamber, usually owing to a weakness of the wall. Most are elongated swellings (*fusiform* aneurysms), but some are *saccular*, especially those of intracranial arteries (berry aneurysms, Chapter 23). The two most common causes of aneurysm are atherosclerosis and **cystic medial degeneration**, a degenerative condition of the vascular wall. Both conditions weaken the wall, which balloons outward owing to intravascular pressure. Rarely, an aneurysm may be the result of local infection (mycotic aneurysm), late stage syphilis (*syphilitic aneurysm,* Chapter 20), or congenital defect, or it may occur consequent to aortic injury from frontal chest trauma, as in a steering wheel injury in an auto accident.

The abdominal aorta is the most common site of an atherosclerotic aneurysm (Fig. 12-12). Abdominal aortic aneurysms usually occur below the renal arteries in men over age 50 who have severe aortic atherosclerosis. Most abdominal aortic aneurysms grow slowly, a few millimeters each year, and they become more dangerous as they enlarge. The most feared complication is rupture, because it is often fatal. More commonly, however, abdominal aortic aneurysms develop thrombi on the internal wall (mural thrombi), which may embolize into the arteries of the legs or intestines, where they can produce ischemia or gangrene. Surgical replacement of the aneurysm by prosthesis is effective treatment.

A vascular *dissection* (**dissecting hematoma**) is a longitudinal tearing within the wall of an artery, most often the aorta, caused by blood that enters the wall through a defect in the lining, usually a tear or ulceration of an atheroma, which allows blood to pulse into the wall and progress (dissect) along tissue planes in the wall until it reenters the main channel downstream (rare) or exits externally (ruptures) with catastrophic hemorrhage. It usually affects older men with hypertension, some of

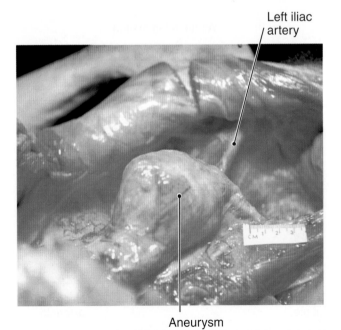

Figure 12-12 **Abdominal aortic aneurysm.** This photo was taken from above the right shoulder of the supine corpse.

whom have cystic medial necrosis, which allows blood to break into the wall.

Vasculitis

Vasculitis is a general term that applies to a group of uncommon diseases that feature inflammation of blood vessels, especially arteries. When small vessels are involved it may be called angiitis; when large arteries are involved it may be called *arteritis*. Several syndromes are recognized, each characterized and named according to its distinctive features, which include pathologic mechanism (autoimmune, infective), tissue most severely affected (nose and sinuses, kidneys, aorta), and the size and type (large or small, artery or vein) of blood vessel. For example, *polyarteritis nodosa* is a generalized autoimmune disease of small arteries that can affect almost any tissue, and *Wegener granulomatosis* is a vasculitis of unknown cause that mainly affects the nose, sinuses, lungs, and kidneys. Substantial clinical and pathologic overlap exists among the various types of vasculitis.

Most vasculitis is of autoimmune origin and almost always involves arteries; veins are rarely affected. Vessels of any size may be involved, from isolated involvement of the aorta to systemic disease of small arterioles.

Vasculitis of *small vessels* is usually **necrotizing vasculitis** (Fig. 12-13): vasculitis with acute inflammation

so intense that the vessel dies (undergoes necrosis). Other vasculitides feature chronic, granulomatous inflammation (Chapter 3). Vasculitis can affect any organ and may cause aneurysm, stroke, renal disease, peripheral vascular insufficiency and gangrene, and DIC (Chapter 11).

Polyarteritis nodosa (Chapter 8) is a distinctive clinical syndrome featuring autoimmune vasculitis of small to medium-size vessels. It usually affects middle-aged adults and causes ischemia and infarcts of downstream tissue. The kidneys are most severely affected but almost any organ may be involved. An example of *large vessel* vasculitis is **Takayasu arteritis**, which is characterized by granulomatous inflammation in the aorta and its main branches. It occurs mainly in women under 40 and results in scarring of the aortic arch and fibrous obliteration of the main branches, which impairs blood flow to the head and arms.

Whereas most *types* of vasculitis are systemic, the most common vasculitis is a local vasculitis—**temporal arteritis** (also called *giant cell arteritis*), characterized by chronic inflammation of the temporal and cranial arteries, including the carotids and ophthalmic arteries. Average age at onset is about 70 years. It usually affects older women, producing headache, scalp tenderness, and stroke or blindness owing to involvement of cerebral or retinal arteries. About 25% of cases occur in conjunction with a polymyalgia rheumatica (Chapter 22).

Thromboangiitis obliterans (Buerger disease) affects small vessels in the hands and feet. It is most common in young cigarette smokers and frequently leads to painful ulcers or gangrene of the fingers and toes. Early cessation of smoking may halt the disease.

Raynaud Phenomenon

Raynaud phenomenon is a common condition, usually of the hands and fingers, but the feet, ears, or nose may be involved. In Raynaud phenomenon small blood vessels exhibit exaggeration of normal vasoconstriction and vasodilation (vasomotor) reactivity to cold or emotional stress. No pathologic lesion is present; that is, the condition is purely functional. Women are affected far more often than men are. Typically one or more fingers blanches at the tip when exposed to cold, after which the fingers may then turn blue (cyanotic). The part may become numb, but pain is uncommon. When rewarmed the part become flushed with blood (hyperemic). Raynaud phenomenon may occur in conjunction with autoimmune diseases (Chapter 8). For example, 80% of patients with systemic sclerosis and 20% with systemic

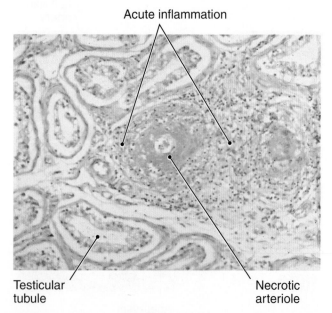

Acute inflammation

Testicular tubule

Necrotic arteriole

Figure 12-13 **Acute necrotizing vasculitis.** This specimen is from a testicular biopsy in a patient with polyarteritis nodosa. The biopsy was performed to confirm a provisional clinical diagnosis.

lupus have Raynaud phenomenon. However, the great majority of patients with Raynaud phenomenon have no underlying disease.

Diseases of Veins

A **varicosity** is an abnormally dilated vein (a **varicose vein**). *Superficial* veins are more often affected than deep ones because they are surrounded by less supporting tissue. Leg veins are most susceptible—hydrostatic pressure (Chapter 5) is greatest there because the column of blood is tallest between the lower leg and the heart. People most affected are those over 50, those who are obese or who must stand for long periods of time, and women, particularly those who have had several pregnancies. Ordinarily, leg varicosities are nothing more than an unsightly nuisance. However, with time, the internal valves of veins, which ordinarily prevent downward backflow and backpressure, become incompetent. As dilation progresses, the column of blood above the varicosity puts more hydrostatic pressure on the vein wall. The most common result is edema of the feet (pedal edema); however, in severe cases blood stagnates and flow is insufficient to maintain proper tissue oxygen supply, which results in skin atrophy and inflammation (**stasis dermatitis**, Chapter 24). In exceptionally severe cases skin ulcers may occur.

Hemorrhoids are varicose veins of the anus and deserve mention because they drain into the portal system and may be seen in conjunction with cirrhosis of the liver and portal venous hypertension (Chapter 16). Varicose veins of the esophageal mucosa (**esophageal varices**) also occur with cirrhosis for the same reason and can rupture and cause fatal gastrointestinal bleeding.

Thrombophlebitis (also called phlebothrombosis), the formation of venous thrombi (Chapter 5), may be accompanied by inflammation of the vein. The *deep* veins of the legs account for 90% of thrombophlebitis; superficial varicose veins are less frequently involved. Any condition that causes increased venous pressure or sluggish blood flow can cause thrombi (Chapter 5) to form, including pregnancy, heart failure, obesity, and prolonged bed rest—patients bedfast from surgery—burns, broken bones or other illness are especially vulnerable. Sometimes thrombophlebitis may be a paraneoplastic syndrome (Chapter 6) that is the first clue to an undiagnosed internal malignancy. Venous thrombi in the legs usually arise silently and can grow up to two feet long without producing clinical signs or symptoms. Not infrequently thrombi break loose and embolize to the lungs, where they may cause infarcts or, if very large, instantaneous death by complete occlusion of the pulmonary artery (Chapter 14).

Tumors of Blood and Lymphatic Vessels

Tumors of blood vessels (**hemangiomas**) or lymphatics (**lymphangiomas**) may occur anywhere in the body, usually in soft tissue. It is difficult to say with certainty if hemangiomas and lymphangiomas are neoplasms, as the names suggest, or hamartomas (Chapter 6), which are abnormal but non-neoplastic accumulations of tissue. Hemangiomas are the more common of the two and usually are found in skin as small, red, blood-filled lesions composed of capillary-size blood vessels (*capillary hemangioma*). Less commonly some are composed of larger vessels (*cavernous hemangioma*) and tend to occur in deeper tissue, such as the brain and liver. Hemangiomas become malignant only very rarely. Lymphangiomas are similar but less common and usually are found in the subcutaneous tissues of the head and neck.

Kaposi sarcoma is a malignant vascular tumor caused by an uncommon type of herpesvirus infection in patients who are immunodeficient (Chapter 8) or are being treated with immunosuppressive drugs. In the United States and Central Africa almost all cases occur in patients with AIDS. In the United States, Kaposi sarcoma is the most common AIDS-associated neoplasm and is a slow-growing tumor that first appears as small, purplish skin lesions in patients with AIDS. For reasons not entirely clear, most United States cases occur in homosexual males with AIDS, but not in other groups of AIDS patients. The number of new cases in the United States has been dramatically reduced by use of anti-HIV drugs. In Central Africa most cases occur in lymph nodes and the tumor is much more aggressive; it is the most common malignant tumor of men in Central Africa.

Angiosarcoma is a rare malignant tumor of vascular endothelial cells that can occur in almost any part of the body. Some occur after irradiation or prolonged exposure to certain chemicals; others arise in areas of chronic lymphedema. ■

CASE STUDY 12.1 *A MAN FOUND DEAD IN HIS OFFICE*

TOPICS
Hypertension
Stroke
Patient compliance with health care
directions

THE CASE

Setting: You are a Field Investigator for the medical examiner's office in a large metropolitan area.

History: You are assigned the case of Leon F., a 52-year-old African-American real estate executive found dead in his office late at night by the cleaning crew. The police report says the deceased was found on the floor beside his desk with a small amount dried blood around a superficial scalp laceration. There was no sign of forced entry or theft.

His family provides you with the name of his physician, who faxes you a lengthy medical record and in a follow-up telephone call tells you he has been treating Mr. F. for five years for hypertension that was difficult to control. The patient's first visit the physician's office was to seek treatment for gastroenteritis, which resolved promptly, but his blood pressure was recorded at 145/91, and he was advised to return for further studies. On the follow-up visit his blood pressure was 146/96. Laboratory and radiographic studies showed no evidence of renal or endocrine disease. The chart records his diagnosis as "essential hypertension." He was put on drug therapy and salt restriction and was advised to stop smoking.

The chart records irregular office visits over the next few years and apparent failure to have his prescriptions refilled despite documented notices that he should return to the office regularly for monitoring and medication adjustment. One entry indicates the patient cut down on cigarettes but was never able to quit except for brief intervals. The last note in the physician's records was 2 years earlier. Records from that visit include an electrocardiogram that revealed evidence of mild left ventricular enlargement, beside which was scribbled "hypertension!" Slight impairment of kidney function was suggested by increased plasma levels of metabolic waste to be excreted by the kidney (creatinine and BUN). Plasma potassium and other electrolytes were normal. On that last visit the physician refilled Mr. F.'s hypertension prescriptions and referred him to a hypertension specialist at the local medical school. As the conversation ends, the physician tells you he does not know if Mr. F. kept his appointment with the hypertension specialist.

You conclude that Mr. F. probably died of natural causes but are not certain enough to recommend the investigation stop without an autopsy. You consult with the medical examiner, who agrees with you and approves an autopsy.

Autopsy findings: Major findings are confined to the cardiovascular system, kidneys, and brain. The adrenal glands are unremarkable, and no tumors are found in any organ. The left ventricle is very large, and there is severe coronary atherosclerosis, with 90% narrowing of the anterior descending coronary artery. A 3 x 3 x 1 cm fibrous scar is present in the anterior wall of the left ventricle. The kidneys are small and granular. The renal arteries are mildly atherosclerotic and show no evidence of significant obstruction. No renal hemorrhages are present. The scalp laceration is superficial and associated with mild scalp hemorrhage. The skull is not fractured. In the midbrain and basal ganglia is a 6 cm hematoma that ruptured into the left lateral ventricle, filling it with blood. Microscopic studies are unremarkable except in the kidney, where there is severe nephrosclerosis.

DISCUSSION

The scalp wound was not severe, and no skull fracture was present, which rules out the possibility of foul play. It is reasonable to conclude that Mr. F. hit his head as he collapsed from intracranial bleeding.

This case is an object lesson in the pathogenesis of hypertension and the consequences associated with it, proving that mild or moderate hypertension is a serious disease. First, the patient was clearly hypertensive—his diastolic pressure was consistently over 90 mm Hg. Second, he was African-American and male, which put him especially at risk—men are more often hypertensive than women are; and African-Americans are more often hypertensive than other Americans are and suffer more serious consequences from it. Third, he was a smoker, which added to the vascular risk. Fourth, he did not take his medicine regularly and did not return for regular follow-up care as recommended, nor did he apparently keep his appointment with the hypertension specialist, which illustrates the problem of patient non-compliance. Patients who do not take their medicine regularly, or at all, are a major problem in health care. Most problematic are those patients who are on drugs that have no immediate, detectable effect on the way the patient feels, which is often the case for anti-hypertensive and cholesterol-lowering drugs. Even former President Clinton stopped taking the statin drug prescribed for him before he had a heart attack in 2004.

This patient's initial workup revealed no evidence of any underlying disease to account for the hypertension, and none was found at autopsy. The enlarged left ventricle suggested the hypertension continued, and the small myocardial scar was evidence of a small, perhaps asymptomatic, heart attack, probably in the 2 years after he was last seen in his physician's office. The kidneys showed severe nephrosclerosis consistent with a long history of hypertension and mildly abnormal renal function tests (increased BUN and creatinine).

Patients with hypertension die prematurely, often from stroke, and this proved true in this case. Mr. F. died ▶

[Case 12-1, continued] suddenly and at a relatively early age from an acute, spontaneous intracerebral hemorrhage, a common site for hypertension-related brain hemorrhage.

POINTS TO REMEMBER

- African-Americans are more often hypertensive than other Americans are; and the hypertension is often more severe.

- Failure of patients to follow medical advice or to take the medicine prescribed for them is a major cause of therapeutic failures.
- Hypertension accelerates atherosclerosis, which causes heart attacks and strokes.
- Stroke is a major cause of death in patients with hypertension.

CASE STUDY 12-1 THE ROAD NOT TAKEN—AN ALTERNATIVE SCENARIO

For all sad words of tongue or pen,
The saddest are these: "It might have been."
JOHN GREENLEAF WHITTIER (1807–1892),
AMERICAN QUAKER POET AND REFORMER, *MAUD MULLER*

THE CASE

With a bit of imagination, we can speculate how Leon F.'s case might have had a happier ending.

Setting: You work in the office of an academic physician who specializes in the treatment of hypertension that other physicians have found difficult to control. Your job is to interview the patients and collect and condense their often lengthy, detailed medical records; many of them have been in the care of myriad physicians and on complex combinations of drugs.

History: Mr. F., a 48-year-old African American real estate executive, is referred by his primary physician because of uncontrollable hypertension. Mr. F. has been treated with a variety of drugs with little or no success and lately has been complaining of vague chest pains. You also learn that he smokes.

Physical examination and other data: Mr. F. is overweight but not obese (BMI 28: weight 195 lb, height 5'10"), and his blood pressure is 148/95. The remainder of the physical examination is unremarkable. A battery of laboratory tests is also unremarkable except for kidney function tests that suggest his kidneys are beginning to be affected by his high blood pressure and are not excreting waste products as well as they should (BUN and creatinine level are mildly elevated).

Clinical course: The physician invites you to stay in the room during her interview with the patient. The physician asks a few questions to confirm the information you have accumulated and then says to the patient. "Sir, there's a lot going on here. You have high blood pressure. It's clearly affecting your heart and kidneys and it's probably responsible for the chest pain you are having. You're overweight and you smoke. And you haven't been good about taking your medicine or keeping your doctor's appointments. You are going to get into very deep trouble if you don't follow directions and take your medicine. In this situation there is no such thing as magic in a bottle. The prescription is as simple as it is difficult: you need to lose weight, start exercising and stop smoking."

Mr. F. nods, grinning sheepishly and says, "Yes, ma'am. I understand. I hate to admit it, but until I got these chest pains, I didn't really take this high blood pressure very seriously. You know, I felt good."

The physician continues, "Yes, sir. I understand, too. However, I presume you are here because you want to deal with these problems, but not even I can help you if you don't help yourself. First, we've got to study your heart to see if it's the cause of your chest pain. In the meantime, we'll be trying some different medicines to control your blood pressure. But most important, all of this isn't going to do much good unless you're willing to change your habits. It's a tough hill to climb, but if you get on board with the program I have in mind for you, we're going to do you a world of good."

Mr. F. smiles ruefully. "Yes, ma'am," he says. "You sound a lot like my wife; she's been hassling me to lose weight and quit smoking since the day we were married. But these chest pains got my attention. The other doctors weren't so direct and emphatic as you have been. I wish somebody had said this to me in these terms years ago. The way you put it, I don't seem to leave me much choice. I've learned my lesson. Sign me up."

Investigation of Mr. F.'s heart reveals moderate coronary atherosclerosis with marked narrowing of one artery too small to warrant catheterization but probably accounting for his chest pain. He is placed on statin drug therapy, which lowers his cholesterol to desirable levels, and his blood pressure is controlled by antihypertensive drugs. Over the next 2 years you see Mr. F. regularly and marvel at his progress. He does not have any more chest pain, he joined a health club, exercises regularly, has lost weight, and has quite smoking. He never misses an office appointment and takes his medicines exactly according to instructions. On his last office visit his blood pressure was 135/83, and he tells you proudly that he is training for a 100-mile bicycle race.

DISCUSSION

The best medical outcomes are achieved by a motivated patient and diligent care by an experienced practitioner. Mr. F. was willing to change his ways and had the willpower to see it through; and he received expert medical advice and treatment. The combination produced a very desirable outcome.

Objectives Recap

1. *Describe the normal functions of endothelial cells*: They control diffusion of substances across the vascular wall into adjacent tissues, and they maintain blood in a smooth, clot-free state.

2. *Classify plasma lipids*: Plasma lipids are classified in two major ways: chemically and by density. Chemically, plasma lipids are either cholesterol or triglyceride, and they circulate attached to a protein (the apoprotein) to form a lipoprotein. Lipoproteins are classified by density into high-density lipoprotein (HDL), low-density lipoprotein (LDL), and very-low-density lipoprotein (VLDL). Each type of lipoprotein contains varying amounts of cholesterol and triglyceride.

3. *Explain why "normal" is not a useful concept in study of plasma lipid levels*: The concept of "normal" is misleading because it is relies on the average cholesterol of presumably healthy people, and the average cholesterol in the United States is unhealthily high. "Desirable" is a better descriptor for healthy levels of plasma lipids.

4. *Explain the difference between atherosclerosis and arteriolosclerosis*: Atherosclerosis is a lifestyle disease of large and medium-size vessels characterized by fatty deposits in vascular walls. Arteriolosclerosis is a disease of small blood vessels mainly seen in diabetes and hypertension; no fatty deposits are involved.

5. *Name the pathologic processes important in the formation of an atheroma*: The important processes are: endothelial damage, lipid accumulation, inflammation, smooth muscle cell migration, and fibrosis.

6. *List the factors that predispose to atherosclerosis, and name some indicators of risk*: Smoking, obesity, lack of exercise, and high-salt, high-fat diets.

7. *Name the most important clinical complications of atherosclerosis*: myocardial infarct, stroke, aneurysm, and peripheral vascular disease.

8. *Discuss the pathologic differences between young and old atheromas*: Young atheromas are danger-ous because they tend to be fatty, soft, and unstable. They are prone to ulceration, hemorrhage, and thrombosis. Old atheromas are fibrotic, hard, and sometimes calcified. They are less dangerous and are stable and may cause downstream ischemia, but they are not prone to thrombosis and sudden occlusion.

9. *Name the two main components that determine blood pressure*: Peripheral resistance and cardiac output.

10. *Name and define the two major types of hypertension*: Essential (primary) hypertension is not associated with any identifiable underlying causative condition. Secondary hypertension is hypertension related to a specific underlying condition.

11. *Name the characteristic kidney findings in hypertension*: Benign nephrosclerosis with hyaline arteriolosclerosis.

12. *Give a clinical definition of hypertension*: Sustained diastolic blood pressure of 90 mm Hg or greater; or sustained systolic pressure of 140 mm Hg or greater.

13. *Name the cause of most aneurysms*: Atherosclerosis, which weakens the vascular wall and allows the affected vessel to dilate.

14. *Name the most common basic mechanism of vasculitis*: Autoimmunity.

15. *Briefly explain Raynaud phenomenon*: It is an exaggeration of normal vasoconstriction and vasodilation reaction to cold or stress manifest by blanching and later cyanosis; it usually appears in the fingers.

16. *Explain the clinical importance of thrombophlebitis*: Thrombophlebitis is a combination of venous thrombosis and vein inflammation. It is a common condition that usually occurs in deep leg veins. Thrombi of any size can embolize. Most travel to the lungs, where they lodge and obstruct pulmonary artery blood flow and can cause lung infarction. A large embolic thrombus can completely occlude the pulmonary artery and cause sudden death.

Typical Test Questions

1. Which one of the following is associated with increased risk of atherosclerosis?
   A. HDL cholesterol <40 mg/dL
   B. LDL cholesterol <100 mg/dL
   C. VLDL cholesterol <30 mg/dL
   D. Triglyceride <150 mg/dL

2. Which one of the following is the site of the initial arterial injury in atherosclerosis?
   A. Endothelial cell
   B. Basement membrane
   C. Muscular wall (media)
   D. Adventitia

3. Which one of the following is the lowest pressure that qualifies as stage 3 (severe) hypertension?
   A. Blood pressure 135/85 mm Hg
   B. Blood pressure 175/105 mm Hg
   C. Blood pressure 185/110 mm Hg
   D. Blood pressure 205/125 mm Hg

4. Which one of the following explains most aneurysms?
   A. Cystic medial necrosis of the wall of the aorta
   B. Atherosclerotic weakening of the vascular wall
   C. Anatomic weakness in the wall of arteries at a branching point
   D. Vasculitis of large arteries

5. Which one of the following is true about thrombophlebitis?
   A. Most instances occur in varicose veins
   B. Most instances occur in the anus and esophagus
   C. Most instances occur in small superficial veins of the legs
   D. Most instances occur in deep veins of the legs

6. True or false? Blood pressure is determined mainly by heart rate.

7. True or false? The innermost part of a blood vessel is the basement membrane.

8. True or false? Plasma lipids circulate attached to C-reactive protein.

9. True or false? Atherosclerosis begins around age 30.

10. True or false? Most aneurysms occur in the abdominal aorta.

Diseases of the Heart

This chapter opens with a review of normal cardiac anatomy and cardiopulmonary blood flow and continues with detailed coverage of major heart diseases. It includes discussions of coronary artery disease, valvular disease, congestive heart failure, congenital heart disease, and other disorders.

BACK TO BASICS
- The Normal Heart
- The Coronary Circulation
- The Cardiac Cycle

ARRHYTHMIAS

CONGESTIVE HEART FAILURE
- Pathophysiology
- Etiology
- Clinical Features

ISCHEMIC HEART DISEASE (CORONARY ARTERY DISEASE)
- Epidemiology of Ischemic Heart Disease
- Causes of Coronary Ischemia
- Angina Pectoris
- Myocardial Infarction
- Chronic Myocardial Ischemia
- Sudden Cardiac Death

HYPERTENSIVE HEART DISEASE

VALVULAR HEART DISEASE
- Rheumatic Heart Disease
- Calcific Aortic Stenosis
- Myxomatous Degeneration of the Mitral Valve

ENDOCARDITIS
- Nonbacterial Thrombotic Endocarditis
- Infective Endocarditis

PRIMARY MYOCARDIAL DISEASES
- Myocarditis
- Cardiomyopathies

CONGENITAL HEART DISEASE
- Malformations with Shunts
- Malformations with Obstruction to Flow

PERICARDIAL DISEASE

Learning Objectives

After studying this chapter you should be able to:

1. Discuss why cardiac arrhythmias decrease cardiac output
2. Define heart failure
3. Explain the Frank-Starling curve and its importance
4. Explain the difference between forward and backward heart failure
5. Explain why and how renin is involved in heart failure
6. Contrast the clinical findings and symptoms of right-heart failure and left-heart failure
7. Name the syndromes of ischemic heart disease
8. Explain why young atheromas are more dangerous than older ones are
9. Explain why prompt intervention may limit the size of an infarct
10. List some complications of myocardial infarct
11. Contrast the symptoms of myocardial infarct and angina
12. Explain the usefulness of cardiac creatine kinase (CK-MB) and cardiac troponin assays in the assessment of chest pain
13. Discuss effects on the heart of chronic hypertension
14. Explain the difference between valvular stenosis and valvular insufficiency
15. Briefly explain the pathogenesis of acute rheumatic fever and rheumatic heart disease

16. Explain the difference between infective endocarditis and nonbacterial endocarditis and know the hazards associated with each
17. Define primary cardiomyopathy and offer several examples
18. Explain why congenital cardiac malformations with left-to-right shunts can cause pulmonary hypertension and late cyanosis

Key Terms and Concepts

BACK TO BASICS
- atrium
- ventricle
- cardiac valve
- excitatory-conduction system
- systole
- diastole

ARRHYTHMIAS
- arrhythmia
- atrial fibrillation

CONGESTIVE HEART FAILURE
- congestive heart failure
- left-heart failure
- uncompensated failure
- right-heart failure

ISCHEMIC HEART DISEASE (CORONARY ARTERY DISEASE)
- ischemic heart disease
- angina pectoris

- myocardial infarct
- coronary thrombosis
- cardiac troponin

VALVULAR HEART DISEASE
- valvular stenosis
- valvular insufficiency
- chronic rheumatic valvulitis
- calcific aortic stenosis
- myxomatous degeneration of the mitral valve

ENDOCARDITIS
- noninfective thrombotic endocarditis
- infective endocarditis

PRIMARY MYOCARDIAL DISEASES
- cardiomyopathy

CONGENITAL HEART DISEASE
- shunt
- coarctation of the aorta

. . . another supper from a sack,
a ninety-nine cent heart attack . . .

TIM MCGRAW (B. 1967), AMERICAN COUNTRY MUSIC SINGER AND ACTOR, *WHERE THE GREEN GRASS GROWS*

Would you please turn on the television? I'd like to see if I'm still alive and how I'm doing.

MURRAY HAYDON (1927–1986), THE WORLD'S THIRD ARTIFICIAL HEART RECIPIENT

BACK TO BASICS

Blood carries life's necessities to cells and returns waste products to organs for disposition. Blood is propelled through the vascular tree by the heart, a tireless bundle of muscle and a complex mechanical and electrical device whose normal function depends on flawless, perfectly timed, interlocked movement of its various parts.

THE NORMAL HEART

The **heart** sits behind the sternum, inside the **pericardial sac** (Fig. 13-1), a loose-fitting, lubricated membrane that allows free and frictionless contact with the **epicardium**, the transparent membrane on the heart surface.

As is illustrated in Figure 13-2, the heart is a pump; actually, it is two pumps, one after the other, although anatomically they sit side by side. The heart has four chambers: the **right** and **left atria**, which sit above the **right** and **left ventricles**. The right atrium, the right ventricle, and the left atrium are thin-walled, low-pressure pumps. Only the left ventricle is a high-pressure pump. The right atrium and right ventricle pump unoxygenated venous blood from the vena cava into the pulmonary artery, through the lungs, down the pulmonary

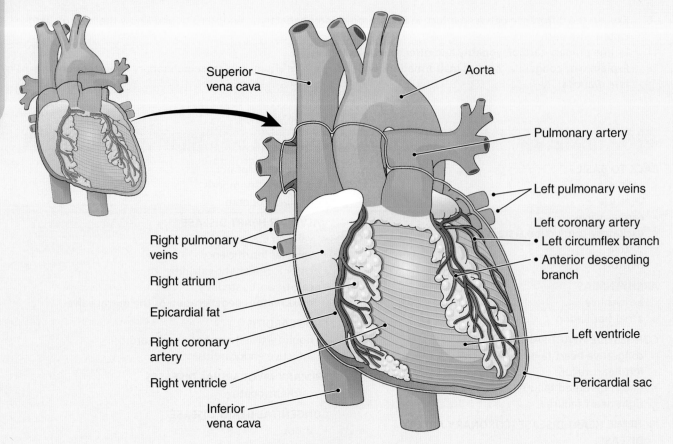

Superior vena cava

Aorta

Pulmonary artery

Left pulmonary veins

Left coronary artery
• **Left circumflex branch**
• **Anterior descending branch**

Right pulmonary veins

Right atrium

Epicardial fat

Right coronary artery

Right ventricle

Inferior vena cava

Left ventricle

Pericardial sac

Figure 13-1 **Normal heart, anterior view.**

veins, and into the left atrium. The robust, muscular left ventricle receives blood from the left atrium and pumps it into the high-pressure aorta.

As it travels through the heart, blood crosses one-way **cardiac valves**, which prevent backflow. Venous (unoxygenated) blood returning from the body flows into the right atrium, where the **tricuspid valve** allows one-way flow into the right ventricle. The **pulmonary valve** allows one-way flow from the right ventricle into the pulmonary artery for delivery to the lungs. Oxygenated blood from the lungs flows to the left atrium, where the **mitral valve** allows one-way flow to the left ventricle. The **aortic valve** allows one-way flow from the left ventricle into the aorta for delivery to the body.

The atria are separated from one another by a thin, fibrous membrane, the **interatrial septum**. The right and left ventricles are separated from one another by a thick muscular wall, the **interventricular septum**. All chambers are lined by a thin, cellular membrane, the **endocardium**, which is a continuation of the vascular endothelium, which lines blood vessels.

THE CORONARY CIRCULATION

The heart is nourished by blood from two coronary arteries, which originate from the root of the aorta behind the aortic valve cusps. The coronary arteries and their major branches travel on the outer surface (epicardium) of the heart, sending *penetrating branches* downward into the myocardium.

In most people the *right coronary artery* wraps around the right side of the heart along the upper edge of the right ventricle before turning downward along the posterior side of the interventricular septum. As it descends it is called the *posterior descending coronary artery*, and it supplies the right ventricle and the posterior aspect of the left ventricle. The *left coronary artery* branches immediately after leaving the aorta, sending the *anterior descending artery* down the anterior aspect of the interventricular septum to supply the anterior septum and left ventricle. The main left coronary continues as the *left circumflex coronary artery*, which wraps around the upper edge of the left ventricle to supply the anterior and lateral aspects of the left ventricle. Considerable varia-

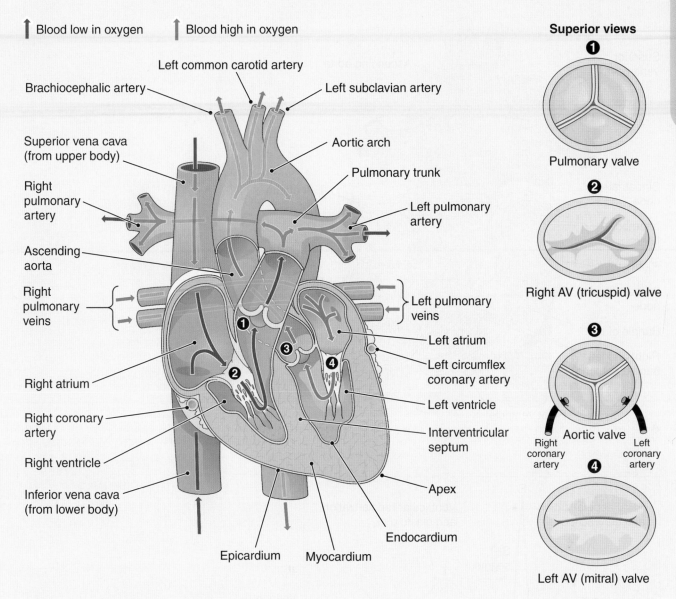

↑ Blood low in oxygen   ↑ Blood high in oxygen

Left common carotid artery

Brachiocephalic artery

Left subclavian artery

Superior vena cava (from upper body)

Aortic arch

Pulmonary trunk

Right pulmonary artery

Left pulmonary artery

Ascending aorta

Right pulmonary veins

Left pulmonary veins

Left atrium

Left circumflex coronary artery

Right atrium

Right coronary artery

Left ventricle

Right ventricle

Interventricular septum

Inferior vena cava (from lower body)

Apex

Endocardium

Epicardium   Myocardium

Superior views

❶ Pulmonary valve

❷ Right AV (tricuspid) valve

❸ Aortic valve
Right coronary artery   Left coronary artery

❹ Left AV (mitral) valve

Figure 13-2 **Cardiac chambers and valves.** Circled numbers on the cutaway of the heart show the location of the valves detailed on the right.

tion can occur in this pattern. Coronary blood returns via *coronary veins*, which gather on the posterior aspect of the heart in the *coronary sinus* before flowing into the right atrium.

THE CARDIAC CYCLE

Each normal beat of the heart is initiated by automatic discharge of an electrical signal from the heart's natural pacemaker in the right atrium, the **sinoatrial (SA) node**. This signal is carried as a wave of electrical stimulation by an **excitatory-conduction system** (Fig. 13-3) composed of specialized myocardial muscle fibers that

distribute the signal throughout the heart in a fraction of a second, causing muscular contraction as it goes. The atria are separated from the ventricles by a nonconductive, insulating fibrous collar that is shaped like a horizontal figure eight, to which the tricuspid and mitral valves are internally hinged (inside the loops of the figure eight, so to speak). In addition to supporting the valves, this collar electrically separates the atria and ventricles and prevents the atrial signal from spreading haphazardly to the ventricles.

After the signal passes down the right atrial wall, it passed through a second node, the **atrioventricular (AV) node**, which sits in the interatrial septum imme-

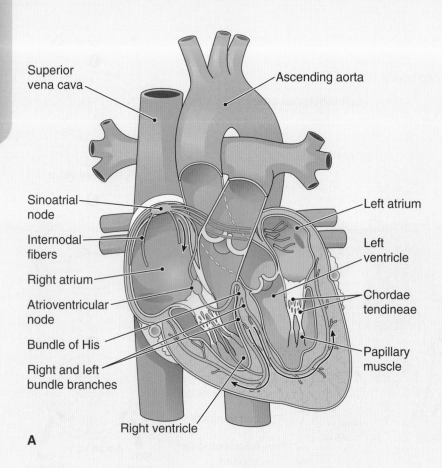

Superior vena cava

Ascending aorta

Sinoatrial node

Left atrium

Internodal fibers

Left ventricle

Right atrium

Atrioventricular node

Chordae tendineae

Bundle of His

Right and left bundle branches

Papillary muscle

Right ventricle

A

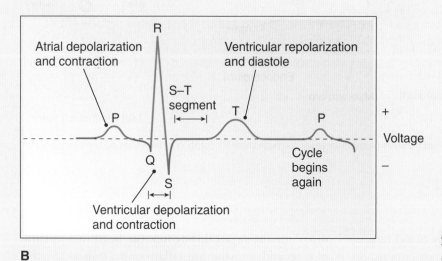

Atrial depolarization and contraction

Ventricular repolarization and diastole

R

S–T segment

P

T

P

+

Voltage

Q

Cycle begins again

−

S

Ventricular depolarization and contraction

B

Figure 13-3 **Electrical activity of the heart. A,** The cardiac excitatory-conduction system (ECS). **B,** Electrocardiogram of a normal cardiac cycle.

diately above the upper end of the interventricular septum. The AV node and other parts of the conduction system are capable of self-excitation at a slower rate than the SA node. If the SA node becomes ineffective or if the signal is blocked before reaching the AV node, the AV node takes over the pacemaker function, but at a

slower rate. After passing through the AV node, the signal passes through a thick bundle of conductive fibers, the **bundle of His**, which penetrates the insulating fibrous collar that separates the atria and ventricles.

Below the bundle of His the conduction system divides into right and left branches before continuing down either side of the interventricular system to the apex of the heart, where fibers first attach to cardiac muscle cells (the **myocardium**). This design causes ventricular contractions to begin at the apex of the heart, ensuring efficient emptying of the ventricle, much like squeezing toothpaste from the bottom of the tube. From the apex the remaining fibers turn upward and spread through the ventricular walls.

The cell membranes of cardiac muscle cells are electrically polarized. That is, they have an electric *action potential*—they are positively charged outside and negatively charged inside. Stimulation causes depolarization and muscle fiber contraction. Repolarization renews the action potential, readying the cell for another wave of depolarization and contraction. As the electrical wave travels through the heart, it causes heart muscle to depolarize, stimulating myocardial cells to contract and relax in sequence and pumping blood through heart chambers and lungs and out the aorta. Cardiac muscle stimulation, depolarization, and contraction occur very quickly and are called **systole**. Relaxation, repolarization, and dilation are called **diastole**. The atria contract together to deliver blood into the relaxed, diastolic ventricles. Immediately thereafter the ventricles contract together in systole to deliver blood to the lungs and body. Then the sequence is repeated. An electrocardiogram (Fig. 13-3B) is an electrical recording of these events.

Heart muscle is striated like skeletal muscle (Chapter 22), but with three significant differences:

- *Cardiac muscle cells are interconnected seamlessly to allow uninterrupted flow of electrical stimulation from cell to cell.* By contrast, skeletal muscle fibers are not electrically interconnected.
- *Cardiac muscle is self-stimulating*; that is, it is capable of automatically initiating contractile waves without outside stimulus; skeletal muscle cannot.
- *Cardiac fibers stay contracted for a few tenths of a second before repolarization.* This is an electrically quiet period in the heart, represented on the electrocardiogram by the S-T segment (Fig. 13-3B), which assures the entire chamber is contracted before any part of it is ready for restimulation, an effect that promotes electrical orderliness. By contrast, skeletal muscle repolarizes instantly.

An **electrocardiogram** is a record of the microvoltage transmitted to skin by each heartbeat. In Figure 13-3B is a typical tracing. Waves are named P, Q, R, S, and T. The P wave is atrial depolarization and contraction. Q, R, and S are ventricular depolarization and contraction. The S-T segment is the period of sustained ventricular depolarization, and the T wave is ventricular repolarization. Repolarization of the atrium is lost in the QRS wave and is not detectable.

MAJOR DETERMINANTS OF DISEASE

- Most heart disease is the result of atherosclerotic obstruction of the coronary arteries.
- Congestive heart failure is mechanical failure of the heart to eject blood delivered to it.
- Metabolic or autoimmune disease may cause heart muscle or valve damage.
- High blood pressure accelerates atherosclerosis and most other cardiac disease.
- Cardiac valves are one-way gates for blood flow and are susceptible to obstruction and regurgitation (incompetence).
- Cardiac valves are susceptible to infection.
- Abnormal embryonic development of the heart produces significant cardiac anatomic malformations.
- Abnormal heartbeat patterns (arrhythmias) can cause cardiac dysfunction or death and can complicate any heart condition.

Arrhythmias

An **arrhythmia**, sometimes called *dysrhythmia*, is an irregularity in the heart's beating pattern. Arrhythmias are mechanically inefficient because they interrupt the normal pattern of filling and emptying of the chambers. Cardiac output decreases because the left ventricle is forced to eject its volume before filling completely. Some arrhythmias are potentially fatal because they threaten complete electrical disorganization of the cardiac cycle, which can cause effective pumping to cease completely. Arrhythmias are caused by myocardial ischemia or myocardial infarct (discussed below), electrolyte imbalance (especially potassium imbalance), stress, caffeine, drugs (especially stimulants, Chapter 10), and congenital defects in the myocardial electrical network.

The regular pacing of the sinoatrial (SA) node in a resting patient is a normal cardiac rhythm and is about 70 beats per minute in most people. *Bradycardia* is a slower beat, usually less than 60/min, which may be normal in fit people, who have high stroke volume.

Tachycardia is a rapid heart rate, usually more than 100/min, but sometimes near 200/min. *Tachycardia is a normal response to work or stress.*

Extra atrial beats (*premature atrial contractions*) are common in healthy people and are not harmful. They are usually the result of stress, lack of sleep, the caffeine in coffee or tea, or drugs frequently associated with common over-the-counter cold medicines. However, patients may feel chest palpitations and become alarmed. Abnormalities in the right atrium can cause *atrial flutter*, a very rapid, organized, *regular* atrial rhythm near 300/min and a *regular* ventricular rate of about 150–200/min. **Atrial fibrillation** is a disorganized, *irregular* atrial rhythm that causes an irregular, rapid ventricular rate near 200/min. Many of the fibrillation signals are filtered out by atrioventricular node before they enter the ventricle to produce a systolic contraction, but enough signals pass to cause a rapid and irregular ventricular beating. This irregular, rapid beating is not efficient because some contractions occur before the left ventricle is maximally filled with blood. The net effect is a serious drop of cardiac output, and patients may complain of dizziness and fatigue. Long-term atrial fibrillation is associated with a risk for development of atrial thrombi, which can embolize to cause brain infarct (white stroke, Chapter 23) or other thromboembolic disease. Ventricular rates in atrial flutter and fibrillation are slower than atrial rates because some beat signals are blocked by the atrioventricular (AV) node.

> Each year heart disease accounts for one third of deaths in the United States, most of which are associated with coronary artery atherosclerosis. If cerebrovascular disease, vascular complications of diabetes, and other vascular diseases are included, the figure is over 40%. After age 40 the lifetime risk for developing symptomatic coronary artery disease is 50% in men and 40% in women.

If the atrial signal is delayed or cannot cross into the ventricle, the condition is called **heart block**. Anatomic abnormalities are a common cause of heart block. For example, a myocardial infarct may damage the conduction system and prevent signal transmission. Digitalis, a drug used in the treatment of congestive heart failure (discussed below), can also cause heart block. *First-degree* block is delay of the atrial signal, but not enough to cause the ventricle to miss beats. *Second-degree* block is delay long enough to cause missed ventricular beats. *Third-degree* block is total block of the atrial signal and is associated with very slow ventricular beating (bradycardia, about 40 beats/min) and marked decline of car-

diac output. Syncope (fainting), associated with third-degree block, is called a *Stokes-Adams seizure*. In some cases third-degree block is associated with ventricular standstill (asystole, cardiac arrest) and death.

Extra ventricular beats (*premature ventricular contractions*) occur in healthy people and are of no consequence unless they occur in patients with known heart disease. They may occur in short runs of 5–10 beats and create chest palpitations and patient anxiety. Rapid, spontaneous ventricular beating at speeds less than 100 beats/min is not associated with decreased cardiac output and usually does not require therapy. **Ventricular tachycardia** is spontaneous, *regular* ventricular beating at over 120/min and is associated with decreased cardiac output and demands treatment, especially if associated with underlying heart disease. Extremely rapid rates can cause fainting and require cardiac resuscitation. **Ventricular fibrillation** is extremely rapid and *irregular* ventricular activity that is associated with negligible cardiac output. It is a complication of myocardial ischemia or infarct and is always fatal unless converted back to normal rhythm by electric shock.

Congestive Heart Failure

Congestive heart failure (CHF) is a condition in which *the heart is unable to eject the volume of blood delivered to it* and becomes engorged with blood. CHF is the endpoint for most serious heart disease: coronary atherosclerosis, hypertension, valve disease, cardiomyopathy, and congenital cardiac malformation. It is a common and serious condition: it affects about 1% of Americans and is often difficult to treat. Half of patients with CHF die within five years.

PATHOPHYSIOLOGY

The most common cause of congestive failure is cardiac muscle damage, usually caused by coronary artery disease. Less common causes are valve defects that result in an *inefficient pumping stroke.* For example, in a patient with aortic stenosis the ventricle must work extra hard to force a normal amount of blood across the valve; or in a patient with aortic regurgitation, the ventricle must pump an extra amount of blood with each stroke in order to make up for the amount that leaks back in diastole.

Before failing, the heart compensates for muscle weakness or valve inefficiency in two ways: 1) sympathetic nervous stimulation and release of adrenal hormones (epinephrine, for example) to increase heart rate and the force of contraction; and 2) cardiac muscle hypertrophy. If these adaptations are unable to maintain cardiac output, then congestive failure occurs.

☞ Congestive Heart Failure

- **The heart is unable to eject the volume of blood delivered to it**
- **In left ventricular failure low cardiac output causes systemic hypoperfusion and pulmonary venous congestion**
- **In right ventricular failure low output causes systemic venous congestion**
- **The most common cause of right-heart failure is left-heart failure**
- **The most common cause of congestive heart failure is cardiac muscle damage from coronary artery ischemia**
- **The low cardiac output of left-heart failure reduces renal blood flow and stimulates the renin-angiotensin-aldosterone system to retain sodium and water.**

In congestive failure as each small increment of blood enters the ventricle but cannot be ejected, the failing ventricle dilates bit by bit as blood accumulates, and the ventricular wall stretches because it is gorged with too much blood. In accordance with the **Frank-Starling Law** (Fig. 13-4), the stretched myocardial muscle fibers react by contracting more forcefully, like a stretched spring pulls ever harder as it lengthens. The result is increased cardiac output. The ventricle regains its ability to eject the blood delivered to it, although the ventricle is dilated and working harder, a state known as **compensated heart failure**, which is clinically asymptomatic.

However, as Figure 13-4 illustrates, stretching muscle fibers works up to a certain point, beyond which further stretching results in weaker, not stronger, contractions—like a spring loses its power if stretched too far. Once fibers are stretched too far the force of contraction weakens, cardiac output falls, and the heart goes into **uncompensated failure**. Cardiac output falls, and blood "backs up" like water behind a dam. *The right and left ventricles can fail independently, but usually they fail together.* Moreover, there are two components of uncompensated failure: *forward failure* and *backward failure*—low ventricular output is the forward component of failure; venous congestion is the backward component.

In uncompensated left ventricular failure (**left-heart failure**) the left ventricle dilates (Fig. 13-5) as it overfills with blood. The forward component (lagging cardiac output) of left-side failure is associated with decreased blood flow to vital organs. The backward component is associated with engorgement of the left atrium, the pulmonary veins, and lungs, associated with increased pulmonary venous pressure that forces fluid into the alveoli, where it accumulates as **pulmonary**

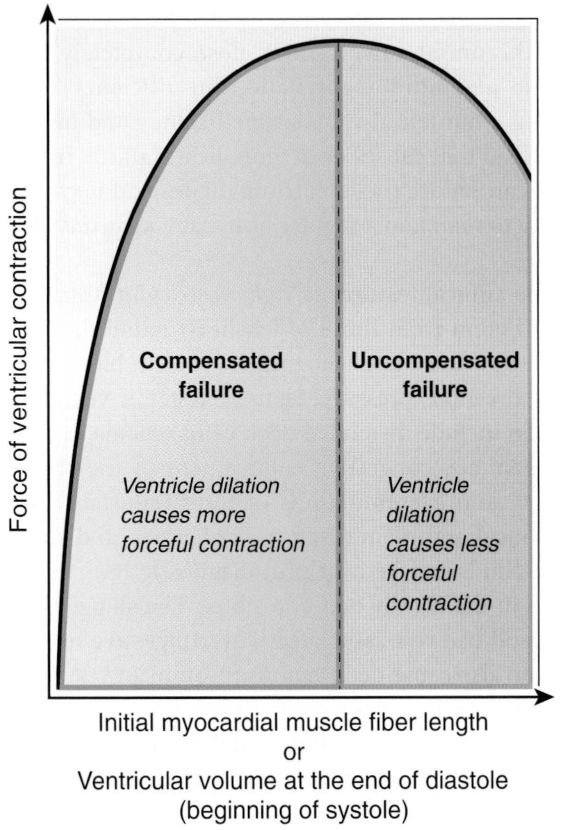

Force of ventricular contraction

Compensated failure	Uncompensated failure
Ventricle dilation causes more forceful contraction	*Ventricle dilation causes less forceful contraction*

Initial myocardial muscle fiber length
or
Ventricular volume at the end of diastole
(beginning of systole)

Figure 13-4 **The Frank-Starling curve.** Up to a point (the apex of the curve), cardiac myocytes contract with more force when stretched. Beyond that point, the fibers contract less forcefully.

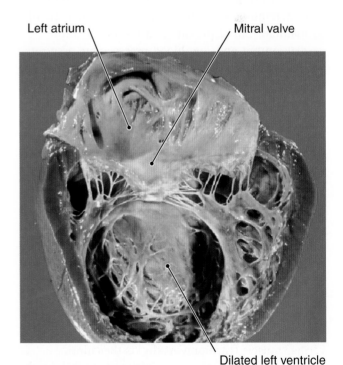

Left atrium   Mitral valve

Dilated left ventricle

Figure 13-5 **Left-heart failure.** The left ventricle is markedly dilated.

edema, accounting for the breathlessness (*dyspnea*) of left-heart failure.

In uncompensated right ventricular failure (**right-heart failure**) the right ventricle dilates (Fig. 13-5) as it overfills with blood. The forward component (lagging cardiac output) of left-side failure is associated with decreased blood flow to the lungs. The backward component is associated with engorgement of the systemic venous circulation, which is associated with enlargement of the liver and spleen as they become overfilled with blood. Increased venous hydrostatic pressure (Chapter 5) forces fluid into tissues and body spaces, where it accumulates as edema of the feet and legs, ascites, and pleural effusion. Pure right-heart failure is uncommon and is usually associated with pulmonary hypertension resulting from lung or pulmonary vascular diseases, a combination known as **cor pulmonale** (Chapter 14). *The most common cause of right-heart failure is left-heart failure*—the failing *left* ventricle leaves pulmonary blood vessels so gorged with blood that the right ventricle cannot force more blood into them.

The **renin-angiotensin-aldosterone system** is also important in the pathogenesis of heart failure. In normal circumstances this system is designed to regulate blood volume and blood pressure (Chapter 12). For example, with serious hemorrhage cardiac output and blood pressure fall, and less blood flows to the kidneys, which stimulates increased secretion of renin and production of more aldosterone by the adrenal cortex. Increased aldosterone production causes sodium and water retention, which increases blood volume in order to maintain blood pressure. In left-heart failure, low cardiac output and low blood pressure are associated with decreased renal blood flow, causing an outpouring of renin and aldosterone and creating a vicious circle: increased fluid retention and expanded blood volume add burden to the failing chamber and worsen the failure. It is from the understanding of these dynamics that drug therapy of CHF is derived. Sodium (salt) restriction and diuretics both reduce blood sodium and blood volume.

ETIOLOGY

The most common cause of *left-heart failure* is damaged cardiac muscle, usually associated with coronary atherosclerosis with ischemia or infarction. Left-heart failure can also be caused by the excess strain of high blood pressure (hypertension, Chapter 12) or aortic or mitral valve disease. Much less commonly, primary disease of cardiac muscle (cardiomyopathy) is the culprit.

Pulmonary hypertension (Chapter 14) can have the same effect on the right ventricle and produce *right-heart failure*. The most common cause of right-heart failure is left-heart failure, but right-heart failure also may be caused by lung disease or tricuspid or pulmonary valve disease. In addition, in some cases of congenital heart disease blood is shunted from the high-pressure left side to the low-pressure right side, which is not equipped to handle the increased load. The volume overload and transmitted pressure from the left side combine to produce failure of the right ventricle.

CLINICAL FEATURES

Congestive heart failure has a widespread ill effect on the body (Fig. 13-6). One of the most prominent clinical features of *left-heart failure* is breathlessness (dyspnea). It is most noticeable when the patient is physically active (exertional dyspnea) or lying down (orthopnea). Chest x-ray typically reveals prominent pulmonary veins (owing to congestion) and an enlarged cardiac silhouette (owing to ventricular dilation). Patients also typically have rapid heart rate, because the heart tries to sustain cardiac output by beating more rapidly. Pulmonary edema, when present, can be detected by hearing fine *rales* (wet, tissue-paper, crinkling sounds) in the lung bases.

With severe *left-heart failure* the left ventricle becomes so dilated (the cardiac wall is pushed so far out) that the mitral valve cannot close completely during systole, and mitral regurgitation (insufficiency) occurs, adding a burden of valvular inefficiency and increased workload that causes even more heart failure. In severe left-heart failure the left atrium dilates and may lose its ability to maintain a regular beat, causing *atrial fibrillation*.

The clinical features of *right ventricular heart failure* are different from those of left-heart failure but derive from the same cause—engorgement with blood and increased venous pressure. Signs of systemic venous congestion include distended neck veins, edema in the feet and genitals, congestive enlargement of the liver and spleen, and accumulations of fluid (*effusions*) in the peritoneal and pleural spaces. Collection and study of these fluids can be a helpful diagnostic tool, as is detailed in the nearby Lab Tools box. The sluggish blood flow and bed rest associated with congestive heart failure can also cause deep venous thrombi and pulmonary embolism (Chapter 5).

Left-heart failure is often fatal because it produces hypoxia, acidosis, and cardiac arrhythmias. *Hypoxia* arises because cardiac output is not sufficient to meet the demands of tissues, and because pulmonary edema interferes with oxygenation of blood in the lungs. *Acidosis* occurs secondary to impairment of CO_2 dis-

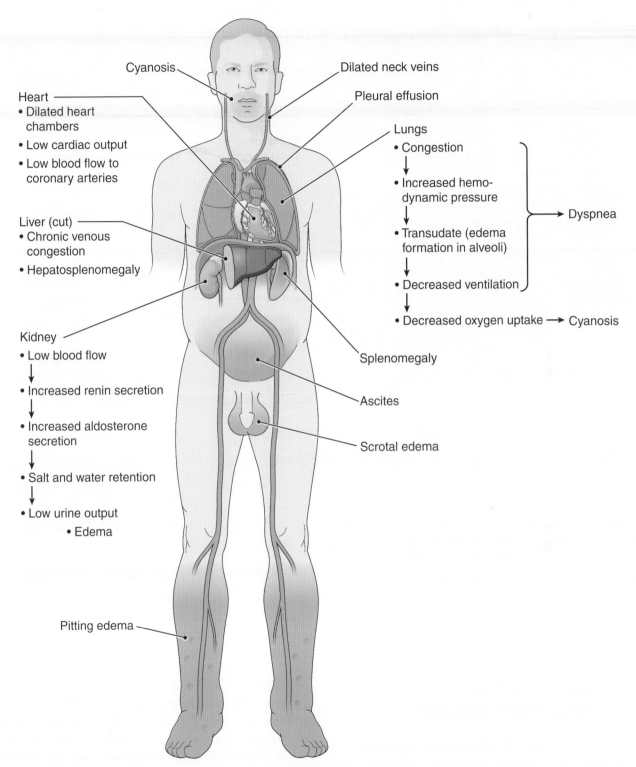

Cyanosis

Dilated neck veins

Pleural effusion

Heart
- Dilated heart
  chambers
- Low cardiac output
- Low blood flow to
  coronary arteries

Lungs
- Congestion
  ↓
- Increased hemo-
  dynamic pressure
  ↓
- Transudate (edema
  formation in alveoli)
  ↓
- Decreased ventilation

→ Dyspnea

- Decreased oxygen uptake → Cyanosis

Liver (cut)
- Chronic venous
  congestion
- Hepatosplenomegaly

Splenomegaly

Kidney
- Low blood flow
  ↓
- Increased renin secretion
  ↓
- Increased aldosterone
  secretion
  ↓
- Salt and water retention
  ↓
- Low urine output
    - Edema

Ascites

Scrotal edema

Pitting edema

Figure 13-6 Clinical findings in congestive heart failure. Left-heart failure (low cardiac output, forward failure) is associated with water retention and general edema, ascites and other effusions, pulmonary congestion and edema, dyspnea, poor ventilation, poor oxygen uptake, and cyanosis. Right-heart failure (backward failure) is associated with systemic venous congestion, peripheral edema, and hepatosplenomegaly.

Pleural and Peritoneal Effusions

Patients with congestive heart failure frequently have pleural or peritoneal effusions, which also may be caused by other conditions such as malignancy or inflammation. Laboratory studies are helpful in the differential diagnosis of the cause of an effusion.

Recall from Chapter 5 that effusions resulting from osmotic or hemodynamic forces are called **transudates** and tend to have low protein content; effusions resulting from malignancy and inflammations have higher protein content and are called **exudates**. The table below details the differences between the two. It is a good rule to obtain culture, Gram stains, and cytologic study for malignant cells on all newly discovered effusions.

Effusion: Exudate or Transudate?

Effusion Characteristic	Transudate	Exudate
Appearance	Clear	Turbid
Color	Pale yellow	Varies
Specific gravity	<1.012	>1.020
WBC	<1,000/cu mm	>1,000/cu mm
Protein	<3.0 g/dL	>3.0 g/dL
Ratio: fluid protein/ blood protein	<0.5	>0.5
Cholesterol	<60 mg/dL	>60 mg/dL
LDH (lactic dehydrogenase)	<200 U/L	>200 U/L
Ratio: fluid LDH/ blood LDH	<0.6	>0.6

charge by pulmonary edema (retained CO_2 is acidic); low cardiac output is also associated with reduced renal blood flow, which deprives the kidney of some of its opportunity to purge acid from blood. Fatal arrhythmias occur when the myocardium becomes irritable following sympathetic nervous system stimulation, the purpose of which is to increase cardiac output by increasing heart rate and contractile force.

Ischemic Heart Disease (Coronary Artery Disease)

Virtually all **ischemic heart disease** arises because of atherosclerotic narrowing or complete occlusion of one or more coronary arteries, which deprives cardiac muscle of blood and results in ischemia or infarction of cardiac muscle. Depending on the degree and character of the obstruction, one of four *clinical* syndromes may occur:

- angina pectoris (cardiac chest pain)
- myocardial infarction
- sudden cardiac death

- chronic ischemic heart disease with congestive heart failure

EPIDEMIOLOGY OF ISCHEMIC HEART DISEASE

Data from the American Centers for Disease Control indicate that as a cause of death "heart disease" rose steadily from 1900, peaked in the late 1940s, and by 1996 had declined to 1900 levels. "Coronary heart disease" was not well recognized enough to be included in death statistics until the mid-1950s. Deaths because of coronary heart disease peaked in the early 1960s and continue to decline. Nevertheless, heart disease, most of it coronary artery disease, remains the number one cause of death in the United States (see the nearby History of Medicine box).

Autopsy studies of American soldiers killed during the Korean War (1950–1953) revealed an astonishing degree of coronary atherosclerosis in these otherwise healthy young men, most of whom were in their late teens or twenties. More recent studies show that *atherosclerosis literally begins in the crib*; however, most coronary artery disease does not become clinically apparent until after age 60 in men and age 70 in women. Coronary disease is more common in males, but women tend to catch up after menopause, when they lose the protective effect of estrogen. In both sexes *age is one of the most important risk factors*—the older you become, the more at risk you are. High levels of LDL cholesterol, low levels of HDL cholesterol, hypertension, smoking, fatty diet, sedentary lifestyle, diabetes, and familial history (genetic influence) are also important.

Atherosclerosis is a lifestyle disease, especially coronary atherosclerosis and its complications: the average patient is overweight, eats a diet high in animal fat, has a big belly, gets little exercise, has high levels of blood cholesterol, and has either diabetes or hypertension, each of which also is largely a lifestyle disease (see The Clinical Side box nearby).

CAUSES OF CORONARY ISCHEMIA

Obstruction to the free flow of blood is the cause of coronary ischemia. Obstruction may be partial or complete, and temporary or permanent. Ischemia can cause pain, arrhythmia, or infarction. Chronic coronary ischemia may cause enough atrophy or slow death of myocardial cells to cause congestive heart failure.

Complete occlusion and myocardial infarction usually occur in conjunction with events in an unstable, young atheroma. The atheroma may fissure, rupture, or hemorrhage, exposing blood to tissue factors that initiate thrombosis and clotting (Chapter 5). Instant occlusion can occur (Fig. 13-7). However, slow complete occlusion by old, fibrotic atheromas may not cause infarction, because alternative (collateral) vessels may develop to supply the affected area. Those atheromas most likely to cause sudden occlusion are young, soft, fatty plaques, which are responsible for 85% of acute coronary occlusions. Prior to occlusion they usually are not large enough to cause ischemia and symptoms, which make them very difficult to detect. Older, sclerotic (sometimes calcified) plaques, while likely to produce ischemia and angina, are not so prone to sudden occlusion and infarction and are easier to identify by diagnostic imaging.

Partial obstruction also can produce ischemia and infarction. Recall from Chapter 5 that an artery does not

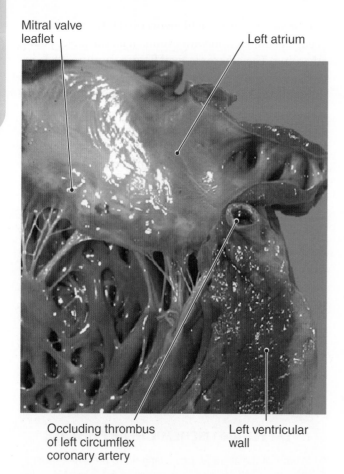

Mitral valve leaflet

Left atrium

Occluding thrombus of left circumflex coronary artery

Left ventricular wall

Figure 13-7 **Acute thrombosis of a coronary artery.** This thrombosis caused infarction of part of the posterior wall of the left ventricle (not visible).

have to be completely occluded to produce ischemia or infarction—a 75% fixed reduction of the coronary lumen may be enough if myocardial demand is high, as during hard exercise. In such cases the partial obstruction is usually attributable to an old, stable atheromatous plaque.

Short-term, partial, *reversible* obstruction also may occur when aggregates of platelets temporarily accumulate on the surface of an atheroma, further narrowing the lumen without proceeding to complete thrombotic occlusion and acute infarction. These aggregates may cause fluctuating chest pain (*unstable angina pectoris*). *Coronary vasospasm* can also cause partial occlusion and ischemia. The source of coronary vasospasm is not clear in many instances, but smoking and cocaine abuse are well-known causes.

ANGINA PECTORIS

Angina pectoris is a distinctive sensation caused by myocardial ischemia. Usually the patient seeks care for a frightening feeling of chest discomfort, described as

smothering, pressing, aching, choking, or heaviness. The sensation occurs beneath the sternum and may radiate to the left jaw, shoulder, elbow, or wrist or even to the back, neck, both arms, or upper abdomen. Dyspnea (shortness of breath) and sweating may occur but are not common. About half of patients show temporary electrocardiographic abnormalities. Laboratory tests and x-ray images do not directly demonstrate the cause of angina, but they may reveal evidence of associated conditions such as diabetes, atherosclerosis, or old myocardial infarction.

Stable angina rises and falls smoothly over a period of a few minutes and is relieved by rest or medication. It may be precipitated by exertion and emotion or by a heavy meal or sudden exposure to cold. It rarely arises spontaneously.

Unstable angina is caused by aggregates of platelets accumulating on an atherosclerotic plaque, and it is a very serious condition that may herald impending myocardial infarction. It is characterized by intensification of existing angina, new onset of angina-at-rest, nocturnal angina, or onset of prolonged angina. Patients with unstable angina, especially angina at rest accompanied by temporary electrocardiographic abnormalities, are at high risk for impending myocardial infarction and need vigorous intervention.

Unremitting angina, angina that does not fluctuate and cannot be relieved by therapy, is caused by myocardial infarction and is accompanied by additional signs and symptoms.

MYOCARDIAL INFARCTION

A **myocardial infarct** (MI) is a circumscribed area of myocardial necrosis caused by ischemia. It is the most important consequence of ischemic heart disease and is the single most common cause of death in industrialized nations. In the United States about 1.5 million persons suffer a myocardial infarct each year; about one third die of it.

Most myocardial infarcts are initiated by *plaque disruption* (rupture, ulceration, hemorrhage) and accompanying *thrombosis* (**coronary thrombosis**) in severely atherosclerotic arteries.

Anatomic Pathology

The *size* of an infarct is largely determined by the *anatomy* of the coronary artery tree and the location of the occlusion. For example, proximal occlusion of an artery is more likely to produce a larger infarct than is distal occlusion of a smaller branch. The coronary distribution varies—the right or left coronaries and their branches supply varying amounts of myocardium from one person to the next; occlusion of a branch supplying a large amount of myocardium produces a correspondingly larger infarct.

Occlusion of the *anterior descending branch* of the left coronary artery, which usually supplies the anterior wall and apex of the left ventricle, is the cause of nearly half of all infarcts. The right coronary artery, which usually supplies the posterior left ventricular wall, is the culprit in about one third of the cases. The left circumflex artery, which usually supplies the left lateral ventricular wall, accounts for the remainder.

The age of a myocardial infarct can be determined by the gross and microscopic findings at autopsy (Fig. 13-8). Coagulative necrosis, characterized by blocks of yellow tissue, appears early and is gradually transformed by the actions of inflammatory cells and by the ingrowth of new blood vessels (angioneogenesis) into granulation tissue (Chapter 4). By eight weeks a mature scar is present.

Infarct Location, Size, and Growth

Coronary arteries run on the surface of the heart and send penetrating arteries downward to supply the

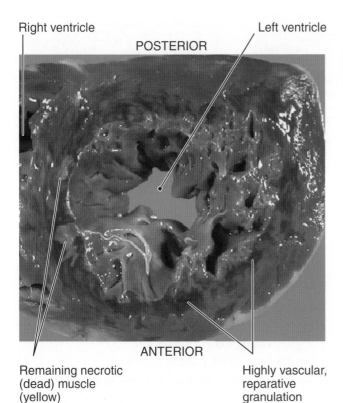

Figure 13-8 Myocardial infarct. Two-week-old infarct of the left ventricle. The infarct completely encircles the ventricle. Note sunken, red granulation tissue with a few remaining islands of yellow, necrotic cardiac muscle not yet removed by the repair process.

myocardium. The last muscle to be supplied is that deepest in the wall—the subendocardial muscle, which is the first to die when an infarct begins to develop. Occlusion of small coronary branches may cause infarction only of subendocardial muscle—a *subendocardial infarct*. As is shown in Figure 13-9, an infarct associated with the occlusion of a larger coronary branch may begin as an area of subendocardial infarction and continue to enlarge for 3 to 6 hours, until it involves the full thickness of the ventricular wall—a *transmural infarct*. It is upon this insight that drug therapy is administered as soon as possible after the diagnosis of an acute infarct is made: if drugs can dissolve the thrombus, flow can be reestablished, and the size of the infarct can be limited.

Anatomic Complications

Complications can occur during the healing process, especially if the infarct is large and transmural. Mitral valve papillary muscles may be infarcted or pulled wide to such a degree by dead, flabby, noncontractile, bulging myocardium that mitral valve backflow (regurgitation) occurs. Infarcted papillary muscles may tear loose completely (rupture), creating the same problem. Moreover, substances from necrotic muscle ooze across the damaged endocardium, attracting platelets and WBC to form a **mural thrombus** (Fig. 13-10), creating substantial risk of cerebral embolization and stroke. Blood dissecting through the soft, dead myocardium can rupture it, causing acute hemopericardium with fatal cardiac smothering (tamponade).

Clinical Features

Myocardial infarction is usually accompanied by severe angina and other symptoms. However, infarction may be asymptomatic and discovered incidentally, for example, by a routine electrocardiogram that shows clear evidence of an old myocardial scar in a patient with no history of an infarct. About 20% of myocardial infarcts are silent, especially in people with diabetes or hypertension, or in the very elderly.

The clinical features of a typical myocardial infarct are distinctive (Fig. 13-11) and include severe, steady, crushing substernal chest pain (unremitting angina) with radiation to the neck, jaw, epigastrium, shoulder, or left arm. Patients often have dyspnea, nausea, and vomiting and sweat profusely. Case Study 13.1 at the end of this chapter presents a typical case. It may be clinically difficult to determine whether a patient is experiencing severe angina or a myocardial infarct. Angina without infarction rises or fluctuates and then

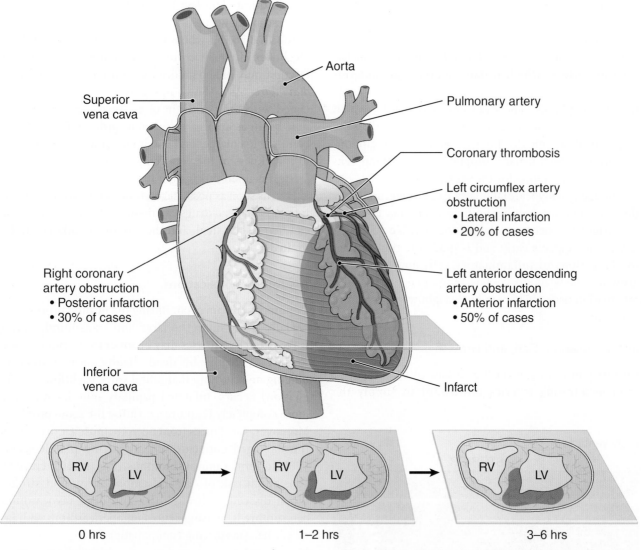

Superior vena cava

Right coronary artery obstruction
• Posterior infarction
• 30% of cases

Inferior vena cava

Aorta

Pulmonary artery

Coronary thrombosis

Left circumflex artery obstruction
• Lateral infarction
• 20% of cases

Left anterior descending artery obstruction
• Anterior infarction
• 50% of cases

Infarct

RV LV   RV LV   RV LV

0 hrs   1–2 hrs   3–6 hrs

Figure 13-9 **Evolution of an acute myocardial infarct.** The area of infarcted muscle is small at the onset and much larger at 3–6 hours.

disappears, or is relieved by coronary vasodilators, especially nitroglycerin. To the contrary, an infarct produces unremitting pain. Blood tests for markers of myocardial infarct are critical: they remain normal in angina but are elevated with infarction.

About half of myocardial infarcts occur without warning; the other half are preceded by episodes of angina. Cardiogenic shock (pump failure) may occur, especially if the infarct is large. Despite the dramatic picture painted here, diagnosing an MI, and differentiating it from other kinds of chest pain (especially esophageal pain due to spasm of gastric acid reflux), can prove challenging.

About 80–90% of MI patients arrive alive at a hospital. Almost all of those who die before reaching a hospi-

tal die of cardiac arrhythmias. Of those who reach a hospital, a minority recover without complication. Most, however, develop one or more of the following clinical complications:

- cardiac arrhythmia (~80%)
- left ventricular failure (~60%)
- thromboembolism (15–50%)
- cardiogenic shock (~10%)
- myocardial, interventricular septal, or papillary muscle rupture (~5%)

Laboratory Diagnosis and Follow-up

Laboratory evaluation is important in the differential diagnosis of chest pain, in the follow-up assessment of the

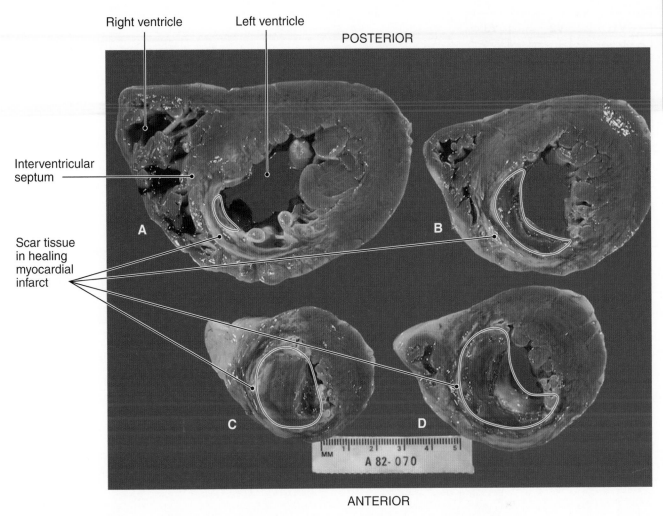

POSTERIOR

Right ventricle

Left ventricle

Interventricular septum

Scar tissue in healing myocardial infarct

A

B

C

D

MM   1   2   3   4   5

A 82- 070

ANTERIOR

Figure 13-10 **Intracardiac mural thrombus (encircled).** Superior view of serial cross-sections. **A,** Section high, near the mitral valve. **B** and **C,** Middle sections. **D,** Section near the apex, where the thrombus fills most of the ventricular cavity.

size of a myocardial infarct, and in the evaluation of recovery and treatment. Dead cardiac muscle cells release enzymes and proteins into blood where they can be measured. The degree of increase of these enzymes in blood is roughly proportional to the size of the infarct. One enzyme is **creatine kinase (CK),** an enzyme found in high concentration in cardiac and skeletal muscle, and in the brain. CK occurs in three combinations: CK-MM from skeletal muscle and heart, **CK-MB** principally from heart, and CK-BB from brain (added together they form total CK). For example, after a myocardial infarct, after severe muscle exertion, or after a stroke, total CK may be elevated, so the trick is to determine the source. Assessment of the relative amount of CK subtypes (MM, MB, or BB) is helpful. CK determination has proven to be a *sensitive,* but not very *specific,* indicator of MI. Another substance that is helpful to assess is troponin. Assessment of blood levels of **cardiac troponin**

(cTn), which is molecularly distinct from skeletal muscle troponin, also has proven to be much more specific than CK in identifying MI. Two types of cardiac troponin have been identified, cardiac troponin I (cTnI) and cardiac troponin T (cTnT). Neither type is present in significant amounts in the blood of healthy people; therefore, detection of even small amounts offers is a *sensitive and specific* indicator of myocardial infarction.

CHRONIC MYOCARDIAL ISCHEMIA

Chronic myocardial ischemia, sometimes called **ischemic cardiomyopathy,** may lead to heart failure as the mass of healthy ventricular muscle deteriorates following infarcts both large and small, clinical or subclinical (asymptomatic), or with the accumulated withering effect of repeated anginal attacks and chronic ischemia. The ventricles become dilated, thin-walled, and flabby,

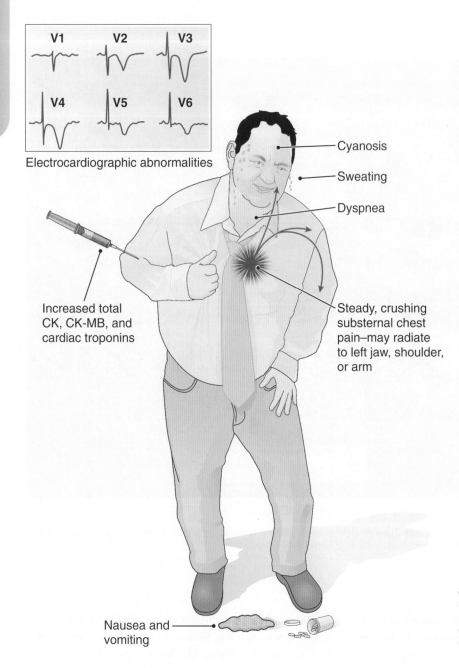

Electrocardiographic abnormalities

Cyanosis

Sweating

Dyspnea

Increased total CK, CK-MB, and cardiac troponins

Steady, crushing substernal chest pain–may radiate to left jaw, shoulder, or arm

Nausea and vomiting

Figure 13-11 **Clinical picture of acute myocardial infarction.** Electrocardiogram abnormalities are characteristic. In blood, total creatine kinase (CK), cardiac creatine kinase (CK-MB), and cardiac troponin are increased.

similar to *dilated cardiomyopathy*, a type of cardiomyopathy with the same features but usually of unknown cause. Most patients with ischemic cardiomyopathy are elderly and present with congestive heart failure.

SUDDEN CARDIAC DEATH

Sudden cardiac death is defined as natural death from cardiac causes within one hour of the onset of symptoms. Sudden cardiac death accounts for about half of all cardiac deaths. Put another way, in these patients death itself is the first symptom of ischemic heart dis-

ease. Patients may or may not have a history of cardiac disease, but the death is sudden and unexpected. Instantaneous death is, perhaps, a phrase that conveys what most physicians and the public have in mind when the topic is discussed. Most sudden deaths are the result of violence; however, a few medical conditions produce an instantaneous (or nearly instantaneous) death—ruptured aortic aneurysm, pulmonary saddle embolus, and ischemic heart disease. *Ischemic heart disease is the most common cause of instantaneous death* in industrialized society, causing more deaths than violence does. Most sudden cardiac death occurs because of cardiac electrical malfunction, either failure to beat (asystole) or complete electrical disorganization (*ventricular fibrillation*), which turns the normal coordinated contractions of the left ventricle into an ineffective mass of squirming muscle.

Hypertensive Heart Disease

The strain imposed by pumping against high blood pressure causes left ventricular hypertrophy, as is shown in Figure 13-12. Hypertrophic myocardium is stiff and has higher-than-normal metabolic requirements, which render the muscle more susceptible to infarction and arrhythmia at any given amount of coronary atherosclerosis and obstruction. Furthermore, stiffness reduces ventricular movement (compliance) and stroke volume and increases the distance over which oxygen and nutrients must diffuse through the ventricular wall. In a vicious circle, chronic hypertension predisposes to coronary atherosclerosis. The end result often is congestive heart failure, myocardial infarction, and cardiac arrhythmia.

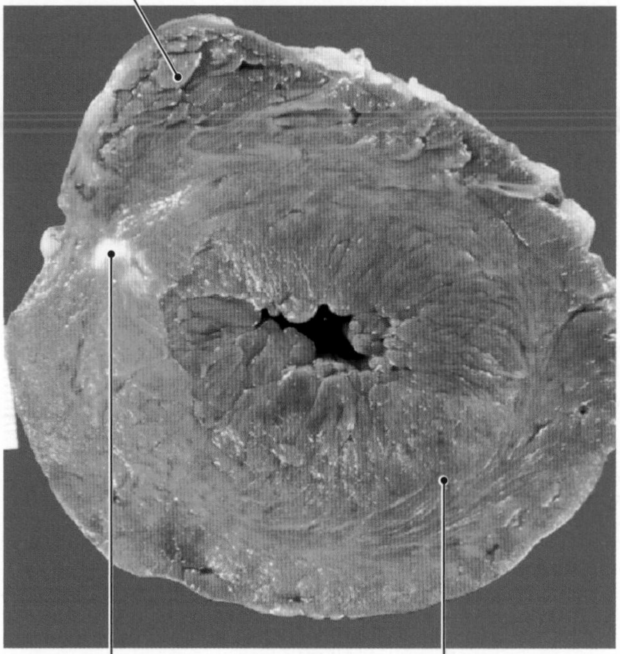

Valvular Heart Disease

Normal cardiac valves are one-way gates. They are subject to two types of mechanical valve malfunctions, both caused by deformities resulting from acute or chronic inflammation. The first is **valvular stenosis**; that is, obstructed flow, usually from stiff or fused valve leaflets. The second is **valvular insufficiency**; that is, regurgitation or backflow, usually associated with valves that do not close properly because they are stiff or deformed by inflammation, or eaten away by bacterial infection. Both stenosis and insufficiency are mechanically inefficient. In some severe cases valves may be both stenotic and insufficient, as is illustrated in Figure 13-13 (see also Fig. 13-16).

Apart from inflammation and infection, some causes of valvular insufficiency include:

- *Syphilitic aortitis*, which weakens and dilates the aortic root and separates the valve leaflets
- *Myxomatous degeneration of the mitral valve* ("floppy mitral valve syndrome," mitral valve prolapse), which is discussed below
- *Ruptured mitral valve chordae tendineae* (a condition in which the chordae tear away from their attachment to infarcted papillary muscles), which cause mitral valve leaflets to flip upward into the atrium with each beat, creating regurgitation (backflow)

Figure 13-12 **Left ventricular hypertrophy.** The left ventricle is thickened because of the strain of chronic hypertension. Also present is a scar from small, old myocardial infarct.

- *Massive left ventricular dilation* that pulls chordae tendineae and mitral valve leaflets down and laterally, preventing valve closure

Post-inflammatory thickening and scarring from chronic **rheumatic heart disease** is a major cause of cardiac valve disease, especially of the mitral valve. Inflamed valve cusps become thick and stiff and do not close or open completely, or valve cusps may fuse together. In some instances the valve cusps may be so diseased that they are fixed in place, and both stenosis and regurgitation occur. Such valves are stenotic in systole and regurgitant in diastole (Fig. 13-13). *Deformed valves also are susceptible to bacterial infection* (infective endocarditis), which may erode the leaflets, creating holes that allow backflow.

RHEUMATIC HEART DISEASE

Rheumatic fever is an acute *autoimmune* disease that occurs in a small percentage of cases of group A streptococcal pharyngitis (Fig. 13-14) but for unknown reasons does not occur with group A streptococcal infections at other sites. Rheumatic fever and rheumatic

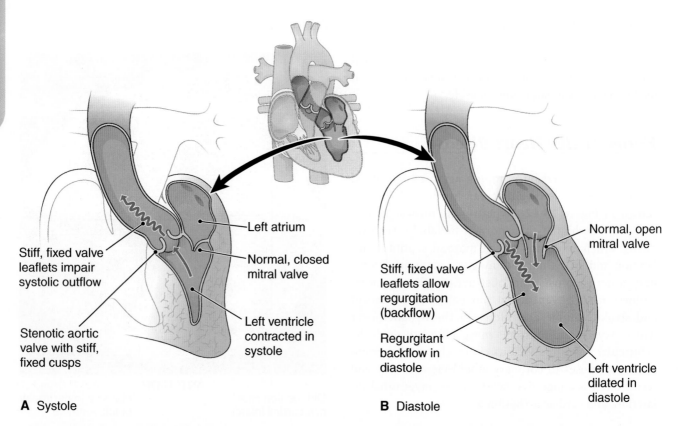

Stiff, fixed valve leaflets impair systolic outflow

Left atrium

Normal, closed mitral valve

Stenotic aortic valve with stiff, fixed cusps

Left ventricle contracted in systole

A Systole

Normal, open mitral valve

Stiff, fixed valve leaflets allow regurgitation (backflow)

Regurgitant backflow in diastole

Left ventricle dilated in diastole

B Diastole

Figure 13-13 **Aortic stenosis and insufficiency.** Severe aortic valve disease can immobilize aortic valve cusps, so that both obstruction to outflow (stenosis) and regurgitant backflow (insufficiency) occur. **A,** Systole: flow across the aortic valve is obstructed. **B,** Diastole: incomplete closure of aortic valve allows backflow.

heart disease are uncommon today because of the effective use of antibiotics.

Recall from our discussion on immune disease (Chapter 8), that *molecular mimicry* is one way in which the immune system can be tricked into attacking self tissues. In molecular mimicry a foreign antigen (streptococcus antigen in this case) is similar to self antigens found in the heart and joints. Antibodies produced against strep antigens attack the invading streptococcus organisms but also attack the similar normal, non-strep, self antigens that reside in heart and joint tissues.

Acute rheumatic fever is a syndrome of *arthritis, valvulitis, myocarditis,* and *pericarditis* that occurs in children 5–15 years old about 2–6 weeks after group A strep pharyngitis. The myocardium, valves, and pericardium are inflamed, producing weak heart sounds, pericardial friction rub, tachycardia, and arrhythmia. A migratory polyarthritis is also present. The disease usually is self-limiting and often not recognized for what it is. Most patients recover completely without long-term ill effect. However, in about 5% of acute cases, severe carditis with congestive heart failure occurs and may be fatal.

Alternatively, the immune attacks may be chronic and subclinical (silent), and the first clinical sign may be chronic *valve disease*, known as **chronic rheumatic valvulitis** (Fig. 13-15). Patients with chronic rheumatic valvulitis rarely have a history of acute rheumatic fever and the diagnosis of chronic rheumatic valvulitis is made in retrospect as a diagnosis of exclusion in the workup of patients with chronic valve disease. Presumably, patients who develop chronic rheumatic valvulitis have been subjected to repeated strep throat infections; however, a history of such infections is rarely obtained.

CALCIFIC AORTIC STENOSIS

Calcific aortic stenosis (Fig. 13-16) occurs when age-related degenerative changes in the aortic valve produce valvular fibrosis, calcification, and deformity. It is the most common cause of isolated aortic stenosis and usually is not manifest until late in life. **Congenital bicuspid aortic valve** (Fig. 13-16) also causes increased valve leaflet wear and tear, leading to calcific stenosis because

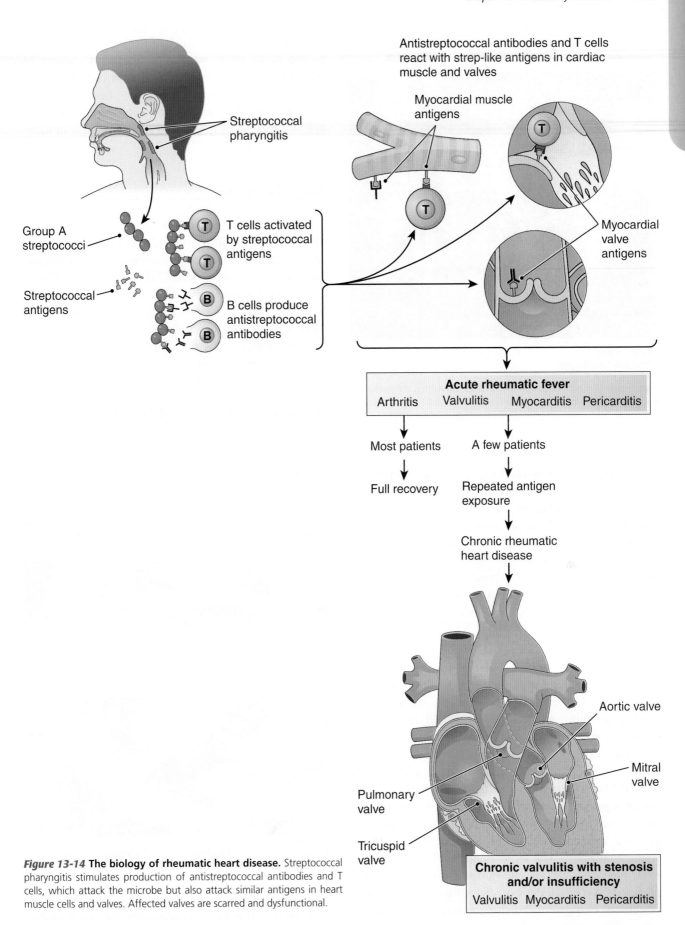

Antistreptococcal antibodies and T cells react with strep-like antigens in cardiac muscle and valves

Myocardial muscle antigens

Myocardial valve antigens

Streptococcal pharyngitis

Group A streptococci

Streptococcal antigens

T cells activated by streptococcal antigens

B cells produce antistreptococcal antibodies

Acute rheumatic fever

Arthritis   Valvulitis   Myocarditis   Pericarditis

Most patients

Full recovery

A few patients

Repeated antigen exposure

Chronic rheumatic heart disease

Aortic valve

Mitral valve

Pulmonary valve

Tricuspid valve

Chronic valvulitis with stenosis and/or insufficiency

Valvulitis   Myocarditis   Pericarditis

Figure 13-14 **The biology of rheumatic heart disease.** Streptococcal pharyngitis stimulates production of antistreptococcal antibodies and T cells, which attack the microbe but also attack similar antigens in heart muscle cells and valves. Affected valves are scarred and dysfunctional.

Autopsy artifact

Thick, scarred mitral valve

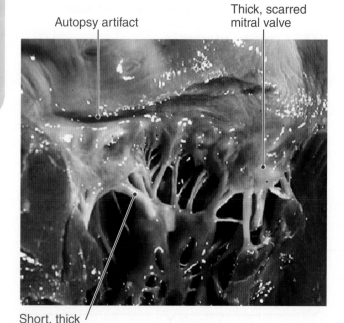

Short, thick chordae tendineae

Figure 13-15 Chronic rheumatic mitral valvulitis. Inflammation and scarring produce a stiff, thick valve and short, thick chordae tendineae. Such valves may be stenotic or regurgitant.

the valves must be stretched with each beat in order for blood to pass (in a normal valve the three leaflets are anatomically designed so that they are merely pushed out of the way and are not stretched with each beat). Clinical features of aortic stenosis include systolic murmur (swishing sound), left ventricular hypertrophy, angina, and syncope (as the brain is starved for blood). Surgical valve replacement is a successful therapy.

MYXOMATOUS DEGENERATION OF THE MITRAL VALVE

Myxomatous degeneration of the mitral valve (also known as *mitral valve prolapse*) is the most common valve disease, affecting about 3% of the United States adult population between ages 20 and 40. It is characterized by an accumulation of interstitial myxoid material in the valve leaflets. The cause is unknown. The result is regurgitant, "floppy" mitral valve leaflets attached to elongated chordae tendineae. Most patients are asymptomatic and suffer no ill effect. Some patients may complain of fatigue, palpitations, or atypical chest pain—a very common symptom often thought to be hypochondriacal. The hypochondriac does not, however, have the late systolic murmur and mid-systolic click that is characteristic of affected patients (the click occurs as elongated chordae tendineae snap tight). Diagnostic imaging confirms the diagnosis. About 3%

will develop a serious complication such as bacterial infection of the valve (bacterial endocarditis), severe mitral insufficiency, valve thrombi with embolic stroke, congestive heart failure, arrhythmias, or sudden death. Patients should be placed on prophylactic antibiotics before dental visits in order to reduce the risk of bacterial endocarditis.

Endocarditis

The growth of vegetations on cardiac valves (or, rarely, other endocardial sites) is called endocarditis. Two types are recognized: *noninfective thrombotic endocarditis* and *infective endocarditis*. Most infective endocarditis is caused by bacteria (*bacterial endocarditis*). Uncommonly, fungi are the cause. Infective endocarditis is far more serious than is noninfective endocarditis, because infective endocarditis may result in erosion of valve leaflets and cause catastrophic valvular insufficiency, or it may cause severe systemic infection.

NONBACTERIAL THROMBOTIC ENDOCARDITIS

Noninfective thrombotic endocarditis (Fig. 13-17) is characterized by valvular vegetations composed of *platelets and fibrinous material*. The lesions contain no

Left coronary artery

Calcium deposit

Anterior valve leaflet

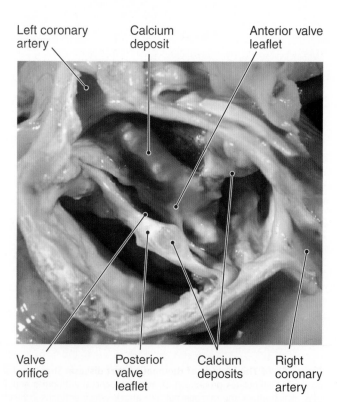

Valve orifice

Posterior valve leaflet

Calcium deposits

Right coronary artery

Figure 13-16 Calcific aortic stenosis. Congenital bicuspid aortic valve. Valve leaflets are thick and crusted with calcium and frozen in position. This valve is both stenotic and insufficient.

Mitral valve with vegetations   Left atrium

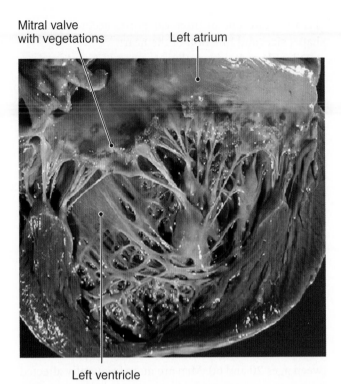

Left ventricle

Figure 13-17 **Nonbacterial thrombotic endocarditis.** Valve vegetations are composed of platelets and fibrin. They are subject to bacterial infection (bacterial endocarditis) and may break away and embolize to distant organs. The cause is unknown.

microorganisms, and affected valves are otherwise normal. The pathogenesis is obscure, but it has been linked to cachexia, deep venous thrombosis, hypercoagulable blood, and malignancies, especially adenocarcinoma. The lesions are often discovered incidentally at autopsy, but they may embolize and cause infarction, notably in the brain. It is important to note, however, that the lesions are susceptible to microbiologic colonization and the added development of infective endocarditis.

INFECTIVE ENDOCARDITIS

Infective endocarditis is almost always caused by bacterial infection (**bacterial endocarditis**) of a valve. The aortic and mitral valves are the valves that are most often infected, with the appearance of ragged masses of organisms known as vegetations (Fig. 13-18). Emboli from these vegetations may break away and seed distant sites, causing an *abscess* or *infarct* of the brain, kidney, or any other organ. The greater hazard, however, is erosion and perforation of the affected valve, with attendant **valvular insufficiency** (regurgitation). Rarely, a previously normal valve may be affected, especially in IV drug abusers; however, most infections occur on previously diseased valves. Examples of susceptible valves include congenital bicuspid aortic valve, valves ravaged

by chronic rheumatic disease, and prosthetic valves. Anything that causes bacteremia can cause transient bacteremia and seed an abnormal cardiac valve and establish infection—teeth brushing, IV-drug shooting, cardiac catheterization, and endoscopic examinations of lungs, joints, and intestine or urinary tract.

Valve infections may be acute or chronic, depending on the infective organism. For instance, staphylococcal infections may cause rapidly progressive valve destruction with devastating regurgitation. Infections by less virulent organisms such as *streptococcus* or *enterococcus* are often referred to as **subacute bacterial endocarditis** (**SBE**) because of their slow course.

The clinical onset of infective endocarditis may be gradual or explosive, depending on the infective agent. Acute infections feature high fever and shaking chills, but subacute infection may present with innocuous appearing low-grade fever, weight loss, and malaise. Cardiac murmurs are usually present, and the spleen may be enlarged if hyperplasia develops associated with chronic bloodstream infection. A valuable clue some-

Left atrium   Mitral valve

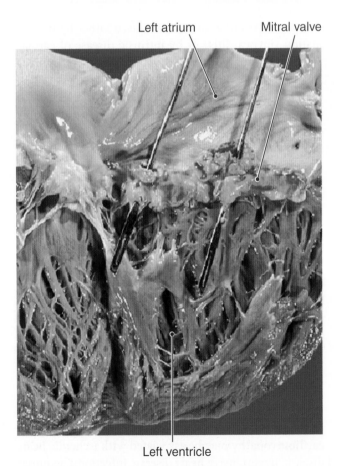

Left ventricle

Figure 13-18 **Bacterial endocarditis of the mitral valve.** Probes demonstrate valve perforations caused by bacterial destruction of valve tissue. This case was associated with severe valvular insufficiency (regurgitation).

times is oral, conjunctival, or subungual (beneath the nail) tiny hemorrhages (*petechiae*) caused by bacterial microemboli. Larger emboli may cause abscesses or infarcts, with specific symptoms, such as brain abscess or stroke, or visual impairment from retinal emboli. Repeated and carefully collected blood cultures may be necessary to establish the diagnosis. Moreover, some patients may be treated with antibiotics for malaise and fever before a diagnosis of endocarditis is considered. Such pre-diagnosis administration of antibiotics can render blood cultures negative when they otherwise would have been positive, thus masking the symptoms of bacterial endocarditis. Infective endocarditis of any type is difficult to treat because heart valves, like the cornea and the lens of the eye, do not have blood vessels, and antibiotics cannot reach the site of infection as easily as in other tissues. Treatment usually requires large doses of intravenous antibiotics over a prolonged period.

Primary Myocardial Diseases

Primary myocardial disease is caused either by inflammation (myocarditis) or by intrinsic disease of cardiac muscle (cardiomyopathy). Several types are recognized according to anatomic and functional characteristics, each of which may result from inflammation, metabolic disorder, autoimmune disease, or muscular dystrophy or other genetic condition. The cause of some cases is unknown.

MYOCARDITIS

In the United States **myocarditis** usually caused by viral infection, especially *Coxsackie A or B* viruses. Some cases result from autoimmune disease—rheumatic fever, for example. Most cases resolve without therapy, but some proceed to chronic congestive heart failure and the syndrome of dilated cardiomyopathy (see below). The diagnosis of myocarditis is usually presumptive, because few diagnostic tests are available to prove myocardial infection.

CARDIOMYOPATHIES

Primary cardiomyopathy refers to intrinsic disease of cardiac muscle. Often the cause is unknown. **Secondary cardiomyopathy** may be associated with ischemic heart disease, hypertensive heart disease, infections, acquired metabolic disturbances, valvular disease, congenital abnormalities, nutritional deficiency, and immune dysfunction. No matter the cause, cardiomyopathies are

classified into one of three categories according to the shape, size, and function of the heart.

Dilated cardiomyopathy, or *congestive cardiomyopathy* (Fig. 13-19), is characterized by progressive cardiac hypertrophy, dilation, and low ejection fraction (the fraction of ventricular blood volume ejected with each beat). Usually the cause is not known, and the case is designated *idiopathic dilated cardiomyopathy*. Viral infection is often suspected. There is a strong association with alcohol abuse, and some cases are clearly associated with chemotherapy. Chronic ischemia of the myocardium caused by coronary artery disease (*ischemic cardiomyopathy*) can produce a clinical syndrome indistinguishable from that stemming from other causes of dilated cardiomyopathy. Peripartum and postpartum cardiomyopathy has been described also. The affected heart is flabby and features weak, ineffectual contractions. The anatomic pathology is characterized by dilation and hypertrophy of all chambers. Dilated cardiomyopathy most commonly presents between ages 20 and 60. Men are more frequently affected than women are, perhaps because more men than women abuse alcohol.

Hypertrophic cardiomyopathy features marked myocardial hypertrophy. About half of the cases result from an autosomal dominant gene defect. Most of the remainder are idiopathic. The condition usually comes to attention in the 30–50 age group because of dyspnea, angina, fainting spells (syncope), or irregular heartbeat.

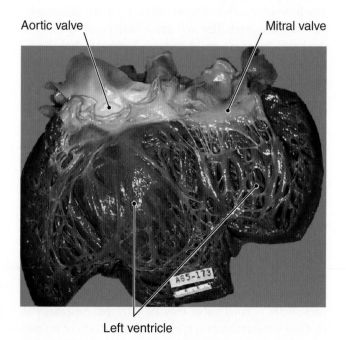

Aortic valve Mitral valve

Left ventricle

Figure 13-19 **Dilated cardiomyopathy.** The markedly dilated left ventricle is so flabby that it lies flat on the examining table.

The first clue that something is wrong may be sudden death, especially in children or young adults, often during or immediately after exertion. As is emphasized in the accompanying Key Point Box, sudden death of young athletes is a well-known phenomenon. The myocardium is stiff, and the left ventricle and septum are markedly thickened. The heart is shaped like, and about as stiff as, one end of a football. The muscular hypertrophy is deforming, so much so that diastolic filling may be chaotic and incomplete, and systolic ejection forceful but ineffective. Left ventricular outflow may be partially obstructed by the very thick upper end of the interventricular septum. In striking contrast to dilated cardiomyopathy, systolic contractions are powerful and hyperactive. Clinical features include myocardial ischemia and angina without coronary artery disease because the thick, stiff heart muscle is difficult to perfuse with blood. Congestive heart failure and arrhythmias are common.

> **Cardiomyopathy is the most common autopsy finding in sudden, nonviolent, unexpected death in young athletes. It accounts for about 40% of such deaths, most of which result from hypertrophic cardiomyopathy.**

Restrictive cardiomyopathy is the rarest cardiomyopathy and is characterized by a stiff, noncompliant ventricle that fills incompletely in diastole. Worldwide the most common cause is *endomyocardial fibrosis*, a mysterious condition of uncertain cause that occurs most commonly in children and is characterized by markedly thickened, porcelain-like endocardium. Other causes of restrictive cardiomyopathy include cardiac amyloidosis, radiation injury, and hemochromatosis. As in hypertrophic cardiomyopathy, the myocardium is stiff, but systole is not forceful. Congestive heart failure is the usual outcome, and other complications and symptoms are similar to those of the other cardiomyopathies.

Congenital Heart Disease

Congenital heart malformations occur in about 8 per 1,000 live births, making them among the most common congenital abnormalities. They may be innocuous and not detected until late adult life, or they may be rapidly fatal. The cause of most congenital heart disease is unknown, but specific genetic and environmental causes can be identified in about 10% of cases and include virus infections (especially first trimester maternal rubella), fetal alcohol syndrome, and cytogenetic abnormalities (especially Down syndrome).

The embryologic heart begins as a tube and becomes an anatomically complete heart by the 10th week of pregnancy. All congenital heart defects, therefore, develop in the first ten weeks. Development has two important characteristics: 1) the primitive heart *expands and twists* in a complicated way that results in the chambers and vessels being the right size and in the correct place, and 2) the *septum* that divides the heart into right and left sides grows internally from one end to the other.

Anatomically, therefore, there are three types of defects: 1) *malrotation defects*, which result in misplacement of a vessel, for example, transposition of the great vessels; 2) *expansion defects*, which result in hypoplastic chambers or vessels, for example, coarctation of the aorta; and 3) *septal defects*, which result in a direct connection between atria or ventricles, for example, interatrial or interventricular septal defects. Combinations of these defects may occur.

A **cardiac shunt** is a defect that diverts blood from one side of the heart or great vessels (from aorta to pulmonary artery, for example) to the opposite side. Blood always flows, of course, from an area of high pressure to one of low pressure. If the low-pressure right side (right atrium, right ventricle, pulmonary artery) is open to the high-pressure left side (left atrium, ventricle, and aorta), oxygenated blood will naturally flow from the left side to the right, producing a **left-to-right shunt**. Other defects or conditions may cause the normally low pressure, unoxygenated right side to have greater pressure than the left, to produce a **right-to-left shunt**. Understanding cardiac malformations and shunts requires study of the path of fetal blood flow in utero, as is detailed in Basics in Brief 13.1.

Congenital cardiac defects are classified as *malformations with shunts* and *malformations with obstruction to flow*.

MALFORMATIONS WITH SHUNTS

Normal fetal circulation is depicted in Figure 13-20A (see also the Basics in Brief box nearby). The major differences from adult circulation are these: 1) oxygenated blood flows in veins (not arteries) from the placenta to the heart; 2) oxygenated and deoxygenated blood is mixed in most of the circulation; and 3) little blood flows through the lungs because blood is shunted away by passing from the right atrium to the left atrium through the foramen ovale, and from the pulmonary artery to the aorta through the ductus arteriosus Normally, both of these fetal shunts close after birth.

Left-to-right shunts (Fig. 13-20) are the most common type of congenital heart defect and feature shunting of blood from the oxygenated, higher pressure left

FETAL BLOOD CIRCULATION IN UTERO

The fetal circulation is depicted in Figure 13-20A. The essence of fetal blood flow in utero is this: *blood is oxygenated in the placenta and is shunted to bypass the fetal lungs.* Oxygenated blood flows up the inferior vena cava into the right atrium, where it divides in two streams. The first stream circulates through the right heart and into the pulmonary artery. The second stream is shunted across the atrial septum directly into the left side of the heart, from which it is pumped into the aorta. The first stream, however, does not go into the lungs from the pulmonary artery; before it reaches the lungs it is shunted to the aorta through the ductus arteriosus. The aorta carries the united streams of blood to the rest of the body.

To study medicine is to confront miracles on a regular basis. Among the most miraculous is this: with an infant's first breath, both the atrial septal shunt and the ductus arteriosus shunt stop diverting blood away from the lungs. The ductus arteriosus clamps down, immediately stopping flow into the aorta from the pulmonary artery, forcing flow into the lungs to be oxygenated by the infant's first breaths. This new flood of blood flows out of the lungs into the left atrium, raising left-atrial pressure to equal right-atrial pressure and effectively ending flow through the foramen ovale, which closes slowly during the first year of life.

side to the lower pressure right side. Left-to-right shunts are especially dangerous because the added volume of flow and higher-than-normal pressure causes high pulmonary artery pressure (pulmonary hypertension), which, if not corrected, can cause right-side heart failure and irreversible (and usually fatal) pulmonary hypertension. Right-side pressure can rise high enough to exceed left-side pressure, causing a reversal of flow and *late cyanosis* as the shunt conveys unoxygenated blood into the systemic circulation.

The three main types of left-to-right shunts are:

- **Atrial septal defect**: Atrial septal defect occurs when there is incomplete closure of the embryonic atrial septum. It presents as a congenital hole in the septum that separates the atria. Even if uncorrected the majority of patients with atrial septal defect do not develop pulmonary hypertension. Atrial septal defect is not to be confused with *patent foramen ovale*, in which the foramen ovale, which usually closes in the first year of life, remains at least partially patent. Patent foramen ovale occurs in about one third of healthy people without ill effect.
- **Ventricular septal defect**: Ventricular septal defect (Fig. 13-21) is incomplete closure of the embryonic ventricular septum and usually is associated with other congenital cardiac anomalies. Small ventricular septal defects may close spontaneously after a few years, or they may exist a lifetime without creating significant problems. Large defects require surgery. Untreated large defects cause pulmonary hypertension because they allow increased flow of blood through the lungs.

- **Patent (persistent) ductus arteriosus**: In utero the ductus arteriosus conveys oxygenated blood from the pulmonary artery into the aorta for distribution to the body. If the ductus arteriosus fails to close at birth, it is called a patent ductus arteriosus, and blood is shunted in the opposite direction from normal, that is, from the aorta to the pulmonary artery. About 90% of patent ductus arteriosus occur as a solitary abnormality, but some are associated with other congenital cardiac defects. Some close following drug treatment; simple surgical closure is effective in the remainder. Closure should be achieved as early in life as is practicable. Unclosed shunts may cause pulmonary hypertension because they allow increased flow of blood through the lungs.

Timely correction of left-to-right shunts is critical. Uncorrected shunts lead to pulmonary hypertension, right heart failure, and death. Heart-lung transplant is the only hope after a certain point because surgical repair of the defect after development of severe pulmonary hypertension would deprive the pulmonary tree of the high pressure necessary to force blood through the lungs. A vicious circle is operating: high blood pressure damages pulmonary arterioles and increases pulmonary resistance, which in turn requires even higher pressure to sustain adequate blood flow.

Right-to-left shunts, which are less common than are left-to-right shunts, result when there is malrotation of the embryonic chambers. They are characterized by *early cyanosis* (cyanosis at birth) as unoxygenated blood from the right side bypasses the lungs and flows into the systemic circulation. The most common right-

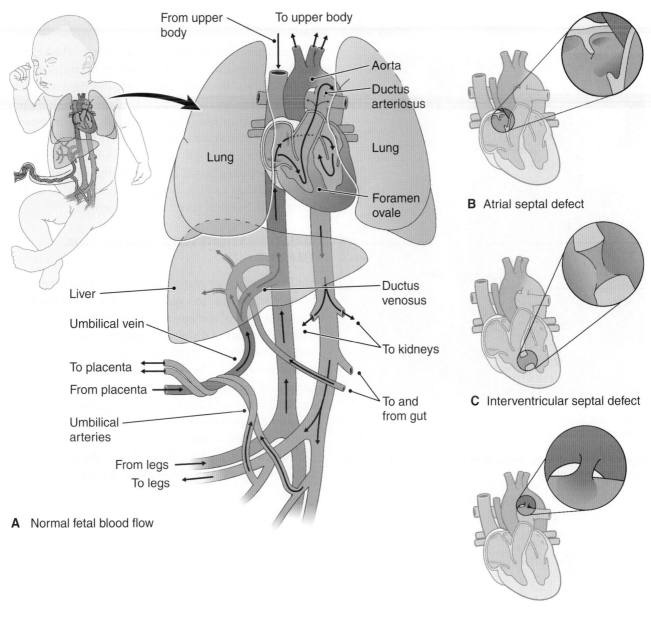

A Normal fetal blood flow

B Atrial septal defect

C Interventricular septal defect

D Patent ductus arteriosus

Figure 13-20 **Left-to-right congenital cardiac shunts.** Blood travels from the high-pressure left side (left atrium, ventricle, or aorta) to the low-pressure right side (right atrium, ventricle, and pulmonary artery). These shunts "short circuit" blood flow by recirculating it through the right heart and lungs, which causes right-side volume overload and abnormally high pressure in the pulmonary blood vessels. Pulmonary hypertension and right-side heart failure may result. **A,** In the normal fetal blood flow, blood is oxygenated in the placenta and bypasses the lungs. **B,** In an atrial septal defect, instead of flowing from the left atrium into the left ventricle and then into the aorta, some blood flows from the left atrium to the right atrium and back through the lungs. **C,** In a ventricular septal defect, instead of flowing from the left ventricle into the aorta, some blood flows from the left ventricle into the right ventricle and back through the lungs. **D,** In patent ductus arteriosus, some blood flows from the aorta into the pulmonary artery and back through the lungs.

to-left shunt is **tetralogy of Fallot** (Fig. 13-22), which consists of:

- *Ventricular septal defect (VSD)*
- *Small pulmonary artery or pulmonary valve stenosis,* which obstructs flow out of the right ventricle and through the ventricular septal defect

- *Misplaced aorta* that overrides (sits low on) the ventricular septal defect and catches venous blood passing through the septal defect from the right ventricle
- *Right ventricular hypertrophy* (which was included in the original set of defects, though it is secondary to the three other primary abnormalities listed above)

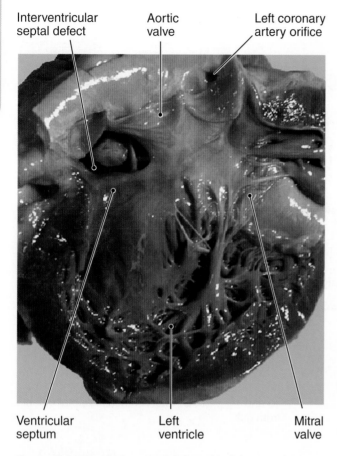

Interventricular septal defect

Aortic valve

Left coronary artery orifice

Ventricular septum

Left ventricle

Mitral valve

Figure 13-21 **Ventricular septal defect.** This defect is at the upper end of the interventricular septum.

Surgical correction is effective if diagnosis is made early.

Transposition of the great vessels is the second most common cause of early cyanotic heart disease. In this condition the aorta rises from the right ventricle and the pulmonary artery from the left, a condition not compatible with life. Those newborns with transposition of the great vessels who do survive birth do so only because they have an additional defect that allows shunting of oxygenated blood from the left side to the right ventricle (which supplies the aorta), or to the aorta itself. Surgical correction is effective.

MALFORMATIONS WITH OBSTRUCTION TO FLOW

Malformations with obstruction to flow occur when embryonic vessels fail to expand properly. **Coarctation of the aorta**, one of the most common congenital cardiac defects, consists of a ring-like fibrous narrowing of the aorta, usually in the aortic arch near the location of the ductus arteriosus. The word *coarctation* is derived from Latin and means drawing or pressing together. It is caused by hypoplasia of a short segment of the fetal aorta and is associated with high blood pressure in the upper extremities and low blood pressure in the legs. Low blood flow to the kidneys (below the obstruction) stimulates renin and aldosterone output, which ex-

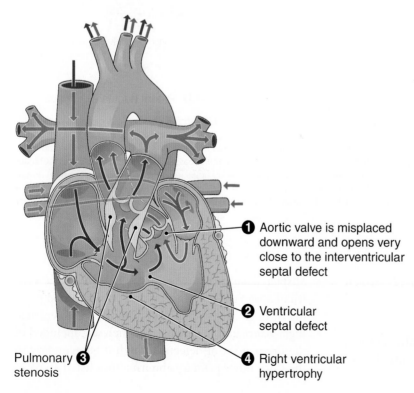

❶ Aortic valve is misplaced downward and opens very close to the interventricular septal defect

❷ Ventricular septal defect

Pulmonary ❸ stenosis

❹ Right ventricular hypertrophy

Figure 13-22 **Tetralogy of Fallot: a right-to-left cardiac shunt.** The defects are: 1) misplacement (rightward shift) of the aortic valve so that the aortic orifice catches unoxygenated blood coming through the 2) ventricular septal defect in a right-to-left shunt because 3) pulmonary artery stenosis obstructs pulmonary blood flow, which increases right ventricular pressure, causing 4) right ventricular hypertrophy.

pands blood volume and elevates blood pressure even further. Hypertension is detected in most patients because blood pressure is always measured in the arm, above the obstruction. Patients also tend to have additional cardiac defects, such as bicuspid aortic valve, aortic stenosis, or septal defect.

In half of cases, coarctation is accompanied by a patent ductus arteriosus. Pressure is higher in the pulmonary artery than in the aorta below the coarctation, so unoxygenated blood flows into the aorta below the obstruction and produces cyanosis of the lower body only, a distinctive sign that prompts early diagnosis and treatment. In the other half of cases, the coarctation is an isolated defect not associated with patent ductus arteriosus or other defects. These patients have upper body hypertension but no other signs or symptoms, and usually diagnosis is not made for many years.

Segments of vessels other than the aorta may also not expand properly during fetal development and are responsible for congenital pulmonary and aortic valve stenosis or hypoplasia of the root of the aorta or pulmonary artery. An example is mild *pulmonary atresia*, which is fairly common and may be compatible with long life.

Pericardial Disease

Pericarditis is most often caused by viral infection, which also may cause an associated myocarditis. Uremia (Chapter 19), a clinical syndrome associated with renal failure, is another common cause. Rheumatic fever and some autoimmune diseases are responsible for most of the other cases. Most cases are characterized by atypical chest pain and an audible friction rub. If a significant inflammatory effusion is present, cardiac malfunction may occur as the pericardial sac becomes tense and impairs diastolic filling. Some cases may progress to chronic scarring and restrictive pericarditis, which may be difficult to distinguish from cardiomyopathy.

Pericardial effusion may occur in noninflammatory conditions—congestive heart failure, blunt precordial chest trauma, metastatic malignancy, or thoracic duct lesions that fill the pericardium with chylous (fatty) lymph fluid. **Hemopericardium** refers to undiluted blood in the pericardial sac and is to be distinguished from bloody effusion and bloody exudate. Hemopericardium may be caused, for instance, by retrograde extension of an aortic dissection or rupture of the myocardium. ■

CASE STUDY 13-1 *"HE'S BEEN HAVING A LOT OF HEARTBURN LATELY"*

TOPICS
Acute myocardial infarction

THE CASE

Setting: You are working the 11 PM to 7 AM shift in a 24-hour walk-in clinic operated in a large Las Vegas hotel that is hosting a big convention.

Clinical history: At 6:30 AM, you first see Mr. Stone, a 55-year-old obese man in a wheelchair, as an aide rolls him into the urgent care cubicle. They are followed by an anxious looking woman, who introduces herself as Mr. Stone's wife. The patient is ashen and in obvious distress, holding an oxygen mask to his face.

His wife says, "He's been having a lot of heartburn lately" and tells you that for the last 2 days the pain had become much worse and was accompanied by "a very bad upset stomach" with nausea and vomiting. He took some antacid medication and felt better the next day and continued with convention activities. The heartburn, nausea, and

vomiting woke him at 6 AM this morning, and his wife insisted he come to the clinic. He agreed because he felt extremely weak, and the pain frightened him for the first time. You ask her some further questions and learn that he has smoked one pack of cigarettes a day for many years, and he recently developed diabetes that is controllable by pills. She also tells you that her husband refused to tell his physician of the chest pain despite her pleas, saying he didn't want to bother the doctor with it because the antacid tablets made the pain disappear.

Your ability to question Mr. Stone directly is limited by his need to keep the oxygen mask to his face, but in between gasps he tells you that he is having severe pain in his chest and that it extends to his left jaw and left elbow.

Physical examination and other data: Mr. Stone is an obese, sweaty, ashen man who is short of breath and in obvious distress. Vital signs: BP 90/60, pulse 110, temperature 97.5° F, respirations 30/min. An electrocardiogram shows numerous abnormal beats and marked S-T segment deviations. Emergency laboratory studies reveal markedly elevated levels of blood glucose, total creatine kinase (CK), cardiac CK (CK-MB), and cardiac troponins. ▶

[Case 13-1, continued]

Clinical course: Shortly after arriving in the clinic, Mr. Stone suffered cardiac arrest and could not be resuscitated.

DISCUSSION

Autopsy records from the Las Vegas medical examiner's office revealed that Mr. Stone had severe generalized and coronary atherosclerosis with thrombosis over an ulcerated, soft plaque in the proximal anterior descending coronary artery. The posterior descending coronary was 90% narrowed by old fibrotic, calcified atherosclerotic plaques. A large myocardial infarct was present, some of it about 4 days old; other areas appeared to be about 24 hours old. The fibrous scar of a small, old myocardial infarct was found in the posterior left ventricle wall. The lungs showed marked acute passive congestion and edema. There were no other significant pathological findings.

This man's infarct occurred in the early morning, a time during which a disproportionate number of acute myocardial infarcts occur because blood is more prone to coagulation and thrombosis during sleep. His diabetes (type 2, adult onset) was related to his obesity, in turn suggesting unhealthy dietary habits and lack of exercise. All of these factors encouraged the development of atherosclerosis, which was accelerated by smoking.

The small infarct that occurred about 4 days before death was heralded by nausea and vomiting, but the pain subsided after the cardiac muscle died. The recurrence of chest pain, nausea, vomiting, and sweating on the morning of admission indicated that he suffered a second infarct at that time. His ashen complexion and low blood pressure resulted from acute cardiac output failure (forward left ventricular failure) and subsequent development of acute passive congestion of the lungs and pulmonary edema (backward left ventricular failure).

An important element of this case was the patient's mistaken assumption that his chest pain was caused by "heartburn," which he self-medicated with nonprescription antacids. When the pain disappeared, he presumed the antacid to be responsible. In retrospect the pain was seen to have been angina, which often disappears naturally, sometimes misleading patients to attribute relief to the antacid medication.

POINTS TO REMEMBER

- Atherosclerosis is a lifestyle disease associated with smoking, obesity, lack of exercise, and high fat diet.
- Prompt treatment of acute myocardial infarcts saves lives.

CASE STUDY 13-1 THE ROAD NOT TAKEN—AN ALTERNATIVE SCENARIO

For all sad words of tongue or pen,
The saddest are these: "It might have been."

JOHN GREENLEAF WHITTIER (1807–1892),
AMERICAN QUAKER POET AND REFORMER, *MAUD MULLER*

THE CASE

With a bit of imagination, we can speculate how this case might have had a happier ending.

Setting: You work at a weight-loss, wellness, and healthy lifestyle business that is part of a fitness center you own with several other professionals who cater to people who want to improve their lives by adopting healthier lifestyles.

Clinical history: Mr. Stone is a 52-year-old obese acquaintance. He is the father of a good friend who has been urging his dad to lose weight and stop smoking.

In the application interview, Mr. Stone confesses that he got a shock recently when one of his best golfing buddies collapsed and died during their regular weekly golf match.

"It really shook me up," he says. "The guy was like me. We're both overweight and smoke, and—this is the thing I just can't get over—he seemed so healthy. We played golf every week, and he could get around better than most of us. I guess you never know."

"That's a point, Mr. Stone," you say, "but you have to admit that the odds favor guys like him and you having heart attacks."

"You're right," he says. "Where do we begin?"

Physical examination and other data: BP 140/88; height 5′7″, weight 211 lb (body mass index 33). His waist measures 44 inches. Laboratory tests reveal: ▶

	Mr. Stone	Reference	Interpretation
Total cholesterol	265 mg/dL	(desirable <200)	High risk
HDL cholesterol	42 mg/dL	(>60)	Increased risk
LDL cholesterol	173 mg/dL	(<100)	High risk
Triglyceride	250 mg/dL	(<150)	Risk uncertain
Fasting glucose	119 mg/dL	(n: <110)	Prediabetic?

[Case 13-1, continued]

Clinical course: A week later you meet with Mr. Stone to discuss his laboratory data and your conclusions. You start by telling him he is "a heart attack waiting to happen." You explain the causes of atherosclerosis—smoking, obesity, abdominal girth, abnormal glucose metabolism, unhealthy cholesterol levels, and hypertension—and the relationship of atherosclerosis to heart attacks. He listens intently, clearly disturbed.

"But, Mr. Stone, it's not hopeless; there is a lot you can do," you tell him, and you go on to explain the program you offer, which includes fitness and dietary instruction, "I quit" classes for smokers, and psychological support for what will be a difficult undertaking.

"Wow," he says, "that's a tall order. But I really don't have an alternative, do I?"

"Not if you want to continue to play golf until you're 90 years old; no you don't," you say.

You refer him to the doctor on your staff, who writes a prescription for a statin drug for cholesterol control, then you enroll him in your weight loss and antismoking programs and begin to track his progress closely. He cuts down to just a few cigarettes a day and begins walking every day for exercise. At first he doesn't lose weight, but with continued encouragement he drops over twenty pounds, which changes his body mass index from "obese" to "overweight." He is very proud and relieved when his fasting blood sugar level falls back into the normal range (<110 mg/dL) and his blood pressure falls to 130/84—not optimal but much better than before. On high-dose statin therapy all of his cholesterol numbers move into the desirable range, but his triglyceride remains slightly elevated, which you explain isn't of much concern and probably will remain high until he drops more weight.

On is most recent visit he tells you of a recent convention trip to Las Vegas. "Your program has been good for my golf game, too," he says. "I won first place in our association tournament."

DISCUSSION

Atherosclerosis is a lifestyle disease caused by a high fat, high salt diet; obesity; lack of exercise; and smoking. Health care professionals can do little unless the patient is motivated to change unhealthy habits. However, most motivated patients with a clearly structured program and advice and support from a professional can achieve their goals.

Objectives Recap

1. *Discuss why cardiac arrhythmias decrease cardiac output*: Arrhythmias are mechanically inefficient because chambers contract (beat) before they are optimally filled with blood.

2. *Define heart failure:* Heart failure is mechanical failure of the heart to eject the volume of blood delivered to it.

3. *Explain the Frank-Starling curve and its importance*: The Frank-Starling curve is a graphical depiction of the relationship between cardiac muscle fiber length and strength of cardiac muscle contraction. Up to a point as cardiac muscle fibers are stretched, they contract with more force; beyond that point contractions weaken. In the failing heart, muscle fibers stretch and contract more forcefully as the heart fills with extra blood. This is a compensatory mechanism that helps the failing heart maintain competence.

4. *Explain the difference between forward and backward heart failure*: The heart fails when it cannot eject the blood delivered to it. A failing left ventricle causes low cardiac output, commonly known as forward failure. Left ventricular output lags, and the unejected blood dams up, congesting the lungs. This in turn makes it difficult for the right ventricle to eject its incoming load of blood. As a result the right ventricle may fail. Right ventricular failure is commonly called backward failure, which produces generalized venous congestion and edema.

5. *Explain why and how renin is involved in heart failure*: Left-heart failure results in low cardiac output, which causes low blood pressure and low blood flow to the kidneys. The kidney responds by secreting additional renin, which stimulates the adrenal cortex to secrete aldosterone. Aldosterone in turn acts on the kidney, causing it to retain sodium (and water), thus expanding its vascular volume. The expanded vascular volume increases cardiac work and makes the cardiac failure worse, lowering cardiac output and causing even more renin secretion in a vicious circle.

6. *Contrast the clinical findings and symptoms of right-heart failure and left-heart failure*: Left-heart failure is characterized by symptoms of pulmonary congestion and edema: shortness of breath, fatigue, tachycardia, an enlarged heart, and congested, edematous lungs. In pure right-heart failure these symptoms are absent (but remember that the most common cause of right heart failure is left heart failure, so both are often present together). The symptoms of right-heart failure are

those of systemic congestion: dependent edema in the feet, legs, and genitals, hepatosplenomegaly, ascites, and pleural effusion. Additional complications of right-heart failure include deep venous thrombi and pulmonary thromboemboli.

7. *Name the syndromes of ischemic heart disease*: Angina pectoris, myocardial infarction, sudden cardiac death, chronic ischemic heart disease (ischemic cardiomyopathy).

8. *Explain why young atheromas are more dangerous than older ones are*: Young atheromas are soft and prone to fissure, rupture, or hemorrhage, each of which may precipitate thrombosis and coronary occlusion. Older, sclerotic (sometimes calcified) plaques, while likely to produce ischemia and angina, are not so prone to sudden occlusion and infarction and are easier to identify by diagnostic imaging.

9. *Explain why prompt intervention may limit the size of an infarct*: Infarcts do not leap into being in an instant; they evolve from smaller to larger. The first muscle to die is at the end of the coronary vascular supply: the subendocardial muscle. The infarct gradually enlarges for several hours until it is complete. Prompt therapeutic intervention to reestablish coronary flow may stop necrosis while the infarct is small

10. *List some complications of myocardial infarct*: Sudden death, congestive heart failure, cardiac rupture, mitral regurgitation, arrhythmia, mural thrombus, thromboembolism, and cardiogenic shock.

11. *Contrast the symptoms of myocardial infarct and angina*: Both angina and the pain of myocardial infarct have similar distribution—substernal with radiation to left arm or jaw or other sites. Angina may be relieved by rest or medication; the pain of a myocardial infarct is unremitting. Additionally, patients with a myocardial infarct may sweat profusely, be nauseated, and vomit, symptoms that do not occur with angina. Dyspnea is common in myocardial infarct but usually does not occur with angina.

12. *Explain the usefulness of cardiac creatine kinase (CK-MB) and cardiac troponin assays in the assessment of chest pain*: These are distinctive molecular elements of cardiac muscle that are washed into the bloodstream in a myocardial infarct and can be detected by laboratory tests. No cardiac muscle damage occurs with angina.

13. *Discuss effects on the heart of chronic hypertension*: The strain imposed by pumping against high pressure causes left ventricular hypertrophy. Hypertrophic myocardium is stiff and has higher-than-normal metabolic requirements, which renders the muscle more susceptible to infarction at any given amount of coronary obstruction. Stiffness reduces ventricular movement (compli-

ance) and stroke volume and increases the distance over which oxygen and nutrients must diffuse through the ventricular wall. Additionally, chronic hypertension predisposes to coronary atherosclerosis. The end result often is congestive heart failure, myocardial infarction, and cardiac arrhythmia.

14. *Explain the difference between valvular stenosis and valvular insufficiency*: A stenotic valve is one in which the valve fails to open fully, obstructing easy passage of blood. An insufficient valve is one in which the valve leaflets have lost part of their one-way gate function—either they do not close completely, or they have defects that allow backflow. Both stenosis and insufficiency are mechanically inefficient.

15. *Briefly explain the pathogenesis of acute rheumatic fever and rheumatic heart disease*: Acute rheumatic fever is an autoimmune disease that occurs in some cases of group A streptococcal pharyngitis, in which antibodies produced against strep antigens also attack the similar self antigens that are found in the heart and joints. The immune attacks may be chronic and subclinical (silent) and cause chronic rheumatic valvulitis.

16. *Explain the difference between infective endocarditis and nonbacterial endocarditis and know the hazards associated with each*: Infective endocarditis is infection, usually bacterial, of the heart valves. It is often associated with intravenous drug abuse, chronic rheumatic valvulitis, or prosthetic valves. Erosion of the valve produces valvular regurgitation (insufficiency), which may occur acutely and catastrophically. Bacterial emboli may cause distant abscesses; for example, in the brain. Nonbacterial thrombotic endocarditis is a condition in which platelets and fibrinous material accumulate on valve leaflets as small vegetations. They are seen in cachexia, internal malignancy, deep vein thrombosis, and other conditions. The risk in these vegetations is that they may become infected or embolize to cause infarction, especially brain infarcts.

17. *Define primary cardiomyopathy and offer several examples*: Primary cardiomyopathy is intrinsic disease of cardiac muscle, which may be caused by inflammation, metabolic disorder, autoimmune disease, or muscular dystrophy or other genetic condition. Some cases are of unknown cause.

18. *Explain why congenital cardiac malformations with left-to-right shunts can cause pulmonary hypertension and late cyanosis*: Pulmonary hypertension arises when increased volume of blood under high pressure is shunted through the pulmonary artery and lungs from the left side of the heart. If pulmonary pressure rises markedly, right-side pressure may exceed left-side pressure and cause reversal of blood flow (and late cyanosis) through the defect.

Typical Test Questions

1. Penetrating branches of the coronary arteries are those that:
   A. Cross the atrioventricular node
   B. Run through the atrial muscle
   C. Extend from the main coronary arteries to the endocardium
   D. Cross the interventricular septum from the left ventricle to the right ventricle

2. Atrial fibrillation is associated with which one of the following?
   A. Rapid, regular ventricular beats
   B. Rapid, irregular ventricular beats
   C. Slow ventricular rate resulting from atrial malfunction
   D. Slow atrial rate resulting from low levels of blood potassium

3. Which of the following is characteristic of compensated ventricular failure?
   A. It may be asymptomatic
   B. Pulmonary edema
   C. Cardiac arrhythmia
   D. Low levels of blood potassium

4. Which of the following is characteristic of stable angina pectoris?
   A. It is relieved by rest or medication
   B. It usually occurs at rest or at night
   C. Patients are at very high risk for immediate myocardial infarction
   D. It is usually caused by coronary vasospasm

5. Which of the following is the most common valve disease?
   A. Bicuspid aortic valve
   B. Chronic rheumatic valve disease
   C. Infective endocarditis
   D. Mitral valve myxomatous degeneration

6. True or false? The greatest hazard of infective endocarditis is stenosis.

7. True or false? About half of cases of hypertrophic cardiomyopathy are caused by a genetic defect.

8. True or false? The cause of most congenital heart disease is unknown.

9. True or false? In congenital heart disease, early cyanosis is a feature of left-to-right shunts.

10. True or false? Most pericarditis is caused by viral infection.

Diseases of the Respiratory System

This chapter begins with a review of normal pulmonary anatomy, ventilation, and gas exchange. Diseases/disorders discussed include asthma, chronic bronchitis, emphysema and other effects of cigarette smoking, pulmonary edema and thromboembolism, pneumonia, tuberculosis, and lung cancer.

BACK TO BASICS
- The Normal Respiratory Tract
- Lung Volume, Air Flow, and Gas Exchange

DISEASES OF THE UPPER RESPIRATORY TRACT

ATELECTASIS (COLLAPSE)

OBSTRUCTIVE LUNG DISEASE
- Asthma
- Chronic Obstructive Pulmonary Disease (COPD)

RESTRICTIVE LUNG DISEASE
- Interstitial Fibrosis Without Granulomatous Inflammation
- Interstitial Fibrosis With Granulomatous Inflammation

VASCULAR AND CIRCULATORY LUNG DISEASE
- Pulmonary Edema
- Pulmonary Thromboembolism

- Pulmonary Hypertension
- Adult Respiratory Distress Syndrome

PULMONARY INFECTIONS
- Pneumonia
- Lung Abscess
- Pulmonary Tuberculosis
- Pulmonary Fungus Infections (Deep Mycoses)
- Other Lung Infections

LUNG NEOPLASMS
- Bronchogenic Carcinoma
- Bronchial Carcinoid Tumor

DISEASES OF THE PLEURA

Learning Objectives

After studying this chapter you should be able to:
1. Describe the pulmonary interstitium
2. Explain spirometry, and name and explain the two spirometric measures critical to understanding lung disease
3. Name two risk factors for laryngeal carcinoma
4. Name the types of atelectases
5. Define asthma, and briefly discuss the underlying pathology
6. Name the two main categories of chronic obstructive pulmonary disease
7. Explain how chronic bronchitis and emphysema differ
8. Define bronchiectasis
9. Briefly define restrictive lung disease, and explain its pathogenesis
10. Name the two basic causes of pulmonary edema, and give an example of each
11. Discuss the consequences of pulmonary thromboembolism
12. Name and discuss briefly the two main anatomic varieties of pneumonia
13. Explain the terms "community-acquired pneumonia" and "nosocomial pneumonia"
14. Explain how lung abscesses differ bacteriologically from most other abscesses
15. Explain the difference between infection by the tuberculosis bacillus and the disease known as tuberculosis
16. Explain why secondary (reactivation) TB differs pathologically from primary progressive TB
17. Classify malignant lung tumors by cell type
18. Explain why small cell carcinoma is placed in a separate category from other lung malignancies

Key Terms and Concepts

BACK TO BASICS
- respiration
- bronchi
- lobe
- bronchiole
- alveoli
- pulmonary interstitium
- pulmonary membrane
- spirometry

ATELECTASIS (COLLAPSE)
- atelectasis

OBSTRUCTIVE LUNG DISEASE
- obstructive lung disease
- asthma
- chronic obstructive pulmonary disease (COPD)
- emphysema
- chronic bronchitis

RESTRICTIVE LUNG DISEASE
- restrictive lung disease
- idiopathic pulmonary fibrosis
- sarcoidosis

VASCULAR AND CIRCULATORY LUNG DISEASE
- pulmonary thromboembolism
- pulmonary hypertension
- cor pulmonale

PULMONARY INFECTIONS
- pneumonia
- tuberculosis (TB)
- granulomatous inflammation
- caseous necrosis
- primary tuberculosis
- primary progressive tuberculosis
- secondary tuberculosis

LUNG TUMORS
- bronchogenic carcinoma

It is better to have bad breath than to have no breath at all.

PROVERB, ORIGIN UNKNOWN

BACK TO BASICS

Respiration is more than breathing. It includes three separate but related functions: 1) ventilation (breathing); 2) gas exchange, the movement of oxygen and carbon dioxide between lungs and tissues via blood; and 3) oxygen utilization, the use of oxygen by cells to release energy. Function of the lungs is called *external respiration*; gas exchange and oxygen utilization in tissues is called *internal respiration*. Impairment of any step in these events can cause disease or death.

THE NORMAL RESPIRATORY TRACT

The normal respiratory tract (Fig. 14-1) is divided into an upper part and a lower part. The airways of both are lined by tall, columnar epithelium with tiny surface hair-like *cilia*. The pharynx, epiglottis, and larynx are lined by smooth squamous epithelium to facilitate swallowing.

The *upper respiratory tract* consists of the nose, sinuses, pharynx, epiglottis, and larynx. Its principal function is to filter, warm, moisten, and channel air. Hair in the nose, cilia in the nasal mucous membrane, and a coat of mucus trap bacteria and particulate matter.

The *lower respiratory tract* consists of the trachea, bronchi, lungs, and pleurae. Its principal function is to oxygenate blood and collect and discharge carbon dioxide (CO_2), produced by energy metabolism. Air enters through the trachea, which divides into right and left main **bronchi**, one for each lung. The bronchi in turn divide into smaller branches, each of which serve one **lobe**—*upper* and *lower* lobes in the left lung, and *upper*, *middle,* and *lower* lobes in the right lung. The smallest bronchial division is the **bronchiole**, each of which serves a small cluster of air sacs, the **alveoli**, which are the final, smallest division of the airway. Blood vessels in the alveolar walls exchange oxygen and carbon dioxide (CO_2) with alveolar air.

As is depicted in Figure 14-2, large *bronchi* are held open by an outer ring of stiff cartilage and are lined by mucous glands, bundles of smooth muscle, and epithelium formed of ciliated cells, mucous cells, and neuroendocrine cells, all of which originate from bronchial stem cells. As bronchi branch into smaller tubes, cartilage and mucous glands gradually disappear until in the bronchioles no cartilage or mucous

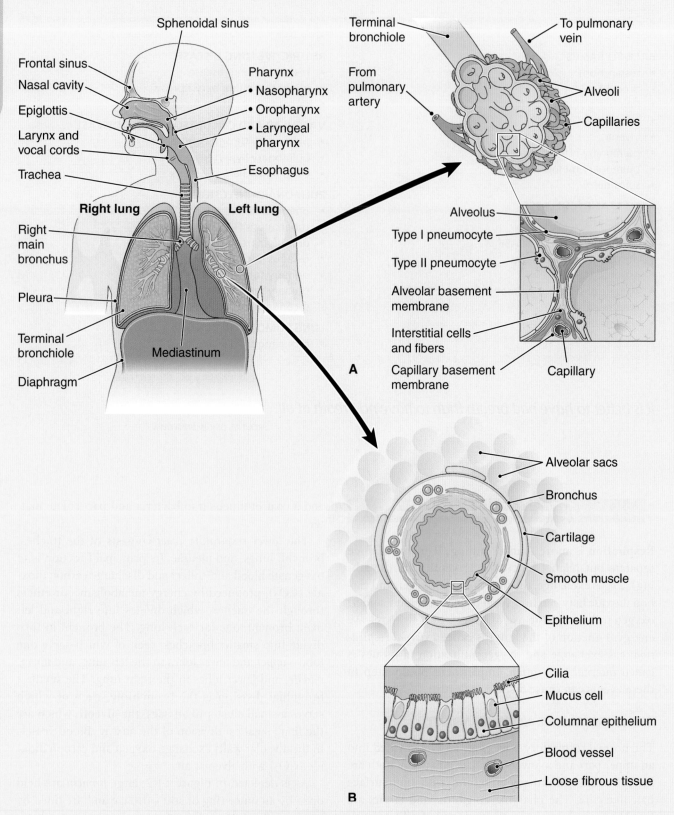

Figure 14-1 **The respiratory system. A,** Alveolar detail. **B,** Bronchial detail.

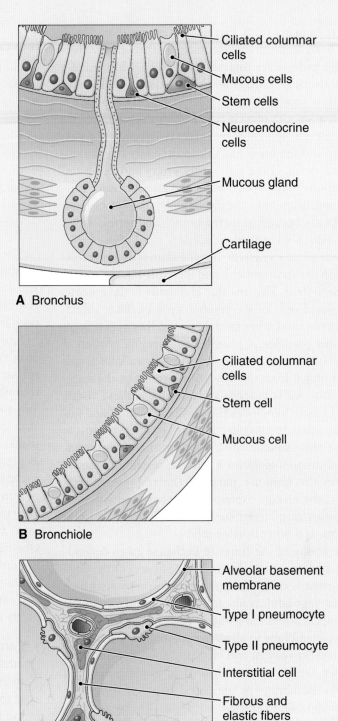

A Bronchus

- Ciliated columnar cells
- Mucous cells
- Stem cells
- Neuroendocrine cells
- Mucous gland
- Cartilage

B Bronchiole

- Ciliated columnar cells
- Stem cell
- Mucous cell

C Alveolus

- Alveolar basement membrane
- Type I pneumocyte
- Type II pneumocyte
- Interstitial cell
- Fibrous and elastic fibers
- Capillary

Figure 14-2 **Microscopic anatomy of bronchi and alveoli.**
A, Bronchi are stiff tubes composed of rings of cartilage and lined by mucous glands, bundles of smooth muscle, and epithelium formed of ciliated columnar cells, mucous cells, neuroendocrine cells, and stem cells (which give rise to all the others). **B,** Bronchioles are smaller, have thinner walls, and are composed of epithelium and smooth muscle; no cartilage or mucous glands are present. **C,** Alveoli are lined by type I and type II (surfactant-secreting) pneumocytes and supported by a basement membrane, beneath which are interstitial cells, fibrous and elastic fibers, and pulmonary capillaries.

glands are present; only epithelium and smooth muscle remain, allowing the bronchioles to dilate or constrict easily.

Alveoli are lined by type I and type II **pneumocytes**. Type I pneumocytes are flat, thin cells that form about 90% of the alveolar surface. Type II pneumocytes secrete **pulmonary surfactant**, a soapy fluid that decreases alveolar surface tension and helps alveoli remain open. The alveolar wall contains capillaries that connect the pulmonary artery, carrying incoming unoxygenated blood, to the pulmonary veins, carrying oxygenated blood back to the heart. Beneath the pneumocytes that line the alveoli is the **pulmonary interstitium**, which is formed of a lacy network of fibrous and elastic tissue, pulmonary capillaries, capillary and alveolar basement membranes, and a few smooth muscle cells and fibrocytes.

The lung is served by two vascular systems: the pulmonary and the bronchial. The pulmonary circulation, which consists of the pulmonary artery and veins and their connecting capillaries in the alveolar wall, provides nourishment to the alveoli only. The trachea and bronchi are nourished by the bronchial arteries, which are branches of the thoracic aorta.

The respiratory system, like the skin, is in direct contact with the environment, and therefore it has a special defense system. The first line of defense is the mucous and ciliated cells of the respiratory epithelium, which trap bacteria and other microbes, as well as pollen, soot, and other particles. A coordinated sweeping motion of the cilia moves mucus upward to be swallowed, spit out, or blown from the nose. Also present in the respiratory mucosa is **mucosa-associated lymphoid tissue** (MALT), which includes the tonsils, adenoids, and numerous other small collections of lymphocytes in the trachea and bronchi. MALT secretes high concentrations of immunoglobulin A into the respiratory mucus to form the **immune paint** of the respiratory tree. Finally, the alveoli contain macrophages (**dust cells**) that scavenge material such as pollen grains, carbon particles, and other inhaled solids.

The ability of the lungs to exchange gases depends on the surface area available. The total area of the alveolar surface is called the **pulmonary membrane**, which in an average adult is about 750 square feet (about the floor area of a four-car garage). The capacity of the pulmonary membrane to allow oxygen and carbon dioxide exchange between air and blood is pulmonary **diffusion capacity**, which can be impaired by any disorder that destroys membrane or limits the ability of oxygen or carbon dioxide to diffuse across it. Destroyed membrane can never be recovered—not by exercise, not by medicines, not by anything short of a lung transplant. Smokers take note.

LUNG VOLUME, AIR FLOW, AND GAS EXCHANGE

For normal ventilation, the lungs must freely exchange oxygen and carbon dioxide, which requires that:

- The alveoli must be open. Disease example: atelectasis, in which an accumulation of pleural fluid compresses the lung and collapses alveoli

- Air must move freely into and out of the alveoli. Disease example: asthma, in which spasm of bronchiolar smooth muscle narrows the airway and restricts air flow
- There must be sufficient pulmonary membrane for gas exchange. Disease example: emphysema, in which smoking has destroyed pulmonary membrane
- The pulmonary interstitium must be thin and delicate. Disease example: interstitial fibrosis, in which an accumulation of fibrous tissue stiffens the lung and prevents free flow of air and also interferes with gas diffusion between blood and alveoli

The total volume of the lungs is about 6 liters. As is illustrated in Figure 14-3, total lung *volume* is subdivided into smaller volumes. A combination of volumes is called a *capacity*. Lung diseases alter volumes and capacities.

Spirometry is a diagnostic procedure that measures lung volumes and capacities, and the flow rate (liters per second) of air going into and out of the lungs. The technique is simple: the patient is given a mouthpiece and tube connected to a measuring device and instructed to breathe normally. Then the patient is asked to take the deepest possible breath and exhale as rapidly as possible. The results are recorded on a graph similar to the one shown in Figure 14-3A.

Lung diseases have typical spirometry patterns. Generalized disease that impairs airflow may be divided into two categories: obstructive and restrictive. **Obstructive disease** (Fig. 14-3B) is characterized by limitation of *airflow*, **restrictive disease** (Fig. 14-3C) by limitation of lung *expansion*. Assigning lung disease to one category or the other requires measuring lung capacity and airflow rate.

- **Forced vital capacity (FVC)** is a *volume* measurement; it is that amount of air expelled from maximum inspiration to maximum expiration, regardless of the time taken to expel it. FVC is measured by asking the patient to take the deepest possible breathe and blow out as much air as possible; no timing is involved.
- **Forced expiratory volume (FEV$_1$)** is a *rate* measurement; the timed measurement of the amount of air that can be expelled from maximum inspiration in the first second of effort. The patient is instructed to take the deepest possible breath and breathe out as hard as possible. The amount of air expelled in the first second is recorded.

The FEV$_1$/FVC ratio is critical in separating obstructive and restrictive lung disease.

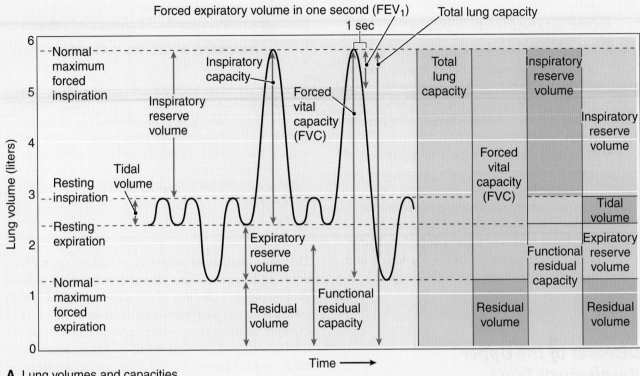

A Lung volumes and capacities

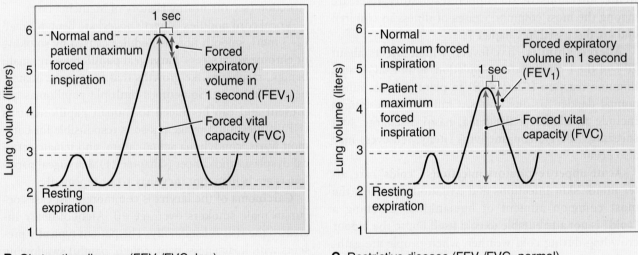

B Obstructive disease (FEV₁/FVC=low)

C Restrictive disease (FEV₁/FVC=normal)

Figure 14-3 **Spirography. A,** Normal spirogram tracings with lung volumes and capacities. **B,** Spirogram in obstructive disease: One-second forced expiratory volume (FEV₁) is low; forced vital capacity (FVC) is normal. **C,** Spirogram in restrictive disease: Both one-second forced expiratory volume (FEV₁) and forced vital capacity (FVC) are low.

In *obstructive disease* the *rate* of air flowing out of the lungs is slowed; therefore the amount the patient can expel is low. What's more, in obstructive disease lung volumes are usually normal, so *the ratio of airflow to lung volume is low*; that is, the *FEV₁/FVC ratio is low.*

To the contrary, in *restrictive disease* the ratio of airflow to lung volume is usually near normal because restrictive disorders limit *both* volume and flow rate pro-portionally, and the FEV₁/FVC ratio remains near the normal range. The ratio may vary slightly up or down, but it is not markedly decreased, as it is in obstructive disease.

Both obstructive and restrictive disease limit CO_2 and O_2 exchange: patients get less O_2 and retain more CO_2 than healthy people. Laboratory study of arterial blood O_2 and CO_2 ("arterial blood gases" in clinical terms) is critical in assessing lung function.

Diseases of the Upper Respiratory Tract

Acute infections of the upper respiratory tract are among the most common causes of illness in children and are discussed in Chapter 7.

Allergic rhinitis (hay fever), which affects about 20% of the United States population, is an exaggerated immune reaction (Chapter 8) to plant pollens, fungi, animal dander, or dust mites. Clinical manifestations include nasal mucosal edema, nasal discharge, and sneezing. Allergic conjunctivitis (itchy, red eyes) may also occur.

Acute upper respiratory infections ("colds") are, after minor skin infections and irritations, perhaps the most common ailment of humankind. Catching a "cold" is not attributable to cold itself but to the indoor crowding during cold weather, when people are gathered together indoors and viruses are easily transmitted by droplets in the air. All "colds" are viral, and symptoms include clear nasal discharge and low grade fever, which resolve spontaneously, usually within a few days, although some infections may last 10–12 days. The appearance of yellow, purulent nasal discharge or ear or sinus pain usually signifies secondary bacterial infection, which warrants antibiotic therapy. Because "colds" are viral, conventional antibiotics are useless; indeed, unwise use of antibiotics to treat upper respiratory infections has promoted the development of strains of antibiotic-resistant bacteria.

Acute pharyngitis ("sore throat") is less common and potentially far more serious than a simple "cold."

The usual case has its origins in a virus infection and is mild, with fever, slight mucosal reddening, painful swallowing, and swelling of the tonsils and neck lymph nodes. Bacterial pharyngitis can be far more serious. For example, acute streptococcal pharyngitis may cause autoimmune reactions that result in either acute rheumatic fever (Chapter 13) or acute glomerulonephritis (Chapter 19). In some cases, inflammation and edema, or the formation of an abscess, can cause airway obstruction (see the nearby History of Medicine box).

Vocal cord nodules (*singer's nodes*) are benign, small (2–3 mm), smooth fibrous nodules caused by smoking or chronic vocal stress. **Laryngeal papillomas** are small, benign, raspberry-like growths that may cause hoarseness or bleeding. Sometimes multiple papillomas are present and can be traced to human papillomavirus (HPV) infection, the agent also is responsible for common warts, condyloma acuminatum, and female cervical dysplasia and cancer (Chapter 21). Laryngeal papillomas are benign, but they may recur repeatedly.

Carcinoma of the larynx is common; most cases occur in male smokers over age 40. Alcohol *abuse* increases the risk substantially. The patient typically presents with hoarseness, pain, cough, painful swallowing (*dysphagia*), or coughing blood (**hemoptysis**). Almost all carcinomas of the larynx are squamous carcinomas arising from laryngeal squamous epithelium. Most are confined to the larynx at time of diagnosis. If the neoplasm has metastasized, the metastases are most likely to be found in neck lymph nodes; distant metastases are uncommon and occur late. Most patients survive beyond five years after surgery or radiotherapy or both.

Atelectasis (Collapse)

Atelectasis is collapse of part of the lung, a condition fatal to politicians. Collapsed lung tissue does not exchange gases properly and invites infection. There are three types of atelectasis:

- *Resorption atelectasis* occurs when a bronchial obstruction prevents air from reaching part of the lung, and the air in the alveoli beyond the obstruction is completely absorbed by blood circulating through the alveoli. The most common cause of obstruction is a mucous plug formed during general anesthesia. Other causes include asthma, bronchitis, and obstructing tumors. A cause in children is aspiration of foreign objects.
- *Compression atelectasis* (Fig. 14-4) occurs when external pressure is exerted on the lung from pleural blood, fluid, or air or from abdominal upward pressure on the diaphragm. Examples include pleural effusion of congestive heart failure, and compression of the posterior lower lobes caused by upward pressure on the diaphragm from patients who are bedridden, who have ascites, or who have had chest or abdominal surgery and are not breathing normally because of pain associated with each breath.
- *Contraction atelectasis* occurs when scars in the lung or pleura constrict, collapsing the lung. Examples include tuberculous lung scars and pleural scars from chronic pleural inflammation.

Compression and resorption atelectases are reversible; contraction atelectasis is not. Severe atelectasis can cause hypoxia, and chronic or recurrent atelectasis invites infection.

In **right middle lobe syndrome**, the right middle lobe undergoes atelectasis because the bronchus is obstructed. Recall that the right lung has three lobes, the smallest of them the right middle lobe, which is sandwiched anteriorly between the much larger upper and lower lobes. The right middle lobe is served by an unusually long, thin bronchus that is particularly prone to obstruction from bronchial mucus or inflammatory debris. Recurrent episodes of atelectasis may evolve into right middle lobe pneumonia or abscess.

Obstructive Lung Disease

In **obstructive lung disease** there is some general barrier to the smooth flow of air through the bronchi. Lung volume is not affected. The problem is getting air *out*, not getting air in. The patient can draw a quick and deep breath, but exhalation is difficult and slow because small bronchioles are constricted, and the patient must breathe in again before the previous breath has been completely exhaled. The result is slow, labored breathing with an audible expiratory wheeze as air whistles through tight bronchi.

Recall from the discussion above and Figure 14-3 that in obstructive disease the one-second forced expiratory volume (FEV_1) is low, and volume (forced vital capacity, FVC) is normal. Therefore, the ratio FEV_1/FVC is low.

ASTHMA

Asthma is a chronic inflammatory disease of small bronchi and bronchioles that is characterized by episodes of bronchospasm and airtrapping. In normal breathing, bronchioles expand slightly with inhalation and constrict slightly on exhalation. In asthma the constriction on exhalation is exaggerated and obstructs air outflow. The pathologic lesion is chronic inflammation, sometimes associated with allergy, but in most cases asthma is triggered by inhaled irritants, such as cigarette smoke or polluted air. Regardless of the initial irritant, with repeated exposure bronchioles become progressively inflamed, irritated, and hyperreactive to irritants.

Asthma can be classified according to the irritant involved.

- *Allergic asthma*: In some patients the irritant is an allergen that stimulates a type I hypersensitivity (ana-

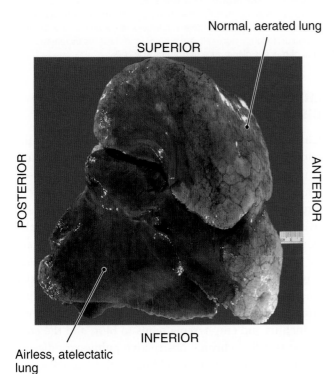

Normal, aerated lung
SUPERIOR
POSTERIOR
ANTERIOR
INFERIOR
Airless, atelectatic lung

Figure 14-4 **Compression atelectasis.** Lateral view of right lung. In this reclining patient pleural fluid compressed the lower and posterior aspects of the right lung, which are dark and airless.

phylaxis) reaction (Chapter 8). Allergic asthma occurs most often in children who have a genetic tendency toward other allergic reactions, a condition known as *atopy*, which is most often manifest by "hay fever" (allergic rhinitis) and skin allergies (atopic dermatitis, Chapter 24).

• *Occupational asthma*: Wood, grain, or textile dust, industrial chemicals, and dozens of other workplace substances can cause asthma or precipitate an acute episode.

• *Exercise-induced asthma*: Exercise, especially in cold air, can stimulate bronchospasm in at least half of patients with asthma.

• *Infectious asthma*: A common precipitating factor in children with asthma is viral acute upper respiratory infection.

• *Others*: Other factors that may precipitate an acute attack include emotional stress, drug reaction (especially aspirin), and severe air pollution.

In many patients with chronic asthma, bronchospasm and chronic inflammation become interlocked and evolve into simple *airway hyperreactivity*, in which bronchospasm is the result regardless of the type of irritant. Similar airway overreactivity can also be seen in some patients, usually smokers, who have chronic bronchitis, a condition known as *chronic asthmatic bronchitis*.

As is depicted in Figure 14-5, the pathology of asthma includes bronchi that have hyperplastic mucous glands, mucous plugs, hypertrophied bronchial smooth muscles, edema, and marked inflammation (typically demonstrating numerous eosinophils).

Most asthma begins in childhood; males are most commonly affected. A typical asthmatic attack begins suddenly, lasts several hours, and features breathlessness, wheezing, tightness in the chest, and spasms of coughing that produce abundant mucus. Drug therapy has two aims, to reduce chronic inflammation and to relieve acute bronchospasm. Steroids and other drugs are administered long term, usually by inhalation, as preventatives to control inflammation. Bronchospasm is relieved by injectable or inhalant drugs (bronchodilators) that block bronchial smooth muscle contractions.

Status asthmaticus is potentially fatal, severe asthmatic bronchospasm. Bronchioles become plugged with thick, sticky mucus that obstructs airflow into and out of the alveoli, and gas exchange falls dangerously. Patients become cyanotic (ashen or blue) from hypoxia and acidotic from retained carbon dioxide. Status asthmaticus is a dire emergency that requires vigorous and prompt treatment.

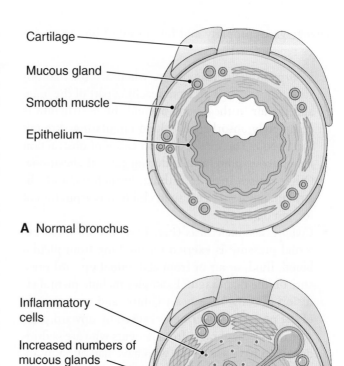

A Normal bronchus

B Bronchus in asthma

Figure 14-5 **The bronchi in asthma. A,** The normal bronchial lumen is wide; normal numbers of smooth muscle cells and mucous glands are present. **B,** In asthma, the lumen is narrow and contains a large amount of mucus; inflammatory cells are present; and there are increased numbers of mucous glands and smooth muscle cells.

CHRONIC OBSTRUCTIVE PULMONARY DISEASE (COPD)

Chronic obstructive pulmonary disease (COPD) is the name applied to several related diseases—emphysema, chronic bronchitis, and chronic asthmatic bronchitis—which have in common chronic bronchial outflow obstruction. Typically, patients with these diseases have overlapping features. Figure 14-6 depicts these relationships, and Case Study 14.1 at the end of this chapter presents a clinical example. Most cases begin as emphysema or chronic bronchitis caused by cigarette smoking. When patients finally seek medical attention after years of smoking, the distinction between chronic bronchitis and emphysema tends to blur, and the condition is called chronic obstructive pulmonary disease (COPD). COPD, with or without asthmatic episodes, slows the flow of air into and out of the lungs, thereby impairing the uptake of oxygen and the discharge of carbon dioxide.

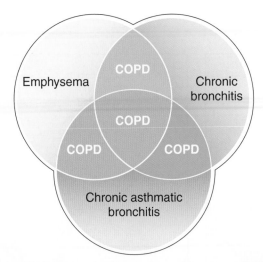

Chronic obstructive pulmonary disease (COPD)

Figure 14-6 **Chronic obstructive pulmonary disease (COPD).** The relationships among emphysema, chronic bronchitis, chronic asthmatic bronchitis, and chronic obstructive pulmonary disease. Most patients have a mixture.

Emphysema

Emphysema is characterized by destruction of alveolar walls and merging of alveoli to form large air spaces. The destruction causes marked decrease of pulmonary membrane surface area and diffusion capacity. Emphysema is a common disease, present in about half of patients coming to autopsy, most of whom had no symptoms. There is a clear relationship to smoking—90% of cases, especially severe emphysema, occur in cigarette smokers. However, only about 10% of smokers develop emphysema; the other 90% do not, and we do not understand why. Nevertheless, half of smokers die from smoking-related illnesses such as cardiovascular disease and cancer.

Cigarette smoke irritates lung tissue and causes inflammation. Inflammatory cells release digestive enzymes as part of their normal activity. These digestive enzymes are normally inhibited by **alpha-1 antitrypsin**, a protein made by the liver, whose purpose is to neutralize these enzymes in order to prevent overactivity and digestion of normal tissue. Cigarette smoke not only inflames the lung, it inhibits alpha-1 antitrypsin, which leaves the enzymes free to digest (dissolve) lung tissue. Pulmonary membrane is destroyed, and diffusion capacity is reduced with every alveolus digested. Of interest, too, is that not only do patients with congenital alpha-1 antitrypsin deficiency (Chapter 7) have a marked tendency to develop early emphysema, but also in these patients, both the age at which emphysema first occurs and its severity are accelerated by smoking.

The gross and microscopic anatomy of emphysema (Fig. 14-7 and Fig. 14-8) features large air spaces throughout the lungs, especially in the apex of each lung. Large air spaces are clearly visible to the naked eye. An unusually large air space is a *bulla* or **bleb**.

Shortness of breath usually is the first symptom of patients suffering primarily from emphysema; however, wheezing and coughing also may be the first symptoms in patients whose initial disease is primarily chronic bronchitis or chronic asthmatic bronchitis. Weight loss in patients with emphysema can be dramatic: the body sheds muscle the lungs cannot support. The typical emphysema patient is an emaciated smoker with severe breathlessness—the chest is barrel-shaped from strained overexpansion, neck muscles bulge with each breath, and the patient sits hunched forward, hands on knees, elbows spread out, breathing out through pursed lips.

Proof of expiratory airflow obstruction requires *spirometry* (Fig. 14-3B), which shows low one-second forced expiratory volume (FEV_1) and relatively normal forced vital capacity (FVC). The FEV_1/FVC ratio is markedly decreased.

Chronic Bronchitis

Chronic bronchitis is a clinical diagnosis that can be made in any patient who has had a chronic cough that *produces sputum* for three consecutive months two years in a row. Although some chronic bronchitis is caused by air pollution, *cigarette smoking is the prime cause*. Smoke

Small pulmonary vessel

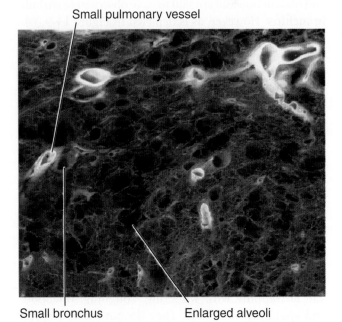

Small bronchus   Enlarged alveoli

Figure 14-7 **Emphysema.** Close-up view. Normal alveoli are too small to be visible to the unaided eye. Merger of alveoli into larger air spaces makes them plainly visible in this specimen.

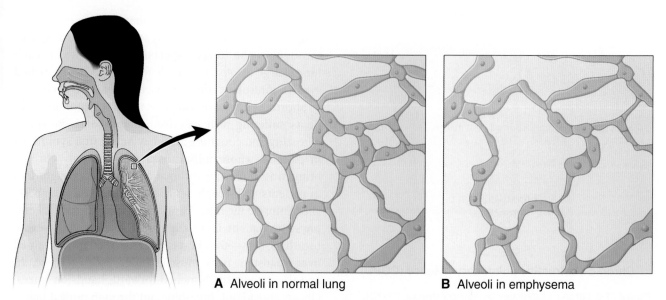

A Alveoli in normal lung   B Alveoli in emphysema

Figure 14-8 **Emphysema, microscopic development. A,** Normal alveoli. **B,** In emphysema, destruction of alveolar walls results in large air spaces with decreased pulmonary surface area for gas diffusion.

irritates the bronchi and stimulates chronic inflammation and marked bronchial mucous secretion. In contrast to emphysema, where the initial lesion is in the alveoli, in chronic bronchitis the initial lesion is in the bronchi.

Patients with **simple chronic bronchitis** have a productive cough but do not have airway obstruction. Some patients with chronic bronchitis have sudden episodes of asthma-like wheezing and are said to have **chronic asthmatic bronchitis.** Others have consistent wheezing and obstruction and are said to have **obstructive chronic bronchitis.** However, as is depicted in Figure 14-9, *virtually all patients with chronic bronchitis also have significant emphysema,* and therefore chronic bronchitis and emphysema are lumped together under the term chronic obstructive pulmonary disease (COPD).

Patients who suffer primarily from emphysema differ clinically from those who suffer mainly from obstructive chronic bronchitis. When loss of diffusing capacity (emphysema) is the main problem, patients are usually thin (because weight loss accompanies loss of pulmonary membrane), barrel-chested, and short of breath, but they remain well oxygenated and pink, an appearance sometimes described as "pink puffer" to contrast them from those with chronic bronchitis.

By contrast, when obstructive chronic bronchitis is the main problem, patients have airflow obstruction and airtrapping with wheezing, coughing, infection, and sputum production. They do not move air well enough for good oxygenation or CO_2 elimination, so they are hypoxic (and cyanotic, blue) and acidotic from retained CO_2. These patients do not lose weight because

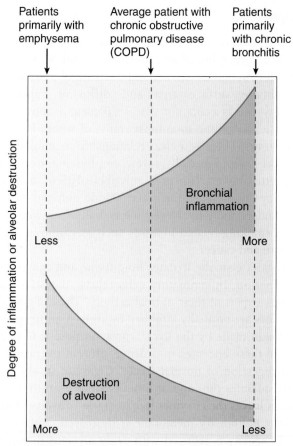

Figure 14-9 **The relationship between emphysema and chronic bronchitis.** Most patients with chronic obstructive pulmonary disease (COPD) have a mixture of bronchial inflammation and alveolar destruction.

they have not lost much pulmonary membrane. Because they are bulkier and cyanotic they are sometimes called "blue bloaters" to contrast them with the "pink puffers" who mainly have emphysema. Most patients fall somewhere between these extremes.

All patients with COPD are at risk for chronic hypoxia (low oxygen), which can lead to pulmonary vasospasm, and they are, as well, at risk for pulmonary hypertension and right heart failure (a combination known as *cor pulmonale*). Death from COPD is usually associated with some combination of hypoxia, acidosis, and right-heart failure. Pneumonia is often the terminal event.

Bronchiectasis

Bronchiectasis (from Greek *ektasis*, for dilated) is characterized by marked, permanent dilation of small bronchi when there is destruction of smooth muscle and elastic supporting tissue of the airway, leaving a dilated, flaccid, pus-filled tube. Both *obstruction* and *infection* are required; either may come first. Obstruction can cause mucous retention, offering a breeding ground for infection; or chronic infection may damage bronchial walls, leading to excess mucous production and mucous retention. In either instance a vicious circle ensues.

Bronchiectasis is not a primary condition; it is always secondary to other, underlying disorders, which include:

- Immunodeficiency states, which encourage infection
- Chronic infections such as tuberculosis, which damage bronchial walls
- Retained bronchial foreign body, which causes mucous retention and infection
- Conditions, such as cystic fibrosis (Chapter 7), that cause generation of thick mucus, which obstructs bronchi

The lower lobes of both lungs typically are involved, especially in airways that are nearly vertical.

The clinical picture in bronchiectasis is dominated by chronic infection and a persistent cough productive of copious amounts of infected, foul smelling, yellow sputum. Life-threatening pulmonary hemorrhage can occur. The severe chronic inflammation can also cause amyloidosis (Chapter 8); microorganisms may spread by blood to cause brain abscess, and cor pulmonale may develop.

Restrictive Lung Disease

Restrictive lung disease is a disease of stiff lungs, which limit both the *volume* of lung expansion and the *rate* of expansion and contraction. Restrictive lung diseases are

chronic inflammatory conditions of pulmonary interstitial tissue that render the lung stiff and inelastic. Recall that the normal interstitium—alveolar walls, capillaries, and supporting tissue—is thin and delicate, a condition necessary for easy gas diffusion. Even a little interstitial disease adversely affects diffusion. As the interstitium thickens, gas diffusion decreases; but of equal or greater importance, less air is moved in and out of the lungs.

As is illustrated in Figure 14-10, interstitial fibrosis is a condition in which there is an accumulation of scar tissue in the interstitium that is the product of chronic inflammation caused by some type of ongoing injury. Some diseases of the interstitium are characterized by *granulomatous inflammation*, a special type of chronic inflammation (Chapter 3), a distinction that serves to separate interstitial lung diseases into two large groups: those with granulomas and those without. Sometimes the cause of the fibrosis is known. For example, interstitial fibrosis can be caused by inhaled materials, such as rock dust from stone cutting or mining (silicosis), or it can occur in association with a collagen-vascular disease such as systemic lupus erythematosus (Chapter 8). However, in many instances the cause is unknown.

Spirometry (Fig. 14-3C) in restrictive disease shows roughly equal declines of one-second forced expiratory volume (FEV_1) and forced vital capacity (FVC). Therefore, the FEV_1/FVC ratio is usually near normal. By contrast, in obstructive disease the ratio is markedly decreased.

Alveolar walls thickened
by interstitial fibrous tissue

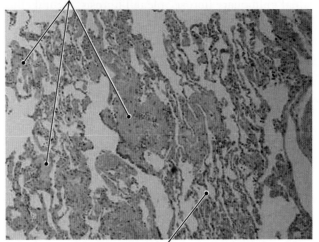

Normal, thin
alveolar wall

Figure 14-10 **Interstitial fibrosis.** Marked thickening of many alveolar walls by dense, scar-like fibrous tissue.

Typically the first symptom of interstitial fibrosis is shortness of breath with exercise; later, patients become short of breath at rest. Breathing is rapid and shallow, and cyanosis appears as disease progresses. Chest x-ray usually reveals a diffuse pattern of streaks, nodules, and shadows in both lung fields. With damage to the pulmonary vascular bed, resistance to blood flow increases, and pulmonary hypertension occurs.

INTERSTITIAL FIBROSIS WITHOUT GRANULOMATOUS INFLAMMATION

Idiopathic pulmonary fibrosis is known by a dozen or more names, a clue that its cause is a mystery. At time of diagnosis most patients are middle-aged adults, but the process presumably has been under way for many years. Men are affected more often than women are. There is a strong suspicion that immune reactions play an important role, and some patients will be found to have collagen-vascular disease as the underlying cause.

Fibrosis begins insidiously and usually presents as shortness of breath. Cor pulmonale, hypoxia, and cyanosis are characteristic of advanced disease. A few cases may regress spontaneously but in most, the prognosis is bleak; median survival is about 5 years. Lung transplant is the only effective therapy.

Pneumoconiosis is a term applied to lung disease caused by inhaled dusts and fumes. Coal dust causes coal worker's pneumoconiosis (black lung disease), and rock or stone dust causes **silicosis**, the most common chronic occupational disease in the world.

Asbestosis is a lung disease caused by inhalation of asbestos particles, which are tiny silicate fibers formerly used in industry, especially for fireproofing and insulation. When inhaled in quantity, asbestos causes interstitial pulmonary fibrosis, pleural fibrosis, pleural effusion, or pleural mesothelioma, a neoplasm of the pleura that can be either benign or malignant. Asbestos per se does not appear to cause lung cancer, but it promotes the development of cancer in smokers because asbestos traps and retains the carcinogens in cigarette smoke.

Most exposure to asbestos occurs in industrial settings; however, improved industrial hygiene has nearly eliminated the risk. In nonindustrial settings asbestos is found as old spray-on insulation on ceilings, walls, and pipes. The risk from undisturbed asbestos in these settings, even in densely occupied public spaces, is virtually zero. Removal is expensive and experts conclude it can be left safely in place if not disturbed.

The clinical picture of asbestosis is similar to that of other interstitial lung diseases except that pleural mesothelioma may develop in some patients with asbestosis.

INTERSTITIAL FIBROSIS WITH GRANULOMATOUS INFLAMMATION

Sarcoidosis is a systemic granulomatous disease of unknown cause that affects many tissues and features granulomatous inflammation. Despite highly distinctive pathology and decades of research, the cause is unknown.

Sarcoid granulomas may develop in any organ, but chiefly they appear in the lungs and mediastinal lymph nodes. Other common sites include skin, mucous membranes of the nose and mouth, the eyes (iritis, glaucoma, and retinitis, Chapter 25), lacrimal glands, and the spleen and liver. Sarcoidosis occurs worldwide, but its incidence varies greatly from place to place, and it occurs ten times more frequently in African Americans than in American whites. Evidence suggests that the cause is a combination of immune dysfunction, genetic susceptibility, and exposure to some type of microbe.

The clinical picture is varied. Many cases are asymptomatic and are initially diagnosed on chest x-ray taken for some other purpose. In others, skin lesions, or enlarged lymph nodes, spleen, or liver offer the first clue. However, most patients seek medical attention for pulmonary symptoms: shortness of breath, cough, chest pain, or hemoptysis.

Sarcoidosis is unpredictable. Two thirds of patients recover completely, many after a course of steroid therapy. Of the remaining one third, most develop lung dysfunction or visual problems. An unfortunate few develop progressive lung disease and usually succumb to pulmonary fibrosis or pulmonary hypertension.

Diagnosis depends on biopsy to demonstrate characteristic granulomas and clinical exclusion of other causes of granulomatous disease, such as tuberculosis.

Hypersensitivity pneumonitis is a T-cell mediated, delayed hypersensitivity reaction (Chapter 8). Also called *allergic alveolitis*, it occurs as a response to inhaled antigens, such as moldy hay and other organic dusts found in occupational settings. Lung biopsy reveals widespread lung granulomatous inflammation. The *acute* form may present as a "flu" syndrome of cough and fever after exposure to the offending dust. A one-time, acute exposure has no lasting consequences; however, chronic exposure can cause interstitial fibrosis.

Vascular and Circulatory Lung Disease

One of the most important differences between the systemic circulation and the pulmonary circulation is the low blood pressure in the pulmonary arterial tree. In the systemic circulation, blood pressure is about 120/80 mm Hg. In the pulmonary circulation, blood pressure is very low—about 25/8 mm Hg, and averages about 15 mm Hg. Resistance in the pulmonary vascular bed is low, too, as it must be for blood to flow normally under such little pressure (Chapter 13).

PULMONARY EDEMA

Normal alveoli contain no fluid. Accumulation of fluid in the alveoli is **pulmonary edema**. Edema can accumulate when hemodynamic forces become altered or lungs sustain injury, allowing fluid to seep into the alveoli from injured pulmonary tissue and blood vessels.

Hemodynamic edema accumulates when there is increased hemodynamic pressure (blood pressure) in the lung vascular bed, most often as a result of left-heart failure (Chapter 13). In left-heart failure the left ventricle cannot eject the blood delivered to it, and blood "backs up," raising hemodynamic pressure in the pulmonary circulation. Low pulmonary blood pressure makes it very difficult for hemodynamic edema to form in the alveoli; however, when pulmonary edema occurs, it resolves slowly and interferes with gas exchange.

Microvascular injury can produce "leaky" capillaries, which exude fluid into the alveoli. Pulmonary capillaries in the alveolar wall can be injured from the alveolar side, for example, by inhaled toxic fumes, or hot gases from a fire, or from the vascular side, for example, by septicemia (blood infection) with release of bacterial endotoxin (Chapter 9), intravenous drug abuse, and many other conditions.

The main symptom of pulmonary edema is shortness of breath. Crackling rales are heard in the lung bases, and chest x-ray usually reveals widespread, splotchy infiltrates. At autopsy the lungs are heavy and wet, and they exude a frothy, slightly bloody fluid.

PULMONARY THROMBOEMBOLISM

Pulmonary thromboembolism (Fig. 14-11) is movement (embolization) of a thrombus from its origin in a vein, through the venous system into the pulmonary arterial system. Pulmonary thromboemboli are common: they cause more deaths (about 50,000) annually than traffic accidents (about 40,000), and they are frequently an undiagnosed incidental finding at autopsy.

Almost all thromboemboli arise from the deep veins of the knee, upper leg, or pelvis (Chapters 5 and 12). Local conditions predisposing to thrombosis and pulmonary thromboembolism include inflammation associated with major surgery; trauma; or infection. General conditions that promote thrombosis and thromboem-

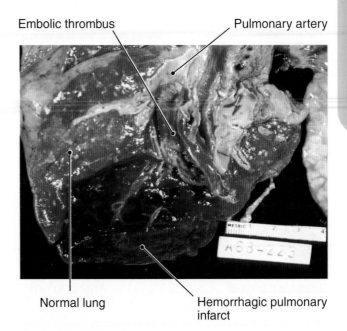

Embolic thrombus — Pulmonary artery

Normal lung — Hemorrhagic pulmonary infarct

Figure 14-11 **Pulmonary infarct.** A thrombus has embolized from the legs to the lung and fills a branch of the pulmonary artery. The dark, hemorrhagic tissue is infarcted lung.

bolism include congestive heart failure, pregnancy, birth control pills, prolonged bed rest, and metastatic cancer (paraneoplastic syndrome, Chapter 10). Two other general causes of venous thrombosis and thromboembolism are: 1) an inherited tendency toward venous thrombosis caused by a genetic defect of the gene that produces coagulation factor V, a condition known as *factor V Leiden* (Chapter 11); and, 2) lupus anticoagulant, an autoimmune antibody that occurs in some patients with systemic lupus erythematosus but is most often found in patients without any other associated disorder. This antibody interferes with laboratory tests of blood coagulation, suggesting the presence of an anticoagulant—thus its designation lupus "anticoagulant." To the contrary, however, lupus anticoagulant promotes venous thrombosis and thromboembolism, and it is other aspects of its activity that cause the laboratory anomalies.

Most thromboemboli are small and do not cause symptoms. Some cause small lung infarcts and are associated with chest pain and dyspnea. About 5% of patients have emboli large enough to completely obstruct the main pulmonary artery as it divides into right and left branches (**saddle embolus**); instantaneous death is the result. There is some evidence to suggest that recurrent, subclinical thromboembolism is one cause of primary pulmonary hypertension.

PULMONARY HYPERTENSION

Pulmonary hypertension is abnormally high blood pressure in the pulmonary vascular tree. It is a dreadful

Alveolus

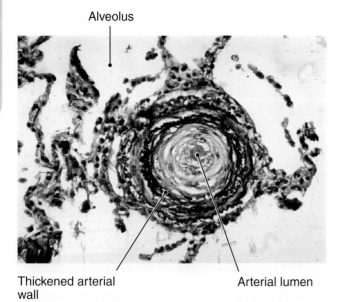

Thickened arterial wall

Arterial lumen

Figure 14-12 **Pulmonary arteriole in pulmonary hypertension.** High pulmonary vascular pressure injures the arterial wall and causes hyperplasia of cells in the wall of the artery.

disease that, once established, feeds on itself in a vicious circle.

The average blood pressure in the pulmonary tree is about 15 mm/Hg. Pulmonary hypertension is defined as sustained systolic pressure over 30 mm Hg or average pressure in excess of 25 mm Hg. As it is in the systemic circulation (Chapter 5), pulmonary blood pressure is a product of vascular resistance and blood flow (cardiac output). The most common cause of pulmonary hypertension is increased pulmonary vascular resistance. Increased pulmonary artery pressure because of increased blood flow from congenital left-to-right shunts (Chapter 13) is less often the problem.

Most cases of pulmonary hypertension are *secondary* to 1) chronic obstructive pulmonary disease or interstitial lung disease; 2) pre-existing heart disease such as shunts or mitral stenosis; 3) collagen vascular diseases, especially systemic sclerosis (scleroderma, Chapter 8); or 4) recurrent pulmonary thromboemboli. In about 5% of cases, the cause is unknown and the diagnosis is primary pulmonary hypertension, which mainly affects young women.

In established pulmonary hypertension the right ventricle is hypertrophic, dilated, and prone to failure (**cor pulmonale**). Microscopic study of the lungs reveals a highly characteristic onionskin hyperplastic thickening of the walls of small pulmonary arteries (Fig. 14-12), which is similar to the onionskin hyperplasia of renal afferent arterioles in systemic malignant hypertension (Chapter 12).

Pulmonary hypertension is characterized by shortness of breath on exertion, exertional chest pain that mimics angina, exercise syncope (fainting), and fatigue. The outlook is bleak; average survival is a few years. Nonsurgical therapy can prolong life a few years; lung transplantation is the only effective therapy.

ADULT RESPIRATORY DISTRESS SYNDROME

Adult respiratory distress syndrome (ARDS) is an acute, catastrophic disease associated with alveolar or pulmonary capillary damage caused by a wide range of conditions. The pathogenesis may be roughly summarized as follows. The offending agent injures vascular endothelium or alveoli. Neutrophils infiltrate the alveolar wall and a protein-rich fluid exudes into the alveolar space. Shortness of breath occurs and rapid breathing dries the fluid into a thick membrane that coats the alveolar wall like glue, stiffening the lung, which limits airflow and interferes with gas diffusion. Hypoxia follows.

At autopsy, pathologic findings in ARDS are striking. Grossly, the lungs look like liver—wet, heavy, dark, and airless. In acutely fatal cases the alveoli are filled with a protein-rich edema fluid. As is depicted in Figure 14-13, inflammatory edema condenses into a thick protein membrane that lines the alveolar walls, a microscopic picture conspicuously similar to that of hyaline membrane disease of the newborn (Chapter 7). After about a week, fibrous repair (Chapter 4) begins in the interstitium and may proceed to interstitial fibrosis.

Protein membrane

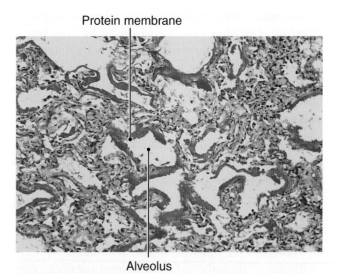

Alveolus

Figure 14-13 **Alveoli in adult respiratory distress syndrome (ARDS).** Edema accumulates in the alveoli as a result of alveolar and pulmonary capillary damage and condenses into a thick protein membrane, which coats alveolar walls and impairs gas exchange. Reprinted with permission from Rubin E. Pathology. 4th ed. Philadelphia. Lippincott Williams and Wilkins, 2005.

The clinical course of ARDS is dreadful—fatality rates are in excess of 50%, especially if associated with bacterial sepsis. Clinical onset is rapid, usually within 24 hours of the initial condition. Shortness of breath and hypoxia are severe. Chest x-rays often show a "white lung" of nearly complete airlessness. Causes are varied: sepsis, smoke inhalation, near drowning, oxygen toxicity, burns, heroin overdose, DIC, pancreatitis, uremia, large bone fracture with bone marrow fat embolism, and bacterial endotoxic shock (Chapter 5). Hypoxia is common and troublesome because the treatment may be worse than the disease: oxygen itself can cause further alveolar damage. The protein-rich alveolar exudate invites growth of microorganisms, and secondary pneumonia is a frequent complication. Most of those fortunate to survive the acute phase regain normal pulmonary function in a few months; some, however, are permanently crippled by diffuse interstitial fibrosis.

Pulmonary Infections

To take a breath is to commit mass murder—of microbes. The airways are specially equipped to resist microbial infection: they have a specialized immune defense and a clearing mechanism to trap and eliminate bacteria, viruses, fungi, and other microbes. The clearing mechanism is a blanket of bronchial mucus that traps microbes and particles, which are swept upward, away from the alveoli and are coughed out or swallowed. The special immune defense is the immune paint (Chapter 8) provided by bronchial patches of B lymphocytes that secrete high concentrations of immunoglobulin A.

PNEUMONIA

Pneumonia is inflammation of the lungs. It is usually acute, and it is usually caused by bacterial infection, although inhaled fumes, gases, and other irritants may be responsible. Pneumonia is surprisingly common, killing about twice as many people per year (80,000) as automotive accidents (40,000). Pneumonia occurs in two *anatomic* forms: *alveolar* and *interstitial*.

Alveolar pneumonia is inflammation, usually acute and usually severe enough to completely fill large numbers of alveoli with inflammatory exudate (Fig. 14-14). Alveolar pneumonia, which is much more common than is inflammation of the pulmonary interstitium (interstitial pneumonia), usually occurs with bacterial infection. As is illustrated in Figure 14-15, alveolar pneumonia also occurs in two anatomic forms.

• *Bronchopneumonia* is characterized by patchy, noncontiguous inflammation, usually involves the alve-

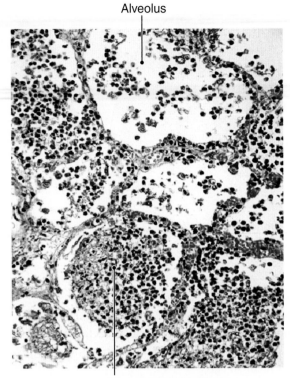
Alveolus

Mix of fibrin and neutrophils
(acute inflammatory exudate)

Figure 14-14 Alveolar pneumonia. Bacterial infection has stimulated an intense acute inflammatory reaction that fills alveoli with neutrophils and strands of fibrin (inflammatory exudate).

oli of more than one lobe, and is most likely to occur in the inferior (basilar) parts of the lower lobes. Grossly, the lungs show patchy areas of wet, poorly aerated, firm tissue that exude a yellowish fluid.
• *Lobar pneumonia* is characterized by intense, consolidated acute inflammation of the alveoli in an entire lobe and is the form that is much more likely to occur in patients with congestive heart failure, COPD, diabetes, or alcoholism. Virtually all lobar pneumonia is caused by *Streptococcus pneumoniae* (also called "pneumococcus"). Lobar pneumonia is usually confined to a single lobe, which appears dramatically different from adjacent, uninfected lobes. Grossly, the affected lobe is uniformly yellowish, firm, and completely solidified and airless.

Interstitial pneumonia is inflammation confined to the alveolar septa; it does not fill the alveoli with inflammatory exudate. The inflammation is diffuse and bilateral and is usually caused by virus infection.

Etiology and Pathogenesis

Of patients treated for pneumonia, about 75% have acute bacterial infection. About half of these have lobar

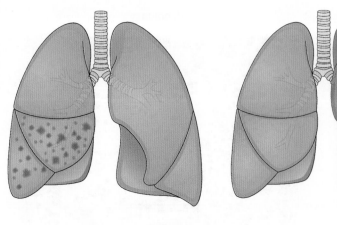

A Bronchopneumonia   **B** Lobar pneumonia

Figure 14-15 **Patterns of acute bacterial pneumonia. A,** In bronchopneumonia, alveolar inflammation is widespread but patchy, leaving some alveoli unaffected. **B,** In lobar pneumonia, all alveoli in the lobe are involved by intense acute inflammation.

pneumonia caused by *S. pneumoniae*. However, viral pneumonia may be as common as bacterial pneumonia, but is usually less severe, and patients do not always seek medical care.

Most bacterial pneumonia is caused by organisms that normally reside in the upper respiratory tract in equilibrium with local tissues. However, if these organisms are aspirated into the lungs, pneumonia may occur. The most important of these upper respiratory bacteria are *S. pneumoniae, Haemophilus influenzae,* and staphylococci. Other bacteria that cause pneumonia are found in feces: the two most important are *Escherichia coli* and *Pseudomonas aeruginosa.*

Microbes find their way into the lungs by 1) inhalation of droplets that originate from the nose or that are in the air; 2) aspiration of gastric contents, food or drink; or 3) blood-borne spread from infection elsewhere, such as the urinary tract or gastrointestinal tract. Most inhaled or aspirated organisms are removed by the clearing mechanism or neutralized by the immune system. But if these defense mechanisms are not working normally, pneumonia may occur. Patients with immune deficiency (Chapter 8) are especially susceptible.

Also susceptible are patients whose clearing mechanism is hampered by:

- *Decreased cough reflex*; for example, patients with severe alcohol intoxication or who are comatose or under general anesthesia.
- *Damage to bronchial epithelium* that impairs ciliary action; for example, patients who have inhaled toxic fumes, smoke, or hot gases or who have a bronchial virus infection.
- *Accumulated secretions*; for example, patients with cystic fibrosis or bronchial obstruction.

- *Pulmonary congestion or pulmonary edema*; accumulations of fluid in the lungs are a perfect culture medium for bacteria.

Clinical Settings

It is helpful to classify pneumonias according to the clinical setting in which they occur because the pathogens are reasonably predictable in each case.

Community-acquired pneumonia is acute pneumonia not acquired in some special circumstance, such as in a hospital, in an immunocompromised patient, or by aspiration of gastric contents. Most community-acquired pneumonia presents as acute alveolar bronchopneumonia or lobar pneumonia. The most common bacterial community-acquired pneumonia is lobar pneumonia caused by *S. pneumoniae*. Other common bacterial causes of community-acquired pneumonia are *Staphylococcus aureus* and *H. influenzae. Legionella pneumophila,* the agent of **Legionnaire disease,** grows in artificial water environments such as air conditioning cooling towers. It is spread by air conditioning systems or by accidental inhalation of contaminated drinking water. If not recognized and treated promptly, it carries a 10% mortality rate.

However, some community-acquired pneumonia is caused by viruses or *Mycoplasma pneumoniae*. Most of these cases are interstitial pneumonia, and they are often called **primary atypical pneumonia** because 1) in most cases the agent cannot be proven; 2) when an agent is identified, it is usually proven to be *Mycoplasma, Chlamydia, Rickettsia,* or a virus; 3) clinically they are less severe; and 4) they cause interstitial rather than alveolar inflammation.

The pathologic findings in primary atypical pneumonia are characterized by scattered, patchy accumulations of lymphocytes and macrophages confined to the alveolar wall. Severe cases, however, can develop a diffuse intra-alveolar exudate with hyaline membranes and ARDS.

Most cases present as an acute, feverish chest illness with minimal sputum production. Complete recovery is the rule. Some cases masquerade as a relatively severe viral upper respiratory infection. At the other extreme it may be a fulminant, fatal infection in immunocompromised patients. Secondary bacterial may occur in elderly or debilitated patients. Chest x-rays, which are important to assess the extent and severity of disease, typically show lower lobe patchy infiltrates that mimic bronchopneumonia. Culture of the causative organism is especially difficult, although in some instances diagnostic antibodies can be identified in the patient's blood.

Nosocomial pneumonia is pneumonia acquired in a hospital. It is common in patients who have other severe disease, are on prolonged antibiotic therapy, or have internal medical devices such as intravascular catheters. Especially at risk are patients on mechanical ventilation. *S. aureus* and fecal bacteria such as *E. coli* are the most common pathogens.

Aspiration pneumonia is caused by aspiration of gastric contents in patients who are comatose or debilitated by stroke. The inflammatory reaction is partially the result of the corrosive effects of gastric acid and partially the result of infection by a mixed flora of bacteria from the mouth. Aspiration pneumonia is serious and carries a relatively high mortality rate. Lung abscess is often a complication.

Clinical Features

Pneumonia is most common in young children and the elderly. It can interfere with oxygenation to cause hypoxia and death. Bacterial pneumonia is usually accompanied by high fever and chills; viral and other interstitial pneumonias are usually less severe. Coughing is a universal symptom. Bacterial pneumonia typically causes production of large amounts of yellow (purulent) sputum, whereas there is little sputum production in interstitial pneumonias. Shortness of breath and rapid breathing are common to all types of pneumonia, and some patients have sharp pain with each breath, caused by inflammation of the pleura, a clinical condition known as *pleurisy*.

Bacterial pneumonia is typically accompanied by a marked increase in the peripheral blood white-cell count, because there is marked increase in the number of neutrophils. In viral or interstitial pneumonias the white-cell count usually is not elevated, but there is an increased percentage of lymphocytes (lymphocytosis). Microscopic examination of sputum is critical—Gram stain can reveal the organism and narrow the possibilities, but sputum culture is required for definitive diagnosis of the etiologic agent.

LUNG ABSCESS

A **lung abscess** is anatomically like any other abscess—a localized area of purulent inflammation with tissue necrosis and liquefaction. However, lung abscesses are different from other abscesses in three ways:

- Lungs abscesses often contain several types of bacteria
- Almost all lung abscesses contain anaerobic bacteria
- Two thirds of lung abscesses contain bacteria normally found in the mouth that do not usually infect other body sites.

The most common cause of lung abscess is aspiration of gastric contents, which usually occurs in patients who are comatose or nearly so, as with stroke or alcoholic stupor. Less commonly, lung abscess is caused by bronchial obstruction or as a complication of bacterial pneumonia.

Lung abscesses may be solitary or multiple. In addition to the usual symptoms of lung infection, they usually cause production of copious amounts of foul smelling sputum. Lung abscesses constantly seed bacteria into the bloodstream, and patients are at risk for infection of the brain or meningitis. Lung abscesses occur with some regularity with bronchogenic carcinoma, so it is wise to suspect bronchogenic carcinoma as the underlying cause in older persons with a lung abscess. Treatment includes antibiotics and surgical drainage.

PULMONARY TUBERCULOSIS

Tuberculosis (TB) is a chronic, communicable bacterial disease caused by *Mycobacterium tuberculosis*, which incites a highly distinctive chronic **granulomatous inflammation** (Chapter 3) with a central area of soft, **caseous necrosis** (from Latin *caseus*, cheese). As is depicted in Figure 14-16, mycobacteria are small, rod-shaped organisms that are commonly spoken of in clinical settings as being "acid-fast" because in the laboratory they stain red with Ziehl-Neelsen stain and retain the color after acid washing. Other species of mycobacteria cause tuberculous disease in animals and under some circumstances may cause human disease. For example, *Mycobacterium avium*—the agent of bird (avian) TB—is the most frequent opportunistic bacterial infection in AIDS.

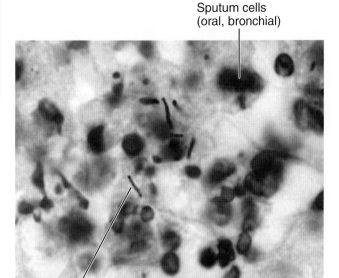

Sputum cells
(oral, bronchial)

Acid-fast bacteria (*M. tuberculosis*)

*Figure 14-16 **Mycobacterium tuberculosis.*** High-power microscopic study of acid-fast stain of sputum. Cells in the background are from the bronchi and mouth.

Pathogenesis

Three points are central to an understanding of the pathogenesis of TB:

- Many people are infected, but few develop disease. About 95% of infections are stopped in the lungs or bronchial lymph nodes by the immune system and become dormant.
- Almost every clinical case of TB is secondary (reactivation) tuberculosis that arises from an initial infection that has been arrested and dormant (latent) for many years, but which reactivates. A few secondary cases arise from a second infection.
- When initially infected, the immune system becomes sensitized (type IV hypersensitivity, Chapter 8) to antigens in *M. tuberculosis*, and the infection is halted. Later, organisms may reactivate if the patient's defenses are affected by AIDS, malnutrition, cancer, or other serious illness. When infection reactivates the patient is already sensitized, and a hypersensitivity reaction to spreading infection causes the caseating granulomas that are characteristic of secondary tuberculosis.

Figure 14-17 depicts the relationships among the different pathogenic pathways for development of tuberculosis. *Infection* implies seeding of the organism by airborne droplet from a diseased person into the lungs of a person not previously infected. The initial lesions in the

lung are known as **primary tuberculosis**. The initial lung lesion is called the **Ghon tubercle**, which may be associated with similar lesions in infected mediastinal (hilar) lymph nodes—a combination known as the **Ghon complex** (Fig. 14-18). In about 95% of newly infected persons the infection is arrested by the immune system after the development of the initial lesions; however, in many patients the organisms are not dead but inactive, and they may persist for many years until patient immunity declines and they re-emerge as *secondary TB* (reactivation TB). However, if the initial infection immediately progresses to active disease, it is known as *primary progressive TB*.

Epidemiology

Tuberculosis was known in ancient Egypt, and it continues to affect nearly 2 billion people worldwide, killing about 2 million each year. Globally, it is second only to AIDS as a cause of infectious disease deaths. In the United States about 15,000 new cases occur, most of them in immigrants from developing nations, where TB flourishes amid poverty, crowding, malnourishment, and chronic disease. In the United States the AIDS epidemic is responsible for many new TB cases, many of them caused by drug-resistant organisms. The nearby History of Medicine box provides additional historical context.

The **Mantoux test** (PPD test) is a skin test for prior infection performed by injecting purified protein derivative (PPD, an extract of TB protein) into the patient's skin, as is explained in greater detail in the nearby box, The Clinical Side. Infected patients have a positive test. Almost all patients with negative test results are not infected, but a few false-negative tests do occur. A positive reaction means only that the patient has been infected, either a few weeks earlier or many years ago. The size of the reaction allows patients to be separated into groups based on their risk for developing active TB.

To get a feel for the magnitude of the TB problem, remember this fact: about 80% of the population in some African and Asian nations have positive skin tests; that is, they are infected. The same population has a high prevalence of AIDS, malnutrition, and other debilitating diseases that lower patient immunity, which promotes reactivation TB. Other debilitating conditions, such as chronic infection, malignancy, diabetes, chronic lung disease, and alcoholism, in previously infected persons also lower resistance and favor the emergence of reactivation TB. In addition, certain ethnic groups have much higher susceptibility to infection—African Americans, Alaskan Inuit, Native Americans, Hispanics, and Southeast Asians.

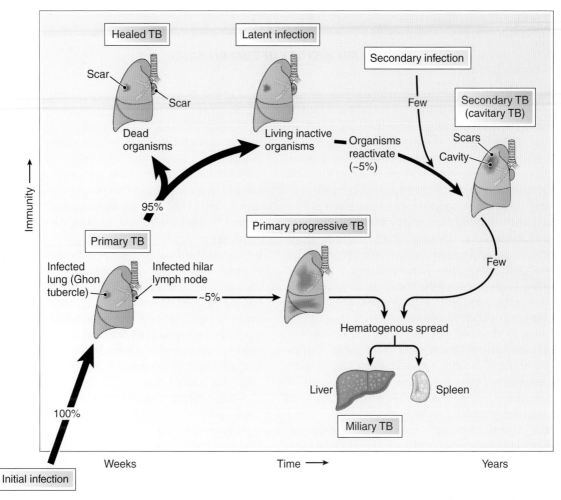

Figure 14-17 The natural history of tuberculosis (TB). Initial (primary) infection rarely progresses to disease because an effective immune response arrests most infections before they spread beyond the initial site (Ghon tubercle), or beyond the lung and a few mediastinal (hilar) lymph nodes. Some initial infections (~5%) spread quickly and widely as primary progressive tuberculosis. Primary progressive tuberculosis produces many small lesions and is called miliary (seed-like) tuberculosis. Most clinical tuberculosis is secondary TB stemming from reactivation of dormant, old infections as microbes escape from their long containment by the immune system. A few cases of secondary tuberculosis arise from a second (new) infection.

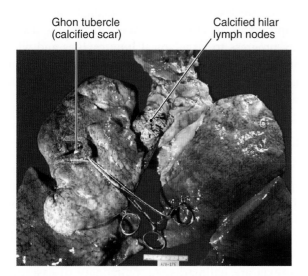

Figure 14-18 Primary (healed) tuberculosis. Forceps point to the Ghon tubercle. This infection was arrested after spreading to nearby hilar lymph nodes. Together these two lesions are known as the Ghon complex.

Pathology

In about 5% of newly infected patients, the infection is not arrested and progresses rapidly to widespread disease, called **primary progressive tuberculosis**. It usually occurs in children, in the immunodeficient, and in elderly or debilitated patients. Typically it occurs as extensive pulmonary tuberculosis, which sometimes is associated with widespread blood-borne spread to other organs, a condition known as **miliary tuberculosis** because various organs contain hundreds or thousands of tiny whitish lesions that look like millet seeds. Patients with primary progressive TB do not develop caseating granulomas like patients do who have reactivation TB, because in primary progressive TB the immune system has not been previously sensitized by infection. The sensitized immune system of patients with reactivation TB causes the development of less numerous, larger lesions with central cores of caseous necrosis.

THE HISTORY OF TUBERCULOSIS

Skeletal remains unearthed in archeological digs demonstrate that TB has been an affliction of humans for millennia. The first written record of TB occurs in the writing of Greek physician Hippocrates, who mentions that *phthisis* (from Greek, *phthinein*, to waste away) was the most widespread of all diseases. *Phthisis* was the scientific term for TB until the 14th century, when it was replaced in English by the term *consumption*, which recognized the fact that patients withered as if flesh was being consumed by an invisible devourer, as indeed it was. Oliver Wendell Holmes, Sr. (1809–1894), American physician, speaker, writer, and father of U.S. Supreme Court justice Oliver Wendell Holmes, Jr., captured the feeling as he described the crumbling of a carriage in "The Deacon's Masterpiece, or the One Hoss Shay":

. . . a general flavor of mild decay,
But nothing local, as one may say."

It was not clear that TB was a contagious disease until the Republic of Lucca, in what is now northern Italy, issued a public edict in 1699 that "The names of the deceased [TB victims] shall be reported to authorities, and measures taken for disinfection."

About the same time (1675) Dutch microscopist Otto von Leeuwenhoek discovered microbiologic life, which he called "animalcules." Leeuwenhoek's discovery that living things could be so small was sensational news that spread widely and later led English physician Benjamin Marten to speculate

in 1720 that TB could be caused by "wonderfully minute living creatures."

The proof of these ideas was slow to come, however. It was not until 1865 that Jean-Antoine Villemin, a French military physician, proved that consumption was infectious by passing the infection from humans to cattle and cattle to rabbits and ended the notion that TB sprang anew in each patient. Soon, in 1882, German microbiologist Robert Koch developed the stain that led him to discover the tubercle bacillus.

Understanding the infectious nature of TB was helpful, but no treatment was available until the dawn of the antibiotic era, when Scottish microbiologist Alexander Flemming discovered penicillin in 1928. Flemming's discovery was not met with immediate enthusiasm, but soon other scientists began to search for other compounds that might have antibiotic properties. In 1943 American microbiologist Selman Waksman discovered streptomycin, which was administered to a critically ill TB patient on November 20, 1944, and resulted in a dramatic cure.

Famous people who suffered from tuberculosis include English poet John Keats, Polish composer Frédéric Chopin, Scottish writer Robert Louis Stevenson, Russian writer Anton Chekhov, Czech writer Franz Kafka, and all of the talented Brontë family of England—the parents and all six of the children, including novelists and poets Charlotte, Emily, and Anne.

Secondary tuberculosis (*reactivation TB*, or *cavitary TB*) accounts for about 95% of clinical tuberculosis. It is the pattern of disease that arises in previously infected and sensitized persons in whom the initial infection was contained by the immune system. Disease may develop within a few months of infection, but it more commonly occurs many years later, when patient resistance is weakened by some other condition and the original organisms reactivate, or the patient is infected a second time. Secondary TB is almost always manifest by lesions in the apex of the lung (Fig. 14-19). Neglected cases may cavitate into airways, seeding bronchial tubes with millions of organisms, which spread more widely in the lungs and are coughed out as a cloud of infective organisms. Wide internal dissemination to other organs may occur also.

The lesions of secondary TB are characterized by *granulomatous inflammation* (Chapter 3) around a central core of caseous necrosis. Body defenses may limit

and heal the lesion, leaving only calcified scars in lung, lymph nodes, or elsewhere. Alternatively, the disease may progress to large apical lung cavities and widespread blood-borne spread with granulomatous inflammation, necrosis, and tissue destruction at any site in the body.

Clinical Course

By its very nature primary infection is asymptomatic except in the 5% of patients in whom the organism overwhelms defenses (in AIDS, for example) and becomes widespread as primary progressive TB.

The usual clinical onset of secondary TB is subtle. Low-grade fever, night sweats, malaise, weight loss, and anorexia are hallmarks. As pulmonary disease progresses, patients begin to cough and produce sputum, which may be bloody. Clinical and x-ray findings may add up to a very high index of suspicion, but positive di-

THE CLINICAL SIDE

THE MANTOUX SKIN TEST (TUBERCULIN SKIN TEST, PPD TEST)

The Mantoux test is a skin test for prior infection and sensitization to the organism *Mycobacterium tuberculosis*. However, the test does not distinguish between active and inactive infection. It is used to evaluate people with symptoms of TB or asymptomatic people who may have been exposed to TB. Some health care workers are screened at the beginning of their careers and regularly thereafter, in order to see if they convert from negative to positive, an occurrence that can indicate recent infection. Routine testing of persons at low risk is not recommended.

The test is performed by injecting a small amount of mycobacterium protein (purified protein derivative, PPD) into the skin of the volar surface of the forearm and observing the reaction at 48 and 72 hours.

About two weeks after infection, the patient's immune system becomes sensitized enough to produce a positive skin test. A positive reaction is indicated by induration (firmness); erythema (redness) does not count. False-negative reactions may occur, for example, in sarcoidosis, Hodgkin disease, and in overwhelming TB infection. People with AIDS or other immunodeficiency disease may have negative skin tests despite being infected. Results are interpreted according to the following table:

Interpretation of the Mantoux Test

Induration	Interpretation	Analysis
None	Negative	Not infected
5–10 mm	Positive	Infected; at high risk for development of active TB. This group includes: • patients with AIDS, or on immunosuppression or steroid therapy; • persons with findings suggesting prior active pulmonary TB; and • people recently in contact with a patient with active TB.
10–15 mm	Positive	Infected; at increased risk for developing active TB. This is a large and varied group, with preexisting risk factors for TB: • recent immigrants • IV drug abusers • TB lab personnel • residents of institutions such as prisons and nursing homes • patients with chronic lung disease • persons with malignancy or other debilitating disease
>15 mm	Positive	Infected; healthy people with no known TB risk factors. Unlikely to develop active TB

agnosis rests on detection of acid-fast organisms in sputum smears or culture of *M. tuberculosis* from sputum.

The Mantoux skin test adds little value in most cases for two reasons: 1) it is usually positive, but it is also positive in a large number of healthy people who have healed primary lesions only; and 2) false-negative tests are rather common: a test could be negative in the absence of a skin reaction (anergy), a common reaction in immunocompromised patients. However, a positive test may be helpful to exclude deep fungus infections, which can mimic TB clinically. In most cases TB remains confined to the lungs, but in AIDS most patients have disseminated (miliary) TB without detectable lung involve-

ment. Such cases may present as a fever of unknown origin (an "FUO" in clinical terms). Diagnosis in these patients may depend on demonstration of acid-fast bacteria in bone marrow or liver biopsy or successful culture of the organism from sputum or biopsy material.

PULMONARY FUNGUS INFECTIONS (DEEP MYCOSES)

Most fungal infections involve epithelial surfaces such as skin or the oral or vaginal mucosa. Examples include vaginitis caused by *Candida albicans* (Chapter 21), and "athlete's foot," "jock itch," and "ringworm" infections caused by *Tinea* species fungi (Chapter 24). However,

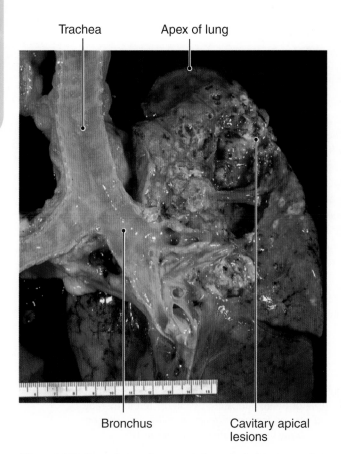

Trachea   Apex of lung

Bronchus   Cavitary apical
lesions

Figure 14-19 **Secondary pulmonary tuberculosis.** Most secondary pulmonary tuberculosis lesions occur in the lung apices.

other fungi cause infection of deeper tissues, the lungs especially, and are known as the **deep mycoses.** Many infections occur in immunocompromised patients. Two kinds of fungi cause deep infection: 1) *yeast-like fungi* that exist as single small round organisms—such as *Candida* species and *Cryptococcus neoformans*—which are opportunistic pathogens that primarily infect patients with diminished immunity; and 2) *dimorphic fungi* that may exist as yeast or as branching, filamentous forms—such as *Histoplasma capsulatum* and *Coccidioides immitis*—which are ordinary pathogens that can produce disease in patients with a normal immune system.

Histoplasmosis, caused by *H. capsulatum,* is one of the most common systemic fungal infections in the United States, and is endemic in the general region of the Ohio River, the central Mississippi River, and along the Appalachian Mountains. It is spread by inhalation of dried bird droppings and clinically mimics TB. Even the pathologic lesions are similar to TB, except that fungi rather than mycobacteria are the cause. Disseminated disease may occur in patients who are severely debilitated by other conditions, or who have immune defi-

ciency. The Mantoux test is usually negative and is helpful in differentiating histoplasmosis from TB in the clinical workup. Positive diagnosis is made by culture, biopsy, or finding high levels of *Histoplasma* antigen or anti-*Histoplasma* antibody in blood.

Coccidioidomycosis is caused by *C. immitis,* a fungus endemic in the western U.S., particularly the San Joaquin Valley of central California, where infection is known as *valley fever.* As with TB, many people are infected by *Coccidioides,* but few become diseased—in the San Joaquin Valley about 80% of the population have a positive skin test for *Coccidioides.* Also as with TB, most infected people remain asymptomatic, but disseminated disease can develop.

Candidiasis is the name of the disease when an infection is caused by *C. albicans,* which is found normally in the mouth of healthy people and is the most common cause of non-skin fungus infections. It most often causes superficial mucosal infections of the mouth (called *thrush,* common in infants), vagina (common vaginitis), and perianal area (diaper rash in infants). Infection of deep organs can occur in immunocompromised hosts; for example, oral candidiasis sometimes extends into the esophagus in patients with AIDS. In immunocompromised patients, *Candida* can invade the bloodstream and spread to the lungs, eye, liver, kidney, heart, or central nervous system.

C. neoformans (**cryptococcosis**) is an opportunistic pathogen that typically infects patients with AIDS, Hodgkin disease, leukemia, and lymphoma. Like histoplasmosis and coccidioidomycosis, cryptococcosis is spread by inhalation and infects the lungs, from which it spreads to other sites, especially the meninges.

OTHER LUNG INFECTIONS

Infections of the larynx, trachea, bronchi, and lungs are among the most important causes of illness in children, and are discussed in Chapter 7.

Cytomegalovirus (CMV), a member of the herpes virus family, may cause a variety of infections. Its name derives from the fact that microscopic examination of infected cells demonstrates an enlarged nucleus that contains a huge, round viral object (inclusion). **Cytomegalovirus pneumonia** typically occurs in patients with AIDS or some other form of immunosuppression. Disseminated CMV infection causes chorioretinitis (retina infection, Chapter 25), gastroenteritis, and pneumonia and can be life threatening.

Pneumocystis **pneumonia** (Fig. 14-20) is caused by *Pneumocystis jiroveci,* a small, fungus-like organism that is an opportunistic pathogen very common in AIDS patients. It does not cause disease in healthy people.

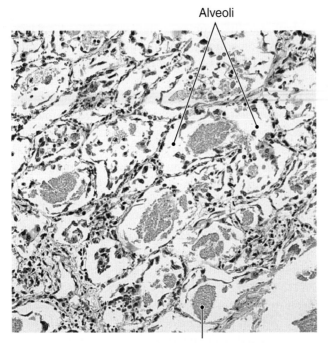

Alveoli

Clouds of *Pneumocystis* organisms

Figure 14-20 Pneumocystis jiroveci **pneumonia.** Microscopic study of the lungs in a patient with AIDS. Clouds of organisms fill the alveoli. Tellingly, little inflammatory reaction is present because of the patient's impaired immune system.

Lung Neoplasms

The most common neoplasm *in* the lung is a *metastasis* from a cancer somewhere else in the body. The most common tumor *of* the lung is *bronchogenic carcinoma* ("lung cancer"), almost all of which arise from the epithelium lining the bronchi. Benign neoplasms of the lung are rare. The most common among them is a *hamartoma* (Chapter 6), which consists of bronchial cartilage mixed with a bit of fat and fibrous tissue. They

are usually perfectly round and small, like a coin, and harmless. They are incidentally discovered on chest x-ray as a solitary "coin" lesion.

BRONCHOGENIC CARCINOMA

Bronchogenic carcinoma is the most common of all human cancers and is the number one cause of cancer death for men *and for women* in the U.S. In 2003 there were about 170,000 new cases of lung cancer and about 160,000 deaths. Why? Cigarette smoking. Current and former cigarette smokers account for about 80–90% of all lung cancers. It is important to note, however, that about 20,000–30,000 cases of lung cancer occur in nonsmokers. Factors include second hand smoke, asbestos and other industrial exposures, and genetic predisposition.

There are two main histologic categories of lung cancer: *small cell* and *non-small cell*. Because small cell carcinoma is so distinctive and lethal, it is separated from the other histologic types, which are lumped together as non-small cell carcinoma. Figure 14-21 illustrates the histologic classification.

> **Lung cancer is the leading cause of cancer death in *both* women and men.**

Etiology and Pathogenesis

Cigarette smoking is the main cause of bronchogenic carcinoma. The evidence is utterly convincing.

- *Statistical evidence* demonstrates a direct relationship between the number cigarettes smoked and the likelihood of developing lung cancer (Chapter 10, Figure 10-8). A common clinical estimate of lifetime cigarette consumption is pack-years: the average number of packs smoked per day multiplied by the number of years smoking. Higher numbers of pack years are associated with increased risk of developing lung cancer.

Tumor	Small cell carcinoma ~20%	Non-small cell carcinoma ~80%			
		Squamous cell carcinoma ~30%	Adenocarcinoma ~30%	Large cell carcinoma ~15%	Mixed pattern carcinoma ~5%
Approximate 5-year survival rate	3-5%	5-8%	10-12%	2-3%	5-8%

Figure 14-21 **Types of bronchogenic carcinoma.** Cell types, prevalence, and five-year survival for bronchogenic carcinoma.

- *Pathologic evidence* shows a direct relationship between the number of cigarettes smoked and precancerous changes in bronchial mucosa: from normal to metaplasia, dysplasia, carcinoma in situ, and finally to invasive malignancy.
- *Experimental evidence* is compelling, too. Cigarette smoke is a cocktail of chemicals capable of inducing cancers in experimental animals.

This evidence has had a positive effect: in 1955 nearly 60% of men in the United States were smokers. In 2005 only 25% smoke, and this dramatic decrease had a positive effect: the number of new lung cancer cases occurring each year in the United States peaked in the early 1990s and has been declining since.

Pathology

Lung cancers are named according to the microscopic appearance (histologic type) of the malignant cells (see Fig. 14-21).

Small cell carcinomas (about 20% of cases) arise from specialized neuroendocrine cells of the bronchial epithelium and have the strongest relationship to cigarette smoking—only about 1% occurs in nonsmokers. Small cell carcinomas are composed of distinctive small, dark cells that look much like large lymphocytes. They are aggressively malignant—most patients have metastases at time of diagnosis, and surgery is ineffective even in patients without demonstrable metastases. Small cell carcinomas are, however, radiosensitive—radiotherapy induces remission in about a quarter of cases. These cancers grow rapidly, invade and metastasize early, and are never resectable for cure. Because of their neuroendocrine cell origin, they are capable of secreting various hormones, such as ACTH and, therefore, can be associated with *paraneoplastic syndromes* (Chapter 6), such as Cushing syndrome. Indeed, it is not uncommon for the first manifestation of small cell carcinoma to emerge from a metastasis or to be some symptom of a paraneoplastic syndrome.

Squamous cell carcinoma (about 30% of cases) is composed of malignant cells that differentiate toward the type of flat cells that normally compose the epithelium of the epidermis, esophagus, and vagina. Tumors arise from areas of bronchial epithelium that have first undergone squamous metaplasia (Chapter 2) and have evolved progressively into malignancy. Squamous cell carcinomas tend to arise centrally in the main bronchi near critical mediastinal structures and therefore may not be as easy to remove surgically as other types. They are most common in men and have a strong association with smoking. Invasive squamous carcinoma is pre-

ceded for years by progressive changes in the bronchial epithelium—first comes metaplasia, then dysplasia, then carcinoma in situ, and finally invasive carcinoma (Chapter 6). After becoming invasive, squamous carcinomas grow comparatively slowly compared to other histologic types, and they have a correspondingly better prognosis. Despite relatively slow growth, sooner or later symptoms occur as the tumor obstructs a bronchus to cause symptoms such as airflow obstruction, atelectasis, or infection. Less commonly, metastasis may cause the presenting complaint, generally enlarged neck lymph nodes or neurologic symptoms from brain metastasis.

Adenocarcinomas (about 30% of cases) are the most well-differentiated lung cancers, and they have a somewhat better prognosis than any of the other types. They tend to arise in the peripheral lung in small bronchi and therefore are easier to remove surgically because they are away from critical mediastinal structures. They are less associated with smoking than other varieties are, and they are the most common variety in women and nonsmokers.

Large cell carcinomas (about 15% of cases) are composed of large, fleshy, round cells that lack differentiation toward any particular type of tissue and probably represent squamous carcinomas or adenocarcinomas that are too undifferentiated to permit specific classification. They have a very poor prognosis and tend to metastasize early.

Clinical Course

Lung cancers are usually clinically silent (asymptomatic), and by the time symptoms appear most are beyond hope of cure. Less than 10% of lung cancer patients survive five years. Unfortunately, often the first symptom occurs as a result of a metastasis; for example, neurologic signs of brain metastasis, hepatomegaly or abnormal liver function tests from liver metastasis, or bone pain from bone metastasis. The presenting complaint may be symptomatic of a paraneoplastic syndrome such as Cushing syndrome resulting from tumor secretion of ACTH (Chapter 18).

Many methods have been tried to screen for lung cancer in an attempt to find them early enough for reasonable hope of cure, but all have failed. Ordinary chest x-ray as a screening tool is discouraged because it leads to a great number of false-positive findings. Recent studies with advanced imaging devices has proven effective at finding very small tumors, but early detection has not decreased the lung cancer death rate. Screening for various types of cancers is discussed further in Chapter 6.

In most lung cancers, clinical staging (Chapter 6) is essential for prognosis and therapy. This is not to say that histologic study is not necessary; it is essential for diagnosis and classification, but the clinical stage of the neoplasm is of paramount importance. Clinical stage is determined by tumor size, local invasion, and metastasis. (Small cell carcinoma is an exception to the rule: survival shows little relationship to the clinical stage at time of diagnosis. Resection has proven ineffective no matter how small the lesion and few are diagnosed when small.)

BRONCHIAL CARCINOID TUMOR

About 5% of lung neoplasms are **carcinoid tumors**, which, like small cell carcinomas, arise from bronchial neuroendocrine cells. Bronchial carcinoid tumors are much less aggressive than are small cell carcinomas, and they are related to similar carcinoid tumors that occur in other organs. In the bronchus they grow slowly, protrude into the lumen, and cause hemoptysis (coughing blood), wheezing, or cough. After surgical resection a majority of patients survive tumor free for five years. A carcinoid tumor may be part of the multiple endocrine neoplasia (MEN) syndrome, which features neoplasms of the parathyroid, pancreas, and pituitary (Chapter 18).

Diseases of the Pleura

The pleural space is a potential space between the *parietal* pleura of the chest wall and the *visceral* pleura covering the lung. The lungs are held to the chest wall and the diaphragm by the capillary attraction force of a thin film of fluid between the two pleural surfaces. With each breath the lungs are filled by the outward pull of the chest wall and the downward pull of the diaphragm. If air enters the pleural space (**pneumothorax**), it breaks the capillary fluid bond and causes collapse (atelectasis) of the lung, roughly equal to the volume of air introduced. Pneumothorax may occur spontaneously in young adult smokers, but it more often occurs in patients with emphysema who have unusually large air sacs (blebs) near the pleura—a bleb that ruptures into the pleural space is a common cause of pneumothorax. Traumatic penetration of the pleura, by a foreign object or the edge of a broken rib, is another common cause.

Pneumothorax is potentially fatal. Some cases resolve spontaneously as the air is slowly resorbed by blood; others require incision of the chest wall and insertion of a suction tube. An especially dangerous variant of pneumothorax is tension pneumothorax—the opening allows air to come in but not to escape, so that air can enter the pleural space but cannot exit, creating an increasingly high pressure that may fatally smother cardiorespiratory function.

Accumulation of fluid in the pleural space is a **pleural effusion** (hydrothorax), which may be either an *exudate* (inflammatory fluid, specific gravity >1.020) or a *transudate* (noninflammatory fluid, specific gravity <1.020). The most common cause of pleural effusion is a transudate produced by congestive heart failure. Most other cases are associated with bacterial or viral infection, pulmonary infarct, or malignant neoplasm in the pleural space. Blood in the pleural space is called *hemothorax*.

Inflammation of the pleura (**pleuritis**) causes a distinctive, sharp, localized pain (*pleurisy*) with each breath. Most cases are caused by extension of inflammation from nearby pneumonia. An effusion (exudate) may occur that has a specific gravity >1.020, identifying it as inflammatory.

Mesothelioma is a rare malignancy of the pleura associated with chronic inhalation of asbestos fibers (asbestosis). ∎

CASE STUDY 14-1 *"CIGARETTE ASTHMA"*

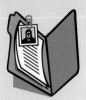

TOPICS:
Chronic obstructive pulmonary disease
The consequences of cigarette smoking
Pneumonia
Nosocomial infection

THE CASE
Setting: You are employed in the pulmonary disease section of a large metropolitan hospital, working a shift in the emergency room seeing patients with pulmonary complaints.

Clinical history: Myrtle M. is a 51-year-old woman who is accompanied to the emergency room by her son, who has been taking care of her for several years because of "lung troubles." She is cyanotic and so drowsy that she cannot give a history. Her son tells you that she has been coming to the pulmonary clinic for many years.

You obtain her old chart from medical records and question her son about her medical history. You quickly learn that years ago she was told by a physician in her small hometown that she was developing "cigarette asthma," and ▶

[Case 14-1, continued] she was advised to quit smoking and lose weight.

Her son says, "She tried, but it was just too hard. She would give up cigarettes for a few days or a few weeks, but then she would gain weight. So she went back to her old ways."

In the last few years she has visited the clinic with increasing frequency. Her son brought her to the emergency room because he became alarmed by her constant sleepiness.

Physical examination and other data: She is cyanotic, short of breath, somnolent, and quite obese—you estimate her to be about 5'4" and 225 lb. She has marked expiratory wheezing, and she coughs a lot, hacking up yellow sputum. Her temperature is 100.5° F, respirations 36, blood pressure 115/75, heart rate 105. Breath sounds are distant, with rales and expiratory wheezes. You order a chest x-ray, arterial blood gases, complete blood count (CBC), blood chemistries, and sputum culture.

A verbal report from radiology says her chest x-ray shows evidence of moderate emphysema and patchy bilateral lower lobe streaks and shadows that suggest bronchopneumonia. The blood gas study shows low pH, high CO_2, and low oxygen. The total white blood cell count is moderately elevated (16,500/cu mm) with an increased percentage of neutrophils and a few immature "band" neutrophils. Hemoglobin levels (18.1 gm/dL) and hematocrit levels (52%) are high. Red cell indices and blood chemistries are unremarkable.

Clinical course: You report your workup to the internal medicine resident, who examines her and admits her to the hospital for antibiotic and bronchodilator therapy, oxygen supplementation, and ventilation assistance.

The next day on rounds you have a chance to study her records in more detail. She began smoking as a teenager and has been smoking two packs a day since she was twenty. Her original visit to your hospital was 12 years ago, when she was seen in pulmonary clinic for coughing, wheezing, and shortness of breath. A spirogram at the time revealed low FEV_1 and normal FVC. Two notations were present on the graph: "obstructive" and "chronic bronchitis." "Still smoking" is a regular chart entry for subsequent visits.

With antibiotics, bronchodilators, and ventilation assistance she becomes more alert, her fever disappears, and she finds it easier to breathe. The admission sputum culture grew mixed flora, probably oral contaminants. An echocardiogram shows mild right ventricular dilation and hypertrophy; the left ventricle and valves appear to be normal.

On the fifth hospital day, she becomes feverish again, respirations become labored, and she becomes difficult to arouse. A chest x-ray reveals widespread changes in both lungs that suggest pneumonia. An emergency bronchoscopy reveals abundant purulent mucus in the airways, which on culture grows penicillin-resistant *Staphylococcus*

aureus. Despite intense antibiotic and respiratory therapy she becomes progressively unresponsive and eventually comatose, and she dies on the tenth hospital day.

DISCUSSION

At autopsy, major abnormalities were confined to the lungs and heart. The right ventricle was moderately dilated and hypertrophic. Grossly, the lower lobes of the lungs were heavy and boggy and showed multiple areas of yellowish induration (firmness) from which a cloudy fluid could be expressed. The upper lobes were pale and airy with enlarged air spaces. Microscopic examination revealed marked mucous gland hyperplasia and chronic inflammation in the walls of small bronchi, and intense acute inflammatory exudate in the alveoli of both lower lobes. A Gram stain revealed gram-positive cocci in the inflammatory exudate.

This patient was an unfortunate and classic example of the ill effects of cigarette smoking: she smoked for a long time and acquired severe COPD from it. Her initial condition was chronic bronchitis with a severe obstructive component (chronic asthmatic bronchitis), which was confirmed by autopsy findings of marked bronchial chronic inflammation and mucous gland hyperplasia. The chronic bronchitis produced obstructive lung disease, which resulted in poor pulmonary gas exchange, hypoxia, and retained CO_2 with acidosis. The high CO_2 levels caused somnolence to such an extent that it alarmed her son, who brought her to the hospital. Her chronic hypoxia stimulated bone marrow production of red blood cells, which raised the hemoglobin and hematocrit levels markedly.

Like most smokers with asthmatic bronchitis, she also had emphysema. On admission she was found to have community-acquired pneumonia. The increased WBC count with neutrophilia and band neutrophils (left shift) suggested that the pneumonia was bacterial, although the initial sputum culture was inconclusive. The reappearance of fever and pneumonia on the fifth hospital day, and sputum culture positive for *Staphylococcus*, strongly suggested that she had developed a second, nosocomial infection after admission. The dense acute inflammatory reaction and gram-positive cocci found in her lungs at autopsy strongly suggested staphylococcal pneumonia, which was confirmed by postmortem culture of the lungs. The clinical diagnosis of emphysema was confirmed by the large air spaces, especially in the apex of each lung. Mild right ventricular hypertrophy and dilation indicated early pulmonary hypertension and cor pulmonale secondary to COPD.

POINTS TO REMEMBER

- Cigarette smoking can cause severe pulmonary disease.
- Fatal pneumonia is a common final event in patients with severe cardiorespiratory disease.
- Nosocomial infections are a hazard to every hospitalized patient. ▶

CASE STUDY 14-1 *THE ROAD NOT TAKEN—AN ALTERNATIVE SCENARIO*

For all sad words of tongue or pen,
The saddest are these: "It might have been."
JOHN GREENLEAF WHITTIER (1807–1892),
AMERICAN QUAKER POET AND REFORMER, *MAUD MULLER*

THE CASE
With a bit of imagination, we can speculate how this case might have had a happier ending.

Setting: You have recently passed your certification exam and have taken a job assisting a solo general practitioner in a small town in far west Texas. Your task is to do just about anything and everything, which on most days includes seeing drop-ins, treating minor emergency injuries, and seeing regular patients returning for uncomplicated follow-up.

Clinical history: Myrtle M. is a 36-year-old woman, a clerk at the local bank, who is one of the first patients you see in your new job. She is jittery and apprehensive and says that over the last few months she has developed pain in her chest. She points to her sternum: "It's right under here," she says. Despite the fact that she appears intelligent and well spoken, she has a difficult time describing the pain—"sometimes" it occurs soon after meals and "sometimes" it occurs with increased physical activity. She says it is not referred to neck, jaw, shoulder, or arm, although "now and then" it is associated with heart palpitations. "It feels like my heart is swelling up," she says, and adds, "Sometimes I get short of breath."

You do a review of systems and find no evidence of other significant problems. When asked about personal information and habits she says she smokes about a pack of cigarettes a day, drinks "a few beers" each week, and takes birth control pills. She does not exercise. She is married and has two children.

Physical examination and other data: She is 5'5" tall and weighs 146 lb. Vital signs are normal. When you ask her to take a deep breath so you can listen to her lungs, she attempts to do so but on inspiration begins to cough and bring up a small amount of sputum. "Sorry," she says, "I have a cigarette cough." You hear some wheezing, but the remainder of the physical exam is unremarkable.

Clinical course: You send her to the lab to collect blood and urine for routine tests and schedule her for a chest x-ray and electrocardiogram. While she is out you consult with the physician. He says he has known her for about 5 years and doesn't think she is a hypochondriac. He adds, "There are several things that worry me about her story. First, the pain is hard to characterize, and I always think about angina when I'm having trouble figuring out chest pain. Yeah, she's a young female, and they're not supposed to get coronary disease, but sometimes it happens. Second, she is a smoker and is taking birth control pills, which is an especially dangerous combination for heart attack risk. I think we ought to refer her to a cardiologist."

The physician joins you to explain your conclusions to her, and you make the necessary arrangements for referral to a distant medical center. In the busy days that follow you forget about her until on coffee break a month or so later the physician asks, "Did you hear what happened to Myrtle M.? I wasn't too concerned about her because her chest x-ray and electrocardiogram came back normal, but she had a heart attack on the treadmill while taking a stress test. She's been hospitalized and is getting out today. We booked her for a follow-up next week."

When she returns to your office the next week she looks much better than when you saw her initially. She has lost some weight, and she says she feels a lot better now than before the heart attack. "I haven't smoked a cigarette in over a month. They were real strict with me over there," she says. "The doctor told me that I had to quit smoking or stop taking birth control pills because the combination was so dangerous. They strongly, real strongly, told me I should choose to stop smoking and get my tubes tied for birth control. It was an easy decision."

You see Myrtle regularly for routine follow-up care and miscellaneous problems unrelated to her heart attack. Fifteen years later when you see her for the last time before departing for a new job, she has not had any recurrence of cardiac trouble and is taking statins to keep her cholesterol low. She has not smoked a cigarette since her heart attack.

DISCUSSION
It is difficult to think of a heart attack as a blessing, but that may be the case in this instance. Sometimes patients resist changing bad health habits, until a serious health problem arises. By then, it is often too late. But in Myrtle M.'s case, it seems likely that she was better off for having had the heart attack because it motivated her to quit smoking; otherwise it seems probable that she would have developed even more serious cardiovascular or lung disease in the next 15 years.

Objectives Recap

1. *Describe the pulmonary interstitium*: The pulmonary interstitium is the tissue lying between alveolar walls; that is, beneath the pneumocytes that line the alveoli. It consists of a thin network of pulmonary capillaries, basement membrane, fibrocytes and smooth muscle cells, and collagen and elastin fibers.

2. *Explain spirometry, and name and explain the two spirometric measures critical to understanding lung disease*: Spirometry measures the volume of air in the lungs and airflow rates. Forced vital capacity (FVC) is a volume measurement: the volume of air expelled between maximum inhalation and maximum exhalation. Forced expiratory volume at one second (FEV$_1$) is a rate measurement: the volume of air flowing out of the lungs by forced expiration in the first second from a start at maximum inspiration.

3. *Name two risk factors for laryngeal carcinoma*: Smoking and alcohol abuse.

4. *Name the types of atelectases*: The types of atelectases are: resorption, compression, and contraction.

5. *Define asthma, and briefly discuss the underlying pathology*: Asthma is a chronic inflammatory disease of small bronchi and bronchioles characterized by airflow obstruction resulting from *bronchospasm*, which is a constriction of bronchioles because of smooth muscle contraction. The pathologic lesion in asthma is *bronchial inflammation*, sometimes associated with allergy, but caused in most cases by inhaled irritants, such as cigarette smoke or polluted air. Irrespective of the initial irritant, allergic or not, with repeated exposure the reaction evolves into progressively severe chronic inflammation.

6. *Name the two main categories of chronic obstructive pulmonary disease*: Chronic bronchitis and emphysema.

7. *Explain how chronic bronchitis and emphysema differ*: Emphysema and chronic bronchitis are obstructive airway diseases; smoking is the usual cause of each. In pure emphysema the problem is coalescence of small alveoli into large airspaces, which markedly decreases the amount of alveolar membrane available for gas exchange. In pure chronic bronchitis the pathologic lesion is bronchial inflammation and hypertrophy of mucous glands with exaggerated mucous secretion, which together combine to produce airway obstruction; the amount of diffusion membrane is not affected.

8. *Define bronchiectasis*: Bronchiectasis is permanent dilation of distal bronchi and bronchioles caused by recurrent necrotizing bronchial infections that destroy supporting tissue of the airway, leaving a dilated, flaccid, pus-filled tube.

9. *Briefly define restrictive lung disease, and explain its pathogenesis*: Restrictive lung disease limits both the *volume* of lung expansion and the *rate* of expansion and contraction. Restrictive lung diseases are chronic inflammatory conditions of pulmonary interstitial tissue that render the lung stiff and inelastic.

10. *Name the two basic causes of pulmonary edema, and give an example of each*: 1) Hemodynamic edema, as in congestive heart failure, and 2) microvascular injury, as with inhalation of toxic fumes.

11. *Discuss the consequences of pulmonary thromboembolism*: Repeated small pulmonary thromboemboli may occlude pulmonary arterioles to produce chronic pulmonary hypertension. Larger emboli may produce lung infarcts. Very large emboli may occlude the pulmonary artery and cause instantaneous death.

12. *Name and discuss briefly the two main anatomic varieties of pneumonia*: Alveolar pneumonia is inflammation, usually acute inflammation, severe enough to completely fill (solidify, consolidate) large numbers of alveoli with inflammatory exudate. Interstitial pneumonia is inflammation that is confined to the alveolar septa and does not fill the alveoli with inflammatory exudate. The inflammation is diffuse and bilateral and is usually caused by viral infection.

13. *Explain the terms "community-acquired pneumonia" and "nosocomial pneumonia"*: Community-acquired pneumonia is acute pneumonia not acquired in some special circumstance, such as in a hospital, in association with an immune deficiency, or because of aspiration of gastric contents. Nosocomial pneumonia is pneumonia acquired in a hospital.

14. *Explain how lung abscesses differ bacteriologically from most other abscesses*: They contain several types of bacteria, most contain anaerobic bacteria, and most contain bacteria normally found in the oral cavity.

15. *Explain the difference between infection by the tuberculosis bacillus and the disease known as tuberculosis*: Infection means only that the lungs have been seeded by the tuberculosis bacillus and the immune system has contained the infection to a small focus in the lung, or to the lungs and nearby mediastinal (hilar) lymph nodes in some cases. Disease implies spread of infection beyond the initial lung or mediastinal lymph node lesions.

16. *Explain why secondary (reactivation) TB differs pathologically from primary progressive TB*: Secondary (reactivation TB) occurs only in patients sensitized by earlier infection. As TB organisms spread the cellular (delayed, type 4) hypersensitivity reaction accounts for the caseous necrosis, which occurs in secondary TB but is not present in primary progressive TB.

17. *Classify malignant lung tumors by cell type*: The two main categories are small cell carcinoma and non-small cell carcinoma, which consists of several other types. Small cell carcinoma is separated from all other types because it is much more aggressive than any other type. Non-small cell carcinoma cell types are: squamous cell carcinoma, adenocarcinoma, and large cell carcinoma.

18. *Explain why small cell carcinoma is placed in a separate category from other lung malignancies*: Because small cell carcinoma arises from neuroendocrine cells rather than bronchial epithelial cells and because it is uniformly lethal (even if discovered early).

Typical Test Questions

1. Among the following, which is the smallest anatomic division of the lung?
   A. Alveolus
   B. Trachea
   C. Lobe
   D. Bronchiole

2. Acute upper respiratory infections are more common in cold weather because:
   A. People are crowded together indoors and infect one another
   B. Cold air restricts bronchial flow and renders people susceptible
   C. Viruses are more active at low temperature
   D. Streptococci are much more contagious in reheated indoor air

3. Which of the following is true regarding emphysema?
   A. The surface area of the pulmonary membrane is decreased
   B. Most have normal or near normal expiratory airflow
   C. Sputum production is a key diagnostic point
   D. CO_2 retention is prominent

4. Which one of the following is true about adult respiratory distress syndrome?
   A. Chronic course leading to pulmonary failure in nearly 100% of cases
   B. Characterized by injury to bronchi and bronchioles

   C. Can be caused by many different underlying conditions
   D. Caused by *Mycoplasma pneumoniae*

5. Which one of the following is true about bronchogenic carcinoma?
   A. It is the number two cancer killer of women behind breast cancer
   B. About half of cases are caused by cigarette smoking
   C. Most squamous cell bronchogenic carcinomas arise in the periphery
   D. Small cell carcinomas of the lung are especially aggressive

6. True or false? Alveolar pneumocytes are part of the pulmonary interstitium.

7. True or false? Obstruction of incoming (inhaled) air is the main problem in obstructive lung disease.

8. True or false? Most interstitial pneumonia is caused by bacterial infection.

9. True or false? Most patients infected with *Mycobacterium tuberculosis* develop primary progressive TB.

10. True or false? Adenocarcinoma is the most lethal type of lung cancer.

Diseases of the Gastrointestinal Tract

This chapter begins with a review of normal gastrointestinal anatomy and digestion. Diseases/disorders discussed include intestinal bleeding and obstruction, gastritis and peptic ulcers, diarrhea, parasitic disease, malabsorption syndromes, ulcerative colitis, Crohn disease, and gastrointestinal tumors.

BACK TO BASICS
- The Mouth and Esophagus
- The Stomach
- The Small Intestine
- The Large Bowel
- Intestinal Bacteria

INTESTINAL BLEEDING

INTESTINAL OBSTRUCTION AND ILEUS

DISEASES OF THE ORAL CAVITY

DISEASES OF SALIVARY GLANDS

DISEASES OF THE ESOPHAGUS

DISEASES OF THE STOMACH
- Gastritis
- Gastric and Duodenal Ulcers
- Carcinoma of the Stomach

NONNEOPLASTIC DISEASES OF THE SMALL BOWEL AND LARGE BOWEL
- Congenital Anomalies
- Vascular Diseases
- Diarrheal Diseases
- Malabsorption Syndromes
- Inflammatory Bowel Disease
- Colonic Diverticulosis and Other Conditions

PERITONITIS

NEOPLASMS OF THE LARGE AND SMALL BOWEL
- Nonneoplastic Polyps
- Neoplastic Polyps (Adenomas)
- Carcinoma of the Colon

DISEASES OF THE APPENDIX

Learning Objectives

After studying this chapter you should be able to:

1. Define melena, hematochezia, and hematemesis, and explain the different implications of slow and rapid gastrointestinal bleeding
2. Explain the importance of stool occult blood tests
3. Distinguish between intestinal mechanical obstruction and ileus
4. Name the cause of most tooth loss and explain its pathogenesis
5. Define achalasia, and offer a short discussion of it
6. Define Barrett esophagus, and discuss its pathogenesis and implications
7. Name some risk factors for esophageal carcinoma
8. Name some conditions associated with *Helicobacter pylori* infection
9. Explain the difference in the pathogenesis of acute gastric erosions and chronic peptic ulceration
10. Explain the cause of Hirschsprung megacolon
11. Name the most common cause worldwide of acute enterocolitis
12. Name some bacteria responsible for epidemic bacterial enterocolitis
13. Explain the pathogenesis of pseudomembranous colitis
14. Among patients with malabsorption syndrome, distinguish between luminal and intestinal malabsorption
15. Characterize and contrast the important differences between ulcerative colitis and Crohn disease

16. Name several extraintestinal manifestations of Crohn disease and ulcerative colitis
17. Explain the pathogenesis of colonic diverticulosis
18. Explain the importance of nonneoplastic polyps of the colon
19. Explain the difference between a tubular adenoma and a villous adenoma of the colon
20. Explain the relationship between colonic adenomas and colonic carcinoma

Key Terms and Concepts

BACK TO BASICS
- digestion
- absorption

INTESTINAL BLEEDING
- hematemesis
- melena

INTESTINAL OBSTRUCTION AND ILEUS
- ileus
- hernia
- intussusception

DISEASES OF THE ESOPHAGUS
- dysphagia
- hiatal hernia
- reflux esophagitis
- Barrett metaplasia

DISEASES OF THE STOMACH
- acute gastritis
- chronic atrophic gastritis

- *Helicobacter pylori*
- stress ulcers
- peptic ulcers

NONNEOPLASTIC DISEASES OF THE SMALL BOWEL AND LARGE BOWEL
- Hirschsprung disease
- enterocolitis
- malabsorption syndrome
- inflammatory bowel disease
- Crohn disease
- ulcerative colitis
- colonic diverticulosis
- diverticulitis

NEOPLASMS OF THE LARGE AND SMALL BOWEL
- tubular adenoma (adenomatous polyp)
- colon carcinoma
- Astler-Coller staging

I would like to be a figment of my own imagination, but belly and bowels will not permit.

MASON COOLEY (1927–2002), AMERICAN WRITER

BACK TO BASICS

Unlike plants, humans cannot make organic molecules and must obtain them from food. The organic molecules in food serve two purposes: they are burned for energy, and they provide the basic building blocks to grow new tissue. Most organic molecules in food are long chains (polymers) of smaller units (monomers). In the gastrointestinal tract the polymers are broken into monomers by the process of **digestion**. The monomers are then transported across the intestinal wall into blood by the process of **absorption**.

As is depicted in Figure 15-1, the gastrointestinal tract consists of the mouth, teeth and tongue, the pharynx, the esophagus, the stomach, and the small and large bowel. The liver and gallbladder (Chapter 16) and pancreas (Chapter 17) also serve digestive functions,

but they are discussed in a later chapter. Functions of the gastrointestinal tract are:

- *Motility*: the ingestion, chewing, and swallowing of food and the movement of food through the bowel by waves of contraction (**peristalsis**)
- *Secretion*: the flow of acid, mucus, and digestive enzymes into the intestinal lumen from glands and mucosa and the secretion of regulatory hormones by the stomach and small bowel
- *Digestion*: the breakdown of food molecules into small, absorbable molecular units
- *Absorption*: the passage of digested food and water into blood and lymph channels
- *Storage and elimination*: the accumulation and ejection of indigestible food as feces

These functions are regulated mainly by the autonomic nervous system (Chapter 23) via the vagus nerve

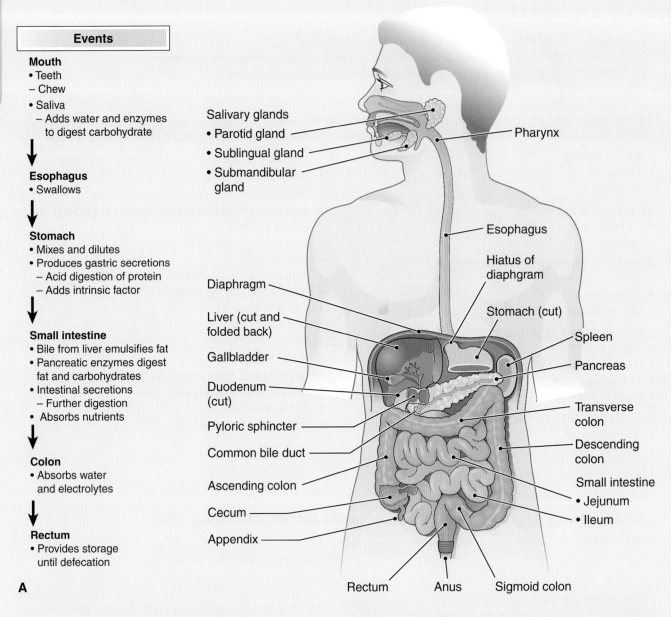

Events

Mouth
- Teeth
  - Chew
- Saliva
  - Adds water and enzymes to digest carbohydrate

↓

Esophagus
- Swallows

↓

Stomach
- Mixes and dilutes
- Produces gastric secretions
  - Acid digestion of protein
  - Adds intrinsic factor

↓

Small intestine
- Bile from liver emulsifies fat
- Pancreatic enzymes digest fat and carbohydrates
- Intestinal secretions
  - Further digestion
- Absorbs nutrients

↓

Colon
- Absorbs water and electrolytes

↓

Rectum
- Provides storage until defecation

A

Salivary glands
- Parotid gland
- Sublingual gland
- Submandibular gland

Pharynx

Esophagus

Hiatus of diaphgram

Diaphragm

Liver (cut and folded back)

Gallbladder

Duodenum (cut)

Pyloric sphincter

Common bile duct

Ascending colon

Cecum

Appendix

Stomach (cut)

Spleen

Pancreas

Transverse colon

Descending colon

Small intestine
- Jejunum
- Ileum

Rectum   Anus   Sigmoid colon

Figure 15-1 Normal anatomy of the digestive system. A, Overview of the digestive system and digestive actions. **B,** Close anatomy of the small bowel. **C,** Microanatomy of an intestinal villus. **D,** Microanatomy of intestinal epithelium.

and ganglia embedded in the bowel wall (myenteric plexus). Also important are hormones secreted by intestinal epithelium.

As is depicted in Figure 15-1, the gastrointestinal tract is a tube that starts at the esophagus and ends at the anus. The tube is composed of concentric layers, which from inside to out are:

- *Mucosa*: the innermost layer of the mucosa is epithelium, which rests upon a basement membrane. In the mouth, esophagus, and the last centimeter of anus the epithelium is composed of layers of flat (squamous) cells; in the stomach, small bowel, and colon

the epithelial cells are tall, columnar cells. Beneath the basement membrane are blood vessels and lymphatics and interstitial tissue, and a thin layer of smooth muscle, the muscularis mucosae.

- *Submucosa*: In the submucosa are accessory glands, specialized lymphoid tissue (mucosa-associated lymphoid tissue, MALT), lymphatics, blood vessels, interstitial tissue, and the autonomic nerve plexus that communicates peristaltic wave commands and other signals.

- *Muscularis*: The muscularis is an outer longitudinal layer and inner circular layer of smooth muscle, which contains another layer of the autonomic neural plexus.

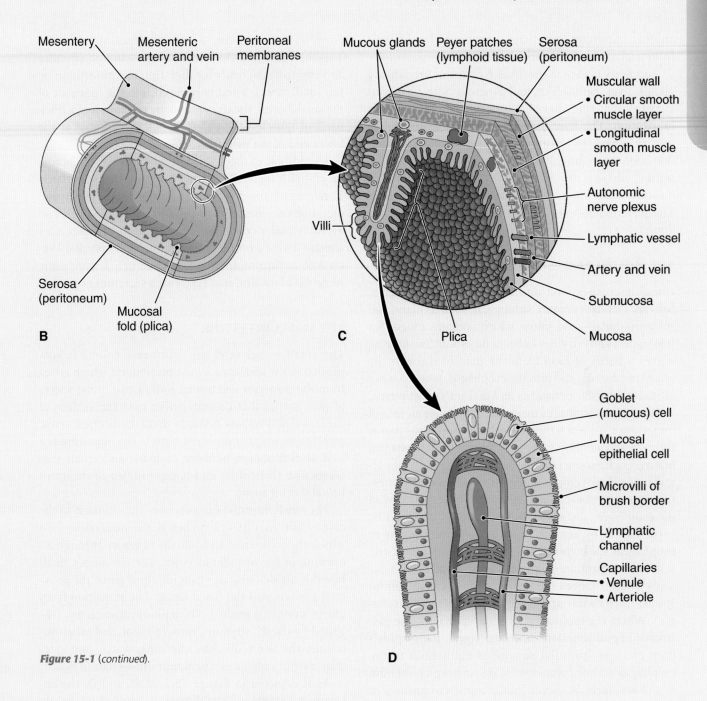

Figure 15-1 (continued).

• *Serosa*: Outermost is the serosa, a layer of flat peritoneal cells.

Digestion of food begins in the mouth and is completed in the small bowel by the action of enzymes, which break large molecules into smaller ones and combine them with hydrogen and oxygen derived from water in a process known as **hydrolysis**. The three basic foodstuffs are carbohydrate, protein, and fat.

Sugars (glucose, fructose, and galactose) are strung together into chains to form *saccharides*, which in turn are strung together to form starch and other complex *carbohydrates*. Specific carbohydrate-digesting enzymes (amylases, saccharidases, and others) break these chains into basic sugar units for absorption.

Amino acids are assembled to form *peptides*, which in turn are assembled to form *proteins*. Protein-digesting enzymes (proteases) break these assemblies into their constituent amino acids for absorption.

Most foodstuff *fat* (lipid) is glycerides, which consists of a molecule of glycerol to which fatty acids are attached. Fat digesting enzymes (lipases) break glycerides into glycerol and fatty acids for absorption. *Cholesterol*, another important lipid that is chemically far different from triglyceride, is absorbed directly.

Accessory organs in the digestive process are salivary glands, liver, gallbladder, and pancreas. Saliva contains enzymes that start digestion and mucus that provides lubrication. The liver makes bile, which contains bile salts that have an ability to make fat soluble in water. Bile is stored in the gallbladder and released into the intestine, where it disperses fat into tiny globules so that it can be acted upon by lipase secreted by the pancreas. The pancreas also secretes amylase to digest carbohydrate.

THE MOUTH AND ESOPHAGUS

Chewing crushes food into manageable, small pieces. Salivary glands—parotid, sublingual, submaxillary, and submandibular—add saliva, which contains mucus for lubrication and enzymes to begin digestion. Swallowing moves a bolus of food from the mouth, through the pharynx (throat), and into the esophagus, where a wave of smooth muscle peristalsis moves it into the stomach.

Where the esophagus meets the stomach is an area of importance. To reach the stomach the esophagus passes through an opening in the diaphragm, the **esophageal hiatus**. Under some circumstances this opening may allow upward movement of part of the stomach or intestines into the chest (**hiatal hernia**). The lowest part of the esophagus, just above the stomach, is encircled by extra bands of smooth muscle to form the **lower esophageal sphincter**, which prevents food and gastric acid from regurgitating upward (gastric reflux). Under some circumstances the sphincter may cause painful spasms (**achalasia**) and difficult swallowing (**dysphagia**). Where the esophagus joins the stomach—the **gastroesophageal junction**—the esophageal lining epithelium changes from flat squamous epithelium in the esophagus to tall columnar, acid-secreting epithelium in the stomach. However, under some circumstances the lower esophageal squamous epithelium may change (undergo metaplasia, Chapter 2) from normal, flat squamous cells to tall, columnar gastric (acid-secreting) cells—a pathologic condition known as **Barrett metaplasia**.

THE STOMACH

The upper (proximal) part of the stomach is the *cardia*; the mid part the *body* (or *fundus*); the distal part the *pylorus*. The stomach produces lubricating mucus and holds food temporarily. The stomach continues the digestive process: gastric glands and epithelium secrete **hydrochloric acid** and **pepsinogen**, which stomach acid converts into **pepsin**, a protein-digesting enzyme. Together, acid and enzyme break protein into peptides and amino acids, ready for digestion and absorption by the small bowel. Food is released into the first part of the small bowel, the duodenum, by relaxation of a thick band of muscle—the *pyloric sphincter*—located at the lower end of the pylorus.

In addition to digestion, the stomach has endocrine functions. It secretes **gastrin**, a hormone that stimulates: 1) release of stomach acid, 2) production of pancreatic digestive enzymes, 3) bile production by the liver, and 4) intestinal peristalsis. The stomach also secretes **somatostatin**, a hormone that inhibits: 1) pituitary release of somatotropin (growth hormone), 2) pancreatic secretion of insulin, and 3) stomach secretion of gastrin.

THE SMALL INTESTINE

The small bowel (and the transverse colon) is suspended in the abdomen by the **mesentery**, which arises from the posterior abdominal wall as two broad sheets of peritoneum that come together over the surface of the bowel and enclose between them the arteries, veins, and lymphatics that serve the bowel. The **omentum** is a fold of peritoneum between stomach and colon that serves as a store of fat and hangs in front of the small bowel like an apron.

The small intestine extends from the stomach to the colon. The first 10–12 inches is the *duodenum*, into which the pancreatic and bile ducts empty through an opening in the *ampulla of Vater*. The remaining small bowel is divided into two roughly equal parts: the proximal *jejunum* and the distal *ileum*. The transition from one to another is gradual. The jejunum absorbs most digested foodstuff, vitamins, iron, calcium, and other nutrients; the ileum absorbs bile salts, water, and electrolytes, but only one critical nutrient—vitamin B_{12}.

As is depicted in Figure 15-1, B, C, and D, the absorptive surface of the bowel is multiplied by its anatomy. First, the mucosa is pleated into large inward folds (plica) of mucosa that provide a foot of bowel with about two feet of mucosa. Second, the mucosa is composed of millions of tiny *villi*, which multiply the absorptive surface many times. Third, the surface of each villus is covered by intestinal epithelial cells, each of which has dozens of *microvilli*, referred to collectively as the *brush border*. Spread among the absorptive epithelial cells are mucus-producing (*goblet*) cells to lubricate intestinal contents. Waves of peristaltic contraction—much weaker than those of the esophagus and stomach—move intestinal contents downward. Also present throughout the small (and large) bowel are patches of lymphoid tissue (*Peyer patches, mucosa-associated lymphoid tissue [MALT]*) that are immunologically active—that is, they secrete high concentrations of immunoglobulin A, the immune paint of the gastrointestinal tract, which protects against invasion of the intestinal wall by bacteria in the gastrointestinal lumen.

THE LARGE BOWEL

The large intestine, or colon (Fig. 15-1A), extends from the end of the small bowel to the anus. The ileum joins the colon at the *ileocecal valve*, a rather narrow one-way gate through which indigestible waste passes. The colonic mucosa contains no villi and has no digestive function. Its function is to absorb water and a few vitamins and to compact feces.

INTESTINAL BACTERIA

Shortly after birth the intestinal tract becomes populated by billions of bacteria from the environment. Most of them inhabit the colon and live there in a natural and mutually beneficial relationship with the body. They are a mixture of bacteria, some of which require oxygen (*aerobic*) and others for which oxygen is toxic (*anaerobic*). Intestinal bacteria are important. First, they produce significant amounts of vitamin K and folic acid. Second, by sheer number they are an important guard against bacterial infection—they are so numerous, and have such a large claim on nutrients, that a large dose (inoculum) of infective bacteria is required to establish a pathologic foothold; ingestion of a few pathogenic bacteria is not likely to establish infection.

MAJOR DETERMINANTS OF DISEASE

- The GI tract is open to the environment
- The GI tract is populated by billions of bacteria
- Breach of intestinal barriers is a common cause of disease
- Mechanical malfunction is a common problem
- The GI tract is richly vascular and subject to hemorrhage
- The colon is host to more neoplasms than any other organ in the body
- Almost all carcinomas of the colon arise from long-preexisting benign polyps

Intestinal Bleeding

Rapid intestinal bleeding can be fatal and is characterized by weakness, fainting, and shock. Intestinal malignancy is often the cause of slow intestinal bleeding, which is often clinically silent and if persistent can cause iron deficiency anemia (Chapter 11).

If blood, either fresh or altered (by stomach acid), is *vomited* the term is **hematemesis**. Vomited *red* blood is usually from the esophagus. Blood from the stomach is usually altered by gastric acid into granular, black material that is accurately described as "coffee grounds." The origin of hematemesis almost invariably is bleeding from the esophagus, stomach, or duodenum. Blood from sites below the stomach usually appears in stool. Unaltered *red* blood *mixed with stool* is **hematochezia** and usually

originates from lesions in the lower colon or rectum. Blood from bleeding hemorrhoids or anal fissures is usually bright red and appears *on*, not *in*, stool. (A note of caution: hemorrhoids and anal fissures are very common; therefore, *never assume* hemorrhoids or an anal fissure is the cause of rectal bleeding until other, more serious lesions [colon cancer] have been excluded. Just because a patient has hemorrhoids does not mean they cannot have colon cancer at the same time.) **Melena** is the passing of black (tarry) stools containing blood altered by intestinal and bacterial digestion. Melena may be caused by bleeding from any intestinal site, including the esophagus. Gastrointestinal bleeding may be caused by tumors, ulcers, inflammation, esophageal varices, vascular malformations, or any one of dozens of other conditions. **Occult bleeding** is clinically unrecognized bleeding, detected by chemical testing of stool. *Gastrointestinal bleeding should be considered to originate in an intestinal malignancy until proven otherwise.* Annual occult blood testing of stool is simple, cheap, and effective: With regular testing over a period of ten or more years, precancerous lesions of the colon can be detected, and about one third of colon cancers can be prevented (see the nearby box, The Clinical Side).

> *Gastrointestinal bleeding is so common and so important that it warrants special attention in every circumstance and should be considered to be caused by intestinal malignancy until proven otherwise.*

The causes of intestinal bleeding are summarized in Figure 15-2. Intestinal bleeding falls into two major categories: upper and lower gastrointestinal bleeding. Up-

THE CLINICAL SIDE

STOOL OCCULT BLOOD TEST

Blood in stool that is invisible to the naked eye can be detected by a simple chemical test. All adults over the age of 30 should be tested regularly. At least three stools should be tested from separate days. Any positive test result warrants further studies to rule out sources of slow bleeding such as colon cancer or colon polyps, diverticula, esophageal varices, peptic ulcer, or other intestinal lesions.

The sensitivity of a single occult blood exam is low, but with repeated examinations using the latest chemical methods, the ability to detect (sensitivity) adenoma or carcinoma rises above 50%. False-negative results are very common because bleeding from polyps or cancers is often limited and irregular. A complete colon exam by direct colonoscopy or radiographic imaging—recommended once every five to ten years for people over age 50 (some say 40)—detects almost all of the tumors missed by occult blood testing.

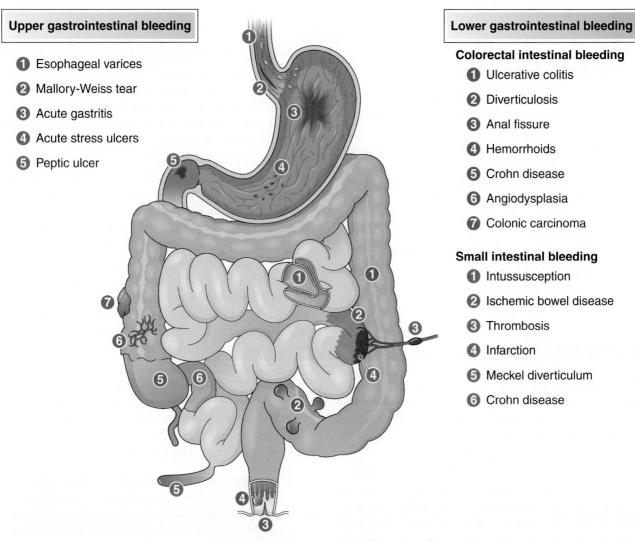

Upper gastrointestinal bleeding	Lower gastrointestinal bleeding
❶ Esophageal varices	**Colorectal intestinal bleeding**
❷ Mallory-Weiss tear	❶ Ulcerative colitis
❸ Acute gastritis	❷ Diverticulosis
❹ Acute stress ulcers	❸ Anal fissure
❺ Peptic ulcer	❹ Hemorrhoids
	❺ Crohn disease
	❻ Angiodysplasia
	❼ Colonic carcinoma
	Small intestinal bleeding
	❶ Intussusception
	❷ Ischemic bowel disease
	❸ Thrombosis
	❹ Infarction
	❺ Meckel diverticulum
	❻ Crohn disease

Figure 15-2 **Causes of intestinal bleeding.**

per gastrointestinal bleeding is from the esophagus, stomach, or the first few centimeters of the duodenum where peptic ulcers usually appear. It may present as hematemesis, hematochezia, or melena. The most common causes of upper gastrointestinal bleeding are, in order, acute hemorrhagic gastritis, peptic ulcer of the duodenum or stomach, esophageal tears caused by vomiting, esophageal varices, and vascular malformations.

Lower gastrointestinal bleeding originates anywhere in the bowel below the first few centimeters of the duodenum. Hematemesis is uncommon; blood usually appears rectally as hematochezia or melena. In persons younger than age 55 the most common causes (not including hemorrhoids and other anal disease), in order, are:

- inflammatory bowel disease or enterocolitis
- colonic diverticulosis
- neoplasms
- colonic angiodysplasia

In people over age 55, the most common causes (not including hemorrhoids and other anal disease), in order, are:

- diverticulosis
- colonic angiodysplasia
- neoplasms
- inflammatory bowel disease or enterocolitis

Intestinal Obstruction and Ileus

Normal intestinal function requires constant peristalsis, which may be interrupted by *mechanical obstruction* or by peristaltic paralysis (**ileus**). In either instance, intestinal contents cannot proceed down the gastrointestinal tract. Obstruction and ileus are serious matters and may quickly become an emergency.

The pathogenesis of ileus is not well understood, but it can be associated with:

- Postoperative state after abdominal surgery
- Appendicitis, gallbladder disease, peritonitis, and other intra-abdominal inflammations
- Intestinal ischemia
- Hypokalemia (low levels of blood potassium)

Clinically, ileus is associated with vomiting, pain, lack of bowel movements (obstipation), and lack of abdominal bowel sounds.

As Figure 15-3 illustrates, the four most common causes of mechanical obstruction are:

- *Hernias*: A **hernia** is a protrusion of bowel through an anatomic space such as the hiatus in the diaphragm,

through which the esophagus passes, or a defect such as a weakened surgical scar. Hernias are a concern because they are common, and because loops of bowel may become trapped in them. The weakness in the abdominal wall or diaphragm allows a pouch of peritoneum to push through the opening, which forms a sac into which loops of small bowel (most commonly), omentum or colon can slide. For example, in the fetus the testes descend to the scrotum from the abdomen, creating a channel (the inguinal canal) through which the spermatic cord passes in adulthood. Intra-abdominal pressure can force the canal open and bowel can slide into it, creating an *inguinal hernia*, illustrated in Figure 15-4. Pressure at the neck of the hernia pouch may impair venous return, causing edema and entrapment (**incarcerated hernia**) of the bowel segment. Ischemia or infarction (**strangulated hernia**) may follow.
- *Adhesions*: Abdominal surgery, infection, or other inflammation may leave bands of fibrous scar tissue (adhesions) in which loops of bowel may become entangled, trapped, and obstructed.
- *Intussusception*: **Intussusception** is a telescoping of bowel, in which the distal (downstream) segment swallows the proximal one. This occurs briefly and regularly in normal people without consequence. Pathologic intussusception may be caused when the swallowed segment becomes trapped; bowel obstruction and infarction are often the result, as is depicted in Figure 15-5.
- *Volvulus*: The intestines are attached to and suspended from the aorta by their blood vessels, which collectively is called the vascular pedicle (stalk) or mesenteric root. A **volvulus** is a twisting of a segment of bowel on its vascular stalk; the result is bowel and vascular obstruction with ischemia or infarction.

Clinically, bowel obstruction is characterized by pain, vomiting, abdominal distention, lack of stools, and hyperactive bowel sounds.

Diseases of the Oral Cavity

The most important congenital abnormality of the oral cavity is *cleft lip* and *cleft palate*, which are malformations that may occur together and are a failure of embryological development.

Figure 15-6 illustrates normal tooth anatomy and the most common dental diseases. **Caries** (tooth decay) is an erosion of tooth enamel caused by bacterial digestion of dietary sugar and other carbohydrates, which produces tooth-destroying acid. Caries was known in an-

Adhesions

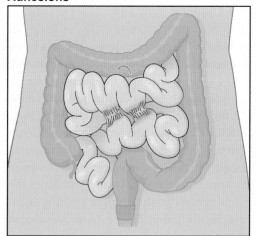

Intussusception

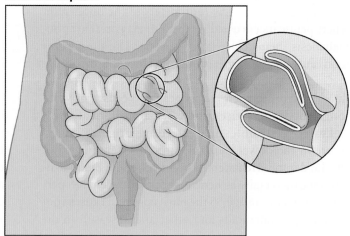

Volvulus

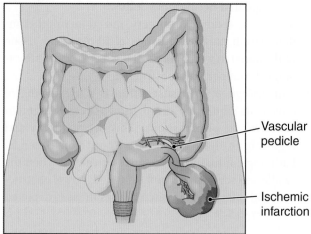

Vascular pedicle

Ischemic infarction

Herniation

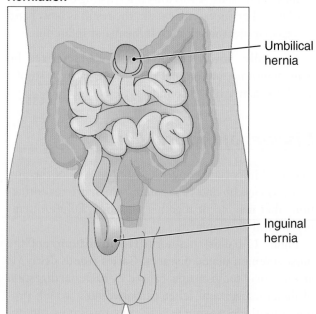

Umbilical hernia

Inguinal hernia

Figure 15-3 Causes of mechanical bowel obstruction.

tiquity and is arguably the most common disease of humankind. It is caused by poor oral hygiene and diet and has an element of genetic predisposition. Bacteria accumulate in **plaque**, a complex film of bacteria, dead cells, and mucus that accumulates at the gum margin. Calcified plaque is **tartar**. Plaque promotes caries and **gingivitis**, inflammation of the superficial gums, and leads to shrinkage and retraction of the gums, which exposes the root to infection. Incidentally, gum retraction—which exposes root and makes the tooth appear long—is the source of the phrase "long in the tooth" to describe an old person or animal.

Gingivitis may proceed to **periodontitis**, a deeper inflammation and infection of soft tissues around the tooth root. Deep-seated inflammation loosens tooth ligaments, allowing deeper bacterial invasion, which may infect the pulp, the soft central tissue of the tooth that contains blood vessels and nerves—which assures that pulp infection is quite painful. Infection of the root produces a *periapical abscess*, which usually requires surgical drainage. Periodontal disease causes far more tooth loss than does caries.

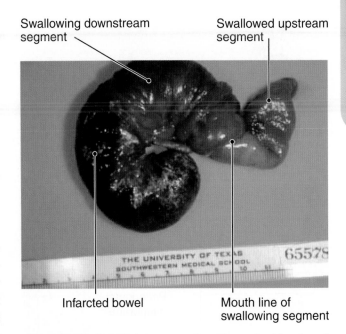

Figure 15-5 **Pathologic intussusception.** The proximal (swallowed) segment is to the right; the distal (swallowing) segment is to the left. The discolored segment is hemorrhagic infarction.

Fluoridation of public drinking water has proven very effective at preventing caries, apparently by producing enamel that is resistant to bacteria. Daily tooth brushing and flossing are most important, however; good oral hygiene is effective at reducing caries, plaque and calculus formation, periodontitis, and lost teeth.

Aphthous ulcers (canker sores) are common, small, painful, shallow ulcers of the oral cavity. They are triggered by stress, fever, or certain foods and occur mainly in children and young adults. They are self-limiting and disappear in about a week. The cause is unknown.

Oral **herpesvirus** infection is very common. The virus is usually passed by kissing; although it can be transmitted sexually (Chapter 20). Initial infection is asymptomatic, but the virus finds a permanent home in the fifth cranial (trigeminal) nerve, which provides sensation to the face and lips. The virus settles in the trigeminal ganglion at the base of the skull and when stimulated by fever, sunlight, cold, trauma, or infection, it multiplies and migrates out nerve axons to erupt in nerve endings in skin or mucosa as a **cold sore** or **fever blister**—a cluster of small vesicles that rupture, leaving a small painful ulcer for a week or two. In children or immunodeficient hosts, the infection may disseminate to cause widespread visceral lesions or encephalitis and death. Genital herpes is usually caused by HSV-2, sometimes by HSV-1, and is passed by sexual contact; otherwise, the pathologic processes are the same.

Candida albicans is a fungus and normal inhabitant of the mouth. It causes disease—variously referred to as

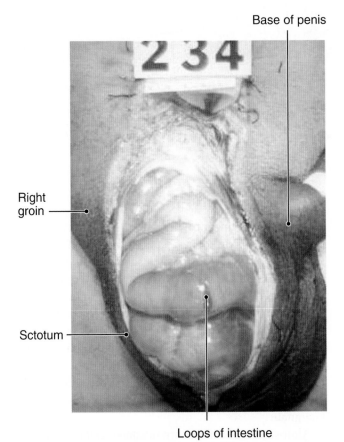

Figure 15-4 **Incarcerated inguinal hernia.** The bowel is trapped (incarcerated) in the scrotum, but it is not necrotic (strangulated).

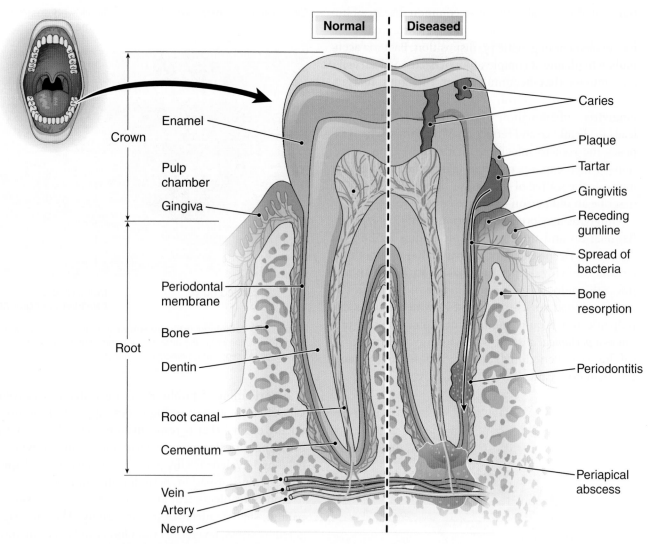

Normal | **Diseased**

Crown

Enamel

Pulp chamber

Gingiva

Periodontal membrane

Bone

Root — Dentin

Root canal

Cementum

Vein

Artery

Nerve

Caries

Plaque

Tartar

Gingivitis

Receding gumline

Spread of bacteria

Bone resorption

Periodontitis

Periapical abscess

Figure 15-6 Normal and pathologic anatomy of a tooth. Caries is caused by bacteria that erode enamel and invade tooth structure. Periodontal disease results from bacterial invasion of gingival pockets around the tooth root.

candidiasis or **moniliasis**—only when normal protective mechanisms are impaired by immune deficiency, diabetes mellitus, antibiotic or steroid therapy, or anemia. Candidiasis of the mouth (where it is called **thrush**) is a fuzzy white membrane or curd composed of matted fungi and acute inflammatory cells. Rarely, infection may extend into the esophagus or disseminate via the bloodstream. *Candida* may cause vaginitis (Chapter 21) in women who are pregnant or taking broad-spectrum antibiotics or oral contraceptives.

Leukoplakia is a clinical term that refers to a small, focal, superficial, white patch of squamous mucosa. When irritated or otherwise damaged, the squamous cells lining the oral cavity undergo metaplasia (Chapter 2) and develop an ability to produce *keratin*, a dense,

protective protein normally found in epidermis (the outer layer of skin). The result is a superficial cap of keratin (*hyperkeratosis*), which is responsible for the white clinical appearance. However, the mere fact that leukoplakia is present says nothing about the squamous cells deeper down, which may be benign or malignant. Leukoplakia is associated with tobacco use (especially pipe smoking or the use of snuff or chewing tobacco), alcohol abuse, and with chronic irritation, as with ill-fitting dentures. In most leukoplakia the pathologic findings are benign, but a few lesions are precancerous or malignant.

Almost all oral cancers are *squamous cell carcinomas*. Most occur in middle-aged to older adults. The most common site is the border of the lower lip, but the floor of the mouth and the lateral aspect of the tongue are also common sites. They are typically associated with poor oral hygiene and with alcohol *abuse* and tobacco use. Many arise from preexisting dysplasia. Despite ease of visibility and access, they are often missed by nondental professionals, who tend to abandon the mouth to dentists and oral hygienists. Nearly all patients with lip cancer survive five years; by contrast, of those with carcinoma of the floor of the mouth, only about one third survive.

Diseases of Salivary Glands

Inflammation of salivary glands is **sialadenitis**, and the etiology is usually viral infection or autoimmune disease. The parotid gland is most often affected. Childhood *mumps* is the most common viral agent. Rarely, mumps may spread from the salivary glands to cause pancreatitis or orchitis (testicular inflammation). Autoimmune sialadenitis is usually seen as a part of **Sjögren syndrome** (Chapter 8), a combination of salivary and lacrimal gland inflammation that damages the glands, drying up tears and saliva and producing dry eyes (*conjunctivitis sicca*) and dry mouth (*xerostomia*). Sialadenitis may also occur as a component of systemic collagen-vascular disease, such as systemic lupus erythematosus (Chapter 8).

Salivary gland tumors are uncommon. Most occur in the parotid gland of older adults, and most are benign. Of the various types of benign and malignant tumors of the salivary glands, the most common is **pleomorphic adenoma**, often called **mixed tumor** because of its varied microscopic appearance. Almost all are benign, but even a benign mixed tumor can be trouble because a branch of the facial nerve passes through the parotid and can be damaged during removal even by the most attentive surgeon. Avoiding the facial nerve and ensuring complete excision becomes a very difficult task—about 10% of pleomorphic adenomas are incompletely removed and recur. The prognosis is good for most salivary gland tumors—average five-year survival is about 80%.

Diseases of the Esophagus

Symptoms of esophageal disease include difficult swallowing, pain, or bleeding. Movement of food from mouth to stomach requires coordinated motor function of the esophagus. Almost all esophageal disease is associated with **dysphagia** (difficult swallowing) or pain, which may be difficult to distinguish from cardiac pain

(angina, Chapter 13). Dysphagia may be caused by hiatal hernia, obstructing scar, tumor (especially esophageal carcinoma), or abnormal peristalsis secondary to neurologic disease such as stroke or parkinsonism (Chapter 23).

Achalasia is spasm of the esophageal sphincter. It is typically chronic and intermittent, and it causes partial obstruction in the lower esophagus near the esophageal hiatus. It produces dysphagia and esophageal pain that can mimic angina. The cause is unknown.

Hiatal hernia is a protrusion of part of the stomach upward into the chest through the diaphragmatic opening (hiatus) that allows passage of the esophagus. Radiographic studies suggest that up to 10% of adults have some degree of asymptomatic hiatal hernia. The majority of these patients are asymptomatic, but about 10% experience dysphagia, pain, or reflux of gastric acid into the lower esophagus.

Severe retching (vomiting), as in bulimia, for example, may cause esophageal *laceration* (also known as the **Mallory-Weiss syndrome**). Lacerations usually occur near the gastroesophageal junction (Fig. 15-7) and can be associated with life-threatening bleeding.

A dilated vein is a *varix*. **Esophageal varices** are like hemorrhoids—dilated veins full of blood (Fig. 15-8). Esophageal veins rarely become enlarged, but when they do it is almost always associated with *cirrhosis of the liver*—a severe scarring (Chapter 16) of the entire liver that obstructs normal flow of portal blood on its

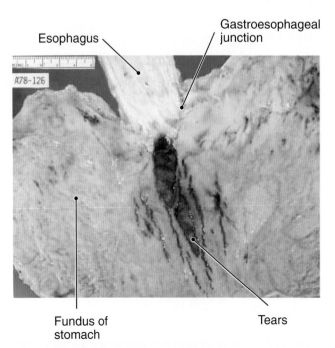

Figure 15-7 **Mallory-Weiss syndrome.** The gastroesophageal tears are from vomiting.

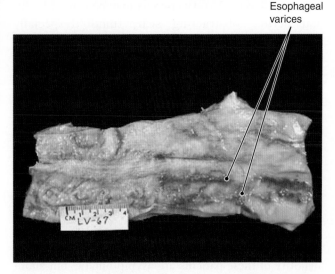

Esophageal varices

Figure 15-8 **Esophageal varices.** Veins in this postmortem specimen are much smaller than during life. The patient had portal hypertension caused by cirrhosis of the liver.

way to the heart from the intestines. Esophageal veins are an important bypass route for blood to get back to the heart if the liver is cirrhotic. Patients known to have cirrhosis can be presumed to have esophageal varices, which are especially dangerous because they produce no symptoms until rupture; and when they rupture, the

bleeding can be horrific and require emergency treatment. Among patients with advanced cirrhosis, half die of ruptured varices, many of them with the first bleeding episode.

Inflammation of the esophagus, which affects about 10% of people in developed countries, is most often the result of gastric acid refluxing upward from the stomach, a condition called **reflux esophagitis**. People over age 40 are most often affected, and the dominant symptom is pain. Complications include bleeding and fibrous scarring (stricture). About 10% of patients with reflux esophagitis develop **Barrett metaplasia** (or Barrett esophagus), a change of lower esophageal squamous epithelium into acid-secreting gastric epithelium, as is depicted in Figure 15-9. Barrett metaplasia is associated with an approximate 40× increased risk for esophageal carcinoma.

Most **carcinomas of the esophagus** arise from the squamous mucosa and are, therefore, *squamous* carcinomas. In the United States, men and African Americans are affected most often. The most important risk factors for esophageal cancer include tobacco *use* and alcohol *abuse*. Other risk factors include Barrett esophagus, achalasia, and dietary deficiencies of certain trace metals and vitamins. Esophageal *adenocarcinomas* are less common; almost all arise in Barrett metaplasia of the lower

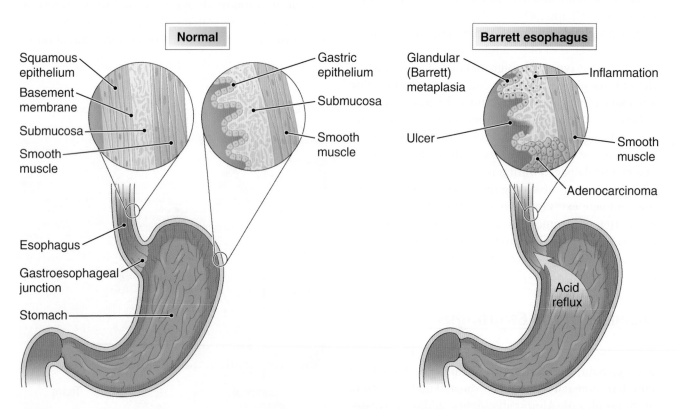

Figure 15-9 **Barrett esophagus.** Normal esophagus is lined by layers of flat, squamous epithelium. Normal stomach is lined by tall, columnar cells. Chronic reflux of gastric acid evokes change (metaplasia) of normal esophageal squamous epithelium into gastric epithelium (Barrett metaplasia). Esophageal ulcers and adenocarcinoma may arise in areas of Barrett metaplasia.

esophagus. Esophageal carcinomas tend to invade and metastasize early; not many patients survive five years after diagnosis. Early detection is best accomplished by careful monitoring of patients with achalasia and chronic esophagitis.

Diseases of the Stomach

Gastric disease may be silent or painful. Gastric pain is usually caused by gastric ulceration. It usually occurs high in the abdomen, just below the end of the sternum and therefore may be mistaken for cardiac pain (angina). Vomiting, also a common symptom, is a reflex that can also be stimulated by many nongastric conditions—intestinal obstruction, brain disease (from increased intracranial pressure), intestinal disease, and acute myocardial infarct.

Gastric bleeding may result in **hematemesis** (vomiting blood). Most gastric hematemesis looks like coffee grounds—a dense collection of small, black clots of altered blood (blood changed by intestinal and bacterial digestion). Esophageal bleeding, on the other hand, usually produces bright red bloody vomiting. If gastric blood passes through the entire gastrointestinal tract, it turns stool black (**melena**), which is spoken of as "tarry stool."

GASTRITIS

Gastritis is inflammation of the gastric mucosa. **Acute hemorrhagic gastritis** is an uncommon, transient inflammation of the gastric mucosa that is associated with intramucosal hemorrhage (Fig. 15-10). The pathogenesis of acute gastritis is poorly understood, a fact emphasized by the variety of conditions that may cause it: aspirin and nonsteroidal antiinflammatory drugs are the most common culprits; other causes include alcohol abuse, heavy smoking, uremia, and shock. Acute hemorrhagic gastritis usually is associated with upper abdominal pain, nausea, and vomiting. It is sometimes associated with multiple *acute superficial ulcers* (discussed below under "Gastric and Duodenal Ulcers"), which may cause severe hemorrhage, and it is an important cause of gastrointestinal bleeding in alcoholics.

> *Infection with* Helicobacter pylori *is the cause of most chronic atrophic gastritis and peptic ulcers.*

However, most gastritis is **chronic atrophic gastritis**, which is asymptomatic and often goes undiagnosed. Over 90% of patients with chronic atrophic gastritis are infected with *Helicobacter pylori*, which is also impor-

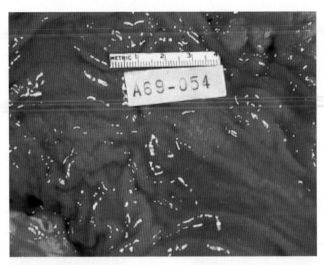

Figure 15-10 Acute gastritis. The inflamed gastric mucosa is markedly hyperemic.

tant in the pathogenesis of peptic ulcer disease and gastric carcinoma. However, it is not clear how *H. pylori* infection causes disease. *H. pylori* infection is common—about half of American adults over age 50 are infected, but only a small percentage develop chronic gastritis or ulcers. Cigarette smoking and alcohol abuse clearly play a role in addition to *H. pylori* infection, and patients with chronic atrophic gastritis have an increased risk of developing gastric carcinoma. Figure 15-11 illustrates that the distal (pyloric) region is most commonly and severely affected. Chronic atrophic gastritis causes few symptoms and therefore may remain undiagnosed until it becomes severe or peptic ulcers or gastric carcinoma appear. Infected patients respond well to antibiotic therapy; reinfection is associated with recurrence of gastritis.

GASTRIC AND DUODENAL ULCERS

Gastric and duodenal ulcers are roundish, discrete defects of mucosa that extend into the submucosa or deeper. There are two types:

- **Stress ulcers** are acute, superficial mucosal defects that tend to be multiple; they are associated with stressful circumstances such as major trauma, brain injury, and acute alcohol abuse.
- **Peptic ulcers** are chronic, recurrent, deep, solitary mucosal defects that were originally presumed to be caused by gastric (peptic) juices and acid. However, we know now that they are mainly caused by infection by *Helicobacter pylori*.

Stress ulcers are often referred to as *erosions* because they are superficial. As is depicted in Figure 15-12, mul-

Esophageal margin

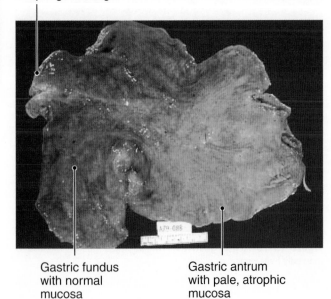

Gastric fundus
with normal
mucosa

Gastric antrum
with pale, atrophic
mucosa

Figure 15-11 **Chronic atrophic gastritis.**

tiple, superficial, discrete lesions are scattered widely across the stomach mucosa. They are associated with stressful clinical conditions such as acute gastritis, severe trauma, sepsis, major surgical procedures, grave illnesses, alcohol abuse, extensive burns, brain trauma

or surgery, and chronic exposure to nonsteroidal anti-inflammatory drugs and corticosteroids. Most patients hospitalized with severe burns, sepsis, or head injury have acute gastric ulcerations, and in these patients gastric hemorrhage can be a serious problem. Oral antacids and blood transfusions are the mainstays of treatment, but the most important index of a favorable outcome is correction of the underlying condition.

Peptic ulcers (Fig. 15-13) are usually found in the *duodenum*, but they also arise in the stomach and esophagus. Infection by *H. pylori* is necessary; however, other factors are also important (only about 10–20% of infected people develop ulcers). Men are more often affected than women are. Associated conditions include chronic gastritis and cigarette smoking, as well as long-term use of aspirin, nonsteroidal antiinflammatory drugs, corticosteroids, and alcohol. Psychological stress, family history, and personality traits also play a role.

About 80% of peptic ulcers occur in the first few centimeters of the duodenum; the remaining 20% occur mainly in the stomach. The lesion is usually solitary and forms a round, sharply demarcated pit a few centimeters in diameter. The ulcer floor is a bed of granulation tissue and inflammatory debris, which is surrounded by a rim of inflamed, edematous mucosa.

Peptic ulcers typically cause a penetrating, burning pain high in the abdomen, but some remain asympto-

Hyperemic (inflamed)
gastric mucosa

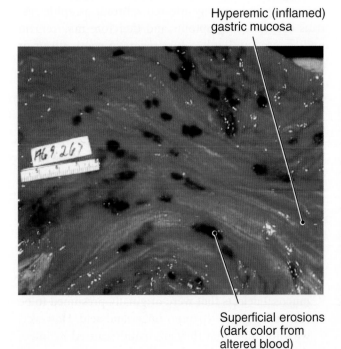

Superficial erosions
(dark color from
altered blood)

Figure 15-12 **Acute gastric stress ulcers.** Multiple superficial ulcers in a patient with brain injury. Altered blood on the ulcer's surface is black.

Dark, altered blood
in base of ulcer

Muscular wall
of stomach

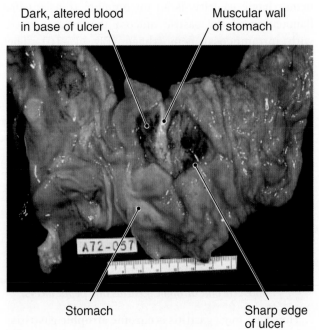

Stomach

Sharp edge
of ulcer

Figure 15-13 **Chronic peptic ulcer of stomach.** The ulcer has been incised to reveal the muscular wall. Note that the ulcer extends down *to* but not *into* muscular wall. Altered blood in the ulcer base is black.

matic until hemorrhage or bowel perforation occurs. The pain typically is relieved by food or antacids. Weight loss, nausea, and vomiting are common. Duodenal ulcers may penetrate into the pancreas, causing acute pancreatitis. A fairly common serious complication is bleeding from erosion of blood vessels in the bowel wall. Perforation, depicted in Figure 15-14, is much less common than is hemorrhage, but perforation is more dangerous and accounts for most deaths from peptic ulcer.

Peptic ulcers are by nature chronic and recurrent—many patients heal completely only to develop ulcers again. Especially noteworthy for recurrence are ulcers associated with the **Zollinger-Ellison syndrome** (Chapter 18), in which pancreatic islet tumors secrete gastrin, which stimulates marked gastric acid production and recurrent ulcers that resist medical treatment. Surgical removal of the tumors is required.

Treatment of peptic ulcers with modern drugs is usually effective and relies mainly on control of gastric acid secretion and antibiotic therapy for *H. pylori* infection.

CARCINOMA OF THE STOMACH

Almost all (95%) malignancies of the stomach are adenocarcinomas (Fig. 15-15). In the 1930s, gastric carcinoma was the number-one cancer killer in the United States, but now ranks far down the list. Worldwide, however, gastric carcinoma still causes about as many deaths as lung cancer does. Regional differences are dramatic: gastric carcinoma is about ten times more common in Japan than the United States.

Risk factors for gastric carcinoma are 1) *H. pylori* infection and chronic atrophic gastritis, 2) a diet high in smoked, pickled, or salt-preserved food, 3) use of nitrite

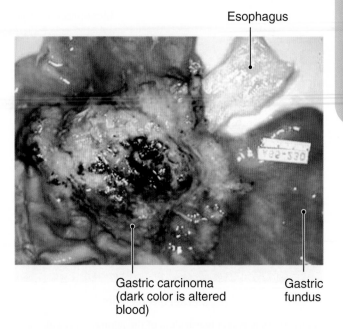

Figure 15-15 **Carcinoma of the stomach.** Altered blood on the tumor's surface is black.

food preservatives, and 4) a diet low in fresh fruits and vegetables.

In keeping with the fact that chronic atrophic gastritis is a predisposing factor and occurs in the gastric antrum (the narrow, distal part), more than half of gastric carcinomas also occur in the antrum. Gastric carcinomas are often asymptomatic—by the time they produce gastric discomfort or weight loss they are usually too advanced for curative surgery. Gastric carcinoma spreads first to regional lymph nodes and the liver; five-year survival is about 10%.

Nonneoplastic Diseases of the Small Bowel and Large Bowel

Bowel neoplasms occur mainly in the colon; conversely, nonneoplastic disease is more common in the small bowel. The most common nonneoplastic diseases are infective or inflammatory, associated with diarrhea, and affect most of the bowel, not just a small segment.

CONGENITAL ANOMALIES

Meckel diverticulum, illustrated in Figure 15-16, is the most common and harmless bowel congenital anomaly. It is an embryologic remnant attached to the jejunum like a large appendix. Rarely, it becomes acutely inflamed like the appendix.

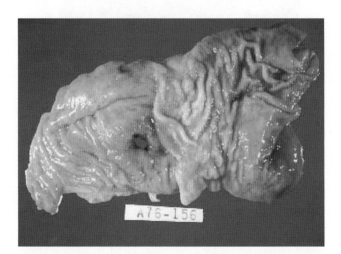

Figure 15-14 **Perforated peptic ulcer of stomach.**

Jejunum   Mesenteric margin

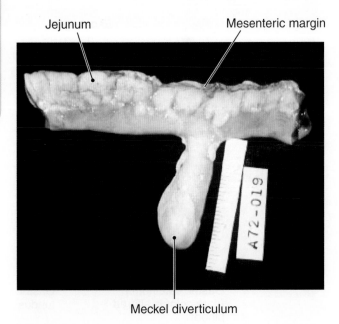

Meckel diverticulum

Figure 15-16 **Meckel diverticulum of the jejunum.** Incidental finding at autopsy.

Congenital *atresia* (complete obstruction) or *stenosis* (partial obstruction) are rare and usually involve the small bowel. **Gastroschisis** is a failure of the abdominal wall to form properly; as a result the intestines are uncovered and protrude outward. A less severe form of the same anomaly is **omphalocele**, in which a smaller amount of bowel protrudes into a membranous sac of peritoneum. Smaller still, and fairly common, is an **umbilical hernia**, a finger-sized opening in the abdominal wall at the umbilicus that is covered by skin and through which bowel may protrude (herniate). Most umbilical hernias close spontaneously early in life.

By far the most important developmental abnormality of the bowel *is congenital megacolon* (**Hirschsprung disease**). It is caused by a genetic absence of the autonomic ganglionic neural plexus, which controls peristalsis in the smooth muscle wall of the colon. The lower colon and rectum are usually involved. Deprived of ganglionic neural control, no peristalsis occurs in the affected segment, feces cannot pass, and the upstream colon distends with fecal material. Hirschsprung disease predominantly affects males and occurs about once in 5,000 live births. The principal threat to life is an overgrowth in the distended segment of toxic bacteria that produce severe intestinal inflammation. Surgical excision of the affected (aganglionic) segment is curative.

VASCULAR DISEASES

The small and large bowel are supplied by the celiac and superior and inferior mesenteric arteries. Obstruction of blood flow from any of these vessels can cause bowel ischemia or infarction (Fig. 15-17). Bowel ischemia is most common in elderly patients with severe generalized atherosclerosis. However, vascular occlusion can also be caused by embolism or vasculitis, or by the twisting of bowel loops (*volvulus*), which strangles flow. Ischemia or infarction can occur without complete vessel occlusion in patients with atherosclerosis of the intestinal vascular supply who also develop low cardiac output, as in shock, myocardial infarction, or congestive heart failure.

Partial or complete vascular occlusion causes abdominal pain and **ileus** (intestinal paralysis; loss of peristalsis). However, with vascular occlusion it is very difficult to make the diagnosis in time to save the bowel. The mortality rate approaches 90%.

Angiodysplasia is a small, tortuous collection of small blood vessels (somewhat like a hemangioma) usually found in the mucosa or submucosa of the right colon or cecum. They are very prone to bleed and account for about 20% of lower intestinal bleeding, especially in older adults. Most are probably congenital defects.

Hemorrhoids are dilated anal veins (varices). As is illustrated in Figure 15-18, they may lie within the anal

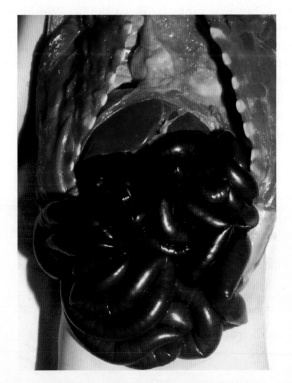

Figure 15-17 **Volvulus with infarction of small bowel.** The intestine in this child twisted on its vascular pedicle and occluded the superior mesenteric artery, which infarcted the entire small bowel. Reprinted with permission from Rubin E. Pathology. 4th ed. Philadelphia. Lippincott Williams and Wilkins, 2005.

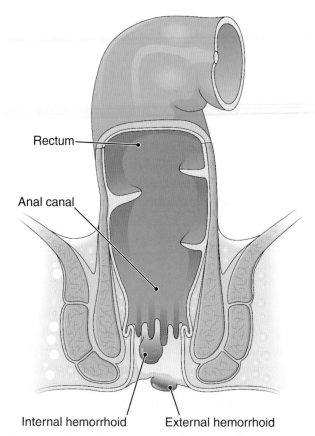

Rectum

Anal canal

Internal hemorrhoid External hemorrhoid

Figure 15-18 **Internal and external hemorrhoids.** Hemorrhoids bleed regularly, leaving bright red blood on the stool surface.

canal (internal hemorrhoids) or protrude from the anal orifice (external hemorrhoids). The anus is richly endowed with nerves, which makes hemorrhoids especially painful. It must have been someone suffering from hemorrhoids who coined a certain well-known term about the anus to describe a vexatious person. Hemorrhoids occur mainly in persons over age 50. Some genetic predisposition is evident, but the principal cause is straining at stool in chronically constipated older adults, or the venous stasis of pregnancy. Rarely, hemorrhoids may result from obstruction of portal blood flow, which is usually caused by cirrhosis of the liver (Chapter 16). Surgical excision of the dilated veins is curative.

The most common complications of hemorrhoids are bleeding and thrombosis, which is especially painful. Blood from bleeding hemorrhoids is *bright red* and appears on the stool *surface*, differing in appearance distinctly from blood from bleeding higher in the gastrointestinal tract. Bleeding from very high in the intestines, such as in the stomach or duodenum, produces black stools (*melena*), from digested blood. Bleeding from lower in the intestines, but above the anus, produces a mix of stool and blood known as *hematochezia*.

However, when hemorrhoids are present and rectal bleeding occurs, *never* assume that the bleeding is *solely* from hemorrhoids. The first episode of rectal bleeding, even in the presence of hemorrhoids, deserves thorough investigation to be certain hemorrhoids are not masking some other disorder, such as colon carcinoma.

DIARRHEAL DISEASES

Given the great variability of normal bowel habits, **diarrhea** is difficult to define with precision. Most patients think of diarrhea as thinner and more frequent bowel movements than normal. A convenient clinical definition is six or more movements per day; nevertheless, diarrhea remains famously difficult to define. **Dysentery** is low-volume, bloody, painful diarrhea.

With diarrhea sometimes comes dehydration. Loss of tissue turgor (fullness) is a useful clinical sign of dehydration, especially in infants and children or anyone unable to speak for themselves. As is illustrated in Figure 15-19, dehydrated tissue, having lost its turgor, does not snap back into place after being pinched into a ridge. Fluid loss shrinks vascular volume, and blood pressure and cardiac output decline. Death may occur in severe cases, especially in children or debilitated people.

Irritable bowel syndrome is, like diarrhea, very difficult to define, and it is common: it accounts for perhaps 30% of referrals to gastroenterologists. It is a functional disorder with no demonstrable pathologic findings, and it is characterized by abdominal pain, bloating, and altered frequency (too few or too frequent movements) or consistency of stool (loose or hard).

Pinched ridge of skin

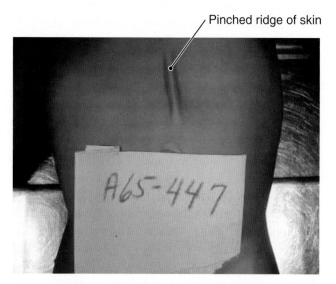

Figure 15-19 **Severe dehydration.** Severe diarrhea caused this case of fatal dehydration in a child. Loss of fluid content causes tissue to lose its ability to snap back into place after being pinched into a ridge.

About two thirds of patients are women, many of whom also have psychiatric disturbances. Temporary relief occurs with bowel movements.

Viral and Bacterial Enterocolitis

Enterocolitis, an inflammation of the bowel associated with diarrhea, is almost always infectious. *Gastroenteritis* is a term used synonymously but erroneously because the stomach is rarely involved. Enterocolitis develops in one of two settings:

- The *equilibrium* of intestinal flora is upset and a normally minor intestinal bacterium overgrows. For example, one of the complications of antibiotic therapy is that it may kill most normal intestinal bacteria and allow overgrowth of *Clostridium difficile*, which secretes a toxin that causes colitis.
- A *pathogen*, such as rotavirus, *Salmonella,* or *Giardia,* is introduced.

Gastrointestinal infections usually produce mild mucosal inflammation and diarrhea. Gastrointestinal infection is second only to the common cold as a regular affliction—about half of the U.S. population suffers a bout of enterocolitis each year. Infective agents vary by region. In developed nations most infections are viral and bacterial; in developing nations *protozoa* and *parasites* are the most common offenders. For adults in developed nations, gastrointestinal infections and the diarrhea that accompanies them are usually nothing more than an unpleasant inconvenience. It is a much different story elsewhere—diarrhea worldwide causes death by dehydration of more than 10,000 persons *per day*, for the most part children in underdeveloped nations.

Enterocolitis may be episodic or epidemic; that is, it may occur in one person, or it may cause widespread waves of illness by transmission from one person to the next. Enterocolitis may be *acute or chronic*, depending on the agent responsible. Viruses and some bacteria tend to produce acute illness; other bacteria, parasites, and protozoa are often associated with chronic or recurrent disease.

Rotavirus is the main cause of acute viral enterocolitis worldwide. It affects infants and young children and is spread by fecal contamination. The *Norwalk virus*, on the other hand, is responsible for nonbacterial, epidemic diarrhea in older children and adults. Norwalk virus is the agent responsible for a series of epidemics on passenger cruise ships in the early 2000s. A typical illness involves 1 to 3 days of nausea, vomiting, pain, and diarrhea that resolves with supportive therapy, mainly fluid replenishment.

Bacterial enterocolitis, which is usually more severe than viral enterocolitis, is produced by one of two mechanisms, depicted in Figure 15-20. The bacterium may form an enterotoxin, either outside the body (Fig. 15-20A), as staphylococci do on unrefrigerated foods; or inside the body, as is the case for *Vibrio cholerae* and some *E. coli* infections (Fig. 15-20B). Alternatively, the organism can invade tissue directly (Fig. 15-20C).

E. coli is a normal inhabitant of the intestinal tract, but some strains are pathogenic and are the cause of food-borne epidemics of diarrhea, which can be fatal in children. Other bacteria can cause epidemics of diarrhea. *Salmonella enterica* has many subtypes that cause a variety of gastrointestinal illnesses called **salmonellosis**, which is transmitted by contaminated food or drink. By far the most common illness is acute enterocolitis characterized by sudden fever, chills, nausea, vomiting, and diarrhea. Diagnosis is confirmed by stool culture of the organism. Less common is **typhoid fever**, a syndrome of slow onset of gastrointestinal and systemic symptoms including fever, headache, sore throat, splenomegaly, bloating, constipation or diarrhea, and skin rash. Diagnosis is confirmed by blood culture of the organism. Some *Salmonella* infections can cause chronic infection and bacteremia with relapsing fever and local infection of bones, joints, heart, pericardium, or lungs. Most *Salmonella* are sensitive to antibiotics. A vaccine is available.

Shigella species cause **shigellosis**, also called *bacillary dysentery*, another epidemic form of enterocolitis. *Campylobacter* species, *Vibrio cholerae* (the agent of **cholera**), and *Yersinia enterocolitica* are also important bacterial agents of enterocolitis.

Diagnosis is confirmed by stool culture. Antibiotic therapy is usually effective, and fluid support is very important. Without proper medical attention, especially in children, death may occur because of dehydration, sepsis, or intestinal perforation.

Pseudomembranous colitis, an uncommon, severe inflammation of the colonic mucosa usually seen in elderly patients, is caused by an enterotoxin produced by *Clostridium difficile*. The usual cause is *broad-spectrum antibiotic therapy*, which in some patients alters the intestinal flora such that *C. difficile*, a normal intestinal inhabitant, overgrows pathologically. *C. difficile* secretes a potent toxin that damages colonic mucosa. The resulting inflammatory exudate forms a membrane of pus and dead tissue that clings to the mucosal surface, hence the name of the condition. Pseudomembranous colitis can affect young or old, and most patients have no history of previous gastrointestinal problems. Diagnosis is confirmed by laboratory detection of *C. difficile* toxin in stool.

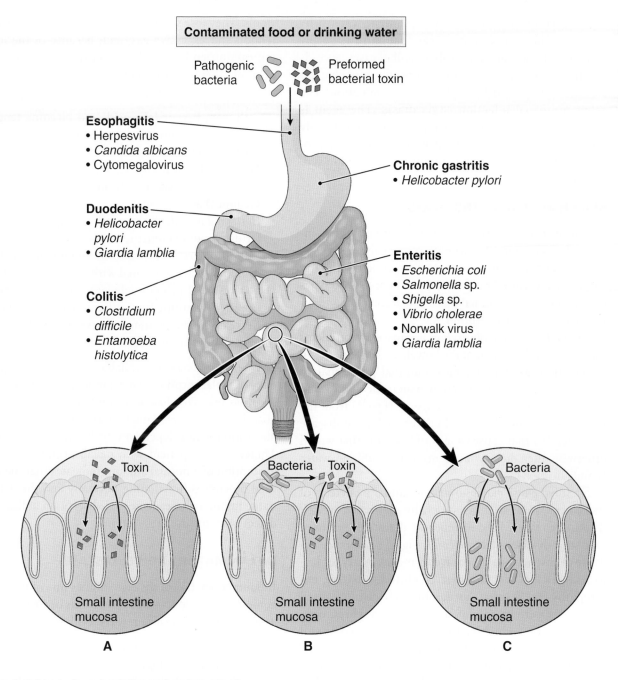

◆ Bacterial toxin from food (formed preingestion)
◆ Bacterial toxin formed in GI tract (postingestion)

Figure 15-20 Mechanisms of bacterial enterocolitis. Diarrhea can be caused by (**A**) bacterial toxin formed in food before ingestion, (**B**) toxin formed in the intestinal tract after infection, or (**C**) direct invasion of infective organisms in the bowel wall.

A somewhat similar condition, **necrotizing entero-colitis**, can affect immature or low birth weight infants in the first week of life. The cause is unknown, and the condition is characterized by acute, necrotizing inflammation involving the small bowel and colon.

Protozoal Infections

Two protozoal infections deserve mention because they are common in developing nations and infect travelers from other lands. Both are spread by food and water contamination. One is **amebic dysentery**, caused by *Entamoeba histolytica*, a protozoan that burrows deeply into the colonic wall and, in about half of cases, spreads up the portal vein to the liver to produce amebic abscesses. It is passed by oral-fecal contamination. The other protozoal infection is **giardiasis**. The agent is *Giardia lamblia*, a noninvasive protozoan that mainly affects the duodenum and small bowel and may produce an acute diarrhea or a chronic malabsorption syndrome.

MALABSORPTION SYNDROMES

Malabsorption syndrome is characterized by poor intestinal absorption of nutrients (especially fats), electrolytes, minerals, and water. Malabsorption with fatty stools (steatorrhea) is called **sprue**. There are two types of malabsorption: luminal phase malabsorption and intestinal phase malabsorption.

Luminal phase malabsorption is caused by problems that occur in the lumen of the bowel, such as absence of pancreatic digestive enzymes. Luminal phase malabsorption is most often caused by pancreatic disease and the absence of a fat-digesting enzyme (lipase) from the pancreas (Chapter 17), or by liver or biliary disease (Chapter 16) that causes a lack of bile salts that would otherwise alter dietary fat to make it soluble in water (emulsification).

Intestinal phase malabsorption is caused by defects of the bowel itself, such as surgically shortened bowel. Another cause is lack of mucosal digestive enzymes. One such disease is lactose (milk sugar) intolerance because of absence of a mucosal enzyme necessary for lactose digestion. Yet another is **gluten-sensitive enteropathy** (*celiac sprue*), an autoimmune disease caused by hypersensitivity to gluten, a protein in wheat, oats, barley and rye, which causes atrophy of mucosal villi and marked decrease of mucosal absorptive surface area. It may present at any time from infancy to adulthood. Removal of gluten from the diet results in dramatic improvement, but patients retain a slight increased risk for intestinal lymphoma and other malignancies. These types of sprue are sometimes collectively called **nontropical sprue**.

Tropical sprue is a poorly understood disease that mimics gluten-sensitive enteropathy—villi are atrophic and absorption is impaired—however, it occurs almost exclusively in persons living in or visiting the Caribbean islands. An infectious agent is suspected because antibiotic therapy is effective, but no causal agent has been identified.

Patients with malabsorption syndrome have bulky, frothy, greasy, yellowish, and especially malodorous stools. They lose weight and suffer from abdominal distention and excessive gas, and, because of the loss of critical nutrients, they also suffer from a variety of diseases of other organ systems:

- *Hematopoietic disorders*: anemia from failure to absorb iron, B_{12}, or folic acid, and bleeding tendency caused by vitamin K deficiency owing to poor intestinal absorption of vitamin K.
- *Musculoskeletal disorders*: weak, brittle bones, and tetany (muscle spasms) from defective calcium and vitamin D absorption.
- *Hormonal disorders*: amenorrhea, impotence, and infertility from malnutrition.
- *Skin disorders*: purpura from vitamin K deficiency; osmotic edema associated with low levels of albumin as a result of protein deficiency; various other skin disorders resulting from other nutrient deficiencies.
- *Nerve disorders*: peripheral nerve disease (peripheral neuropathy) from vitamin A and B_{12} deficiency.

Laboratory tests are available to detect specific varieties of malabsorption. An example is the D-xylose absorption test. D-xylose is a nondigestible sugar that is absorbed and excreted unchanged into urine and whose absorption is not dependent on luminal-phase factors. Therefore, in a patient with malabsorption syndrome, absorption of a normal amount indicates that the intestinal mucosa is functioning normally and the defect is in the luminal phase; decreased absorption indicates the defect is in mucosal absorption.

INFLAMMATORY BOWEL DISEASE

Inflammatory bowel disease implies one of two rather common conditions—*ulcerative colitis* or *Crohn disease*. They are similar in certain ways. Both feature:

- Episodic bloody diarrhea
- Autoimmune etiology
- Tendency to familial clustering (genetic influence)
- Involvement of extraintestinal tissues

However, ulcerative colitis and Crohn disease differ in critical ways, as is indicated in Table 15-1 and Figure 15-21.

Crohn Disease

Crohn disease is a systemic autoimmune disease featuring granulomatous inflammation, which affects the gastrointestinal tract anywhere from the esophagus to the anus. The terminal ileum is most commonly affected. Because of these characteristics it is sometimes called *granulomatous enteritis*, *regional enteritis*, or *terminal*

Table 15-1	*Comparison of Ulcerative Colitis and Crohn Disease*	
Feature	**Ulcerative Colitis**	**Crohn Disease**
Type of inflammation	Nongranulomatous	Granulomatous
Depth of bowel wall involved	Mucosa only	Full thickness of bowel wall
Continuity	Continuous and contiguous	Segmental involvement
Site of bowel involvement	Distal colon and rectum	Anywhere in the gastrointestinal tract, but most often in the small bowel and colon

ileitis. Crohn disease often affects extraintestinal tissues. Onset may occur at any age but most commonly in the teens or young adulthood. Caucasians and females are more often affected than African Americans or males.

In Crohn disease the pathology is characterized by a sharply segmented inflammatory reaction—inflamma-tion is marked in one length of bowel and skips the next length before occurring again. As is shown in Figure 15-22, the full thickness of the bowel wall is involved, from mucosa through to the peritoneal surface, a feature that in gross examination produces bowel segments that are stiff like a rubber hose. Microscopically, there is intense

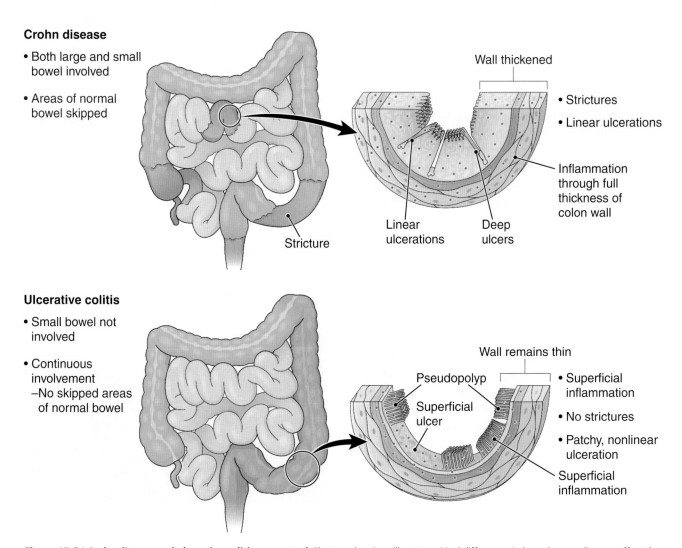

Crohn disease

• Both large and small bowel involved

• Areas of normal bowel skipped

Wall thickened

• Strictures

• Linear ulcerations

Inflammation through full thickness of colon wall

Stricture

Linear ulcerations   Deep ulcers

Ulcerative colitis

• Small bowel not involved

• Continuous involvement
  –No skipped areas of normal bowel

Wall remains thin

Pseudopolyp

Superficial ulcer

• Superficial inflammation

• No strictures

• Patchy, nonlinear ulceration

Superficial inflammation

Figure 15-21 **Crohn disease and ulcerative colitis contrasted.** The two drawings illustrate critical differences in how the two diseases affect the gastrointestinal tract.

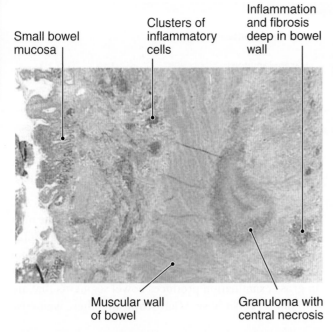

Small bowel mucosa

Clusters of inflammatory cells

Inflammation and fibrosis deep in bowel wall

Muscular wall of bowel

Granuloma with central necrosis

Figure 15-22 **The small bowel in Crohn disease.** The inflammatory reaction extends deep into the bowel wall, where a large granuloma is present.

chronic inflammation with formation of granulomas (Chapter 3). The inflammatory reaction has a burrowing quality that leads to bowel-wall fissures and abscesses.

The clinical onset of Crohn disease may be abrupt and acutely painful, to the point of mimicking an acute surgical abdominal emergency such as acute appendicitis, but in most cases onset is slow and features abdominal pain, diarrhea, and fever that abate only to return after ever shorter periods of relief. Extraintestinal manifestations are fairly common and include arthritis and erythema nodosum (a skin disease featuring hard, red, tender nodules, often associated with arthritis, Chapter 24) and, much less often, *sclerosing cholangitis*, an inflammation and scarring of the hepatic bile ducts (Chapter 16). Some patients have mild disease with few relapses over many decades; others have rapidly progressive disease, with malabsorption syndrome, abdominal abscesses, and inflammatory tracts (fistulae) from bowel into the bladder or perianal skin, or into other loops of bowel. Intestinal inflammation can cause fibrous scarring (stricture) and obstruction, which may require acute surgical intervention. Patients with Crohn disease have a slightly increased risk for carcinoma of the colon. Successful medical therapy usually relies on suppression of the immune system by steroids or other drugs. If medical therapy fails, partial bowel resection may be necessary.

Ulcerative Colitis

Ulcerative colitis is a systemic disease, and is very likely of autoimmune origin—some scientists theorize that dietary or bacterial antigens in the intestinal lumen react with mucosa to cause an autoimmune reaction. Ulcerative colitis affects only the colon, not the small bowel. The inflammatory reaction is most severe in the anus, rectum, and sigmoid colon; however, sometimes the entire colon is involved. In direct contrast to Crohn disease, the inflammation is superficial—it affects the mucosa only and does not involve deeper layers. Inflammation extends continuously; the "skip" areas seen in Crohn disease do not occur in ulcerative colitis. Ulcerative colitis also affects extraintestinal tissues, causing arthritis and bile duct inflammation similar to that of Crohn disease. Ulcerative colitis shows no racial predilection and affects men and women equally. It may arise at any age, but it tends to appear first in the second or third decade of life.

When examined grossly the colon usually shows most intense inflammation in the anus and rectosigmoid. Typically the process spreads as broad, superficial ulcers that merge to leave stranded small polypoid (resembling a polyp) islands of inflamed mucosa (Fig. 15-23). Microscopically the mucosa is ulcerated and chronically inflamed, but the inflammation does not extend deep into the bowel wall (Fig. 15-24), an important diagnostic point that helps to distinguish ulcerative colitis from Crohn lesions in the colon. No granulomas are present.

Polypoid islands of intact mucosa

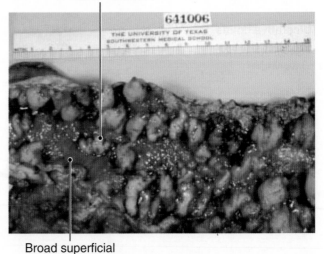

Broad superficial ulcers

Figure 15-23 **The colon in chronic ulcerative colitis.** Polypoid islands of intact mucosa are surrounded by mucosal ulcers.

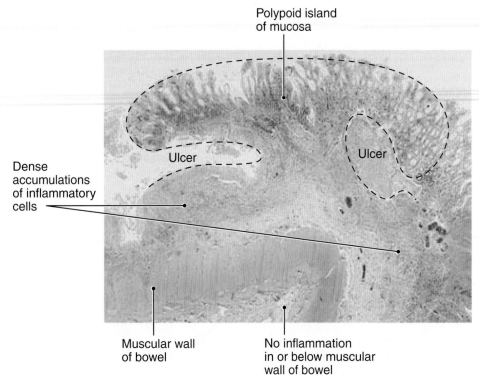

Polypoid island
of mucosa

Ulcer

Ulcer

Dense
accumulations
of inflammatory
cells

Muscular wall
of bowel

No inflammation
in or below muscular
wall of bowel

Figure 15-24 **The colon in chronic ulcerative colitis (microscopic study).** Ulcers undermine the mucosa, leaving polypoid islands of intact mucosa. Dotted line demonstrates polypoid form of remaining mucosa.

As is depicted in Figure 15-25, the clinical picture of ulcerative colitis is one of chronic, relapsing, debilitating disease. Episodes of severe cramping, tenesmus (rectal spasm), and diarrhea may occur abruptly and then remit for weeks, months, or years. Sometimes an explosive episode, bleeding and fluid loss, may produce a medical emergency. Alternatively, a relentless extension of the disease may cause ileus (intestinal paralysis), distention, and necrosis of the entire colon (*toxic megacolon*). Patients also may have erythema nodosum, or pyoderma gangrenosum (a chronic ulcerative skin disease, Chapter 24).

Long-term complications include malnutrition, severe diarrhea and electrolyte disturbances, massive hemorrhage, and toxic megacolon. Patients are also at risk for *sclerosing cholangitis*, an inflammatory disease of bile ducts (Chapter 16). However, the most ominous long-term complication of ulcerative colitis is carcinoma of the colon. A well-defined sequence of progressive mucosal dysplasia, carcinoma in situ, and invasive carcinoma occurs in some cases. Occasionally the risk is great enough to warrant prophylactic complete excision of the colon (total colectomy).

COLONIC DIVERTICULOSIS AND OTHER CONDITIONS

A **diverticulum** is a blind pouch with a mouth opening onto the lumen of a space, in this instance the colon.

Congenital colonic diverticula are rare and represent a blind pouch of normal colon protruding to one side. To the contrary, *acquired* diverticula are very common. As is depicted in the enlargement in Figure 15-26, they have a very thin wall composed of mucosa and submucosa only; no muscle is present, a peculiarity owing to the way they arise: the mucosa and submucosa are extruded *through* the muscular wall at points where small arteries penetrate from the external surface. They are found almost exclusively in the sigmoid colon. The result is multiple small mucosal sacs opening onto the lumen of the colon—**colonic diverticulosis.** An inflamed diverticulum is **diverticulitis.** Figure 15-26 illustrates the anatomy of a diverticulosis and the complications of diverticulitis.

Colonic diverticulosis is uncommon in natives of non-Western countries who eat a traditional diet rich in grains, fruits and vegetables. Western diets contain relatively small amounts of nondigestible bulk, which makes feces more compact and difficult to pass. Straining at stool causes greatly increased pressure in the sigmoid colon and rectum, which forces diverticular pouches to form at weak points, as discussed above. Colonic diverticula are uncommon before age 30 but by age 60 are present in about half of the population in developed nations.

Most diverticula are asymptomatic and are discovered incidentally at autopsy or during colorectal endoscopy or colon x-ray studies. Colonic diverticula con-

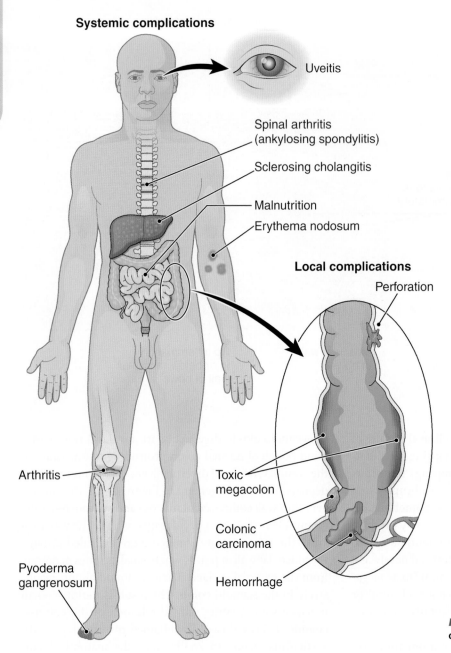

Systemic complications

Uveitis

Spinal arthritis
(ankylosing spondylitis)

Sclerosing cholangitis

Malnutrition

Erythema nodosum

Local complications

Perforation

Arthritis

Toxic
megacolon

Colonic
carcinoma

Pyoderma
gangrenosum

Hemorrhage

Figure 15-25 Complications of ulcerative colitis.

tain feces and may trap seeds or other indigestible matter, which over time irritate the diverticulum and promote infection by colonic bacteria, as Figure 15-27 illustrates. Diverticulitis is characterized by fever, and pain and tenderness in the left lower quadrant of the abdomen. Perforation into the abdominal space can produce peritonitis. Other complications include hemorrhage, abscess, fistulous connections to small bowel loops or bladder, colonic stenosis, and the formation of inflammatory masses that clinically mimic colonic carcinoma on x-ray studies.

Hemorrhoids are common and were discussed earlier. Also common are **anal fissures**, tears in the anal mucosa. Almost all arise from straining to pass large, hard stools. They can be quite painful but usually heal quickly and without therapy. However, they may bleed. Blood from an anal fissure is bright red and appears on toilet tissue or the surface of stool.

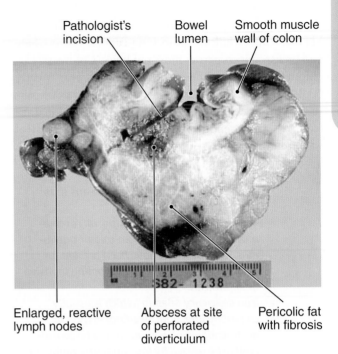

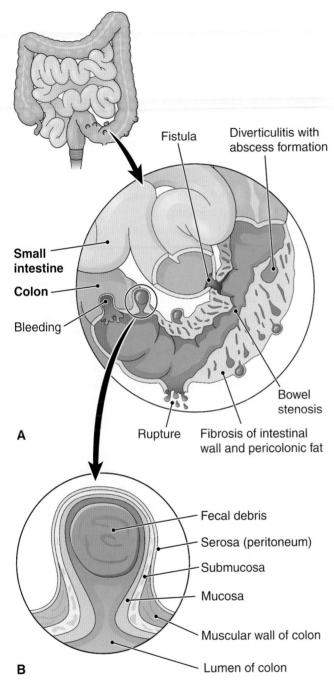

A

Figure 15-26 **Colonic diverticulosis and diverticulitis. A,** Complications of diverticular inflammation (diverticulitis). **B,** Detail of the anatomy of an acquired diverticulum.

B

Figure 15-27 **Acute and chronic diverticulitis.** In this cross-section of the colon, the opened bowel lumen appears at top center. The incision extends from the lumen into an abscess that has obliterated the diverticulum.

Peritonitis

Peritonitis is an inflammation of the lining (peritoneum) of the abdominal cavity. It is usually acute and may either be infectious or sterile and either local or generalized. *Infectious* peritonitis usually arises as a result of bacteria escaping from the bowel, often as a consequence of perforation, as for example with a perforated gastric

ulcer or acute appendicitis with rupture. Ascitic fluid in the abdomen invites peritonitis, especially chronic ascites in debilitated patients (as with alcoholic cirrhosis). It is, in effect, a sac of culture media that awaits bacterial seeding. Other causes of peritonitis include ruptured liver abscess and acute infections of the fallopian tubes (salpingitis). *Sterile* peritonitis occurs with chemical irritation. For example, in acute pancreatitis digestive enzymes may be spilled into the peritoneum, where they incite a severe inflammatory reaction.

In most cases of peritonitis, the inflammation is acute—a purulent inflammatory exudate spreads throughout the abdomen. Healed peritonitis leaves bands of fibrous scar (*adhesions*) that may produce obstruction by snarling loops of bowel.

Neoplasms of the Large and Small Bowel

Tumors of the small bowel are very uncommon and will not be discussed further; however, *the colon is host to more neoplasms than any other organ in the body.* Fortunately, most colonic neoplasms are benign. However, most benign colon neoplasms are premalignant, although it takes many years for them to become fully malignant and capable of metastasis. Unfortunately, *most premalignant intestinal lesions are not discovered in a timely fashion*: in fact, colorectal carcinoma is the number two cancer *killer* behind lung cancer, but prostate and breast cancers garner more publicity. Colorectal carcinoma kills about 50% more people each year (nearly 60,000) than automobile accidents (about 40,000). Virtually without exception, carcinomas of the colon arise from colonic adenomas (benign neoplasms), most of which have been present for about 10–15 years before becoming fully malignant.

> • **The colon is host to more neoplasms than any other organ in the body.**
> • **With extremely rare exception, all carcinomas of the colon arise from colonic adenomas, most of which have been present for about 10–15 years before becoming invasive malignancies.**
> • **Iron deficiency anemia (which is usually caused by intestinal bleeding) in man or postmenopausal woman should be considered to be caused by intestinal carcinoma until proven otherwise.**

NONNEOPLASTIC POLYPS

It is important to distinguish between the neoplastic and nonneoplastic polyps because neoplastic polyps are premalignant; nonneoplastic polyps are not.

Recall that "polyp" is a term that describes a *shape*—a mass rising above a mucosal surface. A sessile polyp is one with a broad, short base; a pedunculated polyp has a relatively long, narrow stalk. The overwhelming majority of intestinal polyps, especially in the colon, are benign **hyperplastic polyps**—small, nipple-like foci of mucosa a few millimeters in diameter. They occur most commonly in the lower colon and rectum of adults and

elderly persons. **Juvenile polyps**, also called *retention polyps*, are nonneoplastic, polyp-shaped glandular malformations a few centimeters in diameter that are most often found as single lesions in children.

NEOPLASTIC POLYPS (ADENOMAS)

A **colonic adenoma** is a benign neoplasm of colonic mucosal epithelial cells; *almost all colon cancers arise from preexisting adenomas*. About 50% of people over age 50 have at least one colonic adenoma; men and women are affected equally; and there is a distinct familial predisposition to develop adenomas.

As Figure 15-28 illustrates, there are two types of adenomas, each with distinctive gross shape and microscopic appearance and with different tendencies to become malignant. The most common kind of adenoma is the **tubular adenoma**, commonly called **adenomatous polyp**. The names derive from the fact that microscopically the tumor glands are simple tubules, and they usually appear grossly as polyps (Fig. 15-29). The second, less common type, is **villous adenoma**, which is a broad-based (sessile) polyp having a villous or fern-like microscopic pattern of epithelial growth. *Villous adenomas have a much higher malignant potential than do tubular adenomas.*

The type of polyp and the degree of microscopic nuclear abnormality (cell atypia) are important in assessing malignant potential, but size is the most important predictor of malignant tendency. For example, malignant change is rare in small tubular adenomas, whereas 40% of villous adenomas larger than 4 cm in diameter have become malignant.

Most adenomas are asymptomatic when small. As they enlarge they tend to bleed, often subclinically, so

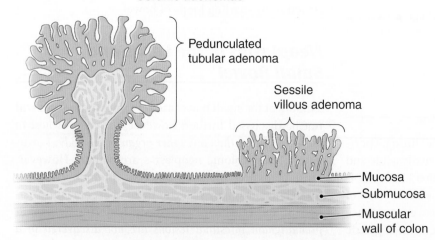

Colonic adenomas

Pedunculated tubular adenoma

Sessile villous adenoma

Mucosa
Submucosa
Muscular wall of colon

Figure 15-28 **Colonic adenomas.** Tubular adenomas are usually pedunculated. Villous adenomas are usually sessile.

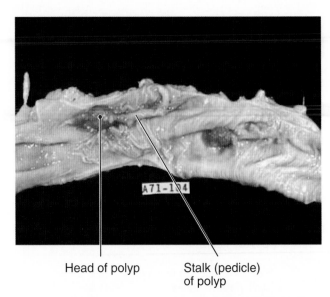

Head of polyp   Stalk (pedicle)
                       of polyp

Figure 15-29 **Pedunculated tubular adenomas of the colon.** These tubular adenomas (adenomatous polyps) have unusually long pedicles.

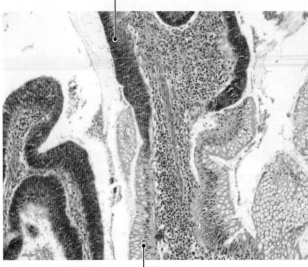

Dysplastic colonic epithelium

Normal colonic epithelium

Figure 15-30 **Dysplastic (premalignant) change in colonic adenoma.** Dysplastic cells have large, dark nuclei and have lost their ability to make mucin.

that iron deficiency anemia may become the first sign of something amiss. For this reason, careful practitioners rely on this rule: *iron deficiency anemia in an adult man or postmenopausal woman is intestinal carcinoma until proven otherwise.*

Familial polyposis syndrome is an uncommon genetic disorder in which the colon contains thousands of small polyps with a great tendency to become malignant. *Hereditary nonpolyposis colorectal carcinoma syndrome (HNPCC)* is a rare genetic disorder that deserves mention because it is the sole exception to the rule that all colon cancers arise from preexisting polyps.

CARCINOMA OF THE COLON

Almost all **colon carcinomas** are adenocarcinomas: gland-forming malignant neoplasms of colon epithelial cells. According to the American Cancer Society, in 2003 163,000 Americans died of lung cancer; 57,000 of colon cancer; 40,000 of breast cancer; and 30,000 of prostate cancer. *The tragedy of colon cancer is that, because virtually all colon cancers arise from adenomas, and because it takes about ten years for an adenoma to become fully malignant, people with colonic adenomas have a curable and diagnosable lesion for about ten years before cancer develops.* Cancer does not leap into being in an instant. Long before development of invasive malignancy, the epithelium in the colonic adenoma becomes progressively dysplastic (Fig. 15-30) and passes through a stage of carcinoma in situ before becoming invasive (see Case Study 15.1 at the end of this chapter).

Colonic carcinoma (Fig. 15-31) is widespread in industrialized nations and is much less common in Asian and African nations. These differences are unexplained. Heretofore, the high colon cancer rate in industrialized nations was attributed to low dietary fiber content, a theory that has been disproved by more recent studies.

There has been a significant change in the pathology and clinical behavior of colorectal carcinomas. Fifty years ago most occurred in the lower-left colon and rectum (the rectosigmoid), but now more occur in the

History of Medicine

FAMOUS PEOPLE WHO DIED OF COLON CANCER

- **Audrey Hepburn**, celebrated film actress; best remembered for her role as Holly Golightly in *Breakfast at Tiffany's.*
- **Vince Lombardi**, legendary coach of the Green Bay Packers, after whom the Super Bowl trophy is named
- **Jackie Gleason**, actor and comedian best remembered for his TV portrayal of New York bus driver Ralph Kramden in *The Honeymooners,* arguably the best TV situation comedy ever produced.
- **Charles Schultz**, creator of the most famous of all American cartoon strips: Peanuts.

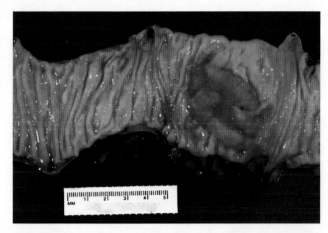

Figure 15-31 **Carcinoma of the colon.** The tumor has raised, rolled edges and a deeply excavated center.

Table 15-2	Clinical Stage and Survival in Colonic Carcinoma (Astler-Coller)	
Stage	**Degree of Tumor Invasion and Spread**	**5-Year Survival**
A	Limited to mucosa	~100%
B_1	Invading muscular wall, negative nodes	~67%
B_2	Full penetration of muscular wall, negative nodes	~54%
C_1	Invading muscular wall, positive nodes	~43%
C_2	Full penetration of muscular wall, positive nodes	~22%
D	Distant metastasis	Very low %

right colon: few are reachable by a fingertip and only about half can be seen by office examination with a sigmoidoscope (which reaches about 60 cm—two feet—into the lower colon). In the right colon they tend to be bulky masses that have plenty of room to grow, produce less obvious bleeding, and do not cause a dramatic change in bowel habits. On the other hand, cancers in the lower-left colon tend to be encircling, constricting, "napkin-ring" lesions that produce more noticeable bleeding or pain and changed bowel habits. Regardless of these patterns, the tumors are microscopically similar. Evidence of the preexisting adenoma is usually obliterated by cancer at the time cancer is found. Most cases are diagnosed because patients become symptomatic with weight loss, overt intestinal bleeding, anemia, metastasis, or pain. By the time patients become symptomatic, most lesions have metastasized.

Colorectal carcinomas grow by direct extension through the bowel wall and spread beyond the colon by invasion of lymphatics and blood vessels. The most common sites of metastasis are lymph nodes, liver (via the portal circulation), lungs, and bones. About a third of cases are beyond cure at the time of initial diagnosis.

The most important prognostic factor in colorectal carcinoma is the clinical stage of the neoplasm at the time of diagnosis. Various schemes have been proposed; the most widely accepted is **Astler-Coller staging**, illustrated in Figure 15-32 and detailed in Table 15-2. The Astler-Coller staging system relies on assessment of the depth of bowel wall invasion by the tumor, the presence or absence of lymph node metastases, and clinical assessment of distant metastasis to liver or other organs.

Colorectal carcinomas secrete a tumor marker, **carcinoembryonic antigen (CEA)**, into the bloodstream. As with other tumor markers, CEA has not proved to be a useful *screening* test because it rarely is elevated when the carcinoma is in a curable stage and because CEA is also produced by other tumors, such as carcinomas of the lung, bladder, prostate, breast, ovary, and urinary bladder, and by other conditions including smoking, cirrhosis, pancreatitis, and ulcerative colitis. Nevertheless, CEA is useful as a monitoring tool to check for tumor regression or recurrence after therapy.

Screening tests for any disease should be inexpensive and sensitive (few false negatives), and they should detect a serious but potentially curable disease. The **stool occult blood test** fits these criteria: it costs a few dollars and screens for a deadly but completely curable disease. A single stool test is not very sensitive, but when used annually over a ten-year period, the test can detect about half of colon cancers and reduce colon cancer deaths by about 30%. However, this leaves many curable tumors undiagnosed. Therefore, there is growing belief that all people over age 50 should have a complete colon exam by colonoscopy or radiographic "virtual colonoscopy" every five years, or every ten years in people with a negative study and no family history of colon polyps or cancers. These exams can detect the great majority of cancers and polyps and reduce the colon cancer death rate by about 60%.

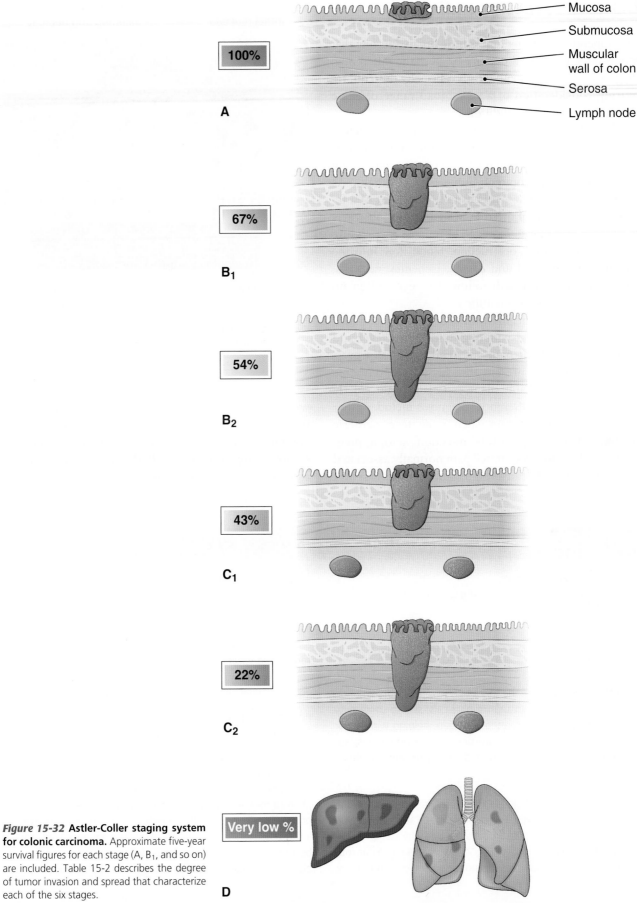

Figure 15-32 **Astler-Coller staging system for colonic carcinoma.** Approximate five-year survival figures for each stage (A, B₁, and so on) are included. Table 15-2 describes the degree of tumor invasion and spread that characterize each of the six stages.

Diseases of the Appendix

The appendix is a functionless little organ, but one that looms large in medical practice because the differential diagnosis of acute appendicitis is especially difficult, requiring consideration of a very broad range of acute medical and surgical conditions.

About 10% of people experience an episode of **acute appendicitis** at some time in their life. Acute appendicitis occurs most commonly in teenagers and young adults and is more common in males than females. As Figure 15-33 illustrates, it is usually the result of a **fecalith**, a small ball of dried fecal matter that obstructs the lumen and blocks drainage of mucus. As pressure increases behind the obstruction, blood flow into the appendix is hindered and edema, ischemia, necrosis, and bacterial overgrowth follow. However, often no anatomic cause can be identified.

The typical case begins with abdominal discomfort, anorexia, nausea, and vomiting followed by fever and right-lower quadrant pain and tenderness. However, many cases do not present the classic picture. Some cases may be remarkably silent, especially in the elderly or debilitated. The differential diagnosis includes other causes of abdominal pain, such as acute mesenteric lymphadenitis, fallopian tube infection, ectopic pregnancy, and the low abdominal pain normally associated with ovulation. Because signs and symptoms vary widely, and because delay of surgical intervention risks the very serious hazard of rupture and peritonitis, it is accepted that 10–20% of abdominal surgery for presumptive appendicitis will find either some other disease process—or nothing. ■

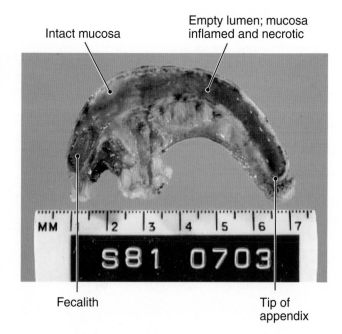

Intact mucosa — Empty lumen; mucosa inflamed and necrotic

MM | 2 | 3 | 4 | 5 | 6 | 7

S81 0703

Fecalith — Tip of appendix

Figure 15-33 Acute appendicitis. A fecalith is wedged into the mouth of the appendix (left).

[Case 15-1, continued] did a digital rectal exam on her regular office visit. Again, the answer is No. You offer to do a simple digital rectal exam, but she says she is pressed for time and promises to mention it do her gynecologist on her next visit.

A week later, you receive her stool test cards in the mail, and test the stool smears for occult blood. All are positive. In a telephone call to the patient, you explain to her that the insurance company will not issue the policy until the source of the bleeding is identified.

After getting the report, the Ms. W. returns to her gynecologist, who performs a rectal exam. Stool on the exam glove finger tests positive for blood. In consultation with the general practitioner for whom you work, Ms. W. is referred to a radiology group for barium enema examination, which reveals a mass in the right side of the colon. She is referred again, this time to a general surgeon, who resects the right half of the colon. The surgeon reports that the peritoneal cavity was smooth and free of metastasis, and no liver metastases were seen. The pathologist's consultation on the surgical specimen reported a grade III adenocarcinoma invading through the full thickness of the wall of the colon. Eleven mesenteric lymph nodes are identified and studied. Two contain microscopic tumor metastases. The tumor is classified Astler-Coller stage C2.

Ms. W. is referred to an oncologist for further treatment. Liver function tests are normal, and imaging of the liver reveals no masses. However, liver metastases are detected 18 months later, and Ms. W. dies in hepatic coma, 3 years after initial diagnosis.

DISCUSSION

This sad story is repeated in one variation or other thousands of times annually in the United States. This woman had everything going for her: career success, apparent good health, and regular private medical care, but it all came to nothing because no one did the simplest of things: check her stool regularly for blood or suggest she have a complete colon exam when she turned 50. The statistics are clear: this woman surely had had a benign colonic adenoma for 10 or 15 years as it slowly evolved into an invasive colon cancer. It is not clear how long the cancer may have been present in a more curable form before invading and metastasizing, but it was probably several years. Altogether, she had had a curable lesion for perhaps 10 or 15 years, but no one found it because they had not bothered to look for it.

Current guidelines call for all adults over 50 (some suggest 40) to have an initial full colon exam by direct colonoscopy or radiographic study and follow-up exams every 5 or 10 years for life. Stool exams for occult blood should be performed annually.

POINTS TO REMEMBER
- With rare exception, all carcinomas of the colon arise from preexisting benign colonic adenomas.
- It takes many years for a colonic adenoma to evolve into invasive cancer.
- Regular stool occult blood tests and full colon exams can prevent many colon cancer deaths.

CASE STUDY 15-1 *THE ROAD NOT TAKEN—AN ALTERNATIVE SCENARIO*

For all sad words of tongue or pen,
The saddest are these: "It might have been."
JOHN GREENLEAF WHITTIER (1807–1892),
AMERICAN QUAKER POET AND REFORMER, *MAUD MULLER*

THE CASE
With a bit of imagination, we can speculate how this case might have had a happier ending.

Setting: You work in the office of a very busy obstetrician-gynecologist; in addition to your many other duties, it is your job to visit with patients about at-home self-collection of stool samples for occult blood testing.

Clinical history: Sheila W. is a 47-year-old self-employed woman who is in the office for the first time for a routine annual gynecologic examination and Pap smear.

You explain the stool sampling procedure in all of its unpleasant detail—using special paper from the kit to catch three separate stools in the toilet bowl, scraping stool onto the tip of a wooden spatula, and smearing each sample onto a stiff cardboard mailer. She grimaces and says, "Ugh. Is this really necessary? I've never had to do this before."

You reply, "Well, I recommend it. You know, cancer of the colon is the number-three cancer killer of women, close behind lung cancer and breast cancer." Then you launch into a well-rehearsed mini-lecture, one you've given hundreds of times, explaining how colon cancers arise very slowly from preexisting polyps, and how polyps and early cancers tend to bleed while they are still 100% curable.

"Okay," she says with a grin, holding up her hands in mock surrender, "You can stop. I give up."

About 10 days, later her specimens arrive in the mail; all three test positive for blood.

The physician calls her and recommends a colon and rectal surgeon, who does a colonoscopy and finds several ▶

[Case 15-1, continued] adenomatous polyps in the colon. The largest one is in the right colon and is several centimeters in diameter. All are removed intact. The pathology report reads as follows:

- *Four polyps from various colonic sites: Benign tubular adenoma*
- *Large polypoid mass from right colon: Tubular adenoma with focal severe epithelial dysplasia (carcinoma in situ);*

no invasive carcinoma identified. Margins of resection are free of atypical epithelial changes.

DISCUSSION

Patients rely on caregivers to know the right thing to do—and to do it. In this scenario the patient was surely spared an early death from colon cancer because she was urged to participate in a messy and unpleasant stool-collection routine.

Objectives Recap

1. *Define melena, hematochezia, and hematemesis, and explain the different implications of slow gastrointestinal bleeding and rapid gastrointestinal bleeding*: Melena is the passage of stool with high content of altered blood, which makes stool black. Hematochezia is the passage of overtly bloody stool. Hematemesis is the vomiting of blood. Rapid gastrointestinal bleeding is usually manifest by hematochezia or hematemesis or signs and symptoms of acute blood loss. Slow gastrointestinal bleeding is often from an intestinal malignancy and tends to be clinically silent and without obvious evidence of blood in the stool. Persistent slow gastrointestinal bleeding is sometimes discovered because of the anemia it can produce.

2. *Explain the importance of stool occult blood tests*: Annual occult blood testing of stool detects many premalignant lesions of the colon before they become malignant and also detects many colon carcinomas early enough for surgical cure.

3. *Distinguish between intestinal mechanical obstruction and ileus*: Normal intestinal function requires constant peristalsis, which may be interrupted by mechanical obstruction or by peristaltic paralysis (ileus).

4. *Name the cause of most tooth loss and explain its pathogenesis*: Periodontitis causes most tooth loss and arises as a result of poor oral hygiene, which allows accumulation at the gum margin of a film of bacteria known as plaque. Bacterial invasion downward into the soft tissues around the tooth root is the cause of periodontitis.

5. *Define achalasia, and offer a short discussion of it*: Achalasia is a spastic condition of the lower esophageal sphincter, which produces a functional partial obstruction in the lower esophagus, causing dysphagia and esophageal pain. The cause is unknown.

6. *Define Barrett esophagus, and discuss its pathogenesis and implications*: Barrett esophagus is a change (metaplasia) of the epithelium of the lowest part of the esophagus from normal squamous epithelium to gastric glandular epithelium. Barrett metaplasia is caused by gastric acid refluxing upward from the stomach (reflux esophagitis). It is painful and can cause bleeding and narrowing because of fibrous scar (stricture). Patients with Barrett metaplasia have an increased risk of esophageal adenocarcinoma.

7. *Name some risk factors for esophageal carcinoma*: Smoking, alcohol abuse, Barrett metaplasia.

8. *Name some conditions associated with* Helicobacter pylori *infection*: Chronic atrophic gastritis, chronic peptic ulceration, and gastric carcinoma (usually in association with chronic atrophic gastritis).

9. *Explain the difference in the pathogenesis of acute gastric erosions and chronic peptic ulceration*: Acute gastric erosions are superficial ulcers of the gastric mucosa that are usually associated with severe trauma, sepsis, major surgical procedures, grave illnesses, alcohol abuse, extensive burns, CNS trauma or surgery, and chronic exposure to nonsteroidal antiinflammatory drugs (NSAIDs) and corticosteroids. Chronic peptic ulceration, a much deeper ulceration of the stomach wall, may burrow into or through the muscular wall. Peptic ulcers are associated with a combination of atrophic gastritis, exposure to gastric juices, and *H. pylori* infection.

10. *Explain the cause of Hirschsprung megacolon*: Hirschsprung megacolon results from a localized, genetic absence of the autonomic ganglionic neural plexus in the colon wall, which controls peristalsis. Deprived of neural control, no peristalsis occurs in the affected segment, fecal movement is impaired, and the upstream colon distends with feces.

11. *Name the most common cause worldwide of acute enterocolitis*: Rotavirus

12. *Name some bacteria responsible for epidemic bacterial enterocolitis*: *Salmonella* sp. causes salmonellosis; *Shigella* sp. causes shigellosis; *Vibrio cholerae* causes cholera.

13. *Explain the pathogenesis of pseudomembranous colitis*: Pseudomembranous colitis occurs with colonic overgrowth of *Clostridium difficile*, which secretes an enterotoxin that causes necrosis of colonic mucosa. The most common cause is broad-spectrum antibiotic therapy that kills normal colonic flora, allowing *C. difficile* overgrowth.

14. *Among patients with malabsorption syndrome, distinguish between luminal and intestinal malabsorption*: Intestinal malabsorption consists of those cases in which a mucosal defect or disease is present that interferes with absorption, or in patients with shortened bowel. Luminal malabsorption is caused by the absence of digestive enzymes or bile salts necessary for hydrolysis or emulsification of ingested foodstuffs (as in patients with pancreatic disease who do not have enough pancreatic enzymes for normal digestion).

15. *Characterize and contrast the important differences between ulcerative colitis and Crohn disease*: 1) type of inflammation: granulomatous inflammation in Crohn disease; nongranulomatous inflammation in ulcerative colitis; 2) depth of inflammation: deep transmural in Crohn disease; superficial mucosal in ulcerative colitis; 3) site of involvement: anywhere in the gastrointestinal tract, but most often in the colon and terminal ileum in Crohn disease; colon only in ulcerative colitis; 4) continuity of inflammatory involvement: discontinuous (skip areas) involvement in Crohn disease; continuous involvement in ulcerative colitis.

16. *Name several extraintestinal manifestations of Crohn disease and ulcerative colitis*: Both may be associated with inflammation in the eye (uveitis), joint disease (various types of arthritis), skin disease, and inflammation of hepatic bile ducts (sclerosing cholangitis).

17. *Explain the pathogenesis of colonic diverticulosis*: Diverticula have a very thin wall composed of mucosa and submucosa only; no muscle is present, a peculiarity stemming from the way they arise: the mucosa and submucosa are extruded *through* the muscular wall at points where small arteries penetrate from the external surface. Colonic diverticulosis is uncommon in natives of non-Western countries who eat a traditional diet rich in grains, fruits, and vegetables. Western diets contain relatively small amounts of nondigestible bulk, which makes feces more compact and difficult to pass. Straining at stool causes greatly increased pressure in the sigmoid colon and rectum, which forces diverticular pouches to form at weak points.

18. *Explain the importance of nonneoplastic polyps of the colon*: Nonneoplastic polyps have no premalignant potential. It is important to distinguish them from colonic adenomas, which are frequently polypoid and are premalignant.

19. *Explain the difference between a tubular adenoma and a villous adenoma of the colon*: Both are benign, premalignant neoplasms. The most common is the tubular adenoma, which has a microscopic pattern of simple tubular glands and is commonly called adenomatous polyp. The second, less common, variety of colonic adenoma is a broad-based, sessile polyp with a fern-like microscopic pattern of epithelial growth that is called villous adenoma. Villous adenomas have a much higher malignant potential than do tubular adenomas.

20. *Explain the relationship between colonic adenomas and colonic carcinoma*: Almost without exception all carcinomas of the colon arise from preexisting benign colonic adenomas that gradually become dysplastic and then malignant over ten to fifteen years.

Typical Test Questions

1. Concerning aphthous oral ulcers, which is true?
   A. Associated with periodontitis
   B. Cause unknown
   C. Caused by herpesvirus
   D. Caused by *Candida*
   E. Associated with poor oral hygiene

2. Which of the following is a condition involving the stomach?
   A. Peptic ulcer
   B. Malabsorption syndrome
   C. *Clostridium difficile* ulceration
   D. Adenomatous polyp

3. Which of the following is associated with increased risk of esophageal carcinoma?
   A. *Helicobacter pylori* infection
   B. Esophageal varices
   C. Herpesvirus infection
   D. Barrett metaplasia
   E. Hiatal hernia

4. Which of the following is a cause of luminal phase malabsorption syndrome?
   A. Chronic pancreatitis
   B. Gluten-sensitive enteropathy (celiac sprue)

C. Whipple disease
D. Tropical sprue
E. Short bowel

5. Which of the following is characteristic of colonic carcinoma?
   A. Usually occurs in the rectosigmoid
   B. Sessile shape
   C. Silent bleeding
   D. Early bowel obstruction

6. True or false? Carcinoma of the colon kills more people annually than breast cancer does.

7. True or false? *Helicobacter pylori* infection is the cause of most malabsorption syndromes.

8. True or false? Barrett esophagus carries an increased risk of carcinoma.

9. True or false? A single stool exam for occult blood can detect most premalignant lesions of the colon.

10. True or false? Most peptic ulcers occur in the stomach.

Diseases of the Liver and Biliary Tract

This chapter begins with a review of the normal anatomy and physiology of the liver and biliary tract. Diseases and disorders discussed include cirrhosis, hepatitis, alcoholic and metabolic liver disease, gallstones and other gallbladder disease, and cancers of the liver and biliary tract.

BACK TO BASICS
- Liver Anatomy
- Liver Function

THE LIVER RESPONSE TO INJURY
- Anatomic Patterns of Liver Injury
- Functional Patterns of Liver Injury

CIRRHOSIS
- Anatomic Types of Cirrhosis
- The Pathophysiology of Cirrhosis
- Clinical Features of Cirrhosis

VIRAL HEPATITIS
- Clinicopathologic Syndromes
- Hepatitis A Virus (HAV) Infection
- Hepatitis B Virus (HBV) Infection
- Hepatitis C Virus (HCV) Infection
- Hepatitis D Virus (HDV) Infection
- Hepatitis E Virus (HEV) Infection
- The Anatomic Pathology of Hepatitis

AUTOIMMUNE HEPATITIS

LIVER ABSCESS

TOXIC LIVER INJURY

ALCOHOLIC LIVER DISEASE
- Fatty Liver
- Alcoholic Hepatitis
- Alcoholic Cirrhosis

INHERITED METABOLIC AND PEDIATRIC LIVER DISEASE
- Hemochromatosis
- Wilson Disease
- Hereditary Alpha-1 Antitrypsin Deficiency
- Neonatal Cholestasis, Biliary Atresia, and Hepatitis
- Reye Syndrome

DISEASE OF INTRAHEPATIC BILE DUCTS
- Primary Biliary Cirrhosis
- Primary Sclerosing Cholangitis

CIRCULATORY DISORDERS

TUMORS OF THE LIVER
- Primary Carcinomas of the Liver
- Cholangiocarcinoma

DISEASES OF THE GALLBLADDER AND EXTRAHEPATIC BILE DUCTS
- Diseases of the Gallbladder
- Diseases of Extrahepatic Bile Ducts

Learning Objectives

After studying this chapter you should be able to:

1. Trace the flow of blood through the liver
2. Name the major functions of the liver
3. Explain the enterohepatic circulation
4. Name the major functional reactions of the liver to injury
5. Explain the difference between conjugated and unconjugated bilirubin
6. Name one cause of unconjugated hyperbilirubinemia and one of conjugated hyperbilirubinemia
7. Define cirrhosis, and name the two most common causes
8. Explain why cirrhosis causes portal hypertension
9. Name two hemodynamic consequences of portal hypertension
10. Outline the main clinical manifestations of cirrhosis
11. Name several clinicopathologic syndromes associated with viral hepatitis
12. Contrast the mode of transmission and clinical course of hepatitis A and hepatitis B infection

13. Name the most important epidemiologic fact about hepatitis C, and name the most common serious consequences of hepatitis C infection
14. Name one common acute and one common chronic change induced in the liver by alcohol abuse
15. Explain the difference between primary biliary cirrhosis and sclerosing cholangitis
16. Name the liver condition most commonly associated with hepatocellular carcinoma
17. Name the two major categories of gallstones, and know which is the most common
18. Name several risk factors that favor the formation of gallstones
19. Discuss some of the most common causes of extrahepatic bile duct obstruction

Key Terms and Concepts

BACK TO BASICS
- portal vein
- hepatocytes
- bile duct
- bile
- bile acids
- bilirubin
- unconjugated bilirubin
- conjugated bilirubin
- jaundice
- cholestasis

THE LIVER RESPONSE TO INJURY
- hepatitis
- cirrhosis
- hepatic failure

CIRRHOSIS
- portal cirrhosis
- biliary cirrhosis
- portal hypertension

VIRAL HEPATITIS
- viral hepatitis
- carrier state
- chronic viral hepatitis
- hepatitis A virus (HAV)
- hepatitis B virus (HBV)
- hepatitis C virus (HCV)

ALCOHOLIC LIVER DISEASE
- fatty liver

INHERITED METABOLIC AND PEDIATRIC LIVER DISEASE
- neonatal cholestasis

DISEASE OF INTRAHEPATIC BILE DUCTS
- primary biliary cirrhosis

TUMORS OF THE LIVER
- hepatocellular carcinoma

DISEASES OF THE GALLBLADDER AND EXTRAHEPATIC BILE DUCTS
- cholelithiasis
- cholecystitis

Two of every three deaths are premature; they are related to the loafer's heart, smoker's lung and drinker's liver.

DR. THOMAS J. BASSLER, PATHOLOGIST; QUOTED BY JAMES FIXX (1932–1984),

IN *THE COMPLETE BOOK OF RUNNING* (Random House, 1977)

▶ BACK TO BASICS

The liver regulates the composition of blood by disposing of waste products (bilirubin, for example), converting substances from one form into another (glycogen into glucose and vice versa), secreting substances into the intestines (bile and cholesterol), and producing plasma proteins (albumin, coagulation factors, and others).

The anatomy of the liver, portal venous system, and bile ducts is illustrated in Figure 16-1. Nutrients absorbed by the intestine do not enter the general circula-

tion directly; instead they flow first to the liver via the **portal vein**. The vein gains its name from the fact that the liver is a gate (a portal or doorway) through which blood must pass before entering the general circulation. This "gate" effect is unique in human anatomy: venous blood goes from one capillary system (the intestine), is collected into a large vein (portal), and passes through a *second* capillary system (the liver) before entering the general circulation. The liver also receives arterial blood from the hepatic artery, which merges with portal blood before flowing through the hepatic vein into the inferior vena cava.

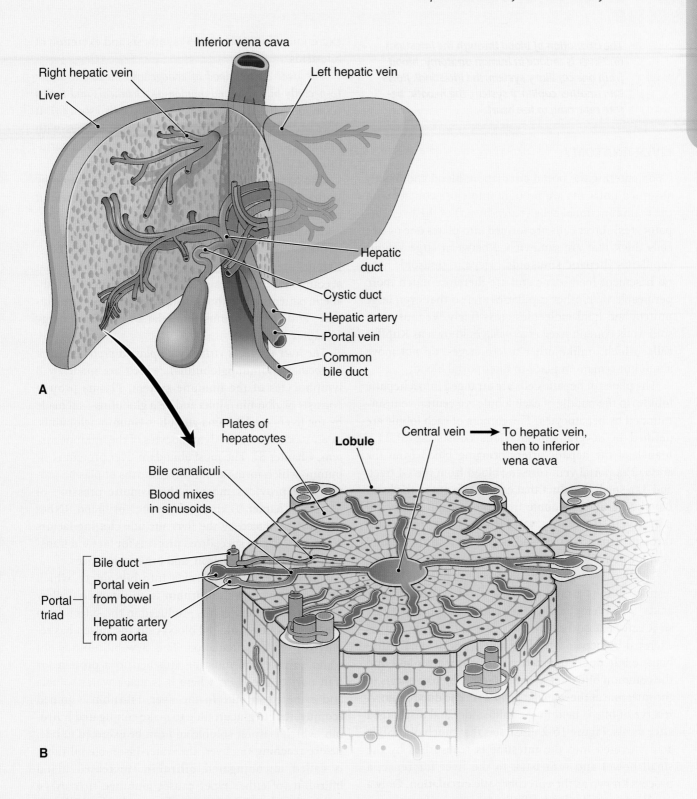

Figure 16-1 The liver, portal venous system, and bile ducts. A, The liver and biliary system. **B,** The hepatic lobule. Blood flows into the central vein from branches of the portal vein and hepatic artery clustered in portal triads at the edge of the lobule. Bile flows in the opposite direction—from the interior of the lobule to bile ducts in the portal triads.

> *The circulation of blood through the intestines and liver is unique in human anatomy: blood from one capillary system, the intestinal, flows into another capillary system, the hepatic, before returning to the heart.*

LIVER ANATOMY

Upon entering the portal circulation, blood and freshly absorbed nutrients are brought into close contact with the main functional cells (*parenchyma*) of the liver (**hepatocytes**). Liver cells are formed into plates one or two cells thick that are sandwiched between large venous capillaries (**hepatic sinusoids**). Hepatic sinusoids have no basement membrane and are therefore much more permeable than other capillaries are, so that even large protein and lipid molecules cross freely. Venous sinusoid walls contain *fixed macrophages* known as **Kupffer cells**, which, unlike other macrophages, do not move about but remain in place to filter portal blood.

The plates of hepatic cells are arranged into a **hepatic lobule**. In the middle of each lobule is a central vein surrounded by hepatocytes. The corners of each lobule are defined by several **portal triads** consisting of 1) a branch of the hepatic artery bringing blood from the aorta, 2) a portal vein carrying blood from the GI tract, and 3) a small **bile duct** that carries bile out of the liver. Blood entering the lobule from the hepatic artery and portal vein flows into venous sinusoids, percolates through hepatic plates, and is collected in the central vein for delivery to the general circulation.

The liver is a large gland that secretes bile into the intestines. **Bile** is a mixture of metabolic waste and **bile acids**, which emulsify (make water soluble) dietary fat so it can be absorbed by the intestinal mucosa. Bile is excreted by hepatocytes into a network of small intrahepatic **bile ducts** that carry it out of the liver and into the **common bile duct** (*hepatic duct*), which connects to the intestine at the *ampulla of Vater* in the duodenum. A reserve of bile is held in the gallbladder and discharged after meals. Figure 16-2 illustrates that much of the bile acid excreted into the intestine is reabsorbed by the small bowel and sent back to the liver for reuse, a process known as the **enterohepatic circulation**. Only a small amount of bile acid finds its way into feces.

LIVER FUNCTION

As is outlined in Table 16-1, the liver has five main functions: 1) detoxification and excretion of metabolic waste, drugs, and hormones; 2) lipid and carbohydrate metabolism; 3) protein synthesis; 4) conjugation and excretion of bilirubin; and 5) synthesis and excretion of bile acids.

The liver clears blood of endogenous metabolic waste (especially bilirubin and ammonia), chemicals and toxins (especially drugs), and hormones (especially estrogen). It does so by excreting them into bile, as it does with bilirubin, or converting them into something not harmful, as it does by converting ammonia to urea.

The liver modulates blood glucose concentration by storing glucose as glycogen and reconverts and excretes it on demand. Additionally, the liver synthesizes triglycerides and cholesterol and, when necessary, burns fat and excretes the *ketones* produced by the process. Ketones are an acidic by-product of fat metabolism that accounts for the acidosis (ketosis) that occurs when diabetic patients are without insulin and cannot burn glucose, and the liver must burn fat to produce energy (Chapter 17).

The liver produces virtually all plasma proteins except antibodies (immunoglobulins), which are made by B lymphocytes of the immune system. Plasma protein consists of albumin, alpha and beta globulins—all made by the liver—and gamma globulins (immunoglobulins, or antibodies, made by lymphocytes of the immune system, Chapter 8). The most abundant liver protein is albumin, which forms about three fourths of plasma protein and provides most of the osmotic pressure of plasma (Chapter 5) that holds water in blood. Other proteins produced by the liver include clotting factors (Chapter 11) and specialized proteins for fat (and transport of fat, hormones, iron, and other substances.

The liver excretes bilirubin into bile ducts, which carry it to the bowel. **Bilirubin** is an intensely yellow pigment, most of which is produced in the spleen from the hemoglobin of old red blood cells the spleen has removed from the circulation. This new bilirubin is not water soluble and must be attached to a protein for transport to the liver, where it is made water soluble and excreted in bile. In the liver, bilirubin is joined (conjugated) to glucuronide to make **conjugated bilirubin**, which is water soluble and can be excreted in bile. Before reaching the liver, the water-insoluble bilirubin is called **unconjugated bilirubin**. Increased blood bilirubin (of either type) causes **jaundice** (*icterus*), a yellow discoloration of skin and sclera that is a hallmark of increased blood bilirubin.

Bacteria in the bowel convert bilirubin into **urobilinogen**, a compound that gives feces its brown color. Patients with jaundice usually have pale stools owing to a lack of urobilinogen. However, some urobilinogen is produced directly by the liver, secreted into blood, and

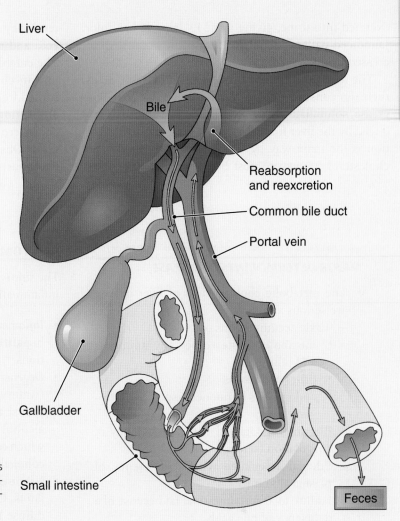

Figure 16-2 The enterohepatic circulation. Bile acids are secreted into bile, absorbed back into blood by the intestine, and recirculated via the portal vein for remetabolism by the liver.

Table 16-1	**Liver Functions**
Metabolic Task	**Hepatocyte Actions**
Detoxification and drug metabolism	• Chemical alteration and excretion of hormones and drugs • Production and excretion of urea and other compounds that are less toxic than the parent compound
Lipid and carbohydrate metabolism	• Conversion of glucose to glycogen and fat • Production of glucose from glycogen and other compounds • Secretion of glucose into blood • Synthesis and secretion of triglyceride and cholesterol into blood • Excretion of cholesterol into bile • Production of ketones from fatty acid
Protein synthesis	• Synthesis and secretion into blood of albumin, transport proteins and blood coagulation (clotting) factors
Conjugation and excretion of bilirubin	• Conjugation of bilirubin with glucuronide and excretion of it into bile ducts
Synthesis and excretion of bile acids	• Synthesis of bile acids by liver cells and secretion of them into bile ducts

excreted into urine, giving urine its faint amber color. Jaundiced patients may have dark urine because of increased urobilinogen.

The *liver produces and excretes bile acids.* **Bile acids**, the main constituent of bile, emulsify fat like soap does grease, solubilizing it for absorption. Bile acids are produced by the liver from cholesterol, and bile acid excretion is the main way by which the body rids itself of cholesterol. However, most bile acids and the choles- terol they contain are reabsorbed by the intestinal mucosa and returned to blood (*enterohepatic circulation*). The enterohepatic circulation is, therefore, very important in cholesterol metabolism. Most cholesterol absorbed from the intestine is not from diet but from reabsorption of bile acids. New drugs lower blood cholesterol by blocking intestinal absorption of cholesterol. Obstruction of bile excretion is referred to as **cholestasis**.

MAJOR DETERMINANTS OF DISEASE

- The metabolic consequences of liver disease are serious and include:
  - Toxic accumulations of:
    - metabolic waste (especially ammonia and bilirubin)
    - drugs and toxins
    - endogenous hormones (especially estrogen)
  - Bleeding, associated with a deficiency of coagulation factors
  - Edema, associated with a deficiency of plasma albumin
  - Failure to absorb intestinal fat because of a deficiency of bile acids
- Viral hepatitis is a common contagious disease
- Cirrhosis is the final endpoint for many liver diseases
- Portal hypertension is the most important consequence of cirrhosis and can be associated with liver failure and severe hemorrhage
- Stones often form in the gallbladder and may pass into and obstruct the bile duct

The Liver Response to Injury

The liver responds remarkably well to injury—it has enormous functional reserve and must suffer a marked decline of capacity before becoming symptomatic. However, because normal liver function is so crucial in metabolism, liver disease looms large in human illness. Laboratory evaluation of blood is critical in the diagnosis and management of liver disease. The nearby Lab Tools box lists and describes the most common lab tests.

ANATOMIC PATTERNS OF LIVER INJURY

The injury to liver prompts one of four consequences: inflammation, degeneration, necrosis, and fibrosis.

- *Inflammation:* Inflammation of the liver is termed **hepatitis**, most of which is caused by virus infections.
- *Degeneration:* Hepatocytes may undergo hydropic (watery) or fatty degeneration (Chapter 2) in response to toxic or autoimmune injury. For example, alcohol abuse typically causes fatty degeneration, which can proceed to injury that is more serious if alcohol abuse continues.
- *Necrosis:* Liver cells may die as blocks of tissue (infarcts, Chapter 2) or as single cells. In some types of diffuse hepatic injuries, such as viral hepatitis and chronic alcohol injury, individual liver cells die one by one, becoming shrunken, dead cells known as **Councilman bodies**.
- *Fibrosis:* Scarring can occur as a result of severe hepatic injury. **Cirrhosis** (discussed in detail below) is a patterned, permanent scarring (fibrosis) of the entire liver from long-standing, severe injury that destroys the normal architecture and replaces it with scar tissue.

FUNCTIONAL PATTERNS OF LIVER INJURY

The direct metabolic consequences of hepatic injury are:

- **Jaundice**: a yellow discoloration of skin and sclerae (Fig. 16-3) caused by an excess of blood bilirubin
- **Cholestasis**: an accumulation of bile acids and cholesterol in blood when there is obstruction of bile flow inside or outside of the liver
- **Hepatic failure**: the loss of hepatic metabolic function severe enough to cause clinical symptoms.

Each of these consequences may be associated with widespread ill effect on the body.

LAB TOOLS

Liver Function Tests

The most useful laboratory tests for liver function are:

- *Enzymes*: The liver is packed with enzymes. In liver disease these enzymes are washed into blood, where they are easily measured. Even mild liver-cell injury can cause minor increases in levels of liver enzymes. Elevation of lactic dehydrogenase (LDH), aspartate aminotransferase (AST), and alanine aminotransferase (ALT) suggests hepatic cellular damage. Alkaline phosphatase levels also may be increased in liver disease, but they tend to rise highest in bile duct diseases. Red blood cells contain some of these enzymes, and in vitro damage (hemolysis) to red cells during specimen collection or handling can cause misleading enzyme level increases.
- *Bilirubin*: The liver metabolizes and excretes bilirubin into the bile ducts. If hemolytic disease has been excluded, increased levels of blood bilirubin usually indicate at least moderate liver disease or bile duct disease.

- *Proteins*: The liver makes albumin and many other plasma proteins. Low levels of plasma albumin and blood coagulation factors are characteristic of moderate to serious liver disease.
- *Coagulation tests*: The liver makes most of the coagulation proteins (factors), and liver disease can cause abnormal (prolonged) prothrombin time and partial thromboplastin time.
- *Hepatitis virus antigens and antibodies*: Each type of hepatitis virus is distinguished by characteristic patterns of virus antigens and antibodies in blood.
- *Autoimmune antibodies*: Antimitochondrial antibodies in blood are characteristic of primary biliary cirrhosis; anti-smooth muscle antibodies are characteristic of chronic autoimmune hepatitis.

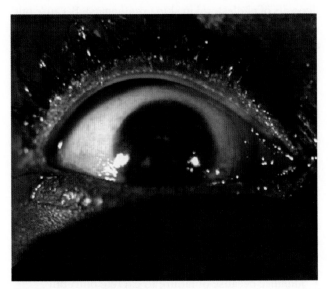

Figure 16-3 **Scleral icterus of jaundice.**

Jaundice and Cholestasis

Jaundice usually becomes visible when blood bilirubin level is >2 mg/dL (normal <1.2 mg/dL). As is illustrated in Figure 16-4, jaundice can be caused by three conditions:

- *the presence of excessive amounts of bilirubin* (prehepatic jaundice), such as accompanies red cell destruction in hemolytic anemia

- *defective liver functioning* (hepatic jaundice), such as occurs with viral hepatitis, drug interference with liver function, or cirrhosis
- *biliary obstruction* (posthepatic jaundice), such as occurs when pancreatic cancer occludes the common bile duct

Prehepatic jaundice causes an increase in blood of water-insoluble **unconjugated bilirubin**. The most common serious cause of increased amounts of unconjugated bilirubin in blood is hemolytic anemia, such as sickle cell disease (Chapter 11).

Increased unconjugated bilirubin can also occur when there is *hepatic malfunction*. For newborns unconjugated hyperbilirubinemia is especially dangerous, because it is toxic to the underdeveloped brain. Because the immature livers of premature infants are unable to conjugate bilirubin effectively, during the first several weeks of life a marked increase of unconjugated bilirubin may cause *kernicterus* (from German: *kern*, nucleus, and *icterus*, jaundice), a severe neurologic condition resulting from toxic deposits of water-insoluble, unconjugated bilirubin in the brain (Chapter 7).

However, the most common cause of increased unconjugated bilirubin in blood is **Gilbert syndrome** (pronounced *jeel-bear*), a very common and harmless condition associated with a mild increase of *unconjugated* bilirubin that is the result of a *genetic enzyme defi-*

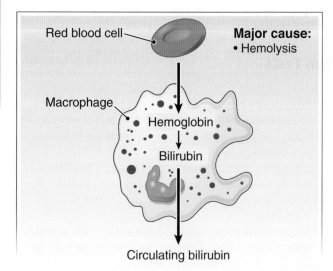

Red blood cell

Major cause:
• Hemolysis

Macrophage

Hemoglobin

Bilirubin

Circulating bilirubin

A Prehepatic jaundice (unconjugated hyperbilirubinemia)

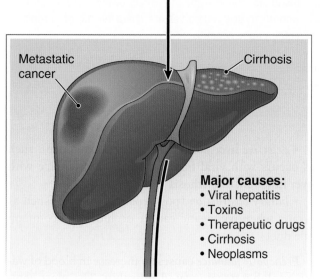

Metastatic cancer

Cirrhosis

Major causes:
• Viral hepatitis
• Toxins
• Therapeutic drugs
• Cirrhosis
• Neoplasms

B Hepatic jaundice (unconjugated or conjugated hyperbilirubinemia)

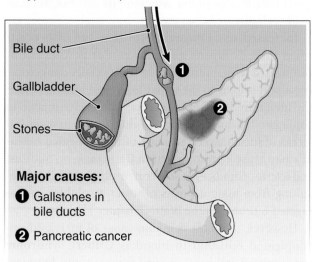

Bile duct

Gallbladder

Stones

❶

❷

Major causes:
❶ Gallstones in bile ducts
❷ Pancreatic cancer

C Posthepatic jaundice (conjugated hyperbilirubinemia)

ciency, which is usually detected accidentally while the patient is being seen for an unrelated illness or when the patient has been fasting for 12 hours or more. A similar genetic syndrome causing increased *conjugated* bilirubin is the *Dubin-Johnson syndrome.*

Jaundice associated with hepatic disorders (hepatic jaundice) may cause an increase in blood of either unconjugated or conjugated bilirubin, because interference can occur either before or after conjugation in the liver.

Jaundice resulting from bile duct obstruction (posthepatic jaundice) is characterized by increased water-soluble, **conjugated bilirubin** in blood because by the time bilirubin enters hepatic ducts all of it is conjugated, and obstruction forces conjugated bilirubin out of the ducts and into blood. Gallstones and pancreatic cancer are the two most common causes of duct obstruction.

Cholestasis is usually accompanied by jaundice and sometimes by severe pruritus (itching) because of the deposition of bile acids in the skin. Cholestasis may result from primary liver disease, drug interference with bile secretion, pregnancy, and a variety of other conditions. Because bile is the means by which the body rids itself of excess cholesterol, blood cholesterol levels may become markedly elevated and associated with yellow deposits of cholesterol in skin (*xanthomas*). Because bile duct epithelium is rich in alkaline phosphatase, a characteristic laboratory finding is marked increase of blood alkaline phosphatase levels, whereas levels of other liver enzymes are usually normal or only mildly increased.

Hepatic Failure

Hepatic failure is the most severe consequence of liver disease—most patients die within a few weeks or months. It may follow sudden injury, as in sudden, severe viral hepatitis (fulminant hepatitis), or it may be the result of chronic injury, as with chronic hepatitis or chronic alcoholism. About 90% of hepatic function must be destroyed before failure occurs.

The clinical features of hepatic failure are:

• *Jaundice* because of failure to excrete bilirubin
• *Ascites* because of increased portal pressure and low blood osmotic pressure
• *Fetor hepaticus*, literally "liver breath," because of an accumulation of volatile waste products such as ammonia

Figure 16-4 Three types of jaundice. A, Prehepatic jaundice causes increased levels of unconjugated bilirubin in blood. **B,** Hepatic jaundice may be caused by interference with the liver's ability to conjugate bilirubin or to secrete it after conjugation; increased levels of blood bilirubin may be of either conjugated or unconjugated type. **C,** Posthepatic jaundice is caused by obstruction of bile flow inside or outside of the liver; increased levels of blood bilirubin are of conjugated type.

- *Hypoalbuminemia* because of diminished hepatic production of protein
- *Hypoglycemia* because of lack of liver glycogen stores
- *Hyperammonemia* because of failure of the liver to convert ammonia to urea
- *Palmar erythema* (*redness of the palms of the hands*), *spider angiomata* (*small skin hemangiomas*), *testicular atrophy, balding,* and *gynecomastia* (*enlarged male breasts*) because of increases in blood estrogen from impaired liver metabolism of estrogen
- *Bleeding disorders* because of deficiency of blood clotting factors made by the liver

Moreover, kidney and brain function can be seriously impaired by liver failure. (A summary of the clinical features of hepatic failure can also be found later in the chapter in Figure 16-10, which appears with the discussion of cirrhosis.)

Hepatorenal syndrome is renal failure owing to acute hepatic failure. The cause is not completely clear—it appears to result from renal vasoconstriction and low renal blood flow, but the kidney is pathologically normal. **Hepatic encephalopathy**, an especially serious complication of hepatic failure, occurs when accumulated ammonia and other unmetabolized waste products exert a toxic effect on the brain. Neurologic signs include rigidity, hyperreflexia, and, rarely, seizures. Fatal coma may occur. A particularly characteristic sign is *asterixis,* a rapid extension-flexion motion of the head and extremities that can be demonstrated by testing for "hepatic flap"—the arms are held extended and the hands dorsiflexed. A pulsating, flapping, or hand waving motion constitutes a positive test.

Cirrhosis

Cirrhosis is the final, common end-stage for a variety of chronic liver diseases. As is illustrated in Figures 16-5 and 16-6, **cirrhosis** is a patterned fibrosis of the entire liver characterized pathologically by a three-dimensional web of interconnecting bands of scar tissue, dividing the liver into small nodules separated from one another by dense fibrous tissue, an architecture that makes cirrhotic livers tense and hard. Cirrhosis is progressive, irreversible, and incurable.

Cirrhosis can be classified by *cause,* such as alcoholic or hepatitic, but regardless of cause there are only two *anatomic* types of cirrhosis:

- *portal cirrhosis,* caused by diffuse liver cell injury
- *biliary cirrhosis,* caused by chronic disease of the biliary tree

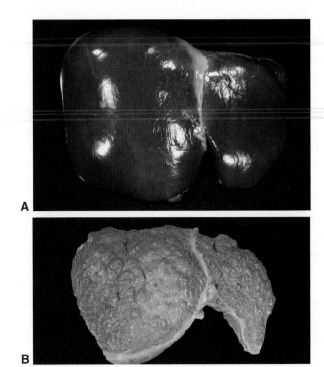

Figure 16-5 Cirrhosis. A, Normal liver. **B,** Cirrhosis. Note the small size of the cirrhotic liver.

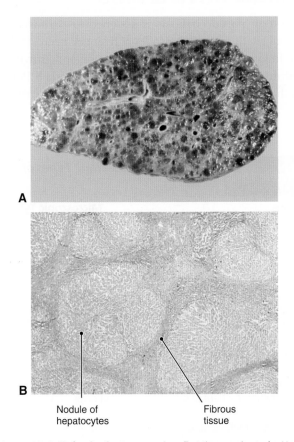

Nodule of hepatocytes   Fibrous tissue

Figure 16-6 Cirrhosis. A, Gross section. **B,** Microscopic study. Note the nodular pattern in both specimens. The liver is divided into nodules by a web of fibrous (scar) tissue. Dark discoloration of some nodules is caused by the accumulation of bile pigment in lobules. The cause of cirrhosis in this patient is unknown.

In early cases, portal and biliary cirrhosis are easy to distinguish by microscopic examination, but as disease progresses the distinctions disappear. In the end the cause of most cases of cirrhosis cannot be determined by study of the liver: clinical findings and history are of paramount importance. However, a few rare types of cirrhosis have highly characteristic microscopic findings. For example, in *hemochromatosis* (discussed below), the body is overloaded with iron, much of which is deposited in the liver. A second example is hereditary alpha-1 antitrypsin deficiency, which is associated with early emphysema (Chapter 14) and distinctive microscopic findings in the liver.

Table 16-2 lists the causes of cirrhosis and the microscopic pattern associated with each. Cirrhosis is among the top 10 causes of death in the western hemisphere, two thirds of it resulting from *alcoholism* and *chronic viral hepatitis*. Less common causes are genetic hemochromatosis, and diseases of bile ducts. In about one third of cases, the cause is unknown (cryptogenic cirrhosis).

ANATOMIC TYPES OF CIRRHOSIS

The term **portal cirrhosis** is assigned to cirrhosis occurring with repeated episodes of liver cell necrosis that are followed by hepatocyte regeneration and growth of fibrous tissue from the area of the portal triad. Portal cirrhosis is by far the most common type of cirrhosis and includes all forms of cirrhosis other than those described immediately below as *biliary cirrhosis*. The majority of portal cirrhosis results from alcoholic liver disease and chronic viral hepatitis.

Far less common is **biliary cirrhosis**, which results from chronic inflammation of bile ducts. *Primary biliary cirrhosis* is an autoimmune disease (Chapter 8) of intrahepatic bile ducts. *Secondary* biliary cirrhosis develops as a consequence of prolonged inflammation of bile ducts, usually associated with obstruction of bile flow because of gallstones lodged in the common bile duct. Another cause of bile duct inflammation and fibrosis that causes biliary cirrhosis is *sclerosing cholangitis*, which is associated with chronic ulcerative colitis (Chapter 15).

THE PATHOPHYSIOLOGY OF CIRRHOSIS

Cirrhosis obstructs free flow of portal blood through the liver and causes **portal hypertension**; that is, high blood pressure in the portal venous system. This obstruction of portal blood flow through the liver diverts (shunts) blood around the liver through alternative (collateral) vessels in the GI tract, spleen, and skin, as is depicted in Figure 16-7.

The hemodynamic consequences of portal hypertension are *ascites*, congestive *splenomegaly* (Fig. 16-8), and various types of prominent veins that result from the shunting of blood around the liver: *esophageal varices* (see Fig. 15-8, Chapter 15), *hemorrhoids*, and prominent veins radiating outward from the umbilicus, known as *caput medusa*—literally snake-head—so named because of its likeness to the female serpent-haired monster, Medusa, from Greek mythology.

Ascites (from Greek, *askos*, for bag) is an intraperitoneal accumulation of watery (serous) fluid. This fluid seeps from portal venules as a result of high portal blood pressure and low blood osmotic pressure caused by low blood albumin owing to low output of albumin by the liver. Ascites becomes clinically evident when about 500 ml of intraperitoneal fluid have accumulated; however, as is depicted in Figure 16-9, fluid accumulation may be massive.

> **Cirrhosis is always associated with portal hypertension.**

CLINICAL FEATURES OF CIRRHOSIS

The clinical features of cirrhosis are summarized in Figure 16-10 and result from four phenomena:

- *Failure to metabolize estrogen and ammonia.* Failing hepatic metabolism of estrogen results in high levels

Table 16-2	Causes and Microscopic Types of Cirrhosis	
Cause		**Microscopic Type**
Alcohol abuse		Portal
Chronic viral hepatitis B or C		Portal
Biliary obstruction		Biliary
Gallstones		
Cystic fibrosis		
Autoimmune disease		
Primary biliary cirrhosis		Biliary
Sclerosing cholangitis		Biliary
Autoimmune hepatitis		Portal
Inherited metabolic disease		Portal
Hemochromatosis		
Alpha-1 antitrypsin deficiency		
Wilson disease		
Cryptogenic (unknown)		Portal

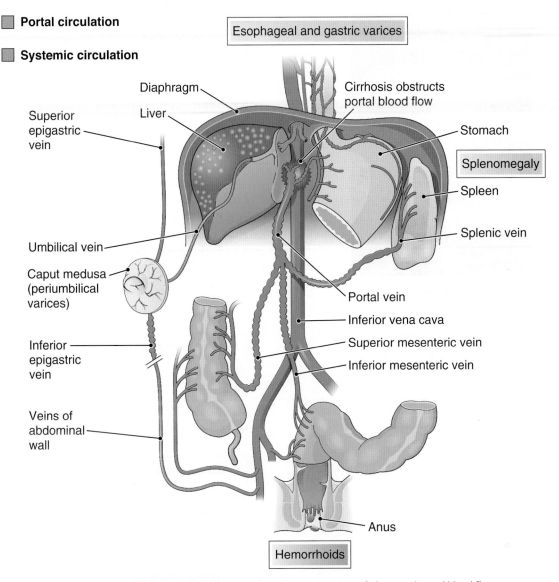

☐ **Portal circulation**

☐ **Systemic circulation**

Esophageal and gastric varices

Diaphragm

Cirrhosis obstructs portal blood flow

Superior epigastric vein

Liver

Stomach

Splenomegaly

Spleen

Splenic vein

Umbilical vein

Caput medusa (periumbilical varices)

Portal vein

Inferior vena cava

Inferior epigastric vein

Superior mesenteric vein

Inferior mesenteric vein

Veins of abdominal wall

Anus

Hemorrhoids

Figure 16-7 **Portal hypertension.** The hemodynamic consequences of obstructed portal blood flow.

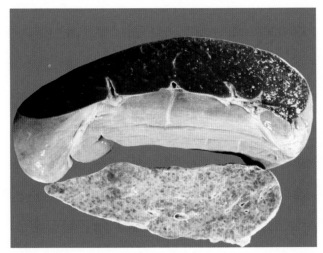

Figure 16-8 **Congestive splenomegaly in cirrhosis.** Both specimens are from the same patient. Note that the spleen *(Top)* is much larger than the liver is; normally the opposite is true.

of blood estrogen, which in men accounts for thinning scalp and genital hair, enlarged breasts (gynecomastia), red palms (palmar erythema), atrophic testes, and spider angiomas—small vascular malformations of skin that feature a tiny central vessel from which spider-like vessels radiate outward. Women may have abnormal menstrual bleeding. Failing hepatic metabolism of ammonia and other waste products accounts for hepatic coma and fetor hepaticus (liver breath).

• *Protein synthesis failure.* Failing hepatic protein synthesis causes decreased plasma albumin, which contributes to ascites and peripheral edema (Chapter 5), and decreased production of blood coagulation factors, which accounts for bleeding tendencies, usually evident as easy bruising (skin purpura).

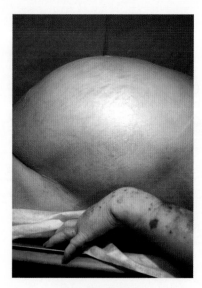

Figure 16-9 Ascites.

- *Excretory failure.* Failing hepatic excretion of bilirubin causes jaundice.
- *Portal hypertension.* Portal hypertension causes hemorrhoids, esophageal varices, splenomegaly, and caput medusa veins radiating from the umbilicus, and contributes to the formation of ascites.

Patients with cirrhosis also lose muscle mass (*muscle wasting*); however, the cause is not clear. In early cirrhosis the liver may be large, but as scarring progresses it always shrinks to less than normal size.

Cirrhosis may go undetected for years. Sometimes the delay is so great that when symptoms appear the original cause may not be apparent. Initial symptoms may be nothing more than anorexia, fatigue, and weight loss. But hepatic symptoms, jaundice especially, are usually present and may appear quite suddenly, mim-

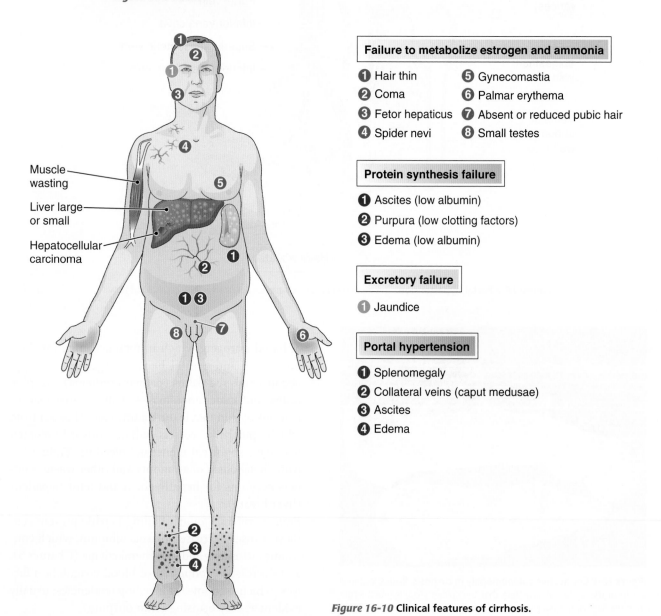

Muscle wasting

Liver large or small

Hepatocellular carcinoma

Failure to metabolize estrogen and ammonia

1 Hair thin   5 Gynecomastia
2 Coma   6 Palmar erythema
3 Fetor hepaticus   7 Absent or reduced pubic hair
4 Spider nevi   8 Small testes

Protein synthesis failure

1 Ascites (low albumin)
2 Purpura (low clotting factors)
3 Edema (low albumin)

Excretory failure

1 Jaundice

Portal hypertension

1 Splenomegaly
2 Collateral veins (caput medusae)
3 Ascites
4 Edema

Figure 16-10 Clinical features of cirrhosis.

icking acute liver disease. The most common causes of death from cirrhosis are hepatic failure, gastrointestinal hemorrhage from esophageal varices, and hepatocellular carcinoma (discussed below).

Viral Hepatitis

Viral hepatitis is infection by one of the several viruses that *preferentially* infect the liver: hepatitis viruses A, B, C, D, and E, which are designated HAV (for hepatitis A virus), HBV, and so on. Other viruses can *incidentally* infect the liver and cause hepatitis, most notably the cytomegalovirus or the Epstein-Barr virus of infectious mononucleosis.

Hepatitis viruses are distinguished from one another according to the following clinical characteristics (summarized in Table 16-3):

• *Mode of transmission*: Is the virus transmitted by oral-fecal contamination, close personal contact, contam-inated water, or blood contamination (needlestick or transfusion)?
• *Length of incubation period*: What is the length of time from infection to symptomatic disease?
• *Carrier state*: After recovery from acute infection, does the virus linger, so that an apparently healthy person continues to infect others?
• *Chronic hepatitis*: Can the virus cause chronic hepatitis?
• *Fulminant hepatitis*: Can the virus cause a sudden, catastrophic hepatitis?
• *Hepatocellular carcinoma*: Is the virus associated with increased risk of hepatocellular carcinoma?

> • **Hepatitis A is a mild, epidemic disease spread by contaminated food and water; it does not cause chronic hepatitis or cirrhosis.**
> • **Hepatitis B and hepatitis C are spread from individual to individual by needles or sexual contact; both can cause chronic hepatitis and cirrhosis.**

Table 16-3 **Characteristics of Major Hepatitis Viruses**

Characteristic	Hepatitis A	Hepatitis B	Hepatitis C
New cases per annum United States (2001)	11,000	8,000	28,000
Transmission Route Mother to child	Fecal-oral No	Parenteral or close contact Yes	Parenteral or close contact ?
Incubation period	3–6 weeks	2 weeks to 6 months	2 weeks to 6 months
Viremia	Very short	Long	Long
Carrier state	No	Yes, uncommon	Yes, common
Chronic hepatitis	No	5–10%	>50%
Increased risk for hepatocellular carcinoma	No	Yes	Yes
Blood markers*	anti-HAV (IgM) anti-HAV (IgG)	HBsAg HBeAg anti-HBs anti-HBc (IgM) anti-HBc (IgG) anti-HBe	HCV-RNA anti-HCV
Vaccine available	Yes	Yes	No

*Marker key: HBsAg, hepatitis B surface antigen; anti-HBc (IgM), anti-hepatitis B core antibody, acute phase (IgM) type

CLINICOPATHOLOGIC SYNDROMES

Viral hepatitis can cause several clinical syndromes or diseases:

- asymptomatic hepatitis
- carrier state
- acute viral hepatitis
- chronic viral hepatitis
- fulminant hepatic failure
- hepatocellular carcinoma

However, not every virus can produce each of these; and some of these disorders can be caused by diseases other than viral hepatitis.

Asymptomatic hepatitis may produce no lasting liver injury and be detected only by accident. The usual circumstance is unexpected abnormal blood tests—abnormally elevated liver enzymes, for example—obtained as part of an annual physical exam or in the course of attention to an unrelated condition.

The **carrier state** exists in a patient who despite being *asymptomatic* harbors the virus and is therefore capable of transmitting the virus to others. The percentage of infected people who become carriers varies greatly from one type of viral hepatitis to another. For example, few patients infected with hepatitis B virus (HBV) become carriers; conversely, many of those with hepatitis C virus (HCV) develop asymptomatic chronic infection and, therefore, fit the definition of carrier.

Acute viral hepatitis is an acute illness that typically progresses through four clinical phases:

- *Incubation* usually lasts a few weeks. Peak *infectivity* occurs about the time symptoms appear.
- The *symptomatic prejaundice phase* is usually marked by constitutional symptoms, including malaise, fatigability, nausea, and anorexia. However, right upper-quadrant pain, low-grade fever, headache, skin rash, vomiting, diarrhea, or muscle and joint aches may occur.
- The *symptomatic jaundice phase* begins as jaundice (icterus) appears and other symptoms fade. The jaundice reflects a rise in conjugated bilirubin. Because conjugated bilirubin is water soluble, it is excreted in urine, causing a brown discoloration. Because less bilirubin is getting into the gut, stools may be pale. With HAV infection, most adults become jaundiced, but most children do not. About half of patients with HBV infection become jaundiced, but patients with HCV infection are rarely jaundiced.
- *Convalescence* begins as jaundice fades, infectivity disappears, and antibodies appear in blood to confer immunity.

Chronic viral hepatitis is defined as viral hepatitis proven by liver biopsy, with six months or more of laboratory or clinical evidence of disease activity. Not all patients with chronic hepatitis have chronic viral hepatitis—autoimmune hepatitis and alcoholic hepatitis, discussed below, are examples. About 10% of patients with hepatitis B infections develop chronic hepatitis, whereas more than 50% of patients with hepatitis C do so. Most patients with chronic hepatitis show few specific clinical signs and symptoms, and the extent of disease is revealed only by laboratory tests.

On the other hand, some patients may be very ill and exhibit a variety of laboratory and clinical abnormalities. Laboratory coagulation tests are often abnormal because liver impairment affects the production of coagulation factors. Increased levels of enzymes by necrotic liver cells are detected in blood. Impaired bilirubin excretion causes increased levels of bilirubin. The immune system (Chapter 8) reacts to the virus infection by producing large amounts of immunoglobulin, appearing in blood as hypergammaglobulinemia. Moreover, about 10% of patients with hepatitis B or hepatitis C infection develop autoimmune disease, usually kidney disease (glomerulonephritis, Chapter 19) or vasculitis (Chapter 12).

Patients with chronic hepatitis may have an enlarged, tender liver because of liver inflammation, and they may have an enlarged spleen (splenomegaly) resulting from portal hypertension and reaction of the immune system to the infection. Appearance of palmar erythema or spider angiomas (owing to failure of the liver to metabolize estrogen) or other signs of liver failure is evidence of severe chronic viral hepatitis.

Fulminant hepatic failure denotes explosively acute liver disease that progresses to hepatic failure and encephalopathy in a very short time, usually a few weeks. *Fulminant hepatitis* (Fig. 16-11) accounts for more than half of cases, most of which are associated with hepatitis A or B infections. Other causes include suicidal doses of acetaminophen, heat stroke, acute fatty liver of pregnancy, wild mushroom poisoning, and adverse reactions to drugs.

Finally, patients with hepatitis B and C infections are at substantially increased risk for development of **hepatocellular carcinoma**.

HEPATITIS A VIRUS (HAV) INFECTION

HAV is the cause of *epidemic* hepatitis, which is primarily spread by oral-fecal contamination of water or food, for instance, contaminated shellfish (oysters, shrimp). Shared food utensils, kissing, handshaking, and sexual activity are less common modes of transmission. HAV

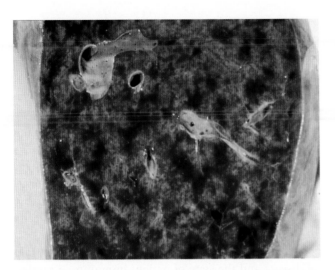

Figure 16-11 Hepatitis with massive hepatic necrosis. Dark spots are hemorrhagic necrosis around central veins; red areas are nonhemorrhagic necrosis.

infection is benign and self-limited (it resolves spontaneously), with an incubation period of 2–6 weeks. It is the most common type of hepatitis infection in the world. Infection is much more common than actual disease is; by mid adult life about half of people in devel-

oped countries have blood **anti-HAV antibodies** as evidence of infection, but few recall being ill. Rates are higher in developing nations, where most children have evidence of infection (anti-hepatitis antibodies in blood) by age ten. About 10,000 new clinical cases are reported each year in the United States; however, because the great majority of cases are asymptomatic, it is likely that hundreds of thousands of unreported infections occur each year. Fatalities are very rare. HAV infection has no carrier state, does not cause chronic hepatitis, and very rarely causes fulminant hepatitis or death. It is most common in poor countries without modern sanitation and hygiene. A vaccine is available.

As is depicted in Figure 16-12A, the virus infects the liver and quickly begins to be shed in feces. It appears transiently in blood (viremia), but the viremia is so short that risk of blood-borne transmission—by transfusion of infected donor blood or accidental needlestick by health care personnel—is very low.

As is illustrated in Figure 16-12B, jaundice, increased liver enzymes in blood, and the appearance of IgM type anti-HAV antibodies are clinical markers of disease progress. Recall from Chapter 8 that IgM antibodies are acute phase antibodies, and IgG antibodies

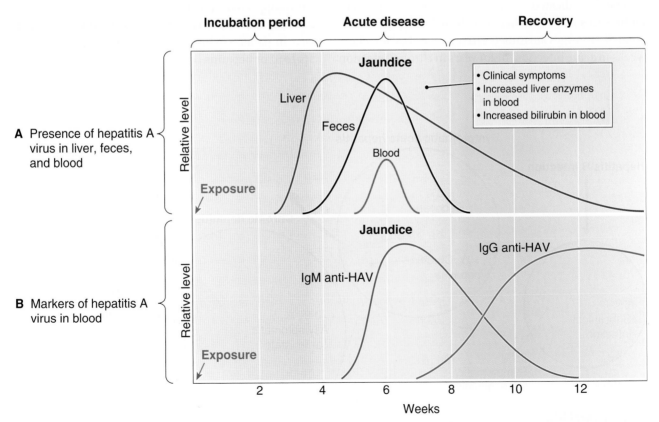

Figure 16-12 Hepatitis A: clinical phases and blood markers of infection. A, Infection of the liver is followed quickly by the appearance of virus in blood and feces. **B,** Jaundice or other symptoms of acute infection are accompanied by the appearance of IgM-type acute phase antibodies in blood. The appearance of IgG-type antibodies signals recovery and immunity against reinfection.

appear later and confer immunity. Anti-HAV (IgM) antibodies are a valuable diagnostic tool to confirm the diagnosis of HAV infection. Vaccination produces immunity by stimulating the production of IgG anti-HAV antibodies.

HEPATITIS B VIRUS (HBV) INFECTION

HBV is a much more serious disease than hepatitis A is. Unlike hepatitis A, it is not spread by food, water, or casual contact—it spreads by needlestick or sexual contact, and it infects hundreds of millions of people worldwide. The incubation period varies greatly: from a few weeks to six months. Outcomes of infection are illustrated in Figure 16-13. In the United States new cases have fallen dramatically to near 10,000 annually because of improved public awareness and vaccination. However, about two thirds of infections are asymptomatic, so the number of actual infections is about three times the number of reported cases. Most symptomatic infections appear as a syndrome of acute hepatitis that resolves quickly with supportive care. A carrier state evolves in less than 10% of infections, most likely in neonates and people with impaired immunity.

As is depicted in Figure 16-14A, the viremia of *acute infection* is indicated by detection in blood of a particular hepatitis B antigen, **hepatitis B surface antigen**, designated **HBsAg**. Hepatitis B viremia may last for many weeks in acute infection, or for years in chronic infection

(Fig. 16-14B) or in asymptomatic carriers (Fig. 16-14C), a critical fact in its infectivity. It is transmitted in blood, saliva, and semen and can be spread by heterosexual or homosexual contact, blood transfusion, renal dialysis, and needlestick accidents among health care workers and intravenous drug users. Some infected mothers infect the fetus in utero or during vaginal delivery. In one third of cases, the method of infection is not known.

Laboratory tests for hepatitis markers (antigens and antibodies) are critical in the diagnosis and management of hepatitis B. HBV *antigens* usually appear first. HBsAg is the first marker to appear and is an indicator of viremia and, therefore, of infectivity.

Anti-hepatitis B *antibodies* are also important markers of disease and the state of patient immunity to reinfection. Significant variation occurs in the type of antibody (acute phase IgM or late phase IgG, Chapter 8), the time at which they appear, and whether or not they disappear or persist, features that reveal much about the state of the infection and patient immunity. Antibody to **hepatitis B core antigen (anti-HBc)** is the first to appear and is useful as an early indicator of HBV infection (Fig. 16-14A). The appearance of antibodies to hepatitis B surface antigen—**anti-HBs**—marks the beginning of recovery and is not usually detectable until viremia (HBsAg in blood) has disappeared. Anti-HBs confers immunity and is the antibody created by vaccination. Anti-HBs does not appear in patients who develop chronic hepatitis B (Fig. 16-14B) or hepatitis B carrier state (Fig. 16-14C).

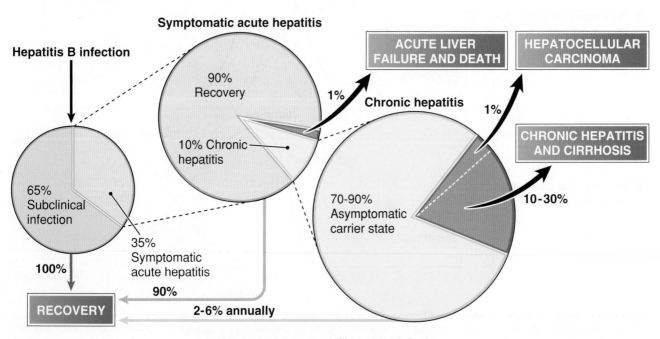

Figure 16-13 Outcomes of hepatitis B infection.

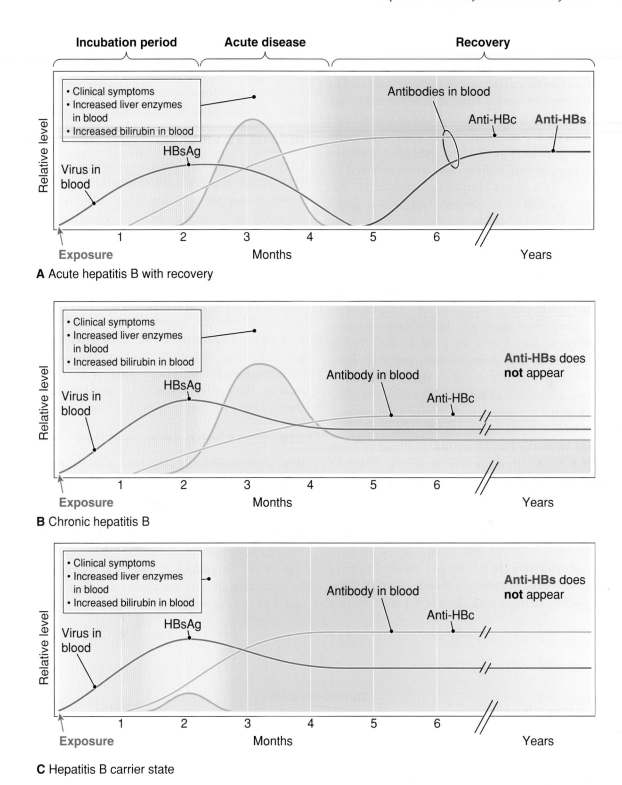

A Acute hepatitis B with recovery

B Chronic hepatitis B

C Hepatitis B carrier state

Figure 16-14 **Hepatitis B: clinical phases and blood markers of infection. A,** Acute infection is characterized by rapid appearance of the virus in blood before symptoms appear, disappearance of the virus from blood, and the appearance in blood of antibodies to hepatitis B surface antigen (HBsAg). **B,** Chronic hepatitis is signaled by continuing jaundice or clinical symptoms, or the continued presence of virus in blood (as is indicated by the detection in blood of HBsAg). **C,** The carrier state is indicated by disappearance of clinical symptoms and the persistence of virus in blood (as is indicated by the detection in blood of HBsAg).

HEPATITIS C VIRUS (HCV) INFECTION

HCV is a major cause of chronic liver disease (chronic hepatitis, cirrhosis, and hepatocellular carcinoma). The incubation period varies from a few weeks to six months, similar to hepatitis B. About 40,000 new cases are reported each year. Nearly 2% of the United States population has blood antibodies, indicating previous infection. In more half of these cases, virus is detectable in the blood, indicating a chronic carrier state. HCV is responsible for half of all chronic liver disease in the United States.

Over half of new HCV infections are a consequence of intravenous drug abuse—the great majority of IV drug users are infected. About 15% of cases can be accounted for by transmission through sexual activity and by infected health care workers, and by neonatal transmission. However, in about one third of cases the manner of infection cannot be determined because the initial infection is usually asymptomatic, and years later, when chronic infection is detected, the patient has no recollection of having had hepatitis. Outcomes of infection are depicted in Figure 16-15. About 3 million people in the United States are chronically infected.

Viremia is marked by detection in blood of virus RNA (**HCV-RNA**). In *acute* infection (Fig. 16-16A), anti-HCV appears promptly as a marker of acute immune response but does not confer immunity. Over half of patients with HCV progress to chronic infection (Fig. 16-16B). Many of these patients remain asymptomatic, but others have relapsing symptoms marked by reappearance of detectable HCV-RNA and elevated levels of liver enzymes and bilirubin in blood. After 20 years about 25%–35% of those with chronic hepatitis develop

cirrhosis. Of those developing cirrhosis a few percent develop hepatocellular carcinoma each year. HCV is a mutating RNA virus with dozens of subtypes, which has frustrated hope for a vaccine. Case Study 16.1 at the end of this chapter focuses on a patient with hepatitis C.

HEPATITIS D VIRUS (HDV) INFECTION

HDV (delta virus) is peculiar—it cannot exist without HBV. It can co-infect at the same time HBV is acquired, in which case the infection takes on characteristics of the usual HBV infection. In most instances of co-infection, the immune system successfully overcomes both of the viruses, and the patient recovers. On the other hand, HDV can infect someone who is already a carrier of HBV, in which case the asymptomatic HBV carrier develops acute hepatitis syndrome, or chronic hepatitis evolves. Most such infections occur among patients who inject illegal drugs, and in patients with hemophilia. Patients in both of these groups have multiple opportunities for infection—first by HBV infection, then by HDV infection on a subsequent injection or transfusion.

HEPATITIS E VIRUS (HEV) INFECTION

HEV infection is rare in the United States, but it is the most common form of epidemic hepatitis in India, where it is more common even than hepatitis A. Like hepatitis A it is transmitted by food and water and causes epidemics from time to time in Asia and Africa. The disease usually is mild and self-limiting, but it is exceptionally dangerous in pregnant women—20% of cases are fatal. It does not appear to have a carrier state and does not cause chronic hepatitis.

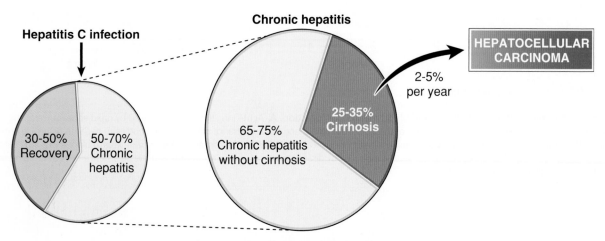

Figure 16-15 **Outcomes of hepatitis C infection.**

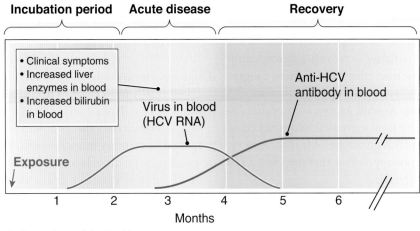

A Acute hepatitis C with recovery

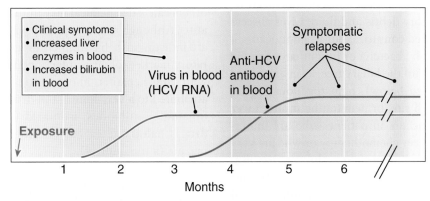

B Chronic hepatitis C with chronic hepatitis or carrier state

Figure 16-16 **Hepatitis C: clinical phases and blood markers of infection. A,** Acute infection with recovery is characterized by permanent disappearance of clinical symptoms and disappearance of the virus from blood (as is indicated by inability to detect hepatitis C virus RNA—HCV RNA—in blood). **B,** Chronic hepatitis is characterized by reappearance of jaundice or clinical symptoms and persistent evidence of the virus in blood, as is indicated by detection in blood of hepatitis C virus RNA (HCV RNA). The carrier state is indicated by asymptomatic persistent evidence of the virus in blood.

THE ANATOMIC PATHOLOGY OF HEPATITIS

A liver biopsy from a patient in the *carrier state* of hepatitis is usually normal, with two exceptions: hepatitis C carriers usually have microscopic evidence of low-grade inflammation, and in hepatitis B carriers the virus particles may be seen as a "ground glass" appearance of hepatocyte cytoplasm.

The microscopic changes seen in *acute hepatitis* are similar among the various types. Hepatocytes show hydropic (watery) degeneration (Chapter 2), and chronic inflammation is present. Necrosis occurs, most often affecting scattered individual cells rather than entire blocks of tissue. Tiny plugs of bile appear between liver cells, indicating that bile flow is obstructed in the smallest bile ducts. In fulminant hepatitis or hepatic failure the inflammatory reaction is overshadowed by extensive blocks of cell necrosis.

In *chronic hepatitis* all of the above changes of hepatitis are present, but the damage is more severe and liver architecture shows considerable disorganization. The inflammatory reaction is more intense, and necrosis is more extensive. A network of scar tissue appears that can evolve into cirrhosis if inflammation persists.

Autoimmune Hepatitis

Autoimmune hepatitis, accounting for about 20% of all cases of chronic hepatitis, is a syndrome of chronic hepatitis not associated with a viral infection, although its microscopic features are indistinguishable from those of chronic viral hepatitis. The clinical picture varies from mild to severe hepatitis, and most patients are young women. As a rule no blood markers of viral hepatitis are present, but a few patients may have false-positive anti-HCV antibody test results. Most patients have high titers of autoantibodies—such as antinuclear, anti-smooth muscle, or anti-mitochondrial antibodies—and in more than half of patients some other autoimmune disease is present, such as ulcerative colitis, Sjögren syndrome, thyroiditis, systemic lupus erythematosus, or rheumatoid arthritis. As with many autoimmune diseases (Chapter 8), there is an increased frequency of association with certain HLA genotypes. Most patients respond well to immunosuppressive therapy, but a few patients progress to cirrhosis.

Liver Abscess

Anatomically, a **liver abscess** is similar to any other abscess (Chapter 3)—it is a focal collection of necrotic and acute inflammatory debris and fluid. Liver abscess is rare in industrialized countries, but when it occurs it is most often caused by bacteria or fungi that reach the liver by direct ascent up the biliary tree, as in ascending cholangitis (discussed below), hematogenous spread from another infected site, or penetrating injury. Liver abscess most often occurs in patients who are immunodeficient or on cancer chemotherapy or who are very old or severely debilitated from chronic disease. Diagnosis is often missed or delayed because symptoms of the abscess are obscured by other serious clinical problems or the patient is too dulled by disability or dementia to respond. Antibiotic therapy may control smaller lesions, but surgical drainage usually is required for larger ones.

On the other hand, in nations with poor sanitary systems, most liver abscesses are caused by infection with *Entamoeba histolytica*, a protozoan parasite that is spread by fecal contamination of unwashed food. Organisms burrow into the intestinal wall and spread up the portal vein to infect the liver.

Toxic Liver Injury

Injury from toxins or drugs should always be suspected in liver disease because the liver metabolizes and excretes most drugs and other exogenous compounds, almost any of which in sufficiently large amounts can cause liver damage. Symptoms of acute toxic injury span the continuum of liver injury from almost imperceptible to fatal, and onset ranges from instantaneous to weeks after exposure. Mild injury may be asymptomatic and detectable only by modest elevations of liver enzymes in blood, whereas severe injury can cause hepatic failure or hepatic coma and death. Patients with drug-

induced or toxin-induced liver disease usually recover upon withdrawal of the agent.

There are two types of liver reactions to drugs and toxins. First are those that are *dose related*; that is, liver damage is certain if enough chemical is present. (Historically most cases of liver toxicity were industrial, but improved occupational safety regulations have nearly eliminated the problem.) Today acute, dose-related liver injury is uncommon. When it happens, it is usually the result of large doses of chemotherapy agents or of suicidal doses of drugs such as acetaminophen (Tylenol ©).

Second, and much more common, is unpredictable toxic injury, where the *damage is out of proportion to the dose*. These reactions, called "idiosyncratic," occur when people cannot metabolize a chemical as well as others can. The chemical may initiate autoimmune hepatitis. Although microscopically, idiosyncratic reactions are indistinguishable from chronic viral hepatitis, laboratory markers of virus infection are present in patients with viral hepatitis. Idiosyncratic reactions have been attributed to a very long list of drugs, among them sulfonamide antibiotics, isoniazid (an antituberculosis drug), halothane (a gas anesthetic), and chlorpromazine (a tranquilizer).

Drugs or toxins may incite neoplastic growth. For instance, oral contraceptives can stimulate the development of large benign liver tumors (adenomas), and chronic industrial exposure to vinyl chloride can cause hepatocellular carcinoma. *Reye syndrome* (discussed in detail below) is a potentially fatal liver and brain syndrome caused by aspirin use in children in some situations.

However, the most important drug affecting the liver is one not mentioned above—alcohol (ethanol).

Alcoholic Liver Disease

They never taste who always drink;
They always talk who never think.

MATTHEW PRIOR (1664–1721), ENGLISH POET AND DIPLOMAT

Alcohol abuse is a fact of antiquity. It is no less true today: alcoholism is the leading cause of liver disease in industrialized countries. About 20 million Americans abuse alcohol (about 10% of adults) and about 25% of hospitalized patients have some alcohol-related problem.

The best evidence linking alcohol to liver disease is epidemiologic: 1) Evidence shows a direct relationship between the amount of alcohol consumed and the development of cirrhosis; and 2) during prolonged short-

History of Medicine

FAMOUS PEOPLE WITH ALCOHOLISM

Historical people who were alcoholic include literary titans Edgar Allen Poe (1809–1849), F. Scott Fitzgerald (1896–1940), Dylan Thomas (1914–1953), and athlete Jim Thorpe (1888–1953). Alcoholism takes nothing from their accomplishments; if anything it makes them all the more remarkable that they triumphed despite the burden.

Poe, most famous for his haunting poem, *The Raven*, died at age 40. Fitzgerald, author of the classic American novel *The Great Gatsby*, died at age 44. Thomas, the Welsh poet most famous for his poem *Do Not Go Gentle into That Good Night*, may have been anticipating his own death at age 39 when he wrote these immortal lines:

Do not go gentle into that good night,
Old age should burn and rave at close of day;
Rage, rage against the dying of the light.

Jim Thorpe, however, lived to age 64. At the 2000 Olympics in Sydney, Australia, Thorpe, a Native American, was voted the greatest athlete of the 20th century, a fact that astonished legions of sports-crazed Americans who had never heard of him. In the 1912 Olympics Thorpe won Gold Medals in the decathlon and pentathlon (which together encompass 16 sports); he played professional baseball, hitting for a lifetime average of .252 in six seasons with the Giants, Braves, and Reds; he played professional football, playing on both offense and defense and scoring 25 touchdowns in one season for the Canton Bulldogs, after which he became president of what would later become the National Football League; in 1950 he was named by the Associated Press as the greatest football professional ever. He was formidable at every sport he tried: basketball, lacrosse, hockey, archery, handball, tennis, boxing, wrestling, bowling, billiards, darts, shooting, golf, gymnastics, and swimming. He even won first place in a school dance contest while a student at Carlisle (Pennsylvania) Indian School. In 1941 on a return trip to Carlisle, Thorpe stood at midfield and drop-kicked a football over the goal. He then turned and placekicked a second ball for a successful field goal at the other end of the field—both at the age of 52 and wearing street shoes.

In a triumph of legalism over justice, Thorpe's Olympic Medals were stripped from him in 1913 because it was found he had played semi-professional baseball, something he did not hide like others, who played under false names. He battled alcoholism the last twenty years of his life and died penniless in 1953.

Thorpe's Olympic medals were restored by the International Olympic Committee in 1983.

---

ages of alcohol there is less cirrhosis—in the United States during Prohibition (1919–1933) and in France during World War II (1939–1945) deaths from cirrhosis declined. As a rule, the amount of alcohol necessary to produce cirrhosis is about 200 grams of ethanol per day—the approximate amount in one pint (near 500 ml) of whiskey, gin, or vodka or two bottles of wine—and consumed regularly for 10–16 years. Even so, only about 16% of alcoholics develop cirrhosis. Women are more prone to develop alcoholic cirrhosis than men are.

Alcohol directly damages hepatocytes, producing three distinct lesions: fatty liver, alcoholic hepatitis, and cirrhosis, which usually occur in sequence.

FATTY LIVER

All alcoholics develop fatty livers. The first sign of alcohol injury is fatty degeneration (Chapter 2) of hepatocytes, also known as steatosis, or **fatty liver**, as is depicted in Figure 10-10 (Chapter 10) and Figure 16-17. In severe cases the liver is large (sometimes two or three times normal), yellow, and greasy. Exactly how alcohol causes fatty liver is unclear, but there is no doubt that alcohol itself is the cause: withdrawal produces complete reversal. For example, a week at the beach downing 8–10 beers a day is likely to produce a fatty liver to go along with the sunburn. But the fat disappears with return to normal habits at home.

Patients with fatty liver are usually asymptomatic, though they may have mild elevations of liver enzyme levels in blood. Elevations of liver enzyme levels indicate that even though fatty liver is fully reversible, hepatocytes are being damaged. Continued damage may lead to increasingly severe liver disease. Evidence of damaged hepatocytes is present in Figure 16-17: Dying hepatocytes appear as small, round, dark cells (*Councilman bodies*), and clumps of damaged protein appear as irregular reddish deposits (*Mallory's alcoholic hyaline*, or *Mallory bodies*).

Not to be forgotten in this discussion is the other damage done by alcohol abuse—social disruption, cancers of the oral cavity and esophagus, pancreatitis, cardiomyopathy, fetal alcohol syndrome, brain damage, and accidents of every kind.

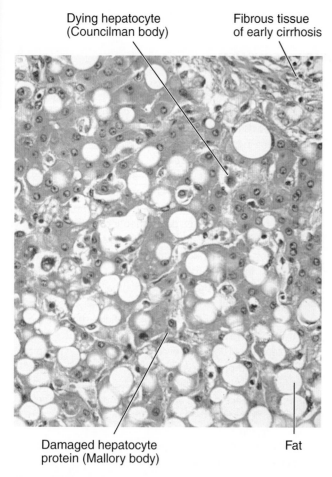

Dying hepatocyte
(Councilman body)

Fibrous tissue
of early cirrhosis

Damaged hepatocyte
protein (Mallory body)

Fat

Figure 16-17 **Alcoholic liver.** Fatty liver (steatosis) and alcoholic hepatitis. Large clear areas are hepatocytes filled with fat. Hepatitis is indicated by necrotic liver cells (Councilman bodies), intracellular degenerative inclusions (Mallory alcoholic hyaline), and fibrosis.

ALCOHOLIC HEPATITIS

Alcoholic hepatitis is a subacute or chronic form of alcohol liver injury characterized by inflammation, hepatocyte necrosis, and early fibrosis, which can progress to cirrhosis if alcohol abuse continues. Why some patients progress from fatty liver to alcoholic hepatitis is a mystery—a patient may have fatty liver for many years without a change in drinking habits but suddenly develop alcoholic hepatitis that eventually progresses to cirrhosis.

Clinical features depend on the degree of liver injury. Occasionally alcoholic hepatitis may appear so suddenly that bile duct obstruction or viral hepatitis is suspected. Malaise, anorexia, right upper quadrant pain, and jaundice are common. Leukocytosis and fever may be present, depending upon the extent of liver cell necrosis. Blood enzyme levels are moderately elevated. Each bout of alcoholic hepatitis carries a 10–20% chance of death, not merely from liver disease, but also

from intestinal hemorrhage, pancreatitis, and other alcohol-related problems. Abnormal clotting tests, low blood albumin, or clinical signs of hepatic failure are a bad prognostic sign because they do not become abnormal until the liver is severely damaged.

Established alcoholic hepatitis may not be reversible even with complete abstention from alcohol. Among those who quit drinking completely, one in five will nevertheless progress to cirrhosis. Patients who continue to drink usually develop cirrhosis within a few years.

ALCOHOLIC CIRRHOSIS

Alcoholic cirrhosis is the final and irreversible stage of alcoholic liver disease and is similar clinically and anatomically to other forms of cirrhosis discussed earlier (Fig. 16-5 through Fig.16-10). It is worth repeating that despite monumental alcohol intake, most alcoholics do not develop cirrhosis—only about 15% do. Alcoholics suffer from the usual consequences of hepatic failure and portal hypertension upon which is piled the train wreck of social ruin, gastric ulcers, cancers of the mouth, throat, and esophagus, encephalopathy, accidents, and pancreatitis. It's enough to kill you. It should be no surprise that alcoholic cirrhosis is one of the leading causes (with chronic viral hepatitis B and C) for adult liver transplantation in the United States.

Inherited Metabolic and Pediatric Liver Disease

Discussed here are diverse and rather uncommon inherited and sporadic liver diseases that primarily affect children.

HEMOCHROMATOSIS

The small intestine avidly absorbs iron, but there is no excretory pathway, especially in men (women regularly shed iron with the blood they lose with each menstrual period). Virtually all body iron reserves are stored in the liver, which therefore is directly affected by iron overload. **Hemochromatosis** is the toxic accumulation of an excessive amount of iron in cells, especially in liver, heart, and pancreas.

Primary (inherited) hemochromatosis is an autosomal recessive disorder caused by abnormally high iron absorption from the intestine. It is surprisingly common: among people of northern European ancestry—about 1 in 10 persons are heterozygous carriers of the faulty gene, and about 1 in 200 persons is diseased (homozygous), making hemochromatosis one of the most common inborn errors of metabolism in the United States. *Secondary* (acquired) hemochromatosis is usually the result of repeated blood transfusions given as treatment for sickle cell anemia, thalassemia, or aplastic anemia. In such cases, iron can be converted to an excretable form by intravenous infusion of chemicals that bind (chelate) iron.

Hemochromatosis usually does not become symptomatic until adulthood because it takes many years to accumulate enough iron to cause damage. Men are affected 10 times more often than women are. As is depicted in Figure 16-18, in fully developed cases iron deposits in the liver cause cirrhosis; in the pancreas, diabetes; in cardiac muscle, heart failure; in skin, brown pigmentation; in joints, arthritis; and in the pituitary, pituitary failure (Chapter 18).

The pathology features excessive amounts of iron deposited in the liver, pancreas, heart (Fig. 16-19), endocrine glands, joints, and skin. Cirrhosis is universal

in untreated cases. In some patients the first complaint is hypogonadism, the origins of which, in these patients, is not well understood. Presumably, it is related to iron deposition in the endocrine glands, including in the pituitary (Chapter 17).

Diagnosis depends on finding clinical features or markedly increased levels of blood iron, ferritin, and transferrin (Chapter 11) in the absence of another known cause. Diagnosis is confirmed by liver biopsy showing marked iron overload. Screening family members of the patient is very important. If the diagnosis of primary hemochromatosis is made early, most patients can expect to live normal lives if the excessive accumulation of iron is removed by periodic bleeding (phlebotomy). Patients with transfusion hemochromatosis who continue to need blood because of their underlying anemia can be treated effectively with injectable chemicals that bind (chelate) iron in a form that allows iron excretion in urine.

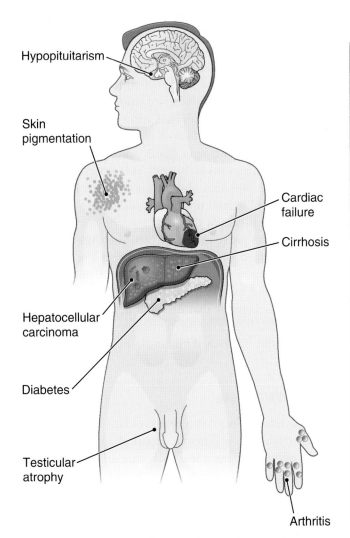

Figure 16-18 Complications of hemochromatosis.

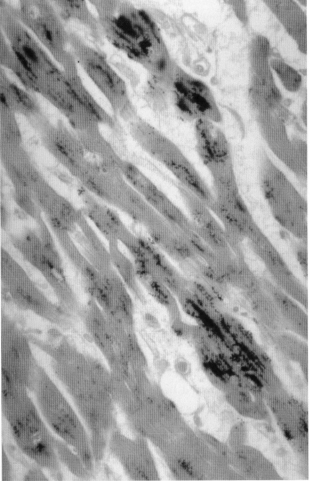

Figure 16-19 Hemochromatosis. Iron stain of myocardium.

WILSON DISEASE

Wilson disease is a rare autosomal recessive inherited disorder of copper metabolism that results in toxic accumulation of copper, mainly in the brain and liver. Copper is absorbed in the gut and excreted in bile. Absorbed copper is carried by albumin to the liver, where it is bound to a copper-bearing protein, *ceruloplasmin*, and secreted back into blood for metabolic distribution. In Wilson disease biliary excretion of copper is decreased, and copper accumulates, with toxic effect, primarily in the liver and brain. Blood levels of copper and ceruloplasmin are low in Wilson disease.

First symptoms may occur at any age but are usually manifest by young adult years. Earliest signs are neurologic—behavioral oddities, psychosis, or tremors and abnormal gait. The liver may show fatty change and chronic hepatitis or cirrhosis, changes that combined with the neurologic symptoms may result in misdiagnosis of alcoholic liver disease. The diagnosis of Wilson disease can be confirmed by liver biopsy slides stained for copper. Copper deposits in the eye also occur in Wilson disease, demonstrated as a brown-green arc (Kayser-Fleischer ring) where the sclera meets the cornea. Early diagnosis is critical. Although many patients given long-term copper chelation therapy do well, in some liver disease is relentless, and liver transplantation offers the only hope.

HEREDITARY ALPHA-1 ANTITRYPSIN DEFICIENCY

Alpha-1 antitrypsin (AAT), a protein made by the liver, inhibits the action of trypsin and other protein-digesting enzymes that are released by neutrophils in acute inflammatory reactions. AAT was discussed in Chapter 14 because of its importance in the pathogenesis of emphysema caused by smoking. AAT *deficiency* is an inherited disorder that results in low levels of AAT activity in the lungs and accumulation of excessive amounts of defective AAT in the liver, which appear in liver cells as distinctive protein globules and damage liver cells by an unknown mechanism.

Only about 10% of patients with AAT deficiency develop clinically significant liver disease. In a minority of patients AAT deficiency appears initially as *neonatal cholestasis* (discussed below). However, in most patients liver disease does not appear until hepatitis or cirrhosis is diagnosed in adolescence or adult life. The lungs are not severely affected unless the patient smokes, in which case early and severe emphysema occurs. Smoking causes inflammation, which results in release of protein-digesting enzymes that are not opposed by AAT, and the diminished AAT activity in the lungs allows the inflammatory enzymes to dissolve alveolar septa to produce emphysema.

In patients with liver or lung disease, the diagnosis is made by finding low levels of blood AAT activity and characteristic microscopic evidence of AAT accumulation in hepatocytes.

NEONATAL CHOLESTASIS, BILIARY ATRESIA, AND HEPATITIS

Almost all newborns, premature infants in particular, have *physiologic jaundice* because of increased *unconjugated* bilirubin for a week or two after birth, until the liver matures enough to produce the glucuronide necessary to conjugate bilirubin. Jaundice associated with other causes usually demonstrates an increase of *conjugated* bilirubin and is termed **neonatal cholestasis** until a definitive cause can be determined. Neonatal cholestasis results from one of two main types of defects: bile duct obstruction, usually termed **primary biliary atresia**, and **neonatal hepatitis**, a collective term for everything else. It is important to realize that these are *clinical terms of convenience* and not specific diagnoses, nor are the diseases necessarily inflammatory. The finding of increased neonatal conjugated bilirubin should stimulate a search for identifiable infectious, toxic, or metabolic disease (of which alpha-1 antitrypsin deficiency is the most common). Affected neonates typically have jaundice, dark urine, light stools, and an enlarged liver. Differential diagnosis is difficult but important because extrahepatic bile duct obstruction is sometimes surgically correctible, and prolonged obstruction can cause severe liver disease or death.

Most cases prove to be idiopathic hepatitis or biliary stenosis, which together probably represent a continuum of diseases from diffuse hepatic inflammation on the one hand to fibrous scarring of bile ducts on the other. This suggests that neonatal hepatitis and biliary atresia result from a common inflammatory process that might better be termed "infantile obstructive cholangiopathy."

REYE SYNDROME

Reye syndrome is a combination of fatty liver and acute brain dysfunction (encephalopathy) in children that most often develops a few days after an acute viral illness treated with aspirin. Onset is heralded by severe vomiting, lethargy, irritability, and hepatomegaly. Jaundice is usually absent initially. About 25% of these youngsters progress to coma. Death may be attributable to liver or to neurologic disease. The cause is unknown, but epidemiologic evidence links it to aspirin administration for viral illness in persons less than 18 years of age. The disease is more complex than simple aspirin toxicity because the doses consumed are far too small to be toxic. Aspirin is now rarely used in the United States to treat childhood fevers, and Reye syndrome is therefore uncommon in the United States.

Disease of Intrahepatic Bile Ducts

Prolonged obstruction in the *extra*hepatic biliary tree results in severe *intra*hepatic damage. The most common cause of obstruction is cholelithiasis (gallstones), discussed below. Other causes of obstruction include biliary stenosis, malignancy in the head of the pancreas, and fibrous strictures (scars) from surgical procedures. Extrahepatic obstruction leads to nonbacterial inflammation in small, intrahepatic bile ducts, which if prolonged leads to a special type of cirrhosis, *secondary biliary cirrhosis*. Obstruction also encourages ascending bacterial infection from the GI tract (*ascending cholangitis*).

PRIMARY BILIARY CIRRHOSIS

Primary biliary cirrhosis is an autoimmune disease that evolves from inflammatory destruction of intrahepatic bile ducts. Nearly 90% of patients also have another autoimmune disease (Chapter 8) such as systemic lupus or Sjögren syndrome, and virtually all have high titers of *antimitochondrial antibody*. As is illustrated in Figure 16-20, biopsy in early disease reveals accumulations of lymphocytes surrounding bile ducts. Later, bile duct scarring occurs and progresses to cirrhosis.

Nearly all patients are middle-aged women who present with cholestasis. They have itchy skin (pruritus) and increased levels of blood cholesterol because of retained bile acids, and their blood alkaline phosphatase level is markedly elevated because of damage to the bile duct epithelium. Jaundice appears late and usually signals that hepatic failure is near. Impaired bile excretion may cause malabsorption syndrome (Chapter 15). Death results from hepatic failure and portal hypertension. The only effective treatment is liver transplantation.

PRIMARY SCLEROSING CHOLANGITIS

Primary sclerosing cholangitis is a chronic liver disease caused by inflammation and fibrosis of intrahepatic and extrahepatic bile ducts. Two thirds of patients have ulcerative colitis (Chapter 15). Less often, other inflammatory bowel disease is present; however, in most of the other third no underlying disease can be found. The

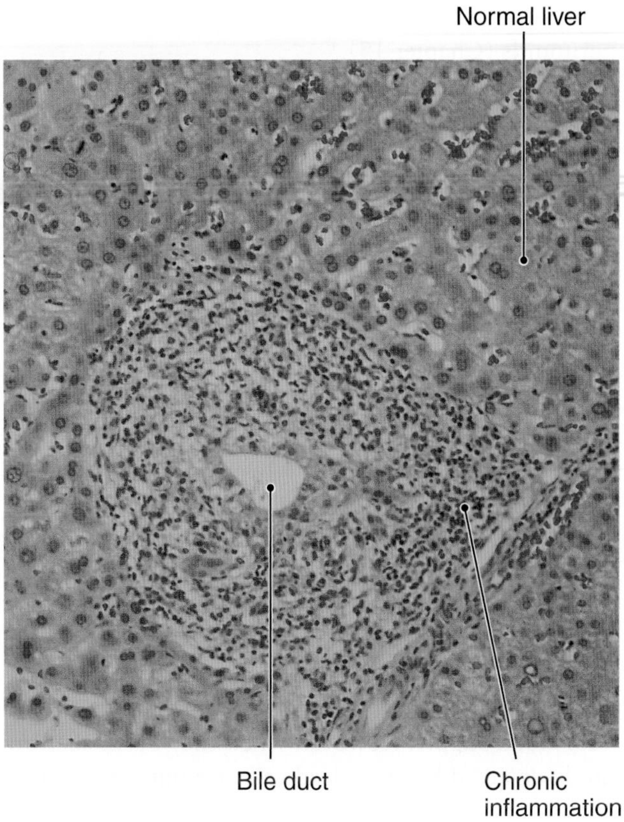

Figure 16-20 **Primary biliary cirrhosis.** Microscopic study of early stage showing a collar of chronic inflammatory cells (lymphocytes) around small bile duct.

pathology of sclerosing cholangitis is characterized by scarring of bile ducts inside and outside of the liver. Microscopically, findings in the liver are distinctive—onionskin fibrosis that encircles and eventually destroys the ducts.

Although most patients with ulcerative colitis are women, most patients with primary sclerosing cholangitis are men under age 40. The typical patient is an adult male with long-standing ulcerative colitis who slowly develops signs and symptoms of liver disease. Few patients have blood autoimmune antibodies. Biliary cirrhosis is the end point. Liver transplantation is the definitive treatment.

Circulatory Disorders

Blood flow may be obstructed in the portal vein as it flows into the liver, as it flows through the liver, or in the hepatic vein as it flows out of the liver.

The portal vein can become obstructed and produce changes similar to the portal hypertension caused by cirrhosis. Obstruction is usually attributable to thrombosis (Chapter 5) associated with intra-abdominal inflammation, such as pancreatitis, abdominal surgery, or peritonitis (Chapter 15).

The most common cause of obstructed blood flow through the liver is *chronic passive congestion*, which is usually associated with right heart failure (Chapter 13), as blood "dams up" trying to enter the heart. Sluggish flow in the liver usually causes minor liver cell damage detectable only by an increase of liver enzyme levels in blood. Cirrhosis with portal hypertension (discussed above) is the most serious cause of obstructed blood flow through the liver.

Blood flowing out of the liver can be obstructed in diseases that involve the hepatic vein. The most common of these is hepatic vein thrombosis (*Budd-Chiari syndrome*), which is usually attributable to diseases associated with an increased tendency for intravascular coagulation and thrombosis—polycythemia vera (Chapter 11), pregnancy, and oral contraceptive use (Chapter 21). Hepatic vein obstruction causes severe congestion and liver cell necrosis. The mortality rate is high.

Liver *infarcts* are uncommon because the liver has a dual blood supply. However, when they occur they are rarely detected because dead cells are quickly replaced by new ones, thanks to the liver's remarkable power of regeneration.

Tumors of the Liver

The most common neoplasm *in* (not *of*) the liver is metastatic carcinoma (Fig. 16-21), usually from a primary malignancy in the colon, lung, or breast.

The most common *benign* tumor of the liver is *cavernous hemangioma*, a vascular mass that is not neoplastic and is composed of dilated blood vessels. Cavernous hemangiomas are usually small and located immediately beneath the fibrous capsule of the liver. *Liver cell adenoma* is a benign neoplasm of hepatocytes and is en-

countered most often in young women taking oral contraceptives. It may become quite large and may rupture, especially during pregnancy, to cause life-threatening intra-abdominal hemorrhage.

PRIMARY CARCINOMAS OF THE LIVER

Hepatocellular carcinoma is a malignant neoplasm of hepatocytes that is usually related to chronic hepatitis virus B and C infections—chronic hepatitis or the carrier state confers a $200\times$ increased risk of hepatocellular carcinoma. Despite the relative rarity of hepatocellular carcinoma in the United States, its incidence in Africa and Asia, where hepatitis B is exceedingly common, makes it arguably the most common malignant tumor of humans. Chronic hepatitis C with cirrhosis is the major cause in industrialized nations. Hepatocellular carcinoma also occurs in association with cirrhosis caused by hemochromatosis and alpha-1 antitrypsin deficiency.

Hepatocellular carcinoma usually grows as a single massive neoplasm (Fig. 16-22). It has a marked tendency to invade hepatic veins and may snake its way up the hepatic vein and far into the vena cava. Hematogenous (blood borne) metastases are common.

The usual patient has preexisting liver disease. Hepatocellular carcinoma may be heralded by a sudden increase of liver size, sudden worsening of ascites, appearance of bloody ascites, or intense abdominal pain. Most patients have increased levels of *alpha-fetoprotein* in their blood, although this is not a specific marker because increases are seen in cirrhosis, other liver dis-

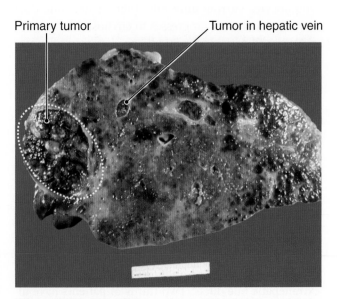

Primary tumor   Tumor in hepatic vein

***Figure 16-22* Hepatocellular carcinoma.** The primary tumor is a single, large mass, which can be seen invading an intrahepatic branch of the hepatic vein. The liver is cirrhotic; cirrhosis is a major cause of hepatocellular carcinoma.

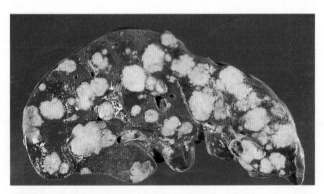

***Figure 16-21* Metastatic carcinoma in liver.** This patient had colon cancer, which metastasized up the portal vein to the liver.

eases, pregnancy, and other conditions. Marked elevations, however, are rarely seen in any disease other than hepatocellular carcinoma. The prognosis for patients with hepatocellular carcinoma is grim; most patients die of tumor in a short period of time. Death usually follows profound wasting (cachexia), hepatic coma, or GI bleeding. HBV vaccinations have proven effective in lowering the incidence of hepatocellular carcinoma in areas where hepatitis B is acquired early in life.

CHOLANGIOCARCINOMA

Cholangiocarcinoma is a malignancy of bile duct epithelium; that is, the cells that line bile ducts. In many aspects, cholangiocarcinoma is very different from hepatocellular carcinoma. Most cases arise without known preexisting risk factors, but known predisposition is associated with two specific conditions: primary sclerosing cholangitis and chronic liver infection with schistosomiasis (parasites seen in Africa, Asia, and South America). Cholangiocarcinoma tends to be more aggressive than hepatocellular carcinoma—patients quickly develop severe cachexia, hepatic coma, and esophageal varices with fatal hemorrhage, and very few survive five years. Legendary American football running back Walter Payton developed cholangiocarcinoma as a consequence of chronic sclerosing cholangitis, and he died when he was but 45 years old.

Diseases of the Gallbladder and Extrahepatic Bile Ducts

Recall that the biliary tree begins as tiny ducts that gradually grow larger as they merge, like rivers leading to the sea, until they form the common bile duct that exits the liver to connect with the duodenum at the ampulla of Vater. The gallbladder, attached to one side of the common bile duct, holds a reserve of bile that is discharged into the common bile duct after meals.

DISEASES OF THE GALLBLADDER

Diseases of the gallbladder are not complicated, and they are very common. Almost all gallbladder and biliary tract disease occurs as a result of inflammation, closely related to the presence of gallstones. There are two major varieties of gallstones: cholesterol stones and pigment stones.

Cholelithiasis (Gallstones)

Stones in the gallbladder or biliary tree are referred to collectively as **cholelithiasis**. Stones in the bile ducts are

referred to as **choledocholithiasis**. The great majority of gallstones form in the gallbladder. Most patients have multiple stones, sometimes several dozen. In the United States about one million new cases are diagnosed each year, half requiring surgery. The surgical mortality rate is less than 1%.

Most gallstones (80%) are **cholesterol gallstones**, which form when bile becomes oversaturated with cholesterol. Why some people develop gallstones and others do not is a mystery; however, there are certain well-known conditions associated with the development of cholesterol stones:

- *Age and gender*: Older people have more gallstones than younger ones do. In their reproductive years, women are three times more likely than men to have gallstones.
- *Weight*: Obese people are much more likely to develop cholesterol stones.
- *Ethnic, hereditary, and geographic factors*: Cholesterol gallstones occur in about 75% of Pima, Hopi, and Navajo Native Americans. A family history of gallstones imparts increased risk. Gallstones are more common in industrialized countries than in developing ones.
- *Drugs*: Oral contraceptives and estrogen therapy increase hepatic uptake and secretion of cholesterol.
- *Acquired conditions*: Any condition that causes decreased gallbladder motility (for instance, pregnancy, rapid weight loss, and spinal cord injury) predisposes to gallstones.

> *About 10–20% of people develop gallstones. The rate is much higher in Hispanics, and in Native Americans in the southwestern United States.*

Figure 16-23 illustrates *pure cholesterol stones*, which are semi-translucent, yellowish, and egg shaped. Cholesterol stones arise only in the gallbladder, but pigment stones may arise in the biliary tree as well.

Pigment gallstones, accounting for the remaining 20% of gallstones, are composed of bilirubin and bile substances other than cholesterol. The greatest risk factor for pigment gallstones is hemolysis of red blood cells, as occurs with sickle cell anemia (Chapter 11), which increases the amount of bilirubin delivered to the liver to be excreted in bile. Other risk factors for pigment gallstones are not so well understood. As is depicted in Figure 16-24, pigment stones are dark brown or black and have multiple flat surfaces.

Gallstones usually do not cause symptoms until they begin to move through bile ducts, and a majority of gall-

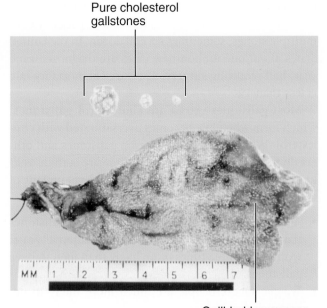

Pure cholesterol
gallstones

Gallbladder mucosa
with heavy deposits
of cholesterol (yellow)

Figure 16-23 **Cholelithiasis (cholesterol gallstones) and chronic cholecystitis.** Normally gallbladder mucosa is green because of staining by normal bile. In this patient cholesterol deposits caused a bright yellow coloration. Microscopic study of the gallbladder wall revealed chronic inflammation.

stones can exist for decades or a lifetime without symptoms. Big stones are usually found in the gallbladder and remain there silently. Very small stones can be passed from the gallbladder or from intrahepatic ducts without symptoms. However, mid-sized stones create most problems because they are small enough to pass from the gallbladder or intrahepatic duct, but are too big to pass out smoothly. Passage of a stone may cause extraordinarily painful cramps—**biliary colic**—in the right upper quadrant or upper abdomen, which is usually accompanied by nausea and vomiting. Fever, which does not occur in uncomplicated cholelithiasis, should arouse suspicion of ascending bacterial infection (ascending cholangitis), which is a threat when stones are passed or become lodged in bile ducts. Other complications include cholecystitis, pancreatitis, perforation, and empyema of the gallbladder.

Because gallstones are often discovered during evaluation of other medical problems, finding asymptomatic stones forces a decision to leave it alone or to do surgery. Individual situations differ and stone behavior is unpredictable—about 2% of silent stones become symptomatic each year. Most patients elect to avoid surgery until symptoms occur.

Cholecystitis

Cholecystitis is inflammation of the gallbladder. **Acute cholecystitis** is the most common major complication of gallstones: more than 90% of cases are associated with stone obstruction of the neck of the gallbladder. Most patients have multiple stones. Bacterial infection usually isn't present but may occur later and cause the lumen of the gallbladder to fill with pus (*empyema*), as is depicted in Figure 16-25. On the other hand, acute

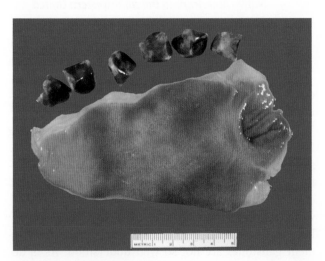

Figure 16-24 **Cholelithiasis (pigment stones) and chronic cholecystitis.** Normally gallbladder mucosa is green because of staining by normal bile. When opened, the lumen contained mucus only; no bile was present, indicating that stones had blocked the cystic duct. Microscopic study of the gallbladder wall revealed chronic inflammation.

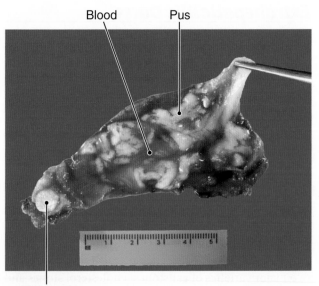

Blood   Pus

Cholesterol stone
lodged in neck of
gallbladder

Figure 16-25 **Acute cholecystitis with empyema.** Gallbladder is filled with blood and pus. Note a pure cholesterol stone lodged in the gallbladder neck where the cystic duct arises.

cholecystitis can occur without stones—about 5–10% of gallbladders removed for acute cholecystitis contain no stones. Most of these patients have other important conditions, such as pregnancy, burns, sepsis, or recent major surgery. In acute cholecystitis the gallbladder is enlarged, tense, and inflamed and in some instances may be necrotic or filled with pus.

Clinically the presentation of acute cholecystitis can vary from persistent, rather mild right upper abdominal pain to severe, crampy pain (colic) associated with fever, nausea, vomiting, prostration, and leukocytosis (increased granulocytes in the peripheral blood, Chapter 3). Jaundice (because of increased *conjugated* bilirubin) suggests obstruction by a stone in the common bile duct. Mild attacks usually resolve in a few days or a week, but about 25% require immediate surgery.

As is depicted in Figure 16-26, **chronic cholecystitis** may develop after numerous episodes of acute cholecystitis, but most often it occurs without a history of acute attacks. Most cases are nonbacterial: in only a third of cases can bacteria be cultured from the bile. Chronic cholecystitis is almost always associated with gallstones, but the exact role stones play is unclear. Obstruction is not necessary. Stones may be the result, not the cause, of the inflammation. At the very least it appears that stones and inflammation coexist in gallbladders for many years.

Clinically, chronic cholecystitis is not as dramatic as an acute attack and is usually characterized by episodes of mild to moderate right upper quadrant pain with nausea, vomiting, and intolerance for fatty foods (because fatty foods stimulate the gallbladder to contract and send bile into the intestine to emulsify the fat). Most cases warrant surgery because complications can be severe—ascending cholangitis, gallbladder perforation with peritonitis, or septicemia (bacterial infection of blood).

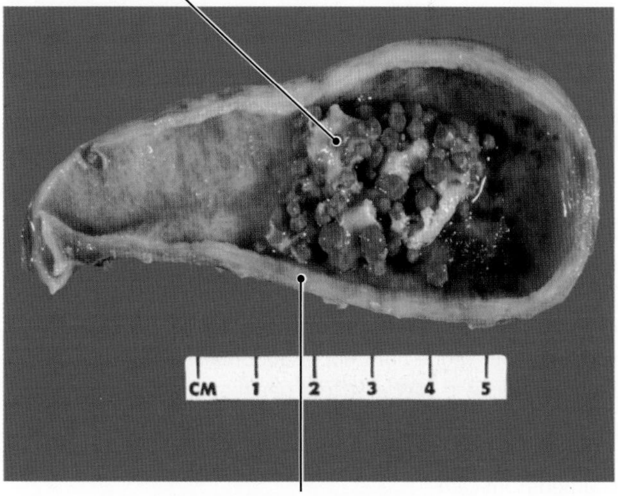

Tumors of the Gallbladder

Tumors of the gallbladder are uncommon. Most common are small benign mucosal papillary growths that occur with gallstones. Carcinomas of the gallbladder are adenocarcinomas and are also associated with gallstones. At the time of discovery most are beyond hope of cure, and five-year survival is less than 5%.

DISEASES OF EXTRAHEPATIC BILE DUCTS

Obstruction is the most important problem of the extrahepatic bile ducts. Figure 16-27 depicts the major causes. Gallstones are by far the most common cause of obstruction. Other causes include cancer of the head of the pancreas, pancreatitis, inflammatory disease of the ducts, and postoperative scarring. In industrialized nations, most gallstones form in the gallbladder, but in Asia there is a much higher prevalence of primary stone formation in ducts. Stones in the bile ducts (*choledocholithiasis*) are the main cause of **ascending cholangitis**, a bacterial infection of the biliary tree caused by intestinal bacteria that travel up the common bile duct into the liver. Not every patient with ductal stones develops ascending cholangitis, but ascending cholangitis almost never occurs without obstruction. Sepsis (bloodstream infection) is the most important clinical complication, far outweighing cholestasis. In its most severe form it may cause general sepsis and intrahepatic abscesses. Other acute complications of ductal stones and obstruction include acute pancreatitis and acute cholecystitis. Chronic obstruction may cause chronic liver disease with secondary biliary cirrhosis.

Extrahepatic **biliary atresia** is an obstruction of extrahepatic bile ducts discussed above in conjunction with *neonatal cholestasis*. Biliary atresia is a pediatric disease (Chapter 7) and, strictly speaking, is not atresia (failure to develop) because most affected infants are born with patent bile ducts that become obstructed and scarred. The cause is unknown. It accounts for over half of children referred for liver transplantation.

Cholangiocarcinomas of the extrahepatic bile ducts are rare and usually fatal, but associated with a somewhat longer survival than hepatic cholangiocarcinomas because they cause obstructive signs and symptoms earlier and are detected earlier. ∎

Pigment stones
and mucus

Thick, fibrotic gallbladder wall

Figure 16-26 **Chronic cholecystitis and cholelithiasis.** Gallbladder contains mucus and numerous pigment stones. No normal bile is present. Note thick gallbladder wall, caused by chronic inflammation and fibrosis.

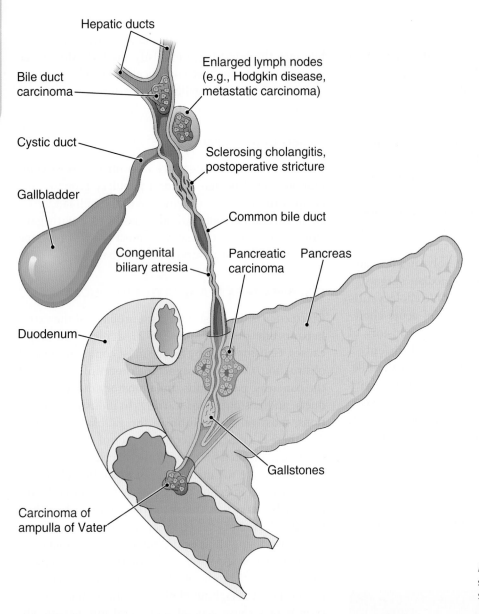

Hepatic ducts

Bile duct carcinoma

Enlarged lymph nodes (e.g., Hodgkin disease, metastatic carcinoma)

Cystic duct

Sclerosing cholangitis, postoperative stricture

Gallbladder

Common bile duct

Congenital biliary atresia

Pancreatic carcinoma

Pancreas

Duodenum

Gallstones

Carcinoma of ampulla of Vater

Figure 16-27 **Extrahepatic biliary obstruction.** The illustration shows the sites and causes of obstruction.

CASE STUDY 16-1 *"I DIDN'T GIVE IT A SECOND THOUGHT"*

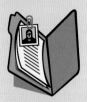

TOPIC
Hepatitis C infection

THE CASE
Setting: You are employed in the office of a liver disease specialist, where one of your tasks is to obtain medical histories and do physical examinations on new patients.

Clinical history: A 48-year-old banker is referred to the office of a liver disease specialist. The entry on her appointment sheet says "hepatitis C?"

The patient is currently asymptomatic, but when she was 22 years old, she underwent a caesarian section that required transfusion of two units of packed red blood cells. About 2 months following this, she experienced an episode of jaundice, dark urine, pale stools, anorexia, nausea, and vomiting with vague right upper abdominal discomfort. An infectious disease specialist told her that she had "non-A, non-B" hepatitis. She was ill for several weeks, but after 3 months was told she was completely recovered and discharged from care.

"I didn't give it a second thought," she adds. "After it was all over, I felt completely normal." ▶

[Case 16-1, continued]

She is in the office now because during a recent change of employment she took an insurance physical examination that revealed mildly increased levels of liver enzymes in her blood. Complete blood count, urinalysis, and other blood chemistries were unremarkable.

Your questioning reveals that she is employed full time and has occasional episodes of fatigue and "the blues." Otherwise, she is in excellent health and has not needed to see a physician except for her annual gynecologic exam and pap smear. She denies having sex with anyone but her husband. She usually drinks a glass of wine with dinner. She has never smoked. In college she "experimented" with marijuana but never injected drugs. She is not taking prescription drugs and denies current illegal drug use of any kind.

Physical examination and other data: She appears her stated age and is articulate and cooperative. She is very anxious about what might be wrong. Vital signs and physical examination are unremarkable. Neither liver nor spleen can be palpated. No jaundice is noted. Her skin shows no evidence of spider angiomata, palmar erythema, or bruises. She does not have hemorrhoids. A vaginal examination is not done.

Clinical course: The blood studies you order show mild increases of liver enzymes and the presence of HCV-RNA. She refuses the offer of liver biopsy but agrees to alpha-2a interferon therapy, which is administered intravenously three times a week for a year under your supervision. At the conclusion of therapy, liver enzymes are normal, and HCV-RNA is no longer detectable. Follow up laboratory studies remain normal for 2 years after therapy, and she is discharged back to the care of her usual physician.

DISCUSSION

This patient became infected with hepatitis C virus from a blood transfusion before the discovery of hepatitis C virus and, therefore, before a way existed to screen blood donors and blood products for infection from what was called at that time "non-A, non-B hepatitis." Modern screening is effective and has reduced the chance of blood product infection to about one case in 2 million transfusions. Although most newly infected patients give no history of transfusion or illicit drug use, among those new HCV infections for which a cause can be determined, most are associated with intravenous drug use.

This patient was unusual in that she developed an acute hepatitis syndrome with the initial infection, whereas most new HCV infections are asymptomatic. At your initial meeting with this patient, her history and lab studies were enough to convince her physicians to treat her without the definitive proof of chronic hepatitis that could have been provided by a liver biopsy.

She had an excellent response to therapy. Only about one fourth of patients are so lucky; most do not respond to therapy. However, of those who do respond well, most do not relapse. She may have been permanently cured; only time will tell.

POINTS TO REMEMBER

- Half of all chronic liver disease in the United States is caused by chronic hepatitis C.
- Blood and blood products for transfusion or injection are safer now than heretofore.
- Blood testing is essential in the diagnosis of viral hepatitis.

Objectives Recap

1. *Trace the flow of blood through the liver*: Venous blood flows from intestinal veins up the portal vein, which divides into progressively smaller vessels to form a second capillary network in the liver. From these hepatic capillaries blood flows into the hepatic vein and then into the inferior vena cava and the main systemic circulation. Arterial blood flows through a second set of capillaries that branch from the hepatic artery, and then mixes with portal blood to flow through the hepatic vein and into the vena cava.

2. *Name the major functions of the liver*: The liver 1) clears blood of toxins, metabolic waste, and hormones; 2) converts glucose into glycogen for energy storage and reconverts it to glucose on demand; 3) produces most plasma proteins, with the exception of antibodies; 4) excretes bilirubin into bile; and 5) produces bile acids and excretes them into bile.

3. *Explain the enterohepatic circulation*: Enterohepatic circulation refers to excretion of bile acids (made from cholesterol) from the liver into the intestine and the reabsorption of most of the bile acids (and their cholesterol) by the intestine for recirculation through the portal system and reuse by the liver. Most cholesterol absorbed by the intestine comes from reabsorbed bile acids, not dietary cholesterol.

4. *Name the major functional reactions of the liver to injury*: Jaundice, cholestasis, and hepatic failure.

5. *Explain the difference between conjugated and unconjugated bilirubin*: Unconjugated bilirubin is not water soluble and is attached to albumin for

transport to the liver, where it is conjugated (joined) to glucuronide and becomes water soluble and can be excreted in bile.

6. *Name one cause of unconjugated hyperbilirubinemia and one of conjugated hyperbilirubinemia*: Unconjugated hyperbilirubinemia can occur with hemolytic anemia, such as sickle cell disease, which can cause increased production of unconjugated bilirubin. Conjugated hyperbilirubinemia occurs when bile flow is obstructed after bilirubin has been conjugated by the liver, such as with bile duct obstruction.

7. *Define cirrhosis and name the two most common causes*: Cirrhosis is a progressive, patterned fibrosis of the entire liver. The most common causes are alcoholism and chronic hepatitis.

8. *Explain why cirrhosis causes portal hypertension*: Portal hypertension occurs when there is obstruction of portal blood flow caused by the choking action of the dense fibrous bands of cirrhosis, which scar and shrink the liver.

9. *Name two hemodynamic consequences of portal hypertension*: The hemodynamic consequences of portal hypertension are ascites, congestive splenomegaly, esophageal varices, hemorrhoids, and radiating prominent periumbilical veins known as *caput medusa*.

10. *Outline the main clinical manifestations of cirrhosis*: 1) Portal hypertension causes hemorrhoids, esophageal varices, splenomegaly, and caput medusa veins radiating from the umbilicus, and contributes to the formation of ascites. 2) Failing hepatic metabolism of estrogen results in high blood estrogen, which in men accounts for thinning scalp and genital hair, female-like breasts (gynecomastia), red palms (palmar erythema), atrophic testes, and spider angiomas—small vascular malformations of skin that feature tiny central vessels from which spider-like vessels radiate outward. Women may have abnormal menstrual bleeding. 3) Failing hepatic metabolism of ammonia and other waste products accounts for hepatic coma and fetor hepaticus (liver breath). 4) Failing hepatic excretion of bilirubin causes jaundice. 5) Failing hepatic protein synthesis causes a decrease in plasma albumin, which contributes to ascites and peripheral edema (Chapter 5), and decreased levels of blood coagulation factors accounts for bleeding tendencies, usually evident as easy bruising (skin purpura).

11. *Name several clinicopathologic syndromes associated with viral hepatitis*: Asymptomatic hepatitis, carrier state, acute viral hepatitis, chronic viral hepatitis, fulminant hepatic failure, hepatocellular carcinoma.

12. *Contrast the mode of transmission and clinical course of hepatitis A and hepatitis B*: Hepatitis A is transmitted by personal contact and oral-fecal contamination of food and water; hepatitis B by transfusion, injection of blood products, renal dialysis, needlestick accidents among health care workers, intravenous drug use, and sexual activity. Hepatitis A is a benign, self-limited disease with no carrier state or chronic hepatitis; hepatitis B is much more serious and may cause symptomatic acute hepatitis, fulminant hepatitis with massive liver necrosis, or chronic hepatitis that may advance to cirrhosis; a small percentage of patients becomes carriers.

13. *Name the most important epidemiologic fact about hepatitis C, and name the most common serious consequences of hepatitis C infection*: Hepatitis C infection is largely the consequence of intravenous drug abuse. It has a high rate of progression to chronic hepatitis and cirrhosis.

14. *Name one common acute and one common chronic change induced in the liver due to alcohol abuse*: The most common acute change is fatty metamorphosis (steatosis); the most common serious chronic change is cirrhosis.

15. *Explain the difference between primary biliary cirrhosis and sclerosing cholangitis*: Primary biliary cirrhosis is an autoimmune disease of intrahepatic bile ducts. Most patients have other autoimmune disease and antimitochondrial antibody in their blood. Primary sclerosing cholangitis is a chronic inflammatory disease of intrahepatic and extrahepatic bile ducts usually associated with ulcerative colitis.

16. *Name the liver condition most commonly associated with hepatocellular carcinoma*: Chronic hepatitis, caused by hepatitis B or hepatitis C infection.

17. *Name the two major categories of gallstones, and know which is the most common*: Cholesterol stones (most common) and pigment stones.

18. *Name several risk factors that favor the formation of gallstones*: Age, gender, and ethnicity. The old have more stones than young, women more than men, Native Americans and Hispanics more than Anglos. Also associated with gallstones are oral contraceptives and estrogen replacement therapy, obesity, hemolytic anemia, and rapid weight loss.

19. *Discuss some of the most common causes of extrahepatic bile duct obstruction*: Gallstones are the most common cause of extrahepatic biliary obstruction. Other causes include biliary atresia in newborn infants, cancer of the head of the pancreas, pancreatitis, inflammatory disease of the ducts, and postoperative scarring. A serious complication of biliary obstruction is ascending cholangitis, a bacterial infection that enters the biliary tree from the intestine.

Typical Test Questions

1. The enterohepatic circulation refers to
   A. Blood flow through hepatic sinusoids
   B. Circulation of bile within the liver
   C. Bile acid absorption from the intestine
   D. Distribution of blood between liver arteries and veins

2. Hepatitis B infection
   A. Is the most common viral hepatitis in the United States
   B. Causes epidemics of infection
   C. Of all hepatitis viruses is most likely to cause chronic hepatitis and cirrhosis
   D. Is transmitted parenterally or by sexual contact

3. Which of the following statements about cirrhosis is false?
   A. It is irreversible
   B. Portal cirrhosis is more common than biliary cirrhosis
   C. Alcoholism produces biliary cirrhosis
   D. The pattern and size of hepatic nodules are not useful in determining etiology

4. Concerning cholelithiasis and cholecystitis, which of the following is false?
   A. Bacterial infection causes most cholecystitis
   B. Cholesterol stones are more common than pigment stones

   C. Ascending cholangitis is closely linked to choledocholithiasis
   D. Most patients with chronic cholecystitis have gallstones in the gallbladder

5. Which of the following is false?
   A. Most liver abscesses worldwide are caused by amebiasis
   B. Most patients with autoimmune hepatitis have anti-mitochondrial antibody
   C. The first stage of alcoholic liver disease is fatty liver
   D. Genetic hemochromatosis can be treated effectively by phlebotomy

6. True or false? Biliary obstruction causes increased conjugated bilirubin.

7. True or false? Esophageal varices are a direct consequence of portal hypertension.

8. True or false? Hepatitis A is usually transmitted by blood transfusion or needlestick.

9. True or false? Cirrhosis is the most common cause of portal hypertension.

10. True or false? Acute cholecystitis is the most common major complication of gallstones.

Diseases of the Pancreas

This chapter begins with a review of the normal pancreas and its digestive and endocrine functions. Major diseases and disorders discussed include diabetes, pancreatitis, and pancreatic cancer.

BACK TO BASICS
- The Digestive (Exocrine) Pancreas
- The Hormonal (Endocrine) Pancreas

DISEASES OF THE DIGESTIVE (EXOCRINE) PANCREAS
- Pancreatitis
- Carcinoma of the Pancreas

DISEASES OF THE HORMONAL (ENDOCRINE) PANCREAS
- Diabetes Mellitus
- Pancreatic Endocrine Neoplasms

Learning Objectives

After studying this chapter you should be able to:

1. Discuss the anatomy of the pancreas, and make a clear distinction between the digestive and the hormonal pancreas
2. Explain the relationship of glucose, glucagon, and insulin to one another and to stored glycogen
3. Name the two most common causes of acute pancreatitis
4. Explain autodigestion in acute pancreatitis
5. Explain why a patient with acute hemorrhagic pancreatitis may develop hypovolemic shock or hypocalcemia
6. Contrast acute and chronic pancreatitis, and describe their relationship to one another
7. Name the most common cause of chronic pancreatitis
8. Discuss the clinical presentation and complications of adenocarcinoma of the pancreas, and give a reasonable estimate of the five-year survival rate
9. Explain the pathogenesis of type 1 diabetes
10. Explain the pathogenesis of type 2 diabetes
11. Name the most important factor in the development of type 2 diabetes
12. Name the two types of diabetic coma and the pathogenesis of each
13. Explain the importance in diabetes of hyperglycemia and glycosylation
14. Explain diabetic microvascular disease
15. Name the leading causes of death in diabetes
16. Name some criteria for the diagnosis of diabetes

BACK TO BASICS

- exocrine
- endocrine
- protease
- lipase
- amylase
- islets of Langerhans
- glucagon
- insulin

DISEASES OF THE DIGESTIVE (EXOCRINE) PANCREAS

- pancreatitis
- carcinoma of the pancreas

DISEASES OF THE HORMONAL (ENDOCRINE) PANCREAS

- hyperglycemia
- type 1 diabetes
- type 2 diabetes
- prediabetes
- glycosuria
- ketones
- diabetic ketoacidosis
- diabetic coma
- glycohemoglobin
- microvascular disease

I'm tired of all this nonsense about beauty being only skin-deep. That's deep enough. What do you want—an adorable pancreas?

JEAN KERR (1923–2003), U.S. AUTHOR AND PLAYWRIGHT, *MIRROR, MIRROR ON THE WALL*

▶ BACK TO BASICS

Anatomically the pancreas is a single organ; however, functionally it is two: an **exocrine** organ that secretes juice into *ducts* that carry it to the intestine, and an **endocrine** (without ducts) organ that secretes hormones directly into blood.

As is depicted in Figures 17-1 and 17-2, the pancreas is a tadpole-shaped organ about 5–6 inches (12–15 cm) long that is embedded in retroperitoneal fat of the mid abdomen and lies across the front of the aorta just below the stomach. The head is nestled in the duodenal loop, and the tail rests near the spleen. Ducts lead from individual pancreatic glands (acini) and join to form the **pancreatic duct**. In most people the pancreatic duct merges with the *common bile duct*, and together they pass through the head of the pancreas before emptying into the duodenum at the *ampulla of Vater*.

The pancreas is exceptional in two respects. First, it is the most inaccessible organ in the body, hidden among soft organs and structures that yield to a pancreatic mass, making pancreatic tumors very difficult to diagnose early. Second, the pancreas has large functional reserves, which means it is also a difficult task to make an early diagnosis of lost pancreatic function.

THE DIGESTIVE (EXOCRINE) PANCREAS

The digestive (**exocrine**) pancreas, which constitutes the bulk of the organ, is composed of acini and ducts. Epithelial cells of the acini excrete about 2–3 liters of alkaline pancreatic juice each day. This juice, a mix of about 20 digestive agents, water, bicarbonate, and mucus, is carried to the duodenum by the ducts. Protein-digesting *enzymes* (**proteases**) are secreted in *inactive* form as *zymogens* (otherwise the digestive juices would digest the organ before getting to the duodenum, a point to remember when reading below about pancreatitis). However, **lipase**, which digests fat, and **amylase**, which digests carbohydrate, are secreted in active form because the walls of the pancreatic ducts are composed of protein and thus are impervious to the action of these two enzymes. As additional insurance against self digestion, while still in the pancreas, pancreatic juice contains protease inhibitors, which become inactive in the intestine. Table 17-1 lists some of the more important pancreatic enzymes.

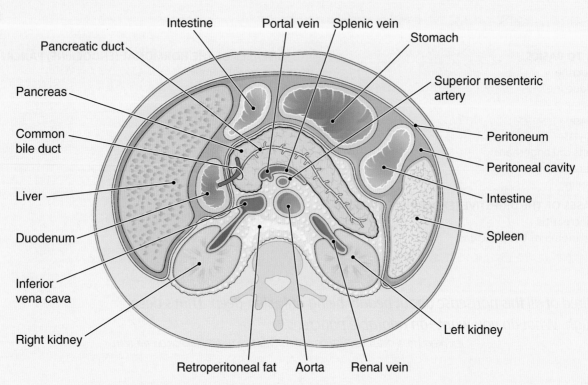

Figure 17-1 **The pancreas and its anatomic relationships.** Cross-section of the upper abdomen.

THE HORMONAL (ENDOCRINE) PANCREAS

The hormonal (**endocrine**) pancreas constitutes a small fraction of pancreatic mass and is composed of thousands of tiny **islets of Langerhans** scattered throughout the gland. The islets are clusters of cells not connected to the ductal system, and they secrete hormones directly into blood. **Hormones** are chemical compounds made in organs or tissues that act on other organs or tissues to stimulate or suppress them. The most important cells in the islets are:

- *Alpha cells*: secrete **glucagon**, a hormone whose main function is to stimulate liver output of glucose by converting glycogen to glucose and forming glucose from amino acids; at very high concentrations it also stimulates breakdown of fat for energy.
- *Beta cells*: secrete **insulin**, a hormone that stimulates cell uptake of glucose from blood, thereby lowering blood glucose levels.
- *Delta cells*: secrete *somatostatin*, a hormone that inhibits glucagon and insulin secretion and slows peristalsis in the gastrointestinal and biliary systems.

As is illustrated in Figure 17-3, the level of blood glucose is controlled by the opposing effects of *insulin* and *glucagon*, the two most important islet hormones.

The most important pancreatic hormone is **insulin**, a "gatekeeper" hormone that acts on muscle and other cell membranes to allow glucose to enter cells, where they can be burned for energy. A mutual push-pull relationship exists between insulin and glucose—a high blood level of glucose causes increased pancreatic secretion of insulin; a low level of blood glucose causes a decrease in insulin secretion. For example, an injection of insulin forces blood glucose levels down because it allows glucose to leave blood and enter cells. Likewise, as blood glucose level rises after a meal, the pancreas secretes more insulin to lower it. Moreover, vigorous exercise burns glucose, lowering blood glucose levels and decreasing beta-cell release of insulin.

A similar but less strong push-pull relationship exists between blood glucose and **glucagon**. It is convenient to think of glucagon as a "backup" system that releases energy from body stores. First, glucagon stimulates the liver to convert stored glycogen (Chapter 16) to glucose

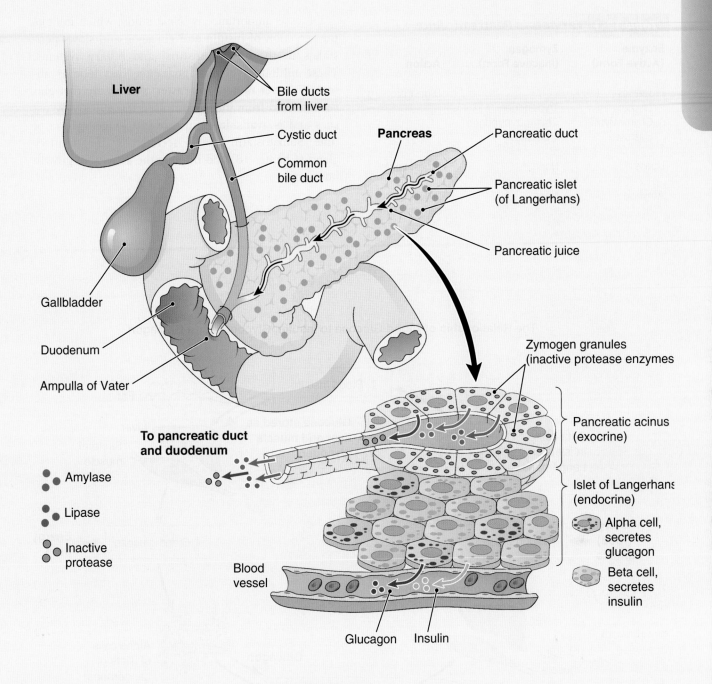

Figure 17-2 Anatomic detail of the pancreas.

and to form glucose from amino acids. For example, in starvation or prolonged fasting, a drop in blood glucose level forces the pancreas to secrete glucagon, which causes liver glycogen to be turned into blood glucose. Second, at high levels glucagon stimulates the break-

down of fat to be used as an energy source if glucose is not available, as occurs with starvation or fasting, or with insulin deficiency (diabetes), when cells cannot burn glucose because glucose cannot get into cells to be burned.

Table 17-1	Enzymes in Pancreatic Juice	
Enzyme (Active Form)	**Zymogen (Inactive Form)**	**Action**
Proteases		Digest proteins
Trypsin	Trypsinogen	
Chymotrypsin	Chymotrypsinogen	
Elastase	Proelastase	
Lipases	None	Digest lipids
Amylase	None	Digest carbohydrates

Of lesser importance is *somatostatin*, which inhibits the secretion of insulin and glucagon and slows peristalsis in the gastrointestinal and biliary systems. These inhibitory actions guarantee that food is absorbed slower rather than faster, and ensure that glucose derived from food is not used too quickly by tissues and is available for use over a longer period of time. Somatostatin is also secreted by the pituitary gland (Chapter 18) and inhibits the activity of growth hormone.

The Relationship of Blood Glucose to Insulin, Glycogen, and Glucagon

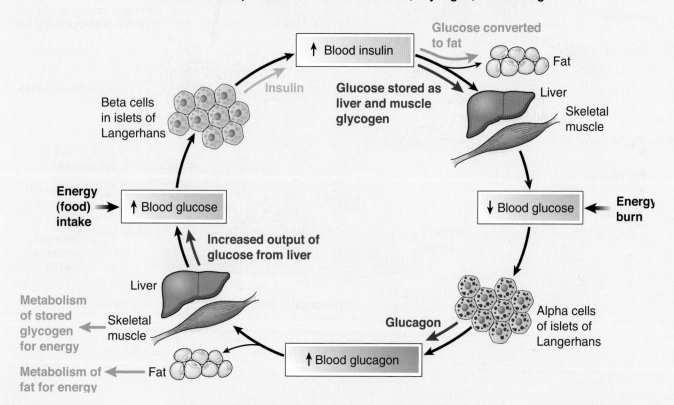

Figure 17-3 Glucose, glycogen, insulin, and glucagon metabolism.

MAJOR DETERMINANTS OF DISEASE

- The pancreas is an integral part of the digestive process, especially fat digestion.
- Disease affecting the digestive function of the pancreas usually does not affect the insulin-producing capacity of the pancreas.
- Normally, pancreatic digestive enzymes are not activated until they reach the duodenum. Premature activation of enzymes causes the pancreas to self-digest, which is a major factor in the development of acute pancreatitis.
- The common bile duct from the liver passes through the head of the pancreas and may be obstructed by disease in the pancreas.
- The pancreas is isolated from other structures; pancreatic malignancies can grow for many years without causing symptoms.

Diseases of the Digestive (Exocrine) Pancreas

A few congenital conditions affect the pancreas and are mentioned here because the digestive pancreas constitutes most of the pancreatic mass. In about 5% of people, the pancreas has two ducts instead of one. In these people, one of the ducts usually drains only a small part of the pancreas and empties directly into the duodenum. The other duct drains most of the pancreas but is often too small for the job, predisposing to duct obstruction and chronic pancreatitis.

Annular pancreas is a congenital deformity in which the head of the pancreas encircles the duodenum and may cause duodenal obstruction.

Ectopic pancreas is embryologically misplaced but histologically normal pancreas that has come to rest in an abnormal place. These "rests" occur in about 2% of people and are usually less than a centimeter in diameter. They occur most often in the submucosa of the stomach and bowel and are rarely symptomatic.

PANCREATITIS

Acute pancreatitis is acute inflammation of the pancreas. **Chronic pancreatitis** is repeated episodes of acute pancreatitis that destroys and scars the pancreas. Figure 17-4 depicts the causes and mechanisms of injury in acute pancreatitis.

Acute Pancreatitis

In *Annals of Surgery* in 1925, in elegantly descriptive language missing from modern medical literature, Dr. B. Moynihan wrote of acute pancreatitis as

> . . . the most terrible of all calamities that occur in connection with the abdominal viscera. The suddenness of its onset, the illimitable agony which accompanies it, and the mortality attendant upon it render it the most formidable of catastrophes.

Normally pancreatic juice flows smoothly out of the ductal system and into the duodenum. Along the way a very small amount, not enough to do damage, diffuses into interstitial fluid and into blood. If more than a small amount of pancreatic juice finds its way from ducts into the substance of the gland, self-digestion of glands, nerves, and blood vessels can occur, causing pain, bleeding, and release of additional enzymes that digest additional tissue in a vicious circle.

Conditions known to be associated with acute pancreatitis are listed below in order of frequency (see also the nearby History of Medicine box, as well as Case Study 17-1 at the end of this chapter):

- *Gallstones.* About half of patients with acute pancreatitis have gallstones (Fig. 17-5), and half of *these* patients suffer a second attack of pancreatitis if the stones are not removed.
- *Alcoholism.* About two thirds of cases are associated with chronic alcohol abuse. It appears that alcoholics have long-standing, smoldering subclinical pancreatitis that may suddenly flare into acute pancreatitis for uncertain reasons.
- *Unknown (idiopathic).* About 10% of cases have no known underlying cause.
- *Other causes.* The list is long and includes virus infections of the pancreas (mumps, for example), blunt trauma to the upper abdomen, thiazide diuretics and other therapeutic drugs, high blood levels of lipids (especially high levels of triglycerides), and high levels of blood calcium (hypercalcemia).

> ☞ *Of patients with acute pancreatitis, half have gallstones and two thirds abuse alcohol.*

The initial lesion of acute pancreatitis is composed of multiple areas of edema, congestion, and acute inflammation. As autodigestion progresses, these foci become progressively inflamed, begin to bleed, and become necrotic and painful (Fig. 17-6). In its most severe form—**acute hemorrhagic pancreatitis**—bleeding is extensive, and the entire pancreas can be destroyed. A common outcome in survivors is the formation of a cyst

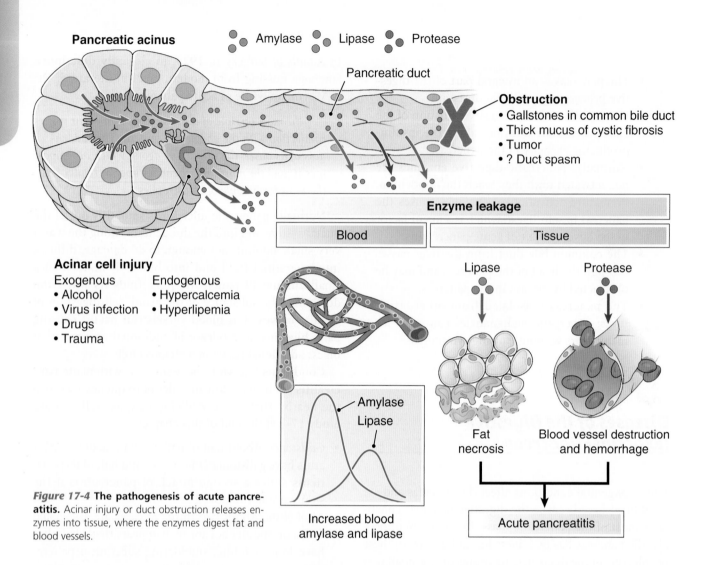

Figure 17-4 The pathogenesis of acute pancreatitis. Acinar injury or duct obstruction releases enzymes into tissue, where the enzymes digest fat and blood vessels.

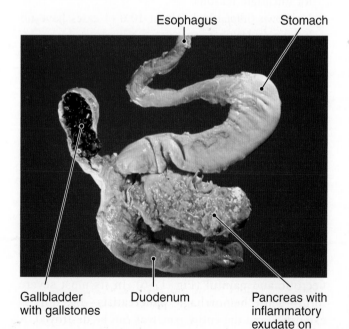

by the fibrous "walling off" of inflammatory fluid and edema. Such cysts can be quite large and are termed **pancreatic pseudocyst** ("pseudo" because the cyst has no lining epithelium).

A typical patient with acute pancreatitis presents with severe upper abdominal pain radiating through to the back. The disease may progress rapidly to catastrophic vascular collapse and shock, caused by pooling of blood and edema in the abdomen. Renal failure (Chapter 19) and acute respiratory distress syndrome (Chapter 14) often develop. In half of patients, the bloody mass of necrotic tissue becomes infected by intestinal bacteria, increasing mortality.

Figure 17-5 Acute pancreatitis. Dissection of esophagus, stomach, duodenum, gallbladder, and pancreas. The gallbladder is full of gallstones, and the surface of the pancreas is covered with an acute inflammatory exudate. Gallstones are an important cause of pancreatitis.

DID ALEXANDER THE GREAT DIE OF PANCREATITIS?

Alexander the Great (BC 356–323)—the celebrated Greek who was arguably the greatest nonreligious leader in recorded history—conquered most of the known Western world before he was 30 years old. His empire included what is now Greece, Turkey, Syria, Lebanon, Israel, Egypt, Iraq, Iran, Pakistan, Afghanistan, and northwest India. At age 32 he died in Babylon—now in southern Iraq—of an acute abdominal crisis that was keenly observed and recorded because of his great power.

His illness featured sudden fever and acute upper abdominal pain and tenderness that erupted after a rich meal and a night of heavy drinking (the modern equivalent of multiple bottles of wine). The initial pain faded, but his abdomen remained tender. Pain and fever returned and fluctuated for several days, during which he bathed in cool water and continued to eat and drink. No skin rash or jaundice was reported. By the 8th day, he was semicomatose and seemed to be paralyzed. His abdomen was soft and nontender. He died on the 11th day.

Scholars have debated his death for more than two millennia. Pancreatitis is among the favorite diagnoses, but good cases have been made for poisoning (either purposeful or some contaminant—lead, perhaps—in the wine), biliary tract infection, malaria, perforated peptic ulcer, and a variety of intestinal infections including typhoid fever.

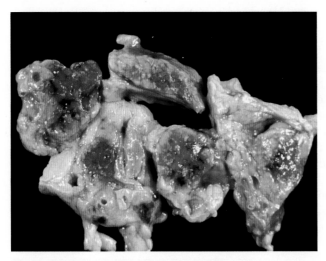

***Figure 17-6* Acute hemorrhagic pancreatitis.** Multiple cross-sections of the pancreas. Pancreatic injury or duct obstruction releases enzymes that digest fat and blood vessels, causing local hemorrhage.

Acute hemorrhagic pancreatitis is a medical emergency, and prompt diagnosis is necessary to differentiate acute pancreatitis from perforated duodenal ulcer (Chapter 15) or acute cholecystitis (Chapter 16). Laboratory tests are critically important diagnostic tools. As is explained in detail in the nearby Lab Tools box, in the typical case, blood levels of amylase rise and fall quickly. On the other hand, blood levels of lipase are slow to rise, and they stay high days or weeks after blood amylase levels have returned to normal. Other laboratory tests are useful to round out the clinical picture. Blood calcium levels may fall as calcium is taken from blood, precipitating as soap (saponification) in areas of pancreatic fat necrosis (Basics in Brief 17-1, nearby, explains the chemistry of soap making). Blood bilirubin levels may rise because of obstructive jaundice, caused as pancreatic edema presses on the common bile duct. Damage to islet cells may cause temporary diabetes.

Acute pancreatitis is reversible: the pancreas may recover fully. However, recurrent acute attacks may produce irreversible chronic disease.

Chronic Pancreatitis

Chronic pancreatitis is the result of recurrent episodes of mild-to-moderate acute pancreatitis, which continue to destroy pancreas until most of it is replaced by scar tissue (fibrosis). In many cases the acute episodes are well documented, but others may present with chronic pancreatitis and no history of prior acute attacks. Despite the close relationship between acute and chronic pancreatitis, they are distinctly different clinical syndromes and have different consequences, as is illustrated in Figure 17-7.

Chronic alcoholism is responsible for two thirds of chronic pancreatitis; of the remainder, most have no known cause. Alcohol stimulates pancreatic enzyme production, but beyond this simple fact little is certain about pathogenesis. Gallstones do not play a role in chronic pancreatitis.

About half of patients have clear evidence of prior episodes of acute pancreatitis. Most of the remainder present with obscure, nagging upper abdominal pain radiating through to the back, which does not initially suggest pancreatitis.

As is depicted in Figure 17-8, in chronic pancreatitis the pancreas is obliterated by dense scar tissue, ducts are dilated, and gritty calcification (from calcium soap formation) may be abundant. Stones can form in pancreatic ducts, but they are not related to gallstones. Late in the course of the disease, severe chronic pancreatitis may destroy enough islets of Langerhans to render the patient diabetic.

LAB TOOLS

Laboratory Tests for Blood Amylase and Lipase in Pancreatitis

Analysis of blood amylase and lipase levels can be very useful in the diagnosis of pancreatitis. As is illustrated in the accompanying figure, after injury, amylase levels rise and fall quickly, whereas levels of lipase rise more slowly and remain elevated longer.

Amylase is found in high concentration in the pancreas and in salivary glands, and even minor inflammation or injury to either one causes release of significant amounts of amylase into the bloodstream. Blood amylase level is, therefore, a sensitive test (Chapter 1) for pancreatic injury; that is, it is very likely to be above normal in pancreatitis or other pancreatic injury. However, it is not a very specific test because it can be increased by salivary gland inflammation or injury.

The opposite is true of lipase, which in pancreatitis or after pancreatic injury is not released as quickly or in such great quantity as amylase. However, damage to no organ other than the pancreas releases enough lipase to cause blood lipase level elevations. Thus, lipase level is a less sensitive and far more specific indicator of pancreatic injury or pancreatitis.

For these reasons, measurement of amylase and lipase levels are usually ordered together because the combination provides high sensitivity and specificity.

Most patients with acute pancreatitis have increased levels of amylase and lipase, but some do not. Amylase level rises within a few hours of pain onset and returns to normal in a few days. Lipase level usually increases slightly on the first day, but to a lesser extent than amylase, and it may remain elevated for a week or so.

Patients with chronic pancreatitis may have normal blood amylase and lipase levels if prior injury has destroyed most of the pancreas.

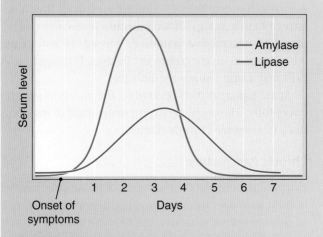

Blood amylase and lipase levels in acute pancreatitis. Whereas amylase levels rise and fall quickly after injury, lipase levels rise more slowly and stay elevated longer.

BASICS IN BRIEF 17-1

HOW TO MAKE SOAP IN THE PANCREAS

Understanding how soap is made will help you understand why patients with pancreatitis can have low blood calcium levels.

Soap and water remove grease (fat or oil) because soap is composed of a unique molecule: one end is made from fat and is soluble in fat; the other end is made from salt and is soluble in water. When soap is added to grease, the fatty end embeds in the grease, leaving the other (water-soluble end) sticking out. When water is added, the water-soluble end of the soap molecule dissolves in the water. The result is that the soap molecule has grease on one end and water on the other, and the flushing action of additional water carries the grease away.

In pancreatitis, soap is made from normal fat found in and around the pancreas and from calcium salts present in biliary and pancreatic juices and blood. Pancreatic juice is alkaline and combines the calcium salts and fat to make soap. Blood calcium levels fall as calcium is consumed in the process.

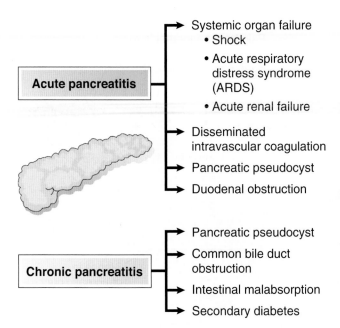

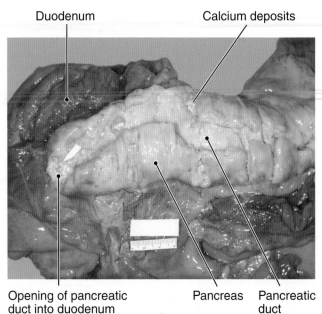

Figure 17-7 **Acute and chronic pancreatitis.** The consequences of the two types of pancreatitis are compared.

Figure 17-8 **Chronic pancreatitis.** The pancreas is abnormally pale, dense, and fibrotic, and the pancreatic duct is dilated from chronic obstruction. The white marker indicates the opening of the pancreatic duct into the duodenum where a pancreatic stone (removed) obstructed the lumen.

The complications of chronic pancreatitis are illustrated in Figure 17-9. In a few patients the first manifestation is diabetes or malabsorption syndrome (fatty stools, Chapter 15) because of a lack of pancreatic digestive enzymes. Weight loss, sometimes dramatic, is common. Chronic pancreatitis is dangerous: within five years about 50% of patients die of their disease. Blood amylase and lipase levels may be elevated during an acute flare-up, but in some cases the gland is destroyed to such an extent that little normal, enzyme-bearing tissue remains and blood amylase and lipase levels are not elevated despite continuing pancreatic damage and inflammation. A very useful diagnostic finding in pancreatitis is radiographic demonstration of calcium deposits or cysts in the pancreas.

It is wise to remember that in children chronic pancreatitis is often a manifestation of *cystic fibrosis* (Chapter 7). Recall that cystic fibrosis is an inherited disease characterized by defective chloride transport across cell membranes. One result is that ductal secretions in all glands—including in the pancreas—are unusually thick and cause ductal obstruction.

CARCINOMA OF THE PANCREAS

In this discussion, **carcinoma of the pancreas** refers only to adenocarcinomas that arise in ducts of the digestive (exocrine) pancreas—tumors of the islets of Langerhans of the hormonal (endocrine) pancreas will be discussed separately.

Carcinoma of the pancreas is common. In men it is the fourth most common cause of death behind lung, prostate, and colon cancers; in women it is fifth behind lung, breast, colon, and ovarian cancer. It usually affects mature to older men and women in equal numbers. It is insidious, causing few symptoms until it has progressed beyond resection for cure. We know little about what causes it except for one thing—smokers have about twice the risk of nonsmokers.

Pancreatic carcinomas are dense, scar-filled tumors, most of which arise in the head of the pancreas and cause jaundice by obstructing the common bile duct. Tumors of the body and tail of the pancreas (Fig. 17-10) have fewer opportunities to invade sensitive structures and may be quite large or have distant metastases at time of discovery. Local lymph nodes and liver are the foremost sites of metastasis.

The clinical picture of pancreatic carcinoma is depicted in Figure 17-11. Upper abdominal pain or back pain is the first symptom; however, by the time pain occurs it is too late—almost all have metastasized. Painless jaundice may be the initial sign if the tumor obstructs the common bile duct. Unexplained weight loss should always suggest a hidden malignancy, especially visceral cancer, and most especially pancreatic cancer. Migratory thrombophlebitis (Chapter 12) that occurs without apparent cause is often a signal of hidden (oc-

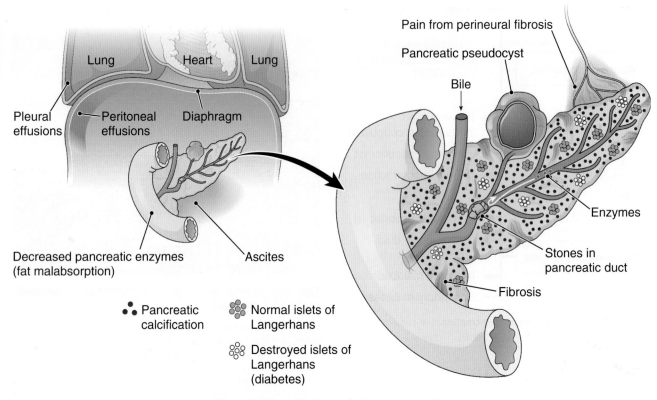

Figure 17-9 Complications of chronic pancreatitis.

cult) cancers and can prove an early diagnostic clue that a pancreatic cancer is present—astute diagnosticians think of pancreatic and other chest and abdominal cancers when investigating unexplained weight loss or thrombophlebitis.

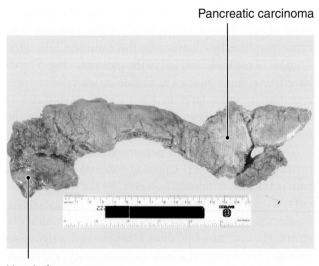

Figure 17-10 Pancreatic carcinoma. This example is in the tail of the gland; most occur in the head.

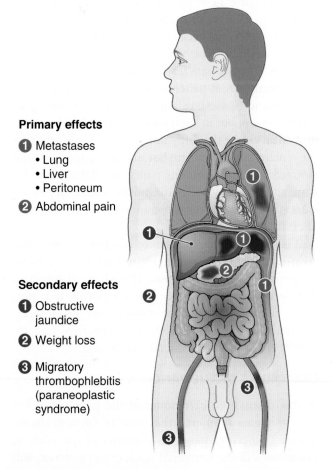

Primary effects

1. Metastases
   - Lung
   - Liver
   - Peritoneum
2. Abdominal pain

Secondary effects

1. Obstructive jaundice
2. Weight loss
3. Migratory thrombophlebitis (paraneoplastic syndrome)

Figure 17-11 Complications of carcinoma of the pancreas.

Half of patients with pancreatic carcinoma die within six weeks of diagnosis. About 10% live one year, and only 1% survive five years.

MAJOR DETERMINANTS OF DISEASE

- The pancreas produces insulin, which is required for glucose metabolism and is essential for life.
- Diabetes occurs when there is a lack of pancreatic insulin or there is tissue unresponsiveness to the action of insulin.
- All of the complications of diabetes result from high blood levels of glucose.
- Disease affecting the insulin-producing capacity of the pancreas does not affect the digestive pancreas.

Diseases of the Hormonal (Endocrine) Pancreas

Those labouring with this Disease, [urinate] a great deal more than they drink, or take of any liquid ailment; and moreover they have always joyned with it continual thirst. . . . The Urine in all . . . was wonderfully sweet as it were imbued with Honey or Sugar. . . .
THOMAS WILLIS (1621–1675), ENGLISH PHYSICIAN, SPEAKING OF DIABETES

Diseases of the hormonal (endocrine) pancreas discussed in this section include diabetes mellitus and pancreatic endocrine neoplasms.

DIABETES MELLITUS

Diabetes mellitus (usually shortened to "diabetes") is a disorder of insulin *action* and *secretion* that results in high blood glucose (**hyperglycemia**). For practical purposes, *hyperglycemia is diabetes and diabetes is hyperglycemia.* Diabetes is defined as a *fasting* blood glucose level 126 mg/dL or more, or a blood glucose level 200 mg/dL on *any* occasion.

There are two types of diabetes. In *type 1* diabetes, the pancreas does not secrete enough insulin, whereas in *type 2* diabetes insulin is produced but is not effective. Each type can be caused by various underlying conditions. The differences in type 1 and type 2 diabetes are summarized in Table 17-2.

In diabetes the pancreas shows relatively little change. In type 1 diabetes the islets of Langerhans show a slight accumulation of lymphocytes owing to the autoimmune (Chapter 8) nature of the disease. In type 2 diabetes the islets are gradually replaced by **amyloid** (Chapter 8), an abnormal protein. The most important pathologic abnormalities caused by diabetes occur outside the pancreas.

Type 1 diabetes (juvenile diabetes) accounts for about 10% of diabetes cases and is caused by an *absolute* deficiency of insulin that results from autoimmune de-

Table 17-2	**Comparison of Type 1 and Type 2 Diabetes**	
Criterion	**Type 1**	**Type 2**
Age at onset	Usually teenage years	Usually mature adult
Rapidity and intensity of onset	Sudden, severe	Slow, subtle
Body weight	Normal to underweight	Overweight or obese
Parents or siblings with disease	<20%	>60%
Autoimmunity	Yes	No
Islet pathology	Minimal inflammation or fibrosis	Amyloid deposits
Beta cells	Marked decrease	Near normal
Blood insulin level	Marked decrease	Normal or increased
Ketoacidosis episodes	Periodic	Rare
Clinical approach	Insulin and diet	Mainly diet or oral drugs; insulin in some patients

struction of the islets by anti-islet cell antibodies. Type 1 diabetes appears most frequently in otherwise healthy people under age 20; however, a few cases occur in adults. The remaining 90% of people with diabetes have **type 2 diabetes** (adult-onset diabetes), which usually appears in obese, mature adults and is initially caused by *resistance to the action of insulin by peripheral tissues*, such as skeletal muscle cells. Figure 17-12 illustrates the age distribution (incidence) of new cases of type 1 and type 2.

The initial diagnosis of type 1 diabetes is usually made because the patient develops diabetic acidosis, characterized by rapid breathing, mental disorientation, and sudden coma. Alternatively, high levels of blood glucose spilling into urine may cause frequent urination, thirstiness, and increased appetite, all associated with calories and water lost in urine.

Patients with type 2 diabetes, however, are often diagnosed following routine laboratory tests that demonstrate high fasting blood glucose, or glucose in the urine. Some are diagnosed in the course of a workup for unexplained weight loss (see the nearby History of Medicine box and Case Study 17-2 at the end of this chapter).

Pathogenesis of Type 1 Diabetes

Type 1 diabetes is a life-long disorder of glucose control that occurs when *autoimmune destruction* of beta cells causes a decrease in or absence of insulin production by

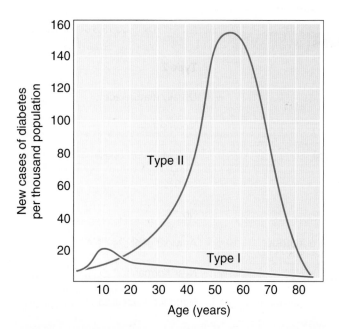

Figure 17-12 Comparison of age distribution in type 1 and type 2 diabetes. The figure shows the age at onset and relative numbers of new cases of both types of diabetes. Type 2 diabetes appears much later and is much more common than type 1 is.

History of Medicine

THE ORIGIN OF THE WORD "DIABETES"

Diabetes is named for one of its distressing symptoms—the passage of large amounts of urine. The word was derived from a similarly pronounced Geek word, *diabetes*, which meant "excessive discharge of urine." The Greek *diabetes* was constructed from two roots, *dia*- meaning "through" + *bainein*, "to go," which referred to the large amount of fluid going through the body. *Diabetes* is first recorded in English in a medical text written around 1425.

In daily usage *diabetes* means *diabetes mellitus. Mellitus* is Latin for "honeyed," which refers to the high glucose content of urine in uncontrolled diabetes mellitus and serves to distinguish diabetes mellitus from *diabetes insipidus. Insipidus* is Latin for tasteless or bland and has the same meaning in English. Diabetes insipidus is a very rare condition (Chapter 23) caused by disease of the pituitary gland that, as in diabetes mellitus, causes production of profuse amounts of urine; however, the urine in diabetes insipidus does not contain glucose and therefore is tasteless or bland.

the pancreatic islets of Langerhans. The evidence for autoimmune pathogenesis is clear: Early in type 1 diabetes the islets are infiltrated by T lymphocytes; in some patients anti-insulin antibodies are present in blood; about 10% of patients have other autoimmune disease such as thyroiditis or pernicious anemia; and immunosuppressive therapy sometimes can ameliorate the disease. There is also a genetic component: some persons are more susceptible than others to the insult (virus infection?) that initiates the disease. Figure 17-13 illustrates the interplay of genetics, environment, and autoimmunity in type 1 diabetes.

Type 1 diabetes tends to run in families, but familial tendency is much greater in type 2 diabetes. Less than 20% of type 1 diabetic patients have a parent or sibling with diabetes; by contrast, about 60% of patients with type 2 diabetes have a parent or sibling with the disease. Type 1 diabetes occurs most often in people of northern European ancestry and is less common among Asian, African Americans, and Native Americans, who tend to get type 2 diabetes.

☞ *For clinical purposes, abnormally high blood glucose and diabetes are one and the same.*

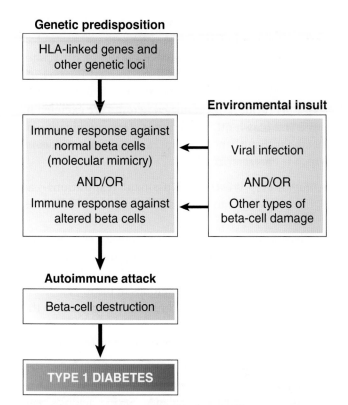

Genetic predisposition

HLA-linked genes and other genetic loci

Environmental insult

Immune response against normal beta cells (molecular mimicry)

AND/OR

Immune response against altered beta cells

Viral infection

AND/OR

Other types of beta-cell damage

Autoimmune attack

Beta-cell destruction

TYPE 1 DIABETES

Figure 17-13 **The pathogenesis of type 1 diabetes.** Type 1 diabetes is caused by autoimmune destruction of beta cells, which is induced by some type of environmental insult in genetically susceptible people.

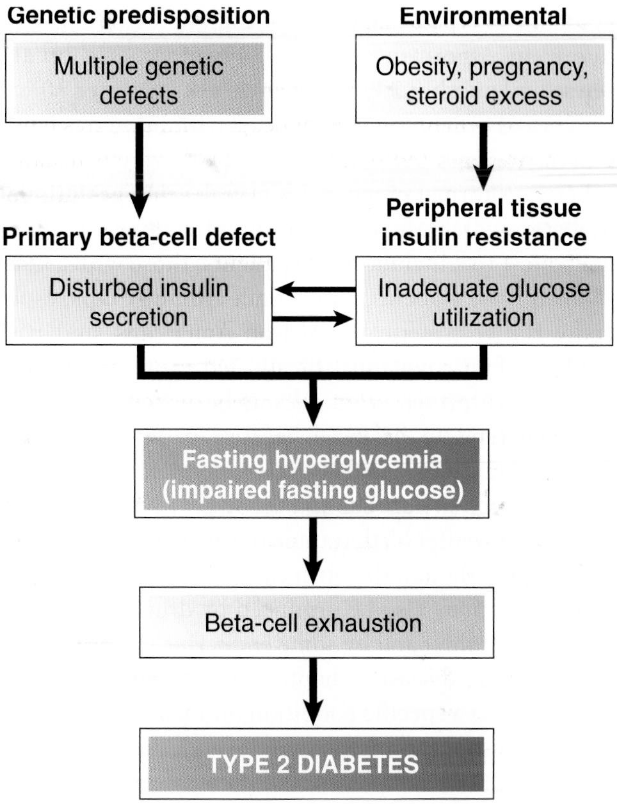

Genetic predisposition

Multiple genetic defects

Environmental

Obesity, pregnancy, steroid excess

Primary beta-cell defect

Disturbed insulin secretion

Peripheral tissue insulin resistance

Inadequate glucose utilization

Fasting hyperglycemia (impaired fasting glucose)

Beta-cell exhaustion

TYPE 2 DIABETES

Figure 17-14 **The pathogenesis of type 2 diabetes.** The primary mechanisms are peripheral tissue resistance to the effect of insulin and strong genetic susceptibility.

Pathogenesis of Type 2 Diabetes

As was mentioned immediately above, the majority of patients with type 2 diabetes have a parent or sibling with the disease. The strong genetic influence toward diabetes is especially evident in some ethnic groups that have very high rates of type 2 diabetes; for example, one third to one half of the population of the Pima tribe of Native Americans in Arizona have diabetes.

The defect in type 2 diabetes is not the destruction of beta cells in the islets of Langerhans: the problem is peripheral (target) cell resistance to the effect of insulin, as is depicted in Figure 17-14.

In patients who develop type 2 diabetes, peripheral tissues begin to resist the effect of insulin as much as 10 years before the diagnosis becomes apparent. As peripheral resistance increases, the pancreas secretes increased amounts of insulin to compensate, and blood glucose levels continue to remain normal or near normal. This early stage is called **prediabetes** and is characterized by *high* blood levels of insulin and blood glucose levels that are normal or slightly increased but not high enough to warrant a diagnosis of diabetes. Some patients may have

abnormal fasting blood glucose levels; that is, above 110 mg/dL (the upper limit of normal) but not high enough to warrant a diagnosis of diabetes (126 mg/dL or more). These patients are classified as having **impaired fasting glucose**, which is an intermediate stage in the natural history of diabetes. Patients with impaired fasting glucose levels are at greatly increased risk of developing type 2 diabetes. About 10–15% of adults in the United States have impaired levels of fasting glucose, and about one third of them will develop diabetes within ten years. Even in this prediabetic stage they are increased risk for vascular disease.

In prediabetes the overworked beta cells ultimately become exhausted, insulin output declines, and blood glucose levels rise high enough for a diagnosis of diabetes.

Increased peripheral resistance (and type 2 diabetes) is secondary to other conditions. *Obesity (Chapter 10) is the cause of 80% of type 2 diabetes.* Precisely how obesity causes insulin resistance is not certain, but the association is clear and strong. Obesity and the multitude of problems associated with it are discussed in Chapter 11. Experts warn that the United States is headed toward an epidemic of type 2 diabetes as a result of the obesity epidemic in American society—23% of Americans are obese and another 34% are overweight (Chapter 10).

Normal pregnancy is associated with limited peripheral insulin resistance, and about 2–3% of women with otherwise normal pregnancies may develop **gestational diabetes**, which usually disappears after delivery. Those at greatest risk include obese patients, those with a family history of diabetes, and certain ethnic groups, especially Native Americans, African Americans, and Hispanics. About one third of affected mothers develop diabetes within ten years. Infants born to women with diabetes tend to be large because maternal glucose crosses the placenta and stimulates fetal insulin output, which causes fat deposits and tissue growth. These large infants may suffer birth trauma or cause maternal injury as they pass though the birth canal.

Diabetes may also be produced by drug therapy (especially steroids) and by some endocrine diseases (usually Cushing disease, Chapter 18). When diabetes is secondary to a specific condition, in most instances the diabetes disappears with correction of the underlying condition. For example, steroid therapy can cause temporary diabetes that disappears upon steroid withdrawal. Some obese patients with diabetes may revert to nondiabetic status if they lose a large amount of weight.

Short-term Complications of Diabetes

In undiagnosed patients or patients whose disease is out of control, blood glucose levels rise above the renal threshold (about 180 mg/dL), and glucose spills into urine (**glycosuria**). Ill effects of glycosuria include wastage of calories (glucose), water, and electrolytes. Urine containing a large amount of glucose has high osmotic pressure, which attracts water, so that urine output rises (*osmotic diuresis*). Frequent urination (**polyuria**) occurs, and increased water intake (**polydipsia**) becomes necessary. Along with the water wastage, the urine is also wasting electrolytes, mainly Na^+, K^+, Mg^{++}, and PO_4^-. Severe dehydration and electrolyte imbalances can occur.

As calories are lost in urine, increased appetite (**polyphagia**) offsets some of the loss, but so many calories are wasted that weight loss and muscle weakness are inevitable. The paradox of a ravenous appetite and weight loss is very suggestive of diabetes, especially after an overactive thyroid (Chapter 18) has been ruled out.

As is depicted in Figure 17-15, *acidosis* may occur and progress to coma if insulin is absent, because of either undiagnosed diabetes or insufficient insulin therapy, or if infection or physical activity increases the demand for insulin. Acidosis arises because in the absence

of glucose, the body must burn fat for fuel. The fat is broken down into fatty acids, which are transported to the liver and converted into **ketones**—small, acidic, glucose-size molecules, which are burned for fuel instead of glucose. The accumulation of ketones lowers blood pH (acidosis). Unburned ketones are excreted in urine and blown off by the lungs. This combination of metabolic disturbances produces **diabetic ketoacidosis**, which is characterized by:

- *Rapid, deep breathing* (**Kussmaul respiration**)—as the lungs labor to expel acid in the form of ketones and CO_2
- *Glycosuria*—as blood glucose levels exceed the renal threshold, and glucose spills into urine
- *Acidosis*—low blood pH owing to ketone buildup
- *Ketonuria*—excretion of ketones in urine
- *Osmotic diuresis*—high urine output as glucose in the urine carries water with it
- *Volume depletion*—as the body loses water in urine

Diabetic acidosis is typically accompanied by nausea and vomiting, which causes further electrolyte and water loss and acid-base imbalance. Severe acidosis may produce **diabetic coma**, most often associated with type 1 rather than type 2 diabetes because glucose metabolism in type 1 diabetes is unstable or brittle—blood glucose levels are very sensitive to and vary greatly with administered insulin, deviations from dietary rules, infection, hard exercise, or other forms of stress. Even mild upsets of physiology, such as diarrhea or vomiting, can rapidly push a patient with type 1 diabetes into a crisis of hypoglycemia or ketoacidosis.

A second type of diabetic coma—**hyperosmolar coma**—can occur if water loss is especially severe and blood glucose levels and osmolality rise extremely high. Hyperosmolar coma is usually seen in elderly or debilitated patients with type 2 diabetes—they may suffer from dementia or other afflictions of age and be unable to medicate themselves properly or to drink enough water to make up for fluid loss from prolonged hyperglycemia and glycosuria. Hyperosmolar coma is not associated with the nausea, vomiting, and rapid respirations that are associated with ketoacidotic coma.

Long-term Complications of Diabetes

Patients with both type 1 and type 2 diabetes suffer from accelerated atherosclerosis, myocardial infarction, stroke, peripheral vascular insufficiency and gangrene, retinal disease (retinopathy), renal insufficiency (Fig. 17-16), and peripheral nerve disease. Infections are a common problem in diabetes; the cause is not clear but defective immune response seems likely. Patients with

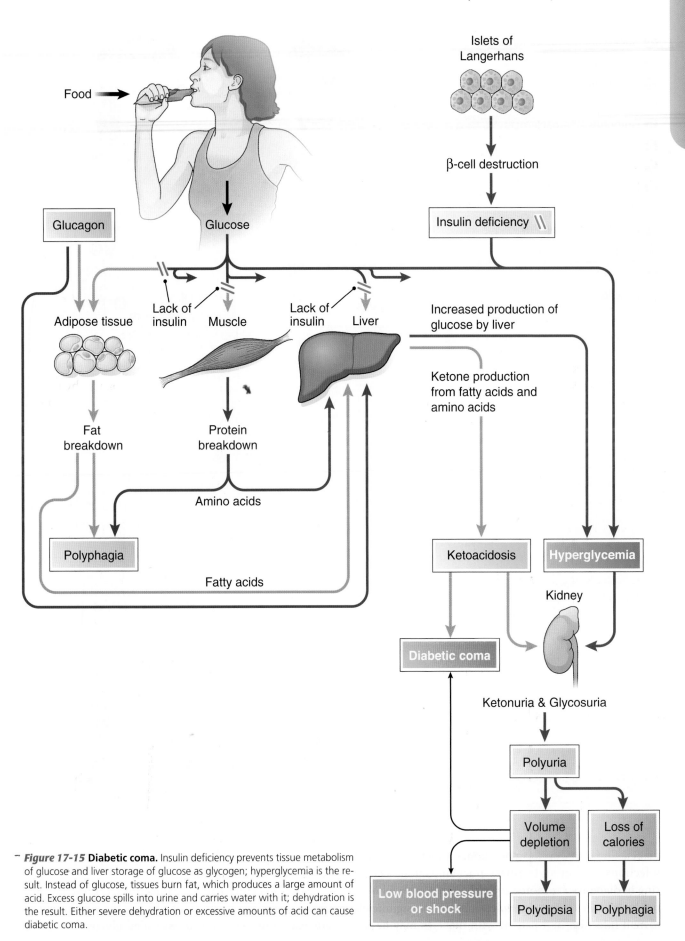

Figure 17-15 **Diabetic coma.** Insulin deficiency prevents tissue metabolism of glucose and liver storage of glucose as glycogen; hyperglycemia is the result. Instead of glucose, tissues burn fat, which produces a large amount of acid. Excess glucose spills into urine and carries water with it; dehydration is the result. Either severe dehydration or excessive amounts of acid can cause diabetic coma.

❶ Stroke (infarct or hemorrhage)
❷ Cataract
❸ Retinopathy
❹ Carotid atherosclerosis
❺ Coronary atherosclerosis
❻ Myocardial infarct
❼ Aortic atherosclerosis
❽ Islet cell changes
❾ Nephrosclerosis
❿ Peripheral neuropathy
⓫ Peripheral atherosclerosis
⓬ Gangrene
⓭ Infections

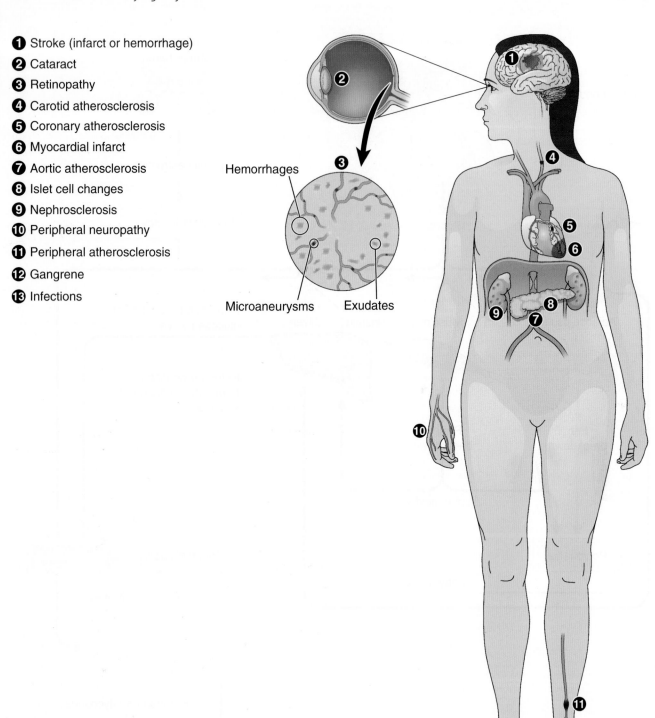

Hemorrhages

Microaneurysms   Exudates

Figure 17-16 Long-term complications of diabetes.

diabetes tend to develop pneumonia, tuberculosis, and infections of skin and urinary tract. Infections occurring in diabetics are more severe than in people who do not have diabetes. For example, an initially insignificant toenail infection in a patient with diabetes may be the

first event in a deadly spiral of deeper infection, gangrene, septicemia, and death.

Hyperglycemia causes damage by several mechanisms, the most important of which is the attachment of glucose to proteins, a process called **glycosylation**. As glucose levels rise, glycosylation and complications increase, which is why treatment of diabetes focuses on keeping blood glucose levels as close to normal as possible. Useful indicators of the degree of glycosylation and glucose control are **glycohemoglobin** (also called *hemoglobin A1C*) and **fructosamine**. Glycohemoglobin is formed by the attachment of glucose to globin, the protein part of hemoglobin; fructosamine is formed by reaction of glucose and albumin. Glycohemoglobin is an index of average blood glucose over the prior two or three months; fructosamine reflects average blood glucose over the prior two or three weeks.

Whether because of glycosylation or another mechanism of damage, the metabolic abnormalities in diabetes cause complications that mainly affect blood vessels and nerves. In *large vessels* the development of atherosclerosis is accelerated, which accounts for the increased risk in diabetes for stroke, heart attack, and gangrene. In *small vessels* (**microvascular disease**) blood flow and diffusion of essential substances is slowed, which accounts for most of the kidney and eye (retina) disease in diabetes. Nerves are also seriously affected by abnormal glucose metabolism—sensory and autonomic nerve dysfunction is among the most common complications of diabetes.

In both types of diabetes, complications are directly proportional to the severity and duration of hyperglycemia. *Strict control of blood glucose levels is associated with fewer complications*: patients have fewer strokes and heart attacks, and less kidney disease, peripheral nerve, and eye disease.

> **High blood glucose levels are the cause of all diabetic complications**

Vascular Disease

Of all body systems, the vascular system is most seriously damaged by diabetes: the aorta and large- and medium-sized arteries suffer from accelerated atherosclerosis (Chapter 12). Impaired blood flow causes ischemia or infarction of downstream tissues and accounts for the high incidence of heart attack, stroke, and lower limb gangrene in patients with diabetes (lower limb amputations are about 200 times more common in diabetes than in patients without diabetes).

Microvascular disease in diabetes is characterized by microscopically distinctive changes in small blood vessels called **hyaline arteriolosclerosis** (Chapter 12). Small vessels in the kidney and retina are most severely damaged. In the kidney, glomeruli and glomerular arterioles are most affected, and the changes are referred to as **diabetic nephropathy**. Retinal blood vessels are similarly damaged, and the changes are referred to as **diabetic retinopathy**.

Kidney Disease

Diabetic kidney disease (**diabetic nephrosclerosis**) is the most common cause of renal failure in the United States, affecting up to 20% of patients with diabetes. Recall from Chapter 12 that nephrosclerosis is a "wear and tear" change that affects everyone but is accelerated by high blood pressure. In patients with diabetes, nephrosclerosis is accelerated to an even greater degree. As is illustrated in Figure 17-17, the diabetic kidney is shrunken and granular, and in some cases the glomeruli are also severely affected by nodular deposits of hyaline material (**diabetic nodular glomerulosclerosis**), which further affects kidney function. Moreover, the renal artery and its main branches are often severely atherosclerotic. Finally, bladder (cystitis) and kidney (pyelonephritis) infections (Chapter 19) are common problems in diabetes.

Eye Disease

Diabetes is an important cause of blindness associated with *cataracts* (opacification of the lens), *glaucoma* (increased intraocular pressure and optic nerve damage, Chapter 25), and *diabetic retinopathy*. Cataracts and glaucoma usually respond well to surgery or drug therapy; however, it is diabetic retinopathy, illustrated in Figure 17-18, that is most devastating. Diabetic retinopathy is a mixture of exudates, hemorrhages, edema, new blood vessel growth (*angioneogenesis*,

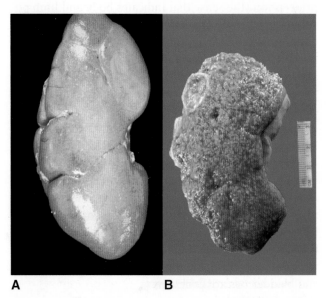

A   **B**

Figure 17-17 **Diabetic nephrosclerosis. A,** Normal kidney. **B,** Diabetic nephrosclerosis. Note the small size of the diseased kidney.

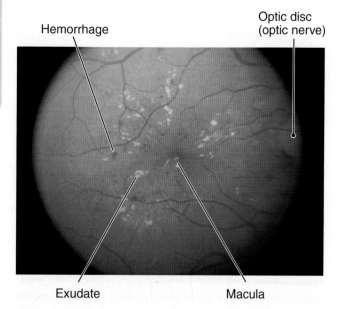

Hemorrhage

Optic disc (optic nerve)

Exudate

Macula

Figure 17-18 Diabetic retinopathy. Funduscopy of the right eye.

Chapter 4), small aneurysms (microaneurysms), and scarring. It is difficult to treat effectively and is the leading cause of blindness in people under the age of 60 in the United States.

Brain and Peripheral Nerve Disease

The entire peripheral nervous system—motor, sensory, and autonomic nerves—is affected by diabetes (**peripheral neuropathy**). Sensory functions are affected more than motor functions are. Initially, patients suffer from nerve irritation, pain, and abnormal sensations, but later they lose the sense of fine touch, pain, and proprioception (the sense that indicates body and limb position). As a result, patients with diabetes often ignore or are unaware of irritation or injury to the feet, an important factor in the development of diabetic foot ulcers and infections. Impaired sensation from lower limb joints can lead to severe wear-and-tear arthritis (neuropathic arthritis or *Charcot joint*) as patients clumsily damage joints without realizing they are doing so. Wristdrop or footdrop can indicate selective paralysis (palsy) of single nerves, but any peripheral or cranial nerve can be affected. A common autonomic dysfunction is *postural hypotension*—light-headedness or fainting—caused by lack of autonomically controlled vascular tone in the legs, which causes pooling of blood in the feet upon rising from a flat or sitting position. Patients with diabetes also have erectile dysfunction and bowel and bladder control problems.

The brain is vulnerable on two counts. First, the accelerated atherosclerosis associated with diabetes affects carotid and intracerebral arteries, which leads to vascular obstruction and stroke (Chapter 23). Second, because the brain is entirely dependent on glucose and cannot burn fat for energy, the cerebral cortex is rendered especially susceptible to necrosis (Chapter 23) from *hypoglycemia*, a serious risk for patients inadvertently taking more insulin than necessary. In patients taking insulin, managing blood glucose levels is a delicate balancing act among insulin dosage, calorie intake, and exercise, and hypoglycemia is an ever-present threat.

Diagnosis of Diabetes Mellitus

Recall that diabetes is defined as *fasting* blood glucose levels of 126 mg/dL or more, or blood glucose levels of 200 mg/dL on *any* occasion, and that a normal *fasting* glucose level is usually defined as 70–110 mg/dL (the range varies slightly from lab to lab). Patients whose fasting results are 110–125 mg/dL have **impaired fasting glucose**. *After a meal*, glucose levels rise above 110 mg/dL but normally do not exceed 200 mg/dL and return to 110 mg/dL or less after 2 hours. *Two hours after a meal*, patients whose blood glucose level is over 140 mg/dL but less than 200 mg/dL are considered to have **impaired glucose tolerance**.

The American Diabetes Association criteria for the diagnosis of diabetes require the classic signs and symptoms of diabetes plus abnormal blood glucose levels, as is illustrated in the nearby Lab Tools box. Other laboratory findings, such as glycosuria, can be suggestive but are not diagnostic.

Patients with impaired fasting glucose levels or impaired glucose tolerance have increased prevalence of atherosclerosis, hypertension, and hyperlipemia, but do not suffer from the diabetic microvascular disease as long as their condition does not proceed to diabetes. About 3% of people with prediabetes become diabetic each year. However, weight loss, exercise, and change of diet may allow a return of glucose metabolism to normal or prevent progression to diabetes.

The diagnosis of **gestational diabetes** is a special case. About 1–3% of pregnant women develop temporary diabetes during pregnancy. An additional small percentage becomes temporarily glucose intolerant. The diagnosis of diabetes is clear if the fasting glucose level is equal to or greater than 126 mg/dL. However, there is no universally accepted standard for diagnosis of gestational diabetes if fasting glucose level is between 110–126 mg/dL. Many caregivers prefer to administer a calibrated oral dose of glucose (**glucose tolerance test**) in order to separate those who are diabetic from those who are glucose intolerant. Standards vary for interpretation of test results.

Laboratory Diagnosis and Management of Diabetes

Blood glucose level is the most reliable diagnostic criterion for the diagnosis of diabetes. *Any* blood glucose level, fasting or non-fasting (called "random" glucose), equal to or greater than 200 mg/dL is diagnostic of diabetes. A *fasting* glucose level equal to or greater than 126 mg/dL is also diagnostic if confirmed by repeat test on a following day. The presence of glucose in urine is suggestive, but not diagnostic.

Patients whose fasting results fall between 110 and 125 mg/dL are considered to have **impaired fasting glucose**. Some experts also consider patients to have impaired glucose metabolism if blood glucose levels are between 140 and 199 mg/dL two hours after a meal. These patients are said to have **impaired glucose tolerance**. For either group and for pregnant women, an oral **glucose tolerance test** (GTT) may be helpful. The GTT test is administered by measuring the fasting blood glucose level, then administering a calculated amount of oral glucose and monitoring the blood glucose level every 30 minutes for 2 hours. However, these results are often not reproducible and must be interpreted differently in pregnant women. This test is losing support in favor of careful documentation of fasting blood glucose measurements.

The accompanying figure illustrates the behavior of blood glucose in several situations. Blood glucose results after a glucose load may vary considerably from one episode to another in the same patient—about one fourth of patients have a diagnostically different result on repeat testing. Reliable results require meticulous patient preparation and rigorous adherence to test protocol.

Other laboratory tests are useful in the *management* of diabetes. Because avoiding diabetic complications requires tight control of blood glucose level, and because blood glucose level reveals only what is happening to the patient at the moment, other tests are necessary to gain a longer term view of the effectiveness of glucose control. **Fructosamine** is a plasma protein-glucose combination that forms and is broken down at a modest pace and roughly correlates with average blood glucose levels over the *prior two or three weeks*. **Glycohemoglobin (hemoglobin A1C)** forms and dissipates more slowly and is a reliable indicator of *average* blood glucose levels over the *prior 2 or 3 months*. Results may indicate the need for different therapy or for patient counseling. Patients sometimes profess that they work very hard to control their blood glucose level, but their fructosamine and glycohemoglobin results may reveal that their blood glucose is out of control most of the time.

Finally, one of the first signs of diabetic nephropathy is **microalbuminuria**, the spilling of very small amounts of albumin into urine. These small amounts are not usually detectable by standard "dipstick" tests and require 24-hour urine collection with quantitative measurement of total albumin excretion per 24 hours.

Normal and abnormal glucose tolerance tests. Diabetes is defined as *fasting* blood glucose levels of 126 mg/dL or more, or a blood glucose level of 200 mg/dL on *any* occasion. Patients with fasting blood glucose levels from 110–125 mg/dL are said to have impaired fasting glucose. Patients whose blood glucose level is 140–199 mg/dL two hours after a meal or ingestion of a standard amount of glucose are said to have impaired glucose tolerance.

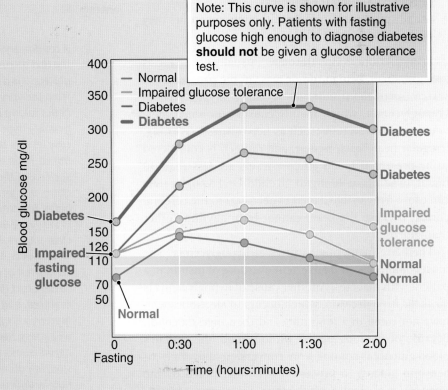

Note: This curve is shown for illustrative purposes only. Patients with fasting glucose high enough to diagnose diabetes **should not** be given a glucose tolerance test.

Treatment of Diabetes

The main thrust of treatment is control of blood glucose levels, which can be monitored by direct measurement of blood levels of glucose and periodic measurement of blood levels of glycohemoglobin. For patients with type 2 diabetes, weight reduction is very important and calls for diet and lifestyle counseling. *Oral hypoglycemic drugs* are useful and work in several ways: some increase insulin secretion by the pancreas, others reduce the amount of glucose released by the liver, improve glucose utilization in target tissue, or block the conversion of dietary carbohydrate into glucose. However, a minority of patients with type 2 diabetes require insulin. Patients with type 1 diabetes always require insulin, which is administered by injection or, more recently, by aerosol inhalation. Patient education about risks, glucose control, diet management, and other aspects of the disease is important in every patient with diabetes.

PANCREATIC ENDOCRINE NEOPLASMS

Other than diabetes, the only significant disease of the endocrine pancreas is tumors of islet cells and related cells that occur in the pancreas and nearby fat. They:

- are rare, far less common than pancreatic carcinoma
- are usually benign but can be malignant
- usually arise from the islets proper or from related cells in fat around the pancreas
- usually produce hormones, although sometimes they may not

Beta cell tumors (**insulinomas**), usually occurring as a single, small, benign tumor mass in the pancreas, *can secrete enough insulin to produce hypoglycemia.* **Hypoglycemia**, which mainly causes autonomic nervous system symptoms such as nervousness, sweating, irregular heartbeats, tremor, and hunger, is considered to be present if blood glucose levels are less than 50 mg/dL in adults or 40 mg/dL in children. Hypoglycemia can cause irreversible damage (necrosis) to the cerebral cortex, because the brain cannot burn anything other than glucose.

There are many other causes of hypoglycemia. The most common is an inadvertent overdose of insulin in a patient with diabetes. Another cause of hypoglycemia is *alcoholic hypoglycemia*, which occurs in alcoholics who have not eaten in a long time and then ingest alcohol. Because of the long period without food, the patient's blood glucose is coming from conversion of liver glycogen into glucose, a process that is interrupted by the toxic effect of alcohol on the liver. Liver output of glucose stops, and the result is hypoglycemia. Alcoholic

hypoglycemia is something to keep in mind when evaluating a stuporous alcoholic patient: It is not always caused by alcohol alone; it can be induced by blood alcohol levels well within the legal limit for driving.

Reactive hypoglycemia is hypoglycemia that follows a meal. There are a few known causes, and most of these occur in children with hereditary enzyme deficiencies. Reactive hypoglycemia is said to occur because insulin production by the pancreas "overshoots" and pushes glucose levels too low; however, the topic is controversial, as is discussed in the Key Point box below, and some experts doubt that it occurs in people who have no other underlying condition.

A second type of hormone overproduction by the pancreas is the *Zollinger-Ellison syndrome*, a constellation of clinical findings resulting from *gastrinomas*, which arise in the stomach, duodenum, and pancreas. The cell of origin is a mystery. Most are microscopically benign, but occasionally they metastasize. They produce large amounts of gastrin, causing marked increases of gastric acid production and recurrent peptic ulcers (Chapter 15) and duodenal ulcers in the duodenum and stomach. These ulcers are identical to peptic ulcers associated with *Helicobacter pylori* infection, except that they may be multiple and are resistant to medical therapy. Surgical excision of the tumor is curative.

Glucagonoma, a tumor of alpha cells, is exceptionally rare and causes mild diabetes, skin disease, and anemia. ■

> *A cautionary note about hypoglycemia: From the text discussion it should be clear that hypoglycemia is a complex physiologic matter. Apart from the very real risk of hypoglycemia in diabetics taking insulin, there are few instances of genuine hypoglycemia; that is, where blood glucose level is documented to be less than 50 mg/dL in an adult or 40 mg/dL in a child. In such cases the underlying cause is usually clear—insulin overdose in someone with diabetes, for example. Documented hypoglycemia is very rare in the absence of diabetes or other clear underlying cause.*
>
> *However, in some circles hypoglycemia is somewhat of a religion, not a disease. In these circles strict diagnostic criteria are usually not required, and undocumented, presumed hypoglycemia is offered as the cause of dizziness, weakness, headaches, cold sweats, trembling, nervousness, irritability, sleeplessness, confusion, impotence, depression, irregular bowel habits, difficulty concentrating or handling stress or fears, and apprehensions.*

CASE STUDY 17-1 "HE DRINKS; I DON'T"

TOPICS
Gallstones
Acute pancreatitis

THE CASE

Setting: You work in the emergency room of a community hospital that is the sole provider for a sparsely populated area on the Great Plains of United States. Your job is to interview "walk-ins" and initiate care and diagnosis, and to contact an appropriate physician.

Clinical history: You are called to the front desk by the reception clerk, who is alarmed by the pain of a woman who has just arrived. At the desk you find an obese woman bent over in a wheelchair and complaining of severe abdominal pain. A man with her introduces himself as her husband and says she was completely normal until a short time previously. You wheel her into an exam room and continue the interview. She is a 41-year-old Native American woman whose pain began 2 hours earlier and has grown steadily more severe. She vomited several times before arriving and describes the pain as "awful." Past medical history and review of systems are unremarkable except for occasional visits to a government clinic for recurrent bladder irritation. She denies drinking alcohol, saying "He drinks; I don't."

Physical examination and other data: Oral temperature 97.9° F; respirations 24; supine BP 110/65, HR 110; sitting BP 90/60, HR 125. The patient is obese and nearly frantic with pain. There is diffuse abdominal tenderness, and she pushes your hand away (guards) when you press on her upper abdomen. Heart and breath sounds are normal, but no bowel sounds are detectable, which arouses concern that she has intestinal paralysis (ileus) brought on by whatever is wrong in her abdomen. Pulses in her arms and legs are normal, and the remainder of the physical exam is unremarkable. She does not appear to be jaundiced.

Clinical course: Concluding that she has an abdominal emergency, you order x-rays of the abdomen, collect blood and urine for laboratory studies, start an IV, and notify the general surgeon on call.

While waiting for the surgeon, you go to radiology and examine the x-rays, which reveal air-fluid levels in bowel loops, confirming your suspicion of ileus. Next, you go to the lab to review results and find the following studies:

Blood tests		
Hematocrit	50% (female normal 35–45)	High
WBC	19,300 (n: <10,500)	High
Neutrophil %	90% (n: 60–70)	High
BUN	37 mg/dL (n: <19)	High
Calcium	6.9 mg/dL (n 9.1–10.6)	Low
Bilirubin	3.1 mg/dL (n: <1.1)	High
ALT (liver enzyme)	302 IU/L (n: <40)	High
Amylase	12,760 IU/L (n: <120)	High
Lipase	26,300 IU/L (n: <165)	High

Urinalysis		
Specific gravity	1.050 (n: 1.003–1.030)	High
Bilirubin	Present (n: Absent)	Abnormal

DISCUSSION

This patient's pain was typical for pancreatitis—severe, upper abdominal, and unrelenting. Gallstones are the most common cause of acute pancreatitis. That the patient was obese and Native American was important: obesity is a major risk for gallstones, especially in women; and Native-American ancestry is also a strong risk factor: about 75% of the adult population in some southwestern tribes of Native Americans have gallstones. The combination of these two factors is a perfect example that much disease is associated with a combination of genetic makeup (Native American) and environmental influence (obesity).

The absence of bowel sounds and the presence of bowel air-fluid levels in the abdominal x-ray indicated bowel paralysis (ileus), further evidence of serious intra-abdominal disease. The diagnosis of pancreatitis was confirmed by sky-high levels of amylase and lipase. Low levels of blood calcium suggested that calcium was being precipitated into areas of fat necrosis around the pancreas.

Initial BP and HR readings showed postural hypotension, which meant she was volume depleted following loss of fluid from the vascular space into the fluid and accumulating as edema in and around the inflamed pancreas. Lab studies confirmed the impression of volume depletion:

- High hematocrit confirmed hemoconcentration following loss of intravascular fluid
- High BUN suggested low renal blood flow and reduced elimination of waste to preserve fluid
- High urine specific gravity confirmed that her body was concentrating urine to save fluid

Blood levels of bilirubin were slightly increased, and bilirubin was present in the urine. This was perhaps a surprise, given the fact that she did not appear to be jaundiced. ▶

[Case 17-1, continued] However, it is easy to miss mild jaundice in people with dark skin. In this setting the jaundice suggested bile duct obstruction that occurred when a swollen, edematous pancreas pressed on the common bile duct as it passed through the head of the pancreas. The slightly increased ALT (alanine aminotransferase) suggested mild liver damage, which could be attributed to common bile duct obstruction.

The surgeon orders rapid IV saline infusion to expand vascular volume and adds antibiotics and calcium to the infusion to avoid pancreatic abscess and hypocalcemia. A gas-

troenterologist is consulted, performs an endoscopy, and removes a gallstone impacted in the ampulla of Vater. The patient has a rocky course for the following ten days but is discharged home after a 3-week hospitalization.

POINTS TO REMEMBER
- Genetic predisposition and environmental influences are important in most disease.
- Gallstones are the most common cause of acute pancreatitis.

CASE STUDY 17-2 *"I DON'T KNOW WHAT'S COME OVER HIM; HE'S ACTING CRAZY"*

TOPICS
Diabetes
Diabetic ketoacidosis

THE CASE

Setting: You work in the emergency room of the main teaching hospital for a medical school. Your job tonight is to interview and examine noncritical patients and order initial laboratory and x-ray studies.

Clinical history: S.B. is a 53-year-old Caucasian man brought to the emergency room by his wife because of weakness and confusion. "I don't know what's come over him; he's acting crazy," she says and gives you the following history. He has been depressed and drinking because he lost his job. She is especially worried that he might have cancer, because he has lost 25 lb recently after being overweight for many years. Yesterday he developed fever, chills, and a cough that produced moderate amounts of yellow sputum. During the night he became short of breath and slept fitfully, getting up many times to urinate, a habit he developed about the time he lost his job several months ago. He vomited several times in the morning but had no diarrhea. When he became weak, confused, and combative, she brought him to the emergency room.

Mrs. B. answers your systems review and past medical history questions. Mr. B. has been a heavy smoker all of his life. For the past few months he has been getting up to urinate four or five times each night. His mother had diabetes and died when she was about 60. He has no siblings. His father died of lung cancer a few years ago. Mr. and Mrs. B. have two healthy adult children. Mr. B.'s main employment has been as a long-haul truck driver, and he has no history of occupational exposures.

You order blood tests, urinalysis, and chest and abdominal x-rays and wheel him into a stall for further examination.

Physical examination and other data: He is a short, moderately obese man who is restless and has been restrained on a gurney. He seems to understand he is in the hospital but not much of anything else. Vital signs are: BP 145/90, pulse 132, respirations 24 with a "driven" or "machine-like" quality, temperature 102° F. Your exam reveals dry mucous membranes and decreased breath sounds and a few rales in the right upper chest. You ask an aide to check with radiology and the laboratory and obtain the following results:

Chest x-ray:	Nearly opaque right upper lobe	
Abdominal x-ray:	Unremarkable	

Blood tests:		
Hematocrit	50% (male normal: 39–49)	Borderline High
WBC count	16.6 106 cells/µl (n: 4.5–10.5)	High
Neutrophils	82% (n: 60–70) with "a few bands"	High
Sodium	136 mEq/L (n: 135–145)	Borderline Low
Potassium	5.1 mEq/L (n: 3.5–5.0)	High
Glucose	626 mg/dL (n: 70–110)	Very high
Creatinine	2.2 mg/dL (n: 0.6–1.2)	High

Urinalysis:		
pH	3.3 (n: 4.8–5.2)	Very low
Ketones	Strongly positive (n: absent)	Abnormal
Glucose	Strongly positive (n: absent)	Abnormal

Clinical course: You call the internal medicine resident to see the patient. She agrees he has pneumonia and diabetes and is in ketoacidosis, and she instructs you to collect ▶

[Case 17-2, continued] sputum for culture and to order blood pH and osmolarity tests and blood cultures. Later you are to add insulin, penicillin, and potassium to the IV fluids. You call the lab, write some orders in the chart, insert a urinary catheter to monitor urine output, and start a saline solution IV at a fast drip.

A lab tech arrives and collects blood cultures and does a bedside arterial pH and osmolarity. Blood pH is abnormally acidic at 7.14 (n: 7.35–7.45), and osmolarity is high at 305 mOsm/L (n: 285–293).

DISCUSSION

That this man had diabetes was abundantly clear from the clinical evidence (remember: diabetes is a clinical diagnosis), and was confirmed by his sky-high admission blood glucose level. He had lost a large amount of weight without trying, and he was getting up many times at night to urinate. Both of these are associated with glycosuria—glucose (calories) was going into the toilet and carrying large amounts of water with it. Confirming laboratory evidence was also clear: he had glucose in his urine.

That he was in diabetic ketoacidosis was also clear. First, he was confused and combative, a sign he was nearing diabetic coma. Second, he had Kussmaul respirations, which have a forced quality somewhat like breathing after hard exercise. Third, his urine and blood pH were abnormally acidotic, and his urine was strongly positive for ketones.

The high WBC, neutrophilia, and left shift were explained by the right upper lobe pneumonia, which probably proved to be lobar pneumonia caused by *Streptococcus pneumoniae* (Chapter 14). Either the sputum or blood culture could prove the point.

The high hematocrit suggested he was dehydrated and hemoconcentrated, a point confirmed by high blood osmolarity. The low blood sodium level resulted from the flushing of salt out in urine because of osmotic diuresis associated with severe glycosuria. The high creatinine could be attributed to two things: low renal blood flow due to dehydration, and diabetic renal disease.

The high blood potassium level resulted from insulin deficiency: potassium cannot enter cells efficiently without insulin; as blood potassium rises it also spills into urine, which causes a total body potassium deficit. Note, however, that despite having high blood potassium, potassium was added to the IV. This is because with insulin treatment, blood potassium moves quickly out of blood and into cells and causes severely low blood potassium levels (hypokalemia) unless supplemental potassium is provided.

The odd thing about this case was that S.B. presented with diabetic ketoacidosis as an adult, a presentation that usually occurs in juvenile (type 1) diabetes. This man could be either a case of type 1 diabetes in an adult or a case of type 2 (adult onset diabetes) presenting with ketoacidosis. Blood insulin assay would answer the question: near normal insulin proves type 2, low insulin type 1. However, the question is somewhat academic: he needed insulin immediately, and he may need it regularly.

Finally, this patient was a cardiovascular time bomb waiting to explode. Despite losing 25 pounds, S.B. was still obese. Although we do not know his blood lipid picture, we can predict that he probably suffers from metabolic syndrome (Chapter 10), which is commonly associated with type 2 diabetes. What's more, he is a smoker and hypertensive, and now he has diabetes.

POINTS TO REMEMBER

- Sometimes a previously undiagnosed adult with diabetes presents in diabetic ketoacidosis.
- Management of diabetic ketoacidosis requires an intimate understanding of the pathophysiology of diabetes.

Objectives Recap

1. *Discuss the anatomy of the pancreas, and make a clear distinction between the digestive and the hormonal pancreas:* The pancreas is a tadpole-shaped organ about 5–6 inches (12–15 cm) long embedded in retroperitoneal fat in the mid abdomen and lying across the front of the aorta. The digestive (exocrine) pancreas is composed of acini and ducts. Ducts lead from individual pancreatic glands (acini) and join to form the pancreatic duct, which empties into the duodenum. Epithelial cells of the acini excrete digestive enzymes into the ductal system, which empties into the duodenum. The hormonal (endocrine) pancreas is composed of many tiny islets of Langerhans scattered throughout the gland. They are not connected to the ductal system, and they secrete hormones directly into the blood.

2. *Explain the relationship of glucose, glucagon, and insulin to one another and to stored glycogen:* The level of blood glucose is controlled by the opposing effects of insulin and glucagon. Insulin acts on muscle and other cell membranes to allow glucose to enter cells to be burned for energy production. A mutual push-pull relationship exists between in-

sulin and blood sugar (glucose): High blood glucose levels cause increased pancreatic secretion of insulin; low blood glucose levels cause decreased insulin secretion. A similar push-pull relationship exists between blood glucose levels and glucagon. Glucagon stimulates the liver to convert stored glycogen to glucose. At high levels glucagon stimulates the breakdown of fat to be used as an energy source if glucose is not available because of starvation or fasting, or with insulin deficiency (diabetes), in which cells cannot burn glucose because glucose cannot get into cells to be burned.

3. *Name the two most common causes of acute pancreatitis*: Gallstones and alcohol abuse.

4. *Explain autodigestion in acute pancreatitis*: Pancreatic enzymes normally are excreted in an inactive form; however, in pancreatitis they are liberated from the ducts, activate prematurely, and begin the digestive process while still in the cell or in the pancreas, causing the pancreas to digest itself and release additional activated enzymes in a vicious circle.

5. *Explain why a patient with acute hemorrhagic pancreatitis may develop hypovolemic shock or hypocalcemia*: Acute hemorrhagic pancreatitis causes massive edema and pooling of blood and fluid in and around the pancreas. Hypocalcemia may occur as calcium soaps are precipitated in areas of pancreatic fat necrosis.

6. *Contrast acute and chronic pancreatitis, and describe their relationship to one another*: Chronic pancreatitis occurs following repeated episodes of acute pancreatitis. Acute pancreatitis is sudden and painful and can be a catastrophic medical emergency associated with shock and death. Chronic pancreatitis is less dramatic, less painful, and less dangerous. It is associated with pancreatic fibrosis, ductal stone formation, and pancreatic calcification. Complications include migratory thrombophlebitis and malabsorption syndrome.

7. *Name the most common cause of chronic pancreatitis*: Alcohol abuse.

8. *Discuss the clinical presentation and complications of adenocarcinoma of the pancreas, and give a reasonable estimate of the five-year survival rate*: Upper abdominal pain or back pain usually is the first symptom. Painless jaundice may be the initial sign if the tumor obstructs the common bile duct. Unexplained weight loss or migratory thrombophlebitis should always suggest a hidden malignancy, especially pancreatic cancer. Only about 1% of patients with pancreatic carcinoma survive five years.

9. *Explain the pathogenesis of type 1 diabetes*: Type 1 diabetes is an autoimmune disease that destroys islets of Langerhans and their ability to produce insulin.

10. *Explain the pathogenesis of type 2 diabetes*: Type 2 diabetes is initially caused by resistance of peripheral (target) cells to the action of normal levels of insulin, necessitating increased pancreatic secretion of insulin. Insulin resistance can be associated with obesity, pregnancy, steroid excess, and other conditions. Later in type 2 diabetes, pancreatic insulin production falls as beta cells "wear out" from insulin overproduction.

11. *Name the most important factor in the development of type 2 diabetes*: Obesity; 80% of type 2 diabetics are obese.

12. *Name the two types of diabetic coma and the pathogenesis of each*: Diabetic coma can occur as a result of acidosis or severe dehydration. Acidosis occurs when insulin is lacking. The acidosis occurs because, with glucose unavailable, the body must burn fat for fuel. Fat is broken down in several steps into ketones, which are acidic molecules that are burned for fuel instead of glucose. The accumulation of ketones lowers blood pH (acidosis), which can lead to coma in extreme circumstances. The coma of severe dehydration occurs in patients with severe, prolonged glycosuria, which wastes water and electrolytes. Urine containing a large amount of glucose has high osmotic pressure, which attracts water; so that urine output rises and coma can occur, resulting from severe dehydration.

13. *Explain the importance in diabetes of hyperglycemia and glycosylation*: High blood glucose levels (hyperglycemia) are the cause of all diabetic complications. Hyperglycemia causes abnormal attachment of glucose to protein molecules (glycosylation). These abnormal molecules accelerate atherosclerosis and are the major cause of diabetic microvascular disease.

14. *Explain diabetic microvascular disease*: Diabetic microvascular disease is a condition of capillaries and other small blood vessels damaged by high blood glucose levels, which slow blood flow and diffusion of critical substances into tissues. It is the major pathologic mechanism of diabetic retinal disease and diabetic kidney disease.

15. *Name the leading causes of death in diabetes*: The most common causes of death are myocardial infarction, renal failure, and stroke.

16. *Name some criteria for the diagnosis of diabetes*: 1) classic signs and symptoms of diabetes such as polyuria, polyphagia, polydipsia, and weight loss; 2) any (random) blood glucose level equal to or greater than 200 mg/dL; 3) fasting blood glucose level equal to or greater than 126 mg/dL; 4) after oral glucose tolerance test 2-hour postprandial blood glucose equal to or greater than 200 mg/dL.

Typical Test Questions

1. Acute pancreatitis is most commonly associated with:
   A. Alcoholism
   B. Trauma
   C. Gastric acid reflux

2. Type 1 diabetes is associated with which one of the following?
   A. Autoimmunity
   B. Young age at onset
   C. Risk of ketoacidosis
   D. All of the above
   E. A and C only

3. Which one of the following is diagnostic of diabetes?
   A. Fasting blood glucose level 120 mg/dL
   B. Fasting blood glucose level 150 mg/dL
   C. Any blood glucose level over 126 mg/dL
   D. None of A, B, or C is diagnostic of diabetes
   E. Each one of A, B, and C is diagnostic of diabetes

4. All of the complications of diabetes are caused by which one of the following?
   A. Circulating ketones
   B. Autoimmunity
   C. Hyperglycemia
   D. Atherosclerosis
   E. None of the above

5. True or false? Blood amylase and lipase levels are elevated only in chronic pancreatitis.

6. True or false? Shock in acute pancreatitis occurs when sympathetic nerve signals relax peripheral vascular tone.

7. True or false? Chronic pancreatitis evolves from repeated attacks of acute pancreatitis.

8. True or false? Carcinoma of the pancreas is usually incurable by the time symptoms occur.

9. True or false? Type 2 diabetes is the result of peripheral insulin resistance.

10. True or false? Diabetic microvascular disease is the cause of diabetic retinopathy.

Diseases of Endocrine Glands

This chapter begins with a review of the normal pituitary gland, thyroid gland, parathyroid glands, and adrenal glands; their interrelationships; and homeostasis and negative feedback loops. Diseases and disorders discussed include overactivity and underactivity of the endocrine glands, as well as tumors and other disorders.

BACK TO BASICS
- Homeostasis
- The Pituitary Gland
- The Thyroid Gland
- The Parathyroid Glands
- The Adrenal Glands

DISEASES OF THE PITUITARY GLAND
- Diseases Affecting the Anterior Pituitary
- Disease of the Posterior Pituitary

DISEASES OF THE THYROID GLAND
- Overactivity of the Thyroid Gland (Hyperthyroidism)
- Underactivity of the Thyroid Gland (Hypothyroidism)

- Goiter
- Thyroiditis
- Neoplasms of the Thyroid Gland

DISEASES OF THE PARATHYROID GLANDS
- Overactivity of the Parathyroid Glands (Hyperparathyroidism)
- Underactivity of the Parathyroid Glands (Hypoparathyroidism)

DISEASES OF THE ADRENAL GLAND
- Diseases of the Adrenal Cortex
- Diseases of the Adrenal Medulla

Learning Objectives

After studying this chapter you should be able to:

1. Explain homeostatic feedback loops
2. Cite an example of change in blood hormone levels in endocrine disease, and explain how feedback is involved
3. Explain mass effect and stalk effect in pituitary disease
4. Name the most common type of functioning pituitary adenoma
5. Explain the difference between acromegaly and gigantism
6. Explain the difference between thyroglobulin and thyroxin binding globulin
7. Define goiter
8. Explain why TSH levels are diminished in Graves disease and other forms of primary hyperthyroidism and why TSH levels are elevated in primary hypothyroidism
9. Name the most common type of thyroiditis, and explain its pathogenesis
10. Name the most common type of thyroid cancer, and give an approximate 5-year survival figure
11. Offer a brief profile of the laboratory abnormalities in primary hyperparathyroidism
12. List the most important hormones produced by the adrenal medulla and cortex
13. Name the adrenocortical hormone responsible for most of the clinical features of Cushing syndrome
14. Name the most common cause of Cushing syndrome
15. Explain why patients with hypertension caused by primary hyperaldosteronism have low blood levels of renin
16. Explain why patients with Addison disease usually have dark skin
17. Explain why patients with pheochromocytoma may have high blood pressure

BACK TO BASICS
- hormones
- endocrine system
- negative feedback
- homeostasis
- anterior pituitary
- hypothalamus
- pituitary stalk
- metabolic rate
- thyroxine
- triiodothyronine (T$_3$)
- parathormone
- cortisol
- aldosterone
- androgenic steroids
- catecholamines

DISEASES AFFECTING THE ANTERIOR PITUITARY
- mass effect
- stalk effect
- prolactinoma
- acromegaly
- Cushing syndrome

DISEASES OF THE THYROID GLAND
- Graves disease
- goiter
- exophthalmos
- thyroiditis

DISEASES OF THE PARATHYROID GLANDS
- hyperparathyroidism

DISEASES OF THE ADRENAL CORTEX
- Cushing syndrome
- Addison disease

War will never cease until babies begin to come into the world with larger cerebrums and smaller adrenal glands.

H. L. MENCKEN (1881–1956), FAMOUSLY CRABBY AMERICAN JOURNALIST AND LINGUIST

BACK TO BASICS

By definition, endocrine glands (Chapter 2) secrete hormones directly into blood. **Hormones** are chemicals that stimulate or suppress cellular activity in a distant target tissue or organ. In this discussion the **endocrine system** is defined as the pituitary gland and the organs it controls—thyroid gland, adrenal glands, testes (Chapter 20), ovaries, (Chapter 21)—and the parathyroid glands. However, other organs can also secrete hormones. For example, the pancreas secretes insulin (Chapter 17), the kidney secretes renin and erythropoietin (Chapter 19), the stomach secretes gastrin (Chapter 16). Excepting the parathyroid glands, all target organs in the endocrine system are controlled by the pituitary gland (the "master gland"). The pituitary gland also influences organs that are not part of the endocrine system: milk formation in the breast, uterus contractions in pregnancy, bone growth in children, and water retention by the kidney. Figure 18-1 illustrates the relationships of the major endocrine glands and their target organs.

HOMEOSTASIS

In the endocrine system, activity of the target organ acts back upon the gland that stimulates it, a characteristic called **negative feedback**, by which the body maintains a balanced physiologic state. Taken together, these self-adjusting, mutually opposing forces keep physiologic function in equilibrium and are known as **homeostasis**. That is, if something tends to deviate upward from the steady state of equilibrium, a homeostatic mechanism forces it back down, and vice versa. For example, if blood sugar levels rise, the pancreas secretes more insulin to reduce it, or if blood sugar levels fall below normal, less insulin is secreted and blood sugar levels rise. For every bodily function—blood pressure, body temperature, blood pH, blood glucose; you name it—self-adjusting mechanisms exist to bring it back to the middle range if it deviates one way or the other.

For example, the relationship between insulin and glucose is a direct, *one-step process*—high blood glucose levels cause greater insulin secretion; low blood glucose levels cause decreased insulin secretion. However, some aspects of pituitary regulation of homeostasis are *a three-*

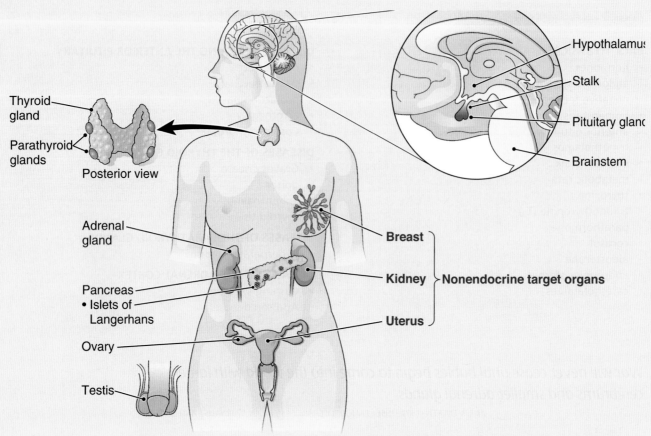

Figure 18-1 Major endocrine glands and target organs.

step process: the brain secretes hormones to influence the pituitary, the pituitary secretes hormones to influence its target organs—the thyroid gland, adrenal glands, testes, and ovaries—which in turn secrete hormones for the final effect on the ultimate target tissue and for negative feedback to the brain and pituitary gland.

However, sometimes a homeostatic mechanism is not capable of correcting a situation that has become unbalanced. For example, in some types of thyroid disease, the thyroid gland escapes pituitary control and operates independently, secreting excessive amounts of thyroid hormone. High blood levels of thyroid hormone act back on the pituitary gland, reducing pituitary output of thyroid-stimulating hormone (TSH). However, because the thyroid gland is acting independently, blood levels of thyroid hormone remain high, and blood levels of TSH remain low.

THE PITUITARY GLAND

The pituitary gland sits at the base of the skull in a bony cradle, the **sella turcica**, arguably the most important

intersection in the body—directly between the ears, encircled by the arteries of the circle of Willis, between the optic nerves, anterior to the brainstem, and between the internal carotid arteries. It consists of two parts—the **anterior pituitary** (the *adenohypophysis*) and the **posterior pituitary** (the *neurohypophysis*). Figure 18-2 illustrates the pituitary gland and the hormones it secretes, which are also tabulated in Table 18-1.

The **hypothalamus**, an area of the brain immediately above the pituitary gland, controls the pituitary via the **pituitary stalk**, which extends directly from the hypothalamus to the pituitary gland. The hypothalamus secretes **releasing hormones** for each of the target organs governed by the pituitary gland. For example, the hypothalamus secretes *thyrotropin-releasing hormone (TRH),* which stimulates pituitary release of TSH from the anterior pituitary. These releasing hormones travel down the pituitary stalk in a plexus of veins to the *anterior* pituitary. In addition to this venous plexus, the stalk contains a bundle of nerve tracts that extend directly from the hypothalamus to the *posterior* pituitary.

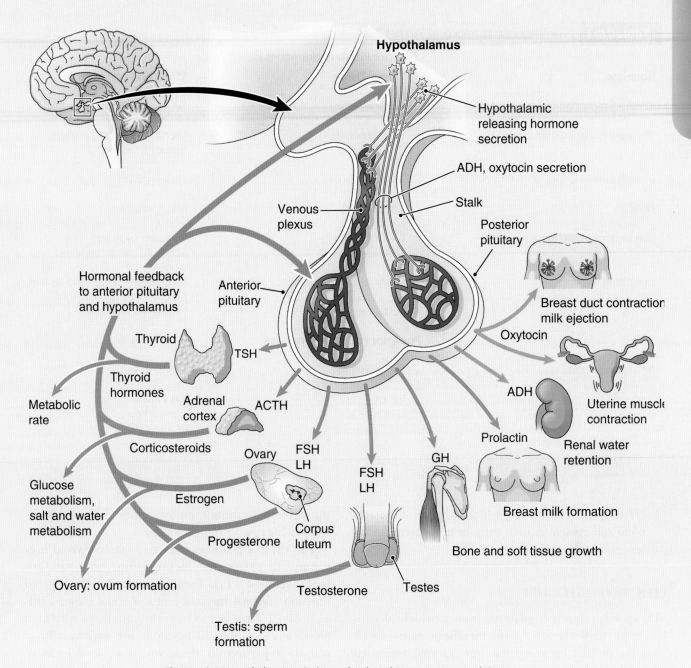

Figure 18-2 Hypothalamus, pituitary gland, and target organs and tissues.

Anterior pituitary hormones affect two types of targets:

- *Organs that have endocrine activity*—adrenal glands, thyroid gland, ovary, and testis—which release their own hormones for final effect, and which interact with the pituitary gland in a negative feedback loop. For example, the hypothalamus stimulates the pituitary gland and then the pituitary stimulates the thyroid gland to release hormones to regulate the rate of cell metabolism. Homeostasis is maintained because

thyroid hormones exert *negative feedback* on the hypothalamus and pituitary gland to decrease release of thyroid hormone. Using the thyroid as an example, Figure 18-3 illustrates how the hypothalamus, pituitary gland, and target organs exist in interlocked in negative feedback loops to maintain metabolic equilibrium.

- *Nonendocrine organs and tissues*—breast, uterus, kidney, bone, and muscle, for which *no negative feedback loop exists.* For example, the anterior pituitary se-

Table 18-1 **Pituitary Hormones and Target Tissues**

Anterior Pituitary Hormones

Hormone	Target Tissue	Effect on Target
Adrenocorticotrophic hormone (ACTH)	Adrenal cortex	Secrete steroid hormones
Thyroid-stimulating hormone (TSH)	Thyroid gland	Secrete thyroxine (T_4) and triiodothyronine (T_3)
Growth hormone (GH, somatotropin)	All body tissues	Tissue growth
Prolactin	Breast glands	Milk formation
Follicle-stimulating hormone (FSH)	Ovary: germ cells Testis: Sertoli cells	Stimulate ovulation Stimulate sperm formation
Luteinizing hormone (LH)	Ovary: granulosa and theca cells Testis: Leydig cells	Form corpus luteum and secrete progesterone and estrogen Secrete testosterone

Posterior Pituitary Hormones

Antidiuretic hormone (ADH)	Kidney tubules	Conserve water
Oxytocin	Breast ducts Uterus	Eject milk Contraction

cretes growth hormone, which directly stimulates bone and muscle growth without influencing an intervening endocrine gland.

THE THYROID GLAND

Thyroid hormones regulate the rate at which physiologic processes proceed—the **metabolic rate**—much like the throttle for an engine. For example, increased thyroid hormone causes, among other things, the heart to beat faster. Just as a rapidly running engine consumes more fuel, a high metabolic rate burns more calories, consumes more oxygen, and produces more heat.

The thyroid gland sits just under the skin in the anterior neck, above the breastbone (sternum), below the larynx, and in front of the trachea. It has two lobes, one on either side of the trachea, which are joined inferiorly by a narrow strip of thyroid, called the isthmus. The thyroid is composed of thousands of tiny spaces (*follicles*), like holes in a sponge, each lined by epithelial cells that synthesize hormone and filled with a gelatinous fluid, the **colloid**. The colloid contains a specialized protein, **thyroglobulin**, which binds thyroid hormones until they are secreted into blood. In this regard

the thyroid is unique among endocrine glands—it stores a big reserve of hormone.

The thyroid gland secretes two major thyroid hormones—**thyroxine** (*tetra*iodothyronine, or T_4) and **triiodothyronine** (T_3). Patients with normal thyroid function (normal metabolic rate, normal blood levels of T_4 and T_3) are said to be **euthyroid**; those with high blood levels of thyroid hormone are hypermetabolic and are **hyperthyroid**; those with low blood levels of thyroid hormone are hypometabolic and are **hypothyroid**.

Critical to understanding thyroid function is an understanding of the homeostatic feedback mechanisms involving the thyroid (Fig. 18-3). Recall the chain of events in thyroid homeostasis: the hypothalamus secretes a releasing hormone (TSH-releasing hormone, TRH), which causes the pituitary gland to secrete TSH, which in turn stimulates the thyroid gland to secrete thyroid hormones, which act back on the hypothalamus and pituitary gland to decrease output of hypothalamic-releasing hormone and TSH.

Most of the hormone secreted by the thyroid gland, and most thyroid hormone in blood, is T_4. However, T_4 lacks the metabolic wallop of T_3, which is secreted in

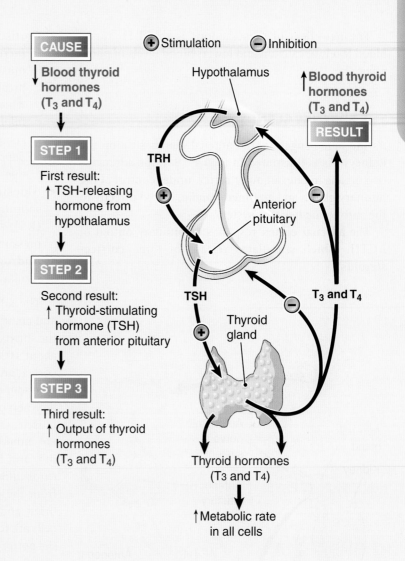

Figure 18-3 **Control of thyroid hormone output.**

lesser quantity and circulates in blood in lower concentration than T_4 does. Both T_4 and T_3 are transported to peripheral tissues attached (bound) to a specialized blood protein, **thyroxine binding globulin (TBG)**. However, to be metabolically active T_3 and T_4 must detach from TBG. Thus, *free T4 and T3 determine metabolic rate.*

THE PARATHYROID GLANDS

Normally, there are four parathyroid glands, one each behind the upper and lower poles of the right and left thyroid lobes; however, they may be embedded in the thyroid gland, and several extra parathyroids can be present in the nearby neck or upper chest. The parathyroids are tiny (about the size of a grain of rice) and tan and contain fat; they can be devilishly difficult to find surgically. *They do not operate under the control of the pi-*

tuitary gland. Rather, their output of **parathormone (PTH)** controls calcium homeostasis in a negative feedback loop with blood calcium: if the blood calcium level falls, PTH secretion increases, and vice versa. PTH acts to raise blood levels of calcium by:

- *Activating bone cells called osteoclasts, whose job it is to resorb bone, thus liberating calcium into blood*
- *Increasing calcium absorption by the intestine*
- *Increasing renal retention of calcium*
- *Increasing urinary phosphate excretion,* which lowers blood phosphate levels. Calcium and phosphate exist in blood in a reciprocal relationship: high levels of phosphate reduce calcium levels; low levels of phosphate raise calcium levels.
- *Activating vitamin D,* which stimulates intestinal absorption of calcium and helps PTH liberate calcium from bones

The net effect of these actions is that PTH raises blood levels of calcium and lowers blood levels of phosphate.

THE ADRENAL GLANDS

As the name suggests, the adrenal glands sit atop the kidneys. As is illustrated in Figure 18-4, the adrenal is two organs in one: an outer *cortex,* under control of the pituitary gland, and an inner *medulla,* linked directly to the autonomic nervous system.

The **adrenal cortex** responds to pituitary output of ACTH, which stimulates release of three **corticosteroids:**

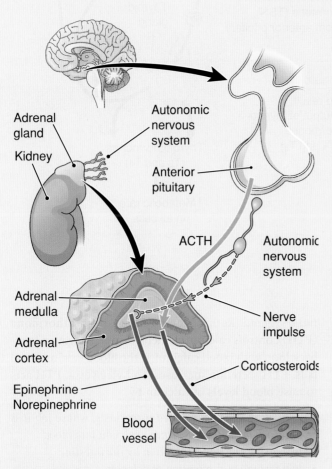

Figure 18-4 **Normal adrenal gland.** The cortex and the medulla secrete hormones directly into blood—the cortex under command of pituitary ACTH, the medulla under command of autonomic nerve impulse.

- **Cortisol** (hydrocortisone), which:
  - *Increases glucose production* by breaking down muscle protein to mobilize amino acids and by breaking down fat to mobilize fatty acids, both of which are converted to glucose by the liver
  - *Inhibits peripheral glucose utilization* to ensure that adequate glucose is available for the brain
  - *Suppresses immune reaction and limits inflammation* to lessen the stress of injury (disease)
- **Aldosterone**, which acts on the kidney to retain sodium (Na^+) and water and excrete potassium (K^+), actions that increase blood volume and blood pressure (Chapter 12).
- **Androgenic steroids**, which are weak versions of similar masculinizing steroids secreted by the testes.

The **adrenal medulla** is functionally, anatomically, and embryologically separate from the cortex. It forms the small central part of each adrenal gland, comprising about 10% of the weight, is completely surrounded by cortex, and is directly connected by nerve fibers to the autonomic nervous system (Chapter 23), the involuntary nervous system (Chapter 23), that acts on cardiac muscle, smooth muscle, and glands to control involuntary functions such as heart rate, blood pressure, sweating, and bowel peristalsis. The medulla is formed of *chromaffin cells,* which are *neuroendocrine cells* derived from the embryologic neural crest that develops into brain and peripheral nerves. Clusters of chromaffin cells are found in the posterior chest and abdomen near the aorta, major blood vessels, the urinary system, and ganglia of the autonomic nervous system, and are called the *paraganglionic system.*

The chromaffin cells secrete **catecholamines**, chemicals that act in various ways to help the body adapt to sudden stress. **Epinephrine**, the most important of these compounds, is released from the medulla upon stimulation by the autonomic nervous system. Epinephrine stimulates heart rate, dilates bronchioles and coronary arteries, constricts peripheral blood vessels, increases mental alertness and respiratory rate, and increases the metabolic rate. **Norepinephrine** is a second catecholamine secreted by the medulla. Its very powerful effect causes constriction of small blood vessels, increasing peripheral resistance and raising blood pressure.

Diseases of the Pituitary Gland

Of the two lobes of the pituitary gland, the anterior is far more often involved by disease. The posterior lobe is an extension of the brain and regulates water retention by the kidney, uterine muscle contraction in pregnancy, and breast duct contraction in nursing mothers. On the other hand, the anterior pituitary affects a much broader array of physiology: it controls function of the thyroid and adrenal glands, sperm and ovum production, bone and soft tissue growth, and breast milk formation. When the pituitary is affected by any disease, patient problems are almost always related to involvement of the anterior pituitary; the posterior pituitary is seldom affected seriously enough to cause clinical symptoms.

DISEASES AFFECTING THE ANTERIOR PITUITARY

Masses, usually neoplasms, are the most common disease of the anterior pituitary and may cause the pituitary gland to be overactive or underactive. Overactivity is much more common than is underactivity, and is usually attributable to a **functioning adenoma** (a benign hormone-secreting tumor) formed from one of the cell types of which the anterior pituitary is composed. Underactivity is usually associated either with a pituitary mass that crushes the normal gland or with gland infarction or other kinds of destruction.

Masses in the pituitary gland can have two consequences independent of their ability to secrete hormone:

- **Mass effect**: the pressure effect of a mass on nearby tissues, which in the pituitary can cause lateral visual field defects (from pressure on the optic nerves) or increased intracranial pressure (headache, nausea, and vomiting). Masses are often detectable by x-ray abnormalities of the bony cradle of the pituitary (sella turcica).
- **Stalk effect**: interference by a pituitary mass with hypothalamic inhibition of pituitary prolactin secretion, thereby allowing abnormal prolactin production.

The most common anterior pituitary mass is an *adenoma. Craniopharyngioma* is a benign cystic tumor that is less common than adenoma and arises immediately above the pituitary gland from an embryologic remnant, damaging the pituitary by downward pressure. Pituitary carcinoma is exceptionally rare.

Overactivity of the Anterior Pituitary (Hyperpituitarism)

Most overactivity of the pituitary gland results from **pituitary adenomas** (Figure 18-5), benign neoplasms that occur only in the anterior pituitary. As is detailed in

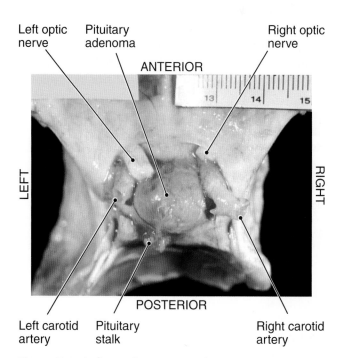

Left optic nerve   Pituitary adenoma   Right optic nerve

ANTERIOR

LEFT   RIGHT

POSTERIOR

Left carotid artery   Pituitary stalk   Right carotid artery

Figure 18-5 **Pituitary adenoma.** View from above, looking down from inside the cranium.

Table 18-2, most adenomas are *functioning adenomas* composed of a single cell type, and they secrete a single hormone. Adenomas occur most frequently in men between ages 20 and 50 years. They occur as solitary lesions that come to attention because of excessive hormone production, mass effect, or stalk effect. Most occur as discrete nodules, but a few are locally aggressive and invade bone, sinuses, or brain.

Prolactinoma is a benign tumor of the anterior pituitary that secretes prolactin, the pituitary hormone that stimulates breast glands to make milk. It is the most common functioning pituitary tumor, accounting for about one fourth of adenomas. In women it causes milk secretions from the breast (*lactation*), cessation of menstruation (*amenorrhea*), infertility, and loss of sexual drive. The diagnosis is much easier to make in menstruating women than in nonmenstruating women or in men. In menstruating women, amenorrhea is a noticeable symptom, whereas nonmenstrual signs and symptoms, which must be relied on for diagnosis in nonmenstruating women or men, are subtle, and the tumor may not become evident until mass effects come to attention. The main symptoms in men are decreased sexual drive and impotence.

Diagnosis is confirmed by finding high levels of prolactin in blood. High levels of blood prolactin, with symptoms similar to those caused by prolactinoma, can be caused by high-dose estrogen therapy, pregnancy, renal failure, thyroid gland failure, lesions of the hypothalamus, and some drugs.

Growth hormone (somatotropin) adenoma is the second most common *functioning* adenoma of the anterior pituitary. Many of these adenomas also secrete prolactin. Often the early clinical manifestations are subtle (for instance, a change of shoe or hat size in an adult),

and they may become quite large before they are diagnosed, often because of mass effect.

Excessive production of growth hormone causes two syndromes: gigantism and acromegaly. **Gigantism**, a general increase in body size, with especially long arms and legs, occurs when a child or teenager develops an adenoma that secretes growth hormone *before* growth plates close at the ends of long bones.

Acromegaly is a syndrome that occurs when abnormal secretion of growth hormone occurs in adults *after* bone growth plates disappear. It is characterized by conspicuous growth of bones in the hand, feet, face, skull, and jaw and growth of viscera, skin, and soft tissue. Patients (Fig. 18-6) have prominent brows and

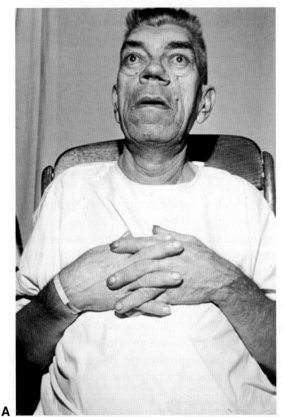

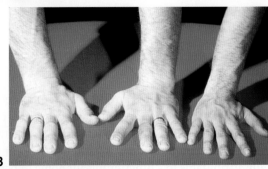

Figure 18-6 **Acromegaly.** Acromegaly is caused by oversecretion of growth hormone in adults, after normal bone growth has stopped. **A,** Note coarse facial features. **B,** Patient's large hands at left; single normal hand at right.

Table 18-2	Adenomas of the Pituitary Gland	
Hormone Secreted	**Frequency**
Prolactin	26%
None (null cell or oncocytoma)	23%
Adrenocorticotrophic hormone (ACTH)	15%
Growth hormone (GH)	14%
Multiple hormones	13%
Follicle-stimulating hormone (FSH) or luteinizing hormone (LH)	8%
Thyroid-stimulating hormone (TSH)	1%

chin, gapped teeth (teeth become separated as the jaw lengthens), and huge feet and hands with thick fingers. However, they are not exceptionally large or tall. Skin and soft tissue growth adds to the coarse facial appearance. Other problems (Fig. 18-7) associated with acromegaly are secondary diabetes (caused by insulin resistance by peripheral tissues) and hypertension, muscle weakness, congestive heart failure, arthritis, and osteoporosis.

ACTH adenoma, an adenoma of the anterior pituitary that secretes adrenocorticotropin (ACTH), accounts for about 15% of pituitary adenomas, and causes

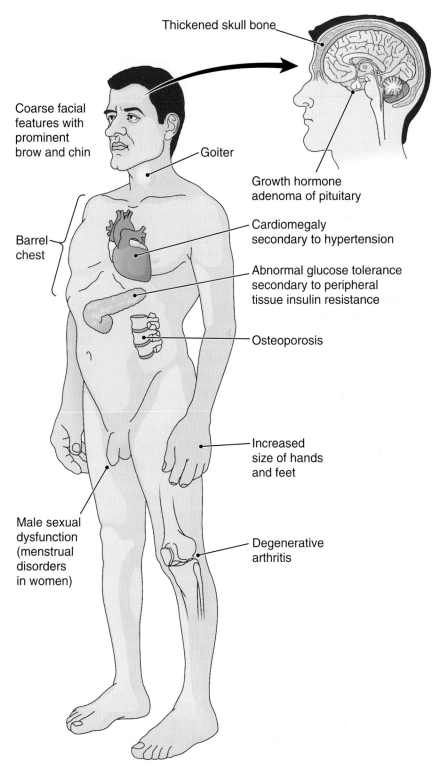

Thickened skull bone

Coarse facial features with prominent brow and chin

Goiter

Growth hormone adenoma of pituitary

Barrel chest

Cardiomegaly secondary to hypertension

Abnormal glucose tolerance secondary to peripheral tissue insulin resistance

Osteoporosis

Increased size of hands and feet

Male sexual dysfunction (menstrual disorders in women)

Degenerative arthritis

Figure 18-7 **Clinical manifestations of acromegaly.**

excessive secretion of cortisol (hydrocortisone) and related hormones from the adrenal cortex. The effects are dramatic and produce a combination of clinical findings known as **Cushing syndrome**—hypertension, obesity, round (moon) facial feature, diabetes, skin marks (striae), excess body and facial hair (hirsutism), and menstrual and mental abnormalities. This syndrome is discussed in detail below with adrenal disease.

Luteinizing hormone adenoma and **follicle-stimulating hormone adenoma** together comprise about 10% of anterior pituitary adenomas. They occur most commonly in middle-aged men and women and produce very little hormonal effect—they almost always come to attention because of mass effect. The rarest adenoma (~1%) is the **thyroid-stimulating hormone adenoma**, which produces symptoms associated with an overactive thyroid gland. It will be discussed below with thyroid disease.

Finally, there are anterior pituitary adenomas that do not secrete hormone. **Null cell adenoma** occurs almost as frequently as prolactinomas do. It comes to attention because it produces a stalk effect that stimulates the remaining normal pituitary to secrete prolactin, or because destruction of the gland by the mass causes pituitary failure.

Underactivity of the Anterior Pituitary (Hypopituitarism)

Most cases of pituitary failure are failure of the anterior pituitary. The posterior pituitary is not often involved.

About 75% of the anterior pituitary must be destroyed for hormonal deficit to become symptomatic. The most common causes of pituitary failure are, in order: mass effect, pituitary destruction caused by vascular ischemia with necrosis (pituitary infarction), and surgical or radiotherapeutic destruction. Usually only one or two hormones are deficient, and sometimes only mildly so. Target organs—adrenal cortex, thyroid gland, testes, and ovary—atrophy, and patients suffer from lack of cortisol, thyroxine, and testosterone or estrogen. Symptoms of hypopituitarism are mild and develop slowly. Patients become easily fatigued, lose weight, and are mildly anemic. Often the effect on organs of sexual function calls attention—patients may develop amenorrhea, loss of libido, atrophic gonads, and impotence. The diagnosis is difficult to make because the symptoms are nonspecific.

Infarction (death of cells because of insufficient blood flow, Chapter 5) of the pituitary gland in pregnancy is **Sheehan syndrome**, illustrated in Figure 18-8. During pregnancy the *anterior* pituitary enlarges, mainly because of an increase in the size of prolactin-secreting

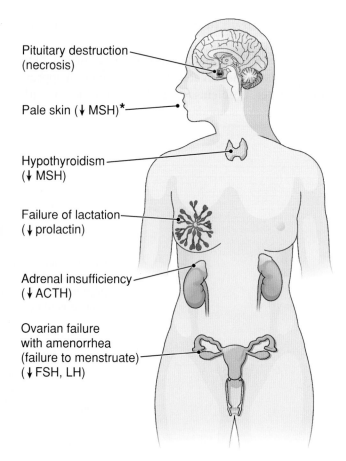

Pituitary destruction (necrosis)

Pale skin (↓ MSH)*

Hypothyroidism (↓ MSH)

Failure of lactation (↓ prolactin)

Adrenal insufficiency (↓ ACTH)

Ovarian failure with amenorrhea (failure to menstruate) (↓ FSH, LH)

* MSH: Melanocyte-stimulating hormone.
MSH is a breakdown product of ACTH.
Excess of MSH produces dark skin.
Deficiency produces pale skin.

Figure 18-8 **Clinical manifestations of Sheehan syndrome.** Sheehan syndrome is caused by pituitary destruction.

cells; however, blood supply to the anterior pituitary does not increase, which leaves it relatively undersupplied with blood. Hemorrhage and shock (Chapter 5) can occur during pregnancy or delivery (Chapter 21), sometimes resulting in blood flow insufficient to maintain the enlarged anterior pituitary. The posterior pituitary usually is spared because its arterial supply is separate from the anterior pituitary and because the posterior pituitary does not enlarge in pregnancy. The diagnosis should be suspected in a woman who does not resume normal menstrual periods after pregnancy (provided, of course, that she is not nursing or pregnant again), or who develops symptoms of thyroid failure (discussed further below with thyroid disease).

DISEASES OF THE POSTERIOR PITUITARY

The posterior pituitary (neurohypophysis) is composed of modified brain cells that connect directly to the hypothalamus, which lies immediately above. The hypothalamus synthesizes *antidiuretic hormone* and *oxytocin* and sends them down the pituitary stalk for storage and release from the posterior pituitary.

Antidiuretic hormone (ADH) acts on renal tubules to stimulate retention of water. ADH deficiency causes **diabetes insipidus**. Insipid means bland or tasteless, as opposed to mellitus, sweet tasting. (The urine of diabetes mellitus tastes sweet; a fact known to antiquity.) Diabetes insipidus is characterized by very high output of very dilute urine (specific gravity < 1.002) because of the absence of ADH secretion, usually caused by destruction of the pituitary gland or conditions affecting the hypothalamus: head trauma, surgery, neoplasm, infarction, or inflammation. One third of cases appear to be caused by sporadic (spontaneous) genetic defects of ADH synthesis. A few cases are caused by a renal defect and have nothing to do with the pituitary gland. Whatever the cause, because patients excrete very large volumes of dilute, nearly colorless urine, dehydration is the consequence. Debilitated patients are at some risk, but most patients can remain hydrated by drinking a lot of water.

Oxytocin stimulates uterine smooth muscle contraction in labor and breast duct smooth muscle contraction to aid lactation. There are no clinical syndromes of oxytocin abnormality.

Diseases of the Thyroid Gland

The thyroid gland regulates the rate of body metabolism by secreting hormones that stimulate the rate at which physiologic processes proceed. Increased amounts of thyroid hormone produce a faster rate of metabolism—more oxygen and calories are burned and more heat is produced. A decreased amount of hormone has the opposite effect. The most common diseases of the thyroid gland are overactivity and underactivity, inflammation, and neoplasms.

OVERACTIVITY OF THE THYROID GLAND (HYPERTHYROIDISM)

An excessive amount of thyroid hormone increases the metabolic rate, producing a condition known as **hyperthyroidism**. Sometimes the term *thyrotoxicosis* is used to refer to the metabolic effect, and *hyperthyroidism* is used to denote the condition of the gland. This distinction is useful in cases with a high metabolic rate caused by overmedication with thyroid hormone—the *patient* is thyrotoxic (hypermetabolic) but the *gland* is not overactive. The terms are sometimes used interchange-

ably, but this text uses hyperthyroidism to refer to both thyroid disease and metabolic effect. The causes of hyperthyroidism are:

- Overmedication with T_3 or T_4 in the treatment of thyroid gland failure
- Increased thyroid gland output of hormone associated with diseases of the thyroid gland (**primary hyperthyroidism**)
- Increased thyroid gland output of thyroid hormone caused by output of thyroid-stimulating hormone (TSH) by the anterior pituitary (*secondary hyperthyroidism*)

Graves disease accounts for 80–90% of all hyperthyroidism and is characterized by:

- Hyperthyroidism
- An enlarged thyroid gland (**goiter**)
- Bulging eyes (**exophthalmos**)—the wide-eyed, staring gaze of Graves disease patients is one of the most distinctive clinical signs in all of medicine
- A minority of patients have a skin disease that affects the skin over the shins and is peculiar to patients with thyroid disease

Primary hyperthyroidism can also occur in other thyroid diseases. Most patients with these other diseases have enlarged thyroid glands (goiter) for unknown reasons. The most common type of goiter is an irregular, lumpy enlargement of the gland, *nodular goiter*. Some nodular goiters become overactive and secrete excessive amounts of thyroid hormone.

Graves disease one of the most common autoimmune diseases (Chapter 8) in the United States; it affects about 1% of the population under age 40. It is particularly prevalent in young women (90% of patients are female), who often also suffer from other autoimmune disease, such as systemic lupus erythematosus. The key immune problem is a unique antithyroid antibody (an immunoglobulin, Chapter 8) that acts like thyroid stimulating hormone (TSH). It attaches to follicle epithelial cells and stimulates them to secrete thyroid hormones; hence, it is named **thyroid-stimulating immunoglobulin (TSI)** and is detectable in blood by a laboratory test. Other autoimmune antibodies act to cause an accumulation of fat behind the eyes, which pushes the eyes out, and results in the remarkable "bug eyed" appearance (*exophthalmos*) of patients with Graves disease.

Less than half of patients with Graves disease have a skin disease that affects the skin over the tibia, which consists of brownish, thick, and scaly plaques. Confusingly, it is called *pretibial myxedema*, although it has nothing to do with the systemic metabolic condition of the same name (*general myxedema*) caused by thyroid failure (*hypo*thyroidism).

The enlargement of the thyroid gland in Graves disease is caused by hyperplasia of the epithelial cells that line thyroid follicles (Fig. 18-9). In Graves disease and other forms of hyperthyroidism that result from an overactive thyroid gland—which, of course, does not include cases caused by overmedication—the thyroid gland is diffusely enlarged and smooth, and so much blood may be coursing through it that with a stethoscope placed over the gland, a swishing sound (*bruit*) can be heard with each heartbeat.

The clinical picture of Graves disease and other types of hyperthyroidism is illustrated in the right half of Figure 18-10. The overly active metabolic state results in weight loss, sweating, heat intolerance, increased appetite, and bowel hypermotility, which can cause diarrhea and poor intestinal absorption of nutrients (malabsorption, Chapter 15). The autonomic nervous system is also overactive and causes nervousness and irritability, tremor, rapid heart rate, palpitations, and overreactive (jumpy) reflexes. Exophthalmos (bulging eyes, proptosis) is a characteristic finding in a majority of patients with Graves disease. *Patients with other forms*

of hyperthyroidism do not develop true exophthalmos—in these non-Graves cases of hyperthyroidism, the upper eyelid retracts and produces an appearance somewhat similar to exophthalmos, but not as dramatic. In true exophthalmos, the eyes can bulge so far outward that the lids cannot close, and the cornea dries and ulcerates. A second characteristic eye sign of hyperthyroidism (of any type) is *lid lag*, a failure of the upper eyelid to retract normally when gaze moves from downward to upward. The result is a brief sleepy-eyed appearance as gaze moves upward.

Laboratory studies are essential for correct diagnosis of thyroidal disease. In patients with Graves disease, blood levels of T_4 and T_3 *are increased* and levels of *TSH are decreased*. In Graves disease the homeostatic mechanism is disrupted because the thyroid gland is secreting large amounts of T_3 and T_4 and will not stop. High blood levels of T_3 and T_4 suppress the hypothalamus and pituitary, and blood TSH level falls.

As is indicated in Table 18-3, blood levels of T_4 and T_3 are increased in hyperthyroidism and decreased in hypothyroidism. If thyroid hormones are high as a result of increased pituitary output of TSH (very rare), then TSH levels would also be increased. However, *the vast majority of hyperthyroidism is caused by primary*

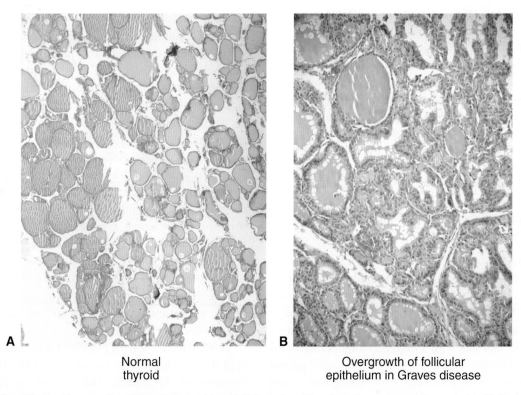

Normal thyroid   Overgrowth of follicular epithelium in Graves disease

Figure 18-9 **Thyroid gland in hyperthyroidism. A,** Normal thyroid. **B,** Hyperthyroidism. Note the overgrowth (hyperplasia) of follicular epithelium.

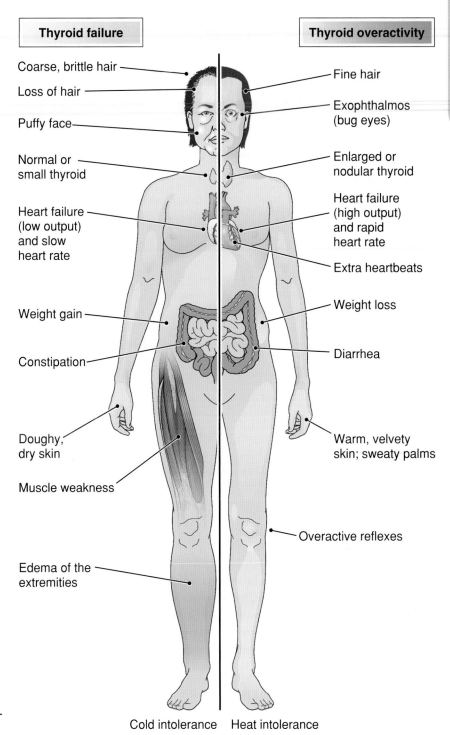

Figure 18-10 Hypothyroidism and hyperthyroidism compared.

thyroid gland hormone output or overmedication with thyroid hormone, both of which suppress pituitary output of TSH and result in low blood TSH levels.

An additional useful tool in diagnosis of thyroid disease is thyroid **radioactive iodine uptake (RAI uptake)**. Patients are given a small dose of radioactive iodine to measure the amount captured by the thyroid in the syn-

thesis of thyroid hormones, which require iodine. Overactive glands take up an abnormally large amount of the administered dose.

Primary hyperthyroidism is treatable with a variety of drugs that in most instances stop the overproduction of thyroid hormones, causing the gland to shrink and the metabolic rate to return to normal. However, some pa-

| Table 18-3 | Laboratory Tests of Thyroid Function |

Condition	Total T$_4$ (µg/dL)	Total T$_3$ (ng/dL)	TSH µU/ml	Radioactive Iodine Uptake by Thyroid in 24 Hours	Comment
Normal	5–12	95–190	0.3–5	10–30%	
Patients with thyroid or pituitary disease, not taking thyroid hormone medication					
Increased thyroid hormone in blood (hyperthyroidism)	↑	↑	↓ in thyroid gland overactivity (primary hyperthyroidism) ↑ in pituitary hyperthyroidism	↑	Thyroid-stimulating immunoglobulin detectable in Graves disease
Decreased thyroid hormone in blood (hypothyroidism)	↓	↓	↑ in thyroid gland failure ↓ in pituitary failure	↓	Assay of TSH-releasing hormone (TRH from hypothalamus) may be helpful
Hypothyroid patients receiving thyroid hormone as replacement medication					
Rx with T$_4$	N	Varies with dose	N to ↓ per dosage	↓	Correct dosage determined by clinical effect
Rx with T$_3$	↓	Varies with dose	N to ↓ per dosage	↓	

Patients with severe nonthyroidal illness such as renal failure, starvation, cirrhosis, and sepsis may have abnormally low thyroid function tests but are clinically normal—they do not have signs or symptoms of hypothyroidism, and, apart from their other disease, appear to have normal thyroid function. This condition is known as the *euthyroid sick syndrome.*

tients may not respond and can be treated with a therapeutic dose of radioactive iodine, which destroys much of the gland, or by surgery to remove it. After treatment, some patients may need supplemental oral thyroid hormone medication to maintain normal metabolic rate.

UNDERACTIVITY OF THE THYROID GLAND (HYPOTHYROIDISM)

Thyroid failure (**hypothyroidism**) is a state in which absence of thyroid hormone causes the body's metabolic rate to slow down. It usually results from thyroid disease (primary hypothyroidism), although, uncommonly, it may be result from failure of the pituitary gland or the hypothalamus to secrete their hormones. In developed nations almost all cases are primary hypothyroidism secondary to thyroid inflammation (*thyroiditis*). Other causes include surgical or radiation ablation, usually as a result of cancer treatment. In developing nations a lack of dietary iodine may be responsible—iodine is neces-

sary for thyroid synthesis of T$_3$ and T$_4$, and in the United States most table salt contains added iodine.

The clinical features of hypothyroidism are illustrated in the left half of Figure 18-10. The clinical syndrome of hypothyroidism in older children and adults is commonly called **myxedema** because of the accumulations of thick (myxomatous) fluid in various organs, especially the skin. (Note: the skin disease sometimes seen in Graves disease is also called myxedema.) Accumulations of this fluid produce bags under the eyes, puffy eyelids, swollen tongue, edema of the vocal cords and hoarseness, swelling of the hands and feet, pleural and pericardial effusions, and weight gain. Hair loss is common, including the outside (lateral) half of the eyebrows. Patients develop a mental dullness that may be misinterpreted as depression. Everything slows down: they are weak and walk with a slow shuffle, their reflexes are slow, they are intolerant of cold, their heart rate is slow, and they are constipated (see Case Study 18-1 at the end of this chapter).

Laboratory findings are also critical to confirm a diagnosis of hypothyroidism (Table 18-3). Most cases are related to thyroid gland problems, and the hypothalamus and pituitary gland cooperate to produce TSH in an effort to get the thyroid gland to respond. Therefore, blood levels of both T_3 and T_4 are decreased, and TSH is usually markedly elevated.

Cretinism is infantile or early childhood hypothyroidism and is a cause of short stature and mental retardation. In developed nations it is now rare because of the addition of iodine to table salt.

GOITER

As is illustrated in Figure 18-11, a **goiter** is an enlarged thyroid gland and is the most common thyroid abnormality—more common than Graves disease or thyroid failure. Remember that the term goiter only describes the *size* of the gland and says nothing about thyroid *function*. Most goiters are not associated with abnormal thyroid function and are called **nontoxic goiter**; however, some goiters may be associated with hyperthyroidism or hypothyroidism.

As the thyroid gland grows into a goiter, thyroid follicles uniformly accumulate colloid to become a simple,

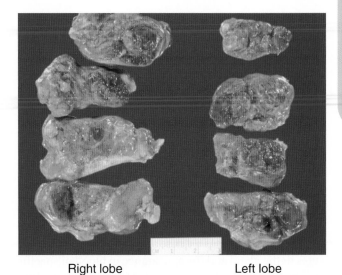

Right lobe　　　　　　　　**Left lobe**

Figure 18-12 **Nodular goiter.** Cross sections of surgically removed thyroid gland reveal an irregular, nodular gland.

or **colloid**, **goiter**, which has a smooth, uniform appearance and which is shaped like, but larger than, a normal thyroid gland. As the gland continues to enlarge, follicles become cystic and irregularly sized and are filled with colloid to become an uneven, lumpy mass known as a **nodular goiter**, which is illustrated in Figure 18-12. In most instances, the cause of goiter is not known. However, in remote, mountainous parts of Africa, Asia, and South America, iodine deficiency is the culprit because iodine supplementation is not available. Without iodine the thyroid gland cannot maintain normal blood levels of T_3 and T_4, and as a result the gland is continually stimulated by TSH, from the pituitary. Goiter that occurs without known cause, called **sporadic goiter**, usually occurs in young women around puberty or in early reproductive years, when there is an increased physiologic demand for thyroid hormones. An enlarged, overactive gland, as seen in Graves disease, is a **toxic goiter**.

Most goiters come to attention because of a mass in the low anterior neck, which may be noticed first by others as the patient takes a sip of a drink and the mass becomes visible, bobbing up and down with the swallow. Goiter may also come to attention because the enlarged gland presses on the trachea and esophagus, causing difficulty breathing or swallowing. Pressure on nerves serving the larynx may cause hoarseness.

THYROIDITIS

Thyroiditis is inflammation of the thyroid gland. Most thyroiditis is **chronic thyroiditis** caused by thyroid autoimmunity (Chapter 8). Thyroiditis usually presents as a painless enlargement of the gland (goiter) that is not

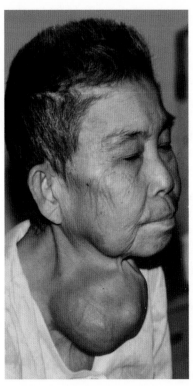

Figure 18-11 **Goiter.** The lumpy appearance of this unusually large goiter and the lack of exophthalmos suggest that it is a nodular, nontoxic goiter. Reprinted with permission from Rubin E. Pathology. 4th ed. Philadelphia. Lippincott Williams and Wilkins, 2005.

associated with thyroid function abnormalities. However, some patients may be hypothyroid if there is destruction of thyroid tissue. Alternatively, early in the disease patients may have a brief period of gland tenderness and slight hyperthyroidism caused by inflammatory disruption of follicles with release of stored hormone. While the thyroid glands of most patients with thyroiditis function normally, the cause of most hypothyroidism is thyroiditis.

Hashimoto thyroiditis is by far the most common type of thyroiditis in the United States. It is a common chronic autoimmune disease and one of the most common causes of goiter and hypothyroidism. The autoimmune reaction causes a dense accumulation of lymphocytes in the gland and the appearance in blood of specific antithyroid antibodies that block TSH and thereby hinder T_3 and T_4 production by the gland. Hashimoto disease has a distinct familial tendency—half of first-degree relatives have antithyroid antibodies in their blood and many have some other type of autoimmune disease, such as systemic lupus erythematosus. As is illustrated in Figure 18-13, the gland is enlarged and overrun by damaging masses of lymphocytes.

Hashimoto thyroiditis occurs almost exclusively in middle-aged women (90% of cases) and presents as a painless enlargement of the gland. At time of diagnosis, most patients have normal thyroid gland function; however, hypothyroidism may occur as inflammation persists and gland is destroyed.

Accumulation of lymphocytes
as part of the autoimmune
reaction
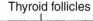
Thyroid follicles

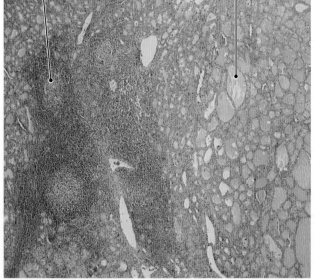

Figure 18-13 **Hashimoto thyroiditis.** Normal thyroid follicles and a collection of lymphocytes involved in the autoimmune reaction.

Subacute (granulomatous) thyroiditis (*de Quervain thyroiditis*) is much less common than Hashimoto disease is. The cause is unknown, but a virus is suspected. Like other forms of thyroiditis it occurs much more commonly in women than men. The pathologic findings in the gland feature a mixture of acute and chronic inflammation. Because the thyroid gland holds a large reserve of hormone, which is released by the inflammatory process, patients may become hyperthyroid for a short period of time as T_4 and T_3 are washed out of the inflamed gland. Over the long term, however, thyroid gland anatomy and function usually return to normal. The clinical picture is one of sudden development of an enlarged, tender thyroid gland with painful swallowing, fever, malaise, and high white blood cell count indicating hyperthyroidism. The condition is self-limited and resolves in 6–8 weeks.

There are several other types of thyroiditis, all uncommon and occurring mainly in women, which feature varying degrees of inflammation, scarring, and goiter.

NEOPLASMS OF THE THYROID GLAND

Although less than 1% of thyroid masses prove to be malignant, all must be investigated. Some important facts about thyroid masses are:

- Solitary masses are more likely than are multiple ones to be neoplastic (adenoma or carcinoma).
- Masses that are "cold," that is, that do not take up radioactive iodine because they are not synthesizing thyroid hormone, are more likely than are "hot" ones to be neoplastic.
- Masses in younger patients are more likely than are those in older patients to be neoplastic.
- Masses in males are more likely than are those in females to be neoplastic.

Most masses prove to be nonneoplastic lumps of nodular goiter; however, a few prove to be neoplasms.

Adenomas

Thyroid adenomas are benign neoplasms of the epithelial cells that line thyroid follicles. They are almost always solitary, round, and discrete. Adenomas most often reveal themselves as a solitary, painless mass in an otherwise normal woman with no evidence of thyroid hormone excess or thyroid failure. Most do not take up radioiodine and are nonfunctional ("cold"). They do not develop into carcinoma.

Carcinomas

Almost all carcinomas of the thyroid gland arise from the epithelium that lines the thyroid follicles. Thyroid carcinoma is uncommon, accounting for about 1% of all cancers. Most occur in adults; females are more affected than males except in the very young or very old. There are no known risk factors for thyroid carcinoma other than radiation, which is discussed in the nearby History of Medicine box.

Only a very small proportion of thyroid nodules are malignant—over 90% of solitary thyroid nodules are lumps in a benign goiter, and most of the others are adenomas. Nevertheless, goiter nodules and adenomas are indistinguishable from carcinoma without biopsy. In most cases fine needle aspiration with pathologic study of harvested cells is a safe and rapid method of making the diagnosis without surgical biopsy.

By far the most common thyroid carcinomas feature a cauliflower-like microscopic growth pattern. They are called **papillary carcinomas** and account for about 80% of thyroid cancers. Fortunately, they grow very slowly, and more than 90% of patients survive five years. Some experts consider small papillary lesions of the thyroid gland to be benign papillomas, but the majority consider all papillary thyroid lesions to be malignant.

Papillary carcinomas are most common in women between 20 and 50 years old. Large tumors and tumors in people over 50 are more aggressive. All papillary thyroid carcinomas have a tendency to lymphatic invasion and metastasis, whereas other tumors of endocrine glands tend toward vascular invasion. Astonishingly, the presence of local lymph node metastases does not affect the long-term prognosis. Positive lymph nodes most often appear as a painless neck mass, but they can appear as a solitary distant metastasis.

Follicular carcinoma is characterized by the production of follicles; no papillary growth is present. It accounts for about 15% of thyroid cancers. When compared to papillary carcinoma, follicular carcinoma occurs in an older age group, is more aggressive, is less likely to spread to lymph nodes, and is much more likely to spread by the bloodstream to lungs, bone, and liver. Most are treated by surgical excision.

Medullary carcinoma, accounting for about 5% of thyroid cancers, arises from specialized nonepithelial cells of the thyroid that secrete *calcitonin*, a hormone important in blood calcium homeostasis. It may occur as a feature of one of the multiple endocrine neoplasia syndromes (MEN), which are discussed later in this chapter and are a family of genetic defects associated with tumors of various endocrine organs. Medullary carcinoma is a microscopically distinctive and clinically aggressive tumor that tends to metastasize via the bloodstream. The five-year survival rate is about 50%.

In contrast to the mild nature of other thyroid carcinomas, **anaplastic carcinoma** of the thyroid gland is among the most aggressive of all human malignancies. It occurs mainly in elderly patients, and most are fatal within a year.

Diseases of the Parathyroid Glands

The parathyroid glands secrete a hormone, parathormone (PTH), which raises blood calcium by its metabolic influence on bones, the kidneys, and the intestines—it mobilizes calcium from bone, decreases renal excretion of calcium, and increases intestinal absorption of calcium. The amount of parathormone secreted by the parathyroid glands is controlled by blood calcium levels: A high blood calcium level causes reduced parathormone secretion; a low blood calcium level causes increased parathormone secretion.

OVERACTIVITY OF THE PARATHYROID GLANDS (HYPERPARATHYROIDISM)

There are three kinds of hyperparathyroidism: *primary, secondary,* and *tertiary,* all of which feature overactivity of the parathyroid glands. Primary overactivity is caused by parathyroid hyperplasia or adenoma; secondary and tertiary overactivity are due to chronic renal failure. The physiologic effects of excessive amounts of parathormone are illustrated in Figure 18-14.

Second only to diabetes mellitus, **primary hyperparathyroidism** is the most common primary endocrine disorder; that is, an endocrine disorder that is not secondary to some other condition, such as Cushing syndrome secondary to overmedication with corticosteroids. It is an important cause of abnormally high blood calcium levels (*hypercalcemia*). Blood calcium measurement is regularly included for patients having blood lab tests performed, so an elevated blood calcium level is often detected incidentally in routine laboratory blood tests. In the general population, occurrence is about 1 in 400 people. Most are women with parathyroid hyperplasia or adenoma. The classic clinical findings, depicted in Figure 18-15, are easily recalled by the phrase "stones, bones, groans, and moans." "Stones"

refers to kidney stones, "bones" to associated destructive bone changes, "groans" to the pain of stomach and peptic ulcers that occur in some cases, and "moans" to the depression that frequently accompanies the disease and is often its first and most prominent manifestation. Muscle atrophy and pancreatitis also may occur.

However, the findings are rarely so dramatic. Most patients have "laboratory disease" only; that is, they are asymptomatic, and blood calcium and PTH are elevated, but not much above normal. Although in many patients the disease lingers in this state indefinitely and does not require surgery, development of symptoms warrants treatment.

The typical laboratory findings are increased blood calcium levels and *increased* blood PTH levels. An important diagnostic point is that PTH levels are *decreased* in other diseases associated with increased levels of blood calcium; for example, the hypercalcemia some-

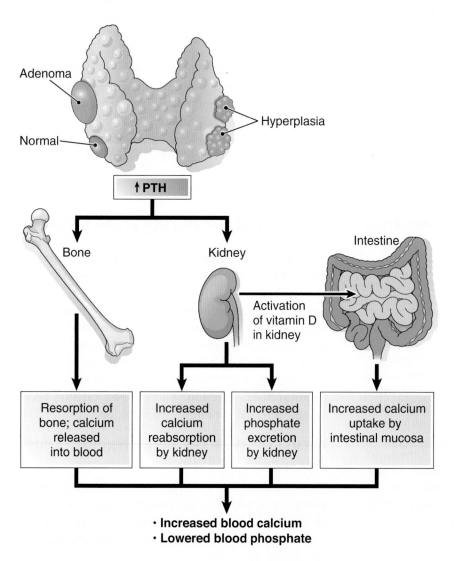

Figure 18-14 Pathophysiology of hyperparathyroidism.

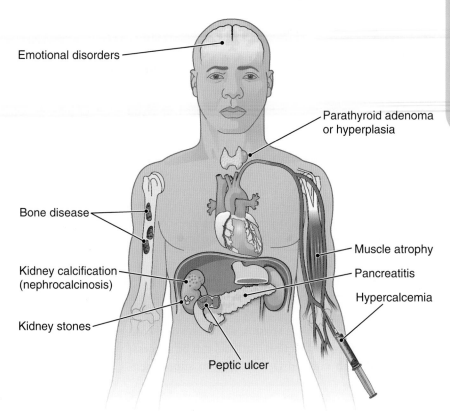

Figure 18-15 **Clinical manifestations of hyperparathyroidism.**

times associated with bone metastases from breast cancer. The accompanying Lab Tools box offers further details.

Secondary hyperparathyroidism, that is, high blood calcium levels caused by some nonparathyroid condition, is almost always associated with hyperplasia of the parathyroid glands induced by the high levels of blood phosphate and decreased levels of blood calcium associated with chronic renal failure. Recall that there is a reciprocal relationship between blood calcium levels and blood phosphate levels—a high phosphate level is associated with a low blood calcium level and vice versa. Chronic renal failure is associated with 1) high blood phosphate levels (because the kidneys fail to excrete it), which 2) pushes blood calcium levels down, causing 3) the parathyroids to secrete increased amounts of PTH to raise blood calcium levels, which in turn causes 4) parathyroid cells to proliferate (hyperplasia) to make more PTH.

Clinical findings are dominated by chronic renal failure—high blood pressure, anemia, edema, low urine output, bleeding problems, diarrhea, and mental problems caused by accumulated waste products. The signs and symptoms of hyperparathyroidism are present, too, with the notable exception that blood calcium levels

may not be increased because high blood levels of phosphate will not allow it to rise (despite high blood levels of PTH). Renal transplant usually corrects the renal failure and cures the hyperparathyroidism. However, sometimes the hyperparathyroidism persists after transplant because one or more of the hyperplastic parathyroid glands becomes autonomous and continues to secrete PTH despite the fact that blood phosphate levels have returned to normal. This condition is referred to as **tertiary hyperparathyroidism** and requires surgical removal of the hyperplastic parathyroid glands.

UNDERACTIVITY OF THE PARATHYROID GLANDS (HYPOPARATHYROIDISM)

Underactive parathyroid glands are much less common than are overactive ones. Hypoparathyroidism is usually caused by inadvertent surgical removal of parathyroid glands during thyroidectomy or removal of the parathyroid glands in surgical treatment of hyperparathyroidism. Less commonly it results from atrophy for unknown reasons (idiopathic atrophy).

The major blood abnormality associated with underactive parathyroid glands is a low blood calcium level, which can cause neuromuscular irritability (tetany):

Hypercalcemia

Calcium is one of the most tightly controlled of blood chemical constituents. Levels even slightly above the upper limit of normal should be taken seriously. The first step is to repeat the test to verify that calcium is, indeed, elevated. Low levels of blood phosphate confirm that an imbalance is present. If a high blood calcium level is confirmed, blood PTH level should be measured; a PTH level above normal confirms the diagnosis of hyperparathyroidism; however, remember that not all such cases are caused by parathyroid gland disease.

Of patients *not in renal failure* with initially unexplained high blood calcium levels, about:

- 50% have hyperparathyroidism.
- 35% have undetected (occult) malignancy, either metastatic to bone or from paraneoplastic effect (Chapter 6), in which a nonparathyroid tumor is secreting PTH (cancer of the kidney is a particular suspect).
- 10% have no detectable disease.

Keep in mind that hypercalcemia of any type can *cause* pancreatitis and renal stones.

tingling sensations, muscle spasms, seizures, vocal cord spasm, and airway obstruction. Patients can be successfully treated with vitamin D and calcium supplementation.

Diseases of the Adrenal Gland

The adrenal gland is two organs in one: an outer *cortex* under control of the pituitary gland, and an inner *medulla* linked directly to the autonomic nervous system. The medulla secretes hormones that increase heart rate, blood pressure, sweating, and bowel peristalsis. The adrenal cortex responds to the pituitary by producing hormones that have a powerful effect on blood volume and blood pressure, glucose metabolism, immune function, and inflammatory reactions.

DISEASES OF THE ADRENAL CORTEX

Disease of the adrenal cortex is usually expressed as oversecretion or undersecretion of cortical hormones, which have a varied and far-reaching effect on metabolism and health, much more so than disease of the adrenal medulla. The most common causes of adrenocortical disease include hyperplasia, atrophy, tumor, inflammation, necrosis, or other destruction.

Overproduction of Cortisol (Cushing Syndrome)

Cushing syndrome is a cluster of clinical signs and symptoms that result from an excessive amount of blood cortisol. As is illustrated in Figure 18-16, Cushing syndrome may result from:

- *Anterior pituitary hyperplasia or tumor* associated with excessive secretion of ACTH, which stimulates

excessive adrenal cortex secretion of corticosteroids (blood ACTH level is high)
- *Secretion of ACTH by nonendocrine tumors* (paraneoplastic syndrome), especially small cell carcinoma of the lung (blood ACTH level is high). Of cases not associated with overmedication with steroid drugs, most are caused by overproduction of ACTH production by a small pituitary adenoma. Because pituitary adenomas were the cause of the first recognized cases, overexcretion of ACTH caused by a pituitary adenoma is properly termed Cushing *disease* (not syndrome) in honor of Harvey Cushing, the American neurosurgeon who first described it.
- *Adrenal cortex hyperplasia or tumor* associated with excessive secretion of corticosteroids (blood ACTH level is low)
- *Overmedication* with corticosteroids, usually owing to treatment of chronic inflammatory disease, especially autoimmune conditions (blood ACTH level is low). Overmedication accounts for the great majority of cases seen in clinical practice.

The pathologic findings in the hypothalamus, pituitary gland, and adrenal glands depend on the cause of Cushing syndrome: a brain lesion in the hypothalamus can stimulate increased amount of hypothalamic-releasing hormone, which can cause increased pituitary output of ACTH. Alternatively, pituitary gland hyperplasia or tumor can cause excessive secretion of ACTH. Both are associated with an increased blood level of ACTH, which stimulates the adrenal cortex and produces bilateral **adrenocortical hyperplasia**. However, in some instances Cushing syndrome is caused by adrenocortical hyperplasia without known cause.

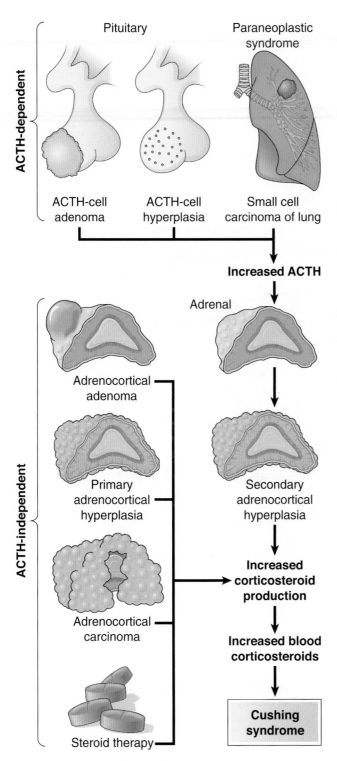

Figure 18-16 **Pathogenesis of Cushing syndrome.**

To the contrary, medical therapy with corticosteroids suppresses pituitary production of ACTH, blood ACTH level is low, and **adrenocortical atrophy** occurs. Because the adrenal cortex may shrink in patients on long-term steroid therapy, patients are weaned off of their drug slowly, in order to give the cortex time to recover.

Adrenocortical adenoma (Fig. 18-17) usually occurs as a single nodule in one adrenal gland. Adrenocortical carcinoma is very rare.

Figure 18-18 illustrates the clinical findings in Cushing syndrome. Most of the symptoms result from increased amounts of blood cortisol; other corticosteroids are increased to a lesser degree but account for some clinical effects. Hypertension and weight gain often develop first and may not be recognized as pathologic until additional features occur. Truncal obesity appears, a "buffalo hump" accumulation of fat collects below the back of the neck (Fig. 18-19A), and the face becomes rounded ("moon facies," Fig. 18-19B). Muscle atrophy produces weak, thin limbs. Secondary diabetes occurs as a result of the effects of cortisol discussed above and is associated with high levels of blood glucose and glucose in the urine. The skin becomes thin and friable: It is easily bruised, and reddish-blue striae develop on the abdomen, hips, and breasts. Increased levels of androgenic steroids cause acne and excessive hair growth, especially facial hair in women. Menstrual abnormalities and mental problems also may occur. Infections are common because cortisol suppresses immunity and the inflammatory response.

When florid clinical signs are present, Cushing syndrome is an easy diagnosis. However, the picture is not so clear in an obese female with acne, "stretch marks," and hypertension—each of which could be of independent causation. The laboratory is an indispensable aid in confirming clinical suspicion. The accompanying Lab Tools box offers more detail.

Overproduction of Aldosterone (Hyperaldosteronism)

Recall that the kidneys and the *renin-angiotensin-aldosterone system* (Chapter 12) are linked in a (homeostatic)

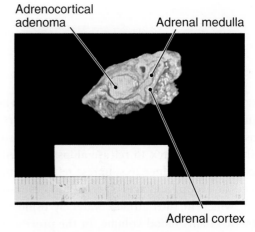

Figure 18-17 **Adrenocortical adenoma.**

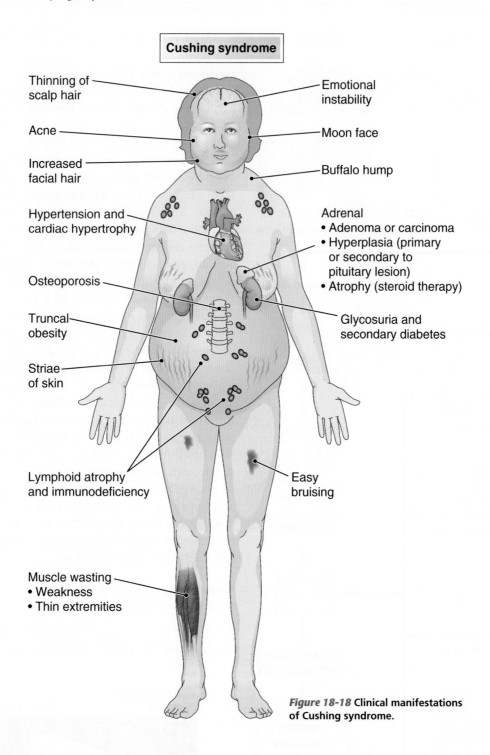

Cushing syndrome

Thinning of scalp hair

Emotional instability

Acne

Moon face

Increased facial hair

Buffalo hump

Hypertension and cardiac hypertrophy

Adrenal
• Adenoma or carcinoma
• Hyperplasia (primary or secondary to pituitary lesion)
• Atrophy (steroid therapy)

Osteoporosis

Glycosuria and secondary diabetes

Truncal obesity

Striae of skin

Lymphoid atrophy and immunodeficiency

Easy bruising

Muscle wasting
• Weakness
• Thin extremities

Figure 18-18 Clinical manifestations of Cushing syndrome.

feedback loop that maintains vascular volume and blood pressure. The kidneys secrete renin, which converts angiotensinogen into angiotensin, which in turn stimulates the adrenal cortex to release aldosterone. Aldosterone acts on the kidney to suppress renin production (the feedback loop) and acts on renal tubules to retain sodium, which in turn attracts water by osmosis and thereby maintains blood volume. In the process of retaining sodium, potassium is excreted into urine by the renal tubules. Therefore, an excessive amount of aldosterone (from any source) causes high blood pressure, low blood potassium levels, and low blood renin level.

Hyperaldosteronism can be caused by adrenocortical disease (*primary* hyperaldosteronism or Conn syndrome), or it can be caused by other conditions (*secondary* hyperaldosteronism). Primary adrenocortical overproduction usually results from cortical adenoma or hyperplasia.

Buffalo hump fat

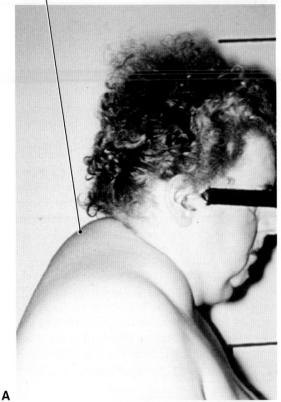

A

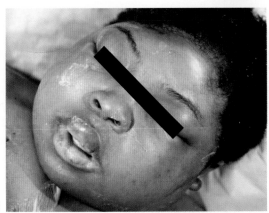

B

Figure 18-19 **Cushing syndrome. A,** Cushingoid obesity, including "buffalo hump" of dorsal fat. **B,** Cushingoid moon facies.

Secondary hyperaldosteronism is usually caused by impaired renal blood flow resulting from renal artery stenosis associated with atherosclerosis (renovascular disease)—low renal blood flow invokes the renin-angiotensin-aldosterone mechanism and causes increased adrenal secretion of aldosterone. The result is high blood pressure, low blood levels of potassium, and high blood levels of renin.

There are, of course, other clinical conditions that increase blood aldosterone, most of them associated with low blood pressure—congestive heart failure and di-

uretic or antihypertension drug therapy, for example. The difference is important: the increased aldosterone in these conditions is the *result*, not the *cause*, of disease.

Adrenocortical oversecretion of aldosterone and renal artery stenosis must be kept in mind when evaluating patients with hypertension; most cases are diagnosed during clinical workups for hypertension. Together the two account for a small percentage of patients with hypertension, but both are surgically curable.

Overproduction of Androgenic Hormones (Congenital Adrenal Hyperplasia)

Congenital adrenal hyperplasia (also called *adrenogenital syndrome*) is a condition resulting from several types of genetic defects that cause enzyme deficiencies in the adrenal cortex. These defects interrupt the chain of events that lead to production of corticosteroid hormones. Genetic enzyme defects can be thought of as a dam in a stream of metabolic reactions: the defect prevents metabolic progress (flow) and causes an accumulation of upstream raw material or a deficit of downstream product. In congenital adrenal hyperplasia the defects cause one of two types of problems:

- An increase of androgenic steroids (accumulation of upstream raw material)
- A decrease of aldosterone and cortisol (deficit of downstream product)

The enzyme deficiency may be mild or severe and result in varying degrees of hormone excess or deficit.

Accumulations of androgenic steroids in the fetus can result in female infants with ambiguous genitalia (Fig. 18-20); male genitalia are unaffected. Males are

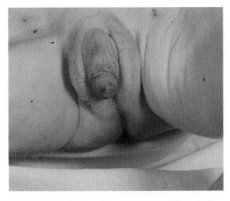

Figure 18-20 **Congenital adrenal hyperplasia (adrenogenital syndrome).** Ambiguous, masculinized (virilized) genitalia in a female infant. Reprinted with permission from Rubin E. Pathology. 4th ed. Philadelphia. Lippincott Williams and Wilkins, 2005.

The Laboratory Diagnosis of Cushing Syndrome

The first step in diagnosing Cushing syndrome is to confirm clinical suspicion by measuring **24-hour urinary cortisol excretion**. Ninety-five percent of patients with Cushing syndrome have increased levels of urinary cortisol.

Normal blood cortisol level varies consistently, peaking at 8 AM and falling to a low point at 4 PM. Although patients with Cushing syndrome have increased blood cortisol levels, normal variations are so large that simple study of blood cortisol levels is not useful.

However, cortisol production in normal persons can be suppressed by oral **dexamethasone**, a potent synthetic steroid that suppresses ACTH production by the pituitary and, therefore, cortisol production by the adrenal gland. However, in patients with Cushing syndrome, cortisol production cannot be suppressed. The **dexamethasone suppression test** exploits this fact for diagnostic purposes.

There are two types of dexamethasone suppression tests:

- In the *high-dose test* a large single dose of dexamethasone is given at 11 PM, and the blood cortisol level is measured the next morning at 8 AM. In normal patients an 8 AM blood cortisol level will be suppressed to below normal range, whereas levels will not be suppressed to below normal in patients with Cushing disease.
- In the *low-dose test* a 24-hour urine is collected on the first day (day 1). On days 2 and 3 the patient is given low oral doses of dexamethasone every 6 hours for 48 hours. On day 4 a second 24-hour urine is collected. In normal patients urinary cortisol excretion is suppressed, but in patients with Cushing syndrome cortisol excretion is not suppressed.

Because steroid hormones normally vary greatly in the course of a day and from day to day and are released from glands in spurts, meticulous attention to test details is essential. Care should be exercised when interpreting the results because the results can be influenced by many factors other than endocrine disease; for example, 24-hour urinary cortisol can be increased because of obesity.

---

usually diagnosed at an older age because of precocious puberty. Older females develop enlarged clitoris, oligomenorrhea, hirsutism, and acne. The growth of both sexes can be stunted by premature closure of the epiphyseal growth plates in long bones (Chapter 22).

Deficits of aldosterone and cortisol result in *"salt wasting"* as sodium is lost in urine owing to lack of aldosterone, which accounts for the clinical findings: an infant with dehydration, low blood pressure, low blood levels of sodium, and high blood levels of potassium and renin. It can be fatal if not diagnosed.

In congenital adrenal hyperplasia the adrenal cortex is markedly thickened: a low level of blood cortisol stimulates the pituitary to produce large amounts of ACTH, which in turn stimulates cortical cell growth (hyperplasia) in a futile effort to produce cortisol. The hyperplastic adrenal cortex and masculinization of genitals give the syndrome its alternative name: *adrenogenital syndrome*.

Underactivity of the Adrenal Cortex (Adrenocortical Insufficiency)

Adrenocortical insufficiency is caused by a lack of adrenocortical hormones, especially cortisol. Almost every condition affecting the adrenal glands affects both glands equally and may be caused by adrenal gland (primary failure) or pituitary gland disease (secondary failure). Primary adrenal gland failure can be acute or chronic, and result from either adrenal gland atrophy or adrenal gland destruction. Secondary adrenal gland failure is caused by failure of the pituitary gland to secrete ACTH. Complete destruction of the adrenal gland without cortisol replacement is uniformly fatal.

Acute Adrenocortical Crisis

Acute adrenal gland failure occurs in three clinical settings and is invariably fatal without quick diagnosis and cortisol replacement.

- *Sudden withdrawal of corticosteroid therapy.* This is perhaps the most common cause of acute adrenal gland failure. Corticosteroid therapy, usually for rheumatoid arthritis or other autoimmune disease, suppresses ACTH secretion by the pituitary gland; and the result is atrophy of the adrenal cortex. Sudden withdrawal of steroid drugs leaves the patient without a replacement source for cortisol.
- *Bilateral acute hemorrhagic infarction of the adrenal glands (Waterhouse-Friderichsen syndrome).* The most common cause is acute *meningococcal meningi-*

tis (Chapter 23). Massive adrenal gland hemorrhage also may occur in septicemia, pregnancy, disseminated intravascular coagulation (Chapter 5), in patients on anticoagulant therapy, or in newborns as a result of birth stress or trauma.

- *Sudden worsening of chronic adrenal insufficiency.* This may occur when a patient with undiagnosed chronic adrenal insufficiency is suddenly stressed by development of an acute infection or has surgery, or it may occur in patients with known adrenal insufficiency who are on steroid therapy, if their dose is not increased during stressful illness.

Clinical signs vary according to the underlying condition, but a typical case is a young person with meningococcal meningitis (Chapter 23), a severe bacterial infection of the covering of the brain. The infection may at first produce relatively mild symptoms—fever, headache, vomiting, and stiff neck—but confusion, weakness, and coma can occur quickly as the infection spreads with a malignant virulence that is characteristic of meningococcus infection. If hemorrhage into the adrenal glands occurs, it can destroy them completely and deprive the patient of the benefits cortisol provides in stressful situations. Confusion and weakness can progress rapidly to profound shock and coma. Death oc-curs quickly if the meningitis is not recognized or adrenal gland hemorrhage is not suspected and antibiotic, corticosteroid, and electrolyte therapies instituted immediately.

Chronic Adrenocortical Insufficiency (Addison Disease)

Addison disease is chronic adrenocortical insufficiency that is invariably fatal without corticosteroid replacement therapy. It is rare, but in recent years it has gained notoriety as it has been revealed that United States President John F. Kennedy suffered from it. See the accompanying History of Medicine box for more details.

Most cases (60–70%) are caused by autoimmune destruction of the gland. Like all other autoimmune diseases, familial tendencies are evident. In about half of cases the autoimmune reaction is confined to the adrenal glands; in the other half other autoimmune disease is present and frequently involves other endocrine organs, causing thyroiditis, Graves disease, or diabetes.

Infectious destruction of the adrenal glands by tuberculosis or fungus infection causes a minority of cases of Addison disease in developed nations, but tuberculous destruction is more common in impoverished areas. Tumor metastases, especially widespread breast

---

History of Medicine

PRESIDENT JOHN F. KENNEDY AND ADDISON DISEASE

In March of 1849, Dr. Thomas Addison read a paper before the South London Medical Society describing peculiar symptoms associated with tuberculosis of the "suprarenal glands." He accumulated more cases of chronic adrenal failure, most due to adrenal tuberculosis, and in 1855, he published them to no acclaim.

Exactly 100 years later, in November 1955, the *Journal of the American Medical Association* (JAMA) published the remarkable case of "a man 37 years of age" who was thought to be the first person with Addison disease to survive major surgery (spinal fusion for terrible back pain). That man was John F. Kennedy. At the time he was a senator from Massachusetts, and he later became the 35th President of the United States.

Kennedy was diagnosed with Addison disease in 1947 by a London physician and maintained on injections of very new and expensive synthetic "cortisteroid" (later called cortisol) pellets injected under his skin.

During the presidential campaign against Richard Nixon in 1960, Kennedy flatly denied he had *Addison disease*. His-tory does not record his ever denying publicly that he had *adrenal insufficiency*. Privately Kennedy must have salved his conscience, and misled the public about his adrenal insufficiency, by relying on a peculiarly narrow definition of Addison disease—that chronic adrenal insufficiency was not Addison disease unless the adrenal glands had been destroyed by tuberculosis (because most of Dr. Addison's original patients had adrenal tuberculosis). In addition to whispers and rumors, one sign of Addison disease was evident to anyone who bothered to look: Kennedy's remarkable bronze "tan," which gave him a misleadingly healthy glow—a distinctly unusual feature for someone who lived in the northeastern United States and was not regularly sun exposed. As this textbook explains, a cardinal sign of Addison disease is deep bronze pigmentation of the skin. However, we may never know the cause of Kennedy's adrenal disease: the official autopsy report released to the public after his assassination makes no mention of the adrenal glands—an inconceivable omission to any pathologist, and explicable only by deliberate exclusion of the anatomic findings.

and lung carcinoma, also may lodge in the adrenal glands and destroy them.

Pathologic changes in the adrenal glands vary according the etiology. In autoimmune adrenal disease the glands may be completely obliterated. In secondary hypoadrenalism—as with chronic steroid treatment—the glands are identifiable but markedly shrunken. In tuberculosis or deep fungus infection (Chapter 9) the glands are so destroyed by the infection that no normal gland can be identified. The same can be true for metastatic tumor in the adrenal glands.

Essential laboratory findings are hyperkalemia (increased levels of blood potassium) and hyponatremia (decreased levels of blood sodium).

The clinical features of Addison disease, illustrated in Figure 18-21, usually appear slowly. Vascular volume depletion and hypotension result in weakness, fatigue, and syncope. Patients may exhibit depression, confusion, and other mental problems. Gastrointestinal complaints include diarrhea, nausea, anorexia, and weight loss. Low levels of blood sugar may occur owing to cortisol deficiency. Patients with Addison disease are physiologically fragile—the stress of minor surgery, trauma, or infection may precipitate an acute adrenal crisis and vascular collapse. In patients with primary Addison disease (that is, of adrenal gland rather than pituitary gland failure) increased pituitary synthesis of ACTH causes increased production of melanocyte-stimulating hormone (MSH), which is a metabolite of ACTH, and a noticeable darkening of the skin. As is illustrated in Figure 18-22 the face, underarms, nipples, and groin are particularly affected.

DISEASES OF THE ADRENAL MEDULLA

The most important diseases of the medulla are neoplasms, many of which produce an excess of medullary hormones (catecholamines). Medullary hyperplasia does not occur. Underactivity of the adrenal medulla is of no consequence. If the entire adrenal gland is destroyed, the effect of lost medullary hormones is minimal; however, loss of *cortical* hormones is devastating.

Pheochromocytomas, although rare, are the most common neoplasm of the adrenal medulla. Some pheochromocytomas arise from chromaffin cells outside the adrenal in the paraganglion system (*paragangliomas*), a division of the autonomic nervous system consisting of a network of chromaffin cell clusters along major blood vessels—the carotid body, located in the carotid artery in the neck, is an example. All pheochromocytomas and paragangliomas secrete catecholamines to some degree, and sometimes it is enough to produce

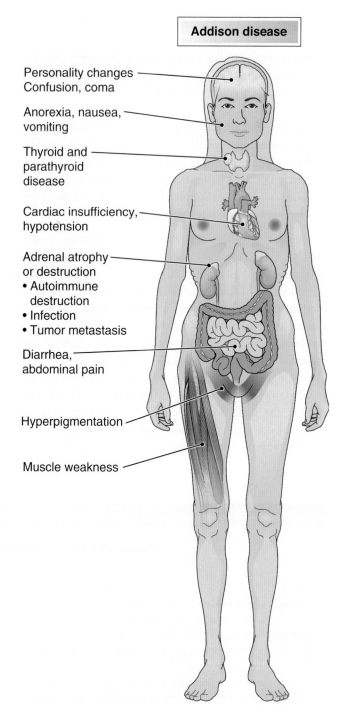

Addison disease

Personality changes
Confusion, coma

Anorexia, nausea, vomiting

Thyroid and parathyroid disease

Cardiac insufficiency, hypotension

Adrenal atrophy or destruction
• Autoimmune destruction
• Infection
• Tumor metastasis

Diarrhea, abdominal pain

Hyperpigmentation

Muscle weakness

Figure 18-21 **Clinical manifestations of Addison disease.**

severe hypertension. About 1 in 1,000 patients with hypertension has a pheochromocytoma or paraganglioma, making them rare but important causes of surgically curable hypertension.

A convenient way to remember clinical characteristics of pheochromocytoma is "the rule of 10s":

- 10% arise outside the adrenal as paragangliomas (in the paraganglion system)

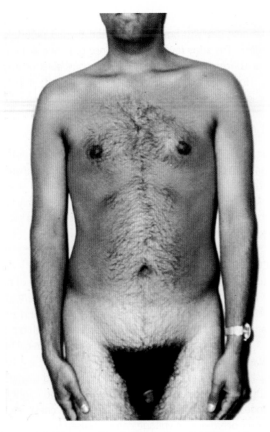

Figure 18-22 **Bronze skin pigmentation of Addison disease.**

The most important clinical sign of pheochromocytoma is hypertension. Most of the time blood pressure is chronically elevated and must be distinguished from essential hypertension (Chapter 12); however, sometimes blood pressure may rise suddenly and dramatically as the result of the release of a large amount of catecholamine, which can be precipitated by exercise, stress, change in body position, or pressure on the tumor. These episodes are characterized by spasms of severe hypertension, chest and abdominal pain, palpitations, anxiety, profuse sweating, facial flushing, and nausea and vomiting. They also can cause stroke, heart attack, or fatal cardiac arrhythmia.

Laboratory procedures are required to make a positive diagnosis. Increased urinary output of catecholamines or their metabolites confirms the diagnosis.

Some pheochromocytomas occur as one tumor among several in the *multiple endocrine neoplasia (MEN) syndromes*. There are several types, each with distinct genetic defects and varying types of endocrine conditions, among them parathyroid hyperplasia and adenoma, islet cell tumors of the pancreas, medullary carcinoma of the thyroid gland, and carcinoid tumors.

Neuroblastomas are malignant tumors of primitive neuroendocrine cells related to chromaffin cells. They can arise in the adrenal medulla, in the paraganglionic system, or in the posterior chest or abdominal cavities close to the autonomic nervous system. They occur almost exclusively in young children and account for about 15% of cancer deaths among children. Their behavior varies remarkably widely: some are aggressively malignant and metastasize to bone marrow and beyond; others mature into benign tumors, and yet others disappear spontaneously. ∎

- 10% of those in the adrenal are bilateral
- 10% are malignant
- 10% arise in children
- 10% occur in association with other endocrine neoplasms, such as the multiple endocrine neoplasia (MEN) syndromes

---

CASE STUDY 18-1 *"I'M RUNNING OUT OF GAS"*

TOPIC
Hypothyroidism

THE CASE

Setting: You are employed in the in-house primary care clinic at the headquarters of a major airline.

Clinical history: The clinic receptionist is a pleasant, somewhat overweight, normally upbeat 63-year-old woman who

frequently asks you questions about her diabetes and minor ailments. Lately she has been complaining to you about feeling tired and down in the dumps and, unusual for her, she has seemed depressed and has been missing work. One day she asks to see you as a patient. When you see her in an exam room she sighs and says, "I'm running out of gas," pausing to gather strength for the next sentence. "I guess I'm just too old for this job."

Your review her chart prior to taking the history and doing an exam. She has a rather full chart, mainly entries regarding adjustments of her diabetes and high blood pressure medicines, but nothing else recently other than a ▶

[Case 18-1, continued] minor vaginal infection and upper respiratory complaints. You ask her to tell you what is most bothersome.

"It's my legs; they are so swollen and heavy even though I'm real regular about my water pills," she says, referring to the diuretics she is taking for blood pressure control and edema in her feet. "I'm just so tired I can't find the energy sometimes to comb my hair. Not that it'll do much good," she says, running fingers through thinning hair to collect some strands, which she holds out to you.

"My hair is falling out, too. I'm just falling apart, I guess," she says with a sigh.

The remainder of the history and review of systems reveals only that she has increased her daily laxative dose lately to avoid constipation.

Physical examination and other data: Vital signs are: BP 135/92, HR 64, respirations 12, thermographic middle ear temperature 97.4. Her eyes, ears, nose, throat, and neck are unremarkable. Her breath and heart sounds are barely audible, and she has a few rales in the lower chest. Her abdomen is soft, and no masses are palpable. Her skin is dry and scaly, especially on her lower legs, where she has moderate pitting edema.

You wonder if she is depressed or has problems she is not telling you about. No diagnosis comes to mind, so you order a battery of laboratory tests and send her for an electrocardiogram and chest x-ray, telling her she can go back to work after the tests are complete. You give her assurance that you will have most of the results in a day or two and will call her when you have all of them.

Later in the day you get some of the results. A complete blood count reveals normal values for red and white cell counts and other cellular determinations. Blood glucose is 318 mg/dL and creatinine is 2.6 mg/dL (n: <1.2). Urinalysis shows moderate amounts of glucose and protein in her urine. Thyroid studies and chest x-ray will not be reported until the next day. The electrocardiogram is unremarkable except for low voltage across all leads.

The next day you find her x-ray and thyroid reports on your desk. The x-ray reveals no evidence of pericardial effusion, a concern because of the low voltage electrocardiogram. However, although there is some congestion in the lower lung fields, there is no evidence of pneumonia. The thyroid studies are: T_4 is 1.1 μg/dL (n: 5.0–11.0), T_3 is 22 ng/dL (n: 95–190), TSH is 17 μU/dL (n: 0.4–6.0).

Clinical course: You quickly conclude she has hypothyroidism and consult with a colleague, who approves thyroid replacement therapy. She responds nicely and soon seems her old self. She loses some weight, most of it probably water, the pedal edema disappears, and her diabetes and blood pressure become easier to control.

DISCUSSION

The thyroid studies in this case were airtight evidence of primary thyroid failure (hypothyroidism)—T_3 and T_4 were low and TSH was elevated, indicating the pituitary gland was fine and working hard to stimulate the thyroid gland to produce T_3 and T_4, but it was not responding. The clinical history was classic, too, for hypothyroidism—the patient had nearly all of the signs: low body temperature and relatively slow heart rate and respirations for someone who might be in congestive heart failure (pedal edema and chest rales). Low electrocardiogram voltage can be caused by pericardial fluid and by hypothyroidism. Then, too, her hair was thinning and brittle, her skin was dry and flaky, especially over her lower legs, she was constipated and weak, and her behavior was dull and depressed.

The elevated creatinine and proteinuria indicated the presence of significant diabetic and hypertensive renal disease (diabetic nephrosclerosis).

POINTS TO REMEMBER
- Sometimes patients, especially older ones, have more than one disease.
- Laboratory tests are very important in the diagnosis of thyroid disease.

Objectives Recap

1. *Explain homeostatic feedback loops:* They are self-adjusting forces that operate to oppose movement of any physiologic function away from its healthy range. If, for example, thyroid hormone deviates upward or downward from the healthy range, the pituitary gland acts to return it. If blood sugar rises too high, the pancreas secretes insulin to lower it. Feedback loops operate in every physiologic system, including, for example, blood pressure, body temperature, and plasma acidity (pH).

2. *Cite an example of change in blood hormone levels in endocrine disease, and explain how feedback is involved:* Sometimes a homeostatic mechanism is incapable of correcting an unhealthy situation. For example, in some types of thyroid disease the thyroid gland escapes pituitary control and operates independently, secreting excessive amounts of thyroid hormone, which causes hyperthyroidism. High blood levels of thyroxine cause the pituitary gland to produce lower amounts of thyroid stimulating

hormone (TSH) in an effort to lower blood thyroid hormone levels. However, because the thyroid is acting independently, blood levels of thyroid hormone remain high, and blood levels of TSH remain low in certain types of hyperthyroidism.

3. *Explain mass effect and stalk effect in pituitary disease*: Mass effect is the result of the pressure exerted by a pituitary mass on the remaining normal pituitary gland tissue and on nearby structures. For example, a tumor may press on the optic nerves to produce visual problems. Stalk effect is an effect of a pituitary mass on the stalk that induces secretion of abnormal amounts of prolactin by the pituitary gland.

4. *Name the most common type of functioning pituitary adenoma*: Prolactinoma.

5. *Explain the difference between acromegaly and gigantism*: Gigantism occurs when abnormal growth hormone secretion occurs before the closure of bone epiphyseal growth plates and is characterized by generalized increase of body size with disproportionately long arms and legs. Acromegaly occurs when abnormal secretion of growth hormone occurs in adults after bone growth plates disappear and epiphyses close. In acromegaly, patients have large hands and feet and other distinctive features but are not otherwise exceptionally large or tall.

6. *Explain the difference between thyroglobulin and thyroxin binding globulin*: Thyroglobulin is a globulin (a protein) in the thyroid gland that binds to thyroid hormones while they are stored in the gland. Thyroglobulin releases thyroid hormones into blood. Thyroxin binding globulin (TBG) is a globulin in blood to which thyroid hormones are attached. TBG transports thyroid hormones from the thyroid gland to target tissues.

7. *Define goiter*: A goiter is an enlarged thyroid gland.

8. *Explain why TSH levels are diminished in Graves disease and other forms of primary hyperthyroidism and why TSH levels are elevated in primary hypothyroidism*: In primary hyperthyroidism or hypothyroidism, the gland itself is diseased and is not secondary to some other condition. In primary hyperthyroidism the gland produces too much hor-

mone; in primary hypothyroidism the gland does not produce enough. In each instance the pituitary secretes increased or reduced amounts of TSH, trying to correct the problem. The result: In primary hyperthyroidism blood, TSH is low; in primary hypothyroidism, TSH is high.

9. *Name the most common type of thyroiditis, and explain its pathogenesis*: Hashimoto thyroiditis. It is a chronic autoimmune disease.

10. *Name the most common type of thyroid cancer, and give an approximate 5-year survival figure*: Papillary carcinoma; about 90% survive after five years.

11. *Offer a brief profile of the laboratory abnormalities in primary hyperparathyroidism*: Blood levels of calcium and parathormone are high; blood levels of phosphate are low.

12. *List the most important hormones produced by the adrenal medulla and cortex*: Epinephrine and norepinephrine from the medulla; cortisol (hydrocortisone), aldosterone, and androgenic steroids from the cortex.

13. *Name the adrenocortical hormone responsible for most of the clinical features of Cushing syndrome*: Cortisol (hydrocortisone).

14. *Name the most common cause of Cushing syndrome*: Steroid drug therapy.

15. *Explain why patients with hypertension caused by primary hyperaldosteronism have low blood levels of renin*: High blood aldosterone suppresses renal secretion of renin.

16. *Explain why patients with Addison disease usually have dark skin*: In Addison disease low blood levels of cortisol causes the pituitary gland to secrete large amounts of ACTH. One of the metabolic breakdown products of ACTH is melanocyte stimulating hormone (MSH), which stimulates melanin production in skin.

17. *Explain why patients with pheochromocytoma may have high blood pressure*: Pheochromocytomas may secrete large amounts of epinephrine and norepinephrine (catecholamines), both of which cause peripheral vasoconstriction, which in turn causes increased peripheral vascular resistance and increased blood pressure.

Typical Test Questions

1. Which one of the following is associated with low blood TSH?
   A. Hypothyroidism
   B. Cushing syndrome
   C. Graves disease
   D. Addison disease

2. Diabetes insipidus is characterized by which one of the following?
   A. Destruction of the anterior pituitary
   B. Lack of antidiuretic hormone (ADH)
   C. Failure of renal tubule to reabsorb potassium
   D. All of the above

3. Which one of the following is a feature of Graves disease?
   A. Autoimmunity
   B. Low blood T_4 level
   C. High blood TSH level
   D. Hypothyroidism

4. Which one of the following is present in all cases of Cushing syndrome?
   A. Increased blood TSH level
   B. Increased blood cortisol level
   C. Increased blood epinephrine level
   D. Autoantibodies

5. Which one of the following is characteristic of hyperparathyroidism?
   A. Low blood PTH level
   B. Increased blood calcium level
   C. Increased blood phosphate level
   D. All of the above

6. True or false? About 90% of patients with papillary thyroid carcinoma survive five years.

7. True or false? Secondary hyperparathyroidism is usually caused by a pituitary adenoma.

8. True or false? Complete destruction of the adrenal gland is fatal in the absence of cortisol replacement therapy.

9. True or false? Pheochromocytomas occur only in the adrenal gland.

10. True or false? Hashimoto thyroiditis is caused by a viral infection of the thyroid gland.

Diseases of the Kidney

This chapter begins with a review of the normal urinary tract, glomerulus, and renal tubules; the formation and flow of urine; the regulation of salt and water balance; and urinalysis. Diseases and disorders discussed include glomerulonephritis and other inflammatory diseases, hypertension, and cancers.

BACK TO BASICS
* Renal Function
* The Normal Glomerulus
* Formation of the Glomerular Filtrate
* Tubular Processing of the Glomerular Filtrate
THE LANGUAGE OF RENAL DISEASE
NORMAL URINE AND URINALYSIS
CLINICAL SYNDROMES OF RENAL DISEASE
INHERITED, CONGENITAL, AND DEVELOPMENTAL
   DISEASE
GLOMERULAR DISEASE
* The Initiation and Progression of Glomerular Disease
* Glomerulonephritis
* Secondary Glomerular Disease

DISEASES OF RENAL VASCULATURE
ACUTE TUBULAR NECROSIS
TUBULOINTERSTITIAL NEPHRITIS
* Obstruction, Reflux, and Stasis
* Pyelonephritis and Urinary Tract Infection
* Drugs, Toxins, and Other Causes of Tubulointerstitial
  Nephritis
RENAL STONES
TUMORS OF THE KIDNEY

Learning Objectives

After studying this chapter you should be able to:
1. List the functions of the kidney
2. Explain the difference between glomerular filtrate and urine
3. Distinguish between renal diseases and syndromes of renal disease, and give an example
4. Explain the difference between azotemia and uremia, and describe what is meant by occult hematuria
5. Explain the difference between nephritic syndrome and nephrotic syndrome
6. Name the pathogenic mechanism responsible for most primary glomerular disease
7. Name the most common type of glomerulonephritis
8. Name the most common cause of renal failure in the United States
9. Give the name of the vascular disease of the kidney that is found in virtually all elderly people
10. Explain why patients with acute tubular necrosis (ATN) have a period of very high urine output
11. Name several causes of tubulointerstitial nephritis
12. Explain the consequences of urinary obstruction and reflux
13. Name the type of microorganisms that cause most acute pyelonephritis
14. List some important facts about chronic pyelonephritis
15. Name the most common type of urinary stone, and discuss some diseases or conditions associated with it
16. Name the two most important malignancies of the kidney

BACK TO BASICS
- renal tubules
- glomerulus
- nephron unit
- glomerular filtrate
- Bowman space

THE LANGUAGE OF RENAL DISEASE
- renal failure
- hematuria
- proteinuria

NORMAL URINE AND URINALYSIS
- urinalysis

CLINICAL SYNDROMES OF RENAL DISEASE
- azotemia
- uremia
- acute nephritic syndrome
- nephrotic syndrome
- occult hematuria
- occult proteinuria

GLOMERULAR DISEASE
- glomerulonephritis

DISEASES OF RENAL VASCULATURE
- nephrosclerosis

ACUTE TUBULAR NECROSIS
- acute tubular necrosis

TUBULOINTERSTITIAL NEPHRITIS
- tubulointerstitial nephritis
- renal ablation nephropathy
- urinary obstruction
- urinary reflux
- hydronephrosis
- pyelonephritis

RENAL STONES
- nephrolithiasis

TUMORS OF THE KIDNEY
- renal cell carcinoma
- transitional cell carcinoma

Drink, sir, is a great provoker of three things . . . nose-painting, sleep, and urine.

WILLIAM SHAKESPEARE (1564–1616), ENGLISH PLAYWRIGHT, MACBETH *(II,iii)*

BACK TO BASICS

Figure 19-1 illustrates the urinary system, which consists of the kidneys, ureters, urinary bladder, and urethra (the figure shows the male urinary tract; the female tract is identical except for the sex organs). The kidney and renal pelvis form the **upper urinary tract**; the ureters, bladder, and urethra form the **lower urinary tract**. The **collecting system** consists of a series of spaces that carry urine from the kidney and hold it for urination. The collecting system consists of the *renal pelvis*, the broad, funnel-shaped space that gathers urine from the kidney and channels it into the *ureter*, a muscular tube that conveys urine to the *bladder*, where it is held until elimination.

RENAL FUNCTION

The most important function of the kidney is to extract waste from blood and excrete it into the collecting system. Urine is carried by the ureters to the bladder, where it is stored until it can be emptied through the urethra. The collecting system is for passive transport and storage; only the kidney is active in the formation of urine and the adjustment of its composition.

The kidney also regulates plasma salt and water concentration, which in turn have an effect on blood pressure (Chapter 12).

The kidney also has an endocrine function. First, it secretes **renin** (Chapter 12), a hormone that aids in the regulation of plasma salt and water concentration and in the maintenance of blood pressure. Second, it secretes **erythropoietin**, a hormone that stimulates the bone marrow to produce red blood cells.

Figure 19-2 illustrates the anatomy of the kidney, which is constructed so that blood vessels are intimately associated with **renal tubules**. One part of each vessel is formed into the **glomerulus**, the filtering apparatus of the kidney. Blood is brought to the glomerulus by the **afferent arteriole** and carried away from the glomerulus by the **efferent arteriole**. The afferent arteriole contains the **juxtaglomerular apparatus**, a cluster of cells that

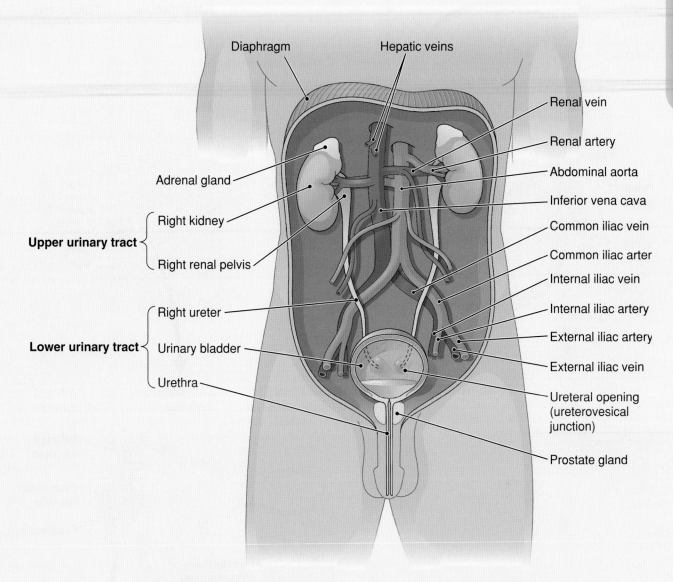

Figure 19-1 The male urinary tract. The female tract is identical except for sex organs.

Labels (top to bottom, left to right):
Diaphragm · Hepatic veins · Renal vein · Renal artery · Abdominal aorta · Inferior vena cava · Common iliac vein · Common iliac arter · Internal iliac vein · Internal iliac artery · External iliac artery · External iliac vein · Ureteral opening (ureterovesical junction) · Prostate gland · Adrenal gland · Right kidney · Right renal pelvis · Upper urinary tract · Right ureter · Urinary bladder · Urethra · Lower urinary tract

senses blood pressure and secretes **renin** to adjust it. Glomerulus, blood vessels, and tubule work together as a **nephron unit**: the glomerulus filters fluid from blood into the tubule. Fluid filtered from blood (the **glomerular filtrate**) first enters a space (**Bowman space**), which surrounds the glomerulus and connects to a renal tubule. As glomerular filtrate moves down the tubule, water and various substances are exchanged between tubular fluid and blood vessels that run alongside the tubule. After passage down the tubule, the remaining fluid is **urine**.

The relationship of the glomerulus, blood vessels, tubules, blood, and urine can be understood best if kidney function is discussed before the anatomy is explained in detail. The kidney has five main functions:

- Excretion (elimination) of metabolic waste
- Adjustment of blood pH (acid-base balance) by excretion of more or less acid
- Adjustment of plasma salt concentration (plasma osmolality) by excretion of more or less salt
- Adjustment of blood volume and blood pressure by secretion of renin (a hormone)
- Stimulation of red blood cell production by secretion of erythropoietin (a hormone)

It is convenient to think of the **glomeruli** as a series of dams around the edge of a salt-water lake (blood) that also contains the nutrients necessary for lake life. Imagine that a large factory sits on the lakeshore and dumps waste and acid into the lake. Think of the lake as

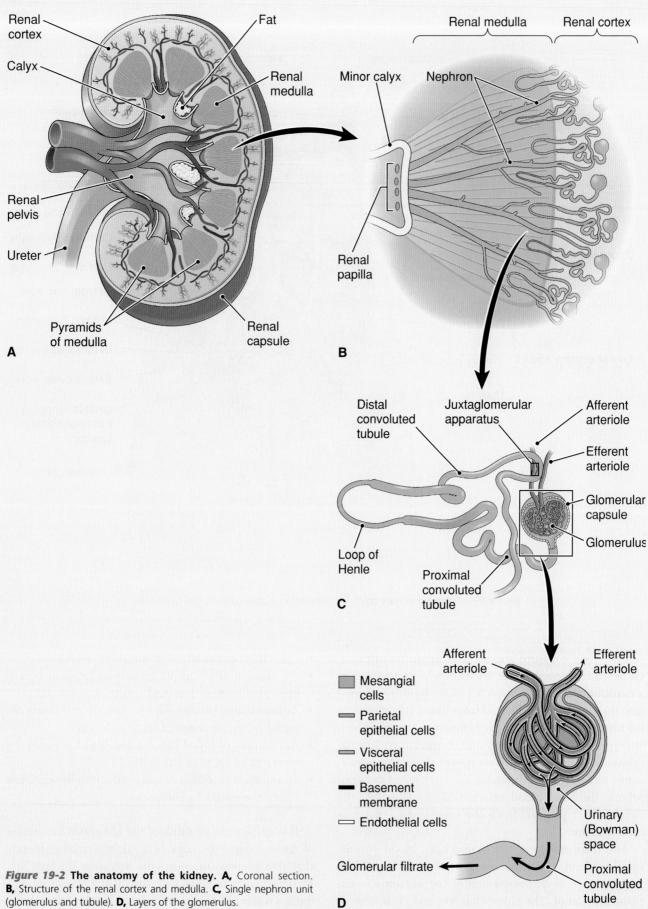

Figure 19-2 **The anatomy of the kidney. A,** Coronal section. **B,** Structure of the renal cortex and medulla. **C,** Single nephron unit (glomerulus and tubule). **D,** Layers of the glomerulus.

containing large fish (red blood cells), smaller fish (plasma proteins), and vital dissolved nutrients such as glucose and amino acids. Further, think of each of these dams as having a fine-mesh screen through which a large amount of water escapes into a pipe. This salty water carries with it nutrients, waste, and acid, but no fish (red cells and protein), because they are too large to pass through the screen.

Now, imagine that the water, salt, acid, glucose, amino acids, and waste (collectively known as the **glomerular filtrate**) that pass through the screen flow into a long pipe (the **renal tubule** associated with each glomerulus) that winds back and forth across the bottom of the lake before emptying into the sewer (the ureter). Imagine further that each pipe is lined by a membrane (the epithelium that forms the renal tubule, the renal **tubular epithelium**) that is in contact with lake water and monitors lake salt and acid content and can exchange water and other substances between water in the pipe and water in lake. This membrane absorbs from the pipe and returns to the lake *all* of the glucose and amino acids, 99% of the water, *some* of the salt and acid, and *none* of the waste, so that the small

amount of water remaining in the pipe (**urine**) contains only the waste and some salt and acid.

Furthermore, imagine that each pipe contains two other special apparatuses. First is the **juxtaglomerular apparatus**, which senses the volume of water and salt in the lake and the pressure at the bottom of the lake. This apparatus secretes a hormone (**renin**), which adjusts the amount of water and salt sucked back up by the lake from the pipe in order to keep the lake at just the right volume, pressure, and salt concentration. Second is another apparatus, precise location unknown, which senses the number of fish (red cells) in the lake, either too few or too many, and secretes more or less of a fish-breeding hormone (**erythropoietin**) into the lake (blood) to maintain the number of fish at a normal level.

THE NORMAL GLOMERULUS

Figure 19-3 illustrates the anatomy of the glomerulus. Blood is supplied to the glomerulus by a relatively large **afferent arteriole**, and leaves through a smaller **efferent arteriole**. That the supply vessel is larger than the drainage vessel ensures that glomerular blood pressure

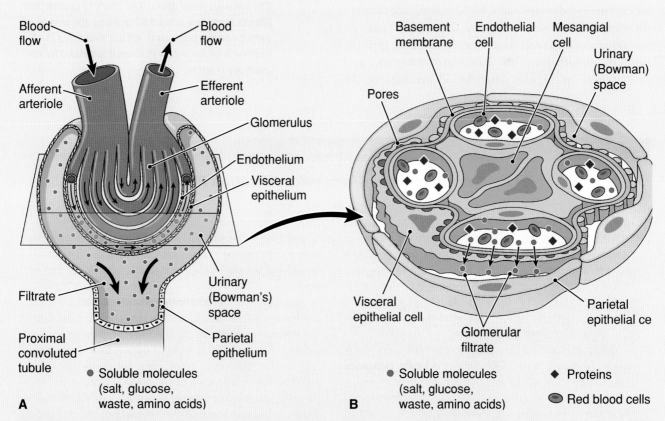

***Figure 19-3* Anatomy of the glomerulus. A,** The relationship of glomerular blood vessels and the Bowman space. Water, salts, glucose, metabolic waste, amino acids, and other small soluble molecules pass from blood into the Bowman space. Red cells and protein molecules are too large to pass. **B,** Fluid and soluble small molecules passing from blood into Bowman space must cross three layers of tissue: vascular endothelium, basement membrane, and visceral epithelial cells.

remains high. Each capillary loop of the glomerulus is composed of a tube of **endothelial cells**. Supporting the glomerular capillary loops are intersitial cells, called **mesangial cells**, which fit between adjacent capillaries in the glomerulus.

Each glomerulus can be conceived of as a fist of capillaries pressed deeply into one side of an inflated balloon, whose wall is composed of **epithelial cells**. The cells of the balloon wall that touch the glomerular capillary fist are **visceral epithelial cells**; the cells of the balloon wall on the other side are the **parietal epithelial cells**. The empty space in between the walls of the balloon is the **urinary (Bowman) space**. Fluid that collects in the urinary space is the **glomerular filtrate**. The neck of the balloon is connected to the renal tubule, which receives the glomerular filtrate.

The **juxtaglomerular apparatus** is a specialized part of the renal tubular epithelium near the glomerulus. It senses blood pressure and blood flow and secretes **renin** as the first step in the *renin-angiotensin-aldosterone* system (Chapter 12), which regulates renal salt excretion as a means to control blood volume and blood pressure.

FORMATION OF THE GLOMERULAR FILTRATE

As Figure 19-3 demonstrates, blood circulating through the glomerulus is separated from the urinary space by several layers of tissue, which are, from inside out: the capillary endothelium, the basement membrane, and the visceral epithelium. High blood pressure in the glomerulus forces fluid through tiny pores in these layers (like the fine mesh screen in our example). Water and dissolved waste, salt (sodium and potassium), glucose, and amino acids cross into Bowman space, where they become the *glomerular filtrate*. Red blood cells and proteins, however, cannot pass because they are too large to pass through the fine mesh of the glomerular layers, a function of the glomerulus known as the *barrier effect*.

Compared to the volume of urine, there is a very much larger volume of glomerular filtrate. Urine output is 1.0–1.5 liters per day; by contrast, the kidney forms about 180 liters per day (125 ml/min) of glomerular filtrate, which means that about 99% of glomerular filtrate is reabsorbed by the renal tubules, leaving 1% as urine. In healthy people, blood contains about 3.5 liters of plasma; therefore, at 125 ml of plasma cleared per minute, it takes about 30 minutes for the entire plasma volume of the body to be filtered or cleared; that is to say, plasma (blood) is cleansed (cleared) completely about 50 times per day. Assessment of glomerular filtration function is an important tool in clinical assessment of renal disease, as is discussed in the accompanying Lab Tools box.

> *The kidneys form about 180 liters of glomerular filtrate each day (about 50 gallons, the size of a very large garbage can). All but 1–2 liters (1–2 quarts) is resorbed by the renal tubules. The remainder is urine.*

LAB TOOLS

Measurement of Glomerular Filtration Rate

The rate at which a substance is removed (cleared, cleaned) from plasma is known as its clearance rate or, simply, its clearance. Clearance is expressed as the volume of *plasma* cleared (cleaned) per unit time. Clearances are an important measure of glomerular function because they depend directly on the rate at which glomerular filtrate is formed: if something interferes with formation of the glomerular filtrate, then less plasma will be cleared.

The gold standard for determining how rapidly the glomerular filtrate is being formed is the **inulin clearance test**, which involves an intravenous injection of inulin, timed collection of urine output, and measurement of blood and urine inulin levels. Inulin is a synthetic sugar that is not metabolized, passes completely from blood into the glomerular filtrate, and is not reabsorbed by the tubules.

Thus, the amount of inulin excreted in urine in a given period of time is the amount of inulin removed from plasma in the same period. Simple calculations allow determination of the volume of plasma cleared of inulin per unit of time

Also useful is the **creatinine clearance test**, which is much more widely used as an indicator of glomerular function because creatinine occurs naturally in plasma and no injection is required. The amount of plasma cleared of creatinine can be assessed by timed urine output measurement and measurement of levels of creatinine in blood and urine. However, creatinine clearance is not as accurate as inulin clearance because some creatinine does not get into urine through the glomerulus (it is secreted into urine by the renal tubules).

TUBULAR PROCESSING OF THE GLOMERULAR FILTRATE

Figure 19-4 demonstrates how the tubule adjusts the glomerular filtrate before it is discharged as urine. As the filtrate passes down the renal tubule, most of the water is reabsorbed into blood under the influence of antidiuretic hormone (ADH, from the posterior pituitary). As was discussed in Diseases of the Endocrine Glands (Chapter 18) the hypothalamus and pituitary sense plasma osmolality (concentration of dissolved salts, mainly sodium and potassium) and secrete more or less ADH to command the kidney to extract more or less water from the glomerular filtrate and add it back to plasma to adjust the amount of plasma water in which the salts are dissolved.

Final fine-tuning of plasma sodium and potassium concentration and acid-base balance is regulated by the influence of aldosterone, which causes plasma sodium levels to rise and potassium levels to fall. Aldosterone stimulates secretion of potassium from blood into the glomerular filtrate in exchange for sodium, which moves from the glomerular filtrate into blood.

The tubule also normally reabsorbs *all* glucose and amino acids; neither is present in normal urine. Glucose appears in urine (*glycosuria*) if the amount of glucose in the glomerular filtrate is more than the tubules can absorb, normally 180–200 mg/dL (the renal "threshold." Glycosuria does not occur in healthy people, but it is a defining characteristic in people with diabetes mellitus (Chapter 17).

Virtually all plasma amino acid passes into the glomerular filtrate, and normally all of it is resorbed back into plasma by the tubules. Amino acids may appear in urine (*aminoaciduria*) if blood concentration exceeds the tubular threshold for amino acid, or if disease impairs the ability of the tubules to reabsorb amino acids. Most aminoaciduria occurs in newborns and infants and is caused by inherited metabolic defects.

After all of these tubular actions on the glomerular filtrate, the remaining fluid is waste—**urine**. The principal waste products in urine are **urea** and **creatinine**, both products of protein metabolism. The accompanying Lab Tools box discusses the importance, in assessing renal function, of measuring both the amount of nitrogen in urea in blood (**blood urea nitrogen**, **BUN**) and the amount of blood creatinine, and discusses how the waste-disposal function of the kidneys is mimicked by artificial dialysis (see also The Clinical Side box on the next page).

Urine also contains toxins and drug metabolites excreted by the kidney. Normal urine is acidic because energy metabolism creates acid, which must be eliminated in urine and breath (as CO_2). Normal urine contains varying amounts of sodium, potassium, and other electrolytes that vary according to diet, exercise, hydration, and metabolism. Finally, urine concentration (specific gravity, **osmolality**) varies according to the body's need to conserve or excrete water in order to maintain normal blood **osmolality**.

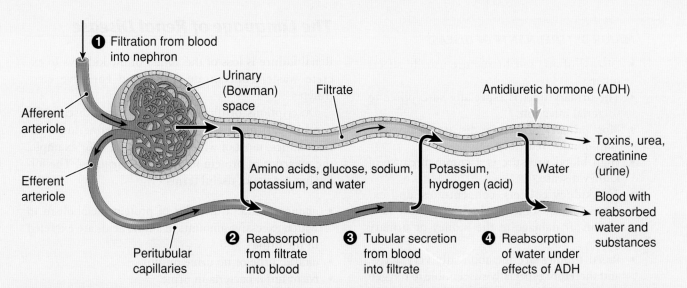

Figure 19-4 **Tubular processing of the glomerular filtrate.** The tubule completely reabsorbs glucose and amino acids and regulates plasma acid-base balance and osmolality by reabsorbing variable amounts of water, electrolytes, and acid. Toxins, creatinine, and urea pass unaltered into urine.

LAB TOOLS

Blood BUN and Creatinine

Blood urea nitrogen (BUN) and **creatinine** are the two most commonly ordered blood tests used to assess renal function.

Urea is produced by the liver from breakdown products of protein and is measured in blood by measuring its nitrogen content (**blood urea nitrogen, BUN**). Urea passes freely from the glomerulus into the glomerular filtrate. Blood urea levels rise with declining renal function. However, patients with large muscle mass or who consume a diet especially high in protein have BUN measurements that are higher than they would be otherwise, but usually not

enough to produce abnormally high levels. For example, a weight lifter with large muscle mass on a high protein diet will have significantly higher BUN than otherwise. Liver disease causes BUN levels to tend downward.

Creatinine also is a product of protein breakdown and passes freely into the glomerular filtrate, but it does not depend on liver metabolism. Blood creatinine level is, therefore, directly related to glomerular function and is a more reliable indicator of renal performance. Blood creatinine level rises as renal function declines—in general every doubling of blood creatinine level indicates a halving of glomerular function.

THE CLINICAL SIDE

THERAPEUTIC DIALYSIS FOR RENAL FAILURE

Patients in acute or chronic renal failure can be sustained by therapeutic dialysis. The two types of dialysis are hemodialysis and peritoneal dialysis.

Hemodialysis involves creating a circuit of blood that passes from the body through a dialysis apparatus (the *dialyzer*) and back into the body again. In a dialyzer blood passes through tubes with thin walls made of a unique (semipermeable) membrane that allows only certain substances to cross into and from blood. The tubes are immersed in the *dialysate*, which consists of water that contains sodium,

potassium, chloride, calcium, and bicarbonate, the concentration of which are varied according to patient needs. Blood cells and protein cannot cross the membrane into the dialysate, but urea, creatinine, acid, and other waste molecules diffuse easily from blood and are washed away.

Peritoneal dialysis involves infusion of dialysate into the peritoneal cavity, where the peritoneal lining acts as the semipermeable dialysis membrane. Dialysate is instilled into the abdomen so that waste can diffuse into it from blood vessels that line the peritoneum. After a suitable interval, usually 6–24 hours, the dialysate is withdrawn and replaced with fresh fluid.

MAJOR DETERMINANTS OF DISEASE

- Disease of one renal structure usually affects others.
- The urinary tract is especially susceptible to bacterial infection.
- Most primary glomerular disease is caused by autoimmune reactions.
- High blood pressure is a common cause of kidney disease.
- The kidney collects, concentrates, and excretes toxins, some of which may cause neoplasms or damage to the kidney or urinary tract.
- Renal tubules are metabolically very active and therefore especially susceptible to oxygen deprivation or toxic damage.

The Language of Renal Disease

Renal failure is loss of the ability of the kidneys to excrete waste, concentrate urine, and conserve electrolytes.

Descriptions of illness caused by renal disease depend in part upon special terms that define urine abnormalities, most of which end in "uria." For example, the presence of protein in urine is *proteinuria*. The following is a list of useful terms:

- *aminoaciduria*: a disorder of protein metabolism in which excessive amounts of amino acids are excreted in the urine
- *anuria*: little or no urine output
- *bacteriuria*: bacteria in urine
- *diuresis*: increased urine output, especially in response to therapy or change in physiologic condition

- **dysuria**: painful urination
- *glycosuria*: glucose in urine
- **hematuria**: intact red blood cells in urine. *Gross hematuria* is visible to the naked eye; *microscopic hematuria* is not grossly visible and requires microscopic examination.
- *hemoglobinuria* (to be distinguished from hematuria): free hemoglobin in urine
- *lipiduria*: fat in urine
- *nocturia*: urination at night. Getting up once is normal; twice is abnormal
- *oliguria*: less than normal urine output
- *polyuria*: more than normal urine output
- **proteinuria**: an excessive amount of protein in urine
- *pyuria*: white blood cells (pus) in urine

Additionally, descriptions of kidney disease depend heavily on clinical signs and symptoms. Recall from our discussion in Chapter 1 that *disease* is a *pathologic* process, such as necrosis, inflammation, or edema; however, by contrast a *syndrome* is a *clinical* picture. Renal disease is usually manifest clinically as one of the following **syndromes**.

- *acute nephritic syndrome* (acute autoimmune glomerular disease with hypertension and hematuria)
- *acute renal failure*
- *azotemia* (renal failure detectable only by laboratory tests)
- *chronic renal failure*
- *nephrolithiasis* (stones in the urinary tract)
- *nephrotic syndrome* (renal failure with marked proteinuria and edema)
- *occult (or microscopic) hematuria* (blood in urine not visible to the naked eye)
- *occult proteinuria* (protein in urine without clinical signs or symptoms)
- *uremia* (renal failure with clinical signs and symptoms)
- *urinary tract infection*
- *urinary tract obstruction*

It is also important to realize that renal disease may appear first as one syndrome and evolve into another syndrome as disease progresses. For example, acute nephritic syndrome may evolve to acute renal failure, which in turn may lead to uremia.

Normal Urine and Urinalysis

Most adults excrete about 1,000 to 1,500 ml of urine per day, urinating about 5–8 times per day and, occasionally, once at night. Urinating twice at night is abnormal.

Urinalysis is laboratory analysis of urine. The best specimen for urinalysis is obtained by catheterization, but for most circumstances a first urine voided upon arising is best because it is the most condensed (highest specific gravity) and gives an indication of the concentrating power of the kidneys. A midstream specimen is best, because mucus, semen, or bacteria from the urethral orifice are washed away first. Specimen collection technique in females is especially important because the specimen can be contaminated by vaginal blood, mucus, or inflammatory exudate. The characteristics of normal urine are listed in the nearby box, Basics in Brief 19.1 (see also the nearby History of Medicine box).

Specimens should be collected in specially prepared, clean, disposable containers that should never be reused. Specimens for culture should be collected in a sterile container. All specimens should be tested quickly, refrigerated, or preserved by a special additive. If left standing at room temperature for more than a short time, all urine characteristics begin to change, and bacteria proliferate, adding to the change by their metabolism; for example, urine glucose can be reduced by bacterial use for fuel.

Typically, urine is tested in large laboratories by automated analyzer, or in the office or at bedside with a strip of stiff paper (*dipstick*) containing bands of chemicals that test for various urine characteristics (Fig. 19-5). The specimen is then centrifuged and the sediment studied microscopically for cells, crystals, bacteria, and other formed elements (Fig. 19-6). Below is a brief description of some of the more important urine abnormalities:

- *Bacteria*: Urinary tract sterility is maintained by the flushing action of urine flow and antimicrobial properties of the epithelium that lines the urinary tract. Routine urinalysis dipstick tests also test for evidence of bacterial infection by testing for urine *nitrite* and *leukocyte esterase*. *Nitrite* is produced in urine by gram-negative bacterial metabolism and suggests infection. Likewise, the detection of leukocyte *esterase* suggests high numbers of leukocytes, an indicator of infection. Urine positive for either must be examined microscopically for bacteria and cultured if necessary. However, both nitrite and leukocyte esterase tests have significant numbers of false-positive and false-negative results, and microscopic examination and urine culture should be performed if laboratory findings do not match clinical suspicions.
- *Bile pigments*: *Urobilinogen* is produced in the intestine by bacterial digestion of bilirubin secreted by the liver. Some of it is reabsorbed and excreted normally in urine. Jaundice because of biliary obstruction is

BASICS IN BRIEF 19-1

NORMAL URINE

First morning voided urine normally has the following characteristics:

- *Odor*: odorless
- *Color and clarity*: crystal clear, light yellow, or amber
- *Specific gravity*: 1.016–1.022
- *pH*: acid, pH about 6.0
- *Bile pigments*: urobilinogen present in small amount; bilirubin absent
- *Protein*: present in very small amounts, usually too small to be detected by routine tests
- *Hemoglobin*: absent
- *Glucose*: absent
- *Ketones*: absent
- *Cells and other formed elements*: Examination of centrifuged sediment may reveal rare red or white blood cells and a few urinary epithelial cells. No bacteria, crystals, or casts are present. (A cast is a cylindrical mass of compacted material—usually red or white cells, protein, or hemoglobin—formed in the lumen of a tubule and flushed into urine. Casts are always pathologic.)

associated with decreased amounts of bilirubin reaching the intestine, which causes urine urobilinogen to decrease or disappear. Urobilinogen is usually increased in other types of jaundice.

- *Bilirubin*: Bilirubin is not normally present in urine. Most types of jaundice are associated with bilirubin in urine (*bilirubinuria*).

- *Color and clarity*: The most common cause of abnormal urine color is medication. Increased urine bilirubin occurs in jaundice and imparts a dark yellow-brown color. A large volume of intact red cells turns urine dark red and opaque (depending on the number of red cells). To the contrary, urine that contains hemoglobin from lysed (destroyed) red cells is red

History of Medicine

LIQUID GOLD

Clay tablets from about 4000 BC mention the examination of urine and offer an inkling of the ancient's ideas about its importance. And it is important: patients who do not make enough of this "liquid gold" soon find themselves in deep trouble from renal failure.

Urine is readily available and easy to collect, and it can be examined at leisure, features that made it a popular choice for study by early physicians, especially for the examination of women, who could not be directly examined because religious beliefs forbade it. Greek physician Hippocrates (460–377 BC) wrote specifically about examination of urine, noting that fever changed its smell. Later, Galen (131–201 AD), a Greco-Roman physician, wrote of his belief that urine revealed the health of the liver. Galen believed that urine was a combination of the body's four "humours"—blood, phlegm, yellow bile, and black bile—and revealed if they were in or out of balance. Galen's ideas on urine, humours, and other medical matters became so entrenched in the an-

cient and medieval worlds that few new ideas were accepted in medicine for over 1,000 years, until the European Renaissance (~1300–1650) launched a revolution in science, politics, religion, art, and every other aspect of human affairs.

Nevertheless, medical advances had to compete with magicians of the time, who relied on the bubble patterns of freshly passed urine to foretell the future. Not content to peer into the darkness of a brass chamber pot, physicians and magicians developed the matula, a glass vessel shaped like the bladder, believing that urine held in a matula was more revealing because it maintained its natural shape. Apart from these well-intentioned fantasies, sometimes the practitioners were right: the ancient Greeks knew that diabetes was characterized by large volumes of urine, and English physician Thomas Willis (1621–1675) bravely tasted urine and learned that diabetic urine was sweet with a sugary substance.

- *Glucose*: Normal urine contains no glucose. By far the most common cause of *glycosuria* is diabetes mellitus; however, many other relatively uncommon conditions are capable of causing glycosuria. Sometimes other sugars can cause a false-positive test for glucose; for example, congenital galactosemia, a treatable genetic disease.

- *Hemoglobin*: Blood in urine occurs in two forms: intact red cells (*hematuria*) and free hemoglobin (*hemoglobinuria*).
  - *Free hemoglobin*: No free hemoglobin (hemoglobin apart from intact red cells) is chemically detectible in normal urine. Free hemoglobin in urine may be caused by free hemoglobin in blood secondary to hemolytic anemia (Chapter 11) or owing to hemolysis of red cells in urine.
  - *Red blood cells*: It is not unusual to find an occasional red blood cell by careful microscopic examination of centrifuged urinary sediment, but there is disagreement about the number required for concern. *Hematuria* (significant numbers of intact red cells in urine) can be caused by renal disease or disease anywhere else in the urinary tract. There are two types of hematuria: *gross*, if blood is visible to the naked eye; and *microscopic* (or occult) if red cells are detectable only by microscopic study.

- *Ketones*: Normal urine contains no ketones. The most important cause of ketonuria is diabetic ketoacidosis, which occurs because people with dia-

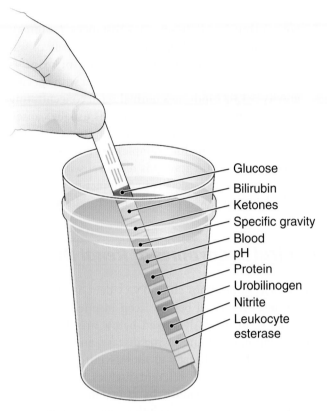

Figure 19-5 Urinalysis. Fresh or refrigerated urine tested by dipstick method. Microscopic examination of urinary sediment is a separate task.

Glucose
Bilirubin
Ketones
Specific gravity
Blood
pH
Protein
Urobilinogen
Nitrite
Leukocyte esterase

and clear. Dietary beets, too, can turn urine red. Cloudy urine is abnormal and usually caused by precipitated chemicals or cells. All cloudy urine should be examined microscopically.

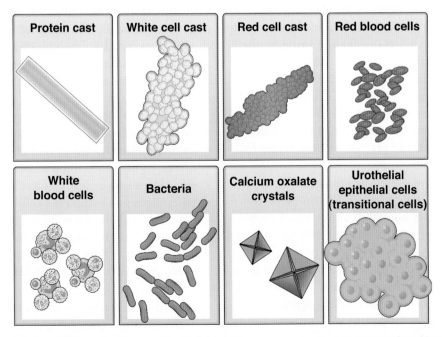

Protein cast   White cell cast   Red cell cast   Red blood cells

White blood cells   Bacteria   Calcium oxalate crystals   Urothelial epithelial cells (transitional cells)

Figure 19-6 Microscopic examination of urinary sediment. Some of the more common formed elements found in urine are shown here.

betes must burn fat instead of glucose. Likewise, patients who are fasting can develop ketonuria because they, too, must burn fat instead of glucose.

- *Microscopic study of centrifuged urinary sediment*: Microscopic study identifies formed elements (Fig. 19.6).
  - *Casts*: Casts, which are cylinders formed by compaction of protein, red or white cells, or epithelial cells in the lumen of renal tubules, always indicate renal disease. For example, a red cell cast indicates that blood in the urine is caused by blood accumulated in a tubule from glomerular disease; free red cells in urine without red cell casts suggests bleeding from some other source in the urinary tract, such as the bladder.
  - *Cells*: Normal urine contains a few urothelial cells from the lining transitional epithelium of the urinary tract. Increased numbers of red cells indicate bleeding somewhere in the urinary tract or contamination, usually from vaginal blood. Increased numbers of white cells indicate infection or contamination, usually from vaginal inflammatory exudate.
  - *Crystals*: Crystals in the urine sediment are not usually an indication of disease. There are many types, which vary according to urine pH, and their presence is rarely of diagnostic value.
- *Odor*: Normal urine is nearly odorless. A foul smell or the odor of ammonia is caused by bacterial metabolism of urea and suggests bacterial contamination of a stale specimen. Ketones in urine (diabetic ketoacidosis) have a distinctive odor.
- *pH*: Normal urine is slightly acidic but may become slightly alkaline (pH >7.0) after meals. Normal pH varies from about 4.5–8.0. Alkaline urine is often caused by bacterial contamination in a stale, unrefrigerated specimen. Strict vegetarian and high-protein diets tend to produce alkaline urine. In generalized acidosis (for example, the acidosis of respiratory failure and CO_2 retention, Chapter 14) the kidneys excrete acid, and urine pH can be very acidic (pH <4.5).
- *Protein*: The kidneys excrete less than 150 mg of protein a day; more is *proteinuria*. Intermittent (transient) proteinuria is normal in about 5% of people. Some spill plasma protein into urine only when erect and not when lying down (*orthostatic* or *postural proteinuria*); others develop *physiologic proteinuria* with vigorous exercise or in association with fever or other temporary conditions. *Persistent proteinuria*, however, indicates renal disease.

- *Specific gravity*: Specific gravity is a measure of the concentration of dissolved substances (solutes), mainly urea and sodium. The specific gravity of water is 1.000. Normal specific gravity of urine is 1.016–1.022. A first-morning specimen with specific gravity >1.022 indicates normal renal concentrating capacity. Increased specific gravity is usually caused by dehydration, but increased amounts of solute (glucose or protein, for example) can also be responsible. Low specific gravity is often caused by excessive fluid intake, especially in conjunction with alcoholic beverages, which have a diuretic effect.

Clinical Syndromes of Renal Disease

Renal disease becomes clinically evident as one of the syndromes discussed below. Keep in mind, however, that the syndromes discussed below are the *clinical* manifestation of an underlying disease, and, as is illustrated in Table 19-1, each of these syndromes may be caused by a number of different diseases.

Azotemia is renal failure that is manifest only by abnormal laboratory tests; no clinical signs of kidney failure are present. It can be caused by almost any type of underlying renal disease. It is always discovered incidentally during examination for some other medical problem or on a routine exam, such as an employment physical. The most commonly detected abnormalities are increased blood urea nitrogen (BUN) and blood creatinine.

Uremia (literally, "urine in blood") is renal failure with clinical signs and symptoms, some of which occur there is accumulation in blood of waste products that should be excreted by the kidney and others of which are caused by failure of other kidney functions. Uremia can be caused by almost any type of underlying renal disease. Patients with uremia typically have:

- *hypertension*, owing to retention of salt and water
- *anemia*, caused by low output of erythropoietin
- *edema*, owing to retention of salt and water
- *oliguria*, caused by low glomerular filtration rate
- other signs and symptoms caused by accumulation of toxic metabolic waste products:
  - *pericarditis* and *gastroenteritis* caused by the irritant effect of toxic products
  - *bleeding/coagulation defects* caused by platelet malfunction
  - peripheral nerve disease (neuropathy) or brain dysfunction (encephalopathy)

Table 19-1   Urinary Tract Diseases and Associated Clinical Syndromes

Results (Clinical Syndromes)	Causes (Diseases)							
	Glomerular	Renal/ Vascular	Tubular/ Interstitial	Obstruction/ Reflux	Pyelonephritis (Infection)	Nephrolithiasis (Stones)	Renal Tumors	Lower Urinary Tract Disease
Azotemia	+	+	+	+				
Uremia	+	+	+	+				
Acute nephritic syndrome	+							
Nephrotic syndrome	+							
Occult hematuria	+	+	+	+		+	+	+
Occult proteinuria	+	+	+			+		
Acute renal failure	+	+	+					
Chronic renal failure	+	+		+	+	+		
Urinary tract infection				+	+	+		+
Urinary tract obstruction				+	+	+	+	+
Nephrolithiasis (stones)				+		+		+

Acute nephritic syndrome, resulting from acute glomerular inflammation (*acute glomerulonephritis*), is characterized by hematuria (either gross or microscopic), hypertension, azotemia, oliguria, and edema and is almost always caused by acute autoimmune (Chapter 8) glomerular disease. The pathologic lesion consists of acute glomerular inflammation and reactive hyperplasia (proliferation) of glomerular cells, which impair blood flow through the glomerulus and reduce renal function. Hypertension is caused by increased renin output, because not enough blood is getting through the glomerulus to reach the juxtaglomerular apparatus. Hematuria occurs when red cells "leak" from damaged glomeruli into the glomerular filtrate. Oliguria is caused by diminished glomerular blood flow and low glomerular filtration rate. An example of acute nephritic syndrome is the acute glomerulonephritis that occurs after some streptococcal sore throats or skin infections, in which antibodies made to attack the strep also attack the glomerulus.

Nephrotic syndrome evolves from various glomerular diseases and is characterized by:

- *marked proteinuria* (>3.5 gm/day), caused by glomerular damage that allows leakage of protein (albumin) across the glomerular barrier from blood into the glomerular filtrate (Fig. 19-7).
- *marked hypoalbuminemia* owing to loss of albumin in urine.
- *marked generalized edema* associated with loss of plasma osmotic pressure caused by low plasma albumin. Loss of water from the vascular space stimulates

aldosterone production, which in turn commands the kidney to conserve additional water.

- *hyperlipidemia and lipiduria* because of low plasma albumin. Low albumin stimulates the liver to increase production of albumin and other proteins, including apoproteins (Chapter 12), which soak up additional lipid to form increased lipoprotein. The result is *hyperlipidemia*, some of which spills into the urine (*lipiduria*).

In children nephrotic syndrome is called **nephrosis** and usually is associated with primary glomerular disease. In adults, however, most nephrotic syndrome is caused by systemic autoimmune disease in which the glomerulus is secondarily involved; for example, diabetic kidney disease is a common cause of adult nephrotic syndrome.

Occult hematuria (microscopic hematuria) is characterized by significant numbers of red blood cells detectable only by microscopic study in normal appearing urine. It is usually found as a surprise on routine urinalysis, and the most common underlying disorder is mild or early glomerular disease. The cause of occult hematuria is not always demonstrable.

Occult proteinuria is protein in urine without clinical signs or symptoms. It occurs in asymptomatic patients and is characterized by protein in urine detectable only by urinalysis. Like occult hematuria, it is discovered incidentally and may have serious or not-so-serious implications. Small amounts of protein may appear in urine with fever, with urinary tract infection, or following strenuous exercise. Some people have proteinuria that appears during the day when the patient is erect and disappears at night (orthostatic proteinuria). The most serious implication of occult proteinuria is glomerular disease or renal damage from hypertension.

Acute renal failure is a combination of acute oliguria or anuria (low or absent urine flow) associated with azotemia (laboratory evidence of impaired renal function). The most common cause is the damage to renal tubules (*acute tubular necrosis*) that occurs during vascular collapse (shock, Chapter 5). Other causes of acute renal failure include toxic damage to tubules from therapeutic drugs or from toxins. Another cause is severe hemolysis (destruction of red cells in circulating blood), which produces a large amount of free hemoglobin that must be excreted by the kidney and can lead to acute renal failure. Similarly, some muscle disorders can liberate into blood a very large amount of myoglobin, a muscle protein similar to hemoglobin, which the kidney must excrete, and which can cause acute renal failure. An example is the muscle necrosis that occurs with heat stoke. Finally, acute glomerular or vascular disease also can cause acute renal failure.

Chronic renal failure, a combination of low urine output and prolonged symptoms and signs of renal failure (uremia), is the end result of all serious chronic renal disease. It progresses to **end-stage renal disease**, a "burned out" final pathologic phase characterized by a shrunken, functionless kidney (*end-stage contracted kidney*) in which evidence identifying the original cause of the disease is obliterated. At any given time about 250,000 people in the United States have end-stage renal disease. Diabetes, chronic glomerulonephritis, and hypertension account for about 75%; the cause of the other 25% is often unknown.

Urinary tract infection (UTI) is a combination of bacteriuria and pyuria caused by infection anywhere in the urinary tract, from kidney to urethra. Infections may be asymptomatic, or they may be associated with fever and dysuria. Acute bladder inflammation (*cystitis*) is a common manifestation of urinary tract infection.

Urinary tract obstruction may be may be acute or chronic. Acute obstruction is usually complete obstruction caused by urethral obstruction in men with prostate disease, and it is a painful medical emergency. Chronic obstruction, which is usually partial obstruction, is caused by tumors, scars, or stones and is usually

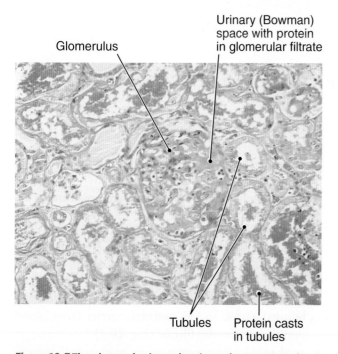

Glomerulus

Urinary (Bowman) space with protein in glomerular filtrate

Tubules   Protein casts in tubules

Figure 19-7 **The glomerulus in nephrotic syndrome.** Urinary (Bowman) space, normally filled with clear glomerular filtrate, contains a large amount of protein-rich fluid, which takes a smooth, red stain. The tubules contain dense deposits of similar, denser red material—protein that has condensed into casts, which will be flushed out as a diagnostic clue in the urine sediment.

associated with stagnation of urine, dilation of the collecting system above the obstruction, and secondary bacterial infection. Severe chronic obstruction can lead to severe renal damage and renal failure.

Nephrolithiasis is the formation of stones in the kidney (*urolithiasis* is formation of stones anywhere in the urinary tract). Although renal stones tend to cause hematuria (gross or microscopic), they most often come to attention because their passage through the ureter can be exceptionally painful (*renal colic*). Some patients tend to form stones time and again; usually the reason is not clear, but hyperparathyroidism (Chapter 18) should always be suspected.

Inherited, Congenital, and Developmental Disease

One or both kidneys may fail to develop (**renal agenesis**). Bilateral agenesis is incompatible with life; infants are stillborn and usually have multiple other abnormalities. Unilateral agenesis is not serious; the sole kidney enlarges to maintain normal renal function.

Horseshoe kidney is single, fused kidney; the two are joined inferiorly by a thick bridge of normal, functioning renal tissue as a result of abnormal embryogenesis. There are usually no clinical consequences.

Renal dysplasia occurs when there is *in utero obstruction of urinary flow*, usually caused by obstruction of the ureter. The obstruction leads to increased pressure in the embryonic kidney: glomeruli fail to develop, and the kidney enlarges because of dilation of the renal tubules into cysts.

There are other forms of **cystic disease**. *Simple cysts* of the kidney are so commonly found at autopsy that they can be considered a normal variation. As is illustrated in Figure 19-8, most are just a few millimeters in diameter, filled with clear fluid and lined by a glistening, unremarkable gray membrane. Larger ones a few centimeters across, however, may be discovered incidentally in the course of radiographic exams and can pose a diagnostic problem because they appear as a kidney mass, which demands investigation, because any renal mass must be considered neoplastic until proven otherwise.

Several types of genetic renal disease are characterized by multiple renal cysts. The most common is **polycystic kidney disease**, depicted in Figure 19-9. There are two types, both caused by genetic defects. *Adult polycystic disease* is caused by an autosomal dominant genetic defect (Chapter 7) and is fairly common: it accounts for about 10% of patients with chronic renal fail-

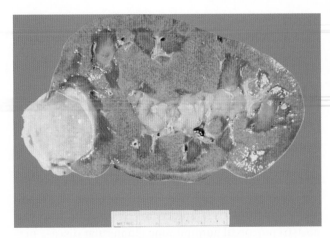

Figure 19-8 **Simple cyst of the kidney.**

ure. Unfortunately, it usually does not become symptomatic until after age 30, by which time many patients have reproduced and passed the genetic defect to their children. It is characterized by very large kidneys riddled with thousands of expanding cysts that injure the intervening renal parenchyma and produce severe chronic interstitial inflammation and fibrosis (*tubulointerstitial nephritis*). Most patients come to medical attention because of hematuria, chronic urinary tract infection, or hypertension. On the other hand, *childhood polycystic disease* is caused by an autosomal recessive defect and usually appears at birth or in late childhood. It is often associated with liver cysts and biliary ductal

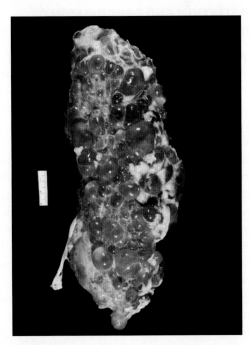

Figure 19-9 **Hereditary polycystic kidney disease.** Specimen from a 33-year-old man.

hyperplasia that leads to a cirrhosis-like scarring of the liver in patients who survive infancy. Most affected infants die in the perinatal period.

Glomerular Disease

Discussion of glomerular disease is bedeviled by the fact that some glomerular diseases are named according to *cause* (etiology), others according to *microscopic findings* in the glomerulus, and still others according to *clinical syndrome* by which they usually present. For example, a patient with streptococcal pharyngitis who gets poststreptococcal autoimmune glomerular disease may be said to suffer from 1) poststreptococcal glomerulonephritis (etiology and pathogenesis), 2) acute proliferative glomerulonephritis (pathologic findings), or 3) acute nephritic syndrome (clinical presentation). Indeed, the patient has all three (see Case Study 19.1 at the end of this chapter). The predictable result is that most glomerular diseases have more than one name, which makes glomerular disease difficult to present to students and difficult for front-line practitioners to remember.

The most common clinical presentations are acute nephritic syndrome and nephrotic syndrome. The most common cause of glomerular disease is an autoimmune reaction (Chapter 8). Pathologic findings vary widely and change as disease progresses.

☞ **All *primary glomerular disease is autoimmune.***

THE INITIATION AND PROGRESSION OF GLOMERULAR DISEASE

Most *primary* glomerular disease is caused by *autoimmune reaction* in the glomerulus. However, glomerular disease can also occur secondary to another disease, such as diabetes or systemic lupus erythematosus (Chapter 8).

The autoimmune reactions of primary glomerular disease are usually one of two types: 1) deposition in the glomerulus of *circulating antigen-antibody complexes* formed elsewhere (type III hypersensitivity reaction, Chapter 8); or 2) direct antibody attack (type II hypersensitivity) on glomerular basement membrane by *anti-glomerular basement membrane antibody*. Figure 19-10 illustrates these reactions. Antibodies of either type can be detected in blood or demonstrated by microscopic technique in glomeruli obtained by kidney biopsy. Electron microscopy, which is capable of very high magnification (near 100,000 ✕), is especially useful in demonstrating the glomerular lesions associated with glomerular disease.

Patients who develop acute glomerular disease (usually called **acute glomerulonephritis**) often recover fully, but in some patients glomerular disease progresses in one of two ways. First, the glomerulus may undergo focal scarring and atrophy, a condition known as **focal segmental glomerulosclerosis**, which is often the consequence of previously diagnosed glomerulonephritis. In some patients focal segmental glomerulosclerosis occurs as a primary lesion of the glomerulus and is considered a separate disease; it may progress to complete destruction of the glomerulus and chronic renal failure. Second, most glomerular diseases, once they have destroyed about one third to one half of glomeruli, are associated with progressive chronic inflammation, with its attendant scarring and destruction of renal tubules (**tubulointerstitial nephritis**), usually leading to chronic renal failure.

GLOMERULONEPHRITIS

Glomerulonephritis (GN) is inflammation of the glomerulus. It may be acute or chronic, and either primary or secondary to some other disease. In our discussion of glomerulonephritis we will use the following framework:

- *Alternative names*
- *Usual presenting clinical syndrome*
- *Etiology and pathogenesis*
- *Pathologic findings in the glomerulus*

There are many types of glomerulonephritis. The discussion below presents only the most important and common ones.

Poststreptococcal Glomerulonephritis

Poststreptococcal glomerulonephritis is acute glomerulonephritis caused by an autoimmune glomerular injury initiated by a particular type of streptococcus (beta-hemolytic streptococcus).

- *Alternative names*: Acute proliferative glomerulonephritis
- *Usual presenting clinical syndrome*: Acute nephritic syndrome
- *Etiology and pathogenesis*: Streptococcal pharyngitis or skin infection, which causes formation of circulating antigen-antibody complexes (Chapter 8) that deposit in the glomerulus.
- *Pathologic findings in the glomerulus*: Increased cellularity of the glomerulus, caused by proliferation of glomerular cells and by the presence of inflammatory cells; clumps of immune complex deposited on basement membrane.

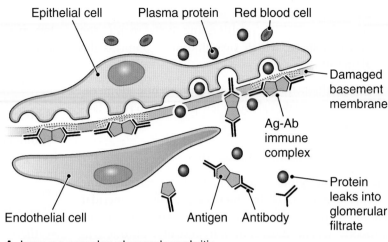

A Immune complex glomerulonephritis
(type III hypersensitivity reaction)

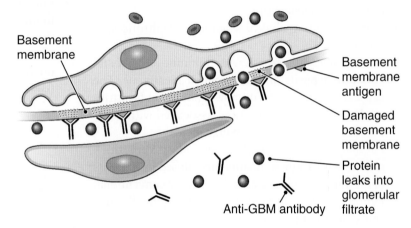

***Figure 19-10* Autoimmune reactions in glomeru-
lonephritis. A,** Circulating immune complexes formed
elsewhere are deposited on the glomerular basement
membrane (GBM). **B,** Antibody attachment to native
antigens in the glomerular basement membrane.

B Anti-GBM glomerulonephritis
(type II hypersensitivity reaction)

Classic acute poststreptococcal glomerulonephritis presents as acute nephritic syndrome with hematuria, hypertension, increased blood BUN and creatinine, low urine output, and edema. It usually affects children and appears several weeks after streptococcal pharyngitis or skin infection. It also may occur after other infections, such as chickenpox, measles, and mumps. In most cases patients recover fully in a few weeks. However, about 10% of poststreptococcal glomerulonephritis cases evolve into a clinical syndrome of *rapidly progressive glomerulonephritis.*

Rapidly Progressive Glomerulonephritis

Rapidly progressive glomerulonephritis is a form of glomerulonephritis that may arise from unknown causes or may be secondary to poststreptococcal glomerulonephritis or other disease affecting the glomerulus. No single mechanism can explain all cases, but most appear to be autoimmune. Regardless of cause, the pathologic picture is characterized by arcs (crescents) of cells that proliferate in urinary (Bowman) space and collapse the glomerulus (Fig. 19-11).

- *Alternative names: Crescentic glomerulonephritis*
- *Usual presenting clinical syndrome:* Sometimes initially presents as acute nephritic syndrome; other cases present initially as renal failure
- *Etiology and pathogenesis:* Some cases are caused by deposition of circulating antigen-antibody complexes in the glomerulus; others have no identifiable immune component. The cause is unknown in half of cases; the other half is a consequence of some known glomerular disease.

- *Pathologic findings in the glomerulus*: Crescent-shaped masses of proliferating cells inside the Bowman space, which surround and compress the glomerulus.

The outlook for patients with crescentic glomerulonephritis is bleak—all but a few progress to renal failure and require dialysis.

Membranous Glomerulonephritis

Membranous glomerulonephritis is an autoimmune disease characterized by thickening of the glomerular basement membrane caused by deposits of autoimmune antibody. It is the most common cause of nephrotic syndrome in adults.

- *Alternative names*: Antiglomerular basement membrane glomerulonephritis.
- *Usual presenting clinical syndrome*: Nephrotic syndrome
- *Etiology and pathogenesis*: Autoimmune antigen and antibody deposits on the basement membrane. The cause of most cases is unknown. Some can be attributed to autoimmune reactions associated with hepatitis B, malaria, drugs, or malignancies.
- *Pathologic findings in the glomerulus*: Very thick glomerular basement membranes caused by deposits of immune complexes, as is depicted by conventional light microscopy in Figure 19-12 and by the fluorescence microscopy in Figure 19-13.

The course of membranous glomerulonephritis is often slow, but it can be unpredictable. About 10% of

cases proceed to renal failure within 10 years; about 25% of patients recover completely and spontaneously with little consequence. However, most progress slowly with persistent proteinuria, hypertension, and progressive loss of renal function.

Minimal Change Glomerulonephritis

Minimal change glomerulonephritis is a disease that affects glomerular epithelial cells with very subtle changes that are not visible by conventional microscopy; however, on electron microscopy characteristic lesions are identifiable.

- *Alternative names*: Lipoid nephrosis
- *Usual presenting clinical syndrome*: Nephrotic syndrome
- *Etiology and pathogenesis*: Unknown; probably autoimmune (responds very well to steroid therapy); sometimes follows infections or allergic reactions.
- *Pathologic findings in the glomerulus*: Nothing by light microscopy; glomerular epithelial cell lesions identifiable by electron microscopy.

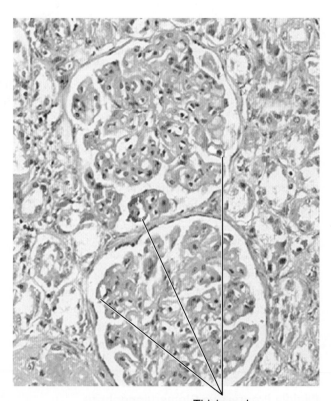

Figure 19-12 **Membranous glomerulonephritis (light microscopy).** Basement membrane is thickened by immunoglobulin deposits.

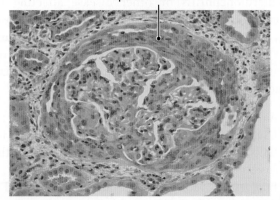

Crescent of proliferating epithelial cells

Figure 19-11 **Crescentic glomerulonephritis.** Crescent of epithelial cells proliferates along the parietal rim of the glomerular space and obliterates the glomerulus. Crescentic glomerulonephritis is an anatomic finding in progressively worsening glomerulonephritis of many types. Reprinted with permission from Rubin E. Pathology. 4th ed. Philadelphia. Lippincott Williams and Wilkins, 2005.

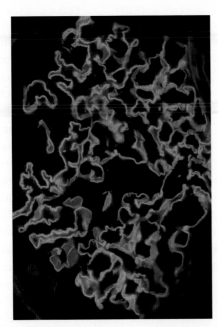

Figure 19-13 **Membranous glomerulonephritis (fluorescence microscopy).** Basement membrane is thickened by a coating of immunoglobulin. Reprinted with permission from Rubin E. Pathology. 4th ed. Philadelphia. Lippincott Williams and Wilkins, 2005.

Minimal change glomerulonephritis is a relatively benign disease that typically occurs in children 2–6 years old, but it can occur in adults. It is the most common cause of nephrotic syndrome in children, and it is characterized by sudden appearance of proteinuria and edema without hypertension or laboratory evidence of renal failure. It responds well to steroid therapy. The alternative name *lipoid nephrosis* refers to the hyperlipidemia and lipiduria that occur in conjunction with nephrotic syndrome. Most patients recover fully after a short course of steroid therapy, but a few go on to chronic renal disease over the next few decades.

IgA Glomerulonephritis

IgA glomerulonephritis is an autoimmune glomerular disease associated with immunoglobulin A deposits in mesangial cells of the glomerulus. It is the most common type of glomerulonephritis worldwide, accounting for 10% of all glomerulonephritis cases in the United States and 40% in Asia.

- *Alternative names: Berger disease*
- *Usual presenting clinical syndrome*: Hematuria
- *Etiology and pathogenesis*: Autoimmune; often first appearing after respiratory or gastrointestinal infection
- *Pathologic findings in the glomerulus*: IgA immune complex deposits in glomerular mesangial cells.

IgA glomerulonephritis occurs mainly in young men age 20–30 years and is characterized by recurrent bouts of hematuria appearing a few days after an acute upper respiratory or gastrointestinal infection. It is to be suspected in young adults with recurrent hematuria for which no other cause can be found. Typically, IgA glomerulonephritis resolves spontaneously for a few months and then recurs. Most children have a benign course and recover completely; however, about half of adults develop chronic renal failure and require dialysis or renal transplant.

Chronic Glomerulonephritis

Chronic glomerulonephritis is the diagnosis applied to "burned out" chronic glomerular disease. Sometimes the cause is one of the glomerular diseases described above. More often, however, the diagnosis is applied to patients with chronic glomerular disease of unknown cause who presumably have had long-standing, smoldering, asymptomatic autoimmune glomerular disease. These cases usually come to attention because of incidental discovery of occult proteinuria or high blood pressure, or because weakness and anemia develop as a result of chronic renal failure. About half of patients on chronic renal dialysis carry a diagnosis of chronic glomerulonephritis.

- *Alternative name*: None
- *Usual presenting clinical syndrome*: Chronic renal failure or occult proteinuria
- *Etiology and pathogenesis*: About half of patients have been diagnosed previously with a particular type of glomerulonephritis; in the other half the cause is unknown.
- *Pathologic findings in the glomerulus*: Some patients have residual microscopic evidence of a particular type of glomerulonephritis. In most, however, the glomeruli are shriveled into small nodular bits of scar tissue that reveal no trace of the original pathogenesis.

The typical patient presents with anemia and fatigue or weight loss, or occult proteinuria. Most patients are hypertensive, and in some patients the kidney disease comes to light in a workup for high blood pressure or edema or during care for heart attack or stroke. Diagnostic workup reveals chronic renal failure, but questioning elicits no history of illness to explain the problem. Renal biopsy shows shrunken, scarred glomeruli, and chronic glomerulonephritis becomes a default diagnosis. The clinical course is progressive but variable. Some patients may go on for many years before dialysis is required, others will have complete renal failure shortly after diagnosis. Dialysis and transplant are the eventual treatments of choice.

SECONDARY GLOMERULAR DISEASE

Diabetic glomerulosclerosis (Chapter 17) is the most common cause of secondary glomerular disease and is the most common cause of renal failure in the United States: about 20% of patients with diabetes develop chronic renal failure. Recall that high blood sugar in patients with diabetes causes formation of glycoproteins, which tend to deposit in the basement membrane of small blood vessels. Glycoprotein deposits in glomerular capillaries interfere with glomerular blood flow and damage the barrier function that prevents protein from entering the glomerular filtrate.

Glomerular disease is often caused by vascular disease. For example, reduced blood flow to the kidney because of atherosclerosis of the renal artery can cause glomerular atrophy; high glomerular pressure in hypertension damages glomeruli; and the vasculitis associated with systemic lupus erythematosus or other systemic diseases can also affect the glomerulus.

Finally, the development of glomerular disease has a tendency to become self-perpetuating due to **renal ablation glomerulopathy**, a vicious circle of renal destruction that begins to appear by the time one third to one half of glomeruli are destroyed by any renal disease. As glomerular disease destroys (ablates) glomeruli, remaining glomeruli must work harder: blood flow through each glomerulus increases; and the amount of glomerular filtrate formed by each glomerulus increases, which in turn increases workload by the associated tubule. This stress on the glomerulus and tubule is so great that the remaining healthy glomeruli are progressively destroyed in a vicious circle of lost glomeruli, increased workload, and additionally destroyed glomeruli. This spiral of destruction leads to the final stage of most renal failure—a shrunken, "burned out," **end-stage contracted kidney**.

Diseases of Renal Vasculature

Benign nephrosclerosis (Chapter 12) is a characteristic change in renal blood vessels and glomeruli that is an inevitable consequence of life because it is a consequence of blood pressure—and blood pressure is necessary for life. Some degree of nephrosclerosis is an incidental finding in all elderly persons coming to autopsy, and is so common that it scarcely warrants diagnosis. *Identical renal changes occur at a much earlier age in patients with hypertension;* the higher the blood pressure,

the earlier the change appears. As is depicted in Figure 19-14, nephrosclerotic kidneys are atrophic and have a granular, finely pebbled surface. The microscopic lesion is smooth, glassy change (hyaline arteriolosclerosis) in the walls of glomerular afferent arterioles, which slowly chokes off glomerular blood supply and reduces the glomerulus to a small ball of fibrous scar tissue. Functional impairment is mild in most patients.

Malignant nephrosclerosis is a much more severe form of nephrosclerosis seen in patients with *malignant hypertension*, which is usually associated with blood pressure over 160/110 mmHg (Chapter 12). The mechanism of damage to renal blood vessels and glomeruli is similar to the mechanism in benign nephrosclerosis, but it happens more quickly. High blood pressure damages the afferent arteriole and strangles blood supply to the glomerulus. This activates the renin-angiotensin-aldosterone mechanism (Chapter 12), which in turn raises blood pressure even more—a perfect vicious circle of high blood pressure, renal destruction, and even higher blood pressure. The relentless pounding of blood pressure causes pressure necrosis (fibrinoid necrosis) of the afferent arteriole and onionskin hyperplasia of cells in the walls of small arterioles (Fig. 19-15), which is a pathologic hallmark of malignant hypertension.

The clinical picture of malignant nephrosclerosis includes 1) renal failure; 2) vascular stress that may present as myocardial infarct, congestive heart failure, or stroke; and 3) increased intracranial pressure that may present as seizures, headache, nausea and vomiting, visual impairments, coma, or mental aberration. Physical exam typically reveals blood pressure >160/110

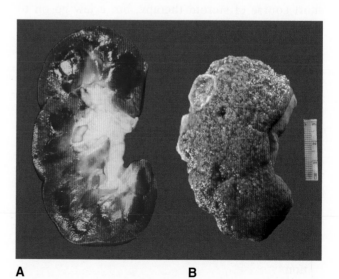

A   **B**

Figure 19-14 **Benign nephrosclerosis. A,** Normal kidney. **B,** Benign nephrosclerosis. The kidney is shrunken and granular.

mg/Hg, pounding heartbeat, and bulging optical discs (papilledema) on retinal exam, as the edematous brain pushes the optic nerves forward. Blood renin is markedly increased. Malignant hypertension is a medical emergency requiring vigorous and prompt intervention. About 25% of patients die within five years.

Renovascular hypertension is elevated blood pressure secondary to renal ischemia; that is, impaired blood flow to the kidney caused by narrowing of the renal artery, usually by atherosclerosis. Renovascular disease accounts for about 2–3% of hypertension cases and should be considered in every clinical workup for hypertension. As with malignant hypertension, impaired renal blood flow invokes the renin-angiotensin-aldosterone mechanism (Chapter 12), which drives blood pressure higher still. Over half of patients are cured by restoration of full blood flow or excision of the affected kidney. However, in some patients long-standing hypertension has caused so much renal damage that restoration of normal blood flow has limited effect.

Acute Tubular Necrosis

Because they consume so much energy processing the glomerular filtrate, renal tubular epithelial cells are especially likely to be damaged or die if renal blood flow

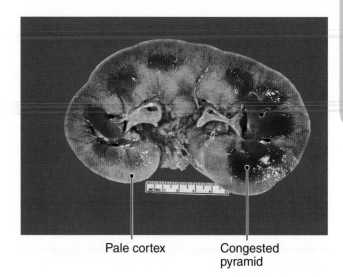

Pale cortex   Congested pyramid

Figure 19-16 Acute tubular necrosis. The paleness of the renal cortex is caused by necrotic tubular epithelium. The pyramids are congested.

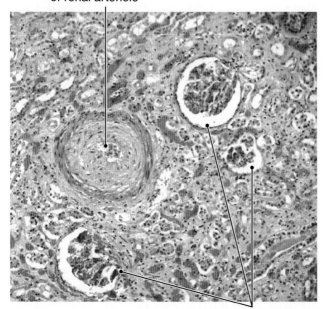

"Onionskin" hyperplasia of renal arteriole

Shrinking glomeruli

Figure 19-15 Malignant nephrosclerosis. The hallmark lesion is onionskin hyperplasia of the renal arteriole.

falls. **Acute tubular necrosis** is extensive necrosis of tubular epithelial cells and is the most common cause of *acute* renal failure. *Ischemic* acute tubular necrosis is usually a consequence of vascular collapse (shock, Chapter 5), which is commonly caused by severe hemorrhage. *Nephrotoxic* acute tubular necrosis is caused by a variety of chemicals that include antibiotics, mercury, and other heavy metals, and by intravenous use of diagnostic x-ray contrast media. As is illustrated in Figure 19-16, the renal cortex is pale, and microscopic study shows necrotic tubules; glomeruli, however, are spared. Unless the basement membrane latticework is destroyed, tubular epithelium regrows quickly, usually within a few weeks. Recovery is usually complete if the underlying clinical condition is corrected quickly.

Patients who survive acute tubular necrosis progress through three distinct clinical phases. The first 24–48 hours (the *initiating phase*) is dominated by the main clinical event, such as hemorrhage or poisoning. Urine output falls dramatically. The *maintenance phase* begins usually within the first few days as patients are given supportive care and dialysis if necessary to tide them over until the tubular epithelium regrows. The *recovery phase* begins with increasing renal output that often rises to a flood of dilute urine, far surpassing normal, as tubular epithelium regrows but has not regained its full ability to resorb most of the huge volume of normal glomerular filtrate. However, urine output falls to normal as epithelium regrows and regains its ability to process glomerular filtrate

Tubulointerstitial Nephritis

One of the major determinants of renal disease is the rule that disease of one element usually affects others. A manifestation of this rule is that sooner or later almost every type of renal disease produces chronic interstitial inflammation and fibrosis among the renal tubules, a pathologic change called **tubulointerstitial nephritis** (Fig. 19-17). Among the most common causes are chronic urinary obstruction, urinary reflux, chronic bacterial infection, adverse reaction to chronic ingestion of certain therapeutic drugs, or reaction to renal toxins. *Renal ablation glomerulopathy*, discussed above, is one of the more common causes of tubulointerstitial nephritis.

OBSTRUCTION, REFLUX, AND STASIS

Just as a healthy nephron unit requires normal flow of blood through the glomerulus and normal flow of glomerular filtrate through the tubule, a healthy urinary system requires normal flow of urine. Normal urine flow depends on an unobstructed collecting system, waves of peristalsis in the ureters to massage urine downward, and on normal function of the ureterovesical junction, which prevents urine in the bladder from regurgitating up the ureters.

Normal urine flow can be impaired by:

* Urinary obstruction
* Ineffective ureteral peristalsis
* Reflux of urine from the bladder into the ureter

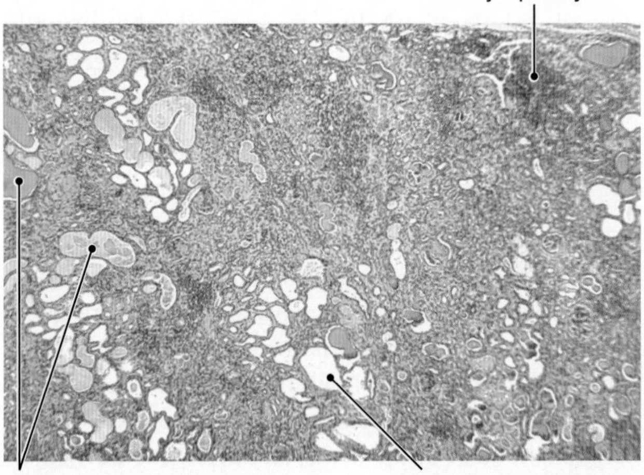

Figure 19-17 **Chronic tubulointerstitial nephritis.** The interstitium is filled with chronic inflammatory cells (lymphocytes). Tubules are dilated and filled with protein casts; tubular epithelium is atrophic. Reprinted with permission from Rubin E. Pathology. 4th ed. Philadelphia. Lippincott Williams and Wilkins, 2005.

Urinary obstruction may occur at any point from the kidney to the urethra, and it may develop suddenly or slowly, be partial or complete, and unilateral or bilateral. Tumors, scars, or urinary stones can obstruct flow at any point from the kidney to the urethra; and nodular hyperplasia of the prostate or urethritis caused by sexually transmitted disease can obstruct flow below the bladder. Normal ureteral peristalsis can be impaired by pregnancy, in which the hormonal environment causes smooth muscle relaxation and dilation of the ureters, or by any condition that impairs neurogenic control of the ureters; spinal cord injury is an example. **Urinary reflux** (regurgitation) from the bladder through the ureterovesical junction also prevents smooth, continuous flow of urine.

Obstruction, ineffective peristalsis, and reflux can cause urinary stasis (stagnation) and renal damage (**reflux nephropathy** or **obstructive nephropathy**) secondary to increased urine pressure in the renal pelvis. As is illustrated in Figure 19-18, *stagnant, high-pressure urine invites infection and damages the kidney directly.*

Figures 19-19 and 19-20 illustrate **hydronephrosis**, a dilation of the renal pelvis and calyces caused by the increased urinary pressure associated with physical obstruction or reflux. Chronic obstruction promotes stagnation, stone formation, and infection and is accompanied by *tubulointerstitial nephritis* and renal atrophy. Most hydronephrosis is associated with undiagnosed chronic *unilateral* physical obstruction in the ureter or renal pelvis. *Bilateral* obstruction above the bladder is rare, and obstruction at the neck of the bladder or below—for example, obstruction caused by urethral stricture or prostatic hyperplasia—usually produces a painfully full bladder that prompts quick attention. If obstruction is diagnosed and relieved promptly, full renal function usually returns. Bilateral hydronephrosis can occur as a congenital condition; it is caused by defective ureterovesical valves (Fig. 19-21).

PYELONEPHRITIS AND URINARY

> ☞ *Normal urinary tract health depends on smooth, brisk, unobstructed flow of urine.*

TRACT INFECTION

Infections are an important cause of urinary tract disease because they are common and tend to recur. Women are more often infected than men are. In women, the urethra is short and open to bacteria that populate the labia and vaginal mucosa, and vaginal delivery may alter pelvic anatomy to cause urinary incontinence or other problems that require surgery or instrumentation, both

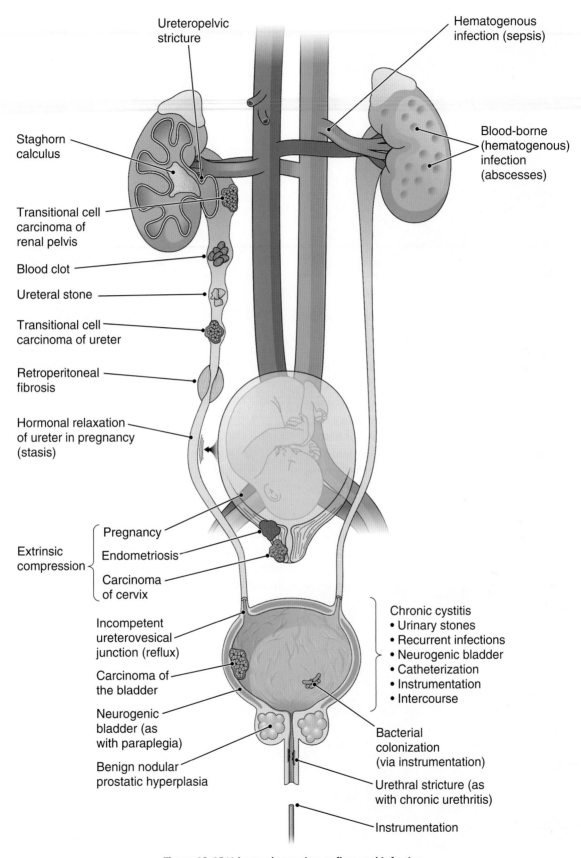

Figure 19-18 **Urinary obstruction, reflux, and infection.**

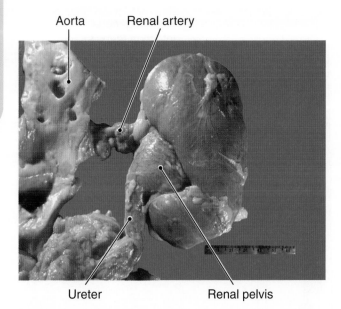

Figure 19-19 **Hydronephrosis.** The renal pelvis and ureter are markedly dilated because there is obstruction lower in the urinary tract.

of which may introduce infection. Bacteria usually infect the kidney by ascending from the urethra into the bladder and up the ureters into the kidneys. Infection is often acquired during sexual intercourse, urinary tract surgery, bladder catheterization, or insertion of instruments into the bladder; however, in many patients the cause of infection is not clear. Urinary tract infections tend to recur, especially those associated with diabetes, urinary stones, or urinary reflux or obstruction.

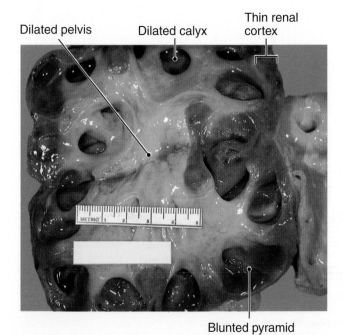

Figure 19-20 **Hydronephrosis.** The pelvis and calyces are markedly dilated and the cortex is very thin, reflecting loss of functional tissue.

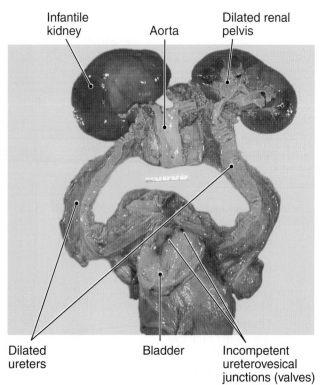

Figure 19-21 **Congenital incompetent ureterovesical junctions.** Urinary reflux has produced dilated renal pelvises and ureters.

Pyelonephritis is bacterial infection of the kidney and is one of the most important diseases of the kidney. Gram-negative fecal bacteria are the usual culprits; *Escherichia coli* accounts for 80% of cases. Most infections occur in women and ascend to the kidney from an infected bladder. **Acute pyelonephritis** is associated with clinical signs and symptoms of acute infection. The clinical presentation of **chronic pyelonephritis** is usually associated with chronic urinary reflux or obstruction. The clinical presentation of chronic pyelonephritis is variable: it may be 1) silent and present for many years, ultimately presenting as chronic renal failure, or 2) it may be symptomatic: flare-ups of acute pyelonephritis interspersed with relatively quiet intervals.

Acute Pyelonephritis

Acute pyelonephritis is almost always secondary to lower urinary tract infection, but it can occur if the kidneys are seeded with blood-borne bacteria (sepsis). Obstruction and reflux are less common causes of infection in acute pyelonephritis than in chronic pyelonephritis. Microscopically, an acute (neutrophilic) inflammatory exudate spreads throughout the kidney. Figure 19-22 illustrates a severe case with multiple small abscesses.

Uncomplicated acute pyelonephritis presents as sudden onset of flank pain associated with fever, high peripheral white blood cell count, and other signs and symptoms of acute infection. The urine is usually packed with white blood cells (pyuria), and bacteria usually can be cultured and seen on microscopic examination of urine sediment. Bladder infection and inflammation (cystitis) are usually associated with frequency and urgency and with painful urination (dysuria). Antibiotic therapy usually is effective, but overwhelming bloodstream infection (sepsis) and renal failure can occur in debilitated patients or in neglected cases.

Chronic Pyelonephritis

Chronic pyelonephritis is chronic bacterial infection of the kidney. It is usually associated with chronic urinary reflux or obstruction and frequently appears clinically as recurrent episodes of acute pyelonephritis with fever, flank pain, dysuria, and pyuria; however, some patients with low-grade infection and reflux or obstruction may be asymptomatic, especially early in the course of disease. Because infection is closely related to obstruction or reflux, it is difficult to separate the pathologic effects of infection from those originating from obstruction or reflux. Whether or not associated with obstruction or reflux, pyelonephritis scars and shrinks the kidney, dilates the collecting system (the pelvis and calyces), and thins the cortex. Microscopic study reveals chronic inflammation and fibrosis throughout (tubulointerstitial nephritis).

Chronic pyelonephritis (with or without reflux or obstruction) is a serious problem that accounts for about 10% of patients on renal dialysis. Most patients are not diagnosed until late in the course of their disease, because chronic pyelonephritis is often asymptomatic and the kidneys have a large functional reserve; that is, most renal capacity must be destroyed before clinical signs or symptoms occur. Autopsy studies show that some patients have convincing anatomic evidence of chronic renal infection but no history of urinary tract infections. However, many of them have evidence of some degree of obstruction or reflux. Interestingly, the presence or absence of bacteria in the urine is not helpful in making the diagnosis of chronic pyelonephritis. Indeed, in clinical practice most patients with bacteria in the urine have infection of the lower urinary tract, not of the kidney.

DRUGS, TOXINS, AND OTHER CAUSES OF TUBULOINTERSTITIAL NEPHRITIS

Acute interstitial nephritis is usually caused by adverse reaction to a therapeutic drug, a type IV immune reaction (T-cell, delayed hypersensitivity, Chapter 8) that begins about two weeks after drug exposure. Antibiotics, nonsteroidal antiinflammatory drugs, and diuretics are the most common offenders. The clinical syndrome includes fever, skin rash, and peripheral blood eosinophilia associated with hematuria, proteinuria, and leukocytes in the urine. About one quarter of patients have a skin rash, and acute renal failure occurs in about half.

Chronic analgesic nephropathy is one of the most common causes of chronic tubulointerstitial nephritis and renal insufficiency in parts of Australia and Western Europe but is rare in the United States. Typically, the patient is an older woman who has ingested for more than three years large daily doses of analgesics that contain some combination of aspirin, caffeine, acetaminophen, codeine, or nonsteroidal antiinflammatory drugs. It can progress to hypertension and chronic renal failure.

Tubulointerstitial nephritis can also be caused by deposits of substances that damage the kidney, including: protein deposits in patients with proteinuria associated with multiple myeloma or related disorders of plasma cells (Chapter 11), deposits of uric acid crystals in gout (Chapter 22), and renal calcium deposits associated with high blood levels of calcium.

Renal Stones

Stones (**calculi, nephrolithiasis**) can form anywhere in the urinary tract, but most form in the kidney. They may be numerous and as small as grains of sand, or they may grow large enough to completely fill the renal

Abscesses

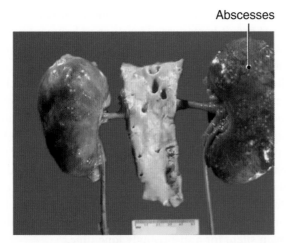

Figure 19-22 **Acute pyelonephritis.** Multiple small abscesses are present. The ureters are normal.

pelvis. Stones are fairly common, affecting about 5% of the population. Most occur in young adults in their twenties or thirties; and men are affected more often than women are. Hereditary predisposition is a strong factor, and patients with some genetic metabolic diseases—gout or aminoaciduria, for example—excrete in urine very large amounts of metabolic products that may crystallize into stones.

Three categories of stones are recognized:

- *Calcium stones* (Fig. 19-23): About 75% of stones are composed mainly of calcium. Typically these stones are hard and dark because blood has accumulated in tiny crevasses of the stone surface, where sharp edges of the stone have gouged urinary epithelium. Most patients have increased levels of *urinary* calcium, but *blood* calcium levels are usually normal. Other patients—such as those with hyperparathyroidism—have increased levels of urine calcium secondary to high blood calcium levels. Whatever the cause, urine becomes supersaturated with calcium, which precipitates and slowly accumulates to form a stone.
- *Infection stones*: Bacterial infection changes urine pH from acidic to alkaline, which causes the formation of stones that are mainly composed of magnesium. About 15% of stones are magnesium stones, which are softer and more breakable (friable) than calcium stones are. Stones and infection are especially problematic because the combination encourages a vi-

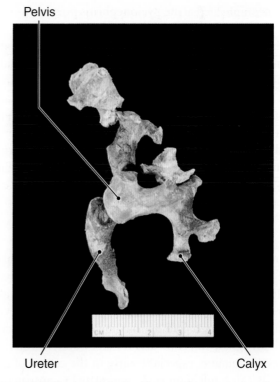

Pelvis

Ureter   Calyx

Figure 19-24 **Staghorn calculus.** The stone forms a nearly perfect image of upper ureter, renal pelvis, and calyces.

cious circle of obstruction and stasis, stone formation, and further obstruction and stasis.

- *Uric acid stones*: About 5% of stones are composed mainly of uric acid. About 25% of patients with gout (Chapter 22) develop uric acid stones; however, most patients with uric acid stones do not have gout or high levels of blood uric acid.

Often the first symptom of a renal stone is hematuria. In other cases, stones are asymptomatic; many are found incidentally by x-ray or routine urinalysis that detects occult hematuria. As a stone or fragment passes down the ureter, it causes a distinctive and very painful syndrome of cramping and flank pain known as **renal colic.** Women who have passed stones and birthed children compare the pain equally. A man who has renal colic invariably says it is painful beyond description; among mothers, he can expect sympathy only from his own. A renal stone too large to pass will remain in the renal pelvis, where it may grow very large and mold itself into the shape of the calyces—called a **staghorn calculus** (Fig. 19-24), which is always associated with hydronephrosis and chronic infection. Large stones may remain silent for a surprisingly long time.

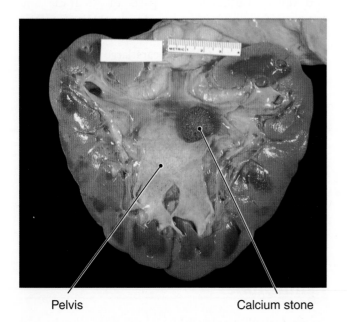

Pelvis   Calcium stone

Figure 19-23 **Nephrolithiasis: calcium stone in the renal pelvis.** Dark brown coloration of the stone is a result of the stone's having absorbed blood altered by urine.

Tumors of the Kidney

As is depicted in Figure 19-25, tumors may occur at any point in the urinary tract. Pediatric renal tumors are discussed in Chapter 7. Most tumors of the kidney are malignant, a sharp contrast to most other organ systems. Most occur in mature or older adults; men are affected more often than women are. Benign renal tumors are rare.

Renal cell carcinoma (*clear cell carcinoma, hypernephroma, renal adenocarcinoma*) is a malignancy of renal tubular epithelium and accounts for 90% of renal malignancies. Most occur in older adults; cigarette smokers have twice the risk of nonsmokers—about one third of renal cell carcinomas are linked to tobacco use. Some renal cell carcinomas are silent for a long time and grow quite large (up to 15 cm) by the time of diagnosis.

Usually hematuria is the presenting symptom, but some tumors may be large enough to find by palpating the flank of a patient presenting with flank pain.

Renal cell carcinomas display an astonishing variety of paraneoplastic syndromes (Chapter 6)—including fever of unknown origin, polycythemia, hypertension, Cushing syndrome, hypercalcemia, and feminization of males or virilization of females. As is illustrated in Figure 19-26, renal cell carcinoma is especially prone to invade renal veins, sometimes extending far into the inferior vena cava. Metastases to lung and bone are common and may be the first sign of the presence of a renal cell carcinoma. Five-year survival is about 75% in patients without metastasis, about 50% in those with metastasis, and about 15% in those with renal vein invasion. Surgical excision of the kidney (nephrectomy) is the preferred treatment.

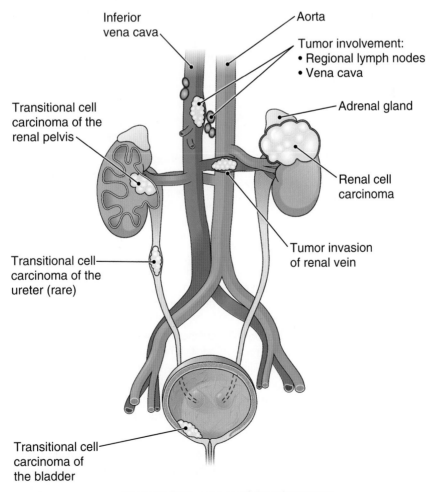

Figure 19-25 **Neoplasms of the urinary tract.**

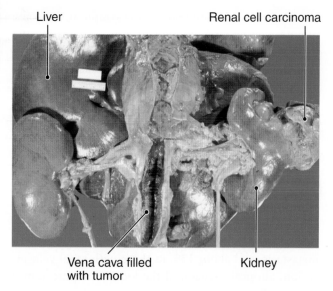

Liver / Renal cell carcinoma

Vena cava filled with tumor / Kidney

Figure 19-26 **Renal cell carcinoma.** Renal vein and vena cava are filled with invasive tumor.

Carcinomas of the renal pelvis account for about 10% of renal malignancies. They arise from the lining epithelial cells of the urinary tract (urothelial cells), which are commonly called transitional cells. Neoplasms of these cells are called **transitional cell carcinomas**. Transitional cell carcinomas tend to occur at multiple points in the urinary tract—about half of transitional cell carcinomas of the renal pelvis are accompanied by a concurrent transitional cell carcinoma of the bladder or history of one. Transitional cell carcinomas of the renal pelvis are usually papillary and friable; they fragment and bleed early—hematuria is often the presenting symptom. Despite their small size they tend to be invasive; only about two thirds of patients survive 5 years. Nephrectomy is the treatment of choice. ■

CASE STUDY 19-1 *"HIS WATER LOOKS LIKE COCA-COLA"*

TOPICS
Streptococcal pharyngitis
Acute glomerulonephritis

THE CASE

Setting: You are spending a week of spring vacation as a substitute for the sole health care professional in a rural health clinic that operates out of the rear of a general store near the entrance to Big Bend National Park in far west Texas. The nearest hospital is 80 miles away.

Clinical history: Your Tuesday morning hike into the nearby hills is interrupted by a call on the community radio net from the clerk at the general store, who watches for patients when the clinic is closed or when personnel are out of the clinic.

You jog back to the clinic to find waiting on the front porch of the store a mother and her child, a boy who looks to be about 10 years old. When you ask "What's the trouble?" she says, describing his urine, "His water looks like Coca-Cola." She goes on to say that in retrospect she thought it might have been discolored the night before, but the light was poor and she couldn't be sure. This morning the boy called her to see the toilet water, which was discolored. She gave him juice and water and waited to observe for herself on his next bathroom trip about 2 hours later.

You locate his chart and scan it quickly, finding nothing notable except unremarkable checkups and immunizations.

You ask the usual questions about recent illnesses and do a review of systems. You explore the possibility of drug use and toxin exposure but find nothing suspicious. The boy's past medical history is unremarkable except for "a cold and sore throat" a few weeks earlier.

Physical examination and other data: Temperature 98.5° F, heart rate 88, respirations 16, blood pressure 145/92. The boy is quiet and not in distress and appears to be of average height and weight. He does not appear anemic or jaundiced, but his face is puffy. When you ask about his face, his mother says she noted it a few days earlier but didn't pay it much attention. She says, "It's spring; it looked like allergies to me." The remainder of the physical examination is unremarkable. He has no rash, enlarged lymph nodes, or abdominal masses.

You collect blood for a complete blood count and chemistries for the office assistant to do the next day. A fingerstick hematocrit is normal at 48%. You give the boy a large glass of water and in an hour he passes a small amount of very dark urine, which is strongly positive for protein and hemoglobin by routine dipstick tests. You centrifuge the urine and study the sediment, and find numerous red blood cells.

Clinical course: You are puzzled—the pieces don't seem to fit together—and focus most of your thoughts on the ▶

[Case 19-1, continued] possibility of drug use or toxin exposure. You phone the hospital that manages the clinic and speak to the physician on call, a well-regarded family practitioner. Together the two of you agree the kidneys are involved but you can't find a diagnosis that explains everything. The family practitioner says he will call a pediatrician colleague and ask her to call you.

In about half an hour, the pediatrician calls and you repeat the clinical history and findings to her. She is quick to say, "This is a classic case of acute glomerulonephritis; I haven't seen one in several years." She outlines a treatment plan of salt restriction and drug therapy with diuretics and antihypertensive medication with careful monitoring of urine output. You dispense the drugs from the limited supply on hand and give the mother a calibrated, disposable urine cup, instructing her to measure his urine output and call you daily. Mother and son return the following Saturday, your last day. His urine shows less hemoglobin and protein than initially, and most of his facial swelling has disappeared. His blood pressure is normal.

DISCUSSION

This child presented a classic case of acute nephritic syndrome secondary to infection. The history of a "cold and sore throat" earlier was significant—although proof is lacking that his earlier sore throat was caused by beta-streptococcus, there was no other reasonable conclusion. If he had also had sniffles at the time, it could have been seasonal "hay fever."

Key to the diagnosis is hypertension, hematuria, and proteinuria, each of which is a striking abnormality in an otherwise previously healthy child. Dark urine, caused by altered blood, is a sign of bleeding high in the urinary tract. Bleeding from lower sites, such as the bladder, usually produces red hematuria. The only other cause of dark urine that might have been considered would have been hemoglobinuria from hemolytic anemia. However, the boy's hematocrit was normal and he was not jaundiced (the liver metabolizes free hemoglobin into bilirubin).

The final clue was the hypertension. Glomerulonephritis restricts renal blood flow and invokes the renin-angiotensin-aldosterone cascade, which increases blood pressure. Pediatric hypertension is rare and most cases are caused by some form of renal disease.

After returning home you learned from a follow-up call that the boy's health had returned to normal and that the blood antistreptolysin O (ASO) titer—sent to a distant laboratory—was reported as increased, confirming the suspicion of strep throat as the culprit.

POINTS TO REMEMBER
• When in doubt about diagnosis or treatment, get help.

Objectives Recap

1. *List the functions of the kidney*: 1) Eliminate waste; 2) regulate plasma osmolality; 3) regulate blood acid base balance; and 4) stimulate red blood cell production.

2. *Explain the difference between glomerular filtrate and urine*: The glomerular filtrate is the large volume of unprocessed fluid that crosses from blood into the urinary space of the glomerulus. Renal tubules absorb 99% of water in the glomerular filtrate, adding and subtracting electrolytes, acid, and other substances. The remainder is urine.

3. *Distinguish between renal diseases and syndromes of renal disease, and give an example*: Disease is a pathologic process such as autoimmune reaction, infarction, inflammation, or edema; by contrast a syndrome is a clinical picture, a collection of clinical signs and symptoms. For example, poststreptococcal glomerulonephritis is an autoimmune glomerular disease that usually presents clinically as the clinical syndrome of acute nephritis.

4. *Explain the difference between azotemia and uremia, and describe what is meant by occult hematuria*: Azotemia is renal failure that is evident only by abnormal laboratory tests. Uremia is a renal failure with clinical symptoms. Occult hematuria is intact red blood cells in the urine in amounts too small to be noticed by gross examination only.

5. *Explain the difference between nephritic syndrome and nephrotic syndrome*: Nephrotic syndrome is marked proteinuria (>3.5 grams/day), hypoalbuminemia, severe generalized edema, hyperlipemia, and lipiduria. Nephritic syndrome is an acute syndrome of hematuria, proteinuria, and hypertension that is associated with acute glomerulonephritis.

6. *Name the pathogenic mechanism responsible for most primary glomerular disease*: Autoimmunity.

7. *Name the most common type of glomerulonephritis*: IgA glomerulonephritis (Berger disease).

8. *Name the most common cause of renal failure in the United States:* Diabetic glomerulosclerosis.

9. *Give the name of the vascular disease of the kidney that is found in virtually all elderly people*: Benign nephrosclerosis.

10. *Explain why patients with acute tubular necrosis (ATN) have a period of very high urine output*: ATN is a syndrome of death of renal tubular epithelial cells. Lack of renal tubular epithelial cells means the tubules cannot absorb the normally very large volume of glomerular filtrate, which is then able to pass through the tubules with little alteration and into the collecting system as urine.

11. *Name several causes of tubulointerstitial nephritis*: Renal ablation nephropathy, acute and chronic pyelonephritis, urinary obstruction or reflux, toxin damage, and chronic analgesic nephropathy.

12. *Explain the consequences of urinary obstruction and reflux*: Obstruction and reflux encourage infection and stone formation and contribute directly to hydronephrosis and tubulointerstitial nephritis.

13. *Name the type of microorganisms that cause most acute pyelonephritis*: Most acute pyelonephritis is caused by ascending infection by *Escherichia coli* and other fecal bacteria that ascend to the kidney from the bladder.

14. *List some important facts about chronic pyelonephritis*: 1) The presence or absence of bacteria in urine is not helpful in making the diagnosis; 2) it is often associated with obstruction or reflux; 3) it may be asymptomatic for a long time; 4) it may be characterized by repeated episodes of fever and other evidence of urinary infection; 5) it is responsible for about 10% of patients on chronic dialysis; 6) it is one of the main causes of chronic tubulointerstitial nephritis.

15. *Name the most common type of urinary stone, and discuss some diseases or conditions associated with it*: Most urinary stones are calcium stones and occur in people with high urinary calcium. Another group of patients are those with high blood levels of calcium (hypercalcemia); for example, those with hyperparathyroidism. Urinary stones often present with urinary bleeding (hematuria) or flank pain (renal colic). Stones predispose to obstruction and infection and chronic tubulointerstitial nephritis.

16. *Name the two most important malignancies of the kidney*: Renal cell carcinoma; transitional cell carcinoma of the renal pelvis.

Typical Test Questions

1. The barrier function of the glomerulus prevents which one of the following from entering the glomerular filtrate?
   A. Glucose
   B. Protein
   C. Amino acids
   D. Creatinine

2. Azotemia is best described as
   A. Glomerulonephritis
   B. Lab findings
   C. Proteinuria
   D. Urinary obstruction

3. Poststreptococcal glomerulonephritis usually presents as
   A. Acute nephritic syndrome
   B. Uremia
   C. Azotemia
   D. Hypocalcemia

4. Which of the following is a cause of renovascular hypertension?
   A. Atherosclerosis
   B. Acute tubular necrosis
   C. Reflux nephropathy
   D. Vasculitis

5. Which of the following is most closely associated with chronic pyelonephritis?
   A. Chronic glomerulonephritis
   B. Urinary reflux or obstruction
   C. Smoking
   D. Uric acid stones

6. True or false? The innermost layer of the glomerulus is vascular endothelium.

7. True or false? Uremia is a syndrome of laboratory results only.

8. True or false? Acute glomerulonephritis is an autoimmune disease.

9. True or false? Urinary obstruction can cause renal damage without infection.

10. True or false? Transitional cell carcinomas are tumors of renal tubular epithelium.

Diseases of the Lower Urinary Tract and Male Genitalia

This chapter begins with a review of the normal lower urinary tract and male genitalia. Diseases and disorders discussed include cystitis, urethritis, epididymitis, and other inflammations; erectile dysfunction and infertility; sexually transmitted diseases; prostate enlargement; and cancers.

BACK TO BASICS

DISEASES OF THE LOWER URINARY TRACT
- Congenital Anomalies
- Urinary Obstruction, Reflux, and Stasis
- Infection and Inflammation
- Neoplasms

DISEASES OF THE MALE GENITALIA
- Erectile Dysfunction and Infertility
- Diseases of the Penis and Urethra

- Diseases of the Scrotum and Groin
- Diseases of the Testis and Epididymis
- Diseases of the Prostate

SEXUALLY TRANSMITTED DISEASE
- Syphilis
- Gonorrhea
- Nongonococcal Urethritis
- Genital Herpes and Other Sexually Transmitted Diseases

Learning Objectives

After studying this chapter you should be able to:

1. Name the component parts of the lower urinary system and the male genital system
2. Explain the importance of the ureterovesical junction in the flow of urine in the lower urinary tract, and know the consequences of malfunction
3. Explain why women have more cystitis than men do
4. Discuss the pathologic and clinical differences between low-grade and high-grade transitional cell carcinoma of the bladder
5. Briefly explain the cause of most erectile dysfunction
6. Discuss the importance of undescended testis
7. Name the two most common malignant tumors of the testis, and briefly discuss the average 5-year survival figure for patients with malignant tumors of the testis
8. Name the most common type of prostatitis and its cause
9. Describe the anatomy of the bladder and prostate critical to the pathologic effect of nodular hyperplasia of the prostate
10. Discuss the location of most prostate cancers, and describe why the location is important
11. Describe the Gleason scoring system for histologic grading of prostate cancer
12. Discuss the role of blood prostate specific antigen (PSA) in the diagnosis and management of prostate cancer.
13. Discuss why syphilis is difficult to diagnose
14. Name some lesions of tertiary syphilis
15. Name the most common cause of nongonococcal urethritis
16. Explain the role of sexually transmitted disease (STD) in the spread of AIDS in Africa and Asia
17. Describe the clinical appearance of genital herpes

Key Terms and Concepts

BACK TO BASICS
- ureterovesical junction

DISEASES OF THE LOWER URINARY TRACT
- ureterovesical valve incompetence
- cystitis
- urethritis
- transitional cell carcinoma

DISEASES OF THE MALE GENITALIA
- erectile dysfunction
- infertility
- undescended testis
- inguinal hernia
- epididymitis
- seminoma
- embryonal carcinoma
- prostatitis

- nodular hyperplasia
- prostatic adenocarcinoma
- Gleason score
- prostate specific antigen

SEXUALLY TRANSMITTED DISEASE
- sexually transmitted disease
- primary syphilis
- chancre
- darkfield microscopy
- secondary syphilis
- condyloma lata
- tertiary syphilis
- gonorrhea
- non-gonococcal urethritis
- genital herpes

Male, n. A member of the unconsidered, or negligible sex. The male of the human race is commonly known (to the female) as Mere Man. The genus has two varieties: good providers and bad providers.

AMBROSE BIERCE (1842–1914?), AMERICAN SATIRIST, JOURNALIST, AND SHORT-STORY WRITER, THE DEVIL'S DICTIONARY

BACK TO BASICS

The *upper urinary tract* consists of the kidney and renal pelvis; the **lower urinary tract** (Fig. 20-1) consists of the ureters, bladder, and urethra. The renal pelves, ureters, and bladder are commonly called the **collecting system**. The walls of the collecting system are composed of layers of smooth muscle and are lined internally by cells, commonly called *transitional cells*. The ureters descend behind the peritoneal cavity (the *retroperitoneum*) on either side of the spine and enter the bladder at a shallow angle to form the **ureterovesical junction**, which acts as a one-way valve to prevent backflow of urine from the bladder into the ureter.

Urine expelled from the bladder by urination (**micturition**) is unchanged from its formation in the kidney. Gravity and ureteral peristaltic contractions (controlled by the autonomic nervous system, Chapter 23) move urine down the ureter into the bladder. Urine is held in the bladder by two sphincters that surround the urethra where it joins the neck of the bladder. The internal sphincter is composed of smooth muscle and is involuntary and controlled by the autonomic nervous system. The external sphincter circles the urethra immediately below the internal sphincter and is composed of skeletal muscle that is under voluntary control. As urine accumulates, the bladder wall stretches and sends signals to the micturition center the lower spinal cord, which activates reflex contractions of the bladder wall and relaxation of the internal, involuntary sphincter. At the same time the stretched bladder sends an "I'm full" signal to the brain, which brings an increasing sense of urinary urgency.

As is illustrated in Figure 20-2, the **male genital system** consists of the testes, epididymis, vas deferens, prostate, seminal vesicles, and the penis. The main function of the male genital system is reproduction.

The **penis** consists of two main parts: the *shaft* and the *glans* (head). The shaft is covered by skin, which folds over the head to form a retractable collar, the **prepuce** (foreskin). The penis contains compartments of spongy vascular (*erectile*) tissue—the *corpus cavernosum* and the *corpus spongiosum*—that become gorged with blood during an erection. An **erection** is the ability to obtain and maintain an enlarged, stiff penis satisfactory for sexual intercourse. During an erection arterial smooth muscles relax and blood flows rapidly into the penis; venous smooth muscles contract and outflow is partially obstructed; and erectile tissue becomes engorged and tense with blood.

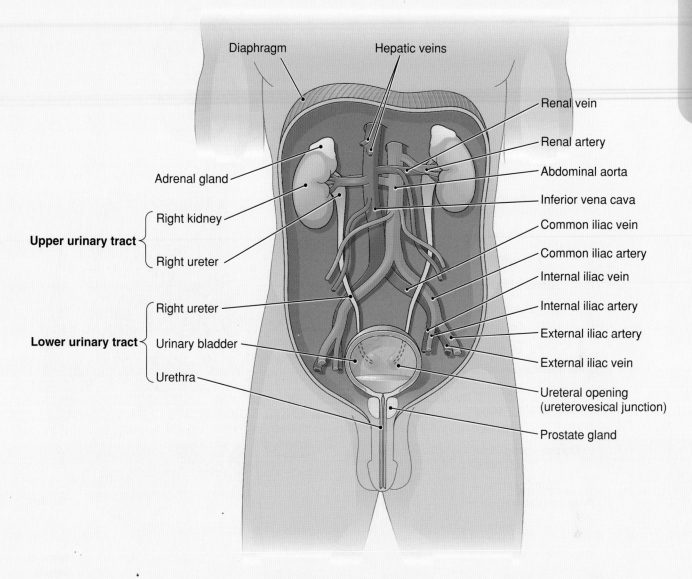

Figure 20-1 **The urinary system.**

In uncircumcised males the glans is covered by moist squamous mucosa, which is protected by the prepuce. *Circumcision*, a common social practice for thousands of years, is removal of the prepuce. In circumcised males the squamous mucosa is unprotected and becomes the anatomic and functional equivalent of the skin covering the shaft of the penis.

The **testis** consists of two compartments: 1) *seminiferous tubules* (90% of testicular mass), where sperm are produced; and 2) *interstitial tissue* that fills the space between the tubules and produces **testosterone**, the primary male hormone responsible for the development and maintenance of male secondary sex characteristics. The **seminiferous tubules** are lined by reproductive cells (germ cells, **spermatocytes**), which divide to form sperm, and specialized partner cells, *Sertoli cells*. **Sertoli cells** regulate and sustain sperm production. Figure 20-

2 also illustrates details of testicular anatomy. On the back side of the testis the seminiferous tubules empty into the **epididymis**, a very long coiled tube that forms an elongated, spongy mass that connects the testis to the *vas deferens*. As sperm migrate through the epididymis they mature and are stored for later ejaculation. The **vas deferens** is a narrow, stiff, heavily muscled tube that travels upward over the pelvic brim and then downward to deliver sperm to the urethra. The vas deferens with its blood vessels, nerves, and supporting tissue is known as the **spermatic cord**.

The vas deferens travels upward from the scrotum, over the bony rim of the pubic bone, and descends into the pelvis, where it merges with the duct from the seminal vesicle shortly before emptying into the urethra. The **seminal vesicles**, glands that lie beside the prostate and bladder, are each about the size of half of a man's

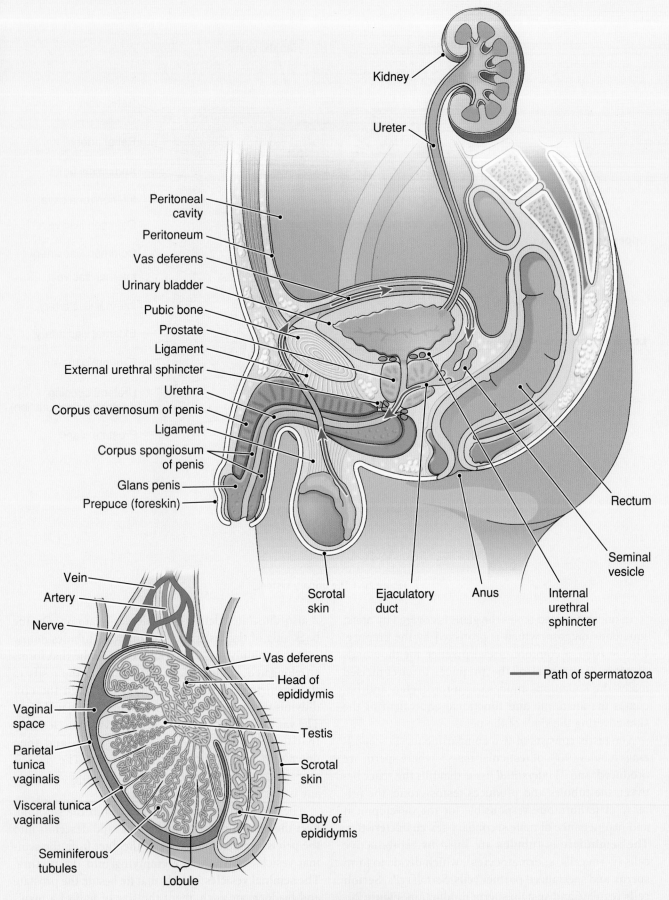

Figure 20-2 **The male genital system.**

little finger and excrete a nutrient fluid into semen. **Semen** is formed of sperm from the testis and nutrient fluids from the seminal vesicles and prostate. In orgasm semen is ejaculated from the penis by muscular contractions of the epididymis, vas deferens, seminal vesicles, and prostate.

The **scrotum** is a sac of skin that holds the testis, epididymis, and proximal vas deferens. The scrotum hangs outside the body in order to keep testicular temperature about 5° F below the temperature of the rest of the body, because sperm will not be produced if testicular temperature is too high (recall from Chapter 7 that failure of the testis to descend into the scrotum from the abdomen is associated with testicular atrophy). Much like the heart lies in the pericardial sac, the testis is contained in a smooth serosal sac, the *tunica vaginalis*, which contains a small amount of lubricant fluid that allows free movement of the testicle in the scrotal sac.

The **testes** produce *spermatozoa* and *testosterone*. As is illustrated in Figure 20-3, sperm are formed from

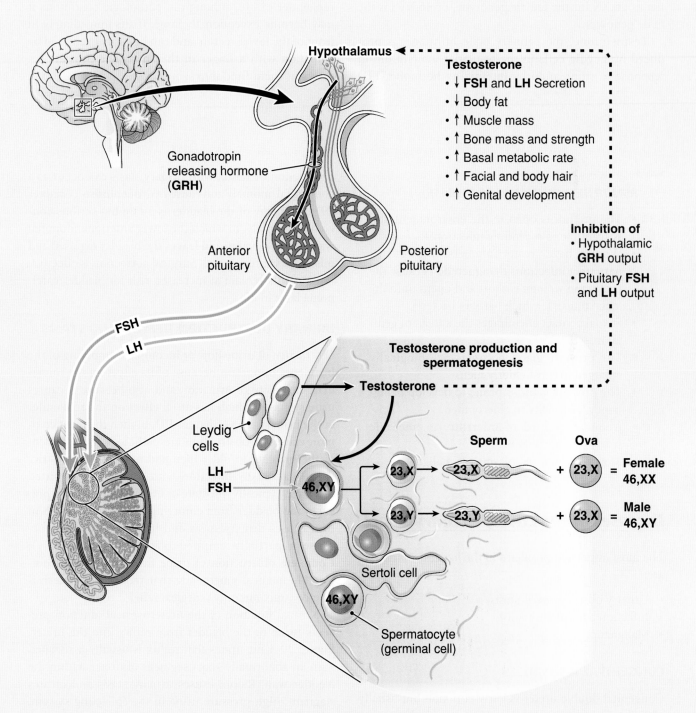

Figure 20-3 **Normal spermatogenesis.**

spermatocytes (germ cells) by meiosis (reduction division), a process discussed in detail in Chapter 7, which halves the number of chromosomes from 46 to 23: each **sperm** (spermatozoan) carries 22 somatic chromosomes plus one sex chromosome, either X or Y, for which the shorthand is 23,X or 23,Y. In like manner each ovum contains 22 somatic chromosomes and an X chromosome. When joined together the combination produces a normal complement of 44 somatic chromosomes plus two sex chromosomes (written as 46,XX for the female genotype, or 46,XY for the male genotype).

Testosterone, the primary male hormone, is produced by **Leydig cells** in the testicular interstitium in response to stimulation by **luteinizing hormone (LH)** from the anterior pituitary. The adrenal cortex also produces some testosterone (Chapter 18). In conjunction with **follicle stimulating-hormone (FSH)** from the anterior pituitary, testosterone stimulates testicular germ cells to mature into sperm and accounts for features such as facial hair, deep voice, increased muscle mass, and other masculine features detailed in Figure 20-3.

The **prostate** gland encircles the urethra at the neck of the bladder. In normal young men it is about the size of a golf ball, and it normally doubles in size during the remainder of life, although in pathologic conditions it may become exceptionally large. It sits immediately in front of the lower rectum and can be easily examined by palpation with a finger in the anus. The prostate secretes nutrient fluid into semen.

MAJOR DETERMINANTS OF DISEASE

- The urethra is open to the environment and susceptible to ascending infection.
- Women have greater numbers of lower urinary tract infections than men do because the urethra in women is short and opens onto the labial mucosa, which harbors bacteria.
- Sexual contact encourages the spread of genital infections.
- The prostate gland becomes pathologically enlarged in most elderly men.
- The prostate gland is prone to develop malignancy, especially in elderly men.
- About one third of infertility is traceable solely to male factors.
- Most testicular neoplasms are malignant.

Diseases of the Lower Urinary Tract

The most important problems in the lower urinary tract are:

- Urinary obstruction or stasis
- Infection and inflammation
- Malignancy

CONGENITAL ANOMALIES

Congenital double ureter is fairly common but usually of little clinical consequence. Ureterovesical junction obstruction or reflux with urinary stasis can occur as a congenital anomaly and cause hydronephrosis (Chapter 19). *Exstrophy* of the bladder is a rare but serious congenital anomaly, in which the lower anterior abdominal wall fails to develop and leaves the bladder exposed and missing its anterior wall. Surgical correction is effective, but patients remain at increased risk for bladder carcinoma later in life.

URINARY OBSTRUCTION, REFLUX, AND STASIS

Obstruction of urine flow or incomplete emptying of the bladder is important because of its effect on the immediate necessity of urination and also because it causes urinary stasis, which has an ill effect on the remainder of the urinary tract (Chapter 19). In men the most common causes of obstruction are pathologic enlargement of the prostate in older men and urethral scars (strictures) caused by infection with sexually transmitted diseases. Typically, prostate or urethral obstruction prevents the bladder from emptying completely, which in turn causes urinary stasis and frequent urination (because a partially emptied bladder refills quickly). Complete obstruction of urine flow is a very uncomfortable medical emergency that requires catheterization or (uncommonly) surgical relief.

Normal function of the ureterovesical junction prevents urine in the bladder from reflux into the ureter. Figure 20-4 illustrates that reflux is usually associated with an abnormally short segment of ureter within the bladder wall. Reflux causes urinary stasis and creates stagnant, high pressure urine in the collecting system, which damages the kidney and encourages infection,

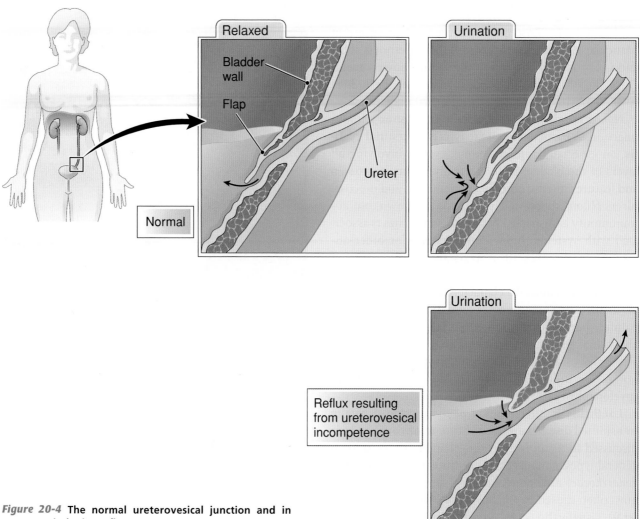

Figure 20-4 The normal ureterovesical junction and in ureterovesical urine reflux.

stone formation, and tubulointerstitial nephritis (Chapter 19).

In women there is an additional cause of lower urinary tract malfunction that can create urinary stasis. **Cystocele** is a downward protrusion of the bladder into the anterior vagina caused by stretching of the vaginal wall from multiple vaginal births. Cystocele prevents complete emptying of the bladder and can be a cause of urine stagnation and inflammation (cystitis).

INFECTION AND INFLAMMATION

Cystitis (Fig. 20-5) is inflammation of the bladder and is a very common problem. *Bacterial* cystitis is usually attributable to infection by gram-negative fecal organisms such as *Escherichia coli*. Viruses, *Chlamydia, Mycoplasma,* and other agents are uncommon causes. As was discussed in relation to renal disease, bacterial infection is often the product of urinary stasis, reflux, or

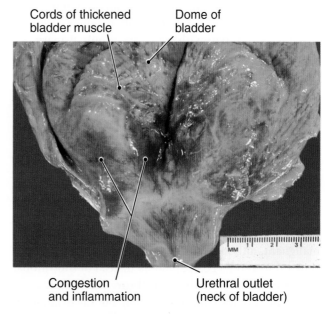

Figure 20-5 Acute cystitis.

insertion of instruments into the bladder for diagnostic examination (cystoscopy) or surgery. Women are at particular risk for cystitis because their urethra is short and is exposed to bacteria in the vaginal environment. Once the bladder is infected, infection of the kidney (pyelonephritis) or prostate (prostatitis) may follow.

Nonbacterial cystitis is bladder inflammation without infection. A particularly severe type is **interstitial cystitis**, an especially painful chronic cystitis involving all layers of the bladder wall. It usually occurs in women and features intense chronic inflammation and mucosal ulcers (*Hunner ulcers*). The cause is unknown, but autoimmunity is suspected because it sometimes is associated with systemic lupus erythematosus or other autoimmune diseases. It is resistant to all forms of therapy.

Cystitis is clinically characterized by 1) frequency of urination, sometimes several times an hour, 2) painful, burning urination (dysuria), and 3) dull low abdominal pain. Some patients may have hematuria. Fever and other signs of systemic infection usually do not occur unless infection spreads to the kidneys (pyelonephritis).

Urethritis is inflammation of the urethra. Sexually transmitted diseases are the most common cause and are discussed in detail later in this chapter. There are two general types: gonococcal urethritis caused by *Neisseria gonorrhoeae*, and nongonococcal urethritis, which is most often caused by *Chlamydia* or *Mycoplasma* (Chapter 9). Usually, however, no pathogen is identifiable because there are no easy ways to identify nongonococcal organisms. In both sexes cystitis is a common complication of urethritis; in men infection may spread to involve the prostate (prostatitis) or epididymis (epididymitis). Recurrent infections in men can produce urethral scarring (strictures) with acute or chronic urinary obstruction.

NEOPLASMS

The urinary collecting system (the renal pelvis, ureter, and bladder) is lined by a special epithelium—the urothelium, which is often spoken of as *transitional epithelium* because it is composed of cells whose shape is about halfway between square (cuboidal) and flat (squamous).

All neoplasms of urothelium are considered to be malignant, although small, early lesions are sometimes called transitional cell papilloma instead of transitional cell carcinoma. **Transitional cell carcinoma** may occur at any point in the collecting system, but the bladder accounts for about 90% of cases (Fig. 20-6).

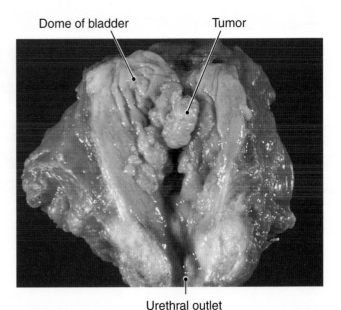

Dome of bladder · Tumor · Urethral outlet

Figure 20-6 **Carcinoma of the bladder.** This tumor has a polypoid or papillary growth pattern.

Transitional cell carcinomas fall into two major groups:

- *Low-grade tumors* are sluggish and slow to invade, and they grow outward into the bladder lumen to resemble a head of cauliflower or broccoli, and are called **papillary transitional cell carcinoma**. They are formed of cells that individually look much like normal transitional cells: they are well-differentiated and have little cellular atypia (Chapter 6). Despite the fact that these tumors are low grade and slow to invade, they tend to recur; that is, *new* primary tumors tend to sprout at other sites in the bladder mucosa. The important point here is that complete removal of the initial tumor does not guarantee that another *new* tumor will not occur at a *different* site in the bladder mucosa. The ten-year survival for patients with low-grade carcinomas exceeds 95%.

- *High-grade tumors* have a different gross and microscopic appearance: they are much less likely to be papillary and are more often flat, ulcerated, or nodular, and have an aggressive microscopic appearance. Like the bladder epithelium in patients with low-grade tumors, the epithelium in patients with high-grade tumors also tends to develop new high-grade tumors at other sites. The ten-year survival for high-grade tumors is about 50%. Survival also depends on the depth of tumor invasion: if the muscular wall is invaded, average five-year survival is about 50%.

Transitional cell carcinomas of the bladder occur most commonly in men over the age of 50. Smoking is the most important risk factor: cigarette smokers are about five times more likely to develop bladder cancer than nonsmokers are.

Painless hematuria is the most common—and often the only—symptom of bladder neoplasms. At time of diagnosis, most transitional cell carcinomas are single and confined to the bladder. Prognosis depends on histologic grade (degree of nuclear atypia and tumor differentiation) and depth of tumor invasion; that is, how deep it has extended into the bladder wall or nearby structures such as the vagina, uterus, prostate, or rectum. Bladder carcinomas tend to recur, and they kill by infiltrative obstruction of the ureters and adjacent pelvic structures rather than by distant metastasis.

The bladder is rarely the site of other tumors, either benign or malignant.

Diseases of the Male Genitalia

The most important problems of the male genitalia are:

- Erectile dysfunction and infertility
- Prostate cancer
- Infections

ERECTILE DYSFUNCTION AND INFERTILITY

About half of men over age 50 at some time experience **erectile dysfunction** (*impotence*), an inability to attain or sustain an erection satisfactory for intercourse. Achieving an erection is a complex physical and mental process; however, all *physical* erectile dysfunction is caused by abnormal blood flow into or out of the penis: either arterial inflow is too slow or venous drainage is too fast. Of men who were able to have satisfactory erections and subsequently cannot, over 90% of cases are associated with physical factors such as atherosclerotic impairment of arterial inflow, disease or injury to nerves controlling penile blood flow, hormone imbalances, or therapeutic drugs. For example, atherosclerosis or other vascular disease may interfere with brisk arterial inflow, or venous outflow may be too rapid. Therapeutic drugs, especially antihypertensives, account for about 25% of erectile dysfunction. Lesions of the brain, spinal cord, or peripheral nerves may be responsible by interfering with neural control of vascular smooth muscle tone and the flow of blood into and out of the penis. About 40% of men undergoing prostatectomy develop some degree of erectile dysfunction, caused by surgical damage to nerves that regulate vascular flow in the penis. Testosterone plays an important physical and mental role, because production declines gradually in older men; testosterone replacement therapy may be effective in some cases.

Infertility is the inability of a couple to conceive after one year of regular intercourse. About 1 in 5 couples in the United States is affected. Factors include sperm disorders (about 35% of couples), ovulatory dysfunction (20%), fallopian tube dysfunction (30%), and abnormal cervical mucus (5%). In about 10% of couples, the etiology cannot be identified.

There are many causes of male infertility. The most common anatomic problem is **varicocele**, a dilation of veins in the spermatic cord and testis. About one third of infertile men (compared to about 10% of fertile men) have varicocele, which causes blood stagnation in the testis and raises testicular temperature enough to impair sperm production. Surgical excision of the dilated veins is effective in about one third of patients.

Sperm may be absent from semen (**azoospermia**) if obstruction of the vas deferens or testicular atrophy exists. However, the mere presence of sperm in semen does not assure fertilization of an ovum: sperm may be attacked by antisperm antibodies in vaginal mucus, or they may lack motility. Even if ejaculate is normal, **retrograde ejaculation** into the bladder can occur and prevent sperm from reaching the vagina.

Female aspects of infertility are discussed in Chapter 21.

DISEASES OF THE PENIS AND URETHRA

Congenital abnormalities of the urethral opening (the meatus) occur in about 1 in 300 male infants. Sometimes the urethra opens as an elongated slit on the underside (**hypospadias**) or top side (**epispadias**) of the penis. Either may be associated with incontinence, infection, obstruction, or other congenital abnormalities such as undescended testis (Chapter 7) or inguinal hernia.

Phimosis is an inability to retract the foreskin over the glans. It is important because an unretractable prepuce promotes poor hygiene, infection, inflammation, and scarring and may encourage the development of squamous carcinoma. If an affected prepuce is forcibly retracted it may become trapped, a condition called **paraphimosis** that produces severe glans congestion, edema, pain, and acute urinary obstruction.

Inflammation of the glans is **balanitis**, and although much of it caused by sexually transmitted diseases (STD), most cases result from poor personal hygiene in uncircumcised males. **Balanitis xerotica obliterans** is an inflammatory disease of unknown cause associated with a white, sclerotic patch of skin at the tip of the glans, which may constrict the urethral opening. **Peyronie dis-**

ease is a fibrosing condition of the *tunica albuginea*, the fibrous sheath that surrounds the corpus cavernosum. **Priapism** (from *Priapus*, the Greek god of male procreative power) is a painful, persistent erection in the absence of sexual desire. It may occur if red blood cells become trapped in the corpus cavernosum, as they do in sickle cell disease, or if venous outflow from the penis is obstructed, as can occur with prostatitis or cystitis.

Neoplasms of the penis are uncommon; most are squamous carcinomas that arise in the squamous epithelium of the glans and occur in uncircumcised males over age 40. Poor personal hygiene and *human papillomavirus* (HPV) infection play a role. As is illustrated in Figure 20-7, **Bowen disease** is a squamous carcinoma in situ that has a distinctive clinical and microscopic appearance identical to Bowen disease of the nipple, vulva, and oral cavity. Untreated, about 10% of cases progress to invasive carcinoma.

DISEASES OF THE SCROTUM AND GROIN

During fetal life the testes descend from the abdomen through the inguinal canal into the scrotum. The most important congenital abnormality of male genitalia is **undescended testis** (*cryptorchidism*), a condition illustrated in Figure 20-8, in which one or both testes fail to complete the journey and remain in the abdomen or

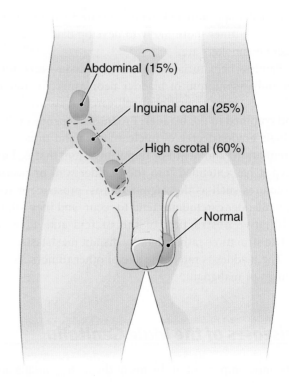

Figure 20-8 Undescended testis (cryptorchidism). An undescended testis may be found in the abdomen, in the inguinal canal, or high in the scrotum. Percent figures indicate the proportion of cases at each location.

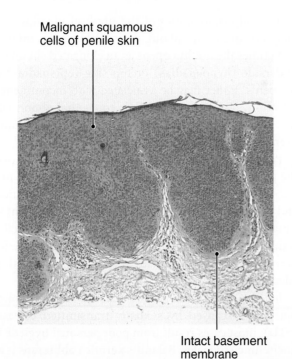

Figure 20-7 Bowen disease of the penis. In Bowen disease (squamous carcinoma in situ), the epithelium is composed entirely of malignant cells. No malignant cells have crossed the basement membrane.

comes to rest in the inguinal canal. Early discovery of the problem and surgical anchoring of the testis in the scrotum is necessary—an undescended testis that remains in the abdomen confers at least a 10× risk for testicular malignancy. Because the scrotal temperature is about 5° F cooler than the rest of the body, the added warmth of the abdomen causes testicular atrophy and infertility if the testes are not surgically placed in the scrotum.

Inguinal hernia (Chapter 15) is a protrusion of bowel into the inguinal canal or scrotum, which occurs as normal intra-abdominal pressure forces open the canal through which the testis descended into the scrotum in fetal life.

"*Jock itch*" is an inflammation of the scrotum or inguinal skin caused by a dermatophyte fungus similar to fungi that cause scalp *ringworm* and *athlete's foot*. **Varicocele** is scrotal varicose veins, which may cause scrotal enlargement and infertility. The scrotum may also be come enlarged if there is accumulation of fluid in the sac of the tunica vaginalis that surrounds the testis, a condition known as **hydrocele**. **Spermatocele** is a cyst of the epididymis that contains sperm and is formed by dilation of the epididymal tubule. It enlarges gradually with continued sperm production.

DISEASES OF THE TESTIS AND EPIDIDYMIS

Inflammation of the testis (**orchitis**) is rare. Mumps is the most common cause—about 25% of adult males with mumps develop orchitis. Inflammation of the epididymis (**epididymitis**) is much more common than orchitis. Acute bacterial epididymitis is usually a complication of urinary tract infection, prostatitis, or urethritis, especially gonorrhea or other sexually transmitted diseases. Nonbacterial epididymitis is fairly common, and the cause is unknown.

Most testicular neoplasms are malignant, and they are the most important cause of painless enlargement of the testis. They occur most commonly between the ages of 15 and 40. They fall into two main groups:

- Tumors of germ (sperm-producing) cells (95%); virtually all are malignant
- Tumors of other cells (5%); virtually all are benign

Sperm begin as primitive, undifferentiated (unspecialized) germ cells and develop through several intermediate stages into fully differentiated sperm. Tumors can arise from primitive germ cells or from cells in any of the intermediate stages of sperm development. Moreover, because germ cells can differentiate into *any* type of adult or embryonic cell, germ cell tumors can contain perfectly formed adult tissue or primitive embryonic tissue. For example, a *differentiated teratoma* (Chapter 6) is a benign neoplasm composed of multiple mature (differentiated) tissues, including tissues not normally found in the organ in which it arises. For example, a benign teratoma might contain normal skin, hair, brain, or thyroid tissue. Teratomas rarely may become malignant. *Embryonal carcinoma* is a tumor of very primitive, undifferentiated germ cells, which is very aggressive and tends to metastasize widely. Figure 20-9 illustrates the cells of origin and the types of tumors that develop in the testis.

The most common testicular malignancy is **seminoma** (Fig. 20-10), a tumor of germ cells. Seminomas are the most primitive of the germ cell malignancies, but despite their primitive nature, seminomas grow

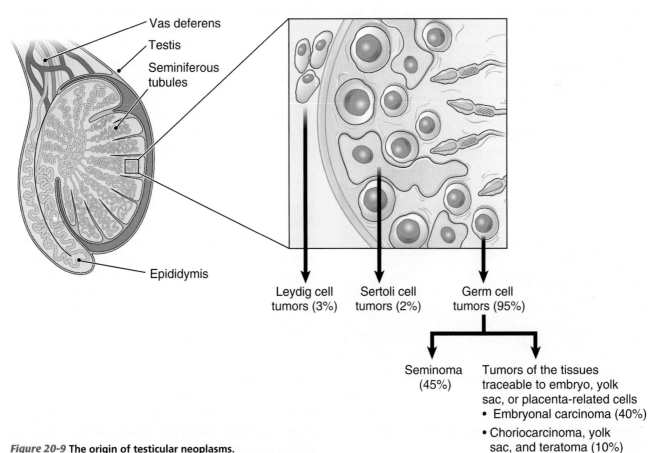

Figure 20-9 **The origin of testicular neoplasms.**

more slowly and metastasize later than other germ cell malignancies. One reason for their slow growth is that they are held in check by the immune system—they incite a brisk immune response and are characterized microscopically by dense accumulations of lymphocytes among the tumor cells. Seminomas respond well to radiation therapy.

Other germ cell malignancies are formed from germ cells that have evolved into primitive embryonic tissue (*embryonal cell carcinoma*), embryonic yolk sac (*yolk sac carcinoma*), or placenta (*choriocarcinoma*). About half of germ cell malignancies contain more than one type of malignant cell. **Embryonal carcinoma**, which is almost as common as seminoma, is composed purely of primitive embryonic cells. Embryonal carcinomas tend to metastasize earlier than seminomas do, both to lymph nodes and by blood vessels to lung, liver, and brain.

Treatment of testicular malignancies depends on hormonal therapy, chemotherapy, and radiotherapy. Several decades ago testicular malignancies were usually fatal. Now, however, thanks to modern chemotherapy and radiotherapy, the five-year survival rate for tumors confined to the testis is about 98%; and five-year survival for patients with distant metastasis is nearly 75% (see the nearby History of Medicine box). Nevertheless, early diagnosis improves the chance of cure. Health care providers should ensure their male patients know not to disregard an enlarged testis.

Nongerm cell tumors are uncommon and almost always benign. In the interstitium between testicular seminiferous tubules (Fig. 20-9) are Leydig cells, which produce testosterone and give rise to **Leydig cell**

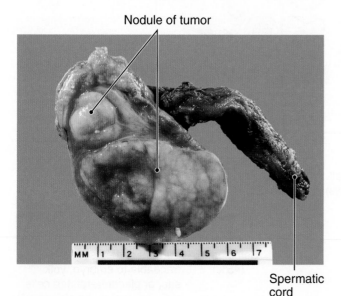

Nodule of tumor

Spermatic cord

Figure 20-10 **Seminoma of the testis.** This tumor has grown to occupy the entire testis.

tumors. Within seminiferous tubules are Sertoli cells, which support and control sperm production and give rise to **Sertoli cell tumor**.

DISEASES OF THE PROSTATE

Knowledge of prostate anatomy, illustrated in Figure 20-11, is important in understanding prostatic diagnosis and treatment. Recall that the prostate encircles the urethrae where it joins the neck of the bladder, placing it in a perfect position to choke urinary flow. It is also immediately in front of (anterior to) the rectum, so that the back (posterior) side of the gland is easily palpated by digital rectal exam. Benign enlargement (nodular hyperplasia) occurs in the central area of the prostate, which encircles the urethra. On the other hand, prostate cancer usually develops in the posterior part of the gland, a fact that makes prostatic cancers easily palpable by digital rectal exam by medical practitioners.

Nonneoplastic Disease

Prostatitis is a common affliction of men. There are three varieties of prostatitis: *acute bacterial prostatitis, chronic bacterial prostatitis,* and *chronic nonbacterial prostatitis.* Diagnosis is based on clinical features and whether or not inflammatory cells or bacteria are present in prostatic secretions, which can be pressed from the gland into the urethra by digital rectal massage of the prostate.

Acute or chronic *bacterial* prostatitis is usually caused by *Escherichia coli* and other fecal bacteria and is commonly associated with recurrent episodes of lower urinary tract infection because the prostate serves as a reservoir of organisms that are difficult to treat effectively. Antibiotic therapy is usually successful in the short term, but often the infection recurs.

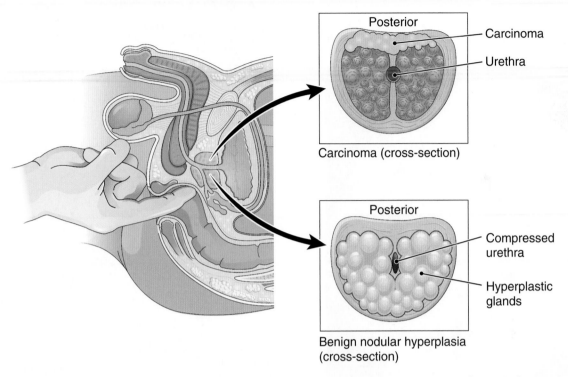

Figure 20-11 **Prostate anatomy.** Benign nodular hyperplasia mainly involves the center of the gland; carcinoma usually arises in the posterior region.

Chronic *nonbacterial* prostatitis is more common than bacterial prostatitis is. Cultures and other tests are negative and the cause remains unknown, but *Chlamydia* and related organisms are suspected.

The clinical picture of acute prostatitis includes varying degrees of urinary obstruction, painful urination, frequency, urgency, and perineal, scrotal, or low back pain. The prostate may be enlarged and tender, and the infection may be accompanied by fever and leukocytosis. In chronic prostatitis the symptoms are similar but less dramatic.

Nearly all men, if they live long enough, develop an enlarged prostate, or prostate cancer, or both. This enlargement is caused by **nodular hyperplasia** of prostate glands and the fibromuscular supporting tissue around the glands. Nodular hyperplasia is very common; it is present in about 20% of 40-year-old men and 90% of those seventy or older. However, only about 10% of men develop clinical symptoms.

The development of nodular hyperplasia is clearly influenced by estrogen and testosterone, but the mechanisms are unclear.

Figure 20-12 illustrates that in nodular hyperplasia the prostate gland is enlarged, sometimes very large. The gland is tense and rubbery, and the cut surface ex-

hibits multiple bulging nodules of hyperplastic glands, as is illustrated by Figure 20-13.

The most common symptoms are those of urinary obstruction: frequency, urgency, nocturia (getting up once at night to urinate is normal, more than once is not), difficulty starting the stream (hesitancy), intermittent interruption of the stream while voiding, and a narrow stream. Many of these symptoms are caused by incomplete emptying of the bladder, a condition that predisposes to urinary stasis and infection (Chapter 19), as is illustrated in Figure 20-14. Treatment varies with the severity of symptoms and the size of the gland. Drug therapy may reduce gland size and improve symptoms over a period of months, but definitive therapy is surgical: either a "boring out" of prostatic tissue through the urethra, an operation much like digging a tunnel, or open surgical removal of the gland.

Prostatic Carcinoma

Prostatic adenocarcinoma (typically called prostate cancer or prostate carcinoma), a malignancy of prostate gland epithelial cells, accounts for all but a tiny fraction of prostatic malignancies. According the American Cancer Society, in 2005 prostate cancer was the most

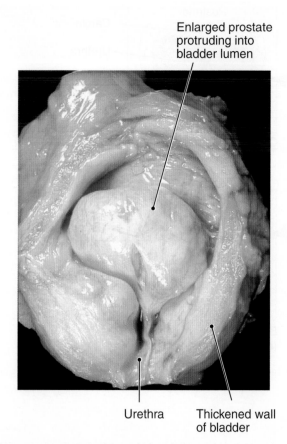

Enlarged prostate protruding into bladder lumen

Urethra   Thickened wall of bladder

Figure 20-12 **Nodular hyperplasia of the prostate.** The gland is massively enlarged, and the middle lobe protrudes into the bladder. Note the hypertrophied bladder wall, which is caused by chronic urinary obstruction.

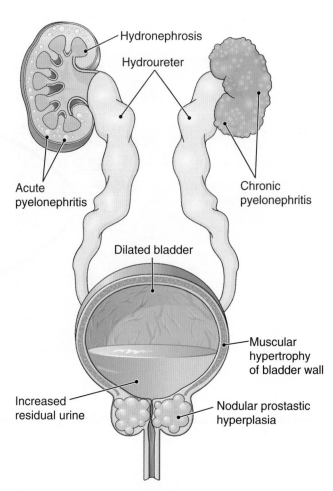

Hydronephrosis

Hydroureter

Acute pyelonephritis

Chronic pyelonephritis

Dilated bladder

Muscular hypertrophy of bladder wall

Increased residual urine

Nodular prostatic hyperplasia

Figure 20-14 **Consequences of chronic urinary obstruction.** This figure illustrates the results of chronic urinary obstruction caused by nodular hyperplasia of the prostate.

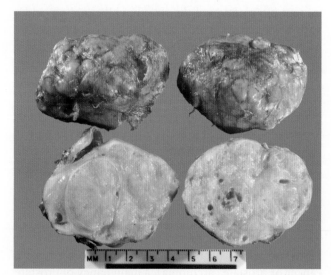

Figure 20-13 **Nodular hyperplasia of the prostate.** This cross section of gland was surgically excised for marked nodular hyperplasia and urinary obstruction. Note the irregular nodules of hyperplastic prostatic tissue.

common of all cancers in the United States, occurring about 10% more often than breast cancer in females. About 1 man in 6 develops prostate cancer in the course of his lifetime, but only about 1 in 30 die of it. Peak incidence of new adenocarcinomas occurs in men 60–70 years old. With the exception of skin cancers, carcinoma of the prostate is the most common cancer in men, far more common than lung or colon cancer. As advancing age and other disease take their toll, surviving men have an increased prevalence of prostatic cancer—if very early cases are included it is estimated that nearly half of men over age 80 have carcinoma of the prostate, but only about 10% of these develop symptoms. However, as a cause of cancer *death* among men, cancer of the prostate ranks second behind lung cancer and slightly ahead of colon cancer. These facts are easier to understand if one keeps in mind that prostate cancer is very common but not as lethally aggressive as lung or colon cancer.

It is now apparent that latent (undetected) cancer is more common than previously suspected. With modern imaging and microscopic techniques, increasing numbers of very early cancers are being discovered. However, very early diagnosis has not resulted in a clear-cut decline in the death rate from prostate cancer. Apparently some prostate cancers are so sluggish that they can exist for a very long time without causing harm, and a debate is under-way about what, if anything, should be done about some small, early tumors in elderly men. That is, should they be treated or should the approach be "watchful waiting," a strategy based on the arguable point that in very early cases in elderly men no treatment is available that is capable of extending life, or of doing more good than harm. Studies are under way to answer this question, and recent results suggest that "watchful waiting" can be the best strategy for some men with prostate cancer, especially older men with small, low-grade cancers and low blood PSA levels.

Multiple factors play a role in the development of prostatic carcinoma. *Hormonal* influence is clear. First, we know from modern medicine and historical evidence that men who were castrated before puberty do not develop carcinoma of the prostate (the nearby History of Medicine box offers an insight into the ancient practice of castrating young boys to be eunuchs). Second, we know that growth of carcinoma of the prostate is inhibited by therapeutic castration and by administration of therapeutic estrogen; and we know that administration of testosterone accelerates tumor growth. *Genetic* factors also play a role—prostate cancer is twice as common in African Americans as in whites. *Environmental* influence is clear—the incidence of prostatic cancer increases in men moving permanently to high-risk nations, such as the United States, from lower risk nations such as China or Japan.

As is illustrated in Figure 20-15, most prostate cancers arise in the posterior portion of the gland and are easily reached by digital rectal exam. However, the location of most cancers in the posterior part of the gland means that as they grow they do not press on the urethra and, therefore, do not cause obstructive symptoms until they are fairly far advanced. Nodular hyperplasia is much more likely to cause symptoms, a fact ensuring that many carcinomas are discovered incidentally during evaluation of patients as candidates for surgery to treat obstructive symptoms caused by nodular hyperplasia.

Gleason Scoring

Microscopic grading of prostatic carcinoma is standardized and offers valuable prognostic and therapeutic information. Pathologists examine microscopic slides of tissue taken from the gland by biopsy or surgical excision of the gland and formulate a **Gleason score** based on histologic grading of the tumor, which can vary from one part of the tumor to another. The best differentiated (least aggressive) and the most poorly differentiated (most aggressive) areas of the tumor are graded on a 1 to

History of Medicine

EUNUCHS

A *eunuch* is a castrated man; a man whose testicles have been removed. The word derives from Greek *eun*, for *bed*, and *oksein*, meaning *to keep*; thus a bedchamber guard or attendant.

The creation of eunuchs was a practice in ancient Egypt, China, India, and part of the eastern Mediterranean until a few hundred years ago. Castration before puberty ensured that certain male characteristics would not develop: the penis, if it was not removed with the testicles, ceased to grow, sexual desire never appeared, muscle mass did not develop, the voice remained high, and facial and body hair did not develop.

The practice was most widespread in ancient royal courts, where eunuchs were employed as keepers of royal female bedchambers, a practice that reached its peak in Constantinople (modern Istanbul, Turkey) during the Ot-

toman Empire (1250–1918). The last royal Chinese eunuch was born in 1903 and castrated at age 8 for the royal court during the last years of the Manchu Dynasty. He died at age 93 in 1996.

This custom was not universally a practice of royalty. Beginning around 1650 in Italy, young boys wanting to sing in the opera were castrated (becoming a *castrato*) to maintain a pure, high voice. The last Italian *castrato* lived long enough to be recorded in 1904 and died in 1922.

The Carrib Indians (for whom the Caribbean Islands are named and from which the word *cannibal* is derived) made a habit of castrating young male captives, well aware that early castration kept their flesh fattier and prevented the muscles from becoming tough and wiry. The Carribs fed the captives richly until they were to be sacrificed and eaten.

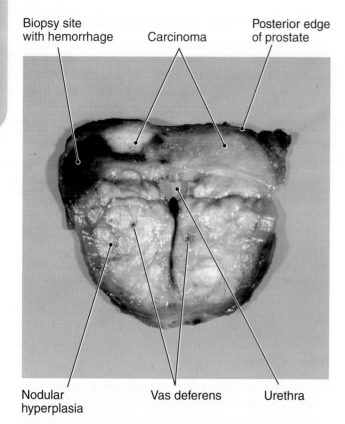

Biopsy site with hemorrhage   Carcinoma   Posterior edge of prostate

Nodular hyperplasia   Vas deferens   Urethra

***Figure 20-15* Carcinoma of the prostate.** Most of the gland is occupied by nodular hyperplasia, as it is in most patients who have prostatic carcinoma. Note the uniform, non-nodular nature of the posterior aspect of gland, which is involved by prostatic carcinoma. Hemorrhage is at the site of a needle biopsy performed two days earlier.

5 scale, where 1 = very well differentiated and 5 = very poorly differentiated. The scores are summed, so that the best possible score is 2 (for the least aggressive appearing tumors), and the worst is 10 (for the most aggressive appearing tumors). For example, a patient with a tumor that has an area of tumor that is grade 2 and another area that is grade 4 would have a Gleason score of 6.

Clinical staging is based on whether or not the tumor involves both sides of the gland, has invaded beyond the prostatic capsule into adjacent tissues, or has spread to nodes or distant sites. Staging is superior to grading as a guide to prognosis and therapy, but grading is more important in prostatic cancer than in other cancers because there is a fairly good correlation between high Gleason scores and poor prognosis.

Clinical Aspects

Prostate specific antigen (PSA) is a protein made by the prostate, which circulates at low levels in normal blood. Prostate cancer can cause an increase in levels of blood PSA. However, *blood PSA level should be interpreted with great caution* because:

- PSA level can be increased with prostatic nodular hyperplasia and other benign conditions
- PSA level can be normal in patients with prostate cancer

Therefore, it very unwise to rely on PSA as the *sole* diagnostic test. Every man having a screening PSA should also have a digital palpation of the prostate—prostatic carcinoma is very firm to the touch, much firmer than normal or hyperplastic prostate tissue. Many prostate cancers missed by PSA can be detected by this simple examination.

> **Never** rely on blood prostate specific antigen **(PSA)** as the **sole** screening test for prostatic cancer. **Always** do a digital rectal examination also to feel the prostate gland for the suspicious hard tissue that is characteristic of prostate cancer.

Experts frequently cannot agree on how to interpret blood PSA levels. To understand why, it is critical to recall our discussion from Chapter 1 about test sensitivity and specificity. Blood PSA has poor sensitivity; that is, there are many false negatives—men with cancer but who do not have blood PSA high enough to cause alarm. As a general rule, the higher the blood level of PSA, the more likely it is that prostate cancer is present. Blood PSA as a test for prostate cancer also has poor specificity: there are many men who have increased blood PSA because of nodular hyperplasia of the prostate, but who do not have prostate cancer. The result is that blood PSA increases gradually with age because of nodular hyperplasia, and it is difficult, therefore, to define where "normal" ends and "abnormal" begins. Nevertheless, a rapid increase of blood PSA is alarming and warrants close investigation, but experts disagree on how to define "rapid" as it applies to rising blood PSA level.

About 10% of carcinomas of the prostate are discovered incidentally in tissue removed during surgery for nodular hyperplasia. Most, however, are discovered by digital rectal examination and assay of blood PSA, but it remains distressingly common for patients to present with symptoms of advanced disease—urinary obstruction or bone metastasis. For example, a patient with bone metastasis may have unusual back or bone pain, which results in x-rays that reveal evidence of bone metastasis. Prostate cancer metastatic in bone stimulates *new bone formation*, which results in highly characteristic radiodense (white on x-ray) bone lesions, a finding that in an adult male is virtually diagnostic of metastatic prostatic carcinoma. Early bone metastases of prostate cancer can be detected by total body bone scan after injecting the patient with a radioactive molecule containing phospho-

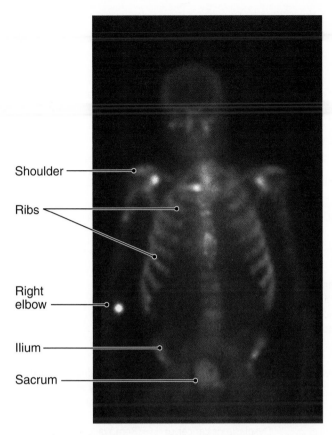

Shoulder

Ribs

Right
elbow

Ilium

Sacrum

Figure 20-16 **Radioactive bone scan.** Prostate cancer captures certain radioactive material injected intravenously and reveals its location by emitted radiation. In this patient the cancer, which appears white to the camera, is detected in the shoulder, ribs, right elbow, ilium, and sacrum.

rus. The phosphorus is taken up by areas of highly active bone metabolism, which in an adult male is almost always new bone growth stimulated by metastatic prostate cancer, unless the patient has bone injury or other focal bone disease. Lesions emit radioactivity, which is captured by a special camera (Fig. 20-16).

Treatment for early prostatic carcinoma relies on surgery, external beam radiation or implantation into the prostate of radioactive metal "seeds." Hormonal therapy in the form of surgical or chemical castration or estrogen administration is useful for advanced disease. For patients with tumor initially confined to the gland, 10-year survival is about 90%. A minority of patients with advanced disease survive 10 years.

Sexually Transmitted Disease

The sexual revolution is over and the microbes won.
P. J. O'ROURKE (B. 1947), AMERICAN HUMORIST
AND POLITICAL COMMENTATOR, *GIVE WAR A CHANCE*

Sexually transmitted disease (STD) is disease communicated by sexual contact. Some diseases are trans-

mitted *only* by sexual contact; infection by the bacterium *Neisseria gonorrhoeae* (gonorrhea) is an example. Others *may* be sexually transmitted; AIDS (Chapter 8) and hepatitis B and C (Chapter 16) are examples. Sexually transmitted diseases are among the most common diseases worldwide, and they are largely preventable. The Clinical Side box nearby discusses methods for preventing STD transmission. Important aspects of sexually transmitted diseases are summarized in Table 20-1.

> The risk of acquiring sexually transmitted disease is directly proportional to the number and variety of sexual contacts.

SYPHILIS

Also called *lues* (lew-eez), **syphilis** was first recognized in epidemic form in late 15th century Europe. The nearby History of Medicine box offers a brief recap of the history of syphilis, and Case Study 20-1 at the end of this chapter details a clinical case. Up to the mid 20th century, it was feared as the ultimate price to pay for a sexual dalliance because it was incurable and often led to dementia, severe disability, or death. However, much of the fear disappeared with the discovery in the 1930s that it was completely curable by penicillin. For over fifty years the treatment of choice has been a single intramuscular injection of 2.4 million units of benzathine penicillin G.

THE CLINICAL SIDE

PREVENTION OF SEXUALLY TRANSMITTED DISEASE

Sexually transmitted disease (STD) is common and largely preventable. The only certain way to prevent STD is by not having sex. For those having sex, the best way to prevent STD is to have sex with only one person who is not having sex with others—limiting the number of sex partners is very important. Those who ignore this fact often find themselves in STD clinics. For example, patients treated in STD clinics report an average of 3 partners in the prior three months and dozens of partners over their lifetime.

Male condoms are very effective at preventing most STDs, including HIV/AIDS; however, genital herpesvirus (HSV) and human papillomavirus (HPV) infection sometimes can be spread by pubic, groin, or other anatomic contact. Other protective devices (dental dams and female condoms, for example) can also be used.

After sexual contact, urination and thorough genital washing with soap and water also decrease the risk.

Table 20-1   *Sexually Transmitted Diseases**

Disease	New Cases per Year	Agent	Lesions	Associated Conditions and Complications	Therapy
Chlamydia	1.5 million	*Chlamydia trachomatis*	Urethritis, cervicitis	Arthritis Females: salpingitis, infertility Neonates: conjunctivitis, pneumonia	Antibiotics
Gonorrhea	430,000	*Neisseria gonorrhoeae*	Urethritis, mild cervicitis	Arthritis *Males*: prostatitis, epididymitis *Females*: salpingitis, infertility *Neonates*: conjunctivitis	Antibiotics
Syphilis	8,000	*Treponema pallidum*	*Primary*: chancre *Secondary*: skin disease, condyloma lata, lymphade-nopathy	*Tertiary*: dementia, aortic aneurysm, aortic valvular insufficiency	Penicillin
Genital herpes	640,000	Herpesvirus	Vesicles, ulcers	Recurrences *Neonates*: fatal infection from mother	Antiviral drugs reduce frequency and length of eruptions
Human papillomavirus infection	4.6 million	Human papillomavirus	Cauliflower-like, gray, soft excrescence	Dysplasia or cancer of the cervix	Removal or destruction; recurrences common; some types cause cervical cancer
Trichomoniasis	1.9 million	*Trichomonas vaginalis*	*Males*: mild urethritis *Females*: vaginitis or asymptomatic carrier state	None	Special antimicrobials
HIV infection	15,000	Human immuno-deficiency virus	Initial skin rash	Opportunistic infections, tumors	Anti-HIV drugs

*New case data are for <u>sexually active 15-24 year olds,</u> United States, 2000.

History of Medicine

WHO WAS SYPHILUS?

The name of the disease we know as *syphilis* springs from a long, elegant poem, "The Shepherd of Atlantis," written in 1530 by Girolamo Fracastoro (1478–1553), an Italian who studied astronomy, geology, philosophy, and medicine—he was the Pope's physician—and was, like Leonardo da Vinci, a renaissance man of the Renaissance. An epidemic of syphilis was recognized in Naples in the mid-1490s, shortly after Columbus returned from the New World, leading many to conclude that his sailors brought it back from their voyage (a point still debated). Syphilus is the proper name of the syphilitic shepherd in Fracastoro's poem.

Why write a poem about an awful disease? It was, in its way, a scientific paper: he describes the dementia, paralysis, and death of advanced cases of syphilis, but on the other hand, he did not recognize that it was sexually transmitted. However, Fracastoro's main purpose was political. It was the tradition of the day to name diseases after your enemies, and syphilis was variously known as the "Spanish disease," the "German disease," or the "French disease," depending, of course, on who was doing the naming, Fracastoro, an Italian, wrote it in a way that absolved Italians of responsibility and laid blame on the French.

Syphilis is very difficult to diagnose after the initial lesion (an ulcer, the *chancre*) disappears. Syphilis can affect almost any organ or tissue in the body and is famous as "the great imitator" of other diseases—among others in a long list, it can cause dementia, hepatitis, skin disease, heart disease, aneurysms, hair loss, oral and genital ulcers, and enlarged lymph nodes. With the advent of "the sexual revolution" in the 1960s and 1970s, syphilis incidence surged again and remains a serious public health problem because it often goes undiagnosed for years, by which time irreparable damage may have occurred to the infected person or to infants born to infected mothers.

Syphilis is caused by the delicate spirochete (corkscrew-like) *Treponema pallidum*, a bacterium whose only natural host is *Homo sapiens*. It is communicated across minute breaks in skin or mucosa during sexual intercourse or, in the case of congenital syphilis, across the placenta from an infected mother. Kissing, food, or toilet seats are not means of spreading syphilis. Immediately after being implanted, the spirochete spreads rapidly throughout the body and infects blood vessels, causing a chronic arteritis (Chapter 12).

Untreated syphilis develops through four stages: *primary*, *secondary*, *latent*, and *tertiary*. The hallmark lesion of **primary syphilis** is the **chancre**, a hard, moist, painless ulcer, illustrated in Figure 20-17, which ap-

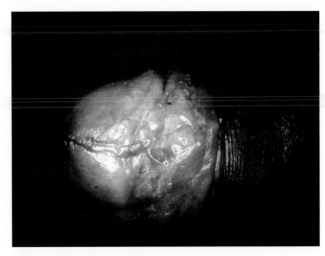

Figure 20-17 **Primary chancre of penis.** A darkfield exam of fluid expressed from the chancre revealed many spirochetes.

pears at the site of implantation about 2–4 weeks after infection and teems with spirochetes. The lesion is usually on the penis; or sometimes on the scrotum, groin, anus, or mouth. Fluid expressed from the lesion contains spirochetes that can be demonstrated microscopically by a special technique, **darkfield microscopy**, which is explained in the nearby Lab Tools box. Although an untreated chancre usually disappears spontaneously in a few weeks, by which time organisms

LAB TOOLS

How Do I Know If a Patient with a Genital Ulcer Has Syphilis?

Diagnosis of primary syphilis (in the *chancre* stage) is a challenge as old as scientific medicine. Perhaps the greatest challenge is to remember syphilis when encountering genital, oral, or anal ulcers. Laboratory blood tests and culture of the lesion are useless because antibodies are not present at the same time as the chancre, and *Treponema pallidum* cannot be cultured. The only way to make a positive diagnosis of syphilis when a chancre is present is to examine fluid pressed from the lesion to see if spirochetes are present. Unlike most other bacteria, *T. pallidum* does not colorize with ordinary bacterial stains, and it is too small and thin to be seen otherwise by the usual microscopic techniques. The *only* way to detect *T. pallidum* in a chancre is by darkfield examination of exudate taken from the chancre. Fluid is pressed from the lesion and placed on a slide for examination with a specialized microscope usually available only at public health facilities.

Darkfield microscopy differs in a simple but important way from *direct* light microscopy, the technique used for most microscopic examinations. With *direct* light mi-

croscopy the observer looks *directly* into the light source, and the object of study lies between the light source and the eye, so that the object is seen against a *bright* background. However, spirochetes in fluid from a chancre cannot be seen by looking directly into the light: they are too tiny and too thin to be seen.

Darkfield microscopy relies on a different technique: light is directed into the specimen from the side, so that no light shines *directly* into the microscopist's eyes; the background remains dark and the microscopist sees only light *reflected* from objects (spirochetes or inflammatory debris, for example). This is the same principle at work in a dusty barn: look at the darkened ceiling and no dust motes are visible except those that float through a stream of light coming into the barn. The motes are visible only because they reflect light into the observer's eye.

Darkfield examination is not widely available because it requires that the patient be present, is cumbersome and time consuming, and requires special expertise.

have spread throughout the body, some chancres may persist for months. As with any infection, syphilis induces the immune system to produce antispirochete antibodies, which are useful in diagnosis, but *do not confer immunity against reinfection in the future, nor do they eliminate the current infection.*

In untreated syphilis the *chancre* resolves spontaneously to be followed in 75% of patients by the syndrome of **secondary syphilis**, a combination of lymphadenopathy (enlarged lymph nodes) and skin rash that tends to occur most noticeably on the palms of the hands and the soles of the feet. These lesions can mimic almost any skin disease, and syphilis should be suspected when puzzling skin lesions are accompanied by generalized lymphadenopathy. The skin lesions swarm with infective organisms, which can be seen with dark-field microscopy. In moist areas of the body, such as the axillae, groin, inner thigh, and anogenital region, broad-based, cauliflower-like epidermal growths, **condyloma lata** (Fig. 20-18), may develop and become quite large. Both treponemal and nontreponemal antibodies are strongly reactive in secondary syphilis. Untreated secondary syphilis spontaneously regresses and gives way to *latent syphilis.*

Latent syphilis is syphilis that is hidden or subclinical. The disease goes underground, so to speak, except for the presence of blood antisyphilis antibodies. Latent syphilis lasts for many years, during which time *T. pallidum* is damaging blood vessels and brain in the de-

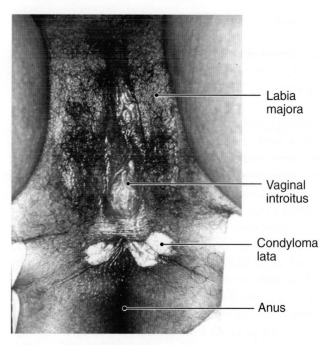

Figure 20-18 Condyloma lata of syphilis. A woman with condyloma lata of the perineum at the posterior edge of the vaginal introitus.

structive work that becomes clinically evident later as *tertiary* syphilis.

In about one third of patients, the disease reemerges 5–20 years later as **tertiary syphilis**. Most tertiary syphilis affects the cardiovascular system and usually presents as syphilitic aortitis, which is illustrated in Figure 20-19. Inflammation of the aortic wall results in

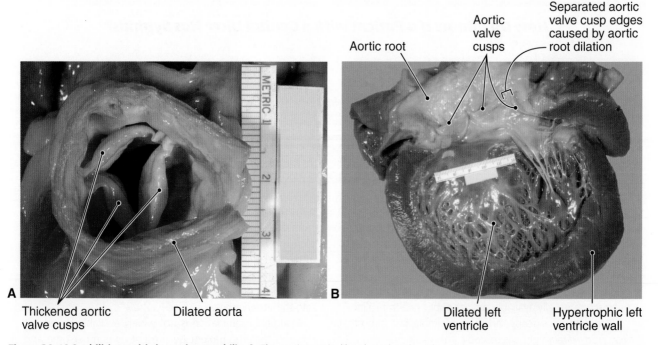

Figure 20-19 Syphilitic aortitis in tertiary syphilis. A, The aortic root is dilated, so that the valve does not seal properly during diastole (regurgitation), and the valve leaflets are thickened because of chronic inflammation and scarring. **B,** Marked left ventricular dilation and hypertrophy caused by aortic regurgitation associated with dilation of aortic root.

aneurysmal dilation of the proximal aorta or to dilation of the aortic root where it attaches to the heart. Dilation can stretch the aortic valve to the point that valve leaflets cannot close, and valvular insufficiency (regurgitation) occurs (Chapter 12). As detailed in the nearby History of Medicine box, research on tertiary syphilis led to the infamous Tuskegee syphilis experiment.

Neurosyphilis is the term for the effects of syphilis on the nervous system. The nervous system is infected in all patients with tertiary syphilis, but only in about 10% does it become the main site of clinical problem. Chronic meningitis may occur and is ordinarily asymptomatic or produces mild symptoms of headache and stiff neck. In some patients the posterior (dorsal) nerve roots of the spinal cord are affected, inducing a sensory defect and abnormal gait, a syndrome known as **tabes dorsalis.** Finally, chronic infection of the brain may cause atrophy of the cerebral cortex, illustrated in Figure 20-20, which produces a dementia known as **general paresis.**

In patients with tertiary syphilis, spirochetes are difficult to demonstrate because they are embedded in solid tissues, and darkfield examination requires fluid.

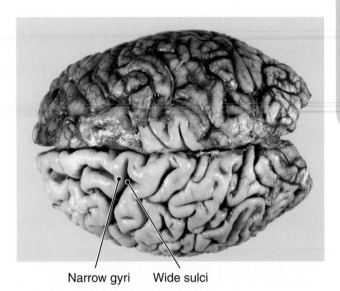

Narrow gyri   Wide sulci

Figure 20-20 **Brain in general paresis.** Note the narrow, atrophic gyri and widened sulci in this case of dementia caused by tertiary syphilis.

Tissue biopsy is required, but it is tricky to identify the organisms.

Risk of sexual transmission is greatest in the primary and secondary stages; transmission is rare after five years. *T. pallidum* can cross the placenta to cause **congenital syphilis.** Because signs of maternal syphilis may be difficult to detect, and because fetal effects may be devastating or fatal, serologic testing for syphilis is mandatory in pregnancy. Nearly half of all pregnancies in women with untreated syphilis abort.

T. pallidum infection causes production of two types of antibodies in blood—those directed specifically against *T. pallidum* (**antitreponemal antibodies**) and others that react with nontreponemal antigens and are called **reagins.** Tests for *antireagin antibodies* (the VDRL and RPR tests; see nearby Lab Tools box) are widely used as initial screening tests because they are cheap, quick, and reliable. Tests for antitreponemal antibodies (FTA-ABS) are used as a follow-up to verify positive reagin tests. Both types of antibodies are useful for diagnosis, however, neither antibody produces immunity, and neither fights the infection; they are mere passive markers. Both types usually remain in blood for a long time—reagin antibodies usually disappear in a few years, but antitreponemal antibodies may persist for life. For further discussion about tests for syphilis, refer to the accompanying Lab Tools box.

Detection of *antitreponemal antibody* is a very reliable indication that the patient has syphilis or has had syphilis (treated or untreated) at some time. Although

Serologic Tests for Syphilis (STS)

A serologic test for syphilis is a test for syphilis antibodies in serum (the fluid remaining after blood clots; it is the same as plasma but contains no fibrinogen, which was consumed in the clotting process). Infection with *Treponema pallidum* produces antitreponemal and nontreponemal (reagin) antibodies.

The two most common tests for syphilis are tests for *reagin antibody*—the Rapid Plasma Reagin (RPR) test and the Venereal Disease Research Laboratory (VDRL) test. These tests are sensitive, inexpensive, and easy to perform and are widely used as initial (screening) tests for syphilis. Antibodies detectable by these tests usually appear in blood shortly after the chancre has disappeared; therefore, a negative test in a patient with a chancre does not rule out syphilis. However, 100% of patients test positive in secondary syphilis. These antibodies may remain positive for a long time after successful therapy, making it very difficult to diagnose second—or third or fourth—reinfections because the test is already positive. On the other hand, about 15% of positive *reagin* tests (not anti-treponemal tests) are falsely positive because of circulating syphilis-like antibodies produced by autoimmune disease, virus infec-

tions, pregnancy, drug abuse, and a long list of other conditions.

The amount of antibody present in blood can be quantified (titered) by diluting plasma until the test is no longer positive. The titer is reported as the greatest dilution at which the test remains positive. For example, a patient with a low amount of antibody might have a titer of 1:2, meaning that plasma diluted in half was positive, but further dilution caused the test to be negative. A patient with a higher titer might still be positive at an eight-fold dilution (a titer of 1:8). Antibody titers tend to decline over time.

Positive VDRL or RPR tests must be confirmed by detection of *antitreponemal antibodies*, such as the Fluorescent Treponemal Antibody (absorbed) test (FTA-ABS). Treponemal tests are more complex, more time consuming, more expensive, and both more sensitive and specific. Positive VDRL and RPR tests that are not confirmed by an antitreponemal test are considered to be false positive. False-positive antitreponemal tests are rare and usually the result of specimen mix-up, lab error, or other nonpatient factor. Antitreponemal antibody usually remains present in blood for life.

false-positive and false-negative test results occur in antitreponemal antibody tests, they are uncommon.

Detection of *antireagin* antibodies, which means only that infection *may* be present or may have occurred in the past, demands a follow-up test for antitreponemal antibodies. Because antireagin antibodies occur in other conditions, especially autoimmune disease (Chapter 8), tests for reagin antibodies are prone to be falsely positive in some other diseases. Such false-positive test results are called **biologic false positives**, to distinguish them from laboratory error. *A false-positive test result for syphilis may be the first clue to underlying autoimmune disease.* Moreover, some of these antibodies interfere with standard laboratory blood coagulation tests (Chapter 11), making it appear (falsely) that the patient is on an anticoagulant drug. Because these antibodies were first detected in patients with systemic lupus erythematosus, they are sometimes called *lupus anticoagulant* antibodies. Patients with these antibodies are at increased risk for thrombophlebitis (Chapter 5) and spontaneous abortion (Chapter 7).

GONORRHEA

Gonorrhea is a sexually transmitted bacterial disease caused by the gram-negative (red-staining) diplococcus *Neisseria gonorrhoeae*, also known as the **gonococcus**. Only *Chlamydia* causes more *reportable* (to public health authorities) communicable disease in the United States. Note, however, that although human papillomavirus infection is the most common of all sexually transmitted disease and is much more common, it is not reportable to authorities.

Humans are the only natural reservoir for *N. gonorrhoeae*. Like syphilis, gonorrhea is communicated only by intimate contact with the mucosa of an infected person, usually during sexual intercourse. The organism provokes an intense acute, purulent inflammatory reaction.

The incubation period is 2–14 days. The clinical picture consists of urethral discharge with frequent, painful urination. In men, untreated cases may cause prostatitis or epididymitis. Urethral strictures may develop in men but are rare in women.

Infection of nongenital sites is uncommon; however, male homosexuals may develop gonococcal pharyngitis or anal infection (proctitis).

Infected mothers may pass the infection to their newborn infants as the fetus passes through the vaginal canal. The affected neonate may develop purulent conjunctivitis, an important cause of blindness in the preantibiotic era that can now be eliminated by the routine use of antibiotic eye ointments in the eyes of all newborns.

Gonococcal infection is proved by culture or by finding gram-negative *intracellular* diplococci in the neutrophils of acute inflammatory exudate collected from urethra, as is illustrated in Figure 20-21. Most strains of gonococci are very sensitive to antibiotics, but resistant strains are becoming more common. Patients with gonorrhea are often concurrently infected with *Chlamydia*, which is so common that patients with gonorrhea should be treated simultaneously for *Chlamydia*.

NONGONOCOCCAL URETHRITIS

Nongonococcal urethritis is a very common infection, especially in young men. A variety of organisms are responsible. *Chlamydia trachomatis* is the most common—about 5% of college-age and young adult men are infected; for minority males the rate is about 10%. Other nongonococcal agents of urethritis include *Ureaplasma urealyticum*, *Mycoplasma hominis*, and *Trichomonas vaginalis*. In women, *Trichomonas* is a common cause of vaginitis, but both men and women may be asymptomatic carriers, who can infect others. These organisms

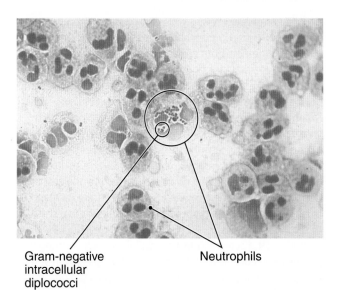

Gram-negative intracellular diplococci

Neutrophils

Figure 20-21 **Gram stain of urethral exudate in gonorrhea.** Note the numerous neutrophils and *intracellular* (phagocytized) gram-negative (red) diplococci in the cytoplasm of a neutrophil.

share several things in common: They are not gonococci, they cause sexually transmitted disease, and it is difficult to document them as the infectious agent by culture or other diagnostic procedure. The urethritis caused by *C. trachomatis* is clinically indistinguishable from gonorrhea and, indeed, most patients with gonorrhea are also infected with *Chlamydia*. All of these agents can be treated effectively by antibiotics.

In contrast to *N. gonorrhoeae*, *Chlamydia* and other non-gonococcal organisms cannot be easily identified by laboratory methods, but new molecular laboratory techniques show promise of improving laboratory diagnosis.

GENITAL HERPES AND OTHER SEXUALLY TRANSMITTED DISEASES

Genital herpes infection caused by *Herpes simplex virus* (HSV) affects about one in ten Americans, especially teenagers. Like cold sores (fever blisters), which are also caused by HSV infection, genital herpes is a relatively innocuous infection with very few serious consequences. HSV is passed by contact with the mucosa or broken skin of an infected person. It is not passed by ordinary daily contact.

Clinically, herpes appears as a localized crop of small blisters, which are mildly irritating. After a few days they crust, and disappear in about a week. Infected cells have nuclei with large, round, very distinctive inclusions, which can be seen microscopically in study of blister fluid. Eruptions of blisters may occur in the urethral meatus or at virtually any site on the genitalia. Anal infection is common in homosexual men. Eruptions tend to recur at the same site because during quiet periods the virus hibernates in the roots of nerves innervating the site. Eruptions may occur every few months and with time occur with less intensity and frequency. Systemic infection, sometimes fatal, may occur in immunocompromised patients, such as those with AIDS.

Human papillomavirus (HPV) is the most common of all sexually transmitted diseases. HPV is a family of viruses that cause benign skin warts (Chapter 24), especially in children, where it is passed by casual skin-to-skin contact. However, other types are passed mainly by sexual contact. In males these types causes genital warts (**condyloma acuminatum**), which appear as small, fleshy, pink, cauliflower-like growths near the urethral meatus or, in uncircumcised men, on the inside of the prepuce. Condyloma acuminatum is anatomically similar to *condyloma lata*, a lesion caused by *T. pallidum*, the infective bacterium of syphilis. Dysplasia and cancer of the cervix are caused by infection by certain high-risk strains of HPV; however, the risk to the average infected woman is very low because repeated infection is required to produce dysplasia or malignancy (Chapter 21; see also the nearby History of Medicine box). The risk of dysplasia or cancer of the penis in men is smaller than the risk for cervical dysplasia or cancer in women.

Molluscum contagiosum is a fairly common and innocuous STD. It is a viral disease that in adults is transmitted mainly by sexual contact; however, in children it can erupt at any point on the body and is contagious from casual contact. Lesions erupt on the skin of the genitals, thighs, or buttocks as small, pearly nodules that look at first like a small abscess. However, when opened there is no pus; the lesion is a cyst filled with cheesy white material.

Other sexually transmitted diseases that are common worldwide but rare in the United States include 1) *lymphogranuloma venereum* (LGV), caused by certain strains of *Chlamydia trachomatis*; 2) *chancroid* (soft chancre) caused by the bacterium *Haemophilus ducreyi*; and *granuloma inguinale* (donovanosis), cause by the bacterium *Calymmatobacterium granulomatis*.

The genital lesions produced by these and other STDs are important in the spread of AIDS, especially in Africa and southeast Asia—AIDS is more easily spread to people who have a venereal disease because the virus can pass through mucosal lesions. ■

CASE STUDY 20-1 *"A SPIDER BIT ME"*

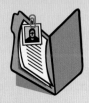

TOPIC:
Syphilis

THE CASE

Setting: You have recently taken a job in the health clinic of a medium-security state prison. You like the work because, among other things, you hear some interesting stories and meet people you otherwise would not encounter. Your duty today is to hold "sick call" for inmates.

Clinical history: D.W. is a 27-year-old man who appears to be in good health. He has been in prison for 9 months and has several more years left on his sentence. "A spider bit me," he says, pointing to his crotch. He reports previous good health except for the usual childhood illnesses. He admits that before coming to prison he "popped some pills" and "snorted" cocaine a few times but denies intravenous drug abuse. His prison health chart indicates that he is developmentally delayed and takes medication for bipolar disorder, but otherwise his history, physical, and admission lab work were unremarkable. He denies having sex since he arrived in prison and denies having sex with men on the outside, saying he had a monogamous sexual relationship with a girlfriend for a year before coming to prison.

Physical examination and other data: His vital signs are normal, and he does not appear to be in distress. He is uncircumcised and has an 8 mm cm shallow, raw area on the shaft of his penis. The glans and prepuce are unremarkable. Bilateral inguinal lymphadenopathy is present. No needle marks or other skin lesions are present. The remainder of the physical examination is normal.

Clinical course: You prescribe a topical antibiotic ointment and discharge him from clinic. However, 3 weeks later he shows up again at sick call, this time complaining of a skin rash. Physical exam reveals that the penile lesion has healed, but he now has a generalized rash. Moreover, his inguinal lymph nodes remain enlarged, and you find new groups of enlarged lymph nodes under his arms and along the side of his neck. Recalling an orientation lecture about sexually transmitted diseases in prison inmates, you give yourself a mental kick in the seat and now suspect that the original penile sore was a chancre (primary syphilis) and the rash and enlarged lymph nodes represent progression of the disease to secondary syphilis.

You order a screening test for syphilis, which is strongly positive. You consult with a colleague who agrees with you that the patient probably has secondary syphilis. You prescribe a dose of intramuscular benzathine penicillin G and tell the patient to return in a week. ▶

[Case 20-1, continued]

A week later you find that the rash has almost disappeared and the enlarged lymph nodes have nearly melted away. When you further question D.W. about the spider bite, he tells you that he didn't actually see a spider; he "just felt something crawling around down there" and concluded the sore was because of a spider bite. You resolve to ask more detailed questions next time and to think of syphilis every time you encounter a penile lesion.

Later the positive screening test is confirmed by a strongly positive antitreponemal antibodies test on a blood specimen sent to the state lab.

DISCUSSION

In the 1990s, the number of *new* cases of syphilis in the United States declined 90% to about 7,000 cases per annum. However, in 2003, the number of new cases began increasing slightly. Rates in women continue to decline, but many more men are being infected, suggesting an increase among homosexual men. Rates of syphilis infection are relatively high in prison inmate populations.

Diagnosing syphilis is difficult because it can cause such varied symptoms and because the primary lesion occurs long after sexual contact and disappears quickly. Moreover, patients are frequently reluctant to disclose the sexual behavior that is important for making a correct diagnosis of sexually transmitted disease. Because a chancre appears a few weeks after sexual contact, and this man has been in prison for 9 months, you know he did not give truthful answers to your questions about sexual contacts in prison. Syphilis is particularly difficult to diagnose in women because the primary lesion may occur in the vagina or on the cervix.

Fortunately, syphilis is very sensitive to penicillin—a single, large injection of slowly absorbed penicillin is curative.

POINTS TO REMEMBER

- Some patients do not give truthful answers to medical questions, especially questions about sexual habits and practices.
- Syphilis is difficult to diagnose.
- Always think of syphilis when finding a genital sore in a male.
- The incidence of syphilis is high in prison inmates.

Objectives Recap

1. *Name the component parts of the lower urinary system and the male genital system*: The lower urinary system consists of the ureters, bladder, and urethra. The male genital system consists of the testis, epididymis, vas deferens, seminal vesicles, prostate, and penis.

2. *Explain the importance of the ureterovesical junction in the flow of urine in the lower urinary tract, and know the consequences of malfunction*: The ureterovesical junction acts as a one-way gate to prevent reflux of urine from the bladder into the ureter. Reflux causes urinary stasis and creates stagnant, high-pressure urine in the collecting system, which damages the kidney and encourages infection, stone formation, and tubulointerstitial nephritis.

3. *Explain why women have more cystitis than men do*: Because the urethra in women is much shorter than the urethra in men, and in women the urethra opens onto a mucosal surface that frequently contains pathogenic bacteria.

4. *Discuss the pathologic and clinical differences between low-grade and high-grade transitional cell carcinoma of the bladder*: Low-grade tumors are always papillary and are formed of cells with minimally atypical features. The ten-year survival ex-

ceeds 95%. High-grade tumors tend to be flat, nodular, or ulcerated and have an aggressive microscopic appearance characterized by marked cellular atypia. High-grade lesions have a much greater tendency to recur than do low-grade lesions. High-grade lesions have a ten-year survival of about 50%.

5. *Briefly explain the cause of most erectile dysfunction*: Abnormally low arterial blood flow into the penis or abnormally rapid venous blood flow outward. Causes include diabetes, atherosclerosis, neurologic disease, hormone imbalances, or therapeutic drugs.

6. *Discuss the importance of undescended testis*: An undescended testis that remains in the abdomen will not produce sperm and is at greatly increased risk for development of testicular malignancy.

7. *Name the two most common malignant tumors of the testis, and briefly discuss the average five-year survival figure for patients with malignant tumors of the testis*: Seminoma and embryonal cell carcinoma are the two most common malignant tumors. The five-year survival rate for tumors confined to the testis is about 98%. Five-year survival for patients with distant metastasis is nearly 75%.

8. *Name the most common type of prostatitis and its cause*: Chronic nonbacterial prostatitis is the most common type of prostatitis; its cause is usually not clear, but *Chlamydia* is often suspected.

9. *Describe the anatomy of the bladder and prostate critical to the pathologic effect of nodular hyperplasia of the prostate*: The prostate encircles the neck of the bladder at its connection to the urethra. Enlargement of the prostate by nodular hyperplasia squeezes the urethra and obstructs the free flow of urine.

10. *Discuss the location of most prostate cancers, and describe why the location is important*: Prostatic carcinoma usually occurs in the posterior part of the gland, an area accessible to diagnostic palpation by digital rectal examination. However, the posterior location of most cancers means they do not cause symptomatic urinary obstruction until late in the disease.

11. *Describe the Gleason scoring system for histologic grading of prostate cancer*: Gleason's score is based on the histologic grade of the tumor—the most (best) differentiated and least (poorest) differentiated areas of the tumor are graded on a 1 to 5 scale: 1 = very well differentiated, with minimal cellular atypia; 5 = poorly differentiated, with marked cellular atypia. The scores are summed so that the best possible score is 2 and the worst is 10.

12. *Discuss the role of blood prostate specific antigen (PSA) in the diagnosis and management of prostate cancer*: Many prostate carcinomas are discovered by finding an elevated blood PSA level. The problem is this: many of those cancers might have been discovered earlier by digital rectal examination. It is unwise to rely on PSA as the *sole* screening test—a negative test (normal blood PSA) result conveys a false sense of security.

Furthermore, PSA level may be elevated in nodular hyperplasia, prostatitis, and other prostatic disease and is therefore best used as an additional test with digital rectal examination of the prostate.

13. *Discuss why syphilis is difficult to diagnose*: First, caregivers fail to think of it. Second, laboratory tests usually do not become positive until after the hallmark chancre has disappeared. Third, darkfield examination of fluid expressed from a chancre is not readily available outside of public health facilities. Fourth, the skin lesions of secondary syphilis mimic many other skin diseases. Fifth, if not diagnosed in the primary or secondary stages, when diagnosis is easiest, syphilis enters a long quiet stage (latent syphilis) that has few signs or symptoms. Sixth, tertiary syphilis mimics many other diseases. Seventh, blood tests for syphilis remain positive after initial infection and successful treatment; therefore, blood tests have limited usefulness in detection of current infection.

14. *Name some lesions of tertiary syphilis*: Some of the lesions of tertiary syphilis are aortic aneurysm, aortic valvular insufficiency, chronic meningitis, and brain atrophy with dementia.

15. *Name the most common cause of nongonococcal urethritis*: Chlamydia.

16. *Explain the role of sexually transmitted disease (STD) in the spread of AIDS in Africa and Asia*: Sexually transmitted disease is very common in Africa and Asia. Genital lesions associated with sexually transmitted disease offer easy entry of the HIV virus into the bloodstream of affected persons.

17. *Describe the clinical appearance of genital herpes*: Usually a localized crop of small blisters that are mildly irritating and disappear in about a week. Recurrences tend to be at the same site and with time become less frequent and less intense.

Typical Test Questions

1. Normal sperm can have which one of the following chromosome sets?
   A. 46,XX
   B. 23,XX
   C. 23,XY
   D. None of the above

2. Syphilis is associated with which one of the following?
   A. Condyloma acuminatum
   B. Balanitis xerotica obliterans
   C. Aortic aneurysm
   D. Hydrocele

3. Nodular hyperplasia of the prostate mainly affects which portion of the gland?
    A. Central
    B. Posterior
    C. Anterior
    D. Lateral

4. For men with prostate cancer, which of the following is true?
    A. Most men who have prostate cancer die of it.
    B. About one man in thirty develops prostate cancer.
    C. The peak incidence is in men 40–60 years old
    D. Prostate cancer in men is more common than breast cancer is in women.

5. Bacterial cystitis is usually caused by which one of the following?
    A. *Neisseria gonorrhoeae*
    B. *Treponema pallidum*
    C. *Escherichia coli*
    D. *Trichomonas vaginalis*

6. True or false? An untreated undescended testis will atrophy.

7. True or false? Patients with gonorrhea are also commonly infected with *Chlamydia*.

8. True or false? Cancer of the prostate and nodular hyperplasia do not occur together in the prostate at the same time.

9. True or false? Papillary carcinomas of the bladder are usually more aggressive than flat or nodular tumors.

10. True or false? Erectile dysfunction in most men is caused by psychological factors.

This chapter begins with a review of the normal female genitalia and breast, including overviews of ovulation, fertilization, menstruation, pregnancy, lactation, and menopause. Diseases and disorders discussed include sexually transmitted disease, ectopic pregnancy, infertility, endometriosis, placental disease, and dysplasia and cancers.

Section 1: Diseases of the Female Genital Tract

BACK TO BASICS
- The Pituitary-Ovarian Cycle
- Ovulation
- The Menstrual Cycle

MENOPAUSE

SEXUALLY TRANSMITTED DISEASE

VAGINITIS AND OTHER VAGINAL CONDITIONS

VULVAR DISEASE

DISEASES OF THE CERVIX
- Ectropion, Polyps, and Cervicitis
- Dysplasia and Carcinoma of the Cervix

DISEASES OF THE ENDOMETRIUM AND MYOMETRIUM
- Abnormal Endometrial Bleeding
- Endometriosis
- Endometrial Polyps, Hyperplasia, and Adenocarcinoma
- Other Conditions of the Uterus and Pelvis

DISEASES OF THE FALLOPIAN TUBE

DISEASES OF THE OVARY
- Nonneoplastic Ovarian Cysts
- Tumors of the Ovary

DISEASES OF REPRODUCTION
- Infertility
- Ectopic Pregnancy and Abortion
- Placental Disease

Section 2: Diseases of the Breast

BACK TO BASICS

INFLAMMATORY DISEASE

FIBROCYSTIC CHANGE

BENIGN TUMORS

BREAST CANCER
- Types of Breast Cancer
- Factors Affecting the Risk of Developing Breast Cancer
- Prognostic Factors for Patients with Breast Cancer
- Clinical Presentation and Behavior
- Diagnosis and Treatment

DISEASES OF THE MALE BREAST

Learning Objectives

After studying this chapter you should be able to:

1. Explain why women tend to develop osteoporosis after menopause
2. Name the most common sexually transmitted disease of women and the problems associated with it
3. Describe the developmental characteristics of the transformation zone of the cervix and its importance in cervical pathology
4. Explain the importance of human papillomavirus (HPV) in cervical dysplasia and carcinoma
5. Discuss the importance of annual Pap smear screening
6. Differentiate between pathologic and functional uterine bleeding
7. Explain why failure to ovulate may cause dysfunctional uterine bleeding
8. Explain why endometriosis may cause infertility

9. Define "fibroid" tumor of the uterus
10. Name the cause of tuboovarian abscess
11. Name the cell of origin of most ovarian tumors and the three main types of carcinoma of the ovary
12. Explain why ectopic pregnancy is dangerous
13. Name the three diagnostic components of preeclampsia (toxemia), and explain how eclampsia is different
14. Name the key difference between nonproliferative and proliferative fibrocystic change of the breast, and explain why the difference is important
15. Name the most common tumor of the breast
16. Name the cell from which most breast cancers arise
17. Explain how the behavior of lobular carcinoma is different from that of ductal carcinoma
18. List the most important pathologic factors that affect the prognosis of patients with breast cancer

Key Terms and Concepts

BACK TO BASICS
- Graafian follicles
- corpus luteum
- menses

SEXUALLY TRANSMITTED DISEASE
- human papillomavirus
- nongonococcal infections

VAGINITIS AND OTHER VAGINAL CONDITIONS
- moniliasis

VULVAR NEOPLASMS AND RELATED CONDITIONS
- vulvar dystrophy
- vulvar intraepithelial neoplasia

DISEASES OF THE CERVIX
- dysplasia
- cervical intraepithelial neoplasia
- transformation zone
- cervical erosion

DISEASES OF THE ENDOMETRIUM AND MYOMETRIUM
- pathologic uterine bleeding
- dysfunctional uterine bleeding
- endometriosis

- endometrial hyperplasia
- leiomyoma

DISEASES OF THE FALLOPIAN TUBE
- salpingitis
- ectopic pregnancy

DISEASES OF THE OVARY
- follicle cysts
- cystadenoma
- cystadenocarcinoma

DISEASES OF REPRODUCTION
- abortion
- hydatidiform mole

FIBROCYSTIC CHANGE
- fibrocystic change
- epithelial hyperplasia

BENIGN TUMORS OF BREAST
- fibroadenoma

BREAST CANCER
- ductal carcinoma
- lobular carcinoma
- carcinoma in situ

Section 1: Diseases of the Female Genital Tract

Female, n. One of the opposing, or unfair, sex.

AMBROSE BIERCE (1842–1914?), AMERICAN SATIRIST, JOURNALIST, AND SHORT-STORY WRITER, THE DEVIL'S DICTIONARY

BACK TO BASICS

The external female genitalia (the **vulva**) are illustrated in Figure 21-1 and consist of the **mons pubis, labia majora, labia minora, clitoris, external urethral orifice,** and the vaginal opening, the **introitus**. The mons pubis and labia majora are the most directly exposed to the environment and are covered by *skin*, which has a surface layer of durable, keratinizing squamous epithelium supplemented by hair follicles and sweat and sebaceous glands. The labia minora, clitoris, and vagina are more

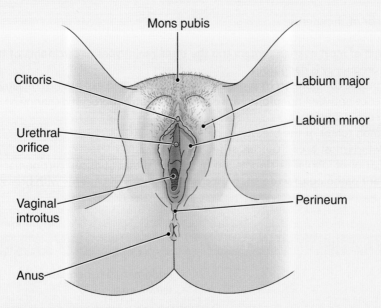

Figure 21-1 **The external female genitalia.**

protected and are covered by delicate nonkeratinizing squamous *mucosa* moisturized by lubricating mucous glands (**Bartholin glands**).

Figure 21-2 illustrates the **vagina, uterus, fallopian tubes,** and **ovaries** and their anatomic relationships in the pelvis. As is shown in the detailed view of the internal female genitalia in Figure 21-3, the **body** of the uterus is the intra-abdominal portion of the uterus; the **fundus** is the upper end of the body. The uterus protrudes into the pelvis and is covered by cells of the peritoneum, which lines the abdominal cavity and folds over the uterus to form the **broad ligament** on each side, forming a pocket deep behind the uterus (the **cul-de-sac**). The uterus is stabilized in the pelvis by other ligaments: the **uterosacral ligament** posterolaterally and the **round ligament** (see Fig. 21-2), which runs anterolaterally through the broad ligament to the pelvis wall.

The vagina is lined by squamous mucosa and connects the vaginal opening (the *introitus*) to the lower end of the uterus, the **cervix.** The cervix is composed of smooth muscle. The part protruding into the upper end of the vagina is called the **ectocervix.** The vaginal opening of the cervix is called the **cervical os** (the cervical "mouth"). The cervical os opens onto a short **endocervical canal,** which is lined by mucinous epithelium that secretes mucus to form a protective plug that protects the endometrium from vaginal organisms; sperm are specially equipped to penetrate this mucus barrier.

The ectocervix and vagina are covered by squamous epithelium, which is moisturized by mucous glands

in the cervix and vaginal wall. The endocervix, endometrium, and fallopian tubes are lined by glandular (columnar) epithelium. The transition point from squamous to glandular (columnar) epithelium occurs in the cervical os and is known as the **squamocolumnar junction,** an important anatomic landmark in the development of cervical cancer.

The uterine wall, the **myometrium,** is composed of smooth muscle. In the center of the uterus, the endometrial cavity connects to the endocervical canal directly below. The endometrial cavity is lined by **endometrium,** the tissue into which fertilized ova implant. The endometrium is composed of two types of tissue—supportive stromal cells, and glands formed of columnar epithelium.

The **fallopian tubes** lead from each corner of the uterus outward to the ovaries. The end of each fallopian tube, the **fimbriated extremity,** flares widely over each ovary with numerous finger-like folds that are lined by undulating cilia that sweep ova, fertilized or not, into the fallopian tube. Ciliated cells in the fallopian tube sweep the ovum into the endometrial cavity. Conception usually occurs in the abdominal cavity near the ovary or in the fimbriated end of the fallopian tube, so a fertilized ovum must make a trip to the endometrial cavity before it implants.

The **ovaries** lie within the broad ligament close to the fimbriated end of the fallopian tube and are attached to the uterus by the *ovarian ligament* and to the lateral pelvic wall by the *round ligament.* The surface of the ovary is covered by a layer of altered peritoneal cells known as the **surface epithelial cells,** which are the

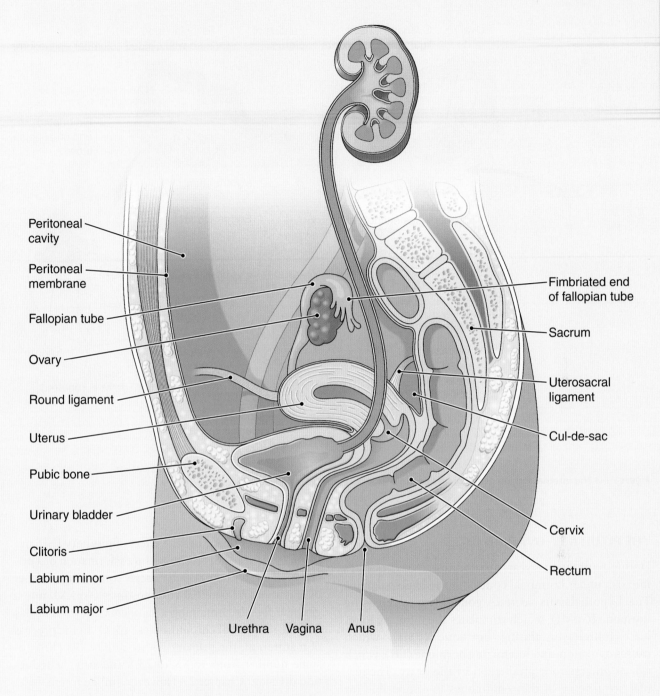

Peritoneal cavity

Peritoneal membrane

Fallopian tube

Ovary

Round ligament

Uterus

Pubic bone

Urinary bladder

Clitoris

Labium minor

Labium major

Fimbriated end of fallopian tube

Sacrum

Uterosacral ligament

Cul-de-sac

Cervix

Rectum

Urethra   Vagina   Anus

Figure 21-2 **The vagina, uterus, fallopian tubes, and ovaries.**

source of most ovarian tumors. The ovary proper is composed of germ cells (**oocytes**), supporting connective tissue **stromal cells**, and specialized cells (**granulosa cells** and the **theca cells**, which secrete hormones and support ovulation).

At birth an infant girl's ovaries have about 2 million *oocytes*—all she will ever have. By puberty the number

has decreased to about 400,000. During her entire reproductive life only about 400 of these will become ova. The remainder die naturally (apoptosis) after menopause. Each *oocyte* contains 46 chromosomes and is nested in the center of a small group of granulosa cells. The oocyte and its rim of granulosa cells together are called the **primary follicle**.

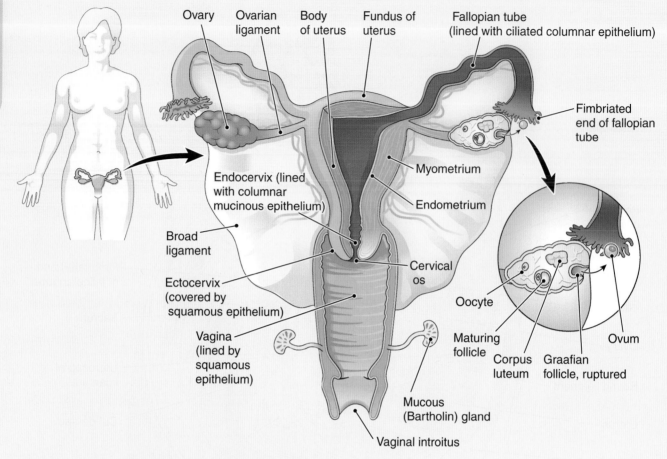

Figure 21-3 **The internal female genitalia and pelvis.** A sagittal section is shown here.

THE PITUITARY-OVARIAN CYCLE

During reproductive years the ovaries convert oocytes into ova under hormonal control of the hypothalamus. The hypothalamus secretes **gonadotropin-releasing hormone** (GnRH), which stimulates the pituitary to release **follicle-stimulating hormone** (FSH), which causes ovulation, and **luteinizing hormone** (LH), which causes progesterone production by the ovary. The regular sequencing of these hormones is responsible for the menstrual cycle.

Under stimulation of FSH, oocytes mature into ova and undergo reduction division (meiosis), in which the number of chromosomes in each cell is reduced to 23 (one half of each of the original 23 pairs). Continued stimulation by FSH causes some primary follicles to mature into small cysts called **graafian follicles**, which contain a maturing ovum in the center. At the edge of this expanding cyst is a rim of granulosa cells and theca cells, which secrete follicular fluid and **estrogens**, hormones that promote growth of the endometrium and the development and maintenance of female secondary sex characteristics.

Figure 21-4 illustrates the effect of pituitary FSH and LH in ovulation. FSH stimulates transformation of a *primary follicle,* with its *primary oocyte* containing a full set of maternal and paternal chromosomes (46,XX), into a *graafian follicle* containing a *secondary oocyte* that has half the number of chromosomes (23,X). In the process of maturation, the primary oocyte reduces its chromosome number from 46,XX to 23,X (meiosis, or reduction division, Chapter 7). However, unlike in the male, where each sperm gets an equal share of both chromosomes and cytoplasm, in the ovary one of the two secondary oocytes gets all of the cytoplasm and the remaining secondary oocyte dies. This uneven division of cytoplasm ensures an abundance of cytoplasmic nutrients for life of the ovum after it is fertilized by sperm, which contains no cytoplasm.

OVULATION

Under continued FSH stimulation the graafian follicle enlarges until it ruptures and releases its ovum (**ovulation**) into the peritoneal cavity. Then under the influence of LH the follicle develops into a **corpus luteum**, a

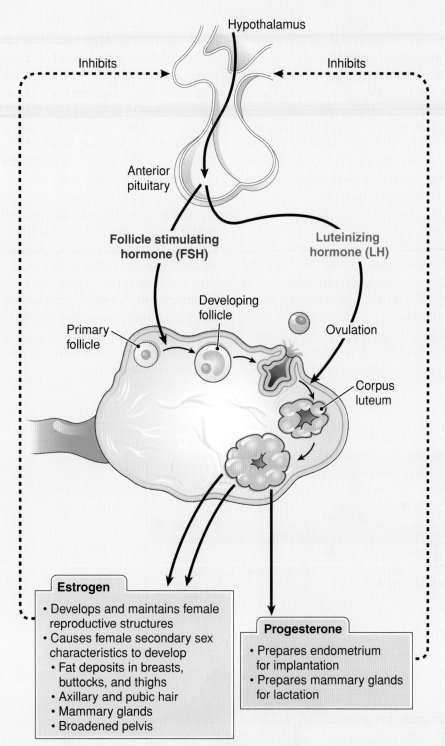

***Figure 21-4* Effects of pituitary FSH and LH in ovulation.** The hypothalamus stimulates the pituitary gland first to release FSH, then LH. FSH stimulates ovarian follicle development, ovulation, and follicular estrogen secretion, which in turn stimulates endometrium to grow (the proliferative phase). Next, LH stimulates formation of the corpus luteum from the ruptured follicle after ovulation. The corpus luteum secretes progesterone, stimulating endometrial glandular development and glycogen accumulation and readying the endometrium for implantation. If pregnancy does not occur, the corpus luteum atrophies to become a corpus albicans, and menstruation occurs.

yellow endocrine body that secretes mainly progesterone and lesser amounts of estrogen to prepare the endometrium for implantation of a fertilized ovum. If pregnancy does not occur, luteinizing hormone falls and the corpus luteum disappears (involutes). However, if pregnancy occurs the corpus luteum persists. Sometimes the ovaries develop more than one graafian follicle at a time, and the additional follicles persist as unruptured cysts (**follicle cysts**), which are so common as to be considered normal; however, they may grow to several centimeters in diameter.

THE MENSTRUAL CYCLE

While these changes are occurring in the ovary, the endometrium is changing in complementary fashion, as is illustrated in Figure 21-5. At the end of **menses** (menstruation), only a thin layer of endometrium remains. The new menstrual cycle begins as pituitary FSH stimulates follicle growth and follicle estrogen secretion. Estrogen in turn stimulates proliferation of endometrial stroma, a period of endometrial growth known as the *proliferative phase*. After ovulation, LH stimulates conversion of the ruptured follicle into the corpus luteum, which secretes progesterone. Progesterone (aided by estrogen) in turn stimulates the endometrium to secrete large amounts of glycogen (not shown on the figure), a period of endometrial growth known as the *secretory phase*. The endometrium is now lush—richly vascular and packed with energy-rich glycogen-filled glands; fertile soil ready for seed.

If implantation does not occur, the corpus luteum shrinks to a small scar (**corpus albicans**, literally "white body"), and the endometrium dies. Menstrual bleeding follows, as necrotic endometrium and blood are shed into the vagina. However, if implantation occurs the conceptus begins secreting **chorionic gonadotropin**—a hormone that has the same effect as luteinizing hormone—thus maintaining the ovarian corpus luteum throughout pregnancy and ensuring a continued supply of estrogen and progesterone to support the pregnancy.

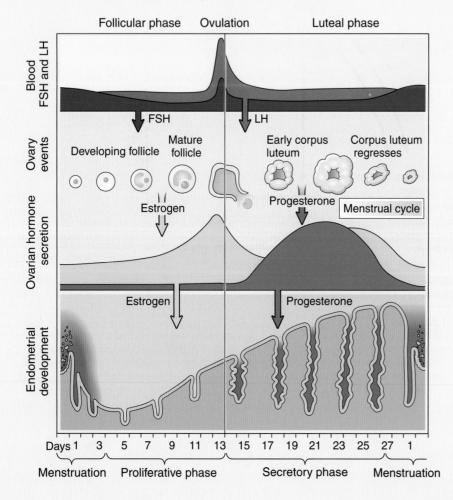

Figure 21-5 Interrelationships among the endometrial cycle, the ovarian cycle, and pituitary and ovarian hormones. Changes in the endometrium are complementary to those in the ovary illustrated here.

Menopause

Menopause is the normal, age-related cessation of ovulation and menstruation. It usually occurs about age 50, resulting from failure of the ovaries to respond to FSH and LH from the pituitary. Ovulation stops, menstruation ends, and levels of blood estrogen and progesterone decline. Some women experience no unpleasant consequences, but most suffer hot flushes (flashes) and other symptoms.

Hot flushes are caused by short-term surges of LH and are characterized by skin blood vessel dilation, a feeling of warmth, skin redness, and sweating. Other symptoms include fatigue, irritability, headache, nervousness, depression, and decline of sexual drive. The marked reduction of estrogen also has a profound effect on the lower genital tract. The covering epidermis and squamous epithelium thins, and all parts decrease in size. Cervical, vaginal, and labial mucous production decline, and vaginal pH becomes alkaline, which encourages infection. Pelvic muscle tone relaxes and urinary incontinence may occur.

Estrogen is necessary for healthy, strong bones. Lack of estrogen is important in the development of **osteoporosis**, a thinning and brittleness of bones that occurs with age, which is a major health risk for menopausal women because it dramatically increases the risk of bone fractures in elderly women. Until recently it was common practice to treat postmenopausal women with supplemental oral estrogen; however, as the nearby box The Clinical Side describes, because of certain long-term risks, estrogen is generally recommended for use only for menopausal women with severe symptoms, usually hot flushes, which do not respond to other therapy. Topical estrogen cream is effective in restoring mucosal integrity and mucous production in the vagina.

MAJOR DETERMINANTS OF DISEASE

- The external genitalia, the vagina, and the cervix are open to the environment and subject to infection.
- Sexually transmitted disease is an important cause of female genital disease.
- Ovarian malignancy is difficult to detect early.
- Disturbed menstrual function is common.
- Female genital health is estrogen dependent.
- Lack of regular Pap smears is an important factor in death from cancer of the cervix.
- Pregnancy has health risks.

THE CLINICAL SIDE

LONG-TERM ESTROGEN REPLACEMENT THERAPY

Long-term estrogen replacement therapy in postmenopausal women was formerly widespread because it helps maintain bone strength and reduces hot flushes. Postmenopausal decline of estrogen renders women, especially small Caucasian women, susceptible to traumatic fractures or spontaneous collapse of vertebral bodies from stresses that might not injure males of similar age or younger females. Estrogen replacement has a proven ability to reduce the incidence of bone fractures and to relieve postmenopausal functional symptoms such as hot flushes and night sweats. As one husband put it, "If you don't believe in spontaneous combustion, get in bed with my wife."

However, the practice of long-term estrogen therapy has declined recently because new concerns have arisen that for most women it carries a small but definite increased risk for breast cancer, thrombophlebitis, heart attack, and stroke. However, the issue is not completely settled, with the most recent information suggesting that women who begin estrogen replacement therapy near the time of menopause suffer fewer heart attacks, whereas women who do not begin therapy until well after menopause probably derive little benefit. It is indisputable, however, that estrogen replacement decreases risk of fracture and controls hot flushes and night sweats, which can be so unpleasant to some women that they conclude the risks are acceptable in order to gain relief.

The bottom line is this: the burden of disease appears to be as great with replacement therapy as without it. There are other means of preventing fractures—exercise, for example. However, estrogen remains the gold standard for treatment of hot flushes. The data and the issues are complex, and health care providers should familiarize themselves with the details and inform their patients of the benefits and risks.

Sexually Transmitted Disease

Among the most important diseases of the female genitalia is **sexually transmitted disease** (STD), which is disease transmitted by sexual contact. STD, syphilis in particular, is discussed in additional detail in Chapters 9 and 20.

Some STD is transmitted *only* by sexual contact; others, hepatitis B and C, for example, *can* be transmitted sexually and by other means. The same diseases affect men and are discussed in additional detail in Chapter 20; however, in women the anatomic distribution is different (Table 21-1).

Syphilis, herpes, granuloma inguinale, chancroid, and *lymphogranuloma venereum* behave in women much the same as they do in men (Chapter 20).

Gonorrhea is infection by the bacterium *Neisseria gonorrhoeae*. Gonorrhea, which in men mainly causes painful urethritis, is less symptomatic in women but may have consequences that are more serious because it primarily affects the fallopian tubes. About 1 in every 200 college-aged and young adult women is infected with gonorrhea, and most are asymptomatic. In women, acute infection may involve the vagina, cervix, or fallopian tubes and when symptomatic is characterized by vaginal discharge, lower pelvic pain, and dysuria. Repeated or untreated infections may result in chronic fallopian tube infection (salpingitis) with tubal obstruction, infertility, or pregnancy that implants in the fallopian tube (ectopic pregnancy) because the pathway to the uterus is obstructed by inflammation and scarring. Infected mothers can infect the fetus with gonorrhea as it passes through the vaginal canal. Penicillin is effective therapy.

Human papillomavirus (HPV) is a family of over 100 viruses that cause a variety of skin and genital lesions. Some types of HPV cause common skin warts, especially in children, and are passed by casual skin-to-skin contact. Other types are passed mainly by sexual contact and cause both benign and malignant neoplasms. HPV genital infection is common: over 4 million *new* HPV infections are reported in men and women in the United States each year, and about 5–10% of the United States population is infected at any given time. Infection rates are much higher in Mexico, South America, Africa, and Southeast Asia. Rates are highest in young adults and decline rapidly in older adults, as the number of sexual partners declines. A recently developed vaccine promises to decrease infection rates.

Sexually transmitted HPV produces two different but related lesions in women: *condyloma acuminatum* and *squamous carcinoma* of the vulva, vagina, or, most commonly, of the cervix. **Condyloma acuminatum** is the more common of these two lesions. It is a benign, cau-

---

Table 21-1   *Anatomic Pattern of Sexually Transmitted Infections* of the Female Genitalia*

	Location and Expression of Infection				
Agent	**Vulva**	**Vagina**	**Cervix**	**Endometrium**	**Tubes/ovaries**
Herpes virus	Herpetic vesicles and ulcers				
Human papillomavirus	Condyloma acuminatum Dysplasia, carcinoma in situ, invasive carcinoma				
Molluscum virus	Molluscum eruptions				
Treponema pallidum	Solitary ulcer (chancre)				
Neisseria gonorrhoeae	Vulvovaginitis in children and adolescents		Acute cervicitis		Acute salpingo-oophoritis
Chlamydia trachomatis			Acute cervicitis		Acute salpingo-oophoritis
Trichomonas vaginalis		Acute vaginitis, cervicitis			
Candida albicans*	Acute vulvovaginitis				

*Candida is a normal inhabitant of the vagina, but may cause infection under certain circumstances.

liflower-like growth of the cervical, vaginal, or vulvar squamous mucosa. It is not to be confused with the similar *condyloma lata* of secondary syphilis. Genital HPV may be passed to infants at vaginal delivery, and infected infants may develop multiple, life-threatening papillomas of the upper respiratory tract. HPV infection produces a distinctive microscopic change that is visible microscopically in squamous cells seen in biopsy or Pap smear material.

Squamous carcinoma of the cervix is a possible consequence of repeated HPV infection. Most HPV infection is detectable by Pap smear, can be treated effectively, and has no lasting physical effect. However, repeated infections over many years may produce **dysplasia** of the cervical epithelium (Chapter 6), a precancerous change that explains the close relationship between sexual habits and cervical cancer—carcinoma (and HPV infection) is associated with early age at first intercourse and unprotected sex with multiple partners.

In women as in men, other infective agents, generally discussed as **nongonococcal infections**, are common causes of STD. *Chlamydia* is a common offender and behaves in women much the same as gonorrhea does. About 5% of college-aged and young adult women are infected. Clinical diagnosis is challenging because many patients, men and women, are asymptomatic carriers. Although early detection is desirable because a single dose of antibiotic is curative, *Chlamydia* is difficult to culture, and other diagnostic techniques are technically difficult and expensive. Most patients are treated based on clinical evidence, not laboratory proof.

Trichomoniasis is caused by an ameba-like organism (*Trichomonas vaginalis*) that is present normally in the vagina of about 10% of otherwise healthy women. It is much more pathogenic in women than in men; even so, most infected women are asymptomatic and form a natural reservoir of infection. Symptomatic infection causes vaginal discharge and burning and is usually precipitated by a change in the vaginal environment that causes the organism to flourish. Examples include pregnancy and the loss of normal vaginal bacterial flora (which inhibit *T. vaginalis* growth) following antibiotic therapy for an unrelated condition. Treatment with special antimicrobials is effective.

Molluscum contagiosum is an innocuous, self-healing viral disease that causes eruptions of small (a few mm) white nodules on the skin of the genitals or on the thighs or buttocks. The eruptions look like small, white abscesses but without the redness and tenderness of an abscess, and they contain a pearly, cheesy material instead of pus.

Vaginitis and Other Vaginal Conditions

Vaginitis is a common, usually transient inflammation that is uncomfortable but typically not serious. It is often caused by microbes normally residing in the vagina, which become pathogenic under certain conditions that cause a change of the vaginal environment—diabetes, antibiotic therapy that alters the normal microbial flora, AIDS and other immunodeficient states, and pregnancy. In other instances the offending agent is introduced by sexual intercourse. One of the most common agents is *Candida albicans*, the agent of **moniliasis (candidiasis)**. *Candida* is found in about 5% of healthy females, so that infection presumes some predisposing condition or sexual transmission of a strain alien to the patient's normal vaginal environment. Trichomoniasis is another cause of vaginitis.

Bartholin glands are lubricant mucinous glands of the posterior vulva that may become cystic or infected (**Bartholin abscess**), especially by gonococci, *Chlamydia*, and staphylococci.

Vulvar Disease

The vulva is affected by several *nonneoplastic* inflammatory conditions that are often associated with white, flat lesions called **leukoplakia** (literally, "white patch") by clinicians. However, the epithelial cells beneath these white, scaly lesions can be benign, dysplastic, or frankly malignant. Skin diseases are the cause of most leukoplakia, and the white patch is a benign, hyperplastic overgrowth of surface squamous epithelium caused by chronic itching and rubbing that causes a skin condition known as **lichen simplex chronicus** (Chapter 24).

Lichen sclerosus (chronic atrophic vulvitis) is a nonneoplastic condition that leads to chronic atrophy, scarring, and contracture of the vulva. The cause is unknown. It is characterized by atrophic, whitish, parchment-like skin dotted with patches of leukoplakia. Lichen sclerosus occurs in all age groups, but it is most common in postmenopausal women and may progress to marked shrinking and constriction of the vulva. Despite the fact that lichen sclerosus is a nonneoplastic disease, about 2% percent of women with lichen sclerosus eventually develop vulvar squamous carcinoma.

Neoplastic lesions are the most important diseases of the vulva. *Condylomas* are broad-based, cauliflower-like, benign anogenital warts composed of hyperplastic or squamous epithelium. Two types are recognized—

condyloma lata, seen in secondary syphilis (Chapter 20), a rare condition in the United States nowadays, and the much more common **condyloma acuminatum**, which is caused by certain strains of HPV that are *not* associated with a high risk of dysplasia. Condyloma acuminatum is a fairly common lesion that occurs anywhere in the anogenital region as single or multiple growths, as is illustrated in Figure 21-6. It is contracted through sexual contact and is not premalignant.

There are two types of *vulvar squamous dysplasia and malignancy*—one associated with high-risk strains of *HPV* infection, the other with *lichen sclerosus* and the squamous hyperplasia that sometimes accompanies it.

The most common type of vulvar neoplasia is **vulvar intraepithelial neoplasia** (VIN, or *vulvar dysplasia*). VIN is uncommon and occurs mainly in women over 60; lesions tend be multiple and sometimes are widely separated on the vulva. Most of these lesions are squamous dysplasia or carcinoma and, like dysplasia and cancer of the cervix, are associated with infection by certain strains of HPV that are known to carry a high risk of inducing squamous dysplasia and carcinoma. They begin as flat, whitish or pigmented areas of squamous hyperplasia and progress slowly, often taking decades to pass through progressively severe stages of dysplasia before becoming frankly malignant. When they finally reach the stage of full malignancy, they tend to be aggressive,

poorly differentiated squamous carcinomas. A few vulvar carcinomas arise in association with lichen sclerosus and are not related to HPV infection.

Early diagnosis and surgery are effective: the five-year survival for invasive carcinoma of the vulva, whether associated with HPV or not, is about 75% for patients whose lesions are treated while less than 2 cm in diameter. If diagnosis and treatment are delayed until the tumor is greater than 2 cm in diameter, only 10% survive five years.

Diseases of the Cervix

Figure 21-7 illustrates the microanatomy and maturation of the cervix, knowledge of which is critical in the understanding of cervical disease. The endocervical canal is lined by glands composed of tall columnar epithelium; the vagina and ectocervix are lined by flat squamous epithelium—where they meet is the **squamocolumnar junction** (Fig. 21-8), which is within the cervical os at birth and in the normal adult. However, during puberty the ectocervix is transformed by metaplasia (Chapter 2) from flat squamous cells into tall, columnar glandular cells. The result is that the squamocolumnar junction is displaced outward. With sexual maturity the glandular epithelium reverts to squamous, and the squamocolumnar junction is restored to its original lo-

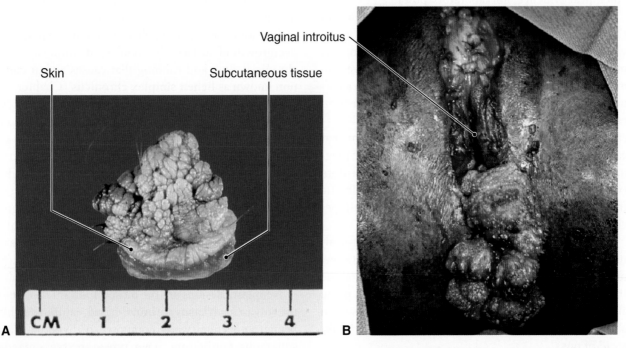

Vaginal introitus

Skin   Subcutaneous tissue

A CM 1 2 3 4   B

Figure 21-6 **Condyloma acuminatum.** These growths are caused by low-risk human papillomavirus (HPV) infection. **A,** Typical small condyloma. **B,** Multiple condylomas of the vulva.

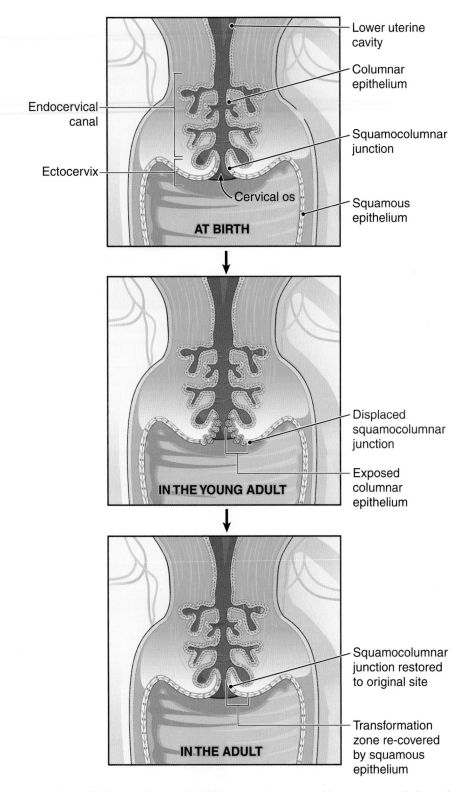

Figure 21-7 **Changes in cervical epithelium with age.** At birth the ectocervix is covered by squamous epithelium. About the time of puberty some of the squamous epithelium is transformed into glandular epithelium of the type normally found in the endocervix. The area undergoing this change is called the transformation zone. Most dysplasia and cancer of the cervix originate in this zone.

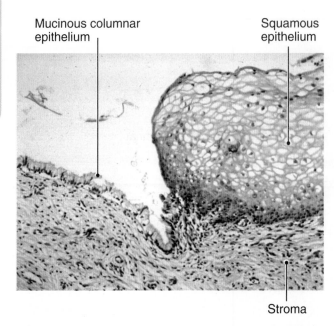

Mucinous columnar epithelium

Squamous epithelium

Stroma

Figure 21-8 **The squamocolumnar junction of the cervix.** Columnar, mucinous endocervical epithelium (left) meets ectocervical-type squamous epithelium (right). Reprinted with permission from Rubin E. Pathology. 4th ed. Philadelphia. Lippincott Williams and Wilkins, 2005.

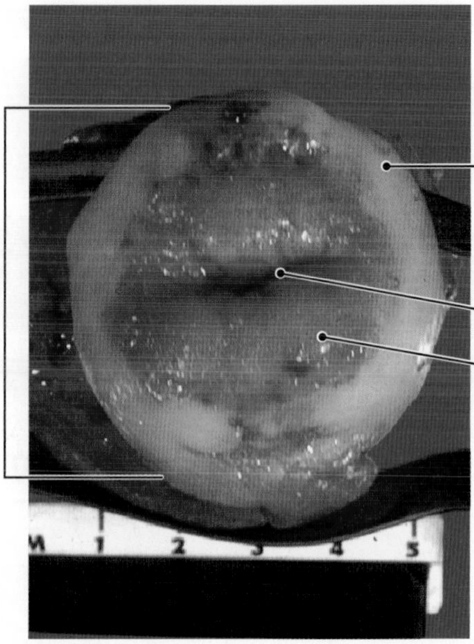

Ectocervix

Normal ectocervical squamous epithelium

Cervical os

Ectropion, or "erosion"

Figure 21-9 **Ectropion ("erosion") of the cervix.** Endocervical glandular epithelium has reappeared in the transformation zone in an adult woman. The rough, red appearance led early observers to believe it involved ulceration (erosion of the mucosa) and inflammation, hence the common clinical name, "cervical erosion."

cation. The area of temporarily transformed ectocervical epithelium is known as the **transformation zone.** *Virtually all dysplasia and carcinoma of the cervix arises in the transformation zone.*

ECTROPION, POLYPS, AND CERVICITIS

Ectropion (literally, "turning outward") of the cervix is the presence of endocervical glandular mucosa on the ectocervix. As was illustrated in Figure 21-7, ectropion is normal in young women and is easily visible on speculum examination of the cervix as a cuff of red, rough epithelium around the cervix, illustrated in Figure 21-9. Ectropion is normal in pregnancy, may remain post-partum, and may also occur in women taking birth control pills. Because ectropion resembles ulcerated (eroded) and inflamed mucosa, early physicians presumed the covering epithelium had been denuded—hence the common clinical term: **cervical erosion.** Ectropion is best considered a normal variant, like big feet or green eyes; however, it may cause spotting after intercourse and can easily be treated by applications of weak acid, which destroys the glandular epithelium and encourages return of squamous cells. Erosion plays no role in the development of cervical cancer or dysplasia.

Endocervical polyps (Fig. 21-10) are not neoplasms. Instead they are protrusions of endocervical mucosa into the endocervical canal and are often visible on speculum examination. They are usually less than 2 cm,

and they tend to occur in chronically inflamed cervices. They are not premalignant.

Acute **cervicitis** is relatively uncommon; *chronic cervicitis* is very common but usually asymptomatic. Acute cervicitis is usually caused by gonococcal or chlamydial

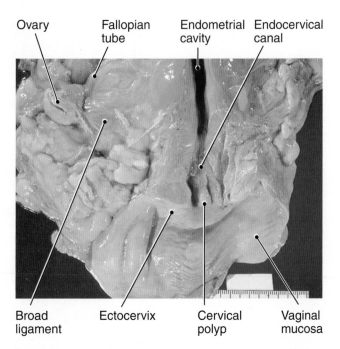

Ovary

Fallopian tube

Endometrial cavity

Endocervical canal

Broad ligament

Ectocervix

Cervical polyp

Vaginal mucosa

Figure 21-10 **Endocervical polyp.** A small polyp sits in the endocervical canal of this hysterectomy specimen.

infection or by post-partum infection with staphylococci or streptococci. Both acute cervicitis and chronic cervicitis are associated with purulent vaginal discharge (*leukorrhea*) and are treatable with antibiotics.

Microscopic examination of the cervix reveals that most women have at least some degree of *chronic cervicitis*, but it is rarely symptomatic. Chronic cervicitis is caused by local events—it is distorted in childbirth, irritated by tampons, trampled during intercourse, swarmed by vaginal microbes, and all the while must remain accessible and patent for upward passage of sperm and downward menstrual flow. The most common clinical manifestation of chronic cervicitis is mild vaginal discharge. Chronic cervicitis is also responsible for causing mildly abnormal (but benign) cells to appear on Pap smears.

DYSPLASIA AND CARCINOMA OF THE CERVIX

In 1930, cancer of the cervix and endometrium was the leading cause of cancer death for women in the United States (separate statistics were not maintained for endometrium and cervix). By 2000 the rate had been cut by nearly 90%, largely because widespread adoption of regular cervical cytology (**Pap smear**) exams led to a decline of cervical cancer, as is detailed in the nearby History of Medicine box.

Human Papillomavirus, Dysplasia, and Cancer of the Cervix

With rare exception, all cancer of the cervix is transmitted by certain *high-risk subtypes (types 16 and 18)* of **human papillomavirus**, which damage DNA (Chapter 6) and induce cells to grow uncontrollably. Repeated episodes of HPV infection can induce dysplasia or, ultimately, cervical cancer. The chance that a *single* HPV infection will culminate in cancer is virtually zero. *It is critical to realize that only a tiny percentage of women infected with HPV will ultimately develop cancer, and even then only after repeated infections over many years.*

Dysplasia refers to a *premalignant* state of cervical epithelium that features cells with abnormal nuclei but that is not yet malignant. That is, it is on the way to malignancy but is not yet malignant. *Carcinoma in situ can be conceived of as the severest form of dysplasia.* "Dysplasia" is a word widely used in casual clinical discussions, but it is not sufficiently precise for communication between clinician and pathologist, or between the pathologist examining a biopsy and a cytologist examining a Pap smear. Hence, in biopsy reports dysplasia is called **cervical intraepithelial neoplasia** (CIN), which is classified into multiple categories, as is detailed in Table 21-2.

History of Medicine

HOW THE PAP SMEAR GOT ITS NAME

The Pap smear, which has reduced the incidence of cervical cancer by 90%, is named after George Papanicolaou, affectionately called "Doctor Pap" by colleagues because of his jawbreaker name. He was born and received his medical training in Greece and later earned a PhD in Germany before coming to New York in 1913, where he passed through Ellis Island as an almost penniless immigrant among the flood fleeing Europe in advance of World War I. His first job in the United States was as a rug salesman. He played the violin in restaurants before landing a job as an assistant anatomist at Cornell University, where he remained until a few years before his death in 1962.

Dr. Papanicolaou's achievement is a powerful example of the unexpected benefits of basic research that initially may seem to have little practical application. Dr. "Pap" was studying the reproductive physiology of guinea pigs when he noticed cyclical changes in the vaginal discharge.

Applying his observations to humans he found similar changes, but purely by coincidence he also noticed abnormal cells in women with uterine cancer, an insight that Dr. Papanicolaou instantly foresaw as having far-reaching consequences, which he later describe as one of the "most thrilling experiences" of his life. He presented his findings in 1923, but they met with little interest in the medical community, which considered his method an unnecessary addition to existing diagnostic technique.

Dr. Papanicolaou persisted for twenty years, however, and in 1943 he published his famous paper showing how cervical cancers, the most deadly cancer of women at the time, could be easily detected earlier by his simple technique. Thus was born the "Pap" smear. However, the natural resistance to change inherent in daily medical practice and the primitive manner of professional scientific communication in those days resulted in slow adoption of the Pap smear, which did not become common in medical practice until the 1950s.

Table 21-2	Squamous Dysplasia of the Cervix: Comparison of Naming Schemes	
Dysplasia	**Cervical Intraepithelial Neoplasia (CIN)**	
Slight dysplasia	CIN-I	
Moderate dysplasia	CIN-II	
Severe dysplasia or carcinoma in situ	CIN-III	

There are multiple risk factors for cervical carcinoma. Among the most prominent are:

- Early age at first intercourse
- Multiple sexual partners
- A male partner with multiple female sexual partners

These risk factors were a puzzle until the role of HPV became clear: each risk factor correlates positively with *repeated* HPV infection. That is to say, cervical DNA must suffer "multiple hits" (repeated injury) before it tips over into malignancy. In addition, factors other than HPV are at work—some patients are genetically predisposed to develop cervical cancer; and patients who smoke or who are immunodeficient are at increased risk.

As is illustrated in Figures 21-11, 21-12, and 21-13, HPV induces characteristic changes (Chapter 6) of infected squamous cells—the nuclei become large, dark, and angular, and a clear cytoplasmic "halo" surrounds the nucleus. If damage persists (if reinfection occurs) these changes become more pronounced and involve increasing amounts of the epithelium until the entire thickness is occupied by severely atypical cells and the lesion is fully malignant but has not invaded across the basement membrane. Untreated carcinoma in situ may penetrate the basement membrane to become invasive carcinoma. HPV-related changes are usually confined to the transformation zone of the cervix, which is easily visualized (Fig. 21-14) by speculum exam for biopsy or Pap smear examination.

Diagnosis and Management of Dysplasia and Cancer of the Cervix

Most HPV infections disappear without permanent ill effect, somewhat like the common cold and other virus infections. Even if dysplasia has developed, most of it disappears of its own accord without treatment. However, *the more advanced the dysplasia, the more likely it is to per-*

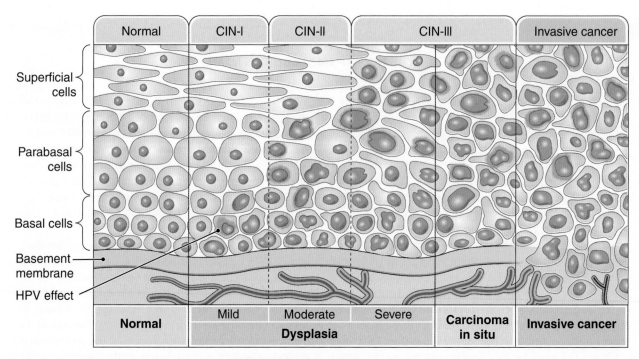

Figure 21-11 Development of dysplasia and carcinoma of the cervix. Repeated human papillomavirus (HPV) infections convert normal epithelium (left) into increasingly severe dysplasia until malignant epithelium breaks through the basement membrane to become invasive cancer, capable of metastasis by invasion of blood vessels and lymphatics.

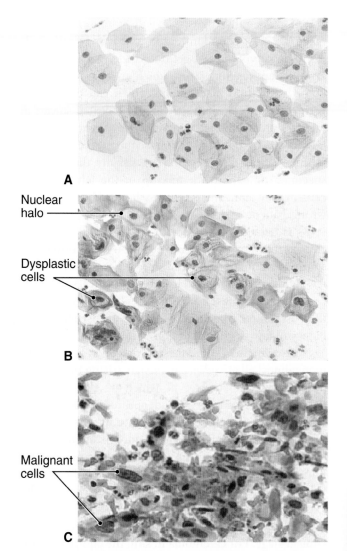

Nuclear halo

Dysplastic cells

Malignant cells

Figure 21-12 Pap smears. A, Normal. Large, flat cells with small nuclei. **B,** Dysplasia. Large, dark nuclei indicate damaged DNA; cytoplasmic halo indicates human papillomavirus (HPV) effect. **C,** Malignant. Compact cells with huge, irregular, dark nuclei indicate malignancy.

sist or become more severe. Even if a CIN-I lesion (mild dysplasia) progresses, it may take many years before it becomes invasive carcinoma. Nevertheless, *all dysplasia deserves immediate treatment and close follow-up.*

> *A single human papillomavirus (HPV) infection does not automatically produce dysplasia or cancer; repeated exposure (sexual contact) and reinfection over many years are required.*

Progression is slow from a milder degree of dysplasia to a more severe degree. The peak age incidence for CIN-III is in patients in their thirties, and the peak age incidence for invasive squamous carcinoma is in patients in their forties, suggesting it takes in the neighborhood of 10 years for CIN-III to develop into invasive

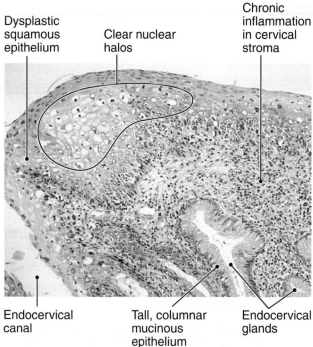

Dysplastic squamous epithelium

Clear nuclear halos

Chronic inflammation in cervical stroma

Endocervical canal

Tall, columnar mucinous epithelium

Endocervical glands

Figure 21-13 Dysplasia of the cervix (biopsy specimen). The presence of many cells with large, irregular, dark nuclei indicates DNA damage and dysplasia. Clear nuclear halos in some cells are evidence of human papillomavirus infection.

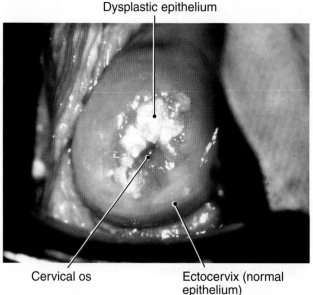

Dysplastic epithelium

Cervical os

Ectocervix (normal epithelium)

Figure 21-14 Dysplasia of the cervix (vaginal speculum view). An acid wash highlights dysplastic epithelium, which turns white.

carcinoma. This slow pace is, however, no reason postpone regular Pap smear examinations.

CIN-I and CIN-II lesions (mild or moderate dysplasia) are usually treated by superficial excision of the affected epithelium or by freezing, laser vaporization, electrocautery, chemical peeling, or other means of destroying superficial tissue. CIN-III lesions are usually treated by a surgical "coring out" of a cone of cervix (cone biopsy) so that a pathologist can examine the tissue to be sure all of the malignant epithelium has been removed and that no areas of invasion are present.

Most invasive carcinomas of the cervix are **invasive squamous carcinomas** that arise in women over the age of fifty from preexisting, asymptomatic HPV-induced dysplasia or carcinoma in situ. One of the earliest and most frequent signs of invasive carcinoma is vaginal bleeding, one of the many reasons intermenstrual or postmenopausal vaginal bleeding deserves careful investigation in every instance. Invasive carcinoma becomes progressively more symptomatic as it invades vagina, pelvis, and bladder, producing pain, dysuria, and other symptoms.

> ☞ *Half of women with invasive cervical cancer have never had a Pap smear, or have not had one in over ten years.*

As with other cancers, microscopic grading is essential to gain an estimate of the innate aggressiveness of the tumor, but clinical staging at time of diagnosis is the best gauge of prognosis and guide to therapy. Stages I–IV are defined depending on extent of local invasion, extent of pelvic involvement, and lymph node or distant metastasis (see Table 21-3 for details).

Fortunately invasive carcinoma is increasingly rare and could be virtually eliminated if every woman had regular Pap smears. However, Pap smears are not perfect—the false-negative rate for a single smear is about 20%; in other words, in patients with dysplasia there is a 20% chance that the smear will be reported as normal. The most common reason is that dysplastic cells from the cervix did not get onto the slide; a blameless error called *sampling error*, which arises from the random distribution of cells and which can occur even with correctly collected specimens. Repeated smears at regular intervals greatly increase the chance that the lesion will be detected on subsequent smears. False-positive smears are rare and are usually the result of specimen or paperwork mix-up in the lab or office, causing the abnormal cells to be attributed to the wrong patient.

As is detailed in the nearby box The Clinical Side, clinical rules vary for the investigation of abnormal Pap smears. For mildly abnormal smears a repeat smear in a few months may suffice. However, for smears that suggest dysplasia, most patients and physicians consider the best course of action to be careful inspection and biopsy of any suspicious lesion of the cervix.

Nonsquamous carcinomas of the cervix are uncommon; almost all are *adenocarcinomas* arising from mucinous cells of the endocervix, which are also related to HPV infection. Endocervical adenocarcinomas are especially troublesome because they are as aggressive as squamous carcinoma but much more difficult to detect—they originate in the endocervical canal and are not easily seen by visual examination of the cervix. What's more, they shed few cells that can be detected by Pap smear.

Therapy for carcinoma of the cervix depends on the clinical stage. For carcinoma in situ, the choice is surgical removal by cone biopsy; for invasive carcinoma, hysterectomy is usually recommended (Fig. 21-15). Advanced cases may call for surgery, radiation, and chemotherapy.

Table 21-3	Squamous Carcinoma of the Cervix: Stage and Five-Year Survival	
Clinical Stage	**Definition**	**5-year Survival Rate**
0	Carcinoma in situ	100%
I	Invasive, confined to cervix or uterine corpus	90%
II	Invasion beyond cervix but not reaching lateral pelvic wall or lower third of vagina	70%
III	Invasion to lateral pelvic wall or lower third of vagina	35%
IV	Extension beyond the pelvis: involvement of bladder or rectum or distant metastasis	10%

THE PAP SMEAR

The mainstay of cervical cancer prevention is the Pap smear. However, newer tests detect the presence of human papillomavirus (HPV) in cervical specimens, and a debate is under way about the best use of this new technology.

Typically, Pap smears are collected using a spatula or brush to scrape cells from the cervix. The cells are then smeared on a small glass slide and quickly treated with alcohol to preserve them until they reach the laboratory. An alternative method, "thin prep" technology, is gaining popularity. Collected cells are placed in a special solution, which is mechanically spread onto a slide in a uniform layer that is easier to examine microscopically. In both cases the cells are stained to give them color and then examined microscopically by specially trained and certified laboratory personnel (pathologists, cytotechnologists).

Microscopic findings are reported using the following classification, called the **Bethesda System**:

- Negative or Within Normal Limits ("WNL")
- Atypical Squamous Cells of Undetermined Significance ("ASCUS")
- Low-Grade Squamous Intraepithelial Lesions ("LSIL")
- High-Grade Squamous Intraepithelial Lesions ("HSIL")
- Carcinoma

With the exception that patients with "Carcinoma" findings are virtually certain to have invasive cancer, there is not a *strict* correlation between the degree of Pap smear abnormality and biopsy findings. Nevertheless, there *is* correlation; for example, patients with "LSIL" smear findings are less likely to have severe dysplasia or carcinoma in situ (CIN-III) than are patients with "HSIL."

Follow-up after the smear is reported depends on many factors, and recommendations vary from one group of experts to another. In general, women under age thirty (the group with most human papillomavirus infections) who have "WNL" smears should have a repeat smear annually. Women over the age of thirty who have had three consecutive "WNL" smears can safely reduce the frequency of Pap smears to one every three years.

In general, women whose smears are reported as "atypical squamous cells of uncertain significance" (ASCUS) should return for a repeat smear in a few months. Some experts recommend HPV molecular testing of cervical cells in ASCUS patients and further diagnostic tests on those proven to have HPV infection. Women whose smears are reported as "low-grade squamous intraepithelial lesion" or "high-grade squamous in-

traepithelial lesion" should have **colposcopy** (visual inspection of the cervix through a low power microscope), and any visible lesion should be biopsied. Women with "Carcinoma" smears should have immediate colposcopy and biopsy.

There is more to the Pap smear than you may think.

- *The Pap smear evaluation is a medical consultation*, just the same as if a surgeon is asked to see a patient with possible appendicitis, and it is imperative that some statement of the patient's medical history accompany the request.
- *All Pap smears are examined in a chain of command* that includes a pathologist, who must examine certain abnormal smears and make a formal diagnosis.
- *False-negative test results are common* (about 20% of women with dysplasia have a negative test result, usually resulting from sampling error); false-positive results are very rare.
- *Abnormal Pap smears are not diagnostic*; they merely raise the index of suspicion. That is, every abnormal smear requires further clinical examination or biopsy to prove the presence or absence of dysplasia or cancer.
- *Inadequate specimens are common*: specimens that are improperly collected may not have adequate numbers or types of cells; specimens can be improperly preserved, or cells can be obscured by excessive blood.
- *The report should contain the following critical elements*, which are illustrated in the accompanying figure:
  - *Identifying information*: 1) Names of the patient, person collecting the smear, cytotechnologist, and pathologist; 2) Patient's age, birth date, and social security number or other unique identifier; 3) Tracking information, such as the number assigned to the smear, when it was collected, and how it was examined and reported.
  - *Whether or not the specimen is satisfactory*: If the smear does not contain an adequate number of epithelial cells, it is ruled unsatisfactory, and another smear should be collected.
  - *The source of the smear* (usually from the cervix; from the vagina in a patient without a uterus).
  - *Findings*:
    - If there is evidence of infection; if so, what kind.
    - Whether the results are considered normal or abnormal; and if abnormal, a statement about the type of abnormality found (Bethesda System).
  - *Recommendation for follow-up*; for example, biopsy or re-smear.

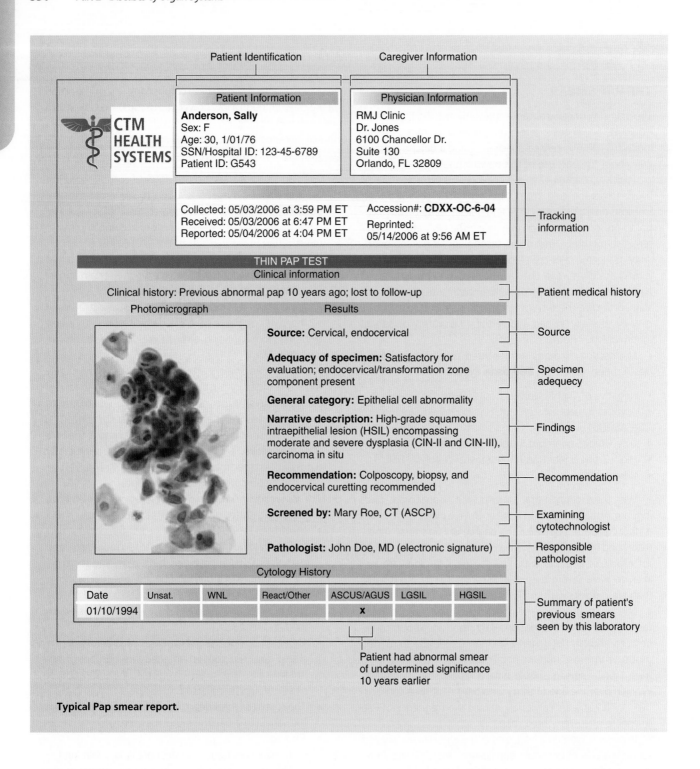

Patient Identification   Caregiver Information

Patient Information	Physician Information
Anderson, Sally Sex: F Age: 30, 1/01/76 SSN/Hospital ID: 123-45-6789 Patient ID: G543	RMJ Clinic Dr. Jones 6100 Chancellor Dr. Suite 130 Orlando, FL 32809

CTM HEALTH SYSTEMS

Collected: 05/03/2006 at 3:59 PM ET
Received: 05/03/2006 at 6:47 PM ET
Reported: 05/04/2006 at 4:04 PM ET

Accession#: **CDXX-OC-6-04**
Reprinted:
05/14/2006 at 9:56 AM ET

— Tracking information

THIN PAP TEST
Clinical information

Clinical history: Previous abnormal pap 10 years ago; lost to follow-up — Patient medical history

Photomicrograph   Results

Source: Cervical, endocervical — Source

Adequacy of specimen: Satisfactory for evaluation; endocervical/transformation zone component present — Specimen adequecy

General category: Epithelial cell abnormality

Narrative description: High-grade squamous intraepithelial lesion (HSIL) encompassing moderate and severe dysplasia (CIN-II and CIN-III), carcinoma in situ — Findings

Recommendation: Colposcopy, biopsy, and endocervical curetting recommended — Recommendation

Screened by: Mary Roe, CT (ASCP) — Examining cytotechnologist

Pathologist: John Doe, MD (electronic signature) — Responsible pathologist

Cytology History

Date	Unsat.	WNL	React/Other	ASCUS/AGUS	LGSIL	HGSIL
01/10/1994				x		

— Summary of patient's previous smears seen by this laboratory

Patient had abnormal smear of undetermined significance 10 years earlier

Typical Pap smear report.

Diseases of the Endometrium and Myometrium

Understanding the physiology of the menstrual cycle is critical to an understanding of endometrial disease. The simple fact that the endometrium sheds monthly during reproductive years and is atrophic thereafter is a very important fact: it makes the endometrium unusually re-sistant to infection and especially susceptible to hormonal abnormalities.

Most acute inflammation of the endometrium (**endometritis**) occurs postpartum or post-abortion and is usually associated with retained fragments of placenta after delivery or retained products of conception after a spontaneous abortion. Removal of the retained tissue results in prompt resolution.

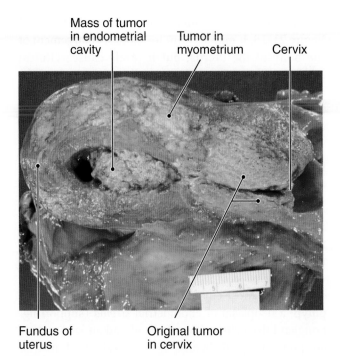

Figure 21-15 **Invasive carcinoma of the cervix.** Extensive involvement of the cervix, endometrium, and uterus is evident.

ABNORMAL ENDOMETRIAL BLEEDING

Menstrual problems and abnormal vaginal bleeding are the most common reasons women seek gynecologic care.

Amenorrhea is the absence of menstruation, and it may be primary or secondary. *Primary* amenorrhea (failure of the ovary itself) may be caused by a genetic disease, such as *Turner syndrome*, a sex chromosome abnormality (Chapter 7) in which the ovaries do not function. *Secondary* amenorrhea (failure of ovarian hormonal support) may be caused by pituitary-hypothalamic disorders, psychological stress, eating disorders, severe weight loss, or intense athletic training. **Dysmenorrhea** is painful menstruation. Most women feel some discomfort with menstruation, and occasionally it interferes with normal activity. In most instances it is not associated with anatomic disease.

There are several clinical types of abnormal endometrial bleeding:

- **menorrhagia**: excessive bleeding at the time of regular menstrual flow
- **metrorrhagia**: irregular bleeding between periods
- **polymenorrhea**: frequent, short cycles, less than 3 weeks
- **oligomenorrhea**: few, long cycles, longer than 6 weeks
- **ovulatory bleeding**: occurs at ovulation; it is usually minor and may be associated with lower abdominal

pain as the graafian follicle ruptures through the ovarian surface.

Abnormal endometrial bleeding is a serious matter because it may indicate endometrial, vaginal, or cervical carcinoma or other grave problem.

Abnormal endometrial bleeding falls into two broad categories. Bleeding associated with pathologic lesions is called **pathologic uterine bleeding**. It is relatively uncommon and can be caused by complications of pregnancy (abortion, ectopic pregnancy, retained products of conception), by tumors of the myometrium, or by endometrial polyps, hyperplasia, or tumors.

By definition, **dysfunctional uterine bleeding** is abnormal uterine bleeding *not* associated with a specific anatomic cause. Dysfunctional uterine bleeding falls into four categories:

- *Ovulatory failure* (**anovulatory cycle**): If ovulation does not occur, no corpus luteum forms and no progesterone is produced. Therefore, the proliferative endometrium that grew between menstruation and ovulation does not receive the expected support from a corpus luteum, and it sloughs away as a bloody drainage at an unexpectedly early time in the cycle (about midway, immediately after ovulation should have occurred). Anovulatory cycles are common and may be caused by a failure in the pituitary to secrete LH, adrenal or thyroid hormonal abnormalities, malnutrition, severe psychological or physical stress, or obesity.
- *Inadequate progesterone production by the corpus luteum*: The corpus luteum may not produce enough progesterone, or it may wither early. If there is not sufficient progesterone to support the secretory endometrium, it will die. The result is bleeding at an unexpected time.
- *"Pill"-induced bleeding*: Early contraceptive formulations contained estrogen and progesterone in amounts that caused unexpected bleeding. Modern oral contraceptives contain a balance of hormones that rarely cause abnormal bleeding.
- *Long-term estrogen replacement therapy*: Though estrogen replacement therapy for postmenopausal women is much less common now than heretofore, it can cause irregular bleeding.

ENDOMETRIOSIS

Endometriosis is deposits of endometrium outside of the uterine cavity (Fig. 21-16). It consists of accumulations of normal endometrium in abnormal places—most often in the ovaries (80% of cases), fallopian tubes,

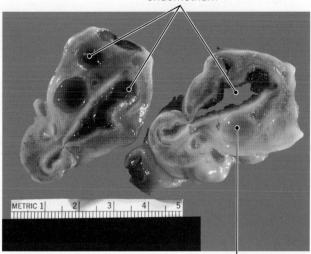

Deposits of hemorrhagic endometrium

METRIC 1 2 3 4 5

Follicle (graafian) cyst

Figure 21-16 **Endometriosis of the ovary.** Hemorrhagic, cystic deposits of endometrium are visible in this ovary. Note the small follicle cyst.

or pelvic peritoneal surfaces. On occasion it occurs in the lungs, liver, or lymph nodes.

Endometriosis is an important clinical condition: it affects 3% of women of reproductive age and is often the cause of infertility, pelvic pain, and dysmenorrhea. Figure 21-17 illustrates places where endometrial deposits tend to occur. How endometrium comes to be located in these odd places remains unknown. This displaced endometrium undergoes cyclic menstrual changes and bleeding in parallel with uterine endometrium. The bleeding occurs into tissues, inciting inflammation and fibrosis, which accounts for most of the symptoms and associated problems. Deposits vary from a few millimeters to several centimeters and contain a mixture of endometrium, blood, inflammatory cells, and fibrosis. Typical of ovarian endometriosis are cysts termed "chocolate cysts" because they contain collections of dark brown, syrupy altered blood.

Clinical symptoms depend on the anatomic sites involved—painful defecation may reflect deposits low in the posterior pelvic peritoneum; dysuria may result from deposits in the dome of the bladder; infertility may reflect blocked fallopian tubes. Half of all women with dysmenorrhea (painful menstruation) have endometriosis; in one third of infertile couples the woman has endometriosis.

Endometrium also may be found deep in the wall of the uterus. This condition, called **adenomyosis**, represents an extension of endometrium (both glands and stroma) deep into the myometrium, as is illustrated in Figure 21-18. It may account for modest enlargement of the body of the uterus, but it rarely causes clinical symptoms, because it is hormonally inert and does not bleed. It is a pathologic curiosity most often encountered as a pathologic diagnosis in a uterus removed for other reasons.

ENDOMETRIAL POLYPS, HYPERPLASIA, AND ADENOCARCINOMA

Adenomas (benign tumors of glandular organs) and other benign tumors of the endometrial epithelium are not known, probably because menstruation washes them away before they have time to form.

There are, however, benign growths of the endometrium. Most common is the benign **endometrial polyp**, a neoplasm of endometrial *stroma* (supporting, nonglandular cells). These have abundant stroma and are populated with benign cystic glands. Endometrial polyps are not premalignant, they may occur at any age, but they are most common near menopause. They make themselves known by causing abnormal uterine bleeding.

Endometrial hyperplasia (Fig. 21-19) is an overgrowth of endometrial glandular *epithelium* that can proceed to endometrial adenocarcinoma. Hyperplasia and carcinoma are more common in women with conditions that tend to result in high levels of blood estrogen. Causes of excessive estrogen production include:

- *Obesity*: The most significant risk factor is estrogen synthesized in fat cells. Women who are 50 lb overweight have ten times the risk of women who are not overweight.
- *Estrogen replacement therapy* in postmenopausal women.
- *Reproductive characteristics that cause increased levels of blood estrogen*: Some women have irregular periods because of failed ovulation (anovulatory cycles), which is associated with a prolonged estrogen effect that is not moderated by progesterone. (These women also are less likely to ever become pregnant.) Excessive estrogen is thus unrelieved by the tide of progesterone from the corpus luteum in a normal cycle or from the placenta during pregnancy.
- *Estrogen-secreting tumors of the ovary*. This condition is rare.

Diabetes and hypertension are additional risk factors for endometrial hyperplasia that are unrelated to estrogen effects.

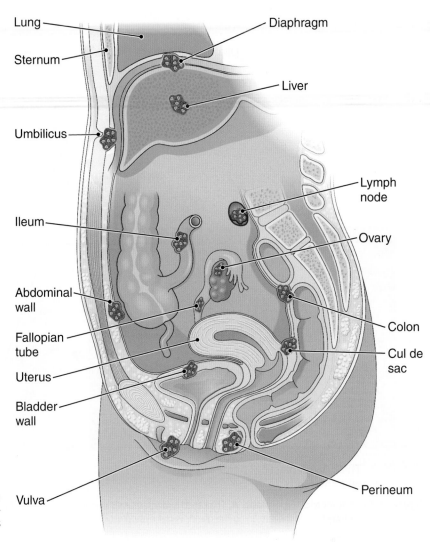

***Figure 21-17* Endometriosis.** The drawing shows some of the sites where endometrial deposits can occur. Most deposits occur in the pelvis and genitalia.

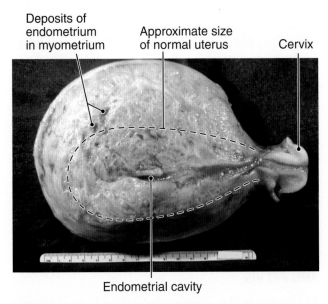

***Figure 21-18* Adenomyosis.** The enlargement of this uterus is caused by endometrial implants in the myometrium. Dotted lines indicate the normal size of the uterus.

Three types of endometrial hyperplasia are recognized, but they are part of the same process:

- **Simple hyperplasia** (sometimes called *cystic hyperplasia*). Microscopically, individual cells are not unusual (they are not atypical), and the glands are simple tubes that are often cystically dilated. If untreated, about 1% of these cases progress to *uterine cancer* (**endometrial adenocarcinoma**) in 10 years.
- **Complex hyperplasia.** The glands are folded and tightly packed, but individual cells show no atypia. If untreated, about 3% of these cases progress to endometrial adenocarcinoma in 10 years.
- **Atypical hyperplasia.** The glands are twisted, complex, and crowded and individual cells have abnormal nuclei (nuclear atypia). If untreated, about 25% of these cases progress to endometrial adenocarcinoma in 4 years.

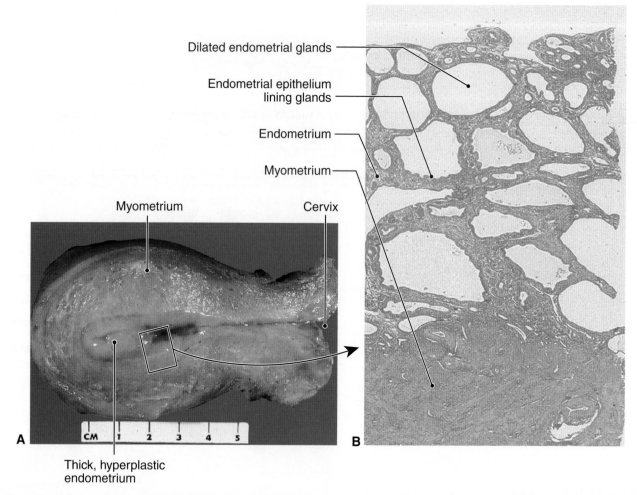

Dilated endometrial glands

Endometrial epithelium
lining glands

Endometrium

Myometrium

Myometrium   Cervix

A   CM   1   2   3   4   5   B

Thick, hyperplastic
endometrium

Figure 21-19 Endometrial hyperplasia. A, Thickened endometrium is evident in this uterus. **B,** Microscopic examination reveals simple, cystic hyperplasia. The endometrial epithelium lining the glands is not hyperplastic.

Effective use of Pap smears has so reduced the incidence of *cervical* cancer that *uterine* cancer (Fig. 21-20) is now the most common cancer of the female genital tract. Unfortunately, there is no useful screening test for uterine cancer: Pap smears are not useful because malignant endometrial cells are rarely shed in sufficient numbers to be detectable by Pap smear.

Uterine cancer occurs most frequently in women around 60 years old. Usually first among clinical signs is abnormal vaginal bleeding. *Vaginal bleeding in a postmenopausal woman must always be thoroughly investigated*; it never should be presumed to be functional or innocuous. There are few other clinical signs of endometrial cancer—in stage I the uterus may be slightly enlarged, scarcely a reliable sign of cancer when so many other more common conditions could be responsible.

The only effective screening technique for endometrial cancer is an annual pelvic examination. Endome-

trial biopsy is a reliable diagnostic tool, but it is an invasive and expensive procedure and cannot be considered a routine test.

Uterine cancers are somewhat slow growing and metastasize late, usually after first invading the muscular wall of the uterus (the myometrium) and then outward into nearby pelvic structures such as ovaries, fallopian tubes, and bladder.

Surgical excision of the uterus, fallopian tubes, ovaries, and pelvic lymph nodes is preferred therapy. Clinical stages and 5-year survival percentages are illustrated in Figure 21-21.

OTHER CONDITIONS OF THE UTERUS AND PELVIS

The uterine wall is composed of a thick layer of smooth muscle that tends to form benign smooth muscle tumors, **leiomyomas** (commonly called **fibroids**), which

Fallopian
tube

Ovary

Ovarian
ligament

Endometrial
adenocarcinoma

Ovary

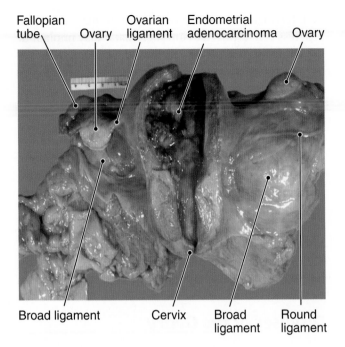

Broad ligament

Cervix

Broad
ligament

Round
ligament

Figure 21-20 **Endometrial carcinoma.** In this hysterectomy specimen showing the uterus, tubes, and ovaries, the opened uterus reveals a ragged mass of cancer filling the endometrial cavity.

are the most common benign tumors of women and occur in a third to half of all women. Genetic influence is important—leiomyomas are much more common in African-American women than in others. Leiomyomas grow larger under the influence of estrogen and oral contraceptives and shrink after menopause. Multiple tumors are often present (Fig. 21-22) and may occur in such numbers and grow to such size that they cause abnormal uterine bleeding or infertility by distorting the endometrial cavity. Rarely, they may become enormous: neglected cases have been documented that have reached more than 100 lb. They are often detected at routine pelvic exam but may become symptomatic initially by abnormal uterine bleeding, pain, or a sensation of pelvic heaviness. They are composed of compact, round masses of normal smooth muscle cells and are not premalignant.

Leiomyosarcoma is a rare malignant smooth muscle tumor that can arise from smooth muscle anywhere in the body, but in the uterus it arises directly from uterine smooth muscle cells, not from a preexisting leiomyoma. Leiomyosarcoma is usually quite large and advanced when discovered, and it is usually fatal.

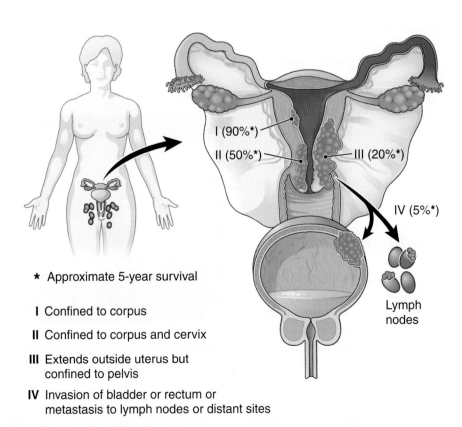

I (90%*)

II (50%*)

III (20%*)

IV (5%*)

Lymph
nodes

* Approximate 5-year survival

I Confined to corpus

II Confined to corpus and cervix

III Extends outside uterus but confined to pelvis

IV Invasion of bladder or rectum or metastasis to lymph nodes or distant sites

Figure 21-21 **Staging of endometrial carcinoma.** Approximate 5-year survival percentage is (%) shown for various stages.

Body of uterus

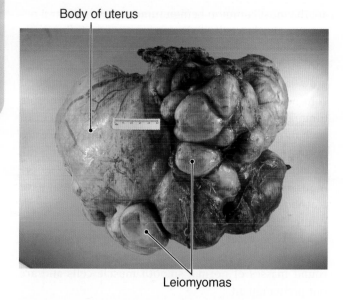

Leiomyomas

Figure 21-22 **Multiple leiomyomas of the uterus.**

Normally the uterus sits immediately behind the pubic bone and tilts slightly forward. When not in this position, the uterus is said to be *malpositioned*. It may be displaced to the rear or excessively tilted (flexed) backward or forward. These abnormal positions have a debatable role in painful menstruation, painful intercourse, and infertility.

There is, however, no debate about **pelvic relaxation syndrome**. Pelvic ligaments may become so relaxed by age and multiple vaginal deliveries that the uterus may slide downward into the vagina (**uterine prolapse**), sometimes so far that the cervix protrudes from the external vaginal opening (introitus). Alternatively, when straining at stool the rectum may bulge forward into the vagina (a protrusion called **rectocele**), which may interfere with bowel movements. The bladder also may bulge downward into the anterior aspect of the vagina (a protrusion called **cystocele**), which interferes with urination.

Diseases of the Fallopian Tube

Pelvic inflammatory disease (PID) is inflammation of the fallopian tubes. PID is also known as **salpingitis**, and it is almost always infectious and sexually transmitted (Chapter 20), Nongonococcal infections, such as *Chlamydia* and *Mycoplasma*, are the most common cause of salpingitis. Repeated infections may produce severe inflammation and scarring that may incorporate the ovary into a single inflammatory mass called a **tuboovarian abscess** (Fig. 21-23). Such inflammation and associated scarring may so impede progress of sperm

that fertilization is impossible, or it may slow the progress of a fertilized ovum such that it may implant in the fallopian tube before reaching the endometrial cavity. The result is an **ectopic pregnancy** (discussed in detail below).

Lower abdominal pain is the primary symptom of salpingitis. Fever and elevated WBC count are common with acute infection but may be absent with chronic disease. Tenderness on pelvic exam is common, and pus may drain from the cervical os. Acute cases respond well to antibiotics, but inflammation and scarring may be so severe in recurrent or chronic infections that only surgical removal of the tubes and ovaries can provide relief.

Endometriosis is the only other fairly common affliction of the fallopian tubes. It also may produce tubal scarring, which can cause infertility or ectopic pregnancy.

Diseases of the Ovary

The most common abnormalities of the ovary are nonneoplastic cysts and neoplasms, most of which also tend to be cystic. Inflammation of the ovary is almost always secondary to inflammation of the fallopian tube caused by sexually transmitted disease.

NONNEOPLASTIC OVARIAN CYSTS

Follicle cysts are enlarged, unruptured graafian follicles (from which, in normal ovulation, an ovum is

Dilated fallopian tube filled with pus

Proximal end of fallopian tube

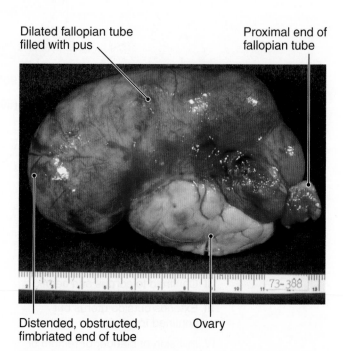

Distended, obstructed, fimbriated end of tube

Ovary

Figure 21-23 **Tuboovarian abscess.** Such an abscess is one result of sexually transmitted disease. It is most often caused by nongonococcal infection of the fallopian tube.

ejected). **Luteal cysts** are formed of graafian follicles that rupture and reseal in the luteal phase and accumulate fluid to become cystic. Follicle cysts and luteal cysts are so common they might as well be considered normal variants, like large feet in a small person. These common cysts are smooth walled and filled with thin, clear (serous) fluid. They are small, usually less than a centimeter, but they may grow to 4–5 cm, and they may account for pelvic pain or a palpable mass discovered on pelvic examination.

Polycystic ovary syndrome (*Stein-Leventhal syndrome*) occurs in about 5% of women in their reproductive years and features hormonal abnormalities and ovaries with a thick, fibrous rind on the surface, beneath which are numerous follicle cysts. The cause is unknown. Most patients are insulin resistant, similar to patients with type 2 diabetes. Other biochemical abnormalities include excessive androgens (masculinizing hormones), abnormal levels of blood lipids, and high blood insulin levels.

Clinical features include obesity, oligomenorrhea (diminished menstrual bleeding), hirsutism, and acne as a result of excess androgens, and *infertility*, caused by chronic inability to ovulate. Women with polycystic ovary syndrome have a markedly increased risk for cardiovascular disease, and nearly half develop glucose intolerance or type 2 diabetes.

Research has shown that diabetes management techniques such as weight reduction and the administration of oral hypoglycemic agents can reverse the hormone abnormalities and infertility associated with polycystic ovary syndrome and can improve glucose and insulin metabolism and reverse blood lipid abnormalities, too.

TUMORS OF THE OVARY

The ovary contains three kinds of cells: 1) *germ cells* for reproduction; 2) hormone-producing *stromal cells*, which form the bulk of the ovarian mass and support ovulation and pregnancy, and 3) surface *epithelial cells* derived from peritoneum. Each type of cell produces several distinctive neoplasms (Fig. 21-24). While carcinoma of the endometrium is the most common cancer of the female genital tract, it is carcinoma of the ovary that causes the most deaths. Ovarian carcinomas are silent, lethal neoplasms.

Following are some rules of thumb to keep in mind about ovarian *masses* and *neoplasms*:

- Most ovarian *masses* are benign cysts
- About 65% of ovarian *neoplasms* arise from the surface epithelium
- About half of ovarian *neoplasms* are bilateral

- About 90% of ovarian *malignancies* are carcinomas of the surface epithelium

Tumors of the Surface Epithelium

The surface epithelium of the ovary is a thin membrane of flat, inactive cells derived from peritoneum. When neoplastic, however, they are transformed into tall columnar cells that may secrete fluid. Tumors of the surface epithelium comprise about 65% of all ovarian tumors and may be benign or malignant. They are usually *cystic* and if benign and cystic are called **cystadenoma**, or if malignant and cystic are called **cystadenocarcinoma**. They are often *bilateral* and rarely exhibit hormonal activity.

There are three main types of surface epithelial tumors:

- **Serous tumors**, which resemble the epithelium lining the fallopian tube, secrete a watery, nonmucinous fluid and are usually cystic and have a papillary growth pattern (Figs. 21-25 and 21-26).
- **Mucinous tumors**, which resemble the epithelium lining the endocervix, secrete thick mucin and are usually cystic and have a papillary growth pattern (Fig. 21-27).
- **Endometrioid tumors**, which resemble the epithelium-forming endometrial glands, may secrete small amount of nonmucinous fluid but tend to be solid rather than cystic. Endometrioid tumors resemble endometrial (uterine) carcinoma, and about one third are accompanied by simultaneous endometrial carcinoma (which is *not* metastatic from the ovary; it is a second primary cancer).

Neoplasms of the surface epithelium are classified into one of three categories according to their potential to spread:

- *benign*
- *borderline malignant*
- *malignant*

Regardless of type, or whether benign or malignant, ovarian neoplasms rarely cause symptoms (pain, vaginal bleeding, or pelvic fullness) until large. At the time of diagnosis more than half of malignant tumors have invaded adjacent organs or spread to the peritoneal cavity and are beyond hope of cure. For frankly malignant tumors, the 5-year survival is 35%; 10-year survival is about 10%. Benign tumors are curable by excision. For borderline malignant tumors with no capsular invasion, the five-year survival rate is near 100%. Table 21-4 summarizes some important facts about tumors of the surface epithelium and other ovarian tumors.

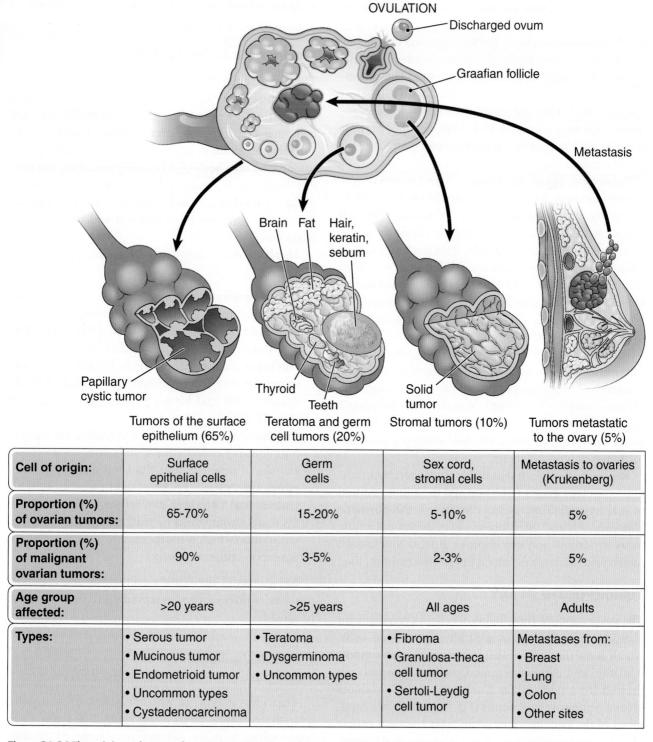

OVULATION

Discharged ovum

Graafian follicle

Metastasis

Brain Fat Hair, keratin, sebum

Papillary cystic tumor

Thyroid

Teeth

Solid tumor

Tumors of the surface epithelium (65%)

Teratoma and germ cell tumors (20%)

Stromal tumors (10%)

Tumors metastatic to the ovary (5%)

	Tumors of the surface epithelium (65%)	Teratoma and germ cell tumors (20%)	Stromal tumors (10%)	Tumors metastatic to the ovary (5%)
Cell of origin:	Surface epithelial cells	Germ cells	Sex cord, stromal cells	Metastasis to ovaries (Krukenberg)
Proportion (%) of ovarian tumors:	65-70%	15-20%	5-10%	5%
Proportion (%) of malignant ovarian tumors:	90%	3-5%	2-3%	5%
Age group affected:	>20 years	>25 years	All ages	Adults
Types:	• Serous tumor • Mucinous tumor • Endometrioid tumor • Uncommon types • Cystadenocarcinoma	• Teratoma • Dysgerminoma • Uncommon types	• Fibroma • Granulosa-theca cell tumor • Sertoli-Leydig cell tumor	Metastases from: • Breast • Lung • Colon • Other sites

Figure 21-24 The origin and types of ovarian tumors. The table summarizes important facts about frequency and age ranges.

Tumors of Germ Cells (Teratomas)

A *teratoma* is a tumor that contains tissues not normally found in the organ from which it arises. **Ovarian teratomas** arise from germ cells and comprise about 20% of all ovarian neoplasms. Most are cystic and contain skin and hair, hence the common name—**dermoid cyst** (skin-like cyst, Fig. 21-28). Most are unilateral and benign, arise in girls or young women, and do not grow larger than softball size. Some are discovered incidentally during pelvic exam or on radiographs that disclose odd images in the pelvis; teeth, for example.

Fallopian tube   Uterus

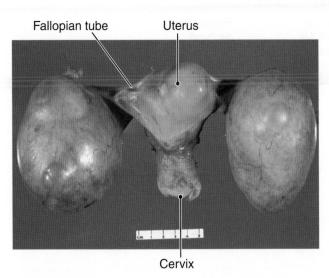

Cervix

Epithelial papillations   Secondary cysts

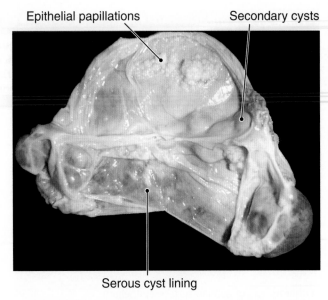

Serous cyst lining

Figure 21-25 Bilateral serous cystadenocarcinoma of the ovaries. Ovarian tumors are often bilateral.

Figure 21-26 Cystic serous tumor of the ovary, borderline malignant. Nearly 100% of these patients survive if papillary growth does not reach the external surface.

Pathologically dermoid cysts are malodorous cysts lined by skin and filled with pasty sebaceous material and matted long hair. Because of the omnipotent nature of germ cells, literally any type of tissue can be found—teeth, bone, cartilage, brain, retina, thyroid, stomach. For reasons that escape understanding, dermoid cysts may be associated with infertility and they occur most often in the right ovary.

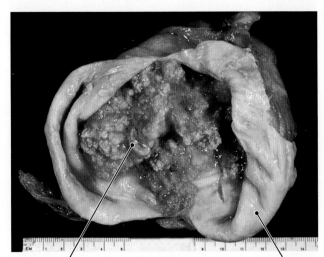

Papillary tumor mass
projecting into cyst cavity

Cyst lining

Figure 21-27 Mucinous cystadenocarcinoma of the ovary. Papillary epithelial growth fills the cyst cavity. Note the glistening of mucous secretions.

Among other germ cell tumors are **dysgerminoma**, the ovarian counterpart to testicular seminoma, and **choriocarcinoma**, a malignant tumor identical to the placental tumor of the same name.

Other Ovarian Tumors

Ovarian stromal cell tumors comprise about 10% of ovarian tumors. Most are **ovarian fibromas** (Fig. 21-29) and are solid, white, unilateral, and benign. **Granulosa-theca cell tumor** is usually yellow and solid and produces large amounts of estrogen similar to the corpus luteum, after which it is named. It is sluggishly aggressive and has the capacity to invade locally, but it rarely metastasizes.

A tumor formed by metastatic spread to the ovary from cancer in another organ is called a **Krukenberg tumor** and comprises about 5% of ovarian tumors. The ovary is more often the site of metastasis than its size and vascular supply would imply, suggesting that the hormonal environment is especially conducive to implantation of malignant cells circulating in blood. Breast, lung, and gastrointestinal carcinomas are the most frequent culprits.

Clinical Aspects of Ovarian Tumors

Ovarian cancer is the second most common gynecologic malignancy after endometrial carcinoma. However, ovarian cancers cause more deaths because they are so difficult to detect early: The pelvis is roomy enough to accommodate them easily, and they do not secrete hor-

Table 21-4 *Characteristics of Selected Ovarian Tumors*			
Tumor Type	**Frequency As % of All Ovarian Tumors**	**Frequency As % of Malignant Ovarian Tumors**	**% That Are Bilateral**
Serous	65%	45%	
Benign: 60%			25%
Borderline: 15%			30%
Malignant: 25%			65%
Mucinous	65%	10%	
Benign: 80%			5%
Borderline: 10%			10%
Malignant: 10%			20%
Endometrioid	65%	20%	40%
Other tumors of ovarian surface epithelium	65%	15%	Varies
Teratoma and other germ cell tumors	20%	Rare	Rare
Benign: 95%			
Malignant: 5%			
Stromal tumors (granulosa cell, thecoma)	10%	Rare	Rare
Carcinoma metastatic to the ovary	5%	5%	>50%

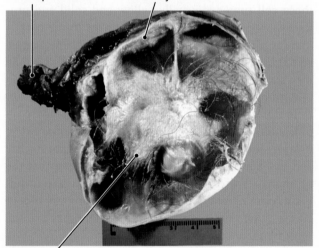

Fimbriated end of fallopian tube

Wall of cyst lined by skin

Mass of hair and sebaceous material

Figure 21-28 **Benign ovarian cystic teratoma (dermoid cyst).** Note hair and sebaceous material.

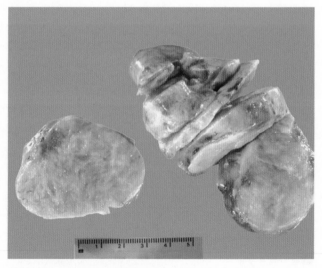

Figure 21-29 **Ovarian fibroma.** A fibroma is a solid, white tumor of ovarian stroma.

mones that might call attention by their effect on other organs. Nevertheless, many ovarian tumors secrete an *antibody* to a cancer antigen, **anti-CA-125**, and detection of this antibody can be a clue to the presence of ovarian cancer. However, it is not suitable as a *screening* test because false-negative test results are very common.

Ovarian cancer ranks fourth as a cause of cancer death in women, behind cancers of the lung, breast, and colon. About 5% of cases are associated with inheritance of the BRCA gene, which is also related to breast cancer and is discussed later in this chapter.

Typically, symptoms of ovarian cancer are slow to become noticeable because the requirements of pregnancy include space for something large to grow in the female pelvis. About a third are discovered during routine gynecologic exam or during an examination for an unrelated problem. At the time of discovery, more than half of malignant ovarian tumors have spread beyond reasonable hope of cure. Despite the great variety of ovarian neoplasms, the symptoms they produce are much the same: a feeling of pelvic heaviness or fullness, dysuria, frequency or other urinary complaint, pelvic pain, and painful defecation. Some tumors fill enough of the abdomen that increased girth is the presenting complaint.

Clinical staging is the best guide to therapy, and prognosis depends on confinement to the ovaries, local spread, peritoneal seeding, or distant metastasis. Surgery is the treatment of choice; chemotherapy is also useful.

Diseases of Reproduction

Birth, n. The first and direst of all disasters.
AMBROSE BIERCE (1842–1914?), AMERICAN SATIRIST, JOURNALIST, AND SHORT-STORY WRITER, *THE DEVIL'S DICTIONARY*

Under this heading we will discuss things that go wrong in the chain of events in reproduction: 1) infertility; 2) abnormal implantation of the fertilized ovum; 3) premature death of the fetus (*abortion, miscarriage*); 4) diseases of the placenta; and 5) pathologic effects of pregnancy on the mother.

INFERTILITY

Male aspects of infertility are discussed in Chapter 20.

Infertility is the inability of a couple to conceive after 1 year of regular intercourse. About 1 in 5 couples in the United States is affected. Causes include sperm disorders (about 35% of couples), ovarian dysfunction (20%), fallopian tube dysfunction (30%), and abnormal

cervical mucus that is "toxic" to sperm (5%). In about 10% of cases, the cause cannot be identified.

The causes of infertility in women are varied and include:

- Obstruction of the fallopian tube caused by chronic salpingitis (the most common cause, usually owing to sexually transmitted infection). (See Case Study 21-2 at the end of this chapter.)
- Large uterine leiomyomas that distort the endometrial cavity so that implantation cannot occur.
- Abnormal cervical mucus can be "toxic" to sperm.
- Some ova are resistant to conception, especially those in older women.
- Irregular or infrequent ovulation significantly decreases the opportunity for fertilization.
- Hypothalamic or pituitary disease may cause a lack of hormonal support for implantation and fetal development.

Systemic factors, too, are clearly important. For example, immune reactions may interfere with conception, implantation, and fetal development.

ECTOPIC PREGNANCY AND ABORTION

Fertilization typically occurs not in the uterus but in the abdominal cavity near the ovary or in the fallopian tube. The conceptus is swept into and down the fallopian tube by the waving motion of ciliated cells lining the fallopian tube. Mechanical obstruction of this process by inflammation, scarring, or endometriosis may cause the conceptus to implant outside the uterus, producing an **ectopic pregnancy** (Fig. 21-30). In about half of cases, some mechanical obstruction can be identified; in the other half the cause is unknown. About 90% of ectopic pregnancies occur in the fallopian tube, the remainder occur on the surface of the ovary or in the pelvis or abdominal peritoneum.

Early development of the fetus and placenta is normal in most ectopic pregnancies, so that an early ectopic pregnancy may be physiologically and medically indistinguishable from a normal one: menses stop, the patient gains weight, and her breasts enlarge and may become tender, and so on. The diagnosis can be readily confirmed by ultrasound imaging of the pelvis in a patient with high levels of blood chorionic gonadotropin.

In a normal pregnancy, the placenta, which is naturally invasive, burrows into the uterine wall seeking the maternal blood supply. In an ectopic pregnancy, the placenta burrows into the wall of the fallopian tube or other tissue, which disrupts blood vessels and causes hemorrhage. Sometimes acute hemorrhage occurs and

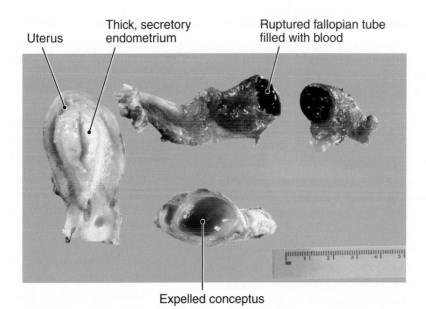

Uterus | Thick, secretory endometrium | Ruptured fallopian tube filled with blood

Expelled conceptus

Figure 21-30 **Ectopic pregnancy in a fallopian tube.** The uterus is small and lined by thick, secretory endometrium ready for implantation of the conceptus, which has implanted in the fallopian tube. As the conceptus grew it ruptured the wall of the tube and was expelled, causing sudden hemorrhage.

causes acute abdominal pain with hemorrhagic shock that can prove fatal.

Abortion is interruption of pregnancy before 20 weeks or 500 grams fetal weight. Abortions can be *spontaneous* or *induced*. Spontaneous abortion ("miscarriage") is involuntary and has no known cause; induced abortion is voluntary. Abortions are further classifiable as:

- *Complete*: All products of conception are expelled from the uterus
- *Incomplete*: Some products of conception are expelled, and some remain in the uterus
- *Threatened*: Bleeding through the undilated cervical os, raising fear that a spontaneous abortion might occur.
- *Missed*: The fetus dies but is not expelled.

The cause of most spontaneous abortions is obscure: about 15% of known pregnancies end in spontaneous abortion and an additional 30% of women abort without being aware they were pregnant. In sum, nearly half of all pregnancies end with spontaneous abortion. Many of these are associated with genetic defects (Chapter 7).

PLACENTAL DISEASE

Normal implantation of the conceptus (fertilized ovum) takes place in the upper part of the uterine cavity. When the placenta implants in the lower segment of the uterus the condition is known as **placenta previa**. As a result, the placenta may cover the internal cervical os, through which the fetus must eventually pass. Placenta previa is prone to hemorrhage because the lower uterine segment does not expand naturally with fetal growth, and when stretched in late pregnancy or during labor the placenta tears and severe hemorrhage can occur.

The placenta is naturally invasive—it must burrow into the endometrium and superficial myometrium to establish close contact with maternal blood vessels for exchange of gases and nutrients. Sometimes the placenta invades too deeply into the myometrium and does not separate spontaneously from the uterine wall after delivery, a condition known as **placenta accreta**. After delivery an accreted placenta does not peel easily away from the uterine wall. Serious bleeding may occur, and manual extraction of the placenta is required.

Tumors and Tumor-like Conditions of the Placenta

Abnormal fertilization may induce neoplastic or semi-neoplastic change in the chorionic epithelium, which covers placental villi. Three overlapping neoplasms are recognized. *Hydatidiform mole* is the least aggressive; *invasive mole* is of intermediate malignancy; and *choriocarcinoma* is frankly malignant. All secrete human chorionic gonadotropin (hCG). Increasing levels of serum hCG parallel tumor aggressiveness.

Hydatidiform mole (Fig. 21-31) takes its name from Greek *hydatis*, meaning watery, and Latin *moles*, meaning mass, and is a benign tumor-like overgrowth of placental cells caused by abnormal combinations of ovum and sperm. These peculiar combinations of ova and sperm cannot properly be considered fetuses, although some hydatidiform moles may develop rudimentary normal fetal parts. Most are caused by fertilization of an ovum with no nucleus by one or more sperm, which produces a conceptus with one, two, or more sets of male chromosomes and no female genetic material.

The typical hydatidiform mole is a watery mass of swollen, grape-like (hydropic) chorionic villi that microscopically are covered by hyperplastic chorionic epithelium. About 90% remain benign, about 10% are locally aggressive (*invasive mole*), and a small percentage becomes frankly malignant (*choriocarcinoma*).

In the United States, hydatidiform mole occurs about once in every 1000 pregnancies. The incidence in Asian countries is much higher for unknown reasons. Moles tend to occur before age 20 or after age 40 and present with painless vaginal bleeding about three months after conception. Examination of a patient with a mole usually reveals a uterus that is unexpectedly large, too large for the length of the pregnancy. No fetal heartbeat can be detected, and there is no ultrasound image of a fetus in the uterus. Abnormally high levels of chorionic gonadotropin are present in blood and urine because there is a large excess of placental tissue in the uterus. Hydatidiform mole is treated first by endometrial curettage. Persistent high blood chorionic gonadotropin af-

ter curettage suggests possible invasive mole or choriocarcinoma.

Invasive mole occupies the middle ground between hydatidiform mole and choriocarcinoma. It may invade through the uterine wall into the pelvis, but it does not metastasize. Invasive moles are difficult to remove completely by curettage and may require hysterectomy or chemotherapy.

Choriocarcinoma is a malignant proliferation of the epithelial cells that cover normal chorionic villi, and it is similar to the tumor of the same name arising in the testis. It can arise from any form of normal or abnormal pregnancy and is much more common in Asia than in the United States. Like hydatidiform mole, choriocarcinoma tends to occur more commonly before age 20 or after age 40. By the time they are discovered most have metastasized widely to lungs, brain, liver, and kidneys.

Virtually all patients with choriocarcinoma who do not have metastases are curable by chemotherapy. The cure rate for patients with metastases is about 70%.

Other Conditions of the Placenta and Pregnancy

Infection of the fetus, placenta, or amniotic fluid usually ascends the birth canal from the vagina and invades the amniotic fluid through a break in the amniotic membrane. Premature rupture of the amniotic membrane is a common cause of early labor, premature birth, and fe-

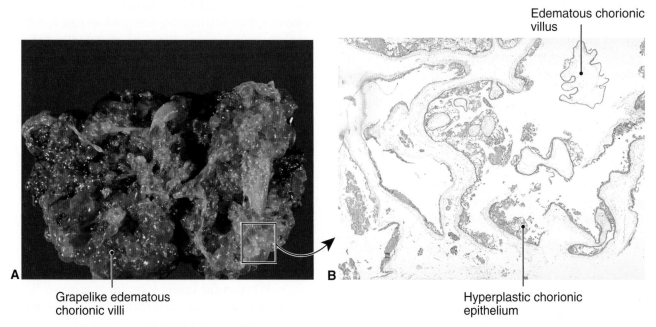

Figure 21-31 Hydatidiform mole. A, Note the grape-like, edematous chorionic villi. **B,** In this microscopic study, note the hyperplastic chorionic epithelium.

tal pneumonia. Blood-borne infection is rare and is usually one of the TORCH infections discussed in Chapter 7. Microbes most commonly involved are *Candida*, *Chlamydia*, and other vaginal organisms.

Toxemia of pregnancy is a syndrome of hypertension, proteinuria, and edema that occurs in the last trimester of pregnancy. Toxemia is also known as **preeclampsia**, a term used to distinguish it from **eclampsia**, a much more serious condition in which patients develop convulsions.

Toxemia appears to be associated with placental malfunction, but the exact mechanisms are not clear. It occurs in about 5% of pregnancies, and older women in a first pregnancy are most vulnerable. Other risk factors include obesity, diabetes, and multiple gestation. Very mild cases of toxemia may not require therapy, but patients with severe disease may develop convulsions, renal failure, stroke, or intravascular blood clotting (disseminated intravascular coagulation, Chapter 11).

Section 2: Diseases of the Breast

I think it's about time we voted for senators with breasts. After all, we've been voting for boobs long enough.

CLAIRE SARGENT (B. 1934), 1992 CANDIDATE FOR
THE UNITED STATES SENATE (ARIZONA)

▶ BACK TO BASICS

The breast (Fig. 21-32) is a modified sweat gland composed of ducts and glands organized into small subdivisions called *lobules*. Breast lobules contain milk-secreting glands, which drain into small ducts that gather into large lactiferous ducts at the nipple. The breast is mostly fat supported by a network of thin fibrous ligaments. Both fibrous tissue and fat are sensitive to female estrogen and progesterone, which accounts for the growth of the breasts at puberty and for the engorgement and occasional tenderness of the breast during the menstrual cycle. The breast has a rich lymphatic network, most of which drains upward and outward to the axilla; lymphatics from the medial aspect of the breasts (between the nipples) drain into lymph nodes inside the chest on either side of the sternum (the internal mammary nodes). During pregnancy, milk-secreting cells develop under the influence of the pituitary hormone prolactin. Milk secretion begins immediately after birth. If the infant does not suckle, glandular epithelium shrivels and milk production ceases.

It is important to understand that the breast is sensitive to estrogen hormones and that different parts of the breast are affected by different diseases. Hormonal influence explains the fact that most breast disease occurs in women, that different diseases predominate at different phases of a woman's life as hormonal influence accumulates or changes, and that carcinoma is 100 times more common in women than men.

MAJOR DETERMINANTS OF DISEASE

- Cancer is the most important disease of the breast.
- Estrogen is critical in the development of breast disease, including in breast cancer.
- Epithelial hyperplasia in any breast disease adds to the risk of developing breast cancer.
- Lobular carcinoma is a strong risk factor for breast cancer in the opposite breast.
- The most important initial determinants of breast cancer behavior are:
  - Whether the cancer is in situ or invasive
  - Whether invasive cancer has or has not spread to lymph nodes

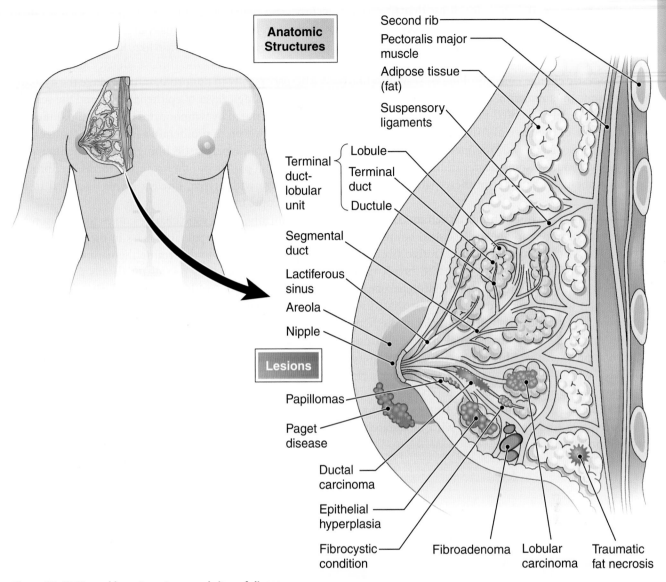

Figure 21-32 **Normal breast anatomy and sites of disease.**

Inflammatory Disease

Acute **mastitis** is an acute infection of the breast. It is uncommon, and almost all cases occur in lactating women. Typically it is bacterial and caused by staphylococcus or streptococcus organisms that gain access through dilated breast ducts plugged with mammary secretions. Staph infection usually produces an abscess; strep infection tends to be more diffuse and produces generalized swelling, tenderness, and pain. *Chronic* breast inflammation and tenderness is usually associated with *fibrocystic change*, a very common condition (discussed below).

Fat necrosis is an unusual type of necrosis (Chapter 2) that occurs only in fat and is especially likely to cause local calcium deposits. The cause of fat necrosis is often unknown, but many cases can be traced to trauma. Fat necrosis heals by scarring and is often stippled with calcium, features that give it a hard, gritty character and an irregular outline that can suggest breast cancer on mammogram. It is most often found in women with large, fatty breasts, most of whom cannot recall any trauma.

Fibrocystic Change

Fibrocystic *change* is now the preferred term for what is still widely called fibrocystic *disease*. The change, no pun intended, was prompted by concerns that patients might be stigmatized by having the word "disease" attached to their diagnosis. In defense of this bit of linguistic nitpicking, it is worth noting that fibrocystic change is so common that, like skin wrinkles associated with age, it is, perhaps, closer to a normal variation than to a disease.

Fibrocystic change consists of breast scarring (fibrosis), chronic inflammation, and cystic dilation of breast ducts. It is widely accepted that fibrocystic change is a consequence of the normal rising and falling of female hormones associated with the menstrual cycle. About 50% of women have some degree of fibrocystic change, but only about one quarter of these patients have any symptoms.

In most cases the duct-lining epithelium consists of a single layer of unremarkable cells, called **nonproliferative fibrocystic change**. Nonproliferative fibrocystic change is not associated with increased breast cancer risk. However, any degree of epithelial hyperplasia in conjunction with fibrocystic change is associated with increased breast cancer risk. If the nuclei of the hyperplastic epithelial cells are normal, the condition is known as **proliferative fibrocystic change**, a finding associated with slight increased breast cancer risk. However, if the nuclei are abnormal (atypical, Chapter 6), the diagnosis is **proliferative fibrocystic change with atypia**, a finding associated with moderately increased breast cancer risk.

Grossly (Fig. 21-33 A) the breast in every type of fibrocystic change is studded by simple cysts a few mm to a few cm in diameter, which are filled with a watery fluid. Accumulation of scar-like fibrous tissue makes the remainder of the breast dense and rubbery. Microscopically in nonproliferative change the cysts are lined by a single layer of epithelial cells, and the scar tissue is infiltrated by lymphocytes (chronic inflammatory cells). However, in proliferative fibrocystic change (Fig. 21-33B) the hyperplastic lining duct epithelium piles up in small papilla or other complex forms. In fibrocystic change with atypia, nuclear atypia as added to the microscopic mix.

Clinically, fibrocystic change comes to attention because it produces a palpable mass in the breast. Breast biopsy is required to determine the nature of the mass and microscopic study reveals the details.

In the breast, **epithelial hyperplasia** of any kind, whether because of fibrocystic change or some other condition, is associated with a small but definite increased risk for the development of breast cancer. Hyperplasia may be mild or it may be florid, and it may occur with or without nuclear atypia. **Proliferative breast disease** is a term that includes conditions, other than fibrocystic change, that are associated with epithelial hyperplasia. For example, intraductal papillomas are cauliflower-like polyps in breast ducts. Risk of cancer is

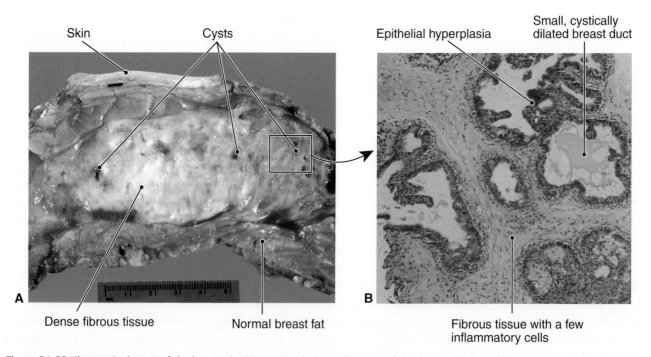

Figure 21-33 **Fibrocystic change of the breast. A,** This gross study shows that most of the abnormal tissue is fibrous. Cysts are relatively inconspicuous in this example. **B,** The microscopic study shows dense fibrous tissue containing dilated ducts lined by hyperplastic epithelium.

► **BASICS IN BRIEF 21-1**

THE DIFFERENCE BETWEEN ABSOLUTE AND RELATIVE RISK

Patients worried about health risks are often presented facts by comparisons of risk. That is, they are told their *relative* risk is X% or Y times greater than normal. But their actual risk (*absolute* risk) often goes unexplained. It is important to explain the difference because *patients tend to overreact to statements of relative risk.* Indeed, anyone who wants to impress others with numbers will use relative risk figures, which brings to mind the following quote:

> *There are three kinds of lies: lies, damned lies, and statistics.*
> BENJAMIN DISRAELI (1804–1881), ENGLISH STATESMAN AND LITERARY FIGURE

Relative risk is the chance of harm from one *situation* compared to another. For example, the relative risk of death by driving 1,000 miles in an automobile is many times that of flying the same distance in a jet airliner.

Absolute risk is the chance of being harmed by a particular risk in a given *period of time* or for a particular *event.* For example, the absolute risk of dying in an air accident during any single jet airline trip is about one in a million.

As a rule, patients who are told they are at twice normal risk (a 100% increase of relative risk) for breast cancer feel they are nearly certain to develop cancer, but it just isn't so, even for a tumor as common as breast cancer.

It is true that a woman with proliferative fibrocystic change has a *lifetime* breast cancer risk about twice that of a woman with normal breasts, but it is still quite unlikely that she will develop breast cancer. And the risks for time frames less than "life" are reassuringly lower. For example, the *lifetime* risk (the *absolute* risk) for breast cancer among women is about 12 cases in 100 women, but the absolute risk that any particular woman in the general population will develop breast cancer in the next 15 years is only 5 in 100. If some factor doubles the *relative* lifetime risk, the *absolute* risk changes from 7 in 100 to 14 in 100—the *relative* risk is doubled, but it is still quite unlikely that the patient will develop breast cancer.

proportional to the degree and extent of epithelial hyperplasia and whether or not microscopic nuclear atypia is present. Compared to women with normal breasts, there is an approximate doubling of breast cancer risk associated with moderate to marked epithelial hyperplasia. A five-fold increase in risk occurs with atypical hyperplasia. A family history of breast carcinoma doubles again the risk in each group. These facts sometimes scare patients more than is warranted, so it is wise to keep in mind that these are relative figures, not absolute, a topic discussed in the nearby box Basics in Brief 21-1.

Benign Tumors

Fibroadenoma is a benign tumor of breast stroma (supporting tissue) rather than of the glands and ducts. It is the most common tumor of the female breast, occurring most often in women in their twenties as a solitary, round mass about 1–5 cm in diameter and composed of dense, fibrous tissue interspersed with compressed breast ducts. It is not premalignant, and simple surgical removal is curative.

Phyllodes tumor is an uncommon, much larger, somewhat aggressive version of fibroadenoma (Fig. 21-34). It may be sluggishly malignant; some recur locally after excision, but metastasis is rare.

Solitary **intraductal papilloma** is a benign neoplasm that most often occurs in the large milk ducts near the nipple. It may call attention because it is palpable, bleeds, or causes a nipple discharge, or because the nipple becomes inverted (retracted). Solitary papillomas, by far the most common, are not premalignant, but multiple papillomas (**intraductal papillomatosis**) are a variety of *proliferative breast disease* and as such carry an increased risk for breast carcinoma.

Breast Cancer

Technically, any malignant tumor of the breast is a breast "cancer" (Chapter 6); however, because almost all malignant tumors of the breast are *carcinomas,* the daily use of the phrase "breast cancer" implies carcinoma of the breast—a malignancy of the breast ducts or glands.

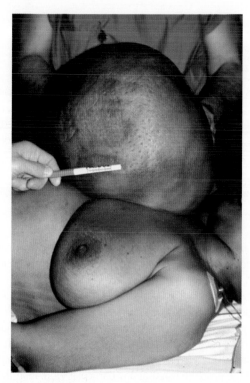

Figure 21-34 **Phyllodes tumor of the breast.** This is an especially large example, which the patient tolerated for an unusually long time.

Sarcomas of the breast are rare, malignant tumors of breast stroma (fibrous tissue, blood vessels, nerves, and fat) similar to malignant tumors of those tissues that occur elsewhere in the body (Chapter 22). Most common is *angiosarcoma*, a malignant tumor of small blood vessels, which arises in a very small percent of women receiving radiation therapy for breast cancer.

In 1986 lung cancer passed breast cancer as the number one cancer killer of women, the result of a marked increase in cigarette smoking by women, which had its start when women went to work in defense factories alongside men during World War II (1939–1945). Annually breast cancer kills about 40,000 women, about as many women as there are total automobile fatalities for both sexes in a year. Many women believe breast cancer is the number one cancer killer and are surprised to learn that more women die each year of lung cancer, and they are further surprised to know that colon cancer is not far behind breast cancer as a cause of death among women.

Although not nearly so lethal as lung or colorectal cancer, carcinoma of the breast is arguably the most feared tumor in all of medicine—it threatens life, deformity, self-esteem, and relationships to a degree unmatched by any other tumor. It is distressingly common. The cumulative risk by age 95 is about 12%; that is, by age 95 about one in eight women will at some time

have had breast cancer. This "one chance in eight" *lifetime* figure leads women to presume that, despite their age, they, too, have one chance in eight of developing breast cancer. They forget they have already lived many cancer-free years (say, 40 of their projected 85 years) already and have not developed breast cancer, so the risk for the *remainder* of their life is much lower. Table 21-5 illustrates the risks for women at various ages over time. Despite improvements in diagnosis and treatment, about one third of women who develop breast cancer die of the disease. By comparison, six out of seven women who develop lung cancer die of it.

TYPES OF BREAST CANCER

Ninety percent (90%) of breast carcinomas are one of two types. **Ductal carcinoma** accounts for about 75–80% of breast cancers and arises from epithelium lining the breast ducts (see Case Study 21-2 at the end of this chapter). **Lobular carcinoma** accounts for 10–15% of breast malignancies and arises from the epithelium of the smallest ducts or from the milk glands themselves. Both ductal and lobular carcinomas exist first as **carcinoma in situ** before becoming invasive, a very important point, because modern techniques allow discovery of breast cancers early in their development, while they are in situ and curable. For example, nearly 90% of breast cancers detected in women 30–39 years old are ductal carcinoma in situ. The distinction between ductal and lobular carcinoma is very important for other reasons: they behave differently and are subject to different types of therapies. The types and frequency of breast cancers are presented in Table 21-6.

Lobular carcinoma is distinctive on several counts: 1) it frequently occurs at *multiple sites* in the affected breast; 2) it appears to have a greater tendency than other breast cancer types to be accompanied by cancer in the opposite breast, though some studies call this into question; and 3) it is associated with an increased

Table 21-5	*Chance of Developing Breast Cancer per Decade of Life**	
Age in Years	**Risk for Decade**
30–39	1 in 229
40–49	1 in 68
50–59	1 in 37
60–69	1 in 26

*Adapted from United States National Cancer Institute (www.cancer.gov)

Table 21-6	Microscopic Types and Frequencies of Breast Cancers	
Histologic Type	**Percent of All Breast Cancers**	
Carcinoma in situ	15–30%	
Ductal	80%	
Lobular	20%	
Invasive	70–85%	
Ductal	80%	
Lobular	10%	
Others	10%	

risk for subsequent development of a *second* breast cancer. In nearly one quarter of patients, lobular carcinoma in one breast is accompanied by concurrent cancer in the opposite breast. Moreover, lobular carcinoma is difficult to diagnose by **mammography** (specialized breast x-rays) because its multifocal, diffuse growth pattern is less likely than ductal carcinoma to form a detectable mass.

Ductal carcinoma is by far the most common cancer of the breast, and, when invasive, it is the most aggressive. Ductal carcinoma in situ is seen with much greater frequency now because early diagnosis by mammography is possible; this accounts for about half of cancers detected by mammography. In contrast to lobular carcinoma, it appears that it is less likely with ductal carcinoma that the opposite breast will be involved with another cancer; however, some studies question this conclusion.

About two thirds of breast carcinomas are invasive ductal carcinoma (Figs. 21-35 and 21-36), often called "carcinoma of no special type" by pathologists because they are not one of the several recognized subtypes of ductal carcinoma. Most of these ductal carcinomas stimulate growth of a very dense, scar-like tissue and are commonly called scirrhous ductal carcinoma (from Greek *skiros*, meaning hard).

Other types of breast cancers account for about 10% of breast cancer cases.

FACTORS AFFECTING THE RISK OF DEVELOPING BREAST CANCER

Breast cancer is caused by the convergence of genetic, hormonal, and environmental influences. The strongest risk factors are:

- *Sex*: Women have about 100× the risk of men.
- *Lobular carcinoma in the other breast*: Other than sex, the strongest of all risk factors is lobular carcinoma in the opposite breast. Lobular carcinoma *in situ* is associated with about a tenfold increased risk for subsequent development of *invasive* carcinoma, either lobular or ductal, in one breast or the other.
- *Family history and genetics*: Breast cancer in family members, especially first-degree relatives (mother, sister, or daughter), increases risk. Although two genes, BRCA-1 and BRCA-2, have been linked to in-

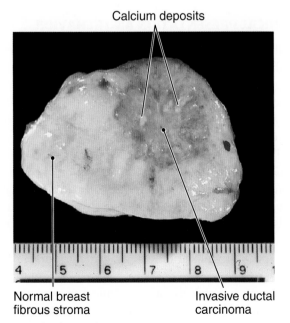

Figure 21-35 Carcinoma of the breast (biopsy specimen). Note the irregular, stellate shape and calcium deposits.

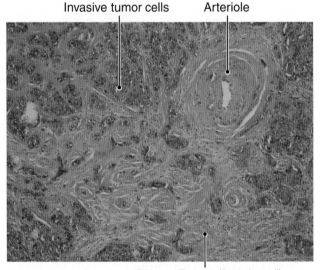

Figure 21-36 Carcinoma of the breast (microscopic study). In this specimen of invasive ductal carcinoma, nests of tumor cells are separated by dense fibrous tissue.

creased breast cancer risk, they are responsible for only a small percent of total breast cancer cases. Screening for BRCA is advisable only in women who have close relatives with breast cancer or a family member with a known BRCA-1 or BRCA-2 mutation.

- *Age*: Breast cancer is uncommon under age 30, but it occurs with increasing frequency with age.
- *Estrogen*: Prolonged exposure to endogenous estrogen is also important—early onset of menses, childlessness, and delayed childbearing increase the risk.

Other, less influential, risk factors include obesity, alcoholism, and cigarette smoking. Exogenous estrogen, as with oral contraceptives and estrogen replacement therapy in postmenopausal women, also causes a small increased risk.

PROGNOSTIC FACTORS FOR PATIENTS WITH BREAST CANCER

The five-year survival rate for women with breast cancer varies from 100% to near 10% depending on multiple factors. The two gravest prognostic signs are clinical: women who present with distant metastasis, or with inflammatory carcinoma, a clinical presentation that includes breast edema, hyperemia, tenderness, and rapid enlargement of the breast. Very few patients in either category survive five years. With the exception of these two clinical presentations, prognosis is determined by pathologic study of the primary tumor and axillary lymph nodes. Listed below are *pathologic factors* that affect prognosis:

- The most important are:
  - *Carcinoma in situ or invasive carcinoma*: This is the most important of all pathologic distinctions. By definition, carcinoma in situ (CIS) cannot metastasize, and risk from CIS is related to the risk of having undetected CIS elsewhere in the same or opposite breast or developing a second cancer at a later time.
  - *Lymph node metastasis*: This is the most important of all pathologic risk factors for *invasive* cancers. If no nodes are involved the 10-year survival rate is near 80%. It falls to near 15% if four or more lymph nodes are involved.
  - *Tumor size*: This is the second most important factor for *invasive* cancers. The 5-year survival rate is 98% for women with invasive cancers less than 1 cm in diameter. Larger tumors are usually associated with lymph node metastasis, but if no metastases are present the survival rate is 96% for women with tumors less than 2 cm.

  - *Invasion of skin or chest wall*: Some neglected or advanced breast cancers invade underlying chest wall muscles and become fixed (immobile). Invasion of skin may cause dimpling or retraction of skin or the nipple.
- Less important prognostic factors are:
  - *Histologic type of carcinoma*: The 30-year survival rate for invasive lobular carcinoma is near 60%; for invasive ductal carcinoma it is near 20%.
  - *The histologic grade of the carcinoma* (the degree of tumor differentiation, Chapter 6): Well-differentiated cancers have a better prognosis than poorly differentiated ones do.
  - *The rate of tumor cell division and the presence of extra sets of chromosomes (aneuploidy)*: Tumors cell that multiply rapidly or that have extra sets of chromosomes, features that can be assessed by laboratory study of the tumor, have a poor prognosis.
  - *The presence or absence of estrogen and progesterone or HER2/neu receptors on tumor cells*: The presence of estrogen and progesterone receptors is a somewhat favorable sign because it suggests that the tumor is dependent on estrogen or progesterone and may not grow as rapidly if deprived of either by removing the ovaries (oophorectomy) or by chemotherapy. Patients with the HER2/neu receptor have a somewhat poorer prognosis than those without it. However, its main importance is not as an indicator of prognosis but, rather, as a guide to therapy with drugs aimed specifically at this receptor.

CLINICAL PRESENTATION AND BEHAVIOR

Half of breast cancers occur in the upper outer quadrant of the breast; a quarter occurs centrally near the nipple (Figs. 21-37 and 21-38). Eighty percent (80%) of breast cancers are discovered accidentally by the patient after they become 3–4 cm in diameter, by which time one third have lymph node metastasis.

Two unusual clinical presentations warrant special notice. First is **inflammatory carcinoma**, an uncommon condition in which the breast and skin are inflamed and swollen, and extensive lymphatic invasion by tumor cells has caused the skin to become thickened and rubbery. Breast cancers presenting in this fashion have a very poor prognosis: only a few patients survive five years.

Second is **Paget disease**, a clinical presentation of breast cancer in which the nipple and areola are involved by an inflamed, tender, red, cracked, oozing, crusted lesion that looks like eczema, an inflammatory

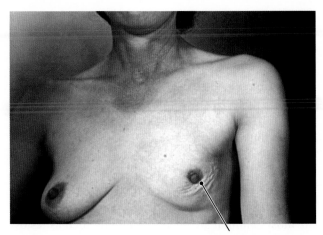

Skin, areola, and
nipple retraction

Figure 21-37 **Carcinoma of the breast (clinical appearance).** The
photograph shows an advanced case that has invaded the skin, causing retraction of the skin, areola, and nipple.

skin disease (Chapter 24). However, Paget disease is
caused by *in situ* extension of cells to the nipple from an
underlying ductal carcinoma, which itself may be either
in situ or invasive.

Breast cancers spread (metastasize) first to the nearest lymph nodes: those in the upper outer quadrant of
the breast spread to the axilla; those between the nipples
spread to the internal mammary nodes beneath the sternum; and some tumors spread to lymph nodes in the
lower neck just above the clavicle (supraclavicular
nodes). Ultimately, however, blood-borne metastasis
may occur. The most common sites of metastasis are
lung, bone, and liver, but no site is exempt. One of the
most threatening and depressing features of breast cancer is that sometimes a decade or more after an apparent
cure, tumor may suddenly emerge in some distant site.

DIAGNOSIS AND TREATMENT

As with other cancers, for many years the conventional
wisdom has been that early detection of breast cancer is
the best way to achieve cure—find the cancer and eliminate it before it has time to spread. Patient breast self-
examination, clinical breast examination by trained
health care professionals, and mammography have been
widely promoted and used to detect breast cancers at
earlier and earlier stages. Early detection of breast cancer and improved treatment has resulted in a 25% decline in the death rate from breast cancer in the United
States since 1990. However, mammography does not replace careful breast examination by a professional:

10–20% of breast cancers detected by physical examination were missed by an earlier mammogram.

Biopsy is required for conclusive diagnosis.
Radiographically guided needle biopsy under local
anesthetic is now widely used and effective, but open
surgical biopsy may be required if needle biopsy is inconclusive. Tissue from the initial biopsy or later surgery should be assayed for the presence or absence of
estrogen and progesterone receptors. Patients with receptors have a somewhat better prognosis because they
respond better to anti-hormone therapy. Treatment can
be delayed for a few weeks in order to accomplish a
thorough workup for distant metastases, which at a
minimum should include physical examination for en-

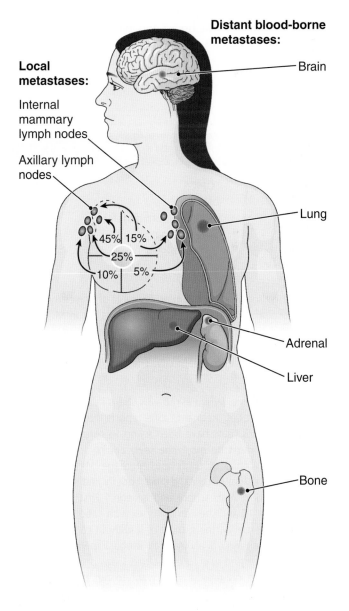

Figure 21-38 **Sites of breast cancer origin and metastasis.**

larged lymph nodes or liver, radiographic imaging of chest, liver, and bones, and blood assay for *carcinoembryonic antigen* (CEA, Chapter 15), a protein secreted by some breast cancers. Elevated levels of CEA suggest distant metastasis.

Treatment depends on factors discussed above and is too complex to discuss in detail. Bilateral mastectomy is often the treatment of choice for lobular carcinoma because of its tendency to involve both breasts. Standard treatment of ductal carcinoma in situ is simple mastectomy or wide local excision (lumpectomy). Invasive cancers demand a more aggressive approach, which at a minimum includes lumpectomy and exploratory biopsy of axillary lymph nodes for possible metastasis. Small tumors can be excised by lumpectomy, sparing the remainder of the breast. Larger tumors sometimes can be shrunk by chemotherapy and excised in the same fashion, but removal of the breast and axillary lymph nodes may be required. Radiation and chemotherapy may also be employed.

Diseases of the Male Breast

Gynecomastia means literally "female breast," but actually is the term for enlargement of the male breast resulting from an increased amount of breast-gland tissue. It is usually bilateral, but, rarely, it may be unilateral. Most of the enlargement is from increased fibrous stroma, not breast ducts and glands. The most common cause is increased levels of blood estrogen associated with cirrhosis (Chapter 16), because in cirrhosis, the liver is unable to metabolize estrogen normally. Many different drugs can cause gynecomastia. Among the most common are anabolic steroids such as testosterone, digitalis, estrogens, theophylline, calcium channel blockers, and chronic marijuana use.

About 1% of breast cancers occur in men. They usually occur later in life in men than in women, and about half of patients have lymph node metastases at time of diagnosis. Otherwise they resemble and behave like tumors in women. ■

CASE STUDY 21-1 "I CAN'T GET PREGNANT"

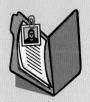

TOPICS
Infertility
Sexually transmitted disease
Chronic salpingitis
Cancer of the cervix

THE CASE

Setting: You work in the infertility clinic of university referral hospital. Your last patient of the day is Susan M., a 34-year-old woman you recognize as a television news reporter introduced recently to local audiences after moving from a smaller market in a distant city. The referral note says "Infertile?"

Clinical history: When asked why she is in your office she says, "I can't get pregnant." She reports that she and her husband of 3 years have been trying to conceive without results. "It must be me," she says, adding that her husband has a child by a previous marriage. When you ask about her sexual history she smiles briefly and says, "I was pretty wild in high school and college." First intercourse was at age 16 and she admits to sex with "about a dozen" different sexual partners, most of it without condoms. "It's ironic," she says. "I always had irregular periods when I was younger and was forever afraid I was pregnant when I didn't start on time. Now I want to get pregnant and can't."

You review her history and exam from Internal Medicine; she is reported to be in excellent general health. A note says, "Pelvic and Pap not done; for fertility clinic to do."

"When did you have your last Pap smear?" you ask.

"Oh," she says, "it's been nearly ten years, I imagine; I've moved around so much in this TV job I never quite got around to it."

Then using charts and diagrams you explain to her the details of internal female anatomy, the menstrual cycle, conception, the role of the pituitary gland, and so on, pointing out how things can go wrong at each step of the process and bracing her for a lengthy and time-consuming workup to establish the cause, if one can be found. "Sometimes we just can't figure it out," you say in closing.

Physical examination and other data: Vital signs and general exam are unremarkable. Her cervix appears to be inflamed around the os and bleeds easily when you scrape it for a Pap smear. On pelvic examination she has bilateral, slightly tender masses on either side of her uterus, each estimated to be about 6–8 cm in diameter. Initial laboratory blood tests reveal nothing remarkable. You refer her for imaging to check the patency of her fallopian tubes, which reveals bilateral complete obstruction. A laboratory test of cervical mucus is positive for *Chlamydia trachomatis*. The Pap smear report is a complete surprise: "High-Grade Squamous Intraepithelial Lesion." ▶

[Case 21-1, continued]

Clinical course: Cervical conization biopsy reveals carcinoma in situ (CIN-III), with a comment that no invasive carcinoma is present; however, in situ malignant epithelium extends to the biopsy margins.

Because she is so young and her problems so severe—cervical cancer complicated by seemingly incurable infertility resulting from severe chronic salpingitis with bilateral tuboovarian abscesses—her attending physician presents her case for evaluation to a conference of specialists. The unanimous agreement is that exploratory surgery will be recommended to the patient and her husband so that her ovaries and tubes can be inspected to see if there is any hope of restoring fertility. If not, the recommendation is total removal of the uterus, fallopian tubes, and ovaries.

Total hysterectomy is performed. The pathology report shows bilateral tuboovarian abscesses and residual foci of cervical carcinoma in situ high in the endocervical canal; no invasive carcinoma is present.

DISCUSSION

This woman was both fortunate and unfortunate. She was fortunate that her cervical cancer was found while it was still in situ, before it became invasive. However, early and frequent unprotected sex with multiple partners is associated with repeated *Chlamydia* and human papillomavirus (HPV) infections. The former developed into the chronic tuboovarian abscesses that rendered her infertile, and the latter produced cervical cancer, which could have become invasive and claimed her life had it gone undetected.

POINTS TO REMEMBER

- Sexually transmitted disease is a hazard of unprotected sex with multiple sexual partners.
- Patients who have one type of sexually transmitted disease often have other types as well.
- Repeated infection with human papillomavirus, a sexually transmitted disease, is the cause of most cervical cancer.
- Regular gynecologic exams and Pap smears are especially important for women in their reproductive years.

CASE STUDY 21-1 THE ROAD NOT TAKEN—AN ALTERNATIVE SCENARIO

For all sad words of tongue or pen,
The saddest are these: "It might have been."
JOHN GREENLEAF WHITTIER (1807–1892),
AMERICAN QUAKER POET AND REFORMER, *MAUD MULLER*

THE CASE

With a bit of imagination, we can speculate how this case might have had a happier ending.

Setting: You work in the student health clinic at a large university seeing routine "sick call" patients.

Clinical history: Susan M. is a 19-year-old sophomore communications major, whose name you recognize: she is an announcer on the student-run campus radio station that you often listen to in your office.

When you ask about her problem, she says she's been having achy lower abdominal pain for three or fours days. She admits to feeling "icky" but says she took her temperature at the sorority house and it was normal. You inquire about other symptoms and learn she has had irregular menstrual periods for many years; it has been five weeks since her last period began. She adds, "I'm forever worried that I'm pregnant, but thank goodness it hasn't happened." You ask a series of routine health questions and learn that she has been showing a slight, yellowish vaginal discharge for a few days but is in otherwise robust good health and plays soccer on an intramural team.

Physical examination and other data: Vital signs are normal; she is not febrile. Physical examination is unremarkable except for the gynecologic exam. Speculum exam of the vagina and cervix reveals a yellowish discharge in the vagina, issuing from the cervical os. Bimanual palpation of the pelvis reveals no masses, but she has bilateral tenderness in the region of both fallopian tubes. A rapid pregnancy test on urine is negative.

Clinical course: In the postexam interview you explain your conclusion: she has an infection in her fallopian tubes, probably owing to gonorrhea or a related bacterium, and she surely obtained it from a sexual partner. You quickly explain that it can be cured by antibiotics, but that such infections do not build immunity, and she can become infected again if she doesn't practice safe sex.

This news occasions a long discussion in which she tearfully confesses to frequent unprotected sex with multiple partners, conduct that began in high school. You listen patiently, and after a while she collects herself and says sits upright in the chair. "I can't believe this has happened to me," she says. "This is what my father calls 'the clap,' isn't it! If he finds out about it he will die of shame. But it's not ever going to happen again."

You continue to follow her college career on the campus radio station and newspaper as she becomes an outspoken advocate for safe sex practices. You never see her again in the clinic.

CASE STUDY 21-2 *"I HAVE A LUMP IN MY BREAST"*

TOPIC
Carcinoma of the breast

THE CASE

Setting: You work in the office of a general surgeon doing new patient histories and physicals, changing bandages, removing sutures, stitching up cuts, renewing prescriptions, ordering lab work and x-rays, and tending to occasional urgent-care matters. You look at the chart in the exam room door and see that your next patient is new: a 34-year-old woman who filled out the office forms with neat, bold strokes that indicate she is in excellent general health and is in the office because of a "breast lump."

Clinical history: The patient is an articulate woman who is clearly distressed. "I have a lump in my breast," she says, pointing to her left breast with a trembling finger. "I'm really worried because it seems so big—it's like it appeared out of nowhere. I do regular breast self-examination. I've never felt a thing until I was showering yesterday when found it." She has two younger sisters and numerous aunts and female cousins, none of whom has breast cancer.

Physical examination and other data: You do a standard physical exam and find no other problems. She has rather large breasts, but you easily locate a 3-cm, nontender mass in the upper outer quadrant. Careful palpation of the right breast is normal, and there are no palpable axillary nodes on either side.

Clinical course: The surgeon sees her and schedules a bilateral mammogram and an office needle biopsy later in the week. The biopsy reveals poorly differentiated invasive ductal carcinoma. An oncologist is consulted, and the patient agrees to mastectomy and axillary lymph node resection. Prior to surgery you direct a metastatic workup that includes chest, bone, and liver imaging, and blood carcinoembryonic antigen (CEA) assay, none of which suggests metastatic disease.

The patient tolerates surgery well. The pathologic diagnosis on the mastectomy and axillary lymph node resection shows an invasive ductal carcinoma, 3.8 cm in diameter, microscopically poorly differentiated and metastatic to 6 of the 13 axillary lymph nodes submitted for study. Lab reports a week later indicate the tumor is negative for estrogen and progesterone receptors. The patient is treated with radiation and chemotherapy and returns to fully active life within three months. Three years later on a quarterly follow-up visit she is found to have increased blood levels of alkaline phosphatase, an enzyme that is elevated in bone disease, which in this clinical setting suggests possible bone metastasis. Blood CEA is also elevated, which also suggests metastasis. Bone scan reveals evidence of metastases in her spine and skull. She dies 5 years to the day from the time she discovered "the lump" in her breast.

DISCUSSION

This young woman did everything right: she practiced breast self-examination and sought medical care immediately—but it was not enough. The initial character of this tumor was ominous—rapid clinical growth (sudden appearance "out of nowhere"), multiple lymph node metastases at the time of initial diagnosis, lack of estrogen and progesterone receptors, and undifferentiated microscopic appearance. The tumor's ultimate behavior—widespread metastasis in a few years—is in keeping with its initial character. Within 2 years of her death, her mother was found to have lobular carcinoma in situ of one breast and was treated with bilateral mastectomy because of the tendency of lobular carcinoma to be bilateral, and the fact that her daughter had breast cancer, which further increased the mother's increased risk for yet another breast cancer later. Pathologists discovered lobular carcinoma in the mother's contralateral breast specimen. No genetic studies were done on the patient before her death, but studies of her mother, her two surviving sisters, and one aunt revealed that none of them carries the BRCA gene. Five years after her sister's death one of the two surviving sisters elected to have bilateral prophylactic mastectomy.

POINTS TO REMEMBER

- The pathologic character of breast cancer—invasive tumor or in situ, tumor size and degree of differentiation, and the number of lymph node metastasis, if any—is very important in determining prognosis.
- Sometimes even the most alert patient and prompt, careful medical care cannot produce desirable results.

Objectives Recap

1. *Explain why women tend to develop osteoporosis after menopause*: Estrogen is necessary for healthy, strong bones. Lack of estrogen is important in the thinning and brittleness of bones (osteoporosis) that occurs with age, which is a major health risk for menopausal women because it dramatically increases the risk of bone fractures in elderly women.

2. *Name the most common sexually transmitted disease of women and the problems associated with it*: Human papillomavirus infection is the most common sexually transmitted disease of women. Less aggressive strains are responsible for benign, warty genital growths known as condyloma acuminatum; strains that are more aggressive cause dysplasia and carcinoma of the vulva, vagina, and cervix.

3. *Describe the developmental characteristics of the transformation zone of the cervix and its importance in cervical pathology*: The transformation zone of the cervix is an area extending from the cervical os outward for a short distance onto the ectocervix. In puberty it is temporarily covered by glandular epithelium, but in adults it is re-covered by squamous cells. Almost all dysplasia and cancer of the cervix arise in the transformation zone.

4. *Explain the importance of human papillomavirus (HPV) in cervical dysplasia and carcinoma*: Repeated infection with HPV is the cause of dysplasia and carcinoma of the cervix.

5. *Discuss the importance of annual Pap smear screening*: Pap smears are highly effective in detecting early, premalignant lesions of the cervix. Because it takes many years for premalignant lesions to become fully malignant, annual smears offer multiple opportunities for detection of lesions before they become potentially lethal.

6. *Differentiate between pathologic and functional uterine bleeding*: Functional uterine bleeding is abnormal bleeding not attributable to a particular anatomic disorder. Pathologic uterine bleeding is bleeding caused by endometrial hyperplasia, adenocarcinoma, or other anatomic disorder.

7. *Explain why failure to ovulate may cause dysfunctional uterine bleeding*: If ovulation does not occur, no corpus luteum is formed and no progesterone is produced to convert proliferative endometrium to secretory endometrium. The result is premature bleeding as the proliferative endometrium dies and sloughs away early for lack of progesterone support.

8. *Explain why endometriosis may cause infertility*: Deposits of endometrium may obstruct the fallopian tube and impede movement of sperm, ovum, or conceptus, preventing either conception or implantation in the endometrium.

9. *Define "fibroid" tumor of the uterus*: It is a benign smooth muscle tumor of the myometrium, a leiomyoma.

10. *Name the cause of tuboovarian abscess*: Repeated infection by sexually transmitted disease, especially *Chlamydia*.

11. *Name the cell of origin of most ovarian tumors and the three main types of carcinoma of the ovary*: Most arise from surface epithelial cells. The three main types are serous, mucinous, and endometrioid carcinomas of the ovary.

12. *Explain why ectopic pregnancy is dangerous*: Because it may produce serious, even fatal, intraabdominal hemorrhage.

13. *Name the three diagnostic components of preeclampsia (toxemia), and explain how eclampsia is different*: Preeclampsia (toxemia) consists of hypertension, proteinuria, and edema; eclampsia is preeclampsia plus seizures.

14. *Name the key difference between nonproliferative and proliferative fibrocystic change of the breast, and explain why the difference is important*: Epithelial hyperplasia occurs in proliferative but not in nonproliferative disease. Epithelial hyperplasia is associated with an increased risk of breast cancer.

15. *Name the most common tumor of the breast*: Fibroadenoma.

16. *Name the cell from which most breast cancers arise*: The breast duct epithelial cell.

17. *Explain how the behavior of lobular carcinoma is different from that of ductal carcinoma*: Lobular carcinoma frequently occurs at *multiple sites* in the affected breast; it has a tendency to be accompanied by *cancer in the opposite breast;* and it is associated with an increased risk for subsequent development of a *second* breast cancer. Additionally, lobular carcinoma is difficult to diagnose by mammography because its multifocal, diffuse growth pattern is less likely than ductal carcinoma to form a detectable mass.

18. *List the most important pathologic factors that affect the prognosis of patients with breast cancer*: 1) Carcinoma in situ or invasive carcinoma; 2) lymph node metastasis; 3) tumor size; 4) invasion of skin or chest wall.

Typical Test Questions

1. Which of the following is the site of origin of most cervical cancer?
   A. Endocervical canal
   B. Transformation zone
   C. Ectocervix
   D. Cervicovaginal junction

2. Which of the following is associated with proliferative-phase endometrium?
   A. Estrogen
   B. Progesterone
   C. Corpus luteum
   D. Glycogen accumulation

3. Which of the following is the most dangerous cervical lesion?
   A. CIN-I
   B. Carcinoma in situ
   C. Ectropion
   D. HPV infection

4. Which of the following is associated with endometrial hyperplasia and carcinoma?
   A. Tuboovarian abscess
   B. Leiomyoma
   C. Obesity
   D. Multiple childbirth

5. Consider the following three lesions:
   1 = proliferative fibrocystic disease
   2 = intraductal papillomatosis
   3 = fibroadenoma

   Which of the above is associated with increased breast cancer risk?
   A. 1 but not 2 or 3
   B. 2 but not 1 or 3
   C. 3 but not 1 or 2
   D. 1 and 2 but not 3
   E. 2 and 3 but not 1

6. True or false? Every breast lump should be investigated as if it is cancer.

7. True or false? Breast cancer is the number one cancer killer of women.

8. True or false? CA-125 antibody is an effective screen for ovarian cancer.

9. True or false? Dysmenorrhea is absence of menses.

10. True or false? A single HPV infection usually leads to dysplasia.

Diseases of Bones, Joints, and Skeletal Muscle

This chapter begins with a review of normal bone and bone types, muscle and muscle types, and ligaments and tendons. Diseases and disorders discussed include bone infection and infarction, osteoporosis and fractures, arthritis and joint injury, and tumors and tumor-like conditions.

Section 1: Diseases of Bone

BACK TO BASICS
SKELETAL DEFORMITIES AND DISORDERS OF BONE
   GROWTH
FRACTURES
BONE INFECTION
BONE INFARCT
OSTEOPOROSIS
OSTEOMALACIA
BONE TUMORS
- Bone-forming Tumors
- Cartilage-forming Tumors
- Fibrous Tumors and Tumor-like Conditions
- Other Tumors of Bone

Section 2: Diseases of Joints and Related Tissues

BACK TO BASICS
OSTEOARTHRITIS
RHEUMATOID ARTHRITIS
SPONDYLOARTHROPATHIES
OTHER TYPES OF ARTHRITIS
INJURIES TO LIGAMENTS, TENDONS, AND JOINTS
PERIARTICULAR PAIN SYNDROMES
TUMORS AND TUMOR-LIKE LESIONS OF JOINTS

Section 3: Diseases of Skeletal Muscle

BACK TO BASICS
MUSCLE ATROPHY
MUSCULAR DYSTROPHY
MYOSITIS AND MYOPATHY
MYASTHENIA GRAVIS
TUMORS AND TUMOR-LIKE LESIONS OF SOFT TISSUE

Learning Objectives

After studying this chapter you should be able to:
1. Describe the difference between osteoblast and osteoclast
2. Explain the role of osteoid in bone formation
3. Explain why patients with achondroplasia are short in stature
4. Discuss the pathogenesis of osteoporosis
5. Distinguish between osteoporosis and osteomalacia
6. Name the most common types of metastatic cancer *to* bone and the most common malignant tumor *of* bone
7. Name the joint near which 80% of primary bone tumors occur
8. Explain the pathogenesis of primary osteoarthritis, and describe the pathologic changes in affected joints
9. Explain the pathogenesis of rheumatoid arthritis (RA), and describe the pathologic changes in affected joints
10. Define rheumatoid factor (RF)
11. Explain how the seronegative spondyloarthropathies differ from rheumatoid arthritis
12. Name the distinguishing features that separate fibromyalgia from arthritis and other painful musculoskeletal syndromes

13. Distinguish between disuse atrophy and neurogenic atrophy of skeletal muscle and offer an example of each
14. Differentiate between Duchenne muscular dystrophy and Becker muscular dystrophy
15. Distinguish between myositis and myopathy
16. Explain the molecular pathogenesis of myasthenia gravis
17. Define soft tissue, and name some tumors or tumor-like conditions of soft tissue

Key Terms and Concepts

BACK TO BASICS
- epiphysis
- epiphyseal growth plate
- periosteum
- osteoblast
- osteoid
- osteoclast

FRACTURES
- pathologic fracture
- callus

BONE INFECTION
- osteomyelitis

BONE INFARCT
- aseptic necrosis

OSTEOPOROSIS
- osteoporosis

OSTEOMALACIA
- osteomalacia

BONE TUMORS
- osteosarcoma

BACK TO BASICS
- solid joint
- synovial joint
- synovium

OSTEOARTHRITIS
- osteoarthritis

RHEUMATOID ARTHRITIS
- rheumatoid arthritis

SPONDYLOARTHROPATHIES
- spondyloarthropathy

INJURIES TO LIGAMENTS, TENDONS, AND JOINTS
- sprain
- strain

BACK TO BASICS
- motor unit
- synapse

MUSCULAR DYSTROPHY
- muscular dystrophy

INFLAMMATORY AND OTHER DISEASES OF MUSCLE
- myositis

TUMORS AND TUMOR-LIKE LESIONS OF SOFT TISSUE
- soft tissue

Section 1: Diseases of Bone

When two dogs fight for a bone, and the third runs off with it, there's a lawyer among the dogs.

GERMAN PROVERB

► BACK TO BASICS

The musculoskeletal system makes up about half of normal body weight, gives the human form its shape, provides for the support and protection of organs, and is the framework for body movement. It consists of 1) bones; 2) cartilage; 3) ligaments, which attach bone and cartilage to one another; 4) skeletal muscle; 5) tendons, which attach muscle to bone; and 6) bursae, which are flat, fluid-filled sacs near joints that allow smooth movement where skin, muscles, tendons, or bones rub over one another.

Bones are deceptive. Although they look absolutely rigid, in fact they are slightly flexible (otherwise they would be brittle); they seem to be solid, but in fact are porous and have a hollow core (the medullary cavity); they appear unchanging and inert, but in fact they are metabolic powerhouses that store calcium, phosphorous, and other minerals

Bone has three functions: mechanical, metabolic, and hematopoietic. Mechanical properties are attributable to its light weight and strength, which serve to protect internal organs and act as a framework for the force of skeletal muscle contractions. Metabolic properties relate to its mineral content: bone is 65% mineral and 35% protein, and contains 99% of the body's calcium, 85% of the phosphorus, and 65% of the sodium, all of which are in a constant state of flux between bone, blood, and other tissues. In their core, many bones also house the hematopoietic system (Chapter 11), the bone marrow, which makes red and white blood cells and platelets.

Bones are classified as long, short, or flat. **Long bones** occur in the extremities; **short bones** and **flat bones** constitute the feet, hands, skull, ribs, pelvis, scapula, and spine. The anatomy of normal bones is illustrated in Figure 22-1. The place where bones meet is a **joint**, which can be very tight and allow no movement (as with the joints between the bones of the skull), or it can be loose and allow for a limited degree of movement (the vertebral joints) or a large degree (the shoulder).

The anatomy and growth of bones are exemplified by long bones. At the end of the long bones are the **epiphysis**, a cap of dense bone tissue, which is usually the widest part of the bone. In *growing* long bones the epiphysis contains an internal **epiphyseal growth plate**, a layer of cartilage unrelated to the cushioning cartilaginous plate in the joint space at the end of the bone. The epiphyseal growth plate adds to bone length by forming cartilage on the advancing side, which is turned into bone on the trailing side. The epiphyseal growth plate disappears when bone growth stops in early adult life. Beneath the epiphysis is the **metaphysis**, the broad, funnel-shaped part of a long bone that gradually narrows to become the **diaphysis**, the center shaft of the bone. In the center of the bone is the **medullary cavity**, containing fat and bone marrow.

Bone is covered by a tough, collagenous membrane, the **periosteum**, which contains osteoblasts, nerves, and blood vessels. Beneath the periosteum is **cortical bone**, a shell of dense, hard bone. In the center, loose, spongy **cancellous bone** houses the medullary cavity, which is lined by a layer of bone stem cells, the **endosteum**. In children, the marrow cavity of all bones contains only *red marrow*; that is, marrow that is producing blood cells. However, as the skeleton matures, fat-storing *yellow marrow* displaces red marrow in the shafts of the long bones of the limbs. In adults red marrow remains chiefly in the ribs, the vertebrae, the pelvic bones, and the skull.

Osteoblasts are bone-forming cells; they form bone by depositing a network of protein (collagen) fibers called **osteoid**, binding it with calcium and phosphate to form bone. As they form bone around them, osteoblasts become trapped in tiny pores (*lacunae*) and are called **osteocytes**, which comprise about 90% of all bone cells. *Osteoclasts* are bone-dissolving cells concentrated mainly around the edges of the bone pores in the medullary cavity. Osteoblasts and osteoclasts work together in a continual process of bone absorption, renewal, remodeling, and repair, and in the regulation of blood calcium and phosphorus. The activity of osteoblasts and osteoclasts is regulated by parathyroid hormone and vitamin D (Chapter 18).

In an adult there is but one type of normal bone structure, a layered design, like tree growth rings, called **lamellar bone**. However, in the fetus and until bone growth stops in the early 20s, another type of bone, **woven bone**—a flat, interlaced design somewhat like fabric—exists temporarily as part of the bone growth process. Woven bone can form rapidly and is the method of bone formation in the fetus and in the epiphyseal growth plates of children and young adults. During normal bone growth, woven bone is gradually replaced by denser, stronger, lamellar bone, the type of all bone in normal adults. However, *when seen in an adult, woven bone is always the result of some pathologic process*. For example, fractures heal first by the production of woven bone.

Normal bone growth occurs in one of two ways:

- By **endochondral ossification**, in which cartilage forms first, then is transformed into woven bone, and finally into lamellar bone
- By **intramembranous ossification**, in which interlaced fibrous tissue is transformed directly into woven bone and then into lamellar bone without beginning first as cartilage

Both methods of growth produce **lamellar bone**, which is organized as a network of canals (*Haversian canals*) that carry long cytoplasmic tentacles of osteocytes (plus blood vessels and nerves) to connect one osteocyte in its lacuna (pore) to other osteocytes in their lacunae. The main canals run lengthwise in the bone, and bone tissue grows around them like tree rings to form an *osteon*. Osteons gather together for strength like a bundle of long, thin sticks to form the dense surface casing of cortical bone around a central core of delicate spongy (cancellous) bone.

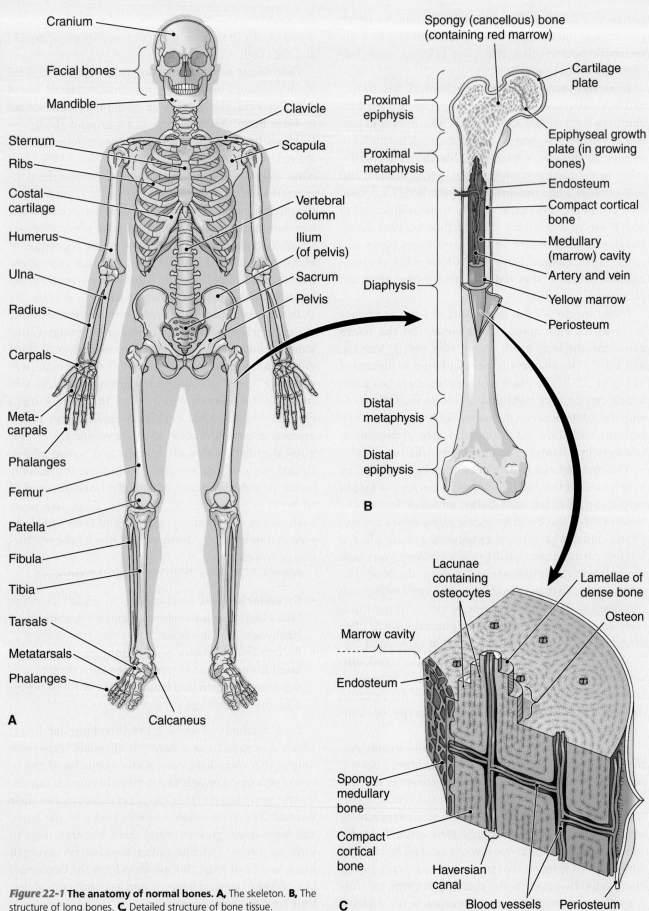

Figure 22-1 **The anatomy of normal bones. A,** The skeleton. **B,** The
structure of long bones. **C,** Detailed structure of bone tissue.

MAJOR DETERMINANTS OF DISEASE

- Bone health requires constant mechanical stress.
- Bones are metabolically active.
- Bones are dramatically affected by hormones and vitamins.
- Bones are affected by bone marrow (hematopoietic) disorders
- Fractures are a major health problem for the elderly.
- Bones are a favorite site for metastatic cancer.

Skeletal Deformities and Disorders of Bone Growth

Disorders of bone growth are characterized by fragile bones and skeletal deformities. Bone marrow disorders (Chapter 11) can affect bone growth, and in children fractures that involve the epiphyseal growth plate can interrupt normal bone growth and limit growth of a limb. As is illustrated in Figure 22-2, abnormal growth of vertebrae can produce *permanent* abnormal curvature of the lumbar and thoracic spine. **Kyphosis**, a very common finding in the elderly, is abnormal forward curvature. **Lordosis** is abnormal backward curvature, and **scoliosis** is abnormal lateral bending of the spine. Other deformities include short stature, bowed legs, and knock-knees.

Of the dozens of disorders of bone growth, only a few are mentioned here. Most bone growth disorders are caused by metabolic or inherited disease. **Achondroplasia** is a genetic syndrome of short-limbed dwarfism caused by failure of epiphyseal cartilage to form normally. The clinical picture is one of a relatively normal trunk to which are attached short arms and legs owing to a disproportionate shortening the long bones of the limbs. The face is small compared to the skull, giving the patient a bulbous appearing forehead. Saddle nose, small jaw, bowed legs, and a swayback (*lordosis*) posture complete the clinical picture. Achondroplasia is not associated with changes in length of life, mental function, or reproductive capacity.

Osteogenesis imperfecta (*brittle bone disease*) is a spectrum of inheritable disorders caused by genetic defects in collagen formation. It is characterized by brittle bones that are easily fractured. Defective middle ear bones cause deafness, and defective collagen also causes abnormal tooth development, floppy heart valves, (Chapter 13) and thin sclerae, which accounts for the semitransparent, bluish sclerae characteristic of these patients.

Paget disease of bone (*osteitis deformans*)—not to be confused with Paget disease of skin or Paget disease of breast—is a surprisingly common bone disease of unknown cause, but evidence strongly points to a chronic virus infection. In the United States Paget disease affects at least one bone in about 3% of people over 40. In Paget disease, bone is formed by osteoblasts and broken down by osteoclasts at an unusually rapid rate, causing the formation of irregular, thick, exceptionally dense bone. Any bone may be affected, but usually more than one bone is involved; the femur, pelvis, and spine are the most common sites. Ultimately, bone resorption and regrowth burn out into a final quiet phase in which bone is deformed and densely sclerotic.

Paget disease is usually asymptomatic and discovered accidentally on x-ray studies (the topic of the nearby History of Medicine box) done for other purposes, or by finding an unexpected increase of blood levels of *alkaline phosphatase*, an enzyme important in osteoblast activity. Pain, deformity, and fractures are the most common clinical problems. About 1% of patients with Paget disease develop an *osteosarcoma* or other malignant bone tumor in the affected bone.

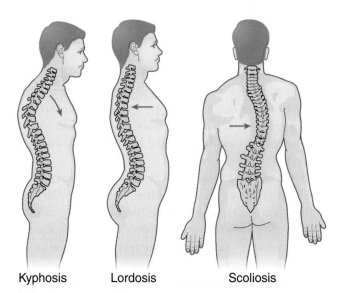

Kyphosis   Lordosis   Scoliosis

Figure 22-2 **Abnormalities of spinal curvature.**

Fractures

Healthy bones require mechanical stress, such as weight-bearing exercise, which stimulates constant osteoblast and osteoclast activity to rebuild and refresh bone. Lack of stress, as with space flight or prolonged

THE DISCOVERY OF X-RAYS

Confronted with crisis deep in the body, ancient physicians surely must have longed to see beneath the skin. Wilhelm Roentgen, a Dutch physicist, not a physician, made it possible to see through the skin when he discovered x-rays as he experimented with electricity by passing an electrical current from one metal pole to another in a vacuum tube. When the current was at low power the apparatus produced ordinary light and other types of rays, which Roentgen focused into a beam and aimed at various materials to see what happened. One such material was a barium compound painted on a panel, which glowed (fluoresced) slightly if he held it very close to the vacuum tube.

On a Friday afternoon, November 8, 1895, he conducted an experiment that initially required the vacuum tube to be covered with tin foil and cardboard to keep all of the light and other rays from escaping. To be sure that nothing was escaping he darkened the room and turned up the current to the apparatus in his vacuum tube. Sure enough, the apparatus was dark; no light or rays could be seen escaping. He was about to turn on the lights when across the room a glow caught his eye—the barium panel was glowing. Roent-gen instantly recognized that some kind of ray—he later dubbed it the x-ray—was passing from the tube, through the foil and cardboard and striking the barium panel, making it glow.

On closer inspection of the fluorescing panel he noticed a dull black line running across it. Looking carefully in the path of the mysterious rays, he discovered a wire, which was absorbing some of the rays. Then he took a simple but profound step—he put a piece of paper in the beam and noticed no interference. Next, he tried a playing card, then a book, finding that the book dimmed the beam slightly. If he had stopped at this point he would have done enough to ensure a lifetime of fame in the world of physics. But he went further and held a small lead disc in the beam, a simple act required his hand to be placed in the beam, an act that ultimately led him to the first ever Nobel Prize in physics. Lead stopped the strange rays completely, and—in a moment that literally changed impossible to possible—he noticed eerily glowing on the panel the unmistakable image of his fingers, the bones clearly visible beneath the hazy outline of his flesh.

---

bed rest, causes bones to dissolve partially and leads to weak, brittle bones. On the other hand, too much mechanical stress causes **fracture**—a broken bone. A **pathologic fracture** is one that results from disease that has weakened bone locally, so that the fracture occurs with normal stress. For example, a patient with a tumor in the femur may suffer a fracture through the lesion while doing something as ordinary as walking.

Fractures are a major health problem for the elderly. The most important risk factors for fracture are:

- Age older than 80 years
- Weight less than 130 lb
- Long term use of benzodiazepines (widely used sedatives)
- No walking for exercise
- Poor vision
- Brain disease that affects physical stability or mental capacity

A single fracture line is a *simple* fracture. A simple fracture line extending all the way across the bone is a *complete* fracture; otherwise the fracture is *incomplete*. Figure 22-3 illustrates the clinical classification of fractures according to the pattern of the break and whether or not bone has broken through skin. A *closed* fracture is one in which bone has not broken through skin. If bone protrudes through skin, the fracture is *open* or *compound*. Multiple fractures in a single site form a *comminuted* fracture. Children's bones are more flexible than adult's bones are and tend to bend or break partially (incompletely), in a manner known as a *greenstick* fracture. Sudden end-to-end force that causes bone to collapse upon itself is an *impacted* fracture, also called a *compression* fracture (especially in vertebrae). Twisting force can cause a *spiral* fracture. Fracture though a bone lesion, such as a bone tumor, is a *pathologic* fracture. Most fractures occur suddenly, but *stress* fracture occurs slowly, after repeated microfractures caused by high stress; for example, in the foot of a long-distance runner.

Force powerful enough to break bone also can damage nearby tissue. Fractures often are accompanied by injury to muscles, blood vessels, nerves, and ligaments, so that often the amount and degree of bleeding and injury is greater than might be expected from a quick glance at an x-ray image.

The healing of a fracture is illustrated in Figure 22-4. A pool of blood (hematoma) accumulates rapidly in the

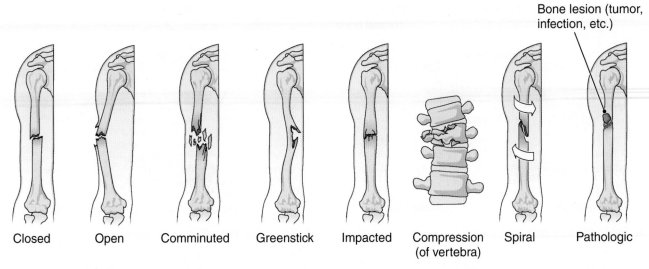

Figure 22-3 **Types of fractures.** A closed fracture is any type of fracture in which the skin is not punctured by broken bone. An open fracture is one with protruding bone. Compression fractures are most common in vertebrae.

fracture site. By the end of the first week fibroblasts, new blood vessels, and woven bone appear in the hematoma. Together they form a rich mixture of granulation tissue (Chapter 4), fibrous (scar) tissue, and soft bone, called a *soft* **callus**, which loosely unites the ends of the broken bone but cannot bear weight. After a couple of weeks soft callus matures into a *bony callus* composed mainly of cartilage and spongy cancellous bone that binds the bone ends more securely and is capable of limited weight bearing. Finally, unstressed spongy bone and excess callus is resorbed and is replaced by dense, lamellar bone, which remodels into the previous anatomic outline under the influence of local stresses.

Diseased bone, as in *osteoporosis* or *osteomalacia* (discussed below), heals poorly. Healing fractures require proper nourishment; the healing of a fracture of a large bone like the femur can consume a surprisingly large number of calories, a demand that some patients cannot easily meet. For example, alcoholics are notable for fracture-prone behavior and poor diet, and thus their fractures may not heal quickly or well. Adequate intake of vitamin D, phosphate, and calcium is especially important. Impaired vascular supply, as in diabetes, also may impair healing.

Bone in some fractures does not unite normally, a condition called *nonunion*, characterized by continued motion across the fracture site. Nonunion can be caused by lack of immobilization, poor blood supply, infection, or poor diet. If this portion of bone continues to be a site of movement (that is to say, if it functions as a "joint"), it is called a *pseudarthrosis* (literally, a false joint). If the

ends of the fracture are allowed to heal in a nonanatomic alignment, at an angle, for example, the fracture is *malaligned*.

Bone Infection

Osteomyelitis is bacterial infection of bone. Traumatic, direct implantation of bacteria into bone is the main cause of osteomyelitis in adults.

To the contrary, most children who develop bone infection do so from blood-borne bacteria from minor infections elsewhere in the body, perhaps a skin or tooth infection. Boys 5–15 years old are most often affected. Pyogenic (pus forming) infections are most common, but bacteria are often difficult to culture and identify with certainty because many patients have been treated with antibiotics by the time culture is attempted. However, *Staphylococcus aureus* accounts for about 80% of *identifiable* bacteria. The epiphysis is most often the site of blood-borne infection because it is the most vascular part of bone, especially in growing long bones of children.

Acute bacterial infection of bone is accompanied by bone necrosis and inflammation. The cause is obvious when infection follows fracture, but in children signs and symptoms may prove subtle, and diagnosis can be difficult. Pain in the affected area is accompanied by typical signs of infection: malaise, fever, chills, and increased white blood cell count. X-rays typically reveal local loss of bone density (osteolytic lesions). Acute

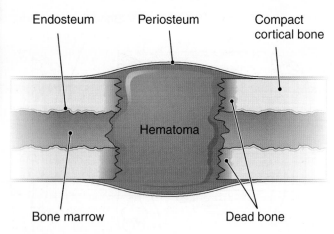

A Fresh fracture with hematoma

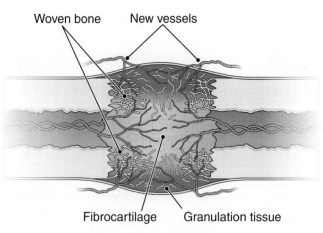

B Soft callus formation (1-2 weeks)

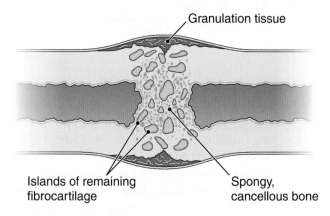

C Bony callus formation (2-4 weeks)

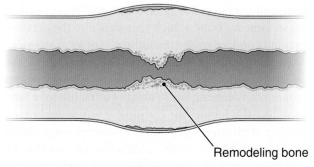

D Remodeling bone (6-10 weeks)

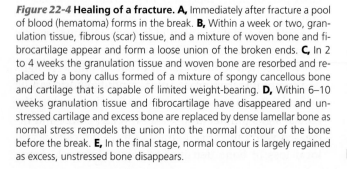

Figure 22-4 **Healing of a fracture. A,** Immediately after fracture a pool of blood (hematoma) forms in the break. **B,** Within a week or two, granulation tissue, fibrous (scar) tissue, and a mixture of woven bone and fibrocartilage appear and form a loose union of the broken ends. **C,** In 2 to 4 weeks the granulation tissue and woven bone are resorbed and replaced by a bony callus formed of a mixture of spongy cancellous bone and cartilage that is capable of limited weight-bearing. **D,** Within 6–10 weeks granulation tissue and fibrocartilage have disappeared and unstressed cartilage and excess bone are replaced by dense lamellar bone as normal stress remodels the union into the normal contour of the bone before the break. **E,** In the final stage, normal contour is largely regained as excess, unstressed bone disappears.

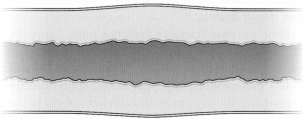

E Healed bone

bacterial osteomyelitis may prove difficult to treat and requires vigorous and prolonged antibiotic therapy. Even so, about 5%–10% of infections become chronic and can serve as a focus of continuing infection that can spread to other parts of the body to cause, for example, bacterial endocarditis (Chapter 13) or generalized blood infection (sepsis). Surgical drainage and wound cleaning (debridement) may be necessary.

Osteomyelitis caused by the tuberculosis bacterium (*Mycobacterium tuberculosis*) remains a problem in developing countries. The AIDS epidemic and increased international travel have brought a resurgence of tuberculosis, including tuberculous bone infections, to the United States.

Bone Infarct

Bone infarcts produce bone necrosis and are often called **aseptic necrosis**, a name retained from the pre-antibiotic era when most bone necrosis was due to bacterial infection, or **avascular necrosis**, reflecting the fact that many infarcts are cause by impaired blood flow. Therapeutic steroids are often the cause of bone infarct, but the mechanism is unclear. In many instances the cause is cannot be related to any event. Some bones are more vulnerable to ischemic necrosis than others: the head of the femur and the carpal bones of the wrist are more often involved than are other bones because of peculiarities of their vascular supply.

Whatever the cause, bone infarcts are mainly a problem of growing children because rapid bone growth requires a lot of blood, and in the elderly because vascular disease may impair blood flow. Necrosis of the head of the femur is a special risk in elderly people following fracture of the femoral neck. Pain is the most common complaint of avascular necrosis. Infarcts that involve joints can lead to severe mechanical arthritis (osteoarthritis, discussed below) as the dead bone within the joint is worn away.

Osteoporosis

Osteoporosis is a condition of increased bone porousness and decreased bone mass; that is, osteoporosis is a *quantitative* defect: bone microstructure is normal but there is not enough of it. Most osteoporosis results from the declining blood estrogen levels that occur in postmenopausal women. Fractures associated with osteoporosis are a major cause of death and debility in the United States and often occur after falls from no more than standing height. Less than one third of these pa-

tients have been evaluated for osteoporosis, which can be easily tested for by simple radiographic study of bone density. The bones most often fractured are weight-bearing ones—vertebrae, femur, and pelvis.

Bone is continually being remade and renewed by a delicate balance between osteoblastic bone formation and osteoclastic bone dissolution. Bone-forming capability is estrogen dependent and declines each year after menopause, tipping the balance toward bone dissolution. Bone mass is also influenced by other factors: age, genetics, physical activity, and diet. The importance of genetic factors can be seen in the fact that African Americans have greater bone mass than Anglos and therefore have less osteoporosis; and women have more osteoporosis than men do. White women have the least bone mass.

Osteoporosis caused by some other condition is secondary osteoporosis. Causes of secondary osteoporosis include cortisone excess (Cushing syndrome, Chapter 18), dietary deficiency of calcium or vitamin D (from malabsorption syndrome, Chapter 15), immobilization from prolonged bed rest, lack of weight-bearing activity because of disability (such as limb paralysis or disease), anticonvulsant medication with diphenylhydantoin (Dilantin), anticoagulant therapy with heparin, or metastatic carcinoma to bone (especially breast carcinoma).

Whether primary or secondary, the precise mechanisms that cause osteoporosis are unclear, but this much is certain: more bone is being resorbed than is being formed. The pathological findings are clear (Figs. 22-5 and 22-6): osteoporotic bones have less bone tissue in them than normal. This stands in contrast to the findings in *osteomalacia*, discussed below, in which bone density declines because it is demineralized, leaving behind soft osteoid protein.

> ☞ *One third of women over age 65 will suffer a fracture associated with osteoporosis.*

As is depicted in Figure 22-7, the typical patient with osteoporosis is an elderly, small-framed white woman. She is likely to be short and stooped: short because vertebrae are collapsed (Fig. 22-8) and stooped owing to spinal kyphosis. Her medical history often includes a recent fall and fracture. Osteoporotic fractures are a major medical and social problem in the elderly, especially of postmenopausal white women; most of these fractures are minor, but many are seriously debilitating. For example, the immobilization required to treat a broken hip may lead to pneumonia and death. About 40,000 people die each year in the United States as a direct or

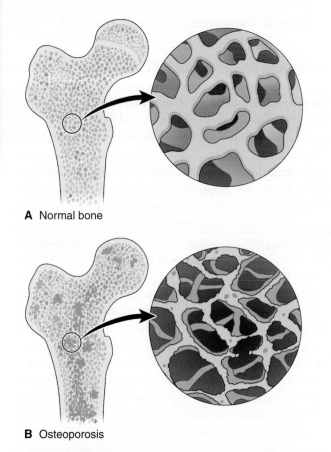

A Normal bone

B Osteoporosis

Figure 22-5 **Osteoporosis. A,** Normal cancellous (spongy) bone. **B,** Osteoporotic bone. Bone organization is correct, but the lattice is thin and less bone mass is present.

OSTEOPOROSIS

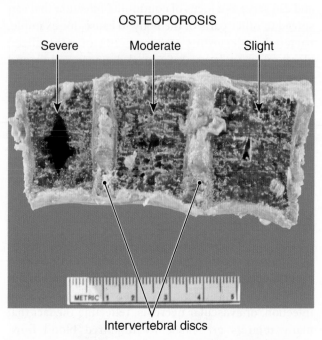

Figure 22-6 **Osteoporosis of the spine.** The degree of severity to which the vertebral bodies are affected decreases from left to right.

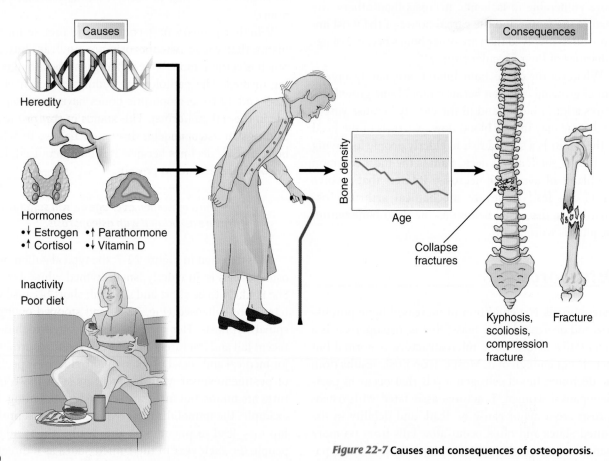

Figure 22-7 **Causes and consequences of osteoporosis.**

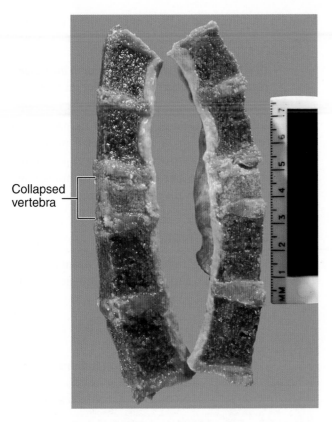

Collapsed
vertebra

Figure 22-8 **Collapse fracture of a vertebral body.** This is a midline section of the spine in a patient with osteoporosis.

indirect result of broken bones related to osteoporosis (about as many as die in traffic accidents).

Early osteoporosis is asymptomatic and cannot be detected by standard x-ray technique until about one third of bone mass has disappeared; however, special radiographic screening devices can detect low bone density before changes are detectable on routine x-rays. Prevention is the best approach for primary osteoporosis; however, new drugs show promise of rebuilding bone in some patients. Correction of the underlying condition is the best therapy for secondary osteoporosis. Exercise and appropriate intake of dietary calcium and vitamin D are essential and can slow bone loss. Estrogen replacement therapy (Chapter 21) which has been proven to be effective, has been sharply curtailed in recent years as an osteoporosis treatment because of concerns about associated health risks.

Osteomalacia

Osteomalacia (literally "soft bones") is defective mineralization (calcification) of bone protein (osteoid); that is, osteomalacia is a *qualitative* defect: osteocytes make a normal or near normal amount of normal osteoid (protein), but the osteoid does not mineralize properly.

Osteomalacia usually results from insufficient intake or poor intestinal absorption of calcium, phosphate, or vitamin D, which are dietary essentials. Additional vitamin D is synthesized in the skin as a result of sunlight exposure, so inadequate sun exposure (polar living, for example) may be a factor. Sunlight also has less effect in the synthesis of vitamin D in dark-skinned people, who are therefore more susceptible to vitamin D deficiency.

Meat and dairy products are the main dietary sources of the calcium and phosphate required for healthy bone mineralization. Although in the United States many foods are supplemented with vitamin D, dietary deficiency is common in underdeveloped countries and is associated with widespread childhood osteomalacia (*rickets*, discussed immediately below).

Small bowel disease (such as Crohn disease) may interfere directly with calcium and vitamin D absorption, or intestinal malabsorption syndromes (Chapter 15) may sweep vitamin D away because it is fat soluble and lost in fatty stools. In either circumstance, the loss of calcium, phosphate, and vitamin D causes compensatory increased secretion of parathormone from the parathyroid glands (hyperparathyroidism, Chapter 18),which causes osteoclasts to increase their bone-dissolving activity.

Osteomalacious bone is susceptible to deformity and fracture. Skeletal deformities are a particular characteristic of **rickets**, a form of osteomalacia caused by vitamin D deficiency in growing children. Typically, children with rickets have bowlegs, delayed dentition and speckled teeth, and a highly characteristic abnormality of the anterior chest wall where the ribs join the sternum: the tips of the ribs are enlarged into nodules that produce a striking, beaded appearance called "rachitic rosary."

Chronic renal failure may cause **renal osteodystrophy**, a variety of osteomalacia similar to that found in patients with hyperparathyroidism (Chapter 18). Failing kidneys do not excrete phosphate properly, and blood phosphate level rises, forcing down blood calcium. Low blood levels of calcium stimulate the parathyroid glands to secrete parathyroid hormone, which in turn stimulates osteoclasts to leach calcium from bone in an effort to increase the blood level of calcium. The result is osteomalacia, caused by demineralization of bone.

Bone Tumors

The most common tumor *in* bone is metastatic cancer. Carcinoma of the prostate, breast, and lung are the three most common malignancies in humans; and all have a predilection for bone metastasis.

Primary tumors *of* bone are uncommon, and the great majority is benign and occurs before age 30. Bone tumors in the elderly usually are malignant. The rarity and diverse histologic appearance of primary bone tumors often make them very difficult for pathologists and radiologists to diagnose correctly.

Excluding bone marrow tumors such as lymphoma, leukemia, and multiple myeloma, bone tumors fall into four groups: tumors that are predominantly composed of bone (tumors whose name usually begins with "osteo . . ."), cartilage ("chondro . . ."), fibrous tissue ("fibro . . ."), and a miscellaneous category. As is illustrated in Figure 22-9, various bone tumors have distinct affinities for certain age groups, particular bones, or parts of bones. For example, most osteosarcomas, malignant tumors of osteocytes, occur in young adolescents near the

knee (in the lower end of the femur or upper end of the tibia).

> **Of primary bone tumors, 80% occur in the lower femur or upper tibia and fibula near the knee.**

Clinically, bone tumors present with pain, as a slowly growing mass, or as an unexpected pathologic fracture. X-ray studies are a very important part of the diagnostic assessment, but biopsy and pathologic assessment is essential for diagnosis and prognosis.

BONE-FORMING TUMORS

Benign bone-forming tumors are not premalignant. They are usually small and of little consequence, except

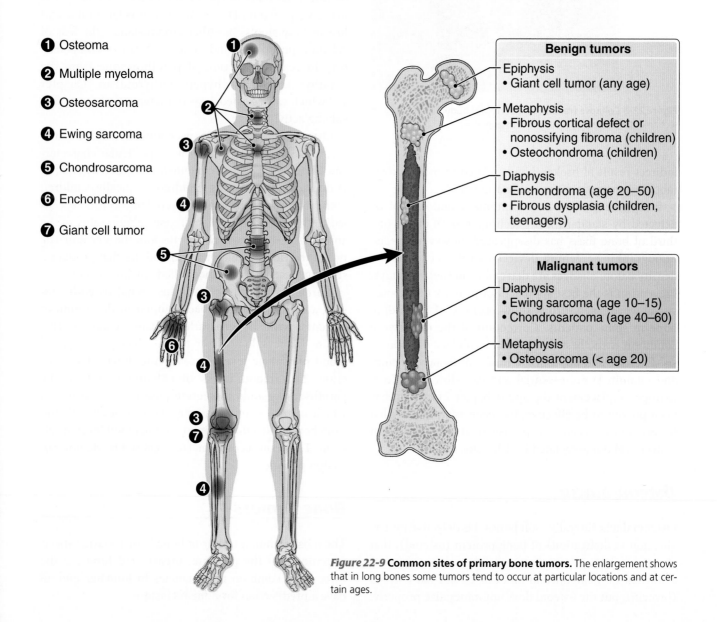

① Osteoma

② Multiple myeloma

③ Osteosarcoma

④ Ewing sarcoma

⑤ Chondrosarcoma

⑥ Enchondroma

⑦ Giant cell tumor

Benign tumors

Epiphysis
• Giant cell tumor (any age)

Metaphysis
• Fibrous cortical defect or nonossifying fibroma (children)
• Osteochondroma (children)

Diaphysis
• Enchondroma (age 20–50)
• Fibrous dysplasia (children, teenagers)

Malignant tumors

Diaphysis
• Ewing sarcoma (age 10–15)
• Chondrosarcoma (age 40–60)

Metaphysis
• Osteosarcoma (< age 20)

Figure 22-9 **Common sites of primary bone tumors.** The enlargement shows that in long bones some tumors tend to occur at particular locations and at certain ages.

that they can be painful or in the skull may press on nerves or other critical structures. Most malignant bone-forming tumors arise de novo and do not originate from benign tumors.

Osteosarcoma (*osteogenic sarcoma*) is a malignant tumor that forms neoplastic bone. Excluding tumors of bone marrow, osteosarcoma is the most common primary tumor of bone. It occurs most often in the metaphysis of long bones—about half occur in the tibia or femur near the knee—a feature probably related to the fact that the metaphysis is where bones grow and where most cell division takes place. Two age groups are most affected: 75% of osteosarcomas occur in patients under 20, and most of the remainder occur in the elderly, many of whom have some underlying condition such as Paget disease or bone irradiation received in the treatment of another condition.

Osteosarcoma usually presents as a painful, enlarging mass. It spreads by the bloodstream, and about 20% of patients have lung metastases at time of initial diagnosis. Surgery and chemotherapy cure about two thirds of patients.

CARTILAGE-FORMING TUMORS

Benign cartilage-forming tumors typically are not premalignant and are seldom of much clinical significance. A fairly common one is *osteochondroma* (also called *exostosis*, Fig. 22-10), a mushroom-shaped bony protuberance capped by cartilage that arises in children and grows on the surface of the metaphysis of long bones. *Enchondroma* is another benign cartilage-forming tumor that tends to grow in the medullary cavity of bones.

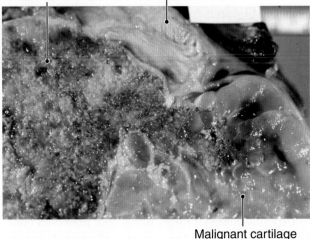

Figure 22-11 **Chondrosarcoma of the sternum.** Most chondrosarcomas arise in the central skeleton—pelvis, spine, shoulder girdle, and rib cage.

Chondrosarcoma (Fig. 22-11) is a malignant tumor of bone that forms neoplastic cartilage. It occurs about half as frequently as osteosarcoma and is the second most common primary malignant tumor of bone. It favors the spine, ribs, pelvis, and vertebrae and occurs most commonly in adults aged 4 to 60. As with osteosarcoma, microscopic grade in chondrosarcoma is of paramount importance in predicting tumor behavior. Fortunately, most are low grade (well differentiated), sluggish tumors for which the 5-year survival is about 80%. For high-grade (poorly differentiated) tumors the survival rate is about 40%. Wide excision is the treatment of choice; chemotherapy is not effective.

FIBROUS TUMORS AND TUMOR-LIKE CONDITIONS

Fibrous cortical defect of bone is a tumor-like condition of bone that occurs in about one third of children over the age of 2 years. It is probably a developmental defect, not a true neoplasm. It occurs as a nodule of benign fibrous tissue, and almost all arise near the knee in the metaphysis of the femur or tibia. They are usually asymptomatic and discovered incidentally on x-rays taken for other purposes. They may be multiple and are usually less than one cm in diameter; however they can grow to baseball size. When large, they are called **nonossifying fibroma**.

Fibrous dysplasia is a benign, nodular growth of fibrous and bone tissue that affects growing bones in children and teenagers. It is probably a developmental abnormality. All components of normal bone are present,

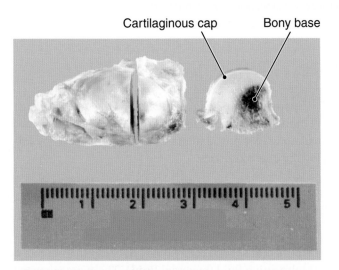

Figure 22-10 **Osteochondroma.** These small bone tumors grow on the epiphyseal surface of long bones and have a characteristic cap of cartilage.

but they do not grow in a coordinated manner into mature bone. They produce instead tumor-like masses of bone in a fibrous matrix. The most troublesome clinical problems are disfigurement and fracture. *Monostotic* fibrous dysplasia affects a single bone and accounts for three fourths of cases. *Polyostotic* fibrous dysplasia affects multiple bones, especially the face and skull, and may be associated with pigmented skin lesions and endocrine abnormalities.

Fibrosarcoma is a malignant tumor of fibrocytes that can occur in bone or other tissues (Chapter 6).

OTHER TUMORS OF BONE

Aneurysmal bone cyst forms tumor-like masses in bone, but it is not a tumor. The cause is unknown. It is composed of large, richly vascular cysts containing pools of blood that expand and erode normal bone, and it may become quite large.

Giant cell tumor (*osteoclastoma*) of bone is so named because it contains large cells with multiple nuclei that have a microscopic appearance similar to normal osteoclasts. Giant cell tumors are rather uncommon, but they are important because they can be locally aggressive. Most occur near the knee in the epiphysis of the femur or tibia and can be locally destructive. Surgical curettage cures about half, but others require additional surgery. A few giant cell tumors metastasize to the lungs.

Ewing sarcoma is a malignant tumor that occurs mainly in children, ages 10 to 15. Genetic factors are important: African Americans are rarely affected. It arises from primitive cells that are small and pose a diagnostic problem because microscopically they look like lymphocytes in malignant lymphoma (Chapter 11). Ewing sarcoma occurs mainly in the long bones and spreads quickly by blood-borne metastasis. Surgery combined with radiation and chemotherapy cures about half of patients.

Multiple myeloma (Chapter 11) is a tumor of plasma cells (B lymphocytes of the hematopoietic system) that frequently grows as localized bone lesions in the cranium, vertebrae, ribs, and sternum.

Section 2: Diseases of Joints and Related Tissues

The joint lubrication was not what it was when I was competing, and I decided that not having arthritis or rheumatism for the rest of my life was a lot more important to me than returning to the track.

EDWIN MOSES (B. 1955), LEGENDARY AMERICAN TRACK AND FIELD ATHLETE,
· EXPLAINING WHY HE CHOSE NOT TO RETURN TO COMPETITION AFTER RETIRING

BACK TO BASICS

A **joint** is the place where two bones meet. **Solid joints** provide for little or no movement; there is no joint space. For example, the bones of the skull are tightly welded by solid joints of fibrous tissue, which allow no movement; the ribs are joined to the sternum by solid joints of cartilaginous tissue, which allow very limited movement. **Fibrous joints** are united by fibrous tissue that allows a narrow range of movement; for example, the intervertebral joints of the spinal column.

Synovial joints (Fig. 22-12) allow the greatest range of motion. The knee, elbow, shoulder, wrist, and hip are examples of synovial joints. Synovial joints have the following characteristics:

- *They contain a space* (the joint cavity) that is enclosed by a sheath of fibrous tissue that binds the outer edges of the bones together and is lined internally by a special membrane (the **synovium**), which is formed of special cells (**synovial cells**) that secrete a lubricating fluid (**synovial fluid**). The synovial membrane lines only the outer edges of the joint space; it does not cover the articular surface.

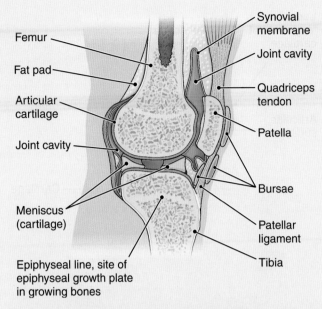

Femur

Fat pad

Articular cartilage

Joint cavity

Meniscus (cartilage)

Epiphyseal line, site of epiphyseal growth plate in growing bones

Synovial membrane

Joint cavity

Quadriceps tendon

Patella

Bursae

Patellar ligament

Tibia

Figure 22-12 Normal synovial joint (sagittal section, knee). Note that in synovial joints the synovial membrane does not cover the articular surface.

- *They contain a plate of cartilage* to cushion movement. This **articular cartilage** is specially constructed to painlessly buffer shock and wear—cartilage lacks blood supply, nerves, and lymphatics and is nourished with oxygen and nutrients from fluid in the joint.
- *The ends of the bones are usually bound together and kept in alignment by strong fibrous straps* (**ligaments**).

The movement of tissues around joints is smoothed by **bursae**, small, closed fibrous sacs lined by synovial cells, which secrete a lubricating fluid that partially fills the sac (much like a collapsed balloon containing a small amount of fluid). Bursae are positioned between tendon and bone or between skin and bony protuberances, such as the elbow, to smooth the movement where tissues rub together.

MAJOR DETERMINANTS OF DISEASE

- Mechanical wear and tear causes osteoarthritis, the most common form of arthritis.
- Arthritis is a common manifestation of autoimmune disease.
- Joints are inherently unstable and subject to injury

Osteoarthritis

Osteoarthritis (*degenerative joint disease*), a mechanical, wear-and-tear condition, is the most common type of arthritis.

Primary osteoarthritis is osteoarthritis that cannot be attributed to some specific circumstance. Secondary osteoarthritis can be attributed to a specific circumstance, such as the osteoarthritis that can occur in the hands of people operating vibrating machinery. While mechanical factors are important in the production of all osteoarthritis, they are not the sole factors. For example, primary osteoarthritis tends to occur in the last joint of the fingers near the tip (the distal interphalangeal joint), a joint that is exposed to very little mechanical stress. Indeed, in patients with arthritis of the hands, involvement of the distal interphalangeal joint of the

hands is a key diagnostic point that suggests osteoarthritis instead of some other diagnosis such as rheumatoid arthritis. Primary osteoarthritis occurs with increasing frequency with each decade of life, presumably owing to the cumulative effect of joint wear and tear. This theory is validated by the fact that primary osteoarthritis mainly affects weight-bearing joints, especially the hip, knee, and spine, and mechanical stress is clearly the cause in most cases of secondary osteoarthritis, where a specific cause is identified.

Secondary osteoarthritis is osteoarthritis that has a specific known cause. Most cases are produced by abnormal stress on a joint. For example, the added joint stress of obesity is a major cause of secondary osteoarthritis in the hip and knee joints. Secondary osteoarthritis is also caused by repeated harsh physical activity. For example, it occurs in the knees of professional football players, and in the arms and elbows of baseball pitchers. Secondary osteoarthritis also can be produced by physical malformations that create abnormal joint stress, such as the secondary osteoarthritis in the lower limbs of persons with an abnormal gait caused by neuromuscular diseases; or in the joints of people with peripheral nerve disease, who cannot feel pain in their joints and traumatize their joints without realizing it as is the case in the lower limbs of patients with diabetic peripheral neuropathy (Chapter 17).

Pathological changes in most cases of osteoarthritis are minimal: they rarely show inflammation except in advanced cases, a fact that reinforces the idea that wear and tear is the cause. Cartilage, which contains no nerves, becomes thin, frayed, or completely worn away (Figs. 22-13 and 22-14) and bones, which are rich in nerves, rub painfully against each other. The irritated bone surfaces become dense and sclerotic, with a hard, ivory-like surface. However, Figure 22-15B illustrates that striking changes may develop in advanced disease, as further stress and degeneration produce subcortical bone cysts and jagged growth of new bone (*joint spurs* or *osteophytes*), which project into adjacent soft tissue and cause inflammation, swelling, and pain.

The most important clinical characteristic of osteoarthritis is that activity-related joint pain is relieved by a short rest, whereas the pain of most other types of arthritis lasts an hour or so despite complete rest. In osteoarthritis, joint motion may produce a grinding effect (*crepitus*) as rough edges of bone and cartilage grate across one another. Early diagnosis is difficult and entirely based on the clinical findings discussed above; x-ray and laboratory findings are minimal. Aspirated joint fluid shows no bacteria and very few, if any, inflammatory cells. In advanced disease x-rays show a narrowing of the joint space, owing to cartilage destruction, and sclerosis of bone on either side of the joint; bone cysts and spurs also may be present. The swollen distal interphalangeal joints of the hands can be quite prominent and are known as *Heberden nodes*. Joints most affected are the hip, knee, and cervical and

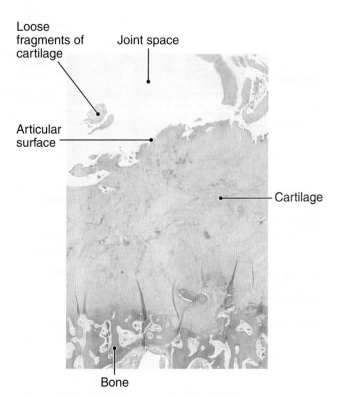

Figure 22-14 **Cartilage damage in osteoarthritis.** The articular surface is jagged and torn from mechanical force. Note that no inflammation is present.

lumbar spine. The most commonly affected joint in the foot is the joint where the big toe joins the foot (first metatarsophalangeal joint), which enlarges and forces the big toe laterally into the other toes (*bunion deformity*).

Rheumatoid Arthritis

Rheumatoid arthritis (RA) is a chronic, systemic autoimmune disease of synovial joints that affects about 1–2% of the adult population. In contrast to osteoarthritis, joints are intensely inflamed (Fig. 22-15C). Women are affected much more often than men are. The root cause of RA is unknown, but the Epstein-Barr virus is suspected of triggering a T-lymphocyte autoimmune reaction (Chapter 7) that attacks the synovial membrane. A distinct genetic tendency is present—about 75% of patients with RA have similar HLA genes (Chapter 8).

> *Eighty percent of rheumatoid arthritis occurs in women.*

The autoimmune inflammatory reaction stimulates growth of blood vessels and fibrous tissue into the sy-

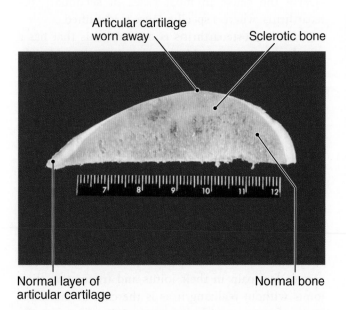

Figure 22-13 **Osteoarthritis of femur head.** The normal cap of articular cartilage is worn and the underlying bone is dense and sclerotic.

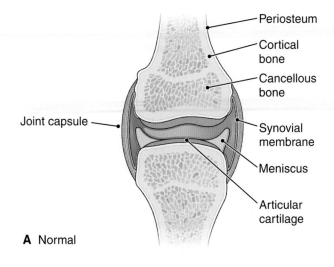

Periosteum

Cortical bone

Cancellous bone

Joint capsule

Synovial membrane

Meniscus

Articular cartilage

A Normal

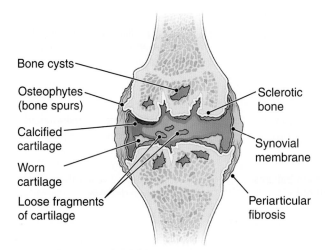

Bone cysts

Osteophytes (bone spurs)

Calcified cartilage

Worn cartilage

Loose fragments of cartilage

Sclerotic bone

Synovial membrane

Periarticular fibrosis

B Advanced osteoarthritis

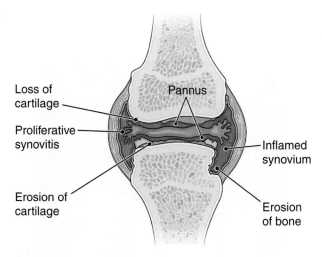

Loss of cartilage

Proliferative synovitis

Erosion of cartilage

Pannus

Inflamed synovium

Erosion of bone

C Rheumatoid arthrits

Figure 22-15 **Joint changes in arthritis. A,** Frontal (coronal) section of normal knee. **B,** Osteoarthritis. Cartilage and bone damage; no inflammation is present. **C,** Rheumatoid arthritis. The joint capsule (synovial membrane) is inflamed, and a pannus of inflammatory tissue has formed across the articular surface.

novium and joint cartilage. As a result, a highly vascular inflammatory membrane (a **pannus**, from the Hebrew word for blanket or bed covering) forms over the cartilage surface (Fig. 22-15) and oozes destructive enzymes and other agents that dissolve the cartilaginous plate. The inflammatory reaction also stimulates a papillary overgrowth of the synovium, known as *proliferative synovitis*. The end result may be complete destruction of the joint, which can undergo fibrous repair that welds together the ends of the bones to produce an immovable joint (**ankylosis**).

The fundamental immune reaction in RA involves T lymphocytes, but B lymphocytes also play a role, as is evidenced by the fact that about 75% of patients with RA have in their blood a circulating antibody complex, **rheumatoid factor** (RF). Although laboratory detection of RF is very helpful, it is not required to establish a diagnosis of RA, because RF can also be found in some patients with other autoimmune diseases or hepatitis B infection. Table 22-1 lists some useful tests in the diagnosis of musculoskeletal disease.

Rheumatoid arthritis usually appears first in patients in their 30s and 40s. It begins subtly with low-grade fever, malaise, and early morning joint pain and stiffness. The most commonly affected joints are where the fingers meet the hand (the metacarpophalangeal joint) and the next joint in the finger (the proximal interphalangeal joint). The wrist, elbow, shoulder, and ankle are also commonly affected, but any joint may be involved. Severe disease of vertebral joints can be especially painful, stiffening, and debilitating.

Especially characteristic of RA are two unique conditions. First is deviation of the bones of the hand toward the radial side of the arm, which is accompanied by deviation of the fingers in the opposite (ulnar) direction to produce the classic **Z deformity** of the hand, illustrated in Figure 22-16. Second, about 30% of patients ultimately develop **rheumatoid nodules** (Fig. 22-17), which are painless 1–2 cm subcutaneous inflammatory nodules not found in other forms of arthritis.

The disease usually progresses to a disabling arthritis over a decade or two, but average life span is reduced only about five years. Fatalities can occur, associated with treatment: GI hemorrhage from chronic administration of aspirin and nonsteroidal antiinflammatory drugs, or with infection resulting from chronic steroid therapy.

Some patients with severe chronic inflammatory disease, including RA, may develop **secondary amyloidosis** (Chapter 7), a condition that is related to the large volumes of antibody (immunoglobulin) produced in response to the autoimmune reaction. The immunoglob-

Table 22-1	**Common Laboratory Blood Tests in Musculoskeletal Disease**	
Test Type	**Primary Disease Association**	**Comments**
To detect inflammation		
Erythrocyte sedimentation rate (ESR)	Inflammation anywhere in the body	Increased in infection, autoimmune disease, polymyalgia rheumatica, some malignancies, anemia, pregnancy, renal failure Low in some diseases of red blood cells Normal in fibromyalgia
C-reactive protein (CRP)	Inflammation anywhere in the body	Increased in same conditions as increased ESR (except for anemia) Also increased in atherosclerosis Normal in fibromyalgia
To detect bone disease		
Alkaline phosphatase (AP)	Osteomalacia, bone tumors and metastases, Paget disease of bone, hyperparathyroidism	Hepatic or biliary disease, normal bone growth, late in pregnancy (from placenta)
To detect disease of joints and related tissues		
Antinuclear antibody (ANA)	Positive in 95% of patients with systemic lupus erythematosus	Also can be positive in rheumatoid arthritis, scleroderma, Sjögren syndrome, and with certain therapeutic drugs
Rheumatoid factor (RF)	Positive in about 70% of patients with rheumatoid arthritis	Also can be positive in other autoimmune diseases
To detect muscle disease		
Creatine kinase (CK)	Myositis, myopathy, trauma	Also can be positive in severe muscular exertion, seizures, heat stroke, myocardial infarction

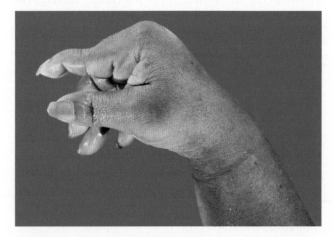

Figure 22-16 Rheumatoid arthritis. The fingers are deviated laterally (toward the ulna, away from the viewer) as part of the typical "Z" deformity of chronic rheumatoid arthritis.

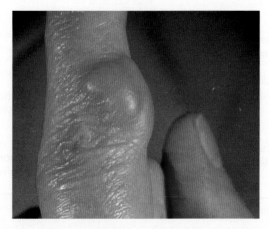

Figure 22-17 Rheumatoid nodule. Rheumatoid nodules are diagnostic of rheumatoid arthritis when found in patients with other clinical features suggesting rheumatoid arthritis. Reprinted with permission from Rubin E. Pathology. 4th ed. Philadelphia. Lippincott Williams and Wilkins, 2005.

ulins are broken down and can be deposited as amyloid protein in kidneys, liver, spleen, and adrenals; RA is a common cause of secondary amyloidosis.

Rheumatoid arthritis also affects tissues other than joints. Heart (myocarditis and pericarditis), blood vessels (vasculitis and infarcts), eyes (scleritis), skin (subcutaneous rheumatoid nodules), lungs (interstitial fibrosis and pleuritis), and skeletal muscle (myositis) are notably susceptible, but no tissue is protected.

Diagnosis of RA is mainly a clinical exercise that depends little on laboratory or other diagnostic tools. History and physical examination are of paramount importance. Joint fluid diagnostic for RA shows chronic inflammatory cells and is free of bacteria and uric acid crystals. (The presence of uric acid crystals is an indication of gout, discussed below.) Rheumatoid nodules and detection of rheumatoid factor in blood confirm the clinical diagnosis if they are present, but their absence does not exclude rheumatoid arthritis as a diagnosis in a patient with arthritis. *Anticyclic citrullinated peptide (anti-CCP)* is an autoantibody present in about half of RA patients, even in the earliest stages of disease. It is more specific than RF and if detected is diagnostic.

Early diagnosis (less than three months from first symptoms) is especially important because immediate, vigorous drug therapy plus physical therapy pay big dividends in the long run. Historically, the most important drugs have been aspirin and other nonsteroidal antiinflammatory drugs and steroids. Pharmacologically produced antibodies (infliximab, for example), which block natural inflammatory molecules, have proven effective.

Rheumatoid arthritis that develops in children or adolescents is called **juvenile rheumatoid arthritis**. It differs from adult RA in several important ways: onset is sudden, systemic, and "toxic," with high fever and prostration. Few joints are involved, and they tend to be large ones such as the knees or hips. RF and rheumatoid nodules are usually absent, and antinuclear antibodies (ANAs) are often found in the blood. As with adult RA, other organs and tissues may be affected. The majority of patients recover fully; few develop chronic, deforming arthritis. Treatment is similar to therapy for adults with rheumatoid arthritis except that in the United States aspirin is not used for fear that it might cause Reye syndrome (fatty liver and acute encephalopathy, Chapter 16).

Spondyloarthropathies

The vertebrae are complex bones, each of which articulates with one another and with the ribs by several joints. The term **spondyloarthropathy** derives from Greek *spondylos*, meaning vertebra, and it describes several related types of autoimmune, genetically influenced, vertebral arthritis that occur in patients who *do not have rheumatoid factor antibody in their blood*; that is to say, they are *seronegative*, and they are often called the *seronegative spondyloarthropathies*.

The spondyloarthropathies are distinctive from rheumatoid arthritis in the following ways: 1) the arthritis is usually confined to the vertebrae and sacroiliac joints; 2) inflammation also involves tendons where they attach to bone; 3) rheumatoid factor is absent from blood; and 4) the cells of most patients carry HLA-B27 antigen (Chapter 8).

The following spondyloarthropathies share overlapping clinical features: the majority of patients are young adults, males are affected much more often than females, infection seems to trigger the onset of disease, and many patients have extra-articular inflammatory conditions such as iritis (Chapter 25) or vasculitis (Chapter 12).

- **Ankylosing spondylitis** (*rheumatoid spondylitis, Marie-Strümpell disease*) is a chronic relapsing arthritis primarily affecting the spine (Fig. 22-18), the sacroiliac joints in particular. Most patients suffer from spinal rigidity and chronic back pain but otherwise usually lead full lives.
- **Reactive arthritis** is arthritis that occurs within one month of an infection somewhere in the body other than the joints; genitourinary (*Chlamydia*) and intestinal infections (*Shigella*, *Campylobacter*) are the

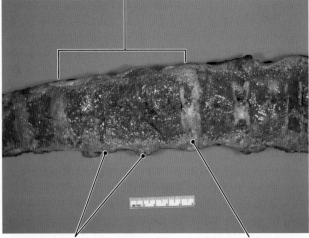

Three vertebrae fused into one

Approximate sites of destroyed intervertebral discs

Intervertebral disc

Figure 22-18 **Ankylosing spondylitis.** Two intervertebral discs have been destroyed and three vertebrae are fused into a single mass.

most common. Low back, ankles, knees, and feet are most often involved.

- **Psoriatic arthritis** is seen in about 10% of patients with psoriasis (Chapter 24). The small joints of the hands and feet are usually first affected, but the spine and sacroiliac joints are often involved later.

Other Types of Arthritis

Primary **gout** is a chronic metabolic disease associated with high blood uric acid levels; joint deposits of uric acid crystals; and inflammatory, nodular subcutaneous deposits (tophi) of uric acid crystals. Uric acid crystals are sharp and incite intense inflammation, which causes a severe acute and chronic relapsing arthritis. The kidney concentrates and excretes uric acid into the urine, and renal deposits of uric acid in the kidney may cause renal failure. There is a strong familial tendency toward the development of gout, but no specific genetic defect has been identified.

Gout can also be *secondary* to other conditions. For example, episodes of gout occur in patients with lymphoma or leukemia, owing to large amounts of uric acid produced when DNA from the nuclei of dead malignant cells is metabolized.

Almost all patients with gout are men. The great toe is affected in 90% of cases and is such a distinctive finding that it has its own name: *podagra* (from the Greek root *pod* for foot, as in *pod*iatrist, a specialist in foot diseases, and *agra*, meaning trapped or seized; thus a short way of saying "foot seizure"). Acute gouty arthritis is characterized by severe inflammation, and affected joints are exquisitely tender. Other joints in the feet and hands are also affected. High serum levels of uric acid accelerate atherosclerosis, and patients with gout have a high incidence of cardiovascular disease.

Treatment includes drugs to increase renal uric acid excretion, and dietary modification. Uric acid derives from purines, a type of organic chemical found in high concentration in animal and fish flesh and certain other foods, consumption of which can aggravate preexisting gout. Alcohol inhibits renal excretion and also should be avoided.

Acute septic arthritis (pyogenic arthritis) is uncommon. In adults the most common organism is the gonococcus, *Neisseria gonorrhoeae*. About 5% of patients with untreated gonorrhea develop acute, septic gonococcal arthritis. Most patients have clear risk factors. For example, corticosteroid therapy and immune disease are associated with weakened immune resistance to infection, and intravenous drug abuse or infected in-

travenous lines or catheters can allow the introduction of bacteria into the bloodstream. Patients with rheumatoid arthritis are particularly at risk because they frequently are debilitated, they often are on steroid drugs, and the rich vascularity of their inflamed joints is a natural seedbed for deposits of blood-borne bacteria. Another well-defined group at risk for acute septic arthritis is children who have a bacterial infection elsewhere in the body—middle ear infection, for example—allowing seeding of a joint with blood-borne bacteria. Half are less than 2 years old, and in most cases only a single joint is involved.

Arthritis is a prominent feature of late stage **Lyme disease**, a summertime bacterial infection caused by *Borrelia burgdorferi*, a corkscrew-like bacterium (spirochete) that is spread from rodents to humans by a deer tick, which is very small and difficult to find once it has burrowed deeply into thick genital, axillary, or scalp hair. Most cases occur in a band of states from Massachusetts to Maryland; another cluster occurs in Wisconsin and Minnesota, and another in California and Oregon.

The initial tick bite is followed by spread of the organism throughout the body, which is accompanied by fever, enlarged lymph nodes near the bite, and an expanding, annular rash with a clear center (*erythema migrans*), signs that are diagnostic to a skilled observer. Arthritis is the dominant feature of chronic infection, but meningitis and myocarditis may also occur.

Although Lyme disease may be suspected in patients with summertime rashes, fevers, aches, pains, and fatigue, infection is difficult to prove. Lab tests for anti-*Borrelia* antibodies may be helpful, but false positives are common.

Polymyalgia rheumatica (PMR) and *giant cell arteritis* are related conditions. PMR is a clinical diagnosis made in the absence of another diagnosis. Symptoms include pain and stiffness in the shoulders, neck, and hips. There is also usually associated fever, malaise, moodiness, mild weight loss, and mild anemia. Observable arthritis—a swollen joint, for example—is usually absent. PMR must be distinguished from arthritis and inflammatory diseases of muscle (discussed below). The diagnosis is confirmed by finding increased levels of C-reactive protein or increased erythrocyte sedimentation rate (Chapter 3), a clear indication that inflammation is present, and by the absence of increased muscle enzymes in blood, which, if present, would suggest disease of muscle. PMR differs from rheumatoid arthritis by the absence of significant joint abnormalities and the absence of rheumatoid factor. About 20% of patients with polymyalgia rheumatica have or will develop **giant cell arteritis** (sometimes called *temporal arteritis*), an autoimmune vasculitis that most often affects the temporal, retinal and cranial arteries (Chapter 11) of elderly women.

Patients with polymyalgia rheumatica respond very well to steroid therapy; failure to respond suggests another diagnosis. In patients with giant cell arteritis, early diagnosis and steroid treatment are necessary to avoid possible blindness from retinal artery occlusion or stroke.

Injuries to Ligaments, Tendons, and Joints

Dislocation is displacement of one bone in a joint such that the articular surfaces no longer meet. **Subluxation** is a lesser degree of separation. Both usually are caused by trauma and can be associated with injury to adjacent soft tissue and joint ligaments and cartilage.

Joint cartilage, ligaments, and tendons may be torn when a joint is forced to move through a greater than normal range of motion. Sports knee and ankle injuries are especially common causes of torn ligaments, tendons, and cartilage. A **sprain** is an injury to a *ligament* induced by stretching it too far. The same injury to a *tendon* is a **strain**. The injury may completely tear the ligament or tendon or pull it away from its attachment (*avulsion*) and require surgical reattachment. Severe tears are accompanied by hemorrhage and swelling. Minor sprains and strains are tender and painful, but no hemorrhage or swelling occurs.

Periarticular Pain Syndromes

Considered here are a group of painful musculoskeletal conditions that are not arthritis but occur in ligaments and muscles near joints.

Back and neck pain are very common and often are not associated with demonstrable pathologic changes. Acute back pain and neck pain are usually caused by acute muscle strain; chronic pain is a much more complex matter that may last a lifetime and sometimes defies anatomic explanation, the principal reason so much quackery and nonsense swarm about the problem. However, there are many causes of acute and chronic back and neck pain that are associated with clear pathologic abnormality—spinal nerve compression, rheumatoid arthritis, metastatic cancer, and vertebral fractures, for example.

Vertebrae are stacked one upon another and separated by *intervertebral discs*, which are cushions of soft, pulpy tissue (the *nucleus pulposus*) encircled by a rind of tough, fibrocartilaginous tissue. With degeneration of the rind (**degenerative disc disease**), which occurs with age, the nucleus pulposus bulges or ruptures (**herniated intervertebral disc**, Fig. 22-19) outward, impinging on spinal nerve roots or on the spinal cord itself. Pressure on spinal nerves or spinal cord tracts can cause pain, numbness, tingling, or paralysis. For example, a herniated disc can press on sensory nerve roots composed of axons that travel in the sciatic nerve, the main nerve to the leg, to cause the clinical syndrome of *sciatica*—pain in the buttock, thigh, or lower leg. Pressure on motor nerve roots can cause partial paralysis that is manifest as *footdrop*, a dragging of the foot due to inability to flex the ankle.

The stack of vertebrae that form the spinal column are interlocked and stabilized by contact at fibrous joints on the arch of bone that surrounds the spinal cord (the joints that are involved, for example, by ankylosing spondylitis and juvenile rheumatoid arthritis). Sometimes, however, the locking mechanism in the vertebral arch fails because of bone degeneration, chronic stress fracture, or intervertebral disc disease, and vertebrae may slip out of alignment, a condition known as **spondylolisthesis** (from Greek *spondylos* for vertebra, and *listhesis* for sliding). Spondylolisthesis usually occurs in the lower back and is often asymptomatic, but it can be associated with pain associated with bone fracture, nerve impingement, or inflammation of vertebral joints that occurs as a result of abnormal joint stress.

Bursitis is inflammation of a bursa and is typically caused by direct trauma or by the stress of repetitive motion. The bursa fills with inflammatory fluid to be-

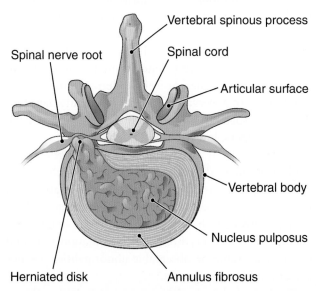

Figure 22-19 **Herniated intervertebral disc.** The central pulp has herniated laterally to impinge on a spinal nerve.

come a tender, fluctuant mass. Rest and nonsteroidal antiinflammatory drugs are usually effective.

Tendonitis is inflammation or pain in a tendon; **tenosynovitis** is inflammation or pain of the synovial sheath through which tendons slide in their motion. Repeated or excessive motion may cause painful syndromes of tendonitis and tenosynovitis. Infiltrates of inflammatory cells are usually not present, and the exact mechanism of the pain in these circumstances is not clear. Pain and tenderness are often located at the point where tendon attaches to bone. The elbow, wrist, shoulder, and knee are most often involved. An example is *tennis elbow*, a painful condition of the ligaments that attach forearm extensor muscles to the lateral epicondyle of the humerus. A related example is *shin splints*, an affliction of runners that is characterized by pain and tenderness along the anterior aspect of the tibia where muscle attaches to bone.

On the other hand, some tendonitis and tenosynovitis is accompanied by clear-cut chronic inflammation and fibrosis. An example is **carpal tunnel syndrome**, a condition of the tendons and tendon sheaths of the ventral wrist in people doing tasks that require repetitive finger and wrist motions. Inflammatory scarring and strictures constrict nerves and blood vessels passing through the wrist, causing pain, swelling, numbness, and discoloration in the hand or fingers. Surgery may be required to open the sheath and release the pressure.

Fibromyalgia is a *clinical* syndrome of muscle and periarticular tendon and ligament pain, tenderness, and stiffness that is not associated with objective signs of disease—laboratory, x-ray, and other studies are normal (see Case Study 22-1 at the end of this chapter). It is one of the most common of all arthritis-like conditions, affecting about 5% of the general population, most often women between ages 20 and 50. Fatigue, sleep disorders, depression, vague feelings of numbness, and headaches are common. Patients may complain that their joints are swollen or feel swollen, although actual swelling is not observable. Patients frequently have tenderness at specific "trigger points" near joints in the neck, shoulders, low back, and thighs.

Diagnosis is by exclusion of other disorders that could account for the patient's symptoms, which include various types of arthritis, polymyalgia rheumatica, and inflammatory diseases of muscle. Fibromyalgia differs from polymyalgia rheumatica in that fever, weight loss, anemia, increased erythrocyte sedimentation rate, and other measurable or observable abnormalities are not present in fibromyalgia.

The lack of objective laboratory tests and other abnormalities raises the question: Is fibromyalgia a psychological condition? Some research suggests that the fault may be in the brain's pain-processing system. Regardless of the cause, the pain, stiffness, and soreness are real enough to patients, and the syndrome is seen by caregivers with enough frequency and consistency that it is now a generally accepted medical diagnosis. However, some skeptics consider it a behavioral disorder. Antiinflammatory drugs are not effective; antidepressants and exercise often help.

Tumors and Tumor-like Lesions of Joints

Neoplasms of joints are rare. They usually occur in soft tissue near the joint, not actually in the joint. They are discussed in the section on Tumors and Tumor-like Lesions of Soft Tissue, in the next section of this chapter.

Ganglion cyst (Fig. 22-20) is a small (usually <1.5 cm), smooth, fluctuant, fluid-filled, simple cyst that arises near a joint or tendon sheath; the wrist is a typical site. Ganglion cyst is a focal myxoid degeneration of connective tissue and lacks an internal lining cell layer (and therefore should be called a pseudocyst). The fluid is oily, similar to synovial fluid. They are innocuous but may be surgically removed if they limit motion, are painful, or are unsightly.

Pigmented villonodular synovitis is a benign neoplasm (despite its name). It arises in patients 20 to 40 years old, and 80% occur in the knee. It can be locally aggressive and invade bone, but it does not metastasize. Surgical excision is usually curative, but some tumors may recur locally. A related neoplasm in tendon sheath is **giant cell tumor of tendon sheath**, which occurs most commonly in the wrist or hand. It, too, may be locally aggressive and require re-excision.

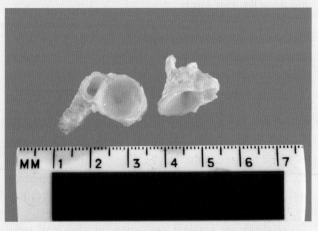

Figure 22-20 Ganglion cyst. These small benign cysts occur near joints, especially the wrist. This particular one was removed because it interfered with wrist motion.

Section 3: Diseases of Skeletal Muscle

Muscles come and go; flab lasts.

BILL VAUGHAN (1915–1977), AMERICAN WRITER AND HUMORIST

BACK TO BASICS

The fundamental element of the neuromuscular system is the **motor unit** (Fig. 22-21), which consists of:

- A lower motor neuron, located in the brain stem or spinal cord and extending via a long cytoplasmic extension (axon) to skeletal muscle
- A motor end plate, the neuromuscular junction, where nerve meets muscle
- A skeletal muscle cell

Skeletal muscles and the nerves that innervate them are composed of permanent cells (Chapter 3), that cannot regenerate, a very important consideration in neuromuscular disease. On the other hand, injured peripheral nerve *axons* (but not whole cells) can regrow, but the process is slow and sometimes not effective.

Signals are sent from the brain by an *upper* motor neuron in the cerebral cortex that connects with a *lower* motor neuron by a long axon, which in turn relays the signal to muscle cells by attaching to them with a special nerve ending known as a **motor end plate**. Where the motor end plate and muscle cell join is the **neuromuscular junction**, which is a special kind of cell union known as a synapse. A **synapse** is a junction between two neurons or between a neuron and a muscle or gland cell, which features a very narrow space (the *synaptic space*) between the signaling nerve cell and the receiving cell (in this instance, muscle).

Signals are transmitted down nerve axons as waves of electrical disturbance in the cell membrane. On arrival at the motor end plate, the signal stimulates release of **acetylcholine** (the neurotransmitter) into the synaptic space. Acetylcholine is a small organic molecule that quickly crosses the synaptic space and interacts with skeletal muscle to cause electrical disturbance of the muscle cell membrane and contraction of muscle fibers. In the process acetylcholine is broken down and immediately reconstituted by an enzyme, cholinesterase, in order for acetylcholine to transfer the next signal across the synapse.

Muscle cells are elongated and have multiple nuclei, which lie at the edge of the cell in order to stay out of the way of muscle fiber contractions. Compared to most other cells, cytoplasm in muscle cells is especially abundant in order to accommodate large amounts of long, thin specialized protein molecules, **actin** and **myosin**, which lie in parallel rows running lengthwise in the cell. The coiling and uncoiling of actin and myosin in response to muscle cell membrane electrical stimulation by acetylcholine accounts for the contraction and relaxation of skeletal muscle.

Muscle fibers are either *type 1*, slow twitch, or *type 2*, fast twitch. Fiber characteristics are detailed in Table 22-2. Type 1 fibers are designed for sustained action; type 2 for short bursts of intensity. Various muscles have different percentages of type 1 and 2 fibers, depending on their task, a fact easily demonstrable in birds. Waterfowl, ducks, and geese, for example, must fly long distances. Their breast muscles, which power their wings for many hours at a time, are type 1 fibers (dark or red muscle), which are packed with energy-providing mitochondria and related chemicals that give them a dark, reddish color. By contrast, turkeys and pheasants are nonmigratory birds that erupt into flight quickly and fly only short distances on flights that last less than a minute and are sustained by short bursts of intense muscle action. Their flight is facilitated by breast muscles that are type 2 fibers (white or pale muscle), with fewer mitochondria than are found in type 1 fibers. Human type 1 and type 2 muscle fibers differ, too, but the distinctions are less obvious. For example, the muscles in the lower leg that are used for walking and running are mainly type 1 fibers; in contrast, the small muscles attached to the eyeball, which control eye movement, are mainly type 2 fibers. Type 1 and type 2 fibers are easily distinguishable microscopically by special tissue stains (Fig. 22-22). Some muscle conditions affect only one type of fiber.

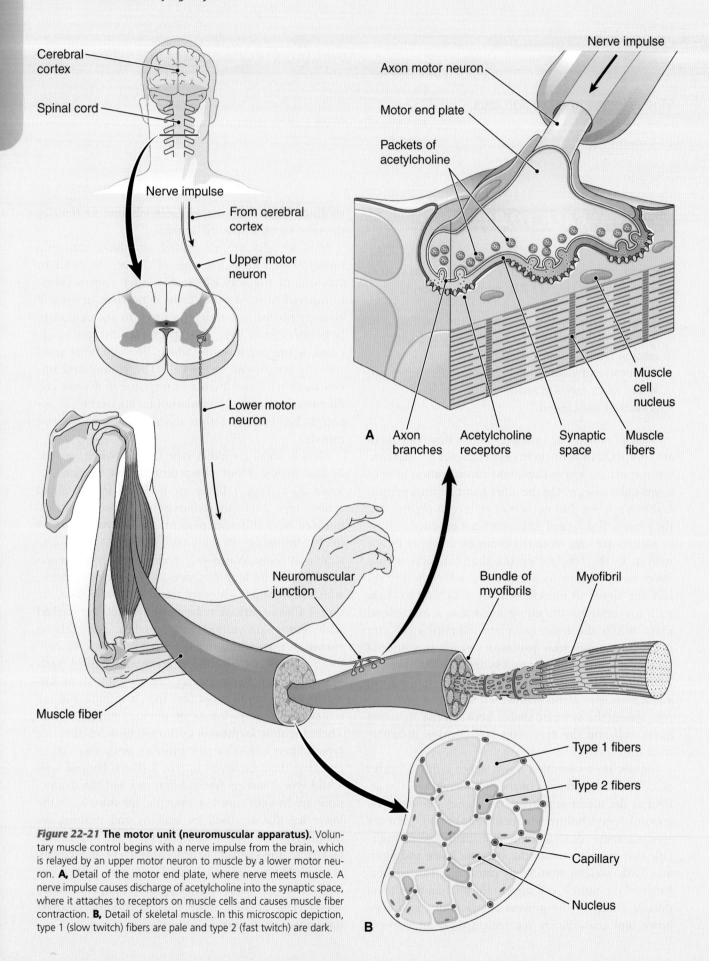

Figure 22-21 The motor unit (neuromuscular apparatus). Voluntary muscle control begins with a nerve impulse from the brain, which is relayed by an upper motor neuron to muscle by a lower motor neuron. **A,** Detail of the motor end plate, where nerve meets muscle. A nerve impulse causes discharge of acetylcholine into the synaptic space, where it attaches to receptors on muscle cells and causes muscle fiber contraction. **B,** Detail of skeletal muscle. In this microscopic depiction, type 1 (slow twitch) fibers are pale and type 2 (fast twitch) are dark.

Table 22-2 *Characteristics of Muscle Fiber Types Compared*

Characteristic	Type I, Slow Twitch	Type II, Fast Twitch
Action	Sustained force or weight bearing	Sudden movement or purposeful motion
Color (from fiber myoglobin content and vascular supply)	Red (dark)	Pale (white)
ATPase stain intensity	Dark	Light
Fat	Abundant	Scant
Glycogen	Scant	Abundant
Example of human muscle with high fiber type content	Neck muscles	Eye muscles

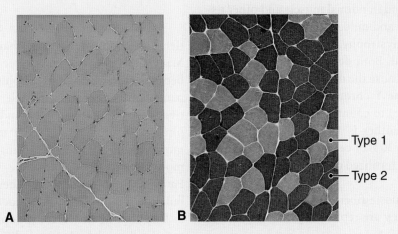

Figure 22-22 Normal muscle. A, Conventional microscopic study. **B,** Special stain demonstrating type 1 and type 2 fibers. Reprinted with permission from Rubin E. Pathology. 4th ed. Philadelphia. Lippincott Williams and Wilkins, 2005.

MAJOR DETERMINANTS OF DISEASE

- Skeletal muscle is composed of cells that cannot regenerate.
- Muscles and their nerves operate as a unit (the motor unit).
- Normal function of the motor unit is dependent on the ability of nerve signals to cross the neuromuscular synapse.
- Muscle health depends on its being connected to a functioning nerve.
- Genetic defect may cause muscle disease.
- Autoimmune disease often affects muscle.
- Muscle is resistant to infection

Muscle Atrophy

Like all other tissues, in order to remain healthy, skeletal muscle must have an adequate blood supply; however, to remain healthy, skeletal muscle, unlike other tissues, must also be connected to (innervated by) a healthy peripheral nerve. **Denervation**, loss of nerve supply, leads to muscle fiber atrophy (**neurogenic atrophy**). Nerve damage associated with diabetes (*diabetic peripheral neuropathy*, Chapter 17) is the most common cause, but peripheral nerve trauma and diseases of the peripheral nervous system (Chapter 23) also can be responsible.

A second type of atrophy is **disuse atrophy**, which occurs in muscles that are inactive because of some reason other than denervation; for example, in bedridden patients or in patients with stroke or other brain disease that affects upper motor neurons and renders patients unable to initiate voluntary movement. Disuse atrophy selectively affects type 2 (fast twitch) fibers only. Cortisol excess (Cushing syndrome) also causes type 2 fiber atrophy.

Muscular Dystrophy

The **muscular dystrophies** are a group of hereditary, progressive, noninflammatory diseases of striated muscle—skeletal and cardiac—associated with muscle weakness.

Duchenne muscular dystrophy is the most common form of muscular dystrophy. It is an X-linked inherited disease (Chapter 7) caused by the absence of *dystrophin*, a normal protein found in normal muscle and other tissues. A less common and milder form of the same type is **Becker muscular dystrophy**, in which dystrophin is present but abnormal. Both diseases occur almost exclusively in males because the defect is present on the X chromosome, and the Y chromosome has no normal matching gene (allele) to counter the defect. In 70% of cases the patient's mother is a clinically normal heterozygous carrier. In 30% of cases the mutations occur spontaneously in the fertilized ovum, and the mother is not a carrier.

Pathologically, muscle fibers atrophy and die, and late in the disease they are replaced by fat and fibrous connective tissue.

The main clinical manifestation of both Duchenne and Becker muscular dystrophy is muscle weakness, especially in pelvic and shoulder muscles (Fig. 22-23). In Duchenne muscular dystrophy the child is slow to take first steps, clear impairment is present by age 5, and pa-

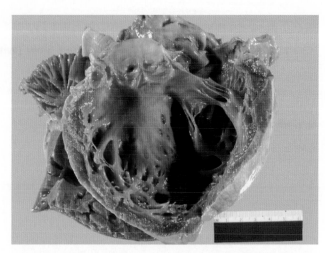

Figure 22-24 The heart in muscular dystrophy. Mechanical weakness of the muscle in this heart has caused congestive heart failure and cardiac dilation.

tients are confined to a wheelchair by the teenage years. Many patients have some degree of mental impairment because of the lack of dystrophin in brain cells. Some patients develop cardiac muscle weakness and congestive heart failure (Fig. 22-24) and die in their 20s of respiratory insufficiency. Becker muscular dystrophy is more variable, in general starting later and progressing more slowly than Duchenne muscular dystrophy. Patients with mild forms of either type may remain ambulatory until well into adulthood.

Diagnosis of muscular dystrophy depends on characteristic clinical findings of shoulder and hip muscle weakness, family history of muscular dystrophy, and markedly elevated levels of serum *creatine kinase*, an enzyme found in very high concentration in skeletal muscle. Special microscopic tissue stains for dystrophin are helpful distinguishing tools—patients with Duchenne muscular dystrophy have no demonstrable dystrophin; however, dystrophin is identifiable in patients with Becker muscular dystrophy. Prenatal genetic diagnosis (Chapter 7) is available by analysis of cells in amniotic fluid or by biopsy of chorionic villi.

Myositis and Myopathy

Myositis is muscle inflammation. The most common type of myositis is muscle infection by a virus in association with viral illness elsewhere in the body. The muscle aches of influenza, for example, are symptoms of mild viral myositis. *Trichinella spiralis* is a parasitic worm usually obtained by eating insufficiently cooked pork. *Trichinella* preferentially infects muscle, causing the disease known as *trichinosis*, which is characterized

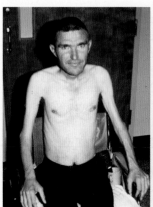
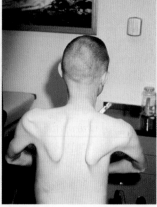

Figure 22-23 Muscular dystrophy. This patient has severe muscle atrophy of the shoulder girdle.

by widespread muscle tenderness and markedly increased levels of blood eosinophils.

Bacterial infection of muscle is very rare unless in association with wounds. It usually occurs in deep, dirty wounds, burns, or illicit drug injection sites. Many of these infections are caused by anaerobic bacteria (Chapter 9). Anaerobic muscle infections include:

- *Gas gangrene* (myonecrosis) is a very serious bacterial infection caused by infection by *Clostridium perfringens*, a large Gram-positive bacillus (rod). The disease gets its name from bacterially produced gas, which imparts a crinkling feel (*crepitus*) to the wound. It may cause extensive local muscle necrosis, hemolysis, shock, and death.
- *Tetanus* is caused by wound infection with *Clostridium tetani*, which secretes a potent neurotoxin that may produce fatal muscle spasms (tetany) and seizures.
- *Ludwig angina* is an infection that usually begins with infected gums and extends to the muscles and soft tissues of the tongue and floor of the mouth.
- *Peritonsillar* or *retropharyngeal abscess* may spread to involve pharyngeal and neck muscles.

Skeletal muscle can be involved by autoimmune disease (Chapter 8) and usually takes one of two forms: *dermatomyositis* and *polymyositis*. **Dermatomyositis** is an autoimmune disease of skin and skeletal muscle, in which the first sign usually is a characteristic rash of the eyelids. Muscle inflammation and weakness follow. All age groups are affected. **Polymyositis** is similar to dermatomyositis, but there is no skin involvement, and most patients are adults. In both diseases proximal muscles are most seriously affected. Symptoms include soreness, weakness, and muscle atrophy, and in both blood creatine kinase is high, and muscles are infiltrated by lymphocytes (Fig. 22-25). Despite their similarities, the pathologic mechanisms are different. In dermatomyositis muscle inflammation is caused by deposition in muscle of circulating antigen-antibody complexes; in polymyositis muscle inflammation is caused by direct muscle damage by T cells.

Myopathy is a term used to describe generalized noninflammatory muscle diseases that are not muscular dystrophy. Some are genetic, but most result from toxic effects of hormones or chemicals. For example, excess thyroid hormone in hyperthyroidism (Chapter 18) or sustained high blood levels of alcohol from binge drinking can induce muscle cell necrosis or muscle weakness. Additionally, a small percent of patients taking the very widely used cholesterol-lowering statin drugs may develop myopathy, which disappears on drug withdrawal.

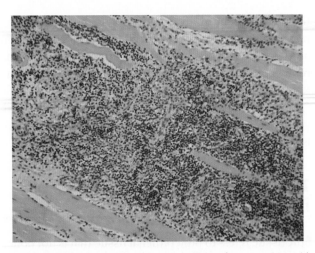

Figure 22-25 **Polymyositis.** This muscle biopsy from a patient with polymyositis demonstrates a dense infiltrate of inflammatory cells (lymphocytes) among muscle cells. Reprinted with permission from Rubin E. Pathology. 4th ed. Philadelphia. Lippincott Williams and Wilkins, 2005.

Rhabdomyolysis is a term used to describe sudden necrosis of skeletal muscle, with release of large amounts of myoglobin into the circulation. Myoglobin circulating in the blood is toxic to the kidneys and is the cause of about 10% of cases of acute renal failure. The urine of most patients turns dark as the kidneys excrete myoglobin. Rhabdomyolysis is always secondary to some underlying serious medical condition. The most common causes are burns and heat stroke; other causes are alcoholic binge drinking, crush injury, muscle contractions during seizures, drug overdose, poisoning, and electrical shock.

Myasthenia Gravis

Myasthenia gravis is an uncommon, acquired autoimmune disease of the neuromuscular junction. Antibodies attach to acetylcholine receptors on the muscle side of the synapse (see Fig. 22-21A), blocking acetylcholine released from the motor end plate and thus interrupting transmission of the nerve impulse. Myasthenia gravis may occur at any age, but usually affects women in the range of 20 to 40 years of age; affected men tend to be older. Drooping eyelids or double vision caused by periorbital and eye muscle weakness are often the first symptoms. Slack facial muscles and difficulty chewing are common complaints. As the disease spreads, proximal limb muscles are next involved; ultimately any muscle may be affected. In advanced stages respiratory failure may occur. Some patients also have other autoimmune disease, lupus erythematosus, for example. The thymus (Chapter 8) is important in the development of myasthenia gravis, but the mechanism is not known—over half of patients have a tumor or hyperplasia of the thymus. If the thymus is abnormal, removal may be beneficial, especially in young women. Removal of circulating antibody by filtering plasma (plasmapheresis) offers relief, sometimes for several years before the disease reappears. All other treatment is symptomatic; no cure is available.

Tumors and Tumor-like Lesions of Soft Tissue

Soft tissue refers to nonepithelial tissue that is not bone, cartilage, brain or nerve, meninges, bone marrow, or lymphoid tissue. By definition it includes fibrous tissue, skeletal and smooth muscle, and fat. Moreover, some tumors that grow in soft tissue are composed of cells that cannot be identified as derived from a particular tissue. Soft tissue tumors may be benign, fully malignant, or somewhere in between—locally aggressive but not capable of metastasis. Nearly half occur in the lower extremity, especially the thigh, and they are well known for the diagnostic difficulty they pose to pathologists.

The cause of most soft tissue tumors is unknown. Radiation-induced sarcoma, Kaposi sarcoma of AIDS, and the neurofibromas of neurofibromatosis (Chapter 7) are exceptions that have clear causes.

Lipoma (Fig. 22-26), a benign tumor of fat cells, is by far the most common soft tissue tumor. Although it may arise anywhere, it is most often seen in subcutaneous fat. It resembles normal fat and is completely benign; it never becomes malignant. **Liposarcomas** are malignant tumors of fat cells. They generally arise in deep tissues and are sluggishly malignant and locally aggressive. They may grow very large.

Neoplasms of skeletal muscle (*rhabdomyoma* and *rhabdomyosarcoma*) are rare. Rhabdomyosarcoma is predominantly a malignancy of infants, children, and adolescents.

Tumors of fibrocytes or fibroblasts (collagen-producing cells) are varied and may occur in any part of the body. They include benign neoplasms (fibromas), highly malignant neoplasms (fibrosarcoma), and tumor-like benign, inflammatory proliferations. For example, **nodular fasciitis** is a benign mass of inflammatory, immature scar tissue that occurs most often on the forearm that microscopically can be deceptively suggestive of malignancy.

A **fibromatosis** is a confined proliferation of fibrous tissue that can be locally aggressive and may recur after

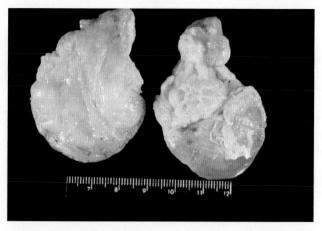

Figure 22-26 Lipoma. Nodular, neoplastic mass of fat excised from the forearm for cosmetic purposes

excision, but does not metastasize. Superficial fibromatoses usually occur in fascia of the palm or sole and present as small, hard, slowly growing nodules. Fibromatoses may occur at almost any location; for example, Peyronie disease is a fibromatosis of the penis. They may recur after simple excision but are not malignant. Fibromatoses in deeper fascia are called *desmoid tumors* and are more aggressive but do not metastasize. An example is desmoid tumor of the abdominal wall fascia. **Sarcomas** of fibrocyte cells occur in several forms.

- **Malignant fibrous histiocytoma** (MFH) is the most common soft tissue sarcoma in adults. Post-irradiation sarcoma is usually MFH. Most occur in the thigh and retroperitoneum; about half metastasize. MFH also occurs in skin, especially on the face, where it is known as *atypical fibrous xanthoma*, a variety of MFH that, for reasons unknown, rarely metastasizes.
- **Fibrosarcoma** occurs most commonly around the knee and thigh and behaves much the same as MFH.
- **Synovial sarcoma** is a malignant tumor microscopically similar to fibrosarcoma that arises near joints in tendons, ligaments, bursae, and joint capsule. Like malignant fibrous histiocytoma and fibrosarcoma, about half metastasize.

Leiomyoma is a benign tumor of smooth muscle that is most often found in the uterus, where it is often called a "fibroid" (Chapter 21). In soft tissue, however, it usually arises from the wall of a subcutaneous blood vessel. It does not become malignant. **Leiomyosarcoma** is a malignant smooth muscle tumor; it is rare and may occur at any location in the body. ■

CASE STUDY 22-1 *"THE DOCTOR TOLD ME I WAS BEING POISONED"*

TOPIC
Fibromyalgia

THE CASE

Setting: You are hiking into the Rocky Mountains on a guided fishing trip to a remote lake. Your guide learns that you are studying health care, and he asks your advice about a personal illness.

Clinical history: JW is a 43-year-old man, a carpenter and mountain fishing guide in the summer and a ski resort real estate salesman in the winter. Along the trail he tells you that since the previous summer he has been having severe aching pains in the back of his neck, in his upper chest and shoulders, and in his hips and knees. You ask some questions at a rest stop. He reports numbness and increased sensitivity to touch in his extremities and adds that his hands feel stiff each morning until he loosens them up. He says he hasn't experienced any weight loss, fever, or swollen joints. He confesses that he worries a lot about his wife's real estate business and their personal finances, and he isn't sleeping well. He also complains of being tired all the time, but he seems energetic on the trail, and his illness hasn't interfered with work. He has no bowel, bladder, or respiratory symptoms.

He has no health insurance and had not seen a physician until the previous Christmas when he was in Florida visiting his daughter, who took him to a physician who collected urine and blood samples to "test for poison." You question him about possible toxic exposures. He drinks city water and doesn't take any medicines or pills other than aspirin and assorted nonprescription pain medicines, none of which seems to help with his pain. You consider lead poisoning and ask questions about possible exposures but come up with nothing suspicious. You inquire about inhalants and learn that he burns wood for heat in the winter and does not have any apparent work or recreational exposures. You also wonder about chronic Lyme disease, but he reports not finding any ticks on his skin after summer outings and has not had any skin rashes. The only thing you come up with is that he handles a lot of lumber treated to make it waterproof; you know from a recent newspaper article that the treatment contains arsenic.

Physical examination and other data: That evening after dinner at his home you do a limited physical examination and find remarkably little. He appears fit and doesn't look anemic. You find no enlarged lymph nodes, rashes, joint abnormalities, or masses, and he appears neurologically normal. On palpation he complains of tenderness in the muscles of his neck.

Clinical course: You suggest he see the physician in his little town, a semi-retired general practitioner who sees patients in a small office in back of his home. He agrees to ask for copies of the doctor's notes and lab reports and to fax them to you. Several weeks later you get a lengthy fax with lab reports but no clinical data. Blood levels of lead, cadmium, arsenic, and mercury are not elevated. Complete blood count and a very long list of blood chemistries (including creatine kinase and thyroxine) are normal. Tests for rheumatoid factor and antinuclear antibodies are negative. Erythrocyte sedimentation rate and levels of C-reactive protein are normal. Lyme disease antibody is not present. In short, nothing is abnormal.

You study the data and your notes and conclude he has fibromyalgia: the clinical symptoms fit, and he has normal lab studies. You call the patient to discuss the matter and learn that his local physician has placed him on antidepressants.

DISCUSSION

This case was typical of many patients who have aches and pains that are difficult to diagnose. Although when a large number of lab tests are ordered, there is always the possibility that a few tests will be abnormal even in a healthy person (Chapter 1). The normal lab test results and lack of other objective abnormalities in this case—fever or weight loss, for example—were the key to the diagnosis of fibromyalgia. Thus, it was possible to exclude rheumatoid arthritis, polymyalgia rheumatica, myositis, and other inflammatory conditions in which physical and laboratory abnormalities are present.

This patient will probably improve on the antidepressant medication prescribed by his physician, but it is unlikely that his symptoms will abate completely, and it is likely that he will have chronic and relapsing symptoms. Patients with fibromyalgia do not respond to the usual pain medicines. They require a comprehensive approach that includes physical therapy, exercise, reassurance, and drug therapy aimed at treating depression and improving sleep.

POINTS TO REMEMBER

• Fibromyalgia is common and is a diagnosis of exclusion after all other possibilities have been ruled out.

Objectives Recap

1. *Describe the difference between osteoblast and osteoclast*: An osteoblast is a bone-forming cell; an osteoclast is a bone-dissolving cell.

2. *Explain the role of osteoid in bone formation*: Osteoid, a specialized protein produced by osteoblasts, is transformed into bone by deposition of calcium, phosphate, and other minerals.

3. *Explain why patients with achondroplasia are short in stature*: Bones grow from the epiphyseal cartilaginous plate at the end of long bones. In achondroplasia, epiphyseal bone growth is genetically defective, and bones are abnormally short.

4. *Discuss the pathogenesis of osteoporosis*: Bones are continually being remade by a delicate balance between osteoblastic bone formation and osteoclastic bone dissolution. Bone-forming capability is estrogen dependent and declines each year as estrogen production declines, ultimately tipping the balance toward bone dissolution. Bone mass is also influenced by other factors: age, genetics, physical activity, diet, and hormones, most notable of which are hormones (estrogen) and genetic factors. For example, African Americans have greater bone mass than Caucasians and therefore have less osteoporosis, and women have more osteoporosis than men do.

5. *Distinguish between osteoporosis and osteomalacia*: Osteomalacia is a qualitative defect of bone microstructure: Bone mass is normal, but it is defectively mineralized. Most osteomalacia is caused by disturbed calcium, phosphate, or vitamin D metabolism. By contrast, osteoporosis is a quantitative defect; bone microstructure is normal, but less bone mass is present.

6. *Name the most common types of metastatic cancer to bone and the most common malignant tumor of bone*: The most common tumor *in* bone is metastatic carcinoma; breast, prostate, and lung cancer are the most common sites of origin. The most common malignant tumor *of* bone is osteosarcoma.

7. *Name the joint near which 80% of primary bone tumors occur*: The knee.

8. *Explain the pathogenesis of primary osteoarthritis, and describe the pathologic changes in affected joints*: Primary osteoarthritis is associated with a genetic predisposition and age-related mechanical wear and tear. Affected joints rarely show inflammatory change. Joint cartilage is thin, frayed, or worn completely away. The underlying bone surfaces become dense and sclerotic. Further stress and degeneration produce subcortical bone cysts and joint spurs (osteophytes), which project into adjacent soft tissue to cause swelling, inflammation, and pain.

9. *Explain the pathogenesis of rheumatoid arthritis (RA), and describe the pathologic changes in affected joints*: RA is caused by an autoimmune reaction that begins in response to some unidentified foreign agent, perhaps the Epstein-Barr virus, that triggers an immune reaction in the synovium. Inflammation and neovascularization of the joint cause release of lytic enzymes that destroy joint cartilage.

10. *Define rheumatoid factor (RF)*: RF is an autoimmune antibody complex that circulates in the blood of most (but not all) patients with rheumatoid arthritis. RF may also be found in some other autoimmune diseases.

11. *Explain how the seronegative spondyloarthropathies differ from rheumatoid arthritis*: 1) the spondyloarthropathies are usually confined to the vertebrae and sacroiliac joints; 2) inflammation also involves ligaments where they attach to bone; 3) rheumatoid factor is absent from blood; and 4) most patients carry the HLA-B27 antigen.

12. *Name the distinguishing features that separate fibromyalgia from arthritis and other painful musculoskeletal syndromes*: Fibromyalgia differs from polymyalgia rheumatica and arthritis in that fever, weight loss, anemia, increased erythrocyte sedimentation rate, and other measurable abnormalities are not present in fibromyalgia. In fibromyalgia no pathologic findings are detectable in the affected tissues, and no objective evidence of disease is present.

13. *Distinguish between disuse atrophy and neurogenic atrophy of skeletal muscle and offer an example of each*: Disuse atrophy occurs in inactive muscle innervated by an intact lower motor neuron; for example, the muscle atrophy that occurs in bedridden patients. Denervation atrophy occurs in muscle whose innervating neuron is diseased or dead; for example, the atrophy that occurs in patients with diabetic peripheral neuropathy or peripheral nerve injury.

14. *Differentiate between Duchenne muscular dystrophy and Becker muscular dystrophy*: Duchenne muscular dystrophy is a severe form of muscular dystrophy caused by a genetic defect that results in the absence of dystrophin, a muscle cell structural protein. Becker muscular dystrophy is a less severe form of muscular dystrophy, in which dystrophin is present but molecularly abnormal.

15. *Distinguish between myositis and myopathy*: Myositis is muscle inflammation. Myopathy is generalized noninflammatory muscle disease that is not muscular dystrophy.

16. *Explain the molecular pathogenesis of myasthenia gravis:* In myasthenia gravis autoimmune antibodies attach to acetylcholine receptors on the muscle side of the neuromuscular synapse. This prevents uptake of acetylcholine, a necessary step in transmission of nerve impulse from nerve to muscle.

17. *Define soft tissue, and name some tumors or tumor-like conditions of soft tissue:* Soft tissue is nonepithelial tissue that is not bone, cartilage, brain or nerve, meninges, bone marrow, or lymphoid tissue; it includes fibrous tissue, skeletal and smooth muscle, and fat. Some soft tissue lesions are lipoma, fibroma, fibromatosis, and various sarcomas.

Typical Test Questions

1. The normal growth of long bones occurs in which part of the bone?
   A. Epiphysis
   B. Metaphysis
   C. Diaphysis
   D. Cortex

2. Bone broken at the site of cancer metastasis is what kind of fracture:
   A. Comminuted
   B. Complete
   C. Pathologic
   D. Compound

3. Which of the following is related to osteoporosis?
   A. Poor blood flow
   B. Fibromyalgia
   C. Rickets
   D. Female sex

4. Rheumatoid factor can be found in which of the following?
   A. Hepatitis B infection
   B. Ankylosing spondylitis
   C. Reactive arthritis following genitourinary or intestinal infection
   D. The arthritis of psoriasis

5. Which of the following diseases is an autoimmune condition?
   A. Muscular dystrophy
   B. Myasthenia gravis
   C. Rhabdomyolysis
   D. Tetanus

6. True or false? Malignant fibrous histiocytoma (MFH) of skin is much less malignant than MFH of other sites.

7. True or false? Becker muscular dystrophy is characterized by abnormal dystrophin.

8. True or false? Acute septic arthritis is a common form of arthritis.

9. True or false? In a patient with apparent rheumatoid arthritis, the presence of rheumatoid nodules confirms the diagnosis.

10. True or false? The head of the femur is especially prone to aseptic necrosis.

Diseases of the Nervous System

This chapter begins with a review of the normal brain, spinal cord, peripheral nerves, and autonomic nervous system; their interconnections; and their connections to other cells. Diseases and disorders discussed include increased intracranial pressure, stroke, brain trauma, and brain hemorrhage; encephalitis and meningitis; degenerative diseases and brain toxins; and benign and malignant tumors.

BACK TO BASICS
- The Central Nervous System
- Vascular Supply
- The Peripheral Nervous System
- The Autonomic Nervous System
- Cells of the Nervous System
- Nerve Cell Connections and Signals

CONGENITAL AND PERINATAL DISEASE
INCREASED INTRACRANIAL PRESSURE
INTRACRANIAL HEMORRHAGE
- Bleeding on the Surface of the Brain
- Bleeding Directly into the Brain

ISCHEMIA AND INFARCTION
BRAIN AND SPINAL CORD TRAUMA
INFECTIONS OF THE CENTRAL NERVOUS SYSTEM
- Infections of the Meninges and Cerebrospinal Fluid
- Infections of Brain Parenchyma

DEGENERATIVE DISEASES
- Degenerative Diseases of Gray Matter
- Degenerative Diseases of White Matter

METABOLIC AND TOXIC DISORDERS
NEOPLASMS
DISEASES OF PERIPHERAL NERVES
- Neuropathies
- Neoplasms

Learning Objectives

After studying this chapter you should be able to:

1. Describe the production, circulation, and absorption of cerebrospinal fluid (CSF)
2. Explain the meaning of the terms gray matter and white matter
3. Name the parenchymal and ancillary cells of the central nervous system (CNS)
4. Explain why increased intracranial pressure is dangerous, and name a specific anatomic result
5. Compare and contrast the anatomic location, the cause, and the effect of subdural and epidural hematoma
6. Name the cause of most spontaneous subarachnoid hemorrhage
7. Explain the anatomic and pathogenic differences between white and red stroke
8. Explain the cause of laminar cortical necrosis
9. Distinguish between brain concussion and contusion
10. Name the cause of most epidemic bacterial meningitis and the population at risk
11. Explain the biochemical dysfunction in parkinsonism, and name some of the conditions causing it
12. Recite some important facts about Alzheimer disease
13. Name the probable cause of multiple sclerosis
14. Discuss why alcoholics develop chronic brain disease
15. List the most common sources of metastatic brain tumor
16. Explain why it is difficult to completely remove most gliomas surgically
17. Name two diseases commonly associated with peripheral neuropathy
18. Explain how Guillain-Barré syndrome can prove fatal

Key Terms and Concepts

BACK TO BASICS
- central nervous system
- peripheral nervous system
- autonomic nervous system
- cerebral hemispheres
- meninges
- cerebrospinal fluid
- subarachnoid space
- gray matter
- white matter
- neuron
- axon
- glia

CONGENITAL AND PERINATAL DISEASE
- neural tube defect
- cerebral palsy

INCREASED INTRACRANIAL PRESSURE
- hydrocephalus

INTRACRANIAL HEMORRHAGE
- red stroke
- epidural hematoma

- subdural hematoma
- subarachnoid hemorrhage

ISCHEMIA AND INFARCTION
- white stroke

DIRECT TRAUMA TO BRAIN AND SPINAL CORD
- concussion
- contusion

INFECTIONS OF THE BRAIN AND MENINGES
- meningitis

DEGENERATIVE BRAIN DISEASES
- Alzheimer disease
- parkinsonism

METABOLIC AND TOXIC DISORDERS OF THE BRAIN
- Wernicke encephalopathy

NEOPLASMS OF THE BRAIN
- glioma

DISEASES OF PERIPHERAL NERVES
- peripheral neuropathy

Brain, n. An apparatus with which we think that we think.

AMBROSE BIERCE (1842–1914?), AMERICAN SATIRIST, JOURNALIST, AND SHORT-STORY WRITER, THE DEVIL'S DICTIONARY

BACK TO BASICS

The nervous system is divided into three parts: 1) the **central nervous system**—the brain and spinal cord; 2) the **peripheral nervous system**—nerves originating from brain or spinal cord, which bring sensory signals (sight, smell, etc.) to the brain and transmit motor (voluntary movement) signals to muscles; and 3) the **autonomic nervous system**, which is connected to the heart, intestines, endocrine glands, and other viscera and controls involuntary functions, such heart rate.

THE CENTRAL NERVOUS SYSTEM

The brain and spinal cord and their relationship to the skull and vertebrae are illustrated in Figure 23-1. The largest part of the brain, the **cerebrum**, is uppermost and is divided into two parts, the right and left **cerebral hemispheres**, which are connected one to the other and to the spinal cord by large internal bundles of nerve fibers called *nerve tracts*. The outermost part of the cerebrum is covered by the cerebral cortex, which contains particular areas that specialize in voluntary motor movement, perception of the five senses, and is the site of abstract thinking, emotion, judgment, and other functions that account for uniquely human behavior. The *midbrain, pons,* and *medulla oblongata,* which are collectively called the *brain stem,* sit below the cerebral hemispheres and above the spinal cord. The brainstem is the main traffic intersection of the brain where bundles of nerve tracts cross from one side to the other, and it is home to numerous nodules of gray matter (called *nuclei*) that control the most basic aspects of human biology such as respiration, wakefulness, aggression, fear, and hunger.

The **cerebellum** sits below and to the rear of the cerebrum. The cerebellum mediates balance, controls fine motor activity, especially rapid, complex, coordinated movements such as writing, and is home to the *proprioceptive sense*—the sense of body and body-part position; for example, knowing where one's arms are without having to look at them.

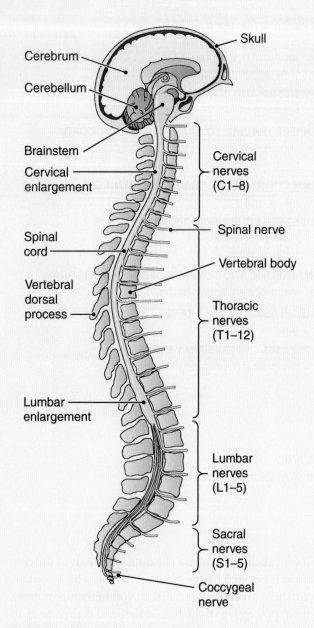

Figure 23-1 **The central nervous systems.**

The brain and spinal cord are enclosed by membranes, the **meninges** (Fig. 23-2). Outermost is the **dura mater**, a tough, thick sheet of fibrous tissue that is tightly stuck to the inside of the skull and surrounds the spinal cord inside the spinal canal. Immediately beneath the dura mater is the **arachnoid**, a thin membrane beneath which is the **subarachnoid space**, containing the cerebrospinal fluid (CSF). The major arteries on the surface of the brain lie in the subarachnoid space. The arachnoid gets its name from the Greek word *arachno* for cobweb, a reference to the web of thin fibers that cross the arachnoid space from the arachnoid to the surface of the brain. The innermost meningeal membrane

is the **pia mater**, a very thin membrane intimately attached to the surface of the brain and spinal cord.

Two extensions of the dura mater form internal membranes to stabilize the brain. The **falx cerebri** (Fig. 23-2) is a vertical fold of dura mater formed into a membrane on the inside of the skull that runs from front to rear, extends downward to separate the right and left cerebral hemispheres, and encloses the **superior sagittal sinus**, an elongated lake of venous blood that runs front to rear under the center of the skull. The **tentorium** (Fig. 23-3 and also see Fig. 23-4A) is a second, horizontal fold of dura in the back of the skull, which separates the cerebral hemispheres above from the cerebellum below.

The brain and spinal cord are filled with and surrounded by fluid. In the center of each cerebral hemisphere are hollow spaces—the right and left lateral (1st and 2nd) **ventricles**—filled with fluid. The **cerebrospinal fluid** (CSF) is a watery substance that circulates slowly and fills the ventricles and all other space in and around the brain and spinal cord. CSF cushions the brain and spinal cord and mediates exchange of substances with the blood. The production, flow, and absorption of CSF are illustrated by Figure 23-3. CSF is made by the **choroid plexus**, a collection of specialized vascular projections into the ventricles. The choroid plexus serves to regulate CSF pressure by the formation of more or less cerebrospinal fluid, which flows through the ventricles and out of the brain through small holes (the **foramina of Luschka and Magendie**) in the roof of the 4th ventricle. Outside of the brain the CSF fills and flows through the arachnoid space. CSF is absorbed out of the arachnoid space and into blood through **arachnoid granulations**, which project into the superior sagittal sinus.

Normal adults have about 150 ml of CSF volume and produce about 500 ml per day, a daily turnover of 3–4 volumes. Because of the rapid rate of CSF production and reabsorption, obstruction of CSF flow or reabsorption causes increased intracranial pressure, which usually has serious consequences.

The internal anatomy of the brain is depicted in Figure 23-4. The outermost layer of the cerebral hemisphere is the **cortex** (from Latin for bark) and is mainly composed of the most specialized cell in the brain—the **neuron**. The cortex is home to the highest brain functions—reasoning, emotion, voluntary motion, and speech. Neurons are grayish; hence the cortex and other deeper, nodular collections of neurons (called *nuclei*) are called **gray matter**.

Long, thin, cytoplasmic extensions of neurons called **axons** are grouped together as *nerve tracts* to carry elec-

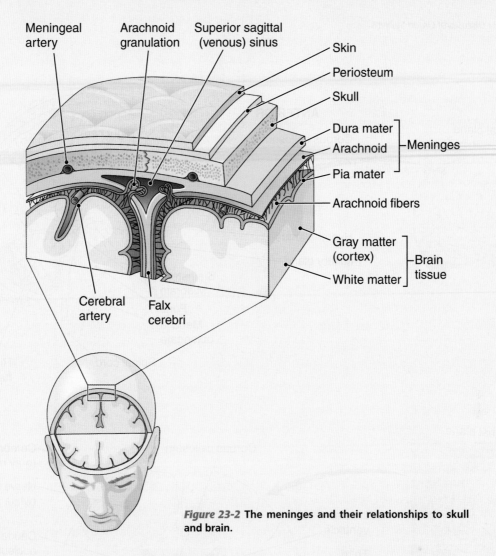

Figure 23-2 The meninges and their relationships to skull and brain.

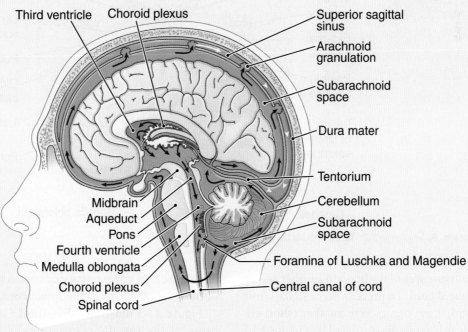

Figure 23-3 Production, flow, and absorption of cerebrospinal fluid (CSF). CSF fills the ventricles and all other space in and around the brain and spinal cord. CSF is made by the choroid plexus, which regulates CSF pressure. CSF flows through the ventricles and out of the brain through the foramina of Luschka and Magendie in the roof of the 4th ventricle. Outside the brain, the CSF fills and flows through the subarachnoid space. CSF is absorbed out of the subarachnoid space and into blood through arachnoid granulations, which project into the superior sagittal sinus.

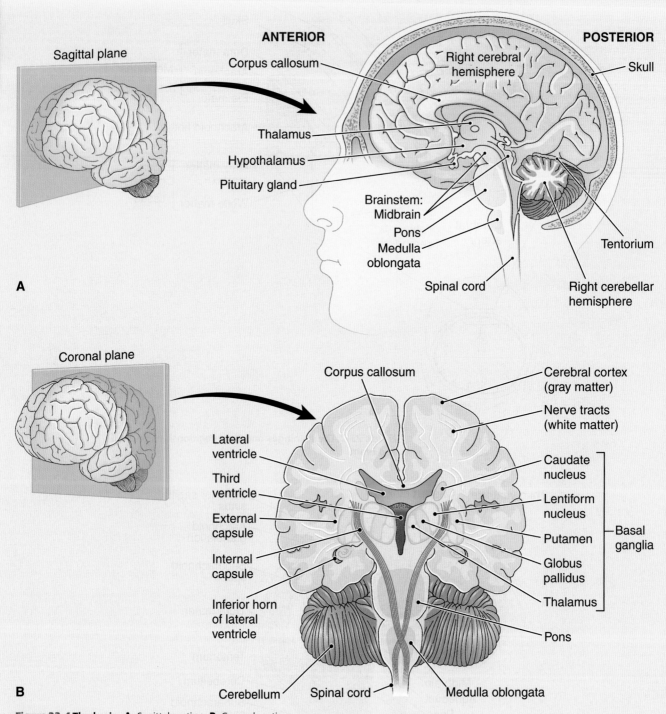

ANTERIOR

POSTERIOR

Sagittal plane

Corpus callosum

Right cerebral hemisphere

Skull

Thalamus

Hypothalamus

Pituitary gland

Brainstem:
Midbrain
Pons
Medulla
oblongata

Spinal cord

Tentorium

Right cerebellar
hemisphere

A

Coronal plane

Corpus callosum

Cerebral cortex
(gray matter)

Nerve tracts
(white matter)

Lateral
ventricle

Third
ventricle

External
capsule

Internal
capsule

Inferior horn
of lateral
ventricle

Caudate
nucleus

Lentiform
nucleus

Putamen

Globus
pallidus

Thalamus

Basal
ganglia

Pons

B

Cerebellum   Spinal cord   Medulla oblongata

Figure 23-4 **The brain. A,** Sagittal section. **B,** Coronal section.

trical signals from one area of the brain to another and up and down the spinal cord. To prevent nerve signals from jumping randomly from one axon to another (short-circuiting, so to speak), axons are insulated by a white, fatty substance called **myelin**. Bundles of axons are white and are called **white matter** and crisscross the brain, running up and down the spinal cord carrying nerve signals. An especially important tract is the **internal capsule**, a very

large bundle of nerve tracts that connects motor neurons of the cerebral cortex to the spinal cord.

Figure 23-5 illustrates that, unlike other organs, because of the specific connections of nerve pathways within the brain and to and from every part of the body, every anatomic part of the brain fulfills a function different from every other part. For example, vision is perceived in the posterior (occipital) cerebral cortex, but

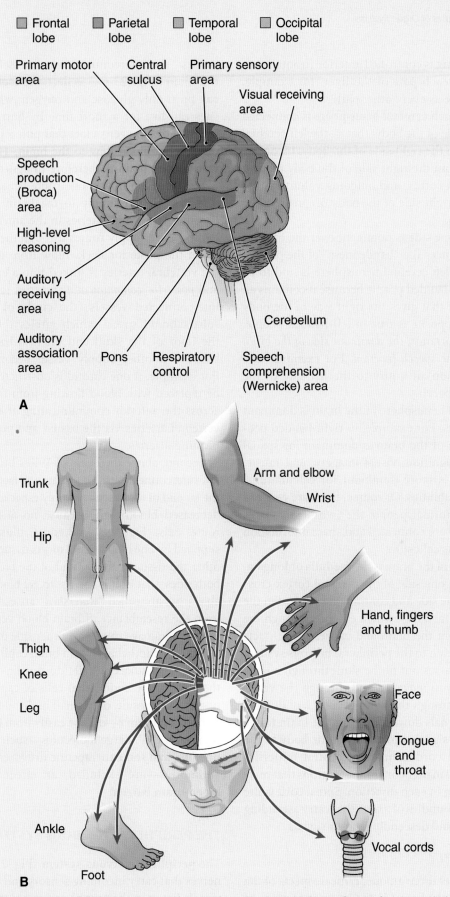

Figure 23-5 Functional anatomy of the brain. A, Map of cortical functions. **B,** Detailed map of motor functions, which reside in the left cerebral cortex in a right-handed person.

high-level reasoning is controlled anterior (frontal) cortex. By contrast, each part of the liver, for example, functions the same as every other part.

The cortex of each cerebral hemisphere is connected to the opposite side of the body; that is, the left cerebral cortex connects to the right side of the body: Incoming sensory signals from the right side of the body register in the left cerebral cortex, and outgoing voluntary motor signals to the right side of the body originate in the left cerebral cortex.

Furthermore, one side is dominant over the other, a feature that influences the "handedness" of the person. For example, the *left* cerebral hemisphere is said to be dominant in *right*-handed people because it contains all of the brain tissue that gives the right side of the body more skill. The opposite is true in left-handed people. Also of great importance, *the dominant side of the brain usually contains the speech function*. For example, in a *right*-handed person an injury to the *left* side of the brain may affect speech.

Moreover, each hemisphere of the brain is dominant for other behaviors. For example, in right-handed people, the right side of the brain is dominant for spatial abilities, face recognition, visual imagery, and music, and the left side is more dominant for calculations, math, and logical abilities. Of course, these are generalizations, and in normal people the two hemispheres work together and are connected and share information through the corpus callosum.

The lowest part of the brain is the **medulla oblongata**, where axons from one side of the cerebral cortex cross over to the opposite side and continue downward in the **spinal cord** (see Fig. 23-1), which extends through the spinal column from the brain and carries nerve tracts that connect the brain to the peripheral nervous system. The spinal cord passes out of the skull through a large opening, the *foramen magnum*, and through the vertebrae, like a pole through the holes of a stack of donuts, carrying motor signals downward from the brain to the body and sensory signals upward from the body to the brain. The spinal cord contains a central butterfly-shaped area of gray matter containing neurons that relay nerve signals going in each direction. Spinal cord white matter consists of bundles of axons that carry ascending sensory impulses and descending motor signals.

VASCULAR SUPPLY

Figure 23-6, depicts three unique, critical aspects of the vascular supply to the brain: 1) the interconnections of vessels at the base of the brain; 2) the relative lack of interconnections elsewhere in the cranium; and 3) the structure of brain capillaries.

First, the interconnections of vessels at the base of the brain (Fig. 23-6A) reflect the fact that the brain can burn only glucose and oxygen; whereas other tissues can live for a short time by burning nonglucose fuel without oxygen, a fact that puts a premium on uninterrupted blood flow to the brain. The vascular network of the brain is therefore designed to allow alternative routes of flow if one route becomes obstructed. The main blood supply to the brain travels through the internal carotid arteries in the anterior neck; a second primary supply routes through the vertebral arteries in the posterior neck. Flow from the carotids and the vertebral arteries is linked into a circle by *anterior* and *posterior communicating* arteries to form a loop of interconnected vessels (the **circle of Willis**) in the subarachnoid space, which circles the brainstem on the floor of the skull and offers a backup source of blood if another supply vessel becomes obstructed. For example, if one carotid is obstructed, lost flow can be replaced with blood flowing from the other carotid across the anterior communicating artery, or from the vertebral arteries via the basilar and posterior communicating arteries.

Second, above the circle of Willis brain arteries have few interconnections. This anatomic fact makes tissue at the far end of the vascular supply especially vulnerable to decreased blood flow because no alternative supply routes exist. Figures 23-6B and C illustrate that tissue supplied by one blood vessel meets tissue supplied by another the tissue at the far end of the blood supply from both sides; that is, it is the last to get blood. Such vulnerable areas are called "*watershed*" areas, the name taken from the resemblance of brain blood vessel distribution to water drainage routes on either side of a ridgeline.

Third, endothelial cells in brain capillaries are joined tightly, and adjacent cells do not have slits between them as do the endothelial cells of capillaries in other tissues. As a result, only small molecules—electrolytes, alcohol, and water—diffuse easily from blood into brain tissue and CSF. Large molecules—such as antigens, antibodies, and some therapeutic drugs, especially certain antibiotics—are excluded, an effect known as the **blood-brain barrier**.

THE PERIPHERAL NERVOUS SYSTEM

The **peripheral nervous system** (Fig. 23-7) consists of nerves that carry incoming sensory and outgoing motor signals between the central nervous system and peripheral tissues. It is composed of 12 pairs (one left and one right) of **cranial nerves** (Fig. 23-7A) that arise from the brain, and 31 pairs of **spinal nerves** (Fig. 23-7B), which

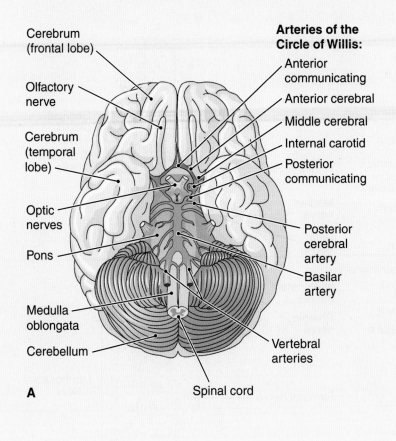

Cerebrum (frontal lobe)

Olfactory nerve

Cerebrum (temporal lobe)

Optic nerves

Pons

Medulla oblongata

Cerebellum

A

Spinal cord

Arteries of the Circle of Willis:

Anterior communicating

Anterior cerebral

Middle cerebral

Internal carotid

Posterior communicating

Posterior cerebral artery

Basilar artery

Vertebral arteries

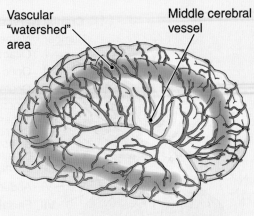

Vascular "watershed" area

Middle cerebral vessel

B Lateral view, right cerebral hemisphere

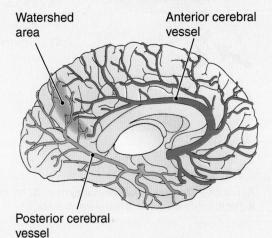

Watershed area

Anterior cerebral vessel

Posterior cerebral vessel

C Medial view, left cerebral hemisphere

Figure 23-6 **Arterial blood supply to the brain. A,** The major vessels and their interconnections in the circle of Willis. **B** and **C,** The vascular supply to the cerebral cortex with emphasis of "watershed" areas.

arise at regular intervals from the full length of the spinal cord.

The cranial nerves include the olfactory (or 1st, for smell), the optic (2nd, for vision), the acoustic (8th, for hearing and balance), and nine other sets of nerves that relay signals back and forth to the tongue (for movement and taste), the face (for movement and sensation), eye muscles, facial muscles, the throat, and other sites.

The spinal nerves connect the remainder of the body—the limbs and trunk—to the spinal cord. Nerves at each level of the spinal cord connect to particular parts of the body on one side or the other: some connect to the right foot, others to the left hand, and so on. After leaving the spinal cord, nerves to the shoulder and arm are woven into two complex networks, the *cervical plexus* and the *brachial plexus*, where fibers from one level of the spinal cord join with fibers from another level to travel to a particular site. Similarly, nerves to the hip and leg are woven into the *lumbosacral plexus*.

Additional details about the motor function of nerves are provided in Chapter 22 and illustrated in Figure 22-21.

THE AUTONOMIC NERVOUS SYSTEM

As is illustrated in Figure 23-8, the **autonomic nervous system** is an involuntary system of nerves that acts on cardiac muscle, smooth muscle, and glands to control functions such as heart rate, blood pressure, sweating and other gland secretions, and bowel peristalsis. The autonomic nervous system has two divisions: *sympathetic* and *parasympathetic*.

The **sympathetic** division is a network of nerve fibers and ganglia that originates from neurons in the thoracic and lumbar spinal cord and reacts to stress by stimulating secretion of epinephrine and norepinephrine from nerve endings and from the adrenal medulla. Because these hormones have an adrenal-like effect, action of

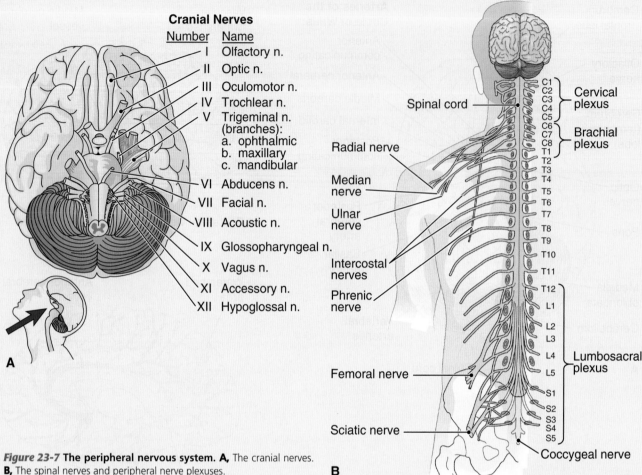

Cranial Nerves

Number	Name
I	Olfactory n.
II	Optic n.
III	Oculomotor n.
IV	Trochlear n.
V	Trigeminal n. (branches): a. ophthalmic b. maxillary c. mandibular
VI	Abducens n.
VII	Facial n.
VIII	Acoustic n.
IX	Glossopharyngeal n.
X	Vagus n.
XI	Accessory n.
XII	Hypoglossal n.

A

Spinal cord — C1 C2 C3 C4 C5 — Cervical plexus
C6 C7 C8 T1 — Brachial plexus
Radial nerve
Median nerve
Ulnar nerve
T2 T3 T4 T5 T6 T7 T8 T9 T10 T11
Intercostal nerves
Phrenic nerve
T12 L1 L2 L3
Femoral nerve — L4 L5 — Lumbosacral plexus
S1 S2 S3 S4 S5
Sciatic nerve
Coccygeal nerve

B

Figure 23-7 **The peripheral nervous system. A,** The cranial nerves. **B,** The spinal nerves and peripheral nerve plexuses.

the sympathetic system is called the **adrenergic** effect. Secretion of epinephrine and norepinephrine affects tissues and organs in what is typically called the "fight-or-flight" response—heart rate and blood pressure rise, the metabolic rate increases, pupils and bronchi dilate, the liver releases glucose, and sweating begins.

The **parasympathetic** division is a network of fibers and ganglia that originates from neurons in the brain and lower (sacral) spinal cord. Stimulation of the parasympathetic system causes release of acetylcholine, which reverses the "fight-or-flight" response. This is called the **cholinergic** effect. Table 23-1 lists the effects of the sympathetic and parasympathetic systems on various organs and tissues.

Neurons of the autonomic system in the brain and spinal cord send axons down cranial and spinal nerves to connect with autonomic **ganglia**, which are small nodules of autonomic neurons connected by axons to end organs. Autonomic ganglia occur in three locations: 1) in a chain along side vertebral bodies of the chest and abdomen (the *sympathetic chain*), 2) in a web of collateral ganglia in the retroperitoneum, and 3) in the end organ.

Sympathetic fibers usually travel with spinal nerves and connect (via a synapse) with autonomic second neurons in ganglia located 1) in an interconnected chain (the *sympathetic chain*) situated alongside vertebral bodies in the chest and abdomen and 2) to a network of other ganglia in the retroperitoneum. Sympathetic fibers also connect directly to the adrenal medulla, which can be thought of functionally as a modified sympathetic ganglion. *Parasympathetic* fibers travel with cranial and sacral nerves and connect to (via a synapse) second autonomic neurons in ganglia located next to or actually within the end organ.

CELLS OF THE NERVOUS SYSTEM

Cells of the nervous system are illustrated in Figure 23-9. The primary functional cell of the central nervous system (CNS) is the **neuron**, which extends one or more short *dendrites* (to connect with other brain cells) and a single long **axon** (to connect with other neurons or effector cells such as skeletal muscle cells). All other cells in the nervous system function in support of the neuron. Neurons have a large central cytoplasmic mass that collectively form the CNS **gray matter**. Neurons

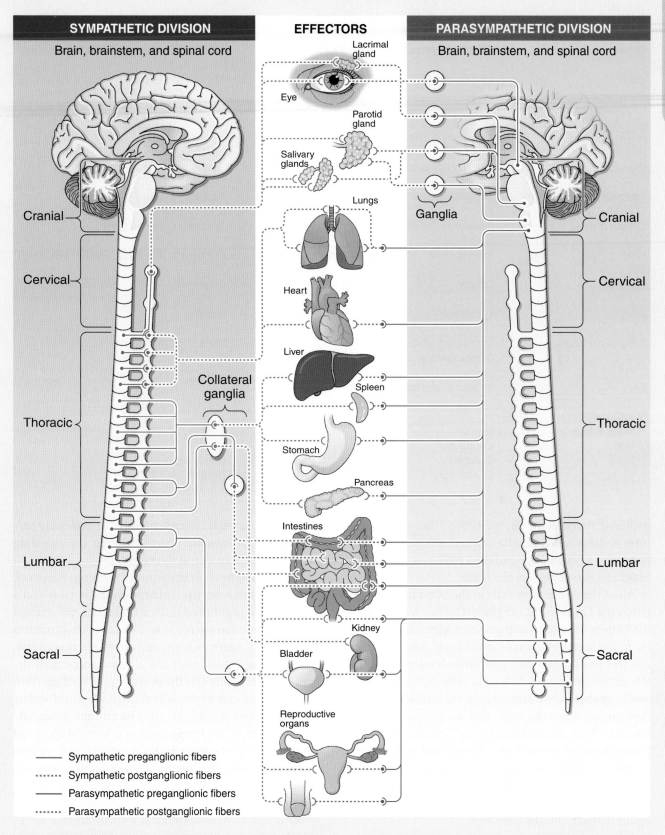

Figure 23-8 **The autonomic nervous system.** See also Table 23-1, which summarizes effects on particular organs. Reprinted with permission from Cohen B. Memmler's The Human Body in Health and Disease. 10th Edition. Philadelphia. Lippincott Williams and Wilkins, 2005.

Table 23-1	The Effects of Autonomic Stimulation on Selected Organs	
Organ	**Effect of Sympathetic Stimulation**	**Effect of Parasympathetic Stimulation**
Iris	Dilation of pupil	Constriction of pupil
Lacrimal gland	—	Formation of tears
Sweat glands	Formation of sweat	—
Digestive glands	Inhibition of secretions	Stimulation of secretions
Intestinal motility	Decrease peristalsis	Increase peristalsis
Urinary bladder	Relaxation and expansion	Contraction and emptying
Heart	Increase in rate and power of contraction	Decrease in rate and power of contraction
Bronchioles	Dilation	Constriction
Penis	Ejaculation	Erection
Adrenal medulla	Stimulation of epinephrine and norepinephrine secretion	None
Liver	Release of glucose	None
Blood vessels to:		
Skeletal muscle	Dilation	Constriction
Skin	Contraction	None
Lung	Dilation	Constriction
GI tract	Contraction	Dilation

gathered together in the peripheral nervous system form nodules called **ganglia**. Axons form the **white matter** of the CNS and are gathered into *tracts* within the brain and *nerves* outside the brain.

All of the nonneuron cells in the brain form the **glia** (from the Greek word for *glue*). The soft framework of the brain is formed by **astrocytes**, which fill a role similar to fibrocytes elsewhere in the body, except that astrocytes produce no collagen. **Oligodendrocytes**, literally cells with few dendrites, are cells that make myelin and wrap themselves around axons to insulate nerve signals passing down the axon; that is, they prevent "short circuits." They are analogous to the *Schwann cells* wrapping peripheral nerve axons. **Ependymal cells** line the cerebral ventricles and the central canal of the spinal cord and have cilia that help circulate CSF. **Microglia** are the scavenger (phagocytic) cells of the CNS and are analogous to macrophages elsewhere.

NERVE CELL CONNECTIONS AND SIGNALS

A **synapse** is a junction between two neurons or between a neuronal axon and another cell, such as a mus-cle cell. A synapse is characterized by an extremely narrow space (the *synaptic space*) between the signaling nerve cell or its axon and the target cell.

The membrane of an undisturbed (resting) nerve cell carries a positive electrical charge on the outside and a negative charge on the inside, a difference that creates potential electrical energy (like a coiled spring contains energy that is spent as it uncoils). In effect, this electrical difference makes each cell a tiny battery with the negative pole inside and the positive pole outside, from which energy can be harvested. This electrical difference, measured in volts, is called **membrane potential**.

Nerve signals are transmitted as a wave of electrical disturbance in the membrane potential that sweeps down the axon to the synapse at the end of the axon. On arrival at the motor end plate, the signal stimulates release of **acetylcholine** (the *neurotransmitter*) into the synaptic space. Acetylcholine is a small organic molecule that rapidly crosses the exceedingly narrow synaptic space and interacts with the target cell to produce an effect. Acetylcholine is then instantly broken down and reconstituted by an enzyme, **cholinesterase**, to be ready for the next signal to cross the synapse.

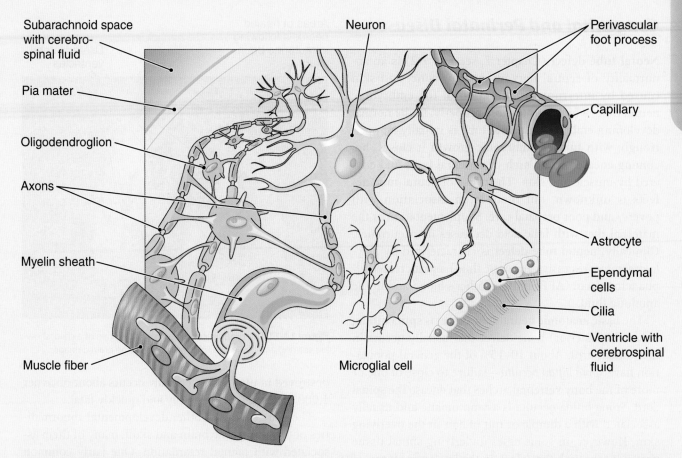

Figure 23-9 Cells of the nervous system. Neurons are the main functional cell of the nervous system and connect with other neurons by axons. Oligodendrocytes wrap axons with a layer of myelin (myelin sheath), which insulates nerve signals from other neurons. Astrocytes are the glue cells that hold the others together. Microglial cells are specialized macrophages.

The relay of signals happens in the following way. For example, let's say the cerebral cortex initiates a signal destined for a muscle that moves a finger. The neuron in the cerebral cortex sends an axon down the spinal cord to connect with a spinal cord neuron. The signal travels down the axon to the spinal cord, where it connects at a synapse with the spinal cord neuron, which in turn sends an axon to the target muscle. The signal is relayed across the synapse from the first neuron to the second and from the second to the muscle in the same way. The end result is muscle contraction in response to the cortical command.

MAJOR DETERMINANTS OF DISEASE

- Brain anatomy is functionally site specific.
- The central nervous system is filled with and surrounded by flowing fluid.
- In the brain are few lymphatic channels; resorption of edema is difficult.
- The brain is encased in bone and has little room to swell or to move.
- All neurologic effects of brain disease are caused by disturbed or lost neuron function.
- Neurons are exquisitely sensitive to oxygen and glucose deprivation.
- Large molecules, such as antibodies, cannot diffuse easily into the brain from blood.
- The brain is frequently affected by atherosclerotic vascular insufficiency.
- Microscopically benign brain tumors can cause death because of critical location.

Congenital and Perinatal Disease

Neural tube defect (Chapter 7, see Fig. 7-2) is an abnormality of central nervous system, bone, and skin caused by interrupted maturation of the embryonic neural tube, which fails to close properly. In the normal developing embryo the neural tube is initially an open trough; with further embryonic growth it closes, becoming encased by an arch of vertebral bone and covered by muscle and skin. The cause of neural tube defects is unknown, but there is an association with poverty and poor prenatal care. Supplementation of the maternal diet with folic acid decreases its occurrence. Clinically, neural tube defect is characterized by *polyhydramnios* (excessive amniotic fluid) and increased alpha fetoprotein (AFP) in the mother's blood and in the amniotic fluid.

The basic anatomic neural tube defect is **spina bifida**, a dorsal (posterior) bone defect that usually occurs in the lumbar area. About 10–15% of the general population have *spina bifida occulta*—failure to close of one or more of the bony vertebral arches that encase the spinal cord. Spina bifida occulta is asymptomatic and usually associated with a dimple or tuft of hair in the overlying skin. However, in some cases underlying spinal tissue protrudes through the defect. In the less severe forms of spina bifida, only the meninges protrude through the opening (**meningocele**); in more severe cases neural tissue also protrudes (**meningomyelocele**). The most common clinical problems are meningitis, lower limb motor or sensory neural defects, and difficulty with bowel and bladder control.

Anencephaly (literally "without a brain"), illustrated in Figure 23-10, is the most serious neural tube defect—the skull fails to develop, and the exposed brain is

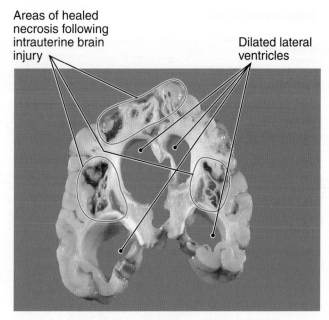

Figure 23-11 The brain in cerebral palsy. The brain of a child, showing scarring and tissue loss following intrauterine brain damage.

destroyed in utero. Anencephaly occurs about once per 1,000 births and is invariably and quickly fatal.

There are dozens of other developmental abnormalities of the embryonic brain and skull, many of them associated with mental retardation. One fairly common condition is *microcephaly*—an unusually small skull and brain that may be caused by cytogenetic abnormalities, fetal alcohol syndrome, and congenital infection by the AIDS virus (HIV). Another developmental abnormality is *agyria* (also called *lissencephaly*), a severe neurological condition in which gyri are absent and the cerebral surface is smooth.

Cerebral palsy (Fig. 23-11) is the term applied to permanent, nonprogressive motor problems (spasticity, paralysis) that arise owing to an insult to the brain before it reaches a certain maturity. Because brain development continues during the first two years of life, cerebral palsy can result from brain injury occurring in utero or before age two. About 75% of cerebral palsy cases arise from unknown prebirth conditions. Some cases are associated with birth trauma. Neonatal risk factors for cerebral palsy include prematurity, low birth weight, and intrauterine growth retardation (Chapter 7). About 15% of cases arise from injury after birth: brain or meningeal infections, hyperbilirubinemia, automobile accidents, falls, or child abuse.

Increased Intracranial Pressure

The brain and spinal cord are completely enclosed by the meninges, which form a sealed sac filled with CSF

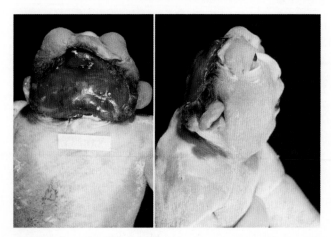

Figure 23-10 Anencephaly. Anencephaly is the most severe neural tube defect.

under pressure that is slightly greater than venous blood pressure. Intracranial pressure is regulated by the production, circulation, and reabsorption of CSF.

Intracranial pressure can increase abnormally with obstruction of CSF flow, impaired reabsorption of CSF, hemorrhage, brain edema, or expanding intracranial mass, usually a tumor. Increased intracranial pressure is pathologic and, like fluid under pressure in any closed space, CSF seeks natural relief by enlarging the space or escaping through any available opening.

In children, because the skull is still growing and bone margins are not fused, increased intracranial pressure is relieved by enlargement of the skull. In adults, however, the skull cannot enlarge, and slowly enlarging masses, such as slowly growing tumors, press on other parts of the brain, causing them to atrophy. For example, slow-growing tumors of the meninges press on nearby brain tissue, causing it to atrophy. However, rapid increases of brain mass or pressure within the strict confines of the adult skull—as with malignant brain tumors, sudden hemorrhage, brain abscess, or brain edema—force the brain to herniate through internal or external openings in several ways, illustrated in Figure 23-12.

Increased pressure usually arises from mass lesions, but it may also be caused by general brain edema. A **subfalcine herniation** is herniation of the lower medial aspect of the affected cerebral hemisphere *horizontally* across the lower margin of the falx cerebri, which may press on the anterior cerebral artery to produce cerebral ischemia or infarct. A **tentorial herniation** is herniation of the ipsilateral (same side) temporal lobe downward and medially through the tentorium. The herniated brain may press on the third cranial nerve, causing dilation of the pupils or impairment of eye motion, or it may press on and obstruct the posterior cerebral artery to cause brain hemorrhage or infarction. A **tonsillar herniation** is herniation of the lower cerebellum, an area known as the cerebellar tonsils, through the foramen magnum. Tonsillar herniation obstructs venous and arterial blood flow in the brainstem and can produce hemorrhage or infarction in the midbrain. Illustrated in Figure 23-13 is a case of pontine hemorrhage, which usually occurs secondary to tonsillar herniation caused by massive intracerebral hemorrhage.

Increased intracranial pressure can also push on one or both of the optic nerves and cause bulging of the op-

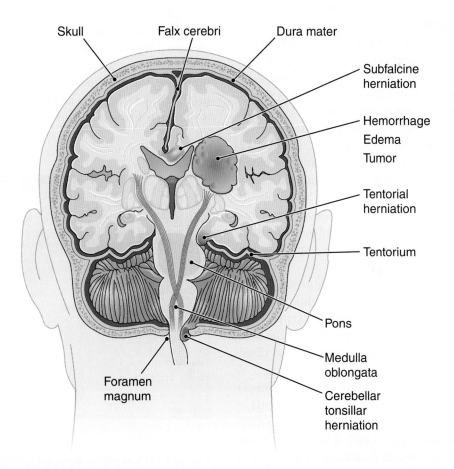

Figure 23-12 **Brain herniations.** Brain edema and intracranial tumor or hemorrhage are the usual causes.

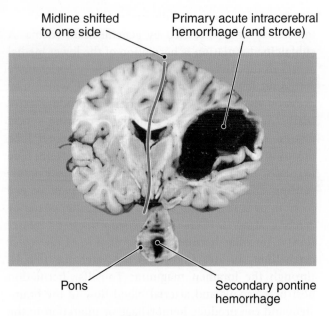

Midline shifted to one side

Primary acute intracerebral hemorrhage (and stroke)

Pons

Secondary pontine hemorrhage

Figure 23-13 Pontine hemorrhage secondary to cerebellar tonsillar herniation. A massive intracerebral hemorrhage (red stroke) in a patient with hypertension has forced the cerebellar tonsils into the foramen magnum, which obstructed blood flow to the pons.

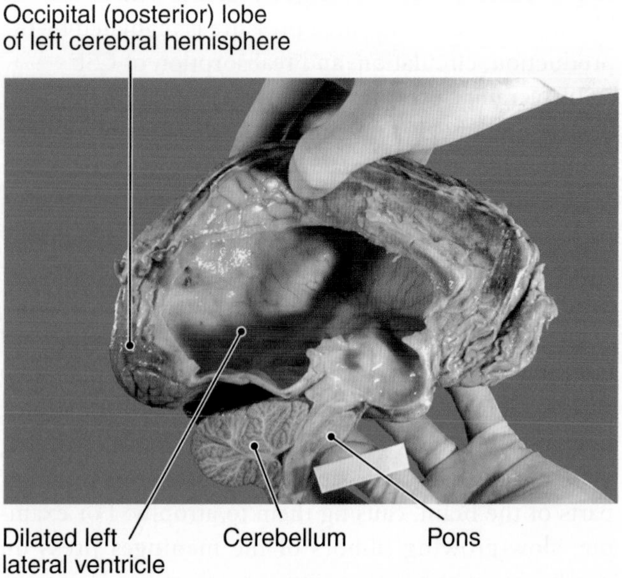

Occipital (posterior) lobe of left cerebral hemisphere

Dilated left lateral ventricle

Cerebellum

Pons

Figure 23-14 The brain in hydrocephalus. In this patient flow of cerebrospinal fluid was obstructed in the aqueduct of Sylvius (not labeled) between the third and fourth ventricles. Increased intraventricular pressure caused ventricular dilation and atrophy of surrounding brain tissue.

tic disc, where the optic nerve enters the eye, a condition known as **papilledema**.

Brain edema also may be caused by a breakdown of blood-brain barrier (*vasogenic edema*), which allows vascular fluid to escape from blood vessels into brain interstitial tissue, or by toxic or hypoxic cell injury (*cytotoxic edema*), which causes cells to swell with fluid (hydropic degeneration, Chapter 2). For example, extremely high blood pressure (malignant hypertension, Chapter 12) can cause brain edema by forcing fluid across the blood-brain barrier and into the brain. Or, extremely low blood sodium levels (hyponatremia) can lower blood osmotic pressure to such an extent that water escapes from blood vessels into the brain. Cytotoxic brain edema can also be a feature of exposure to certain toxins, especially lead and carbon monoxide (Chapter 10).

Obstruction to the flow or reabsorption of CSF causes a condition known as **hydrocephalus**, an abnormal accumulation of CSF in the ventricles (*internal hydrocephalus*, Fig. 23-14) or over the surface of the brain (*external hydrocephalus*). Hydrocephalus is also classified as *obstructive* (or *noncommunicating*; that is, CSF that cannot communicate from one space to another), which is a blockage of CSF flow that can be caused by tumor, scar (gliosis), and other conditions, and *nonobstructive* (or *communicating*), which is failure of CSF absorption by the arachnoid granulations and can be caused by infection or hemorrhage.

In children the brain enlarges and the skull grows to accommodate it by delayed closure of the sutures (seams) between bones. If CSF flow or absorption is blocked and intracranial pressure rises before the sutures fuse, the head may become greatly enlarged (Figure 23-15). On the other hand, if CSF flow or absorption is obstructed in adults, raised CSF pressure can cause

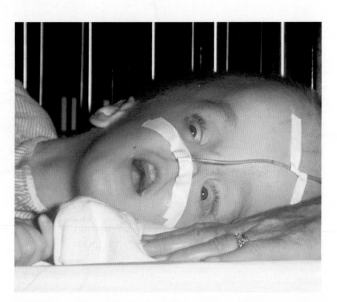

Figure 23-15 Child with hydrocephalus. Before cranial bone sutures close, increased intracranial pressure causes enlargement of the head.

brain atrophy and symptoms that can mimic other brain disease such as multiple sclerosis or parkinsonism.

Finally, diseases that cause brain atrophy—Alzheimer disease, for example—are accompanied by compensatory accumulations of CSF in the ventricles or over the surface of the brain (*hydrocephalus ex vacuo*) to make up for lost brain tissue.

Intracranial Hemorrhage

Intracranial hemorrhage is classified according to its anatomic location: *intraparenchymal* (within the tissue of the brain) or *extraparenchymal* (on the surface of the brain). Extraparenchymal hemorrhage is classified according its relationship to the skull and meningeal layers as *epidural*, *subdural*, or *subarachnoid* hemorrhage. Most intracranial hemorrhage occurs suddenly and without apparent cause; nevertheless, most can ultimately be traced to hypertension, aneurysm, or other specific abnormality.

Any sudden, spontaneous vascular event in the brain is called a **stroke**, or *cerebrovascular accident*. *Apoplexy* is an older, less common term for the same malady (see the nearby History of Medicine box). A stroke may be caused by either hemorrhage into the brain (**red stroke**, 20% of cases) or infarction (**white stroke**, 80% of cases).

BLEEDING ON THE SURFACE OF THE BRAIN

Epidural hematoma is an accumulation of blood beneath the skull and outside the dura mater. It is almost always caused by skull fracture that tears a meningeal artery; hence bleeding is rapid the hematoma forms quickly owing to rapid arterial bleeding (Fig. 23-16). Meningeal arteries are partially embedded in the inner convexity of the skull and covered internally by the dura mater (see Fig. 23-2), so that they have little room to flex and are easily torn by fracture. The most common type of injury associated with epidural hematoma is a temporal skull fracture that ruptures the middle meningeal artery. Bleeding is brisk, with formation of a rapidly enlarging epidural mass that presses inward on the cerebral hemisphere, as is illustrated in Figure 23-17. If bleeding is not stopped quickly and the hematoma drained promptly, epidural hematomas are quickly fatal because of increased intracranial pressure and brain herniation. In a significant number of cases, hematomas present with a distinctive history. The initial trauma is usually severe enough to render the patient unconscious owing to concussion. The patient recovers consciousness for a while before becoming unconscious again, owing to accumulation of the hematoma. This "lucid interval" is a key clinical diagnostic point. By contrast, patients with other types of intracranial bleeding from head injury usually show no lucid interval.

Subdural hematoma (Figs. 23-17, 23-18, and 23-19) is an accumulation of blood beneath the dura mater caused by relatively slow venous bleeding, owing to head trauma that is usually not severe enough to cause skull fracture. Bleeding occurs from small veins that bridge the subdural space from the superior sagittal sinus to the brain surface, and accumulates as a mass that pushes the brain aside. Subdural hematoma differs from

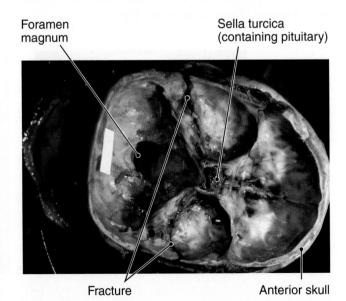

Foramen magnum

Sella turcica (containing pituitary)

Fracture

Anterior skull

***Figure 23-16* Skull fracture.** This patient developed an acute epidural hematoma, caused by bleeding from an artery torn by the fracture.

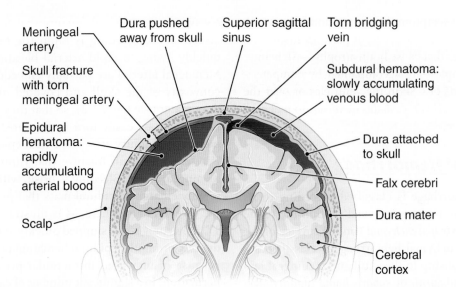

Figure 23-17 **Epidural and subdural hematomas.** Bleeding in epidural hematoma is rapid because of skull fracture and severance of a meningeal artery. Bleeding in subdural hematoma is slow and results from tearing of veins that extend across the subdural (subarachnoid) space.

epidural hematoma in that bleeding in subdural hematoma is slow and venous; epidural hematomas form quickly from brisk arterial bleeding.

In subdural hematoma the trauma may be so mild that it is not recallable by the patient or anyone else, so there may be no history of head trauma. Bleeding may be caused by almost any abrupt motion of the head that results in significant internal shifting of the brain; automobile whiplash is an example. A violently shaken infant, unable to control its head, is another.

Although the bleeding in subdural hematomas is slow, they can be classified as acute or chronic. In cases of *acute* subdural hematoma (Fig. 23-18) the history of trauma is clear. Venous bleeding and symptoms build over a period of several hours or days.

Conversely, a clear clinical history of trauma is rare in *chronic* subdural hematoma. Bleeding is slow, so slow that often by the time of discovery the hematoma has been organized into a sac of golden fluid encapsulated by a rind of fibrous scar tissue. This fluid mass may grow after bleeding has stopped, because the residue of blood-cell debris and protein produces a high internal osmotic pressure that attracts water. As a consequence symptoms may occur so slowly as to be mistaken for dementia or other types of neurologic disease. Elderly patients on anticoagulants for vascular or cardiac valve disease are among the most common clinical presentations.

Subarachnoid hemorrhage is any bleeding into the subarachnoid space. It is usually sudden and not associated with trauma or other precipitating cause. The most

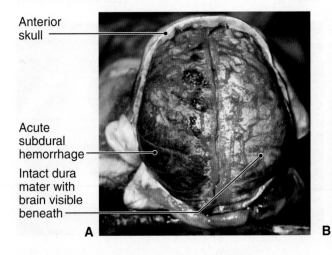

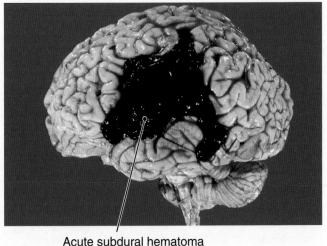

Acute subdural hematoma

Figure 23-18 **Acute subdural hematoma.** This gross autopsy study was done after a mild head injury in a patient taking anticoagulants. **A,** Brain in the cranial case. Blood is visible through the intact dura mater. **B,** The dura mater has been removed from the brain.

Cerebral sulci   Cerebral gyri   Skull

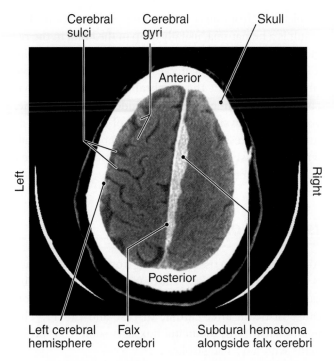

Anterior

Left   Right

Posterior

Left cerebral hemisphere   Falx cerebri   Subdural hematoma alongside falx cerebri

Figure 23-19 Subdural hematoma (radiographic study). Blood is accumulated to the right side of the falx cerebri. Note the blurring of sulci and gyri on the right owing to cerebral edema.

common cause of subarachnoid hemorrhage is trauma. There are two main causes of spontaneous nontraumatic subarachnoid hemorrhage: *saccular (berry) aneurysm,* which develops after birth, and *vascular malformation,* which is congenital.

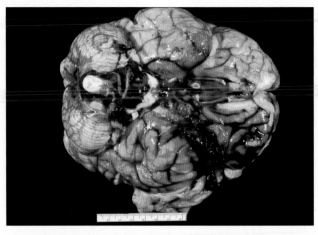

Figure 23-20 Spontaneous subarachnoid hemorrhage. This patient had a ruptured saccular (berry) aneurysm (not visible).

The most common cause of subarachnoid hemorrhage is *spontaneous* rupture of a **saccular aneurysm,** illustrated in Figures 23-20 and 23-21. Less frequent causes are extension of bleeding from another site, tumor, coagulation problems, and trauma. About 1% of the population has a berry aneurysm, most of which are asymptomatic and never cause a problem. The name is well taken—berry aneurysms are often the size and shape of a berry, varying from a few millimeters to over a centimeter. They are caused by ballooning of the vascular wall, the effect of blood pressure at the weakest point of cerebral vessels, where one vessel divides into

Left anterior cerebral artery   Right anterior cerebral artery

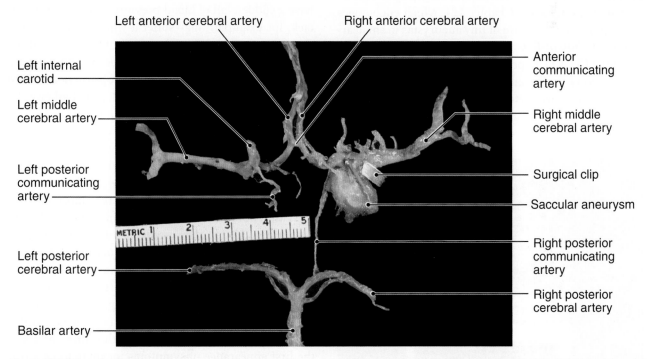

Left internal carotid   Anterior communicating artery

Left middle cerebral artery   Right middle cerebral artery

Left posterior communicating artery   Surgical clip

Saccular aneurysm

Left posterior cerebral artery   Right posterior communicating artery

Right posterior cerebral artery

Basilar artery

Figure 23-21 Saccular (berry) aneurysm. In this dissection of the circle of Willis, the aneurysm arises at the junction of the right internal carotid (not visible), right middle cerebral, and right anterior cerebral arteries. A metal surgical clip was placed at the base of the aneurysm to staunch the hemorrhage.

two in or near the Circle of Willis. Unlike aneurysms elsewhere, saccular aneurysms are not caused by atherosclerosis. Sometimes they grow large enough to produce symptoms by pressing on adjacent structures, such as the optic nerve. When they bleed they usually do so without cause, but some bleeds can be attributed to increased intracranial blood pressure associated with straining at stool or exertion. Clinical onset is sudden and characterized by severe headache that rapidly proceeds to unconsciousness. When hemorrhage occurs the fatality rate is 50%.

Vascular malformations (Fig. 23-22) are congenital malformations that also can cause spontaneous intracranial bleeding. Blood may accumulate in the subarachnoid space or in brain tissue, depending on the location of the malformation. Vascular malformations usually occur on the surface of the cerebral hemisphere and are formed of tangled masses of arteries or veins or a mixture of both. They may not become symptomatic for many years, if ever. In addition to hemorrhage, they can be the cause of seizure disorders (epilepsy).

BLEEDING DIRECTLY INTO THE BRAIN

Bleeding directly into the substance of the brain can be spontaneous or secondary to another condition, such as trauma or a congenital vascular malformation deep inside the brain.

Spontaneous bleeding directly into the substance of the brain is called a **red stroke** and is usually caused by chronic hypertension (Chapter 12), which encourages development and rupture of tiny aneurysms in small arterioles (*Charcot-Bouchard microaneurysms*). Fifteen percent (15%) of hypertension deaths are caused by spontaneous intracranial hemorrhage. Hemorrhage may, however, originate as bleeding occurring in association with coagulation defects, anticoagulant therapy,

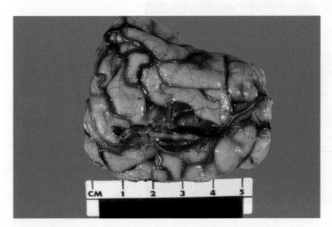

Figure 23-22 **Vascular malformation of cerebral cortex.** This specimen was excised because it was causing epileptic seizures.

or bleeding from an arteriovenous malformation. The result is a hematoma, usually deep in the brain in the region of the basal ganglia and internal capsule (see Fig. 23-4B), the bundle of nerve tracts that carries nerve fibers that connect the cerebral cortex to the spinal cord. Typical clinical onset is sudden, with headache, vomiting, paralysis, and rapid loss of consciousness as intracranial pressure escalates. Most episodes are fatal, with progressively deep coma, spasticity, and fixed pupils. Treatment is supportive.

Ischemia and Infarction

An infarct of brain tissue resulting from vascular disease is called a **white stroke**. White stroke is a crippling disease and in the United States is the third most common cause of death after cardiac disease and cancer. The nearby History of Medicine box lists some U.S. presidents who have had strokes.

Recall from Chapters 5 and 12 that infarcts are caused by ischemia; that is, a lack of oxygen. By far the most common cause of ischemia is obstruction of blood flow. Atherosclerotic narrowing and thrombotic occlusion of the carotid (Fig. 23-23), middle cerebral, or basilar arteries cause most white strokes. However, in some patients white stroke occurs without complete obstruction of blood flow. For example, patients who have atherosclerotic narrowing of cerebral vessels and who have a sudden fall of blood pressure (during a heart attack, for example), may suffer a white infarct because there is not enough blood pressure to force blood beyond the obstruction. After atherosclerotic obstruction, the second most common cause is obstruction caused by an embolus from fragments of ulcerated atherosclerotic plaques, from thrombi in fibrillating atria (as illustrated in Case Study 23-1 at the end of this chapter), or from bits of thrombus that break away from an intraventricular thrombus associated with a myocardial infarct (mural thrombus, Chapter 13). Embolic vegetations from endocarditis also may be the culprit.

Within hours after infarction, brain tissue swells with edema (Fig. 23-24), then gradually softens over the next few days and eventually liquefies (liquefactive necrosis), leaving a filmy residue of scarring (gliosis) and an empty space filled with cerebrospinal fluid (Fig. 23-25).

Speed is of the essence in treating vascular obstruction that produces signs and symptoms of white stroke, and treatment must be initiated within three hours of the first appearance of symptoms for there to be a reasonable chance of recovering lost neurologic function. Mainstays of treatment include anticoagulant therapy

History of Medicine

STROKES IN UNITED STATES PRESIDENTS

There is good evidence that five U.S. Presidents had strokes, two of them while in office. However, sketchy records and relatively primitive medicine make some of the diagnoses speculative. However, study of their illnesses reveals the varied manifestations of stroke.

- *Paralysis, numbness, and motor problems:*
  - *John Quincy Adams* (1767–1848, served 1825–1829) clearly had a sudden episode of paralysis in 1846 at age 78 while serving as an elected member of the House of Representatives after his term as president. Two years later he collapsed again with paralysis and died at age 80.
  - *Woodrow Wilson* (1856–1924, served 1915–1921) had several minor strokes before becoming president. The first episode occurred in 1896 when he was 40—he suffered weakness and numbness in his right arm and was unable to write for a year. Multiple other episodes of right arm weakness and numbness occurred between 1904 and 1915, when he was elected President. In 1919 at age 63 while President he suffered a serious stroke with left hemiplegia diagnosed by his physician as a thrombosis not a hemorrhage—arguably the most serious illness ever suffered by a sitting President. He never fully recovered, and there was debate about its effect on his mental ability. His condition was hidden from the public, and he served out his term in greatly diminished capacity.

- *Sudden collapse:*
  - *John Tyler* (1790–1862, served 1841–1845) probably died of a stroke: he collapsed unconscious but revived for short while before dying at age 72 during the United States Civil War. At the time he was serving in the Congress of the Confederacy.

- *Speech problems:*
  - *Dwight Eisenhower* (1890–1969, served 1953–1961) found himself unable to finish sentences one day in 1957. Examination of the 67-year-old President revealed that he had neither sensory nor motor deficit, and he was diagnosed with aphasia due to occlusion of the left middle cerebral artery. Never a good public speaker, Eisenhower never fully recovered normal speech—he hesitated and stumbled verbally for the remainder of his term in office.
  - *Gerald Ford* (b. 1913, served 1974–1977) developed temporary speech and balance problems at age 87 and was diagnosed with a small brainstem infarct.

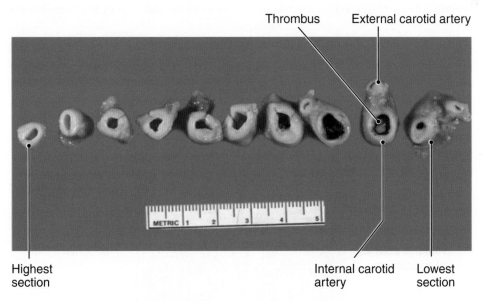

Figure 23-23 **Thrombosis of the internal carotid artery.** Multiple cross-sections were taken from a patient who died of a large cerebral infarct (white stroke).

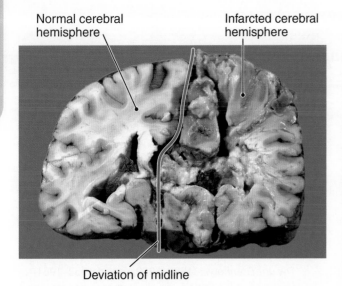

Normal cerebral hemisphere

Infarcted cerebral hemisphere

Deviation of midline

Figure 23-24 Acute white stroke. This acute infarction of a cerebral hemisphere occurred in a patient with thrombosis of the internal carotid artery. Note the deviation of the midline caused by edema of the infarcted tissue.

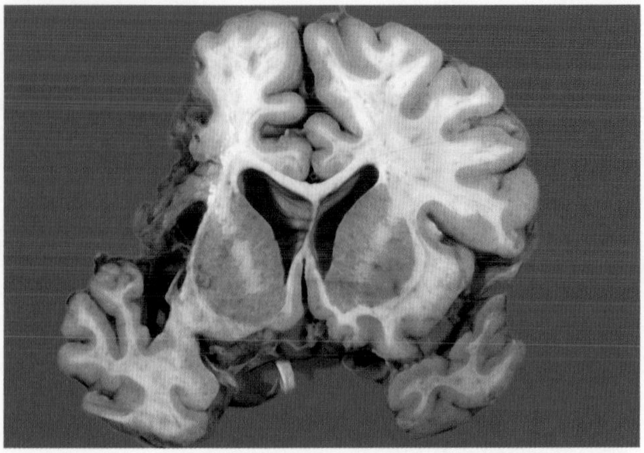

Figure 23-25 Healed infarct of the cerebrum. Long-standing hemiparesis in this patient resulted from a white stroke caused by occlusion of the middle cerebral artery.

with heparin (because it acts rapidly) and drugs to dissolve the thrombus. Success has been reported for arterial catheterization to remove the thrombus.

Clinically, most patients who develop white stroke have a history of diabetes, valvular heart disease, hypertension, or atherosclerotic vascular disease in another part of the body, especially coronary vascular disease. Infarcts cause symptoms related to the particular part of the brain affected. For example, an infarct confined to the motor cortex of the right cerebral hemisphere produces left-side weakness or paralysis. White infarcts oc-

cur rather suddenly, but many are preceded by episodes of dizziness, syncope (fainting), focal weakness, or other neurologic symptoms that last a few minutes or hours, termed **transient ischemic attacks**. About 25% of patients who have a transient ischemic attack have a white stroke within five years.

Infarction is usually a local event related to a specific blood vessel. However, the entire brain can become hypoxic (**global hypoxia**, or global ischemia) if severe generalized hypoxia occurs (Fig. 23-26). Neurons are the most vulnerable cell in the brain because they consume

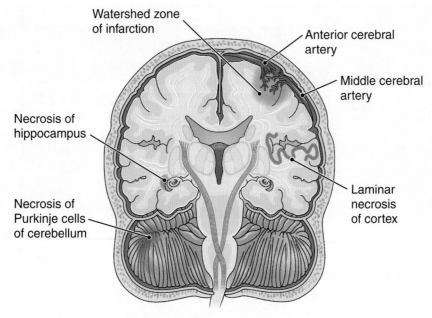

Watershed zone of infarction

Anterior cerebral artery

Middle cerebral artery

Necrosis of hippocampus

Necrosis of Purkinje cells of cerebellum

Laminar necrosis of cortex

Figure 23-26 Consequences of global ischemia. Patients with global hypoxia (ischemia) may develop laminar cortical necrosis, necrosis of the hippocampus and cerebellar Purkinje neurons, and watershed infarcts of the cerebrum.

the most oxygen and are extremely sensitive to oxygen deprivation. The neurons most sensitive to oxygen deprivation are those of the superficial cerebral cortex and certain cells (Purkinje cells) in the cerebellum. When deprived of oxygen, these cells suffer first and undergo necrosis in circumstances that may not cause permanent injury to other brain cells. If the hypoxia is relieved, the rest of the brain may recover, leaving in the superficial cerebral cortex a layer of necrotic neurons, a condition known as **laminar cortical necrosis** (Fig. 23-27). Global ischemia may produce temporary coma or other neurologic deficits, but laminar cortical necrosis is irreversible and is usually associated with permanent coma or death.

Clinical conditions associated with global ischemia include insufficient blood flow in patients with heart failure or shock or who are hypoxic from near drowning or carbon monoxide poisoning (Chapter 10). Children tolerate global hypoxia better than adults do; for example, some children may be submerged in water for half an hour or longer and recover completely. In some instances general hypoxia not severe enough to produce widespread laminar cortical necrosis may produce local rather than general necrosis in tissue supplied by blood vessels narrowed by atherosclerosis. In this circumstance the ischemia may produce infarction in the "watershed" areas (see Fig. 23-6B and C) of the cerebral cortex, which exist in the borderland between two areas supplied by different cerebral arteries. Because the anatomy of superficial blood vessels on each side of these areas resembles water drainage on ei-

ther side of a ridge line, white strokes in these areas are called **watershed infarcts**.

Brain and Spinal Cord Trauma

Brain and spinal cord trauma are major health problems in the United States. Automobile accidents are the most common cause of injury; other causes include assaults, falls, and child abuse. The spinal cord, especially the cervical spine, is vulnerable to force that causes hyperflexion (backward motion) or extension (forward) of the neck. Force may tear ligaments or fracture vertebrae; in either case the cord can be crushed or bruised (contused). Permanent flaccid paralysis below the level of injury is common. Autonomic control of bowel and bladder function may eventually return.

A **concussion** is a period of temporary brain dysfunction following head injury. Concussion is not associated with anatomically demonstrable brain lesions, and radiographic images of the brain are normal. About 10% of concussion victims are rendered unconscious; frequent symptoms include confusion, dizziness, amnesia, nausea, and blurred vision. Repeated concussions, as in boxing or other contact sports, may produce chronic organic brain syndromes, such as the Parkinson syndrome suffered by American boxer Muhammad Ali.

Diffuse axonal injury occurs when sudden, severe twisting motion of the head (as in an auto accident) can stretch brain nerve tracts (white matter) to the point of injury. Gross abnormalities may be minimal, but severe neurologic deficit (dementia or permanent coma, for example) can occur.

Blunt trauma may cause **contusion**, a bruise, usually characterized by hemorrhages in the superficial cerebral hemisphere caused by sudden shift of the brain that brings it into contact with the skull. Blunt force to an immobile head causes injury to brain tissue immediately beneath the site of the blow; however, when a moving head meets an immobile object, injury occurs at the site of the blow (the *coup* injury) and at the rebound site in the brain directly opposite from the initial point of contact (the *contrecoup* injury). The *coup-contrecoup* combination is illustrated in Figure 23-28. The contrecoup injury usually is the more severe of the two and produces more tissue damage and symptoms.

Infections of the Central Nervous System

Infections of the central nervous system are of two principal types: those of brain tissue and those of the

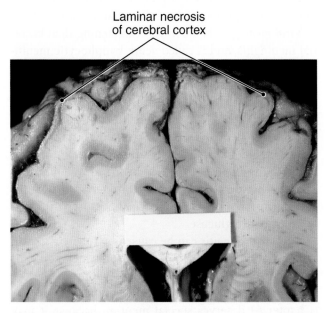

Laminar necrosis
of cerebral cortex

Figure 23-27 **Laminar cortical necrosis.** This patient suffered global cerebral hypoxia secondary to vascular collapse (shock) following traumatic hemorrhage.

Coup injury (primary)   Contrecoup injury (secondary)

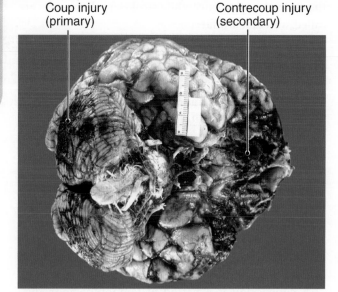

Figure 23-28 **Coup and contrecoup injuries.** This patient received a primary blow (the *coup* injury) to back of head (occiput). At the opposite (frontal) side of the skull is a more severe contusion in the frontal lobes (the *contrecoup* injury) caused by commotion of the brain inside the skull.

meninges and cerebrospinal fluid. Organisms usually localize to a preferred site. For example:

- Aerobic bacteria usually cause meningitis; anaerobic bacteria usually cause brain abscess
- Poliovirus usually infects spinal motor neurons
- Syphilis and *Rickettsia* usually infect small blood vessels

Infections in another part of the body can spread to the brain. The central nervous system may be infected by direct extension from nearby tissue, such as a bacterial invasion from an infected sinus; blood-borne organisms may seed the brain from another site (for example, bacteria may spread from an infected middle ear to the meninges); or viruses can travel along nerve axons from peripheral tissue to the brain (the rabies virus reaches the brain from the bite of a rabid animal in this way).

INFECTIONS OF THE MENINGES AND CEREBROSPINAL FLUID

Meningitis is inflammation of the meninges, and the cause is almost always infection, usually by viruses or pyogenic (pus-forming) bacteria. The accompanying Lab Tools box describes the procedure for obtaining CSF for laboratory examination and summarizes some of the noteworthy findings.

Most *acute purulent meningitis* is caused by aerobic bacteria and may occur at any age, although the type of

bacterium varies with age group:

- *Escherichia coli* infection usually occurs in newborns.
- *Haemophilus influenzae* usually infects children aged 1–3 years.
- *Streptococcus pneumoniae* is most often found as the agent in mature adults and people with basilar skull fracture.
- *Neisseria meningitidis* (**meningococcal meningitis**) causes a very dangerous variety of epidemic meningitis in youth and young adults, especially those living in groups, such as in the military or in university dormitories. It may develop explosively and rapidly progress to septicemia, shock, and death. About one third of all people carry meningococci in the pharynx, but few become infected. Transmission is by airborne droplets. A vaccine is available and recommended for military recruits and college freshmen. Early diagnosis and immediate penicillin therapy are the keys to successful treatment.

The anatomic findings in acute purulent meningitis are typical of acute bacterial infection: pus in the CSF and over the surface of the brain. The clinical signs include fever, headache, stiff neck, and prostration. Rapid diagnosis is paramount, and survival depends largely on the speed with which correct antibiotic therapy is begun.

Findings in the spinal fluid in acute purulent meningitis are characteristic: large numbers of neutrophils, glucose level that is lower than blood glucose (because of bacterial metabolism of glucose in spinal fluid) and high levels of protein (from inflammatory exudate).

Viral meningitis is much less threatening than bacterial meningitis, and is called **acute lymphocytic meningitis** because cells in the CSF are lymphocytes, not neutrophils. Because bacterial cultures are negative, viral meningitis also may be called *aseptic meningitis*. Viral meningitis features a lymphocytic infiltrate in the arachnoid and in the CSF. CSF findings are of paramount importance: the cells are almost all lymphocytes, CSF protein is increased owing to inflammatory exudate; however, in contrast to bacterial meningitis, CSF glucose level is usually normal because viruses do not metabolize glucose.

Chronic meningitis can be caused by tubercle bacilli, syphilis, and fungi. Much of the chronic meningitis today occurs in AIDS patients, many of whom are infected with the fungus *Cryptococcus neoformans*. Syphilis (Chapter 8) deserves special mention because it may produce a variety of lesions and clinical syndromes, two of which are especially notable. Patients with *late*

Laboratory Examination of Cerebrospinal Fluid

Laboratory study of cerebrospinal fluid (CSF) is critical in many diseases of the central nervous system, especially infectious diseases.

Lumbar puncture is indicated in patients suspected of having meningitis and other CNS inflammations, subarachnoid hemorrhage, leukemic infiltration of the meninges, and some neoplastic disorders. If increased intracranial pressure or intracranial mass is suspected, radiographic images should be obtained for further assessment before proceeding because lowering spinal pressure by draining fluid from the spinal canal may cause downward herniation of the cerebellar tonsils, which can cause paralysis or death. Most patients tolerate lumbar puncture well, but some experience headache, and a few have minor bleeding into the CSF.

CSF is usually obtained by inserting a needle between lumbar vertebrae into the subarachnoid space, a procedure first performed in 1891 by Heinrich Quincke, a German physician who thought drainage of CSF might help infants with hydrocephalus. The technique is relatively simple (see the accompanying figure): the patient lies on one side in the knee-chest position and a long, thin needle is threaded between vertebrae and into the subarachnoid space. Typically 2–3 ml of fluid is collected and divided among several sterile tubes for culture, cell count, and chemical/immunologic/molecular studies. A blood specimen should always be collected at the same time: it is important to compare levels of blood glucose and protein with CSF values.

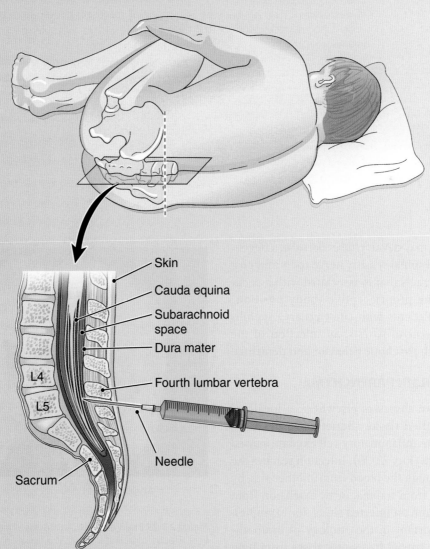

Lumbar puncture. A long, thin sterile needle is inserted between lower lumbar vertebrae in the region of the cauda equina of the spinal cord. Spinal fluid pressure can be gauged, and fluid can be obtained for analysis.

The following is a brief example of some noteworthy findings in CSF (see also the summary in the accompanying table):

- *Color*. Bloody fluid followed by clear fluid after the first few drops indicates bleeding caused by the procedure.

Normal Adult Cerebrospinal Fluid

	Findings
Pressure	70–180 mm Hg
Color	Clear
Total cell count (per µl)	0–5
Cell differential count	Mononuclear cells only (lymphocytes, macrophages, occasional meningeal cells)
Protein (mg/dL)	15–45
Glucose (mg/dL)	50–80

*Newborn CSF may be substantially different

Bleeding associated with disease is characterized by uniformly colored CSF. Fresh pathologic blood is pink, but blood from bleeding 4–6 hours old may be orange or yellowish due to metabolism of blood into bilirubin (Chapter 16).

- *Cells*: The presence of any red blood cells or neutrophils is abnormal. Purulent meningitis is associated with elevated neutrophil counts. Viral meningitis is associated with increased numbers of mononuclear cells (lymphocytes, macrophages). If a tumor is present in the central nervous system, sometimes tumor cells can be identified.
- *Protein*: An increased level of protein is usually a sign of infection, inflammation, degenerative disease, or hemorrhage. Low protein levels are a sign of CSF leakage, the most important cause being basilar skull fracture, in which CSF leaks out through the nose (CSF rhinorrhea).
- *Glucose*: CSF glucose is derived from blood glucose and fluctuates with it; for example, patients with diabetes who have a high blood glucose level will have high CSF glucose level. Low CSF glucose levels may occur with low blood glucose levels, bacterial or fungal infection (caused by metabolism of glucose by inflammatory cells or microbes), or subarachnoid hemorrhage.
- *Culture*: Normal CSF is sterile.

syphilitic meningitis may develop *tabes dorsalis*, a degeneration of the dorsal spinal sensory nerve roots and posterior spinal nerve tracts that is associated with a peculiar gait because the proprioceptive (body position) sense is damaged. Patients with late (tertiary) syphilis also may develop *general paresis*, an infection of the brain associated with psychotic behavior and dementia.

INFECTIONS OF BRAIN PARENCHYMA

Brain abscess is, like abscesses elsewhere, a localized area of dead, liquefied tissue (liquefactive necrosis, Chapter 2) and acute inflammatory cell exudate caused by bacterial infection (Fig. 23-29). Infection reaches the brain by spread through the blood from another site, by direct implantation from trauma, or by extension from nearby infection (from an infected sinus, for example). The lungs are important in the etiology of brain abscess—blood-borne spread frequently arises from lung abscess or from the pus-filled bronchioles associated

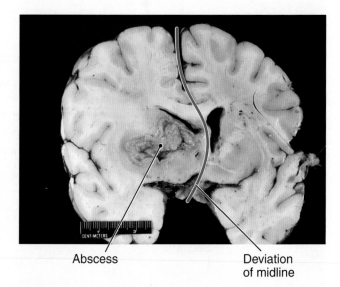

Abscess   Deviation of midline

Figure 23-29 **Brain abscess.** An abscess in the basal ganglia in a patient with bacterial endocarditis. The deviation of the midline resulted from unilateral cerebral edema.

with bronchiectasis (Chapter 14). Patients with cyanotic heart disease (right-to-left shunt, Chapter 13) are susceptible because blood bypasses the sieve of the lungs that otherwise filters out blood-borne bacteria, allowing greatly increased numbers of organisms to circulate in the blood and through the brain. Patients with bacterial endocarditis (Chapter 13) are also at risk for brain abscess.

Whereas brain abscess is a localized infection in patients who usually have another serious illness, viral infections of the brain (*viral encephalitis*) are generalized brain infections that usually affect previously healthy people. However, some viruses affect a particular part of the brain. For example, herpes encephalitis most often affects the temporal lobe, rabies virus infects neurons only, and the *JC virus*, which causes *multifocal leukoencephalopathy*, targets oligodendrocytes. Other brain infections are more common in immunodeficient patients; for example, cytomegalovirus (CMV) encephalitis in AIDS. The HIV virus itself tends to infect the brain as well as the immune system and produces a progressive neurologic disease, AIDS dementia (Chapter 7). *Arbovirus encephalitis*, of which there are multiple subtypes such as *St. Louis* and *Western Equine*, is the most common form of epidemic encephalitis and is spread by mosquitoes, usually in late summer. The measles virus causes a rare chronic, fatal brain disease (*subacute sclerosing panencephalitis*), which usually appears in children who became infected by the measles virus before age 2.

The **spongiform encephalitides** are a group of universally fatal, very rare diseases that deserve mention because of the uniqueness of the infective agent and because they are related to a veterinary disease—mad cow disease—that is widely publicized because of the fear that eating beef may communicate a devastating condition. Spongiform encephalopathy is a progressive, chronic degenerative brain disease caused by **prions** (Chapter 8), which are proteins, not living things like other infective agents. Prions have no DNA or RNA and no metabolism and are altered forms of previously normal proteins that attach to normal brain protein and convert it into additional prions; much like a snowflake grows by adding more ice crystals. The most notable spongiform encephalopathy of humans is **Creutzfeldt-jakob disease** (CJD), a very rare, rapidly advancing, and invariably fatal disease that causes progressive dementia. However, most human CJD appears spontaneously rather than resulting from infectious transmission. A few cases of CJD in humans have been obtained by eating infected beef.

Degenerative Diseases

Degenerative diseases of the central nervous system fall into two main categories: some diseases affect neurons (gray matter) directly, and the axons (white matter) are affected only secondarily; other diseases affect axons (white matter) directly.

DEGENERATIVE DISEASES OF GRAY MATTER

Degenerative diseases of neurons share certain characteristics. They usually

- Have no known cause, though some are inheritable
- Occur in selected areas of gray matter while leaving other areas unaffected
- Feature abnormal protein deposits in affected tissue
- Are associated with dementia

Dementia is a deterioration of mental abilities, such as memory, attention span, and reasoning, that results from brain disease. Dementia is not normal, no matter the patient's age. There are many degenerative diseases of gray matter, some associated with dementia, others that mainly cause paralysis or movement disorders. The most common degenerative disease of gray matter is Alzheimer disease.

Alzheimer disease is a degenerative disease of gray matter in the *cerebral cortex* that is the cause of over half of all cases of adult dementia. It usually occurs in the elderly, and it affects women more often than men. About 1% of people aged 60–64 years are affected, but the prevalence rises rapidly with advancing age and affects up to one third of people over the age of 85.

The cause is unknown; however, about 10% of cases have a familial association. Pathologic findings are distinctive. At autopsy the most notable finding is atrophy of the cerebral cortex: gyri are narrowed and sulci are broad (Fig. 23-30) due to loss of gray matter neurons. Microscopically the cerebral cortex contains pathologically characteristic tangles of abnormal protein fibrils (Fig. 23-31) and deposits (plaques) of amyloid protein (Chapter 7).

The clinical symptoms begin insidiously as memory loss, disorientation, loss of motor skills, and aphasia, and the patient eventually becomes bedfast, mute, and immobile. Death usually occurs in about ten years, from bronchopneumonia. Some drugs show promise of slowing disease progress and offer temporary symptomatic improvement, but treatment is generally supportive.

Parkinsonism is a *clinical syndrome*, a constellation of symptoms arising from degenerative disease in the *basal*

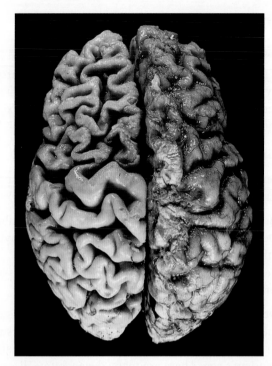

Figure 23-30 Alzheimer disease. Severe frontal lobe atrophy, Gyri are narrow; sulci are wide, especially in the frontal lobes (top). Meninges have been removed on the left, but are in place on the right.

ganglia (see Fig. 23-4B) in the midbrain. Symptoms result from lack of sufficient *dopamine*, a neurotransmitter chemical. When the etiology is unknown, as it is in most people, patients are said to have Parkinson *disease*. However, when the cause is known patients are said to have

Parkinson *syndrome* secondary to a particular cause, such as repeated head injury, which is the cause of parkinsonism suffered by American boxer Muhammad Ali. Parkinsonism can also be caused by vascular disease, toxins, or viral encephalitis.

The fundamental defect in parkinsonism is faulty nerve signal transmission in the basal ganglia. Pathologic findings include loss of pigment in basal ganglia, and the presence in affected neurons of *Lewy bodies*, which are composed of an amyloid-like protein. Lewy bodies, however, can be found in other degenerative brain diseases.

Parkinsonism is a disease of the elderly; most cases begin in people over age 60; men are affected more frequently than women are; and there are no racial differences. Onset is usually slow, but full-blown cases are characterized by tremor, difficulty walking, rigidity, shuffling gait, slurred speech, and a wooden, emotionless facial expression. About 10% of patients with parkinsonism also have dementia. Treatment with L-dopa, a dopamine precursor, may offer temporary relief but does not slow progression of the underlying disease. There is no cure; however, experimental brain implants of cloned cells show promise.

Amyotrophic lateral sclerosis, also known as *Lou Gehrig disease* after the famed New York Yankee baseball player of the 1920s and 1930s who died from it, is a degenerative condition of motor neurons in the gray matter of the cerebral cortex and spinal cord gray matter in mature adults (Fig. 23-32). Renowned English as-

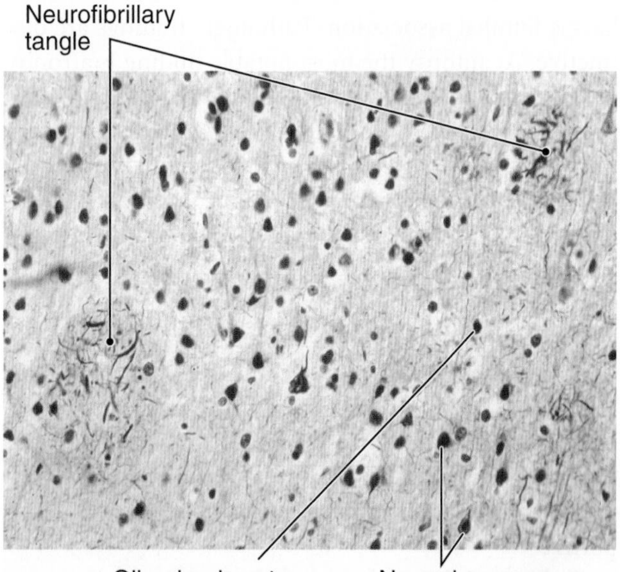

Neurofibrillary tangle

Oligodendrocyte   Normal neurons

Figure 23-31 Alzheimer disease. Characteristic neurofibrillary tangles are visible in this microscopic study.

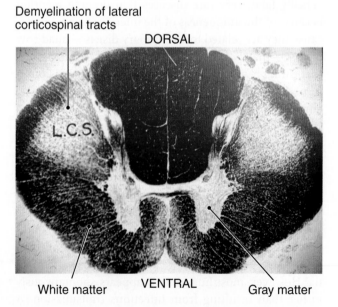

Demyelination of lateral corticospinal tracts

DORSAL

L.C.S.

White matter   VENTRAL   Gray matter

Figure 23-32 Amyotrophic lateral sclerosis (Lou Gehrig disease). In this microscopic study of a cross-section of spinal cord, myelin is stained black. The lateral corticospinal tracts (L.C.S. in the section) are pale due to loss of myelin.

tronomer Stephen Hawking suffers from it. A familial form has been linked to an abnormal gene on chromosome 21. It presents with weakness and muscle twitching (fasciculations) and progresses to interfere with speech, locomotion, and respiratory effort. Cognitive and sensory functions are unimpaired. Death usually occurs because of respiratory failure.

Huntington disease is an autosomal dominant genetic disease (Chapter 7) traced to a defect on chromosome 4 that causes neuron degeneration in the basal ganglia. Most cases are inherited, and it occurs in whites of northern European ancestry. Some new cases occur as spontaneous mutations. Like other degenerative neuronal diseases, it features microscopic deposits of amyloid-related protein in the basal ganglia. Huntington disease does not become symptomatic until well into adult life (aged about 30–40 years). Huntington disease has been traced to a gene that codes for an abnormal protein that interferes with the function of nerve cells in the cortex and midbrain, and it is characterized by dementia and involuntary writhing movements (*chorea*). It is relentlessly progressive and fatal, usually within 10–20 years of first symptoms.

DEGENERATIVE DISEASES OF WHITE MATTER

Recall that nerve fibers (axons) are insulated from one another like electrical wires are insulated by rubber, a feature that prevents signals from crossing to another neuron except at a synapse. *Oligodendrocytes* insulate axons in the CNS; in peripheral nerves it is the function of *Schwann cells*, both of which produce a white, fatty substance, *myelin*, that covers and insulates the axons. Degenerative diseases of white matter cause loss of the myelin sheath of neuronal axons and are called **demyelinating diseases**, which may be acquired or hereditary.

Multiple sclerosis is an acquired chronic demyelinating disease that usually first appears in young adults. It affects the myelin sheath of both motor and sensory neurons in the brain, particularly the optic nerves and white matter near the lateral cerebral ventricles. Women are affected twice as often as men are. Multiple sclerosis is the most common demyelinating disease of the central nervous system and typically waxes and wanes over many years. The etiology of multiple sclerosis is not certain, but there is a definite familial tendency, and evidence is abundant that the immune system is reacting to a triggering antigen, probably a microbe—antibodies to the presumed microbe mistakenly attack self antigen in nerve cells. The pathological lesions are characteristic microscopic foci in white matter that show infiltrates of lymphocytes and macrophages, loss of myelin, and marked decrease of oligodendrocytes.

MS usually first appears in adults 18–40 years old and is famously unpredictable and subtle in its first manifestations—blurred vision or scotomata (spots), tingling, numbness, minor gait disturbances, or stumbling speech. Some patients may decline rapidly and die within a few months of onset. Others, for reasons unknown, may live a normal life span with few consequences, but most become wheelchair-bound over the course of a decade or two. Therapy is supportive, but anti-immune therapy may be beneficial. Laboratory and radiographic changes are minimal: many patients have white matter brain lesions visible by magnetic resonance imaging and abnormal patterns of immunoglobulins (Chapter 8) in their spinal fluid.

The **leukodystrophies** are a group of autosomal recessive genetic demyelinating diseases (Chapter 7) characterized by intrinsic defects of myelin resulting from a DNA coding defect for enzyme proteins important in the production and maintenance of healthy myelin. Lesions are found in the white matter. The leukodystrophies are diseases of infancy and childhood and are uniformly fatal. One such disease is *metachromatic leukodystrophy*, which is caused by a gene defect on chromosome 22. It derives its name from the pinkish alteration it causes in blue dyes used in microscopic study of myelin.

Metabolic and Toxic Disorders

The list of things toxic to the brain is almost endless; illicit drugs and alcohol (Chapter 10) top the list. Chronic alcoholics tend to develop cirrhosis (Chapter 16) and liver failure, one consequence of which is **hepatic encephalopathy**, a brain syndrome of personality changes, confusion, and a depressed level of consciousness as a result of accumulated metabolic products, especially ammonia, that cannot be metabolized properly by the liver.

One of the most perverse effects of chronic alcoholism is malnutrition—ethanol has plenty of calories but nothing of other nutritional value. As a consequence, chronic alcoholics may develop nervous system disease related to nutritional deficiency. The most common brain disorder associated with nutritional deficiency is vitamin B_1 (thiamine) deficiency, which may take several forms. One form is known clinically as beriberi (from the Sinhalese—Sri Lankan, Ceylonese— word *beri*, meaning weakness: beriberi means very weak). Beriberi (Chapter 10) is manifest by motor weakness because of peripheral neuropathy, and general weakness because of congestive heart failure. Other manifestations of thiamine deficiency are two related brain syndromes that occur in chronic alcoholics. **Wernicke encephalopathy**, a syndrome associated with cerebellar atrophy (Fig. 23-33), which features ataxia, tremors, confusion, and paralysis of extraocular muscles, none of which has to do with acute drunkenness but can look a lot like it. Untreated Wernicke encephalopathy may evolve into **Korsakoff psychosis**, a permanent defect of both short and long-term memory that leads patients to confabulate aimless, convoluted tales of explanation that never get anywhere because the patient cannot remember where the conversation should go.

Two other fairly common metabolic conditions of the central nervous system are vitamin B_{12} deficiency and lead poisoning. Patients with *vitamin B_{12} deficiency* (Chapter 10) may develop a demyelinating disease of certain white matter nerve tracts in the spinal cord, a condition known as *subacute combined degeneration of the spinal cord*, which features motor and sensory ("combined") problems characterized by spasticity, weakness, numbness and tingling in the limbs, and loss of proprioception (the ability to sense the position of limbs and other body parts). Patients with *lead poisoning* (Chapter 9) may develop peripheral neuropathy with weakness, numbness, and tingling in the limbs, or seizures brought on by brain edema and increased intracranial pressure.

Most other metabolic conditions of the brain are congenital or genetic, and include:

- *Cretinism* (infantile hypothyroidism, Chapter 18); a syndrome of very serious mental and physical retardation due to lack of thyroid hormone.
- *Phenylketonuria* (Chapter 7), an autosomal recessive, inherited enzyme deficiency associated with toxic accumulation of phenylalanine, which causes mental retardation and seizures.
- *Wilson disease* (hepatolenticular degeneration, Chapter 15), an inherited disease of copper metabolism characterized by mental instability and parkinsonian-like motor symptoms.
- *Neuronal storage diseases*, a group of autosomal recessive genetic enzyme deficiencies (Chapter 7) that include *Gaucher disease* (Chapter 6). Each of these storage diseases features accumulation of normal metabolic products in neurons owing to failure of enzymes to metabolize them in the usual fashion. Patients become symptomatic in infancy; the result is severe neurologic impairment and early death in most cases.

Neoplasms

Brain tumors are relatively uncommon, accounting for about 2% of all cancer deaths. Brain neoplasms are not like other tumors primarily because the difference between benign and malignant is less clear than with other tumors:

- Microscopically benign tumors may produce severe debility or death because of the confined space and critical anatomy of the brain.
- It is difficult to completely remove most tumors in the brain because the visible difference between tumor and normal tissue is minimal, especially at the tumor margin.
- Some brain tumors are located in areas of the brain that are not surgically accessible except by sacrifice of normal brain tissue that is too great to consider.
- Even highly malignant brain tumors rarely spread to other parts of the body: invasion of blood vessels is rare because vascular endothelial cells are so tightly joined to form the blood-brain barrier, and lymphatic spread is rare because there are few lymphatics in the brain.

Half of all intracranial tumors are metastatic carcinoma; the other half originate in the cranium. Metastases mainly are a problem in the elderly because malignant tumors are more common in older people. The

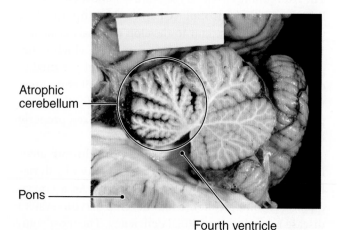

Atrophic cerebellum

Pons

Fourth ventricle

Figure 23-33 **Wernicke encephalopathy.** Cerebellar atrophy in a patient with chronic alcoholism.

three most common sources are lung cancer, breast cancer, and malignant melanoma. Brain metastases rarely occur with carcinoma of the prostate or ovary or sarcomas of any kind. Lymphoma and leukemia also may spread to the brain. Mental or neurologic symptoms caused by brain metastases may be the first manifestation of an occult (hidden) carcinoma. If brain metastasis is suspected, lung carcinoma is the prime suspect, because lung cancer is common and difficult to find before it metastasizes.

Half of brain tumors originate in the cranium and include:

- Tumors of brain cells (glia, neurons, and related embryonic cells): 60%
- Tumors of cranial nerves and the meninges: 20%
- All others: 20% (not including tumors of the pituitary, Chapter 18)

Much as bone tumors tend to occur in certain parts of long bones, primary brain tumors have a tendency to occur in certain parts of the brain and associated tissues (Fig. 23-34). Primary tumors rarely occur in the spinal cord.

Gliomas (*astrocytoma, oligodendroglioma,* and *ependymoma*) are tumors of glial cells and are the most common primary brain tumors. Of gliomas, **astrocytomas** are most common. They occur principally in adults but may be seen at any age. They are classified according to microscopic grade: well-differentiated, intermediate differentiation, and poorly differentiated. Even microscopically benign appearing astrocytomas usually prove fatal. Regardless of initial grade, astrocytomas tend to behave more aggressively with time.

Low-grade (well-differentiated) astrocytomas tend to occur early in life and are the least aggressive, but they usually prove fatal nevertheless. They are difficult, if not impossible, to remove completely because they blend imperceptibly into normal nearby brain tissue (Fig. 23-35) or their location precludes removal because nearby tissue is so critical to life. Average survival is about 5 years.

Intermediate grade (moderately differentiated) astrocytomas are rather uncommon. Average survival is about 3 years.

High-grade (poorly differentiated) astrocytomas comprise nearly half of all primary intracranial tumors and are called **glioblastoma multiforme** (Fig. 23-36).

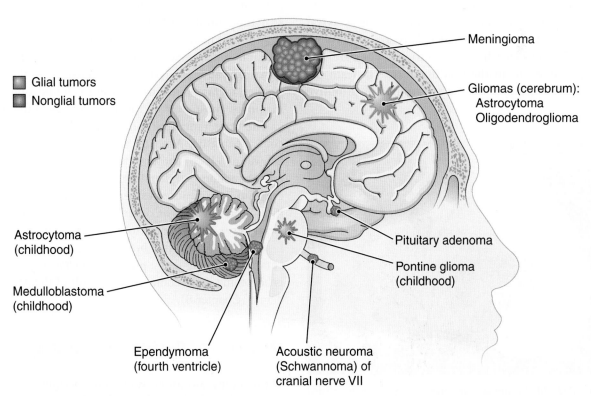

Figure 23-34 **The most common intracranial tumors.**

Well-differentiated
astrocytoma

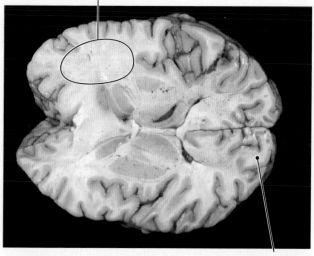

Frontal lobe

Figure 23-35 **Well-differentiated astrocytoma.** Shown here is a horizontal section of a tumor in the occipital (posterior) lobe. Grossly, it is difficult to distinguish the tumor from normal white matter.

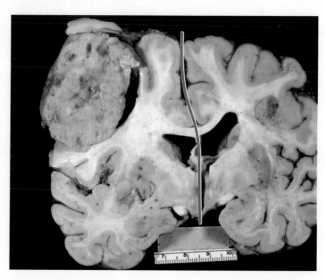

Figure 23-37 **Meningioma.** This tumor originated on the inner surface of the parietal bone of the skull. The underlying brain is atrophic, and the midline is pushed to one side by the expanding mass.

They tend to occur in older adults and are usually fatal within a year.

Oligodendrogliomas are tumors of oligodendroglial cells, the cells that form brain myelin. They are moderately aggressive primary brain neoplasms that usually grow more slowly and less predictably than astrocytomas do. They occur mainly in adults. Average survival is about 5–10 years. *Ependymomas* are tumors of ependymal cells that line the ventricles. They are rare and usually occur in the fourth ventricle beneath the cerebellum. *Medulloblastoma* is a tumor of primitive

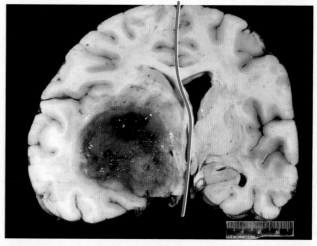

Figure 23-36 **Glioblastoma multiforme.** This poorly differentiated tumor is easy to distinguish from surrounding normal tissue. The midline is pushed to one side by the expanding tumor mass.

embryological cells that occurs almost exclusively in the cerebellum of children. It is highly sensitive to radiation therapy: the ten-year survival rate is about 50%.

Meningiomas are usually benign, very slow growing tumors of the arachnoid membrane that produce problems mainly by mass effect—they press on adjacent structures until headache, seizure, mental aberration, or localized neurologic deficit occurs (Fig. 23-37). For example, a meningioma pressing on the seventh cranial nerve can cause paralysis of facial muscles. As the name implies, meningiomas arise in the arachnoid, one of the meninges; most grow on the inner surface of the skull.

The intracranial portion of cranial nerves may become neoplastic. **Acoustic neuroma** is a tumor of the Schwann cells of the eighth cranial nerve and is the most common peripheral nerve tumor to occur in the cranium. It can cause deafness or a ringing sound (tinnitus) and can press on other cranial nerves, such as the facial nerve, that are near to the eighth cranial nerve.

There are many other brain tumors, each of them uncommon. Among them, *primary lymphoma of the brain* is becoming more common as a result of the AIDS epidemic (Chapter 8).

Diseases of Peripheral Nerves

The anatomy and connections of the peripheral nervous system were detailed earlier in this chapter in Figure 23-1 and Figure 23-5, and in Chapter 22, and Figure 22-21.

Recall that peripheral nerves are composed of axons of neurons located in the brain or spinal cord, and each axon is sheathed by a layer of myelin formed by Schwann cells. Peripheral nerve disease primarily affects either the axon or the Schwann cell that wraps around the axon.

NEUROPATHIES

A **peripheral neuropathy** is any nonneoplastic disease of peripheral nerve and is a malfunction of one or more nerves—sensory or motor signals are interrupted by disease process that causes weakness, paralysis, numbness, tingling, pain, or other sensation. There are dozens of causes of peripheral neuropathies, too many to list. The most prominent associations are with diabetes, AIDS, renal failure with uremia, lead poisoning, and alcoholism. Peripheral neuropathy also occurs as a paraneoplastic syndrome (Chapter 5) in patients with cancer. It also occurs in association with alcoholism, autoimmune vasculitis, and a variety of inherited diseases.

Diabetic peripheral neuropathy (Chapter 17) is the most common peripheral neuropathy. It mainly affects sensory fibers and is caused by vascular disease in small blood vessels serving the affected nerves. Alcoholics may develop peripheral neuropathy from vitamin or other nutritional deficiency or from lying comatose for a long time in an awkward position that compresses a nerve.

Inflammation and infection are important causes of peripheral nerve disease. **Guillain-Barré syndrome** is an acute autoimmune disease caused by antimyelin antibody. It is usually seen following immunization or infection and can be life threatening because it affects motor function and can lead to respiratory muscle paralysis. The motor weakness begins in the distal limbs and moves rapidly upward to involve respiratory muscles in a matter of days or weeks. Death is uncommon, but it may occur in the absence of prompt clinical recognition and ventilatory support. Slow but full recovery is the rule, but some patients may have residual weakness for years.

The *varicella-zoster virus* (VZV, the chickenpox virus), formerly *herpes zoster*, causes **shingles**, a painful infection of sensory nerves that features clusters of small blisters and scabs. It most often involves the trigeminal (5th cranial) nerve, the main sensory nerve of the face, or nerves of the skin of the chest.

Among the most common peripheral neuropathies is **Bell's palsy**, which affects about 40,000 Americans each year (about the same number as die in auto accidents). Bell's palsy is a paralysis of facial muscles resulting from impairment of the facial (7th cranial) nerve that cannot be attributed to a known cause, such as trauma or tumor compression. The presumptive cause is viral infection of the nerve, leading to swelling of the nerve, which causes compression as the nerve passes through tight channels in the temporal bone near the middle ear. Bell's palsy usually affects mature adults and arises suddenly. Most patients recover within a month or two; others require nearly a year. A few patients may suffer permanent paralysis.

Trauma to peripheral nerves may cause death of the axon and Schwann cells distal to the point of injury; that is, from the site of injury out to the target tissue. Axons and Schwann cells can regenerate, but they regrow very slowly, and axonal reconnection to the target organ is not always effective. Within one week of trauma new nerve axons sprout from the proximal point of injury. If the injury is a clean, complete transaction, and the ends of the separated parts are close together, the sprouting fibers stand a good chance of regrowth and reattachment to the target organ. If the ends are too far separated, the sprouting fibers and scar tissue may accumulate into a nodule, a **traumatic neuroma** (amputation neuroma), which can be quite painful. Women who wear high-heeled shoes are prone to develop traumatic neuroma on the ball of the foot (**Morton neuroma**) from repeated nerve compression.

NEOPLASMS

Tumors of the peripheral nervous system arise from neurons of the autonomic nervous system, or from nerve sheath cells (Schwann cells or fibrocytes that reside in the nerve sheath).

Neurons form two types of peripheral tumors: **ganglioneuroma** (benign) and **neuroblastoma** (malignant) (Chapter 18). Both occur most commonly as tumors of the adrenal medulla or, less commonly, sympathetic ganglia.

Schwannomas arise from Schwann (myelin sheath) cells; **neurofibromas** contain both Schwann cells and nerve sheath fibroblasts. Either type may arise from any nerve. Both are benign, and both occur sporadically in adults. A child with either type or an adult with multiple tumors should be investigated for **von Recklinghausen disease** (neurofibromatosis, Chapter 6) an autosomal dominant inherited condition characterized by multiple neurofibromas (Figure 23-38). About 5% of patients with von Recklinghausen disease develop **neurofibrosarcoma**. Malignant tumors of peripheral nerve are rare; von Recklinghausen disease accounts for half of cases. ■

Right nipple

Peripheral nerves Neurofibromas

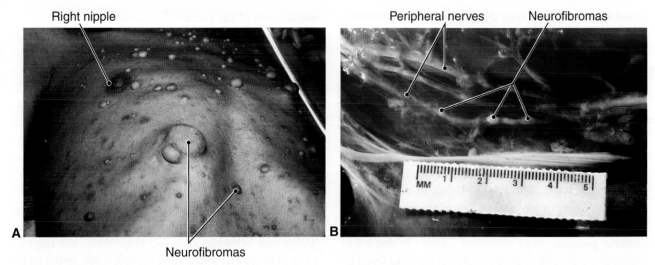

A
B

Neurofibromas

Figure 23-38 **von Recklinghausen disease. A,** Skin of the chest with multiple neurofibromas. **B,** Dissection of forearm showing multiple neurofibromas of peripheral nerves.

CASE STUDY 23-1 "SOMETHING DOESN'T SEEM RIGHT IN MY HEAD"

TOPICS
Stroke

THE CASE
Setting: You are visiting your grandfather, who is hospitalized with a "heart condition" at a large metropolitan medical center. You arrive to find him in good spirits, joking about the need to have his cardiac pacemaker "revved up." The attending physician enters the room and, after the usual pleasantries and limited discussion of the situation, you follow her out the door to ask some question and to ask permission to look at the chart.

Clinical history: You know that your grandfather, 92, comes from a long line of octogenarians and has been in exceptionally good health except for a heart attack in his 60s, after which he gave up smoking and began walking regularly for exercise. Shortly before his 90th birthday he developed atrial fibrillation and was placed on oral medicine to control his heart rate at an acceptable pace and anticoagulant therapy to prevent atrial thrombi (Chapter 12).

His current illness began a few days earlier when he called his physician to report swollen feet. After examination in the physician's office he was hospitalized for congestive heart failure (Chapter 12).

Physical examination and other data: The chart reveals that on admission his vital signs were unremarkable except

irregular, rapid heart rate (96). Chest auscultation revealed a galloping rhythm and crackling rales, suggesting congestive heart failure. The edge of his liver was palpable, and his feet were swollen with 2+ pitting edema (Chapter 4). A chest film showed cardiac enlargement and pulmonary congestion. Laboratory data were normal except for mild elevation of liver enzymes. Cardiac enzymes and troponin (Chapter 12) were normal, indicating no current cardiac muscle damage. An electrocardiogram showed atrial fibrillation. The admission diagnosis was arteriosclerotic heart disease with congestive heart failure and chronic atrial fibrillation.

Clinical course: He was placed on digoxin to slow his heart rate and strengthen cardiac muscle contractions. On the evening of the third hospital day he calls his wife to tell her "something doesn't seem right in my head." You visit the next day and don't see any change apparent in his neurological status; however, about half an hour into the visit you notice he seems to be struggling to find words and is becoming frustrated about it. You help by guessing at the word he is trying to find; once he hears the word he says it and continues with the conversation until it occurs again. You excuse yourself and go to the nursing station and tell the supervisor you think he is aphasic and is having a stroke. The nurse visits the room, agrees with your concern, and calls a resident physician, who quickly confirms the diagnosis of stroke. Over the next few days the language problem gradually improves and the heart failure responds to therapy. He is discharged to home on the seventh day. ▶

[Case 23-1, continued]

The next day he collapses at home and is returned to the hospital. Admission diagnosis is ischemic stroke of the left cerebrum with right hemiplegia (paralysis of one half of the body). He is also completely aphasic (cannot speak) and has difficulty swallowing. He becomes progressively less responsive, then comatose. He dies on the eighth hospital day. You discuss an autopsy with your grandmother, and she consents.

The autopsy reveals a moderately enlarged, dilated heart with large mural thrombi in both atria. There is severe coronary atherosclerosis with marked narrowing of all vessels, but no fresh occlusion. The brain reveals a large fresh, white infarct of the left cerebral hemisphere in tissue supplied by the left middle cerebral artery. Marked cerebral atherosclerosis is present, but no embolus is identifiable. The lungs are congested and edematous, the liver shows moderate chronic passive congestion, and the spleen is congested and enlarged.

DISCUSSION

The underlying problem here was atherosclerosis (Chapter 11). One of the more remarkable facts in the history was that he smoked until he was in his 60s but quit after a heart attack and began exercising and lived nearly 30 more years. Usually nature is not so forgiving, but his long-lived ancestors bequeathed him a wonderful genetic endowment. Chronic myocardial ischemia resulting from coronary atherosclerosis (Chapter 12) eventually produced atrial fibrillation and congestive heart failure. Atrial fibrillation is well known to promote formation of atrial thrombi (Chapter 4). Atrial thrombi are fragile, break apart easily, and embolize. Those in the right atrium embolize to the lungs and are of little consequence because they are small. Those from the left atrium, however, are a different matter. Even a small thrombotic embolus to a cerebral artery can cause a serious, even fatal, ischemic infarct (white stroke), as in this case. That the thrombus was not demonstrable at autopsy is not surprising: it was dissolved by natural thrombolytics in the eight days between the event and death.

The first indication of trouble came from the patient's complaint that "something doesn't seem right in my head." We never learn what it was. The next day he became aphasic, an indication in this right-handed man that he was having a problem in his left cerebral hemisphere, probably in the distribution of the middle cerebral artery, which serves the speech area of the cerebral cortex, a conclusion confirmed by autopsy findings. The initial stroke was small and produced no motor impairment, only aphasia. However, the second stroke was massive and fatal. Both were caused by atrial embolic thrombi.

POINTS TO REMEMBER:
- Complications of atherosclerosis mainly affect the heart and brain.
- One of the consequences of atrial fibrillation is the formation of atrial thrombi.
- Embolic arterial thrombi can cause brain infarction (white stroke).

Objectives Recap

1. *Describe the production, circulation, and absorption of cerebrospinal fluid (CSF)*: CSF is made by the choroid plexus of the lateral (1st and 2nd) and third ventricles. CSF flows downward to the fourth ventricle and exits the ventricular system through openings in the dorsum of the fourth ventricle (the foramina of Luschka and Magendie) into the subarachnoid space, where it bathes the surface of the brain and spinal cord. CSF is resorbed by arachnoid granulations over the cerebral hemispheres.

2. *Explain the meaning of the terms gray matter and white matter*: The cortex and other collections of neuronal cell bodies are gray and are called gray matter. Myelinated nerve fibers are white and are called white matter. In the central nervous system the axons of neurons are gathered to form tracts; in the peripheral nervous system nerves carry incoming and outgoing motor signals.

3. *Name the parenchymal and ancillary cells of the central nervous system (CNS)*: The parenchymal (main functional) cell of the CNS is the neuron. Ancillary cells are astrocytes, which form the structural framework; oligodendrocytes, which contain myelin and wrap the neuronal axons; and microglia, which are the macrophages of the CNS.

4. *Explain why increased intracranial pressure is dangerous, and name a specific anatomic result*: Abnormally high intracranial pressure is dangerous because it can force brain tissue to herniate (protrude) through any available opening in internal membranes or through skull openings. Herniated brain may undergo direct pressure necrosis or may impede vascular flow that results in brain hemorrhage or infarction. One specific example: herniation of cerebellar tissue through the foramen magnum in a patient with massive intracranial hemorrhage.

5. *Compare and contrast the anatomic location, the cause, and the effect of subdural and epidural hematoma*: Subdural hematoma is usually caused

by mild head injury that breaks small venous channels and allows slow accumulation of blood in the subdural space and slow onset of symptoms. An epidural hematoma is usually caused by more severe injury, sufficient to cause skull fracture and tear an epidural artery. Blood accumulates rapidly in the epidural space, and symptoms occur promptly.

6. *Name the cause of most spontaneous subarachnoid hemorrhage*: Berry (saccular) aneurysms are the most common cause of spontaneous subarachnoid hemorrhage.

7. *Explain the anatomic and pathogenic differences between white and red stroke*: White stroke is a bloodless infarct of brain tissue usually caused by arterial ischemia secondary to atherosclerotic blood vessels supplying the brain. Red stroke is spontaneous bleeding into brain tissue and is usually caused by hypertension.

8. *Explain the cause of laminar cortical necrosis*: Laminar cortical necrosis is necrosis of a layer of cells in the cerebral cortex, caused by generalized cerebral hypoxia. When deprived of oxygen, this layer of cells suffers first and most and undergoes necrosis in circumstances that may not cause permanent injury to other brain cells. Global ischemia may produce temporary coma or other neurologic deficit, but laminar cortical necrosis is irreversible and is usually associated with permanent coma or death.

9. *Distinguish between brain concussion and contusion*: A concussion is a period of temporary brain dysfunction following head injury. Concussion is not associated with anatomically demonstrable brain lesions, and radiographic images of the brain are normal. About 10% of concussion victims are rendered unconscious; frequent symptoms include confusion, dizziness, amnesia, nausea, and blurred vision. Contusion is superficial hemorrhage (bruise) in the brain caused by head injury.

10. *Name the cause of most epidemic bacterial meningitis and the population at risk*: The bacterium is *Neisseria meningitidis,* and the population at risk is groups of young adults living in close quarters (as in college dormitories, youth travel groups, or military installations).

11. *Explain the biochemical dysfunction in parkinsonism, and name some of the conditions causing it*: Parkinsonism is caused by motor control abnormalities in the basal ganglia of the midbrain. The affected cells do not transmit signals properly because they do not release normal amounts of the neurotransmitter dopamine. Parkinsonism may be caused by vascular disease, toxins, encephalitis, or repeated head injury, but usually the cause is unknown.

12. *Recite some important facts about Alzheimer disease*: Alzheimer disease causes over half of all cases of adult dementia. It usually occurs in the elderly, and it affects women more often than men. About 1% of people aged 60–64 are affected, but the prevalence rises rapidly with advancing age and affects up to one third of people over the age of 85. The cause is unknown; however, about 10% of cases have familial association.

13. *Name the probable cause of multiple sclerosis*: Multiple sclerosis is probably an autoimmune disease triggered by an as-yet undetected microbe.

14. *Discuss why alcoholics develop chronic brain disease*: Ethanol has plenty of calories and nothing else of nutritional value; as a consequence chronic alcoholics may develop a variety of nervous system disorders resulting from a deficiency of essential nutrients, especially vitamins.

15. *List the most common sources of metastatic brain tumor*: In descending order of frequency: lung, breast, and malignant melanoma of skin.

16. *Explain why it is difficult to completely remove most gliomas surgically*: Most gliomas are difficult to remove completely by surgery because fingers of neoplastic tissue extend microscopically into adjacent normal tissue; excision cannot be done with a wide margin of normal tissue because of the critical need to preserve every possible gram of normal brain.

17. *Name two diseases commonly associated with peripheral neuropathy*: Diabetes mellitus and chronic alcoholism.

18. *Explain how Guillain-Barré syndrome can prove fatal*: If nerves innervating respiratory muscles are severely affected and ventilation is compromised.

Typical Test Questions

1. The primary functional cell of the central nervous system is the:
   A. Axon
   B. Ependymal cell
   C. Neuron
   D. Astrocyte

2. Which one of the following is a pathologic protrusion of brain through the foramen magnum due to increased intracranial pressure?
   A. Cerebellar tonsillar herniation
   B. Subfalcine herniation
   C. Tentorial herniation
   D. Papilledema

3. Which of the following is characteristic of ruptured berry aneurysm?
   A. Subdural hematoma
   B. Subarachnoid hemorrhage
   C. Epidural hematoma
   D. None of the above

4. Which of the following is most likely to cause epidemic bacterial meningitis?
   A. *Neisseria meningitidis*
   B. *Escherichia coli*
   C. *Haemophilus influenzae*
   D. *Streptococcus pneumoniae*

5. Glioblastoma multiforme is a tumor of which of the following cells?
   A. Neurons
   B. Oligodendrocytes
   C. Astrocytes
   D. Microglia

6. True or false? Laminar cortical necrosis is one possible result of generalized brain hypoxia.

7. True or false? White stroke is caused by brain infarction.

8. True or false? Multiple sclerosis is caused by a genetic defect.

9. True or false? Subdural hematoma is usually associated with skull fracture.

10. True or false? The most common form of peripheral neuropathy is caused by diabetes mellitus.

CHAPTER 24

Diseases of the Skin

This chapter begins with a review of the unique language of skin disease, the normal physiology and microanatomy of skin, and the skin's role in body defense. Diseases and disorders discussed include skin conditions, hair loss, eczema, acne, allergies, autoimmune disease, infections and other inflammations, and lesions including malignant melanoma.

BACK TO BASICS
Section 1: Nonneoplastic Diseases of Skin

THE UNIQUENESS OF SKIN DISEASE
GENERAL CONDITIONS OF SKIN
* The Effects of Sunlight
* The Effects of Pregnancy
* Disorders of Hair Growth
THE SKIN IN SYSTEMIC DISEASE
DISEASES OF THE EPIDERMIS
* Disorders of Pigmentation
* Other Diseases of the Epidermis
DISEASES OF THE BASEMENT MEMBRANE ZONE
DISEASES OF THE DERMIS
* Noncontact Dermatitis
* Contact Dermatitis

INFLAMMATORY DISEASES OF SUBCUTICULAR FAT
ACNE
INFECTIONS AND INFESTATIONS
Section 2: Neoplasms of Skin

TUMORS OF THE EPIDERMIS
* Keratoses
* Malignant Tumors of the Epidermis
TUMORS OF SUBEPIDERMAL TISSUE
TUMORS OF MELANOCYTES
* Nevi
* Malignant Melanoma

Learning Objectives

After studying this chapter you should be able to:
1. Differentiate between dermis, epidermis, and subcutis
2. Define eczema, and offer an example
3. List several systemic diseases with important skin findings
4. Explain the pathogenesis of psoriasis
5. Define lichen simplex chronicus
6. Name two characteristics of diseases of the basement membrane zone, and list several diseases
7. Explain the pathogenesis of allergic contact dermatitis, and give an example
8. Explain the pathogenesis of atopic dermatitis, and name one characteristic of susceptible persons
9. Explain how acne vulgaris differs from rosacea
10. Define impetigo
11. Explain the pathogenesis of epidermoid cysts
12. Name the cause of skin warts
13. Name the skin cancer that may originate in a solar keratosis
14. Name the most common skin cancer, and discuss the behavior of skin cancers
15. List several neoplasms or neoplasm-like lesions of the dermis
16. Name the most common benign tumor of melanocytes
17. List several clinical features of malignant melanoma that may be clues to early clinical diagnosis.
18. Explain the importance of accurate microscopic measurements of the thickness of a malignant melanoma

BACK TO BASICS
- epidermis
- basal cell
- melanocyte

GENERAL CONDITIONS OF SKIN
- photoaging
- alopecia

DISEASES OF THE EPIDERMIS
- lentigo
- seborrheic dermatitis
- lichen simplex chronicus

DISEASES OF THE DERMIS
- urticaria
- allergic contact dermatitis
- eczema
- irritant contact dermatitis
- atopic dermatitis

INFLAMMATORY DISEASE OF SUBCUTICULAR FAT
- panniculitis
- erythema nodosum

ACNE
- acne vulgaris

INFECTIONS AND INFESTATIONS
- impetigo

TUMORS OF THE EPIDERMIS
- seborrheic keratosis
- actinic keratoses
- basal cell carcinoma
- squamous cell carcinoma

TUMORS OF MELANOCYTES
- nevus
- malignant melanoma

All the beauty of the world, 'tis but skin deep.

RALPH VENNING (1620–1673), ENGLISH CLERGYMAN, ORTHODOX PARADOXES *(BOOK OF DEVOTIONS)*

BACK TO BASICS

Skin is the largest human organ and our prime defense against the environment. It is, literally, tough as leather; and, yet, it is easily damaged because the surface layer, the epidermis, is only about 0.1 mm thick. Skin thickness varies greatly—it is thinnest around the eyes and genitals and thickest on the back of the chest and on the palms and soles. The skin is also critical in conserving and regulating body fluids and in maintaining body temperature. For example, an early complaint of patients with extensive skin burns is "I'm thirsty" and "I'm cold" because these patients are losing heat and fluid rapidly. The skin is also inhospitable to microbes: the surface layer of epidermis is formed of dead, dry cells that mainly contain an indigestible protein (keratin, the stuff of hair and nails). Finally, the skin is very active immunologically: allergic and immune skin reactions are among the most common afflictions of humankind.

Anatomically normal skin (Figs. 24-1 and 24-2) is composed of two layers—epidermis and dermis—and rests on a bed of subcutaneous fat (the subcutis or panniculus).

The **epidermis** is the surface layer of skin. It is composed of specialized cells, *keratinocytes*, which contain keratin, a stiff protein. The cells of the epidermis are flat and pancake-like and are called squamous cells (from Latin *squama*, for scale). They are layered upon one another like fish scales or the shingles of a roof. The deepest layer is composed of **basal cells** (epidermal stem cells), from which new squamous cells are formed and pushed upward by newer cells forming below. As they rise and mature, epidermal cells flatten and accumulate keratin to form the **stratum corneum**, the layer of dry, dead cells, which are shed imperceptibly every day as they are replaced from below.

The epidermis rests on a **basement membrane**, a thin, acellular film of protein, which separates the epidermis from the dermis below and which plays an important role in skin physiology and disease. The epidermis does not contain blood vessels, nerves, or glands, and it gets its nourishment by diffusion across the basement membrane. In most areas the epidermis is very thin—10–20 cells thick; about 0.1 mm—but it is considerably thicker on the palms and soles because of the extra thickness of the surface layer of dead cells of the stratum corneum.

The epidermis also contains **melanocytes**. These specialized cells, derived from the embryonic nervous system, lie among the basal cells on the basement membrane. They produce melanin pigment and deliver it into nearby basal cells. Skin color is determined by the amount of **melanin** (a dark brown pigment) deposited in basal cells.

Also present among the basal cells of the epidermis are **Langerhan cells**, macrophages from the immune system that capture and present antigen to lymphocytes (Chapter 8).

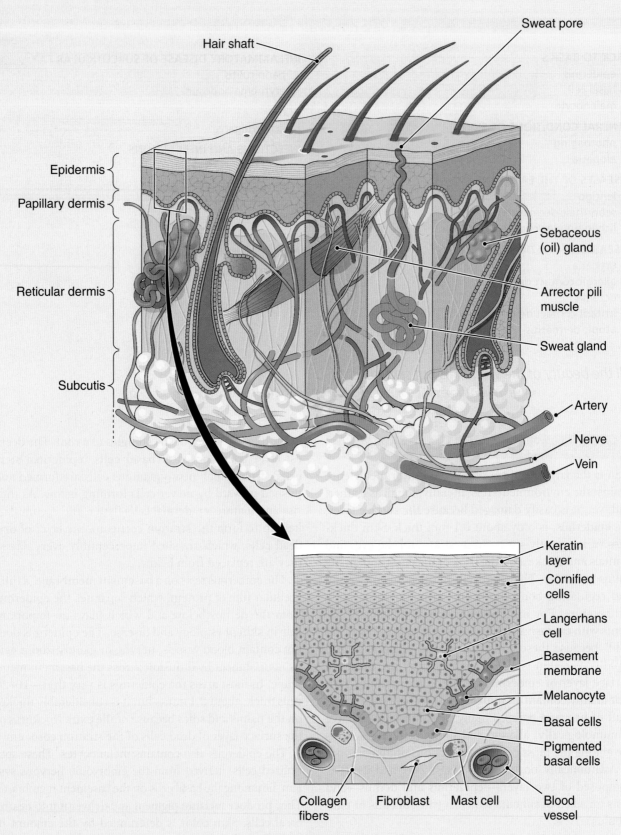

Figure 24-1 **Normal skin.**

Loose keratin (shedding)

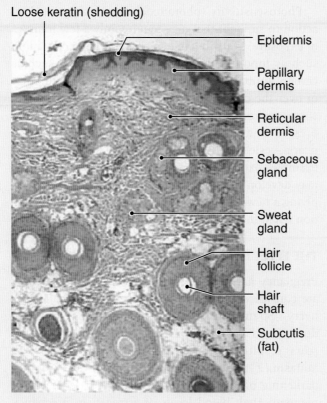

Epidermis

Papillary dermis

Reticular dermis

Sebaceous gland

Sweat gland

Hair follicle

Hair shaft

Subcutis (fat)

Figure 24-2 **Normal skin (low-power photomicrograph).**

The **dermis** is a framework of fibrous and elastic tissue that lies below the basement membrane and is home to nerves, specialized sensory nerve endings, blood vessels, and skin appendages (adnexa), such as sweat and sebaceous glands and hair follicles. The dermis is usually about 1–2 mm thick, which is 10–20× thicker than the epidermis. The superficial dermis is called the **papillary dermis**; it is less dense than the dermis and is the layer most often involved in skin disease. The deepest part of the dermis is the **reticular dermis**, which is dense and is home to hair follicles and skin glands. It is less often involved in skin disease than are other layers of the dermis.

The main cell in the dermis is the fibroblast (or fibrocyte), which produces the collagen and elastin fibers that account for skin toughness and resiliency. Also present in the dermis are dermal dendritic cells, which are similar to epidermal Langerhan cells and have similar immune function. Finally, the dermis is home to specialized sensory nerve endings for pain, touch, heat, and other sensations.

Below the dermis is a pelt of fatty **subcutaneous tissue** (the subcutis), which serves as insulation and cushion and is home to some hair follicles. Below subcutaneous fat is a layer of dense fascia that sheaths the entire body and covers bone, muscle, and other deep structures.

MAJOR DETERMINANTS OF DISEASE

- The skin is more affected by the environment than any other organ.
- Diseases have a tendency to affect particular areas of skin.
- Excessive sun exposure is an important element of many skin diseases.
- Much skin disease is allergic or autoimmune.
- Most skin cancers are very slow growing and are not a threat to life.
- Malignant melanoma is a viciously malignant skin cancer.

Section 1: Nonneoplastic Diseases of Skin

The Uniqueness of Skin Disease

Skin comes into daily contact with countless environmental substances and conditions and is afflicted with more disease than any other organ. About one third of the population of the United States develops a skin condition each year, and skin complaints account for about 10% of annual physician office visits. Many diseases, such as psoriasis, are primary in skin. On the other hand, skin is often secondarily affected by internal dis-

ease; the malar rash of systemic lupus erythematosus (Chapter 8) is an example.

Despite abundance, visibility, and easy access, skin disease is a mystery to many in health care. There are several reasons for this. First, the language of dermatology is peculiar and unfamiliar. Learning a discipline, be it carpentry or pathology, requires learning the specialized language of the field. This is especially true for skin diseases, where words are used regularly that are uncommon elsewhere in medicine—try finding **lichenified** in your average medical textbook index (it is illustrated and defined in Fig. 24-3). But we cannot avoid using clinical dermatologic terms because, for skin disease, gross pathology and clinical description are one and the same. The most common terms are defined and illustrated in Figure 24-3. Second, detailed understanding of skin disease requires a grasp of microscopic pathology, a skill not usually required for clinical practitioners to understand diseases of other organs. There are numerous special terms used in the microscopic pathology of skin disease; they will be used sparingly in this discussion. Finally, the etiology and pathogenesis of many skin diseases are unknown.

General Conditions of Skin

Skin occupies an outsized place of importance in human affairs because it contributes so strongly to appearance, and people care a lot about their appearance. Skin color, uniformity, smoothness, dryness, oiliness, hairiness, and other features are crucial to self-image, so much so that even medically minor skin disease may cause severe patient distress.

THE EFFECTS OF SUNLIGHT

A certain amount of sunlight is necessary for good health—among other things it regulates sleep patterns, and vitamin D metabolism depends on it—but too much can be unhealthy. Most people get the necessary amount of sunlight from normal daily activities. It is, in fact, difficult to *not* get enough sunlight for health, although people experiencing long periods of confinement, such as prolonged hospitalization and imprisonment, may have inadequate exposure. The ultraviolet (short, bluish) wavelengths of sunlight contain higher energy levels than the red, longer wavelengths do, although both can cause acute as well as chronic skin damage. Acute excessive exposure produces sunburn, which is very much like a mild burn produced by a flame. Most **sunburn** results in a first-degree burn (erythema only), but severe exposure can produce second-degree burns (burns with blisters). Chronic sunlight overexposure produces **photoaging**, an excessive wrinkling and sagging.

> *Excessive exposure to sunlight causes premature wrinkling of skin and can ultimately result in skin cancer. Evidence suggests use of protective clothing and sunscreen from childhood into adult life may decrease the incidence of adult skin cancer by 75%.*

Photosensitivity (phototoxicity), an exaggerated reaction to sunlight that may require only a few minutes of exposure, is attributable to an underlying condition, such as lupus erythematosus, to medication, such as certain antibiotics (tetracycline, especially), diuretics, or over-the-counter drugs, or to local use of perfumes, cosmetics, or ointments. Photosensitivity may be expressed as almost any type of skin reaction—as urticaria, vesicles (blisters), or erythema, for instance. For example, patients with systemic lupus erythematosus may develop sunburn in a few minutes, or patients applying a new cosmetic may develop an acute skin reaction when the area is exposed to sunlight.

THE EFFECTS OF PREGNANCY

Pregnancy has effects on skin, some so common they are considered normal. All usually disappear after delivery. "Stretch marks" (*striae*) may appear over the abdomen and breasts, representing superficial dermal scars resulting from the stress of stretched skin. **Melasma** ("the mask of pregnancy") is a temporary darkening of facial skin caused by increased melanin pigment. High blood levels of estrogen in pregnancy can produce *spider angiomas*—small vascular lesions on the face or upper body that have a small, central arteriole and tiny radiating capillary spokes. Pregnancy may also cause mild, temporary hair loss (alopecia) or excess facial or body hair (hirsutism). Each of these conditions fades quickly after delivery.

DISORDERS OF HAIR GROWTH

Fine hairs (*lanugo hairs*) cover the body at birth and are shed quickly and replaced by slightly darker, thicker hairs (*vellus hairs*) that cover the body from childhood onward. *Terminal hairs*, the thick hairs of the scalp and the male face, are usually deeply pigmented. Both vellus and terminal hairs go through a growth cycle, which varies from a few months (eyelashes) to several years (scalp).

The natural life cycle of hair growth has several phases. The growth phase (*anagen phase*) is the longest. It is followed by a very short transitional phase (*catagen phase*) before coming to the final resting phase (*telogen phase*), after which the hair is shed, and the cycle repeats. In the normal scalp about 90% of follicles are in the growth phase, about 1–2% are in the transitional phase, and about 10% are in the resting phase.

Male baldness is a natural consequence of aging that is attributable to the effect of male hormones (androgens), which shortens the growth (anagen) phase of hairs until, ultimately, no hair grows. No inflammation or scarring is

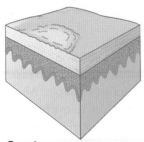

Crust:
A surface collection of dried serum and cell debris (see also Fig. 24-19B)

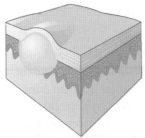

Cyst:
A closed space beneath the epidermis that contains fluid or semisolid material (see also Fig. 24-25)

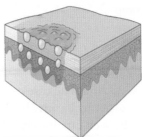

Eczema:
Inflamed, crusted skin with vesicles (see also Fig. 24-18)

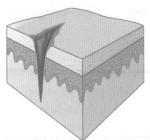

Fissure:
A groove or crack-like lesion

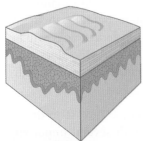

Lichenified:
An area of skin with thickening of epidermis and exaggeration of normal skin lines caused by chronic rubbing or scratching (see also Fig. 24-12)

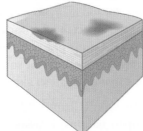

Macule:
A flat, discrete, discolored lesion <1.0 cm (see also Fig. 24-7)

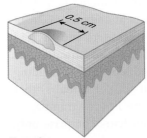

Papule:
A raised, domed superficial lesion <0.5 cm (see also Fig. 24-14)

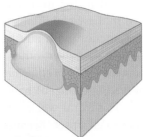

Nodule:
A firm, raised lesion; larger and deeper than a papule (see also Fig. 24-31)

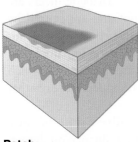

Patch:
A flat, discrete, discolored lesion larger than a macule (see also Fig. 24-9)

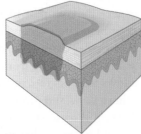

Plaque:
A raised, flat-topped superficial lesion larger than a papule (see also Fig. 24-10)

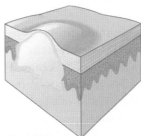

Pustule:
A small superficial abscess

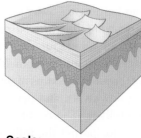

Scale:
A superficial, thin, plate-like flaking off of shedding epidermal cells (see also Fig. 24-10)

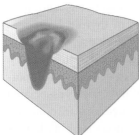

Ulcer:
A cavity not covered by epidermis (see also Fig. 24-5)

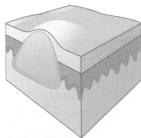

Vesicle/bulla:
A blister filled with fluid; a vesicle is small (<0.5 cm) whereas a bulla is larger (see also Fig. 24-23)

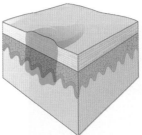

Wheal:
A smooth, slightly elevated lesion that is reddish or pale and usually itchy (see also Fig. 24-17)

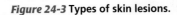

Figure 24-3 Types of skin lesions.

involved. Women, too, naturally experience hair loss as they age, but it begins later and is less severe.

Alopecia is abnormal hair loss. In almost all cases the cause is unknown, but stress seems to be involved. *Alopecia areata* is characterized by well-circumscribed areas of total hair loss, usually on the scalp (Fig. 24-4). *Alopecia totalis* is loss of all scalp hair. *Alopecia universalis* is loss of all body hair, including eyebrows, a condition that affected John D. Rockefeller, Sr., perhaps the richest man in modern world history, whose story is recounted in the nearby History of Medicine box. Hair loss in these conditions is permanent and may occur in conjunction with autoimmune disorders and thyroid disease. However, other types of hair loss are not permanent. *Telogen effluvium* is a sudden, diffuse shedding of resting (telogen) hairs (about 10% of all hairs) that occurs several weeks after severe illness, trauma, or emotional upset. Because telogen hairs comprise only about 10% of scalp hair, and because the loss has usually stopped by the time the patient is examined, the examining clinician usually cannot see much wrong. Much cancer chemotherapy is aimed at interrupting cell growth and can cause temporary hair loss, because one effect of interrupting cancer cell growth is interruption of hair growth. As a consequence roots become thin, and hair breaks away.

Pseudofolliculitis barbae is a common problem in African-American men (and to a lesser extent in African-American women and Anglos), which is caused by the angulated tips of tightly curled shaved hairs turning downward and penetrating the skin to one side of the follicle. The result is an inflammatory papule adjacent to (*para-*) the follicle. It can often be relieved in men by growing a beard.

Hirsutism is the growth of dark, thick hair in women in locations where hair is normally minimal or absent.

Hirsutism is one of the more common consequences of steroid therapy and of adrenal or pituitary disease (Chapter 18); Cushing syndrome is an example. Also, hirsutism is an integral part of polycystic ovary syndrome and certain hormone-secreting ovarian tumors (Chapter 21).

The Skin in Systemic Disease

Many nondermatologic diseases have skin manifestations, far too many to mention here, but it is safe to say that the clinician who knows basic dermatology will be a more astute practitioner than one who does not. Below is a short list of some common systemic conditions that often affect skin:

- *Diabetes* (Chapter 17), a common disease in developed nations, is associated with several important skin conditions that are peculiar to diabetes. Two worthy of specific mention are *Candida* fungal infections of skin, especially of or near the genitals, and diabetic skin ulcers (Fig. 24-5) at pressure points. *Candida* skin infection usually produces a raw, painful, red rash on the genitals or in skin folds around the genitals or buttocks. Diabetic ulcers are especially common in the foot and are caused by poor blood flow secondary to diabetic peripheral microvascular disease (Chapter 17) and impaired pain sensation resulting from diabetic neuropathy, which allows patients to repeatedly traumatize an area that otherwise would prove painful.
- *Thyroid disease* (Chapter 18) affects skin, because thyroid hormone has profound influence on dermal and epidermal cell growth. Overproduction of thyroid hormones is associated with warm, moist, velvety skin, hair loss, changes in finger and toenails, increased skin pigmentation, and waxy translucent plaques over the anterior lower leg (*pretibial myxedema*). Underproduction of thyroid hormones features coarse, yellowish, dry skin; dry, brittle hair; and hair loss (including loss of lateral eyebrow hair).
- *HIV infection* (Chapter 8) is associated with important skin changes. Acute HIV infection is associated with a measles-like rash. Skin infections are common in AIDS, especially virus infections such as herpes simplex and herpes zoster. Kaposi sarcoma (Fig. 24-6) is an AIDS-defining vascular neoplasm of skin caused by a type of herpesvirus that occurs typically as dark red macules, papules, or nodules on the nose, genitals, and extremities. Some AIDS patients may develop severe generalized dermatitis, such as seborrheic dermatitis and psoriasis.

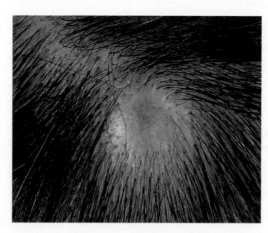

Figure 24-4 **Alopecia areata.**

History of Medicine

JOHN D. ROCKEFELLER, SR.'S HAIR

John D. Rockefeller, Sr., arguably the wealthiest person in world history, lost all of his body hair (*alopecia universalis*) in 1901, when he was 62. Records reveal that he bought bottles of hair restorative in 1886, when he was 47, which could have been related to concern about alopecia or male pattern baldness. In 1893, at age 54, his hair began falling out. During this period he was consumed by worry over finances, not his own—the smoothly oiled machinery of Standard Oil and other enterprises continued to earn prodigious sums—but, paradoxically, he was worried about the finances of charitable enterprises he had endowed. He had fallen into the rich man's trap: the worthy causes he blessed with grants—the University of Chicago among them—were requiring ever grander sums of money. The stress continued throughout the 1890s, and in 1901 his moustache began to fall out; in a few months all his hair was gone—scalp, eyebrows, eyelashes, all of it.

Alopecia universalis is a crushing psychological blow to most who suffer from it—even though it is not connected to other physical ailments—and Rockefeller was no exception. An abstemious Baptist who regarded good health as "a religious duty"—he did not smoke or drink and was famous for his fitness, trim physique, and careful diet—the loss was devastating to him. The change in his appearance was startling; he suddenly looked like a cartoon character, an ogre: shriveled, old, and stooped under the weight of worry about money. For awhile he withdrew from public life. On one occasion he emerged from seclusion to go to a public dinner, one of the few he attended in his life, and seated himself next to Charles Schwab, a friend and president of U.S. Steel. Schwab did not recognize him—Rockefeller had to introduce himself. Later, however, he began to socialize more and sported a wig. He died in his 98th year.

In the 100+ years since Rockefeller's alopecia began, three things remain unchanged: the psychological damage it does to its victims; the absence of a cure; and the scarcity of scientific knowledge about its cause.

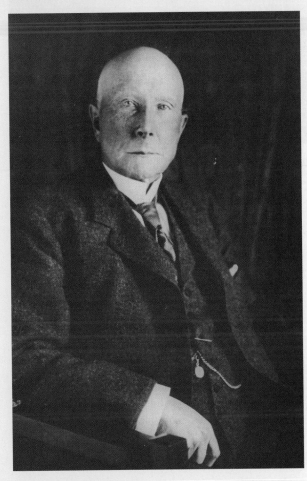

John D. Rockefeller, Sr. This 1904 portrait shows the complete loss of scalp hair, eyebrows, and eyelashes that are characteristic of alopecia universalis. Courtesy of the Rockefeller Archive Center.

- *Blood lipid abnormalities* (Chapter 11) may cause skin *xanthomas*, which are distinctive deposits of lipid. Very high levels of plasma triglyceride (usually above 2,000 mg/dL) may cause *eruptive xanthomas*—dozens of small, yellow-red papules on extensor surfaces (the back of the forearms or the shins) and pressure points such as the elbows, feet, or buttocks. High levels of total plasma cholesterol (usually above 300 mg/dL) may be associated with *nodular xanthomas*—nodular deposits of cholesterol crystals that appear over the elbow, on the palms or soles, or in the Achilles tendon.

High cholesterol levels may also be associated with *xanthelasma*, a flat, bright yellow cholesterol xanthoma in the skin of the eyelids near the nose.

- *Autoimmune disease* (Chapter 8) often produces skin lesions. Patients with systemic lupus erythematosus can be photosensitive and may also have the classic butterfly skin lesion on their cheeks (Fig. 24-7). Skin disease is prominent in systemic sclerosis (scleroderma)—skin progressively becomes waxy, stiff, and shiny, and so tight that the tips of fingers and toes may ulcerate (see Fig. 7-13).

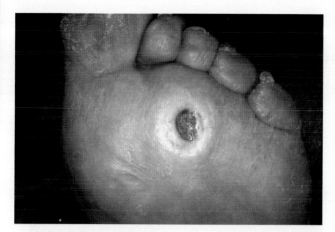

Figure 24-5 **Diabetic ulcer.** Most diabetic ulcers occur at pressure points in the lower extremity.

- *Sarcoidosis* (Chapter 14) is a systemic disease most common in African Americans that features chronic granulomatous inflammation (Chapter 3), chiefly in the lungs and mediastinal lymph nodes. Lesions in skin are small papules that occur mainly around the nose, lips, and eyes.
- *Hematologic diseases* (Chapter 10) that cause low platelet counts (<50,000) can cause tiny skin hemorrhages (petechiae).
- *Neurocutaneous syndromes* are genetic diseases, exemplified by *neurofibromatosis* (Chapter 23), which features clusters of large light brown macules called *café au lait* (coffee with milk) spots. Patients typically also have peripheral nerve tumors that appear as skin nodules (see Fig. 23-42A).

Diseases of the Epidermis

The epidermis is the most often diseased layer of skin because it is in direct contact with the environment. Epidermis contains several types of specialized cells, each of which is subject to certain diseases.

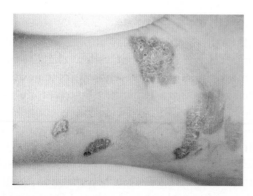

Figure 24-6 **Kaposi sarcoma.** These confluent plaques occurred on the ankle of a patient with AIDS.

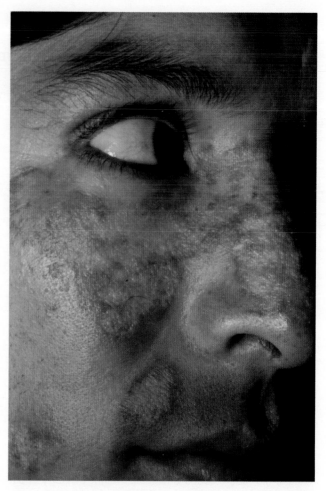

Figure 24-7 **Systemic lupus erythematosus.** Erythematous macules form a butterfly rash on the cheeks and across the bridge of the nose.

DISORDERS OF PIGMENTATION

The most noticeable attribute of skin is its color. The degree of skin pigmentation is perhaps the most important distinguishing and universal attribute of a healthy person, and it has profound social implications in all cultures (see the nearby History of Medicine box). Skin color is shaded from very dark brown-black to light tan in infinitely small increments from one person to the next, depending on the amount of melanin in it.

Melanin is made by melanocytes located in the lower epidermis and is distributed to nearby basal cells of the epidermis, so that most skin pigment is located in the basal cell layer. Pigmentary disorders, therefore, may result from decreased or increased numbers of melanocytes, or greater or lesser melanin production.

> **The color of normal skin is subject to the amount of melanin pigment in it.**

General darkening of the skin may appear as a manifestation of other disease or as a result of drug treatment. In Addison disease (Chapter 18) the adrenals fail and the pituitary secretes large amounts of ACTH in response. Metabolic breakdown of ACTH produces melanocyte-stimulating hormone (MSH), which causes increased melanin production in skin. For example, President John Kennedy's famous tan was not obtained at the beach; Kennedy had Addison disease. Rarely, dark skin is caused by increased levels not of melanin but of other compounds, most notably skin iron deposits associated with hemochromatosis.

Vitiligo (Fig. 24-8) is a common disorder characterized by white macules that may coalesce into large patches of depigmented skin. Melanocytes are absent in affected areas. People of all ages and races are affected. It is seen especially in people with diabetes, Addison disease, thyroiditis, and pernicious anemia and after head trauma. The cause is unknown, but an autoimmune reaction is suspected. **Albinism** is a very rare, genetic lack of melanin pigment owing to an inability of melanocytes to produce melanin pigment. Patients have very white skin and pink eyes (because they lack iris pigment).

A **freckle** (ephelis) is a small macule of increased pigment in basal cells of the epidermis. It is caused by increased sensitivity of melanocytes to sunlight; the number of skin melanocytes is normal. Freckles appear or darken in summer and fade in winter according to sun exposure.

Melasma, a mask of darkened skin or patches of dark skin over the face in pregnant women, is similar to freckling but more generalized. Increased blood estrogen and progesterone make melanocytes more sensitive to the effect of sun exposure. Women who live in sunny climates are especially affected. Melasma fades after the pregnancy ends.

Lentigo (Fig. 24-9) is also characterized by patches of dark skin, but differs from freckles and melasma—lentigo is caused by a localized hyperplasia of melanocytes in skin. Lentigo is not neoplastic. Lesions are usually larger and more deeply pigmented than freckles; and freckles darken with sun exposure, whereas lentigo does not. The common pigmented mole (*nevus*, discussed below) is also composed of a localized collection of melanocytes; however, moles are nodular, and lentigo is macular (flat, nonpalpable).

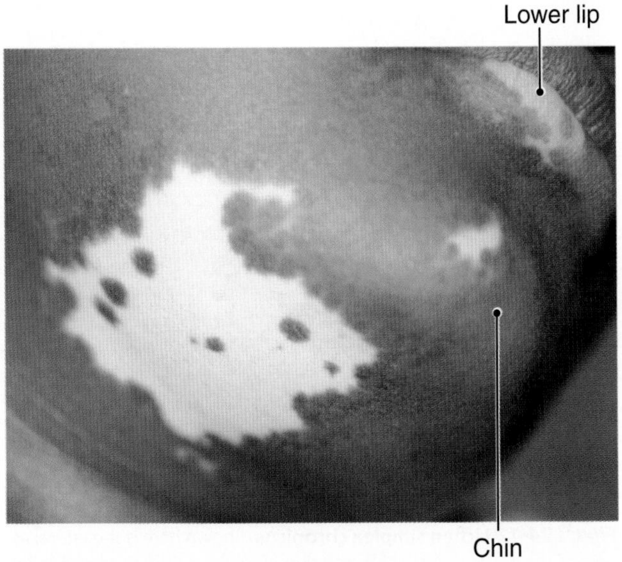

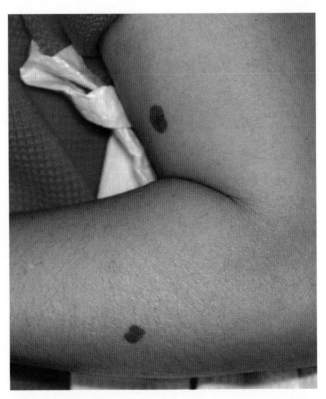

Lower lip

Chin

Figure 24-8 **Vitiligo.** These confluent macules and patches are on the chin and lower lip of an African-American boy.

Figure 24-9 **Lentigo.** The flat, brown patches shown here are typical of the disease.

Postinflammatory pigmentation is local darkening of skin that may follow almost any kind of skin inflammation.

OTHER DISEASES OF THE EPIDERMIS

Psoriasis is an acquired proliferative disease of the epidermis characterized by epidermal hyperplasia that forms salmon-colored, dry, scaly, sharply delineated plaques, illustrated in Figure 24-10. Psoriasis usually appears first in teenagers or young adults. Lesions most often occur bilaterally and with remarkable symmetry on the elbows, knees, and knuckles, but they may spread to involve the low back, scalp, the cleft between the buttocks, glans penis, and nails. The patient's main concern usually is the unsightly nature of the lesions. The cause is unknown, but there is a strong genetic component—one third of patients have a family history of psoriasis. Evidence suggests an autoimmune phenomenon that stimulates excess epidermal growth and is also responsible for the arthritis, enteropathy, myopathy, or other autoimmune phenomena seen in some patients with psoriasis. Skin lesions are treated by methods to slow cell reproduction, such as chemotherapy agents; less severe cases are treated with topical tar compounds or ultraviolet light.

Dandruff is white flakes of dead skin; when accompanied by inflammation the diagnosis is **seborrheic der-**

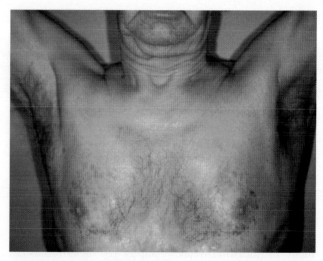

***Figure 24-11* Seborrheic dermatitis.** This severe case is composed of confluent papules and plaques in the oily skin of the chest and axillae. (The face and scalp, not shown, were also involved.)

matitis (Fig. 24-11), a very common dermatitis of oily, hairy skin that typically appears on the scalp, central face, upper anterior chest, and groin as greasy, scaly, red patches. The cause is unknown. Men are more often affected than women are. It may affect newborns (*cradle cap*), children, or adults. For unknown reasons patients with parkinsonism (Chapter 23) may develop severe seborrheic dermatitis; and in HIV-positive patients an outburst of seborrheic dermatitis may be a clue that HIV infection has become serious enough to warrant a diagnosis of AIDS. Dandruff responds well to shampoos that contain selenium or tar.

Lichen simplex chronicus, illustrated in Figure 24-12, is a *pattern* of skin reaction that can occur with al-

Scales

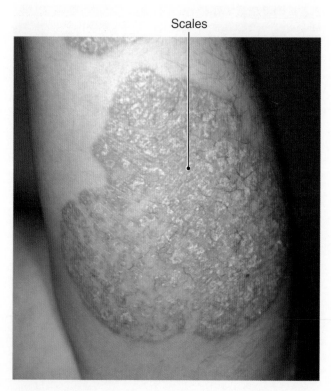

***Figure 24-10* Psoriasis.** The large, erythematous plaque with scales shown here is typical.

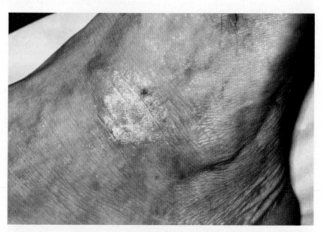

***Figure 24-12* Lichen simplex chronicus.** Shown here is the lateral aspect of the patient's left ankle, the skin of which is thickened and rough from rubbing and scratching subsequent to itching associated with chronic atopic dermatitis.

most any itchy skin disease. It is caused by chronic rubbing or scratching of skin. The result is overgrowth (hyperplasia) of the epidermis, producing thick, rough skin with exaggeration of normal skin lines. The underlying cause usually is an itchy (pruritic) allergic skin disease. Lesions are usually solitary, thick plaques on the back of the neck, scalp, forearm, ankle, inner thigh, or lower leg. It usually occurs in patients with asthma or allergic rhinitis or other atopic disease (type I hypersensitivity reaction, Chapter 8). Treatment is aimed at interrupting the itch-scratch-itch cycle by covering the lesion or by applying topical steroids (see the nearby box, The Clinical Side) or taking antihistamines.

Pemphigus (from Greek *pemphix*, for bubble) is a rare and serious blistering disease caused by an autoimmune antibody attack on the intercellular cement that holds epidermal cells together. People of Mediterranean heritage are at greatest risk. Skin is the primary target, but the oral mucosa may also be affected. As epidermal cells come unglued, fluid accumulates in *intra-epidermal* (above the basement membrane) blisters (small vesicles or large bullae), which rupture to leave weeping, crusted, inflamed patches. Pemphigus usually begins in mature adults and affects the trunk (Fig. 24-13), face, neck, and scalp, sparing the extremities. Skin infection is a frequent complication. Severe cases can be fatal. Systemic steroids and antineoplastic agents are mainstays of treatment.

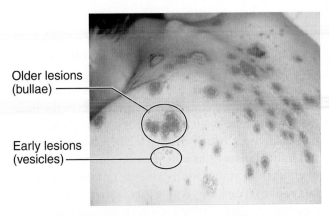

Older lesions (bullae)

Early lesions (vesicles)

Figure 24-13 Pemphigus. Fresh lesions are small, intact vesicles. Older lesions are large, unroofed bullae that are now shallow ulcers.

Diseases of the Basement Membrane Zone

Diseases that affect the basement membrane zone usually form blisters (small vesicles or large bullae) and are often associated with autoimmunity.

Epidermolysis bullosa is a group of rare blistering diseases caused by genetically defective binding of epidermis to dermis at the basement membrane. There are several types of epidermolysis bullosa, all of which are hereditary and share a tendency to blister formation at sites of pressure or minor trauma, usually on the hands and feet. Most varieties of epidermolysis bullosa are cosmetically disturbing but manageable; however, some can be fatal.

Bullous pemphigoid is a chronic blistering disease resulting from an autoimmune autoantibody attack that destroys the basement membrane; fluid seeps into the loosened space to form blisters. It is clinically similar to pemphigus, hence the name *pemphigoid*. Most cases are mild and disappear without therapy, but severe cases may be fatal if not treated. Systemic steroid therapy is effective.

Dermatitis herpetiformis is an autoimmune disease resulting from gluten hypersensitivity. Gluten is a protein found in wheat and other cereal grains that may also cause gluten-sensitive enteropathy (*celiac sprue*, Chapter 15). IgA-gluten immune complexes (Chapter 8) deposit in the superficial dermis and cause acute inflammation, which loosens the attachment of basement membrane and epidermis and allows accumulation of fluid as blisters. Dermatitis herpetiformis appears as a chronic, pruritic (itchy) eruption of papules, clusters of vesicles (which look like herpes, hence *herpetiformis*), and wheals (short-lived, itchy papules and streaks). These lesions gradually appear on the elbows, knees,

THE CLINICAL SIDE

TOPICAL STEROID THERAPY

Topical steroids are very widely used in the treatment of skin disease, and they are divided into classes according to potency: Class I are the most powerful and are synthetic compounds; betamethasone propionate is an example. Class IV are the weakest; hydrocortisone is an example. In any given class there is little other than price to recommend one over the other. Steroid ointment is more potent than steroid cream, but it is oilier and messier. Potency dramatically increases when skin is covered with dressings such as bandages or gloves.

Chronic topical steroid therapy causes skin to become thin and fragile. Elderly persons with thin skin should be advised to be careful and use topical steroids sparingly, and all patients should be so advised when applying steroids to thin skin such as the face, scrotum, or vulva. Although absorption into blood occurs, ill effects, such as diabetes or hypertension, are very rare.

buttock, sacrum, and back of the head in middle-aged adults. Gluten-free diet is effective. Acute episodes can be managed by use of sulfonamide antibiotics (the mechanism is unknown).

Erythema multiforme is an autoimmune reaction in which an antibody attaches directly to cells in the basement membrane zone and destroys them (type II hypersensitivity, Chapter 8). It is a fairly common, acute, self-limited disease, usually seen on the lips and palms of children or young adults as acute eruptions of round target-like red macules with a dark center. About half of cases can be attributed to known environmental agents, the most common of which is herpesvirus infection. However, a long list of drugs and vaccines can also be responsible. When the lesions are more severe and widespread, the condition is called *Stevens-Johnson syndrome*, which is associated with fever. In its most severe form it is characterized by extreme skin damage analogous to an extensive burn and is called *toxic epidermal necrolysis*. Treatment consists of supportive therapy and eliminating or avoiding any known cause.

The skin lesions of **systemic lupus erythematosus (SLE)** have the same pathogenesis as systemic lesions—deposition of circulating antigen-antibody complexes (type 3 hypersensitivity reaction, Chapter 8). Classic skin lesions are merging (confluent), red papules and patches on both cheeks and across the bridge of the nose (the hallmark "butterfly" rash, see Fig. 24-7). Immune complexes are deposited on the basement membrane and typically require exposure to ultraviolet light to cause tissue damage and inflammation.

Chronic cutaneous (discoid) lupus erythematosus is a skin disease with pathogenesis identical to the skin disease of patients with systemic lupus, but in discoid lupus no systemic disease is present. Discoid lupus is confined to sun-exposed skin, especially the face, where the malar "butterfly" rash is typical. Most patients with discoid lupus do not have antinuclear antibody (the characteristic antibody of systemic lupus) in their blood. A small percentage of discoid lupus patients develop systemic lupus after many years.

Lichen planus (Fig. 24-14) is a chronic autoimmune disease of skin or the oral cavity caused by an alteration of epidermal squamous cells on the basement membrane that makes them appear as nonself to the immune system (Chapter 8). Lichen planus in skin is characterized by "the four Ps:" pruritic, purple, polygonal papules on the wrists, ankles, and penis. When it occurs on the oral mucosa, it appears as white patches of leukoplakia (Chapter 15). Lichen planus occurs with greater frequency in patients with other autoimmune diseases such as systemic lupus erythematosus or ulcer-

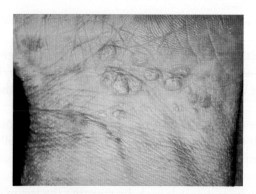

Figure 24-14 **Lichen planus.** These purple, polygonal papules appeared on the volar surface of the patient's wrist.

ative colitis. It usually disappears on its own and rarely deserves therapy.

Diseases of the Dermis

Diseases of the dermis can be divided conveniently into two groups: those caused by contact with an environmental substance, such as an allergen or direct irritant, which is called contact dermatitis, and those not involving contact.

NONCONTACT DERMATITIS

Scleroderma (systemic sclerosis), a chronic systemic autoimmune disease of young women, is characterized by severe fibrosis and tightening of skin (Chapter 8, Fig. 8-12). Raynaud phenomenon (Chapter 12) is almost always present. The gastrointestinal tract, lungs, kidney, heart, and skeletal muscle also may be affected. The normal loose, interwoven character of dermal collagen is replaced by dense bands of collagen that destroy hair follicles and other structures, leaving skin tight and smooth and devoid of hair follicles, sebaceous glands, or sweat glands.

Chronic overexposure to sunlight has an adverse effect on skin; it causes cancers of the epidermis and damages dermal collagen. Microscopically, dermal collagen is fragmented, as if it had been run through a kitchen blender. Too much sun for too long pulverizes the dermis and produces **photoaging** (Fig. 24-15). Skin overexposed to sunlight becomes wrinkled, leathery, and scaly. It is home to premalignant keratoses and carries a marked increased risk for skin cancer. Photoaging is exaggerated by smoking.

Stasis dermatitis accompanies severe varicose veins in the legs. Sluggish blood flow causes local hypoxia and tissue injury, resulting in dermal scarring. Typically, affected skin is swollen, firm, and dark. The epidermis fre-

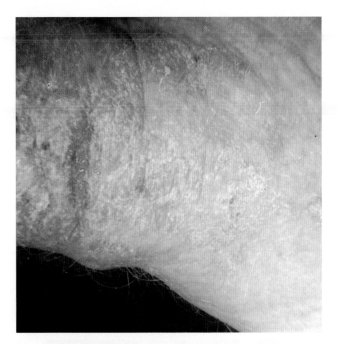

Figure 24-15 **Photoaging.** This wrinkled, leathery, scaly skin is on the dorsum of the right wrist of a farmer.

quently is itchy, red, and scaly. Severe cases may progress to ulceration and infection. Lesions are most notable over the medial ankle and heel (Fig. 24-16).

Granuloma annulare is a disease of the dermis that is characterized by granulomatous inflammatory reaction. The cause is unknown. It presents as annular (circular) red papules, usually on the extremities. It may be generalized in skin, but it is not associated with systemic internal disease. It usually resolves of its own accord in a few months or years.

Urticaria (hives) is a localized, acute allergic reaction (anaphylaxis, type I hypersensitivity, Chapter 8) that causes local vasodilation and increased vascular permeability. The reaction produces short-lived, pale or pink, firm, itchy streaks and papules (Fig. 24-17), which quickly rise and fade in a few hours after exposure to an antigen to which the patient has been previously sensitized. **Angioedema** is similar but affects the deep dermis and subcutis and produces nodular, soft swellings up to several centimeters in diameter. The skin lesions of urticaria or angioedema are usually innocuous, but they can be associated with systemic anaphylaxis that can be life threatening: anaphylactic vascular collapse or asphyxiation from bronchospasm or laryngeal edema. Urticaria and angioedema occur most frequently between the ages of 20 and 40 years. Treatment consists of avoidance of the offending antigen or administration of antihistamines or steroids.

CONTACT DERMATITIS

Contact dermatitis is skin inflammation caused by direct skin contact with some environmental substance. It is a very common skin problem. Given the number of things in daily contact with skin, it is somewhat of a miracle we do not have more of it, but the dry, dead cells in the stratum corneum offer little reactivity. There are two types of contact dermatitis: *allergic* and *irritant*.

Allergic Contact Dermatitis

Allergic contact dermatitis is a delayed-type immune reaction (T-cell–mediated hypersensitivity, Chapter 8) caused by contact with a sensitizing agent. Often the offending agent is a *hapten* (Chapter 8), a small molecule that is not capable of stimulating an immune response unless attached to a large protein molecule. For exam-

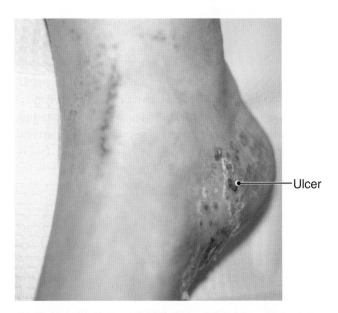

———Ulcer

Figure 24-16 **Chronic stasis dermatitis.** The atrophic, ulcerated skin shown here is on the medial aspect of the ankle of a patient with severe varicose veins (not evident).

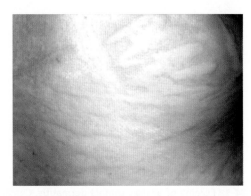

Figure 24-17 **Urticarial wheals.** These pale pink itchy streaks occurred in a patient with allergies.

ple, the sensitizing agent in poison ivy is a hapten. Upon skin contact the hapten attaches to an epidermal protein, which stimulates a T-cell immune reaction. Within a few days sensitized T cells proliferate and travel to the point of contact to incite an inflammatory reaction. The list of sensitizing agents is almost limitless—topical antibiotics, metals (such as nickel or gold in jewelry), cosmetics, nail polish, latex gloves, perfume, chemicals in leather, and so on.

Allergic contact dermatitis is commonly called **eczema** (Fig. 24-18), a clinically useful and widely used description. The word derives from Greek: *ek*—meaning *out*—and *zema*—meaning boiling; hence a boiling out, which provides a vivid indication of the clinical findings in acute eczema—a hot, bubbly skin eruption. *It is important to understand the word eczema is descriptive and is applied to a wide variety of skin diseases* that produce itchy, weepy, crusting, red inflammation, the most common of which is *atopic dermatitis.*

Atopic dermatitis (*atopic eczema, endogenous eczema*), illustrated in Figure 24-19, is a very common dermatitis caused by an immune reaction (type I hypersensitivity, Chapter 8) in genetically susceptible persons. It affects about 5–10% of the United States population, and these people usually have other allergic conditions such as asthma or hay fever. In infants and children atopic dermatitis tends to produce acute, weepy eruptions on the cheeks, scalp, chest, and extensor surfaces. Children often outgrow the disease. In adults the lesions tend to be chronic, less sharply demarcated, dry, and lichenified. Regardless of age, the lesions are usually itchy (pruritic), and symptoms wax and wane with the intensity of the patient's hay fever or other allergies. In adults, atopic dermatitis may be

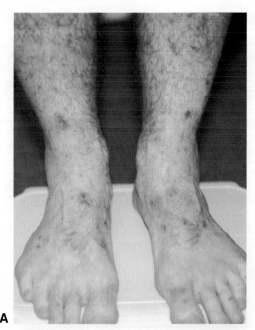

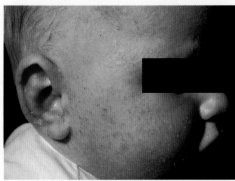

Figure 24-19 **Atopic dermatitis. A,** Chronic atopy: these erythematous plaques and papules appeared on the ankles and feet of an adult. **B,** Acute atopic eczema in a child: the lesions are crusted, maculopapular, and confluent.

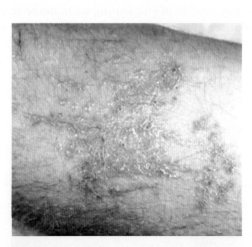

Figure 24-18 **Eczema of allergic contact dermatitis.** Contact with poison ivy has produced a weeping, crusted, erythematous collection of vesicles and papules.

worse in winter months, when the air is dry; however, usually no precipitating agent can be identified. Topical antihistamines and steroids are mainstays of treatment.

Nummular dermatitis is a clinical variant (a pattern) of eczema that occurs as one or more coin-like (nummular) patches. It is not a disease, per se, but merely the clinical appearance of a skin condition.

Irritant Contact Dermatitis

Irritant contact dermatitis is caused by the direct toxic effect certain chemicals exert upon contact with the skin—no allergy is involved. Common offenders include soaps, solvents, acids, and alkalis found in the home and workplace. The lesions are itchy red, scaly papules and patches, but affected skin tends to be dry, not weepy, because vesicles are less common than in allergic contact dermatitis. The irritant effect of the offending chemical is aggravated by friction or rubbing—"dishpan hands" is one example. "Diaper rash" is another, which is caused by chafing diapers, soaps, and prolonged exposure to the wet environment of urine and feces. Treatment is by avoidance of the offending substance and by topical therapy with steroids and soothing ointments.

Inflammatory Diseases of Subcuticular Fat

The fatty layer beneath skin is called subcuticular fat or *panniculus*, a term derived from Hebrew *pannus* for bed or covering. **Panniculitis** is inflammation of subcutaneous fat. The most common form of panniculitis is **erythema nodosum**, an acute disease characterized by red, tender nodules of chronic inflammation and fibrosis in the subcuticular fat on the anterior aspect of the legs. It is most common in young adult women and most often occurs 1) in patients with infections (such as streptococcal infections or tuberculosis), 2) in patients taking certain drugs (sulfonamide antibiotics, oral contraceptives), or 3) in patients with certain illnesses (sarcoidosis, inflammatory bowel disease, and some malignancies); however, in many instances no associated condition is identifiable. Biopsy may be required for diagnosis.

Widespread panniculitis, known as *Weber-Christian disease*, is characterized by skin nodules, fever, fatigue, nausea, vomiting, weight loss, and joint pain. It is often associated with other conditions such as pancreatitis, pancreatic carcinoma, infections, or autoimmune disorders. Sometimes Weber-Christian disease appears as a paraneoplastic syndrome (Chapter 6) associated with an undiagnosed (hidden, occult) visceral cancer.

Acne

Acne is a self-limited inflammatory disorder of hair follicles and associated sebaceous glands. It primarily affects adolescents and is characterized by red papules and pustules that can lead to unsightly scars. There are several types of acne—by far the most common is *acne vulgaris* (adolescent acne), which is the most common skin disease in the United States.

Acne vulgaris (Fig. 24-20) is a disorder of teenagers, but it may persist into adulthood. It is mainly a disease of Caucasians, has a strong genetic component, and begins when hair follicles become plugged by epidermal cells as they are shed daily. The

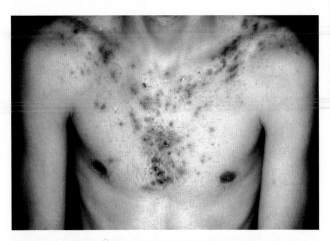

***Figure 24-20* Acne vulgaris.** The confluent (merged), erythematous papules, patches, and pustules shown here occurred on the chest of a teenager.

plugged follicle fills with oily sebaceous gland secretions (sebum) to form a noninflammatory plug called a *comedo*. There are two types of comedos—*whiteheads*, pores that have small, tight openings, and *blackheads*, pores that have large openings, revealing a surface layer of dark, oxidized melanin (not dirt). Oily skin produces more and larger comedos, which are hospitable to growth of *Propionibacterium acnes*, a bacterium that metabolizes sebum and causes rupture of the comedo and an inflammatory reaction in the surrounding skin. The exact cause of the inflammation is unclear. It may be caused by a direct irritant effect of sebum and keratin; or it may be an immune reaction to *P. acnes*; or it may result directly from *P. acnes* infection. The result is collections of red papules and pustules over the face and upper chest and back. Treatment is complex and primarily topical, although oral antibiotics may be useful in severe cases.

Postadolescent acne may arise in adult women, but it seldom occurs in men. Its appearance is related to hormone fluctuations associated with the monthly menstrual cycle. It is less severe than acne vulgaris and is less associated with comedo formation. Lesions appear and disappear quickly as red papules or pustules on the face. When men are affected the lesions usually appear on the chest and back and are longer lasting.

Rosacea (formerly *acne rosacea*) is an inflammatory disorder of hair follicles and sebaceous glands that is frequently mistaken for acne. However, it is confined mainly to fair-skinned women aged 30–50 of northern European descent; it is not associated with comedos, and it has no relationship to hormonal status. Lesions are red papules and pustules on the face, which are not severe enough to cause scarring. Rosacea may be induced by sun exposure or chronic steroid therapy, but the cause is usually unknown. Treatment is topical, but oral antibiotics may prove useful in difficult cases.

Infections and Infestations

Impetigo (Fig. 24-21) is a common, highly contagious, superficial skin infection common in preschoolers. Staphylococcus and streptococcus are the usual infective organisms. Impetigo appears first as transient, small vesicles that quickly unroof to form erythematous patches that are "honey-crusted" with dried exudate. It is usually asymptomatic and heals without scarring in a few weeks, even without treatment. Systemic infection and complications are rare. Topical therapy and systemic antibiotics are standard treatment.

Erysipelas (Fig. 24-22) is a superficial skin infection usually caused by *Staphylococcus pyogenes* or certain

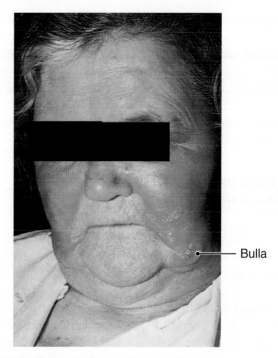

Bulla

Figure 24-22 **Erysipelas.** This patient has large, confluent erythematous plaques. A bulla is present near the angle of her jaw.

types of streptococci. The initial lesion is small, but it soon blossoms into a bright red, intensely painful, swollen area on the leg or face that may feature small blisters. As infection spreads to the lymphatic system it causes fever, malaise, and enlarged, tender local lymph nodes.

Dermatophytosis is a common superficial skin, hair, and nail infection caused by a group of fungi that metabolize keratin. Dermatophytosis includes "athlete's foot," "jock itch," and "ringworm" of the scalp. The infectious agents are *Tinea* species fungi that have evolved an ability to digest keratin in the dead surface cells of the cornified layer of the epidermis, and in nails and hair. Positive diagnosis requires microscopic identification of fungi in scrapings from infected skin (see the nearby box, The Clinical Side). Infections respond well to topical antifungals with the exception of nail infections, which may be difficult to eradicate even with prolonged oral antifungal drug therapy if the infection has spread deep under the nail.

Herpesvirus infection causes common cold sores and genital infections (Chapter 8). **Cold sores** (Fig. 24-23) are painful eruptions of vesicles at the oral mucocutaneous border (where lip mucosa meets lip skin). Typically they are induced by stress, excess sun exposure, or dry, cold air.

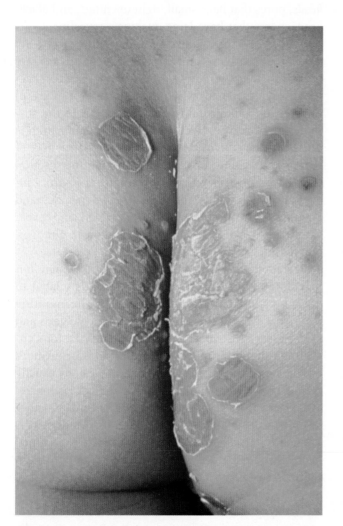

Figure 24-21 **Impetigo.** The confluent erythematous patches of denuded vesicles (small) and bullae (large) have crusted rims.

THE CLINICAL SIDE

THE POTASSIUM HYDROXIDE (KOH) TEST FOR DERMATOPHYTES (SKIN FUNGI)

The KOH test consists of microscopic examination of hair, skin, or nail scrapings after treating the scraping with KOH, which dissolves skin cells and debris, leaving only fungi, if they are present.

Skin specimens are collected by scraping at the active edge of the lesion. Nail scrapings are best obtained from beneath the nail edge with a curette or blade. Hair and associated scale are best obtained with a toothbrush.

A thin layer of specimen is placed on a glass slide. A small drop of KOH is added and covered by a glass coverslip. The KOH is heated by a small flame (a match will do) until bubbling begins.

The preparation is examined microscopically for fungi. In experienced hands it is very accurate.

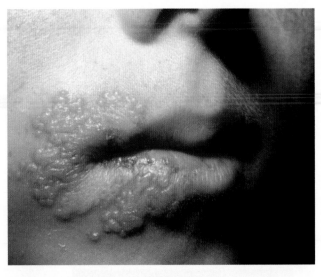

Figure 24-23 **Cold sores (oral herpesvirus).** This patient has an unusually large crop of confluent vesicles.

Section 2: *Neoplasms of Skin*

Skin neoplasms are classified according to the tissue or cells from which they arise:

- *Epidermis*, which includes keratoses, epidermoid cysts, and basal and squamous carcinoma
- *Dermis*, which includes tumors of sebaceous and sweat glands and other adnexal structures; and tumors of subcuticular tissues, which includes lipoma (a tumor of fat), dermatofibroma (a tumor of fibrous tissue), hemangioma (a tumor of blood vessels), and neurofibroma (a tumor of nerves)
- *Immune system* cells in skin, which includes tumors of Langerhans cells, lymphocytes, and others
- *Melanocytes*, the pigment-producing cells of skin, which includes nevi and malignant melanoma

Tumors of the Epidermis

Two of the the most common skin growths are not actually neoplasms, but are tumors only in the broadest sense of the word—that is to say, they are masses. **Skin tags** (Fig. 24-24) are innocent polypoid growths usually a few millimeters in size, but sometimes they may be up to a centimeter or more. They have a simple core of blood vessels and fibrous tissue covered by unremark-

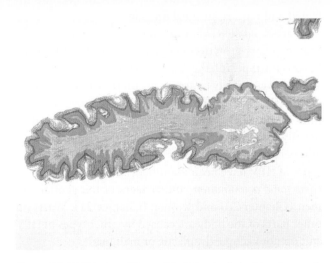

Figure 24-24 **Skin tag (fibroepithelial polyp).** In this microscopic study, both the covering epidermis (which is unremarkable) and the fibrous core are visible.

able epidermis. They are often seen in the body folds of obese persons. Skin tags are not associated with other conditions and rarely deserve treatment except for cosmetic purposes or if they become irritated. **Epidermoid cysts** (*wens*) are not true neoplasms: they form from occluded hair follicles or trapped pieces of epidermis that

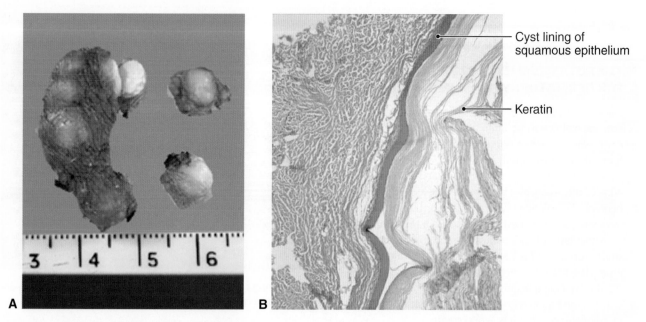

A

B

Cyst lining of
squamous epithelium

Keratin

Figure 24-25 **Epidermoid cysts. A,** The multilobulated large cyst (left) has been opened to expose white, keratinaceous contents. **B,** In this microscopic study, the cyst's unremarkable epidermal lining is visible, as is its content of dead cells shed from the lining.

continue to grow as trapped masses of new squamous cells—they enlarge like a slowly growing tumor as they fill with keratin debris (Fig. 24-25). Epidermoid cysts are innocuous and, like lipomas, are usually removed for cosmetic reasons; however, they can become infected and require surgical drainage.

Warts (*common skin wart, verruca vulgaris*) are common papillary growths of epidermis (Fig. 24-26) caused by certain types of the human papillomavirus (HPV). Warts are especially common in children and in patients with AIDS or other immunodeficiency. They are transmitted by casual skin-to-skin contact. In children they usually disappear spontaneously, but in adults they usually persist and may be difficult to eradicate. Over 100 types of HPV have been identified, some of which cause *condyloma acuminatum*, and cancers of the genitalia in men (Chapter 20) and women (Chapter 21). Warts on other parts of the body are caused by other types of HPV and do not become dysplastic or malignant.

KERATOSES

Seborrheic keratosis (Fig. 24-27) is a very common lesion that usually appears in people over age 40. It is a pigmented, superficial, velvety, dry overgrowth of epidermal cells with a thick, loose layer of surface keratin. It is but one of many pigmented skin lesions (freckle, lentigo, nevus, malignant melanoma, and others). The cause is unknown; unlike most other keratoses, seborrheic keratosis is not premalignant, and it does not deserve treatment except for cosmetic improvement.

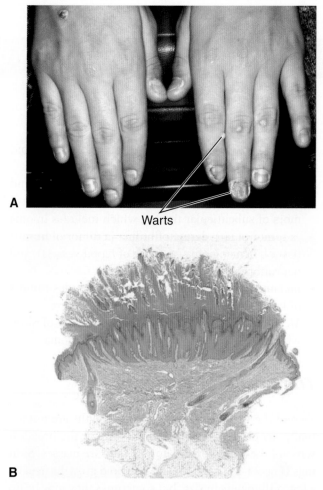

A

Warts

B

Figure 24-26 **Verrucae vulgaris (warts). A,** The multiple papules shown here occurred on the hands of a child. **B,** The microscopic study shows a markedly hyperplastic, jagged overgrowth of epidermis.

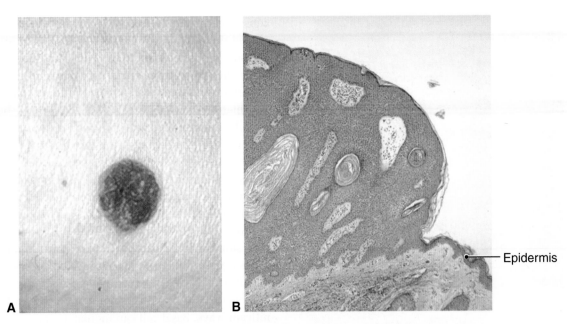

Figure 24-27 **Seborrheic keratosis. A,** This plaque is brown, dry, uniformly pigmented, sharply demarcated, and smoothly outlined. **B,** The microscopic study shows a superficial proliferation of basal cells with small cysts of keratin.

Because seborrheic keratoses are usually deeply pigmented, they must be distinguished from malignant melanoma, another dark skin lesion that can be highly malignant. Some key differences are:

- Seborrheic keratosis is brown but usually not as dark as malignant melanoma, which is often nearly black or contains areas that are deep black
- Seborrheic keratosis tends to have a uniform color, whereas malignant melanoma often varies: deep black in some areas, brown or pink in others
- Seborrheic keratosis has a rough, dull, medium-to-dark brown surface and relatively uniform edges; malignant melanoma is usually smooth and glossy and has areas that are nearly pitch black, with irregular borders, and sometimes with small satellite pigmented spots.

Actinic keratosis (from Greek *aktin* for ray; also known as *solar keratosis*) (Fig. 24-28) is very common and is a forerunner of squamous carcinoma of skin—for practical purposes it can be considered squamous carcinoma in situ. It occurs as a small (<1 cm) discrete, rough, scaly patch or plaque in sun-exposed skin, especially on the face, back of the hand, and back of the neck. Actinic keratosis is especially common in people with lightly pigmented skin; people with deeply pigmented skin rarely are affected. Actinic keratosis often, but not necessarily, progresses to invasive squamous

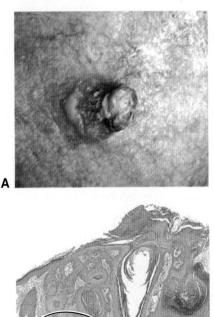

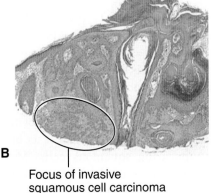

Focus of invasive
squamous cell carcinoma

Figure 24-28 **Actinic (solar) keratosis. A,** The nodule is capped by a thick layer of keratin, while the adjacent skin shows a marked photoaging effect. **B,** This microscopic study shows epidermal hyperplasia with a thick cap of keratin. In the base of the lesion is a focus of invasive squamous cell carcinoma.

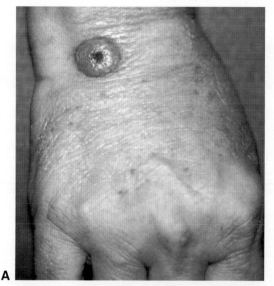

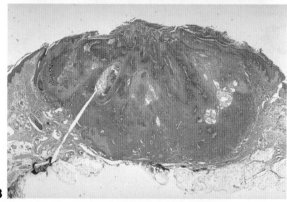

Figure 24-29 **Keratoacanthoma. A,** This rapidly growing nodule appeared on the sun-exposed dorsum of the wrist. Note its volcano-like appearance. **B,** The microscopic study shows hyperplasia of the epidermis and a central core of keratin.

carcinoma. It can be removed safely by simple superficial methods such as curettage, lasering, topical chemotherapy, or freezing.

Keratoacanthoma (Fig. 24-29) is a rapidly growing squamous tumor of sun-exposed skin that can be very alarming. The cause is unknown, but sun exposure is important, and there is a debate about whether or not it is malignant. Keratoacanthoma appears suddenly on sun-exposed skin and grows rapidly as a solitary nodule. The typical lesion is volcano-like, with a central crater plugged with keratin, which rests on a base of malignant-appearing squamous cells. Most regress without therapy; however, those who view them as malignant treat them by excision.

MALIGNANT TUMORS OF THE EPIDERMIS

Malignancies of the epidermal cells are the most common of all cancers, but they so rarely metastasize and

cause death that cancer statistics do not usually included them. There are two types: basal cell carcinoma and squamous cell carcinoma. They have much in common: they arise from epidermis, occur principally in sun-exposed skin, grow slowly, are locally aggressive, and metastasize only rarely. If treated early, both are usually inconsequential. However, neglected lesions near critical structures such as the nose, eyes, or ears can cause significant local problems. Also, keep in mind that squamous cell carcinomas of other organs, such as the lung, are much, much more aggressive than are squamous cell carcinomas of skin.

Basal cell carcinoma (Fig. 24-30) is the most common skin cancer, especially in persons with fair skin. It arises from primitive basal cells located deep in the dermis near the basement membrane. Basal cell carcinoma differs clinically from squamous carcinoma in four significant ways. Basal cell carcinoma:

- rarely appears on the back of the hand
- may occur in skin not exposed to intense sunlight
- may occur as a feature in some genetic disease syndromes

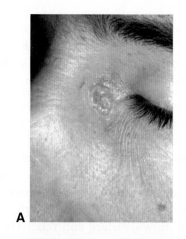

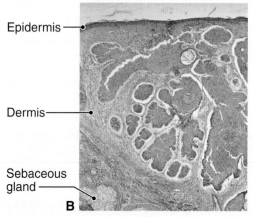

Epidermis

Dermis

Sebaceous gland

Figure 24-30 **Basal cell carcinoma. A,** The pearly plaque/nodule has raised, rolled edges. **B,** The microscopic study shows masses of small, dark basal cells invading the dermis.

• very rarely metastasizes (squamous carcinoma rarely metastasizes, but it does so more often than basal cell carcinoma does)

Microscopically, basal cell carcinoma is composed of groups of round basal cells that contain no keratin, a contrast to squamous carcinoma. Clinically, basal cell carcinoma appears as a pearly, semitransparent, shiny papule or nodule that has a raised, rolled margin and tiny blood vessels arrayed across the surface. Local, complete excision or destruction is curative.

> ⚷ *Basal cell carcinoma is the most common and the least aggressive cancer of skin.*

Squamous cell carcinoma is a malignant tumor of keratinizing epidermal cells that mature toward squamous cells. It is the second most common skin cancer. It usually arises from a preexisting actinic keratosis (see Fig. 24-28) in sun-exposed skin of older persons. Squamous cell carcinomas appear as scaly or ulcerated papules or plaques, or as nodular, hard, cornified nodules that grow slowly. Local destruction or excision is curative.

Tumors of Subepidermal Tissue

Beneath the epidermis are the dermis (which contains fibrous tissue, immune cells, blood vessels, and nerves), subcuticular fat, and skin appendages such as hair follicles, sebaceous glands, and sweat glands. Any of these tissues can become neoplastic.

Most of these neoplasms are *benign*, and they include the following:

• **Lipomas** are tumors of fat cells. They are rubbery, yellow, greasy, moveable subcutaneous masses in the subcuticular fat. They are not premalignant and are clinically distinctive enough not to warrant biopsy except under unusual circumstances.
• **Dermatofibromas** (Fig. 24-31) are innocuous fibrous tumors that appear as small, brownish, sharply outlined, hard dermal nodules. They occur on the legs, arms, and trunk, and they are most common in women over age 20. Treatment is not necessary.
• **Keloids** (Chapter 4, Fig. 4-8) are nodular masses of exaggerated scar tissue that far exceed the degree of injury and the expected repair response. They occur in genetically susceptible persons, usually of African heritage. A common site is the earlobe after piercing.
• **Angiomas** (or **hemangiomas**, Fig. 24-32) are abnormal collections of blood vessels. Some are composed

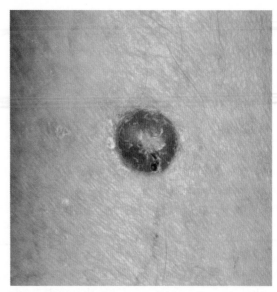

Figure 24-31 Dermatofibroma. The lesion in this patient is typical: a firm, sharply outlined reddish-brown nodule.

of small vessels (*capillary* hemangioma) and others of larger, thin-walled vessels (*venous* hemangioma). *Pyogenic granuloma* (Chapter 4) is an abnormal nodule of blood vessels that occurs in wound repair and for all practical purposes is identical to a hemangioma. Angiomas can occur anywhere in the body, but they are especially common in dermis, where

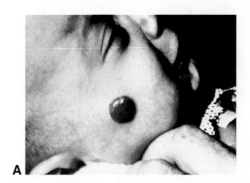
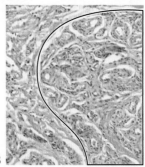

Figure 24-32 Angioma (hemangioma). A, The nodule on the cheek is a compact mass of blood vessels. **B,** A microscopic study shows an otherwise unremarkable mass of small blood vessels.

they appear as small, reddish nodules or flat patches of discolored skin that vary from a few millimeters to several centimeters. It is not clear if angiomas are neoplasms or congenital anomalies; but it rarely matters because almost all are innocuous.

• **Telangiectasis** (Fig. 24-33) is a collection of superficial blood vessels that is less compact and nodular than an angioma. Telangiectasis can be thought of as a local collection of dilated blood vessels that is seen most often in sun-exposed skin. Some, called *spider angiomas*, have a small central vessel with "legs" that radiate outward in spoke-like fashion; they are usually found in association with female hormone excess associated with oral contraceptives, pregnancy, and liver failure (Chapter 16).

• **Nevus flammeus** (port wine stain) is a common congenital, red or purple patch on the neck, scalp, or face that is composed of small, dilated dermal blood vessels. Some fade with time; others can be treated effectively with lasers.

• **Adenomas** of sweat or sebaceous glands and hair follicles are benign growths of specialized glandular ep-ithelium and are uncommon. Most appear as an unremarkable, smooth, tan, small skin nodule.

• **Neurofibromas** are benign tumors of peripheral nerves usually seen in the dermis of patients with von Recklinghausen neurofibromatosis (Chapter 23).

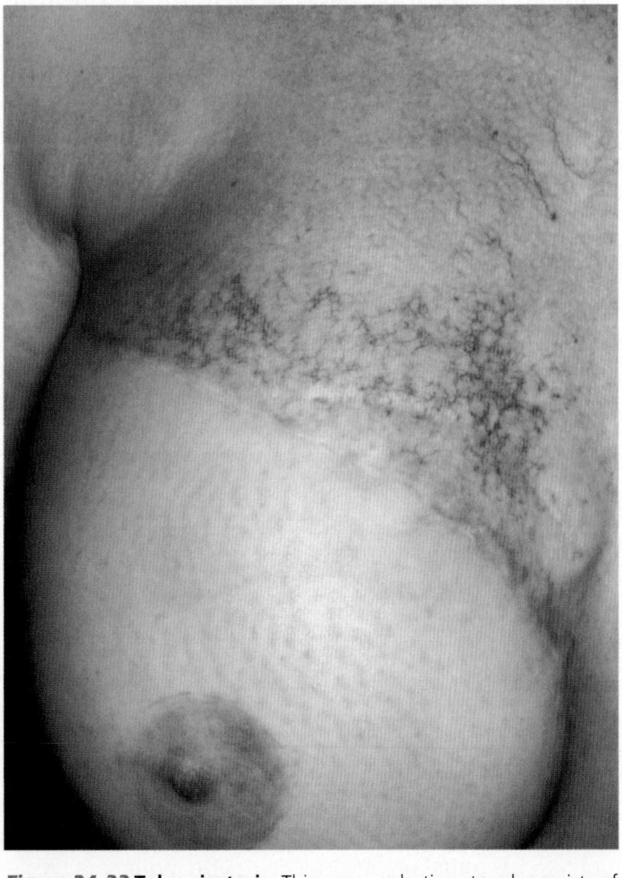

However, some dermal neoplasms are *malignant*, and they include the following:

• **Immune cell neoplasms** can arise from Langerhans cells (special skin macrophages) and T cells. *Histiocytosis X* (Chapter 11) is a sluggishly malignant disease of Langerhans cells; *mycosis fungoides* is T-cell lymphoma of skin. Lymphomas of any type can originate elsewhere and involve the skin secondarily.

• **Kaposi sarcoma** (see Fig. 24-6) is a malignant tumor of vascular endothelial cells caused by a certain type of herpesvirus. It is especially prevalent in people with an immunodeficiency, most notably patients with AIDS (Chapter 8). Before the AIDS epidemic, Kaposi sarcoma was seen, rarely, as a tumor in the skin of the lower legs of elderly men; however, it is much more common now because of the AIDS epidemic. The two groups at highest risk are male homosexuals and intravenous drug users. Kaposi can metastasize widely.

Tumors of Melanocytes

Melanocytes, the pigment-producing cell of the epidermis, are derived from the embryonic nervous system. Tumors of melanocytes are discussed separately from other skin tumors because their behavior is so distinctively different: virtually all deaths from skin malignancy are caused by malignant tumors of melanocytes. Two types of melanocyte tumors occur: the common mole, known scientifically as *nevus*, which is benign, and *malignant melanoma* (also known simply as melanoma).

NEVI

Nevi (Fig. 24-34) are benign tumors of melanocytes, the pigment-producing cells of the epidermis. Nevi are common and usually begin appearing before age 20. They arise as a brown papule about 1 mm in diameter and slowly enlarge and become darker. They usually stop growing when they reach about 5 mm in diameter, and after many years they tend to become pale and flat. In most people the number of nevi gradually declines with age. They are most common in persons with white skin who were exposed to significant amounts of sunlight in childhood. People with deeply pigmented skin rarely develop nevi. A clear relationship exists between the

Figure 24-33 **Telangiectasis.** This nonneoplastic network consists of dilated superficial blood vessels. Most telangiectases occur in sun-exposed skin.

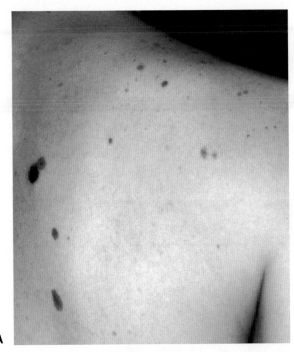

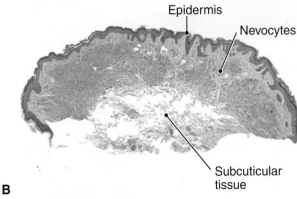

Figure 24-34 **Moles (nevi). A,** The multiple pigmented small (papules) and large (plaques) lesions shown here appeared on the patient's back. **B,** In this microscopic study, nevus cells (benign melanocytes) are evident in the dermis.

amount of sun exposure, the development of nevi, and the development of malignant melanoma. As a rule, a person with a large number of nevi (many dozens, for example) is more likely to develop malignant melanoma than a person with a few nevi; however, because nevi are so common the risk is very small that that any given nevus will become malignant.

A **dysplastic nevus** is a distinctive clinical lesion worthy of note because of its relationship to malignant melanoma. Dysplastic nevi are usually larger (up to 15 mm) than a common nevus and are surrounded by a slowly enlarging collar of irregularly pigmented skin. Dysplastic nevi are controversial because it is debatable how much alarm should be attached to each individual one. However, this much seems clear: people with large

numbers of dysplastic nevi are at a much greater risk of developing malignant melanoma than people with one or two dysplastic nevi. Patients with multiple dysplastic nevi and a family history of malignant melanoma may have a genetic condition, *heritable melanoma syndrome*, which is associated with a very high risk for malignant melanoma. These people should have their skin examined by a dermatologist every year.

All nevi are important, not because they may become malignant but because they must be differentiated from malignant melanoma. Sometimes a malignant melanoma can masquerade clinically and microscopically as an ordinary nevus and escape detection until it has passed the point of being curable.

MALIGNANT MELANOMA

Malignant melanoma (or *melanoma*) is a malignant neoplasm of melanocytes. It is by far the most dangerous skin cancer and the most common malignancy of any kind occurring in women ages 25–29, and it is the subject of Case Study 24-1 at the end of this chapter. The great majority of melanomas arise in skin, but some develop on mucosal surfaces of the vagina, oral cavity, and anus, and others in the eye or the meninges, each of which normally contain melanocytes. These diverse sites seem odd until one recalls that melanocytes are neuroectodermal cells, having common ancestry with nerves. Like squamous carcinomas of skin, malignant melanomas occur most often on sun-exposed skin, and light-skinned persons are more at risk than those with darker skin are. About half of melanomas arise spontaneously, and another half arise from preexisting nevi (common moles), a fact worthy of special note: one of the most important signs of early melanoma is change in the appearance of a common mole. However, moles are so common that there is little risk of an individual nevus becoming malignant.

> ☞ *Malignant melanoma is by far the most dangerous skin cancer.*

The typical malignant melanoma is a pigmented plaque about 1 cm in diameter with irregular borders and varying degrees of pigmentation (Fig. 24-35); for example, some melanomas may have areas of very dark tissue and others of light tan or pink, unpigmented tissue. Figure 24-36 illustrates the growth of a melanoma, which begins as a proliferation of melanocytes in the basal cell layer of the epidermis near the basement membrane. This initial malignant stage is melanoma in situ—growth is confined to the epidermis and has not broken through the basement membrane to invade the dermis,

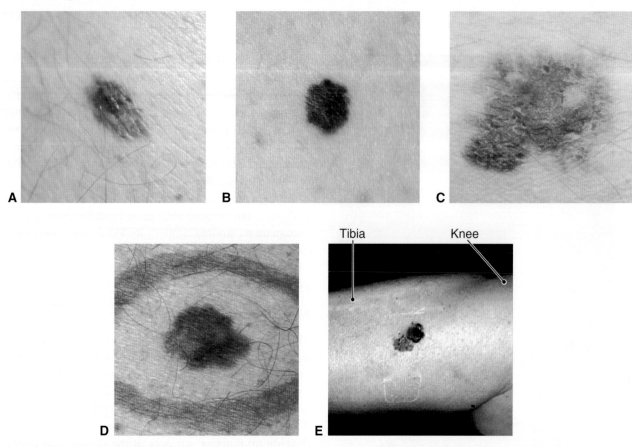

Figure 24-35 Malignant melanomas. Important clues in each of these lesions are as follows: **A,** The irregular border of the lesion and the variation of pigmentation. **B,** The deep black pigmentation and the irregular border. **C,** The very irregular border and the variation of pigmentation. **D,** The pinkish area and the irregular border. **E,** The large size, pinkish area, variation of pigmentation, and irregular border of this neglected lesion on the lower leg.

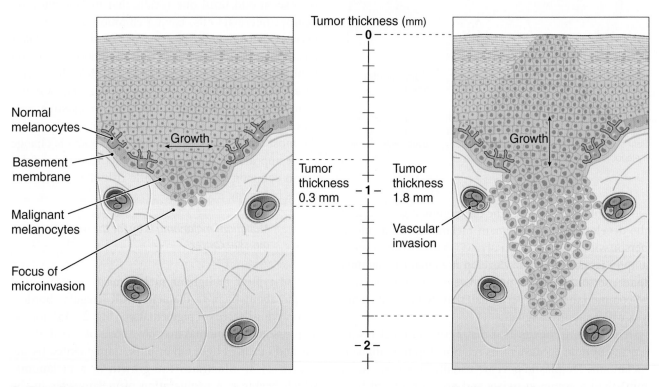

Figure 24-36 Growth of malignant melanoma. A, Superficial spreading phase. Initially, malignant melanoma spreads outward in a radial fashion as an in situ malignancy before penetrating the basement membrane. **B,** Nodular malignant melanoma. Later, the tumor becomes nodular and grows vertically into the dermis.

where it can gain access to blood vessels and lymphatics. After penetrating the basement membrane it invades the upper few tenths of a millimeter of superficial dermis (microinvasion) and spreads outward in the *radial growth phase* called **superficial spreading melanoma**. In the radial growth stage melanoma rarely metastasizes. However, with time the tumor enters the *vertical growth phase* and becomes much more dangerous, as it penetrates deeper into the dermis and becomes nodular (**nodular malignant melanoma**), shown in Figure 24-37.

The metastatic potential of any given melanoma can be estimated by careful microscopic measurements of the tumor, a process known as *microstaging*, which de-

pends on measurements, made to the tenth of a millimeter, of dermal invasion. Microstaging is a reliable guide to prognosis and therapy. For example, the ten-year survival rate with tumors that have less than 1.0 mm of dermal invasion is about 90%; for dermal invasion over 3 mm, ten-year survival is about 30%. At whatever depth, the survival rate for women is somewhat better than for men.

The most important clinical features of melanoma to look for are:

- Rapid enlargement of an existing pigmented lesion
- A nodule in an otherwise flat pigmented skin lesion
- Itching or pain in a previously asymptomatic pigmented lesion
- Development of a new pigmented lesion in adult life
- Irregular borders of a pigmented lesion
- Satellite areas of pigmentation around a pigmented lesion
- Varied coloration in a pigmented lesion, especially spots of pink or gray decoloration or spots that are much blacker than the rest of the lesion
- If a pigmented lesion looks suspicious, it warrants excisional biopsy—the entire lesion should be excised, because excision may prove curative. This also allows evaluation of the entire lesion and avoids disturbing the tumor by cutting directly into it.

Melanomas spread by lymphatic and vascular invasion. One of the most fearsome features about melanoma is its tendency for vascular invasion while still small. Vascular metastases usually appear first in the brain and lungs. Lymphatic metastases also occur but are not as dangerous. The medical community and general public have become better informed about melanoma; lesions are detected earlier and survival rates have improved substantially. ■

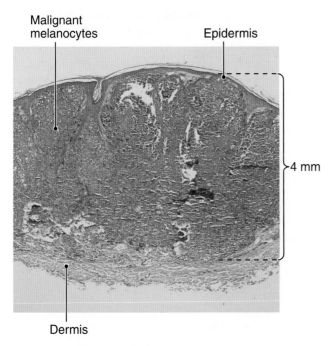

Figure 24-37 **Nodular melanoma.** The tumor has invaded the dermis and is 4 mm thick.

CASE STUDY 24-1 *"SHE FRIES EASIER THAN BACON"*

TOPIC
Malignant melanoma

THE CASE
Setting: After several years of working in a physician's office you are doing a post-graduate year of study in dermatology in a large academic medical center. One day you are

assisting a pathology resident with logging and gross description of skin biopsy specimens, and you recognize the name of a former undergraduate classmate on the requisition slip accompanying the specimen.

Clinical history: The patient is a 29-year-old woman, whom you know to have striking red hair and fair skin. You recall her at picnics and other student outings as always seeking the shade or wearing a big floppy hat and long sleeves because, as her husband, also a student, said, "She fries ▶

[Case 24-1, continued] easier than bacon." The abbreviated history accompanying the biopsy says only "Pigmented lesion from upper back; suture marks superior tip."

Physical examination and other data: The pathology resident dictates the following description of the specimen: *"The specimen is an ellipse of pale skin 3.5 x 2.5 x 0.5 cm. In the center is a roughly circular lesion 1.2 cm in diameter. The periphery is flat and unevenly pigmented—some areas nearly black, others light tan. In the center is a small, irregular, raised lesion about 0.5 cm in diameter; some is pink, shiny and smooth, the remainder black."* The resident slices the entire specimen in bread-loaf fashion and submits it for microscopic study, the pieces numbered sequentially beginning with the suture-tagged end.

You tell the resident that you are acquainted with the patient and her husband, and he asks you to get her chart from medical records, which reveals unremarkable medical history and regular annual physical examinations for the last three years by an internist on the medical staff.

The next day you review the slides on a dual-head microscope and listen as the resident dictates preliminary microscopic findings and diagnosis for later authentication by the senior pathology staff: *"The main lesion is a nodular mass of melanocytes with considerable variation of nuclear size and shape. Occasional mitotic figures are present and many cells have a large, eosinophilic nucleolus. Spreading outward from the main mass are clusters of atypical melanocytes at the dermal-epidermal junction. Tumor extends deep into the dermis. Maximum tumor thickness is 3.9 mm. No lymphatic or vascular invasion is present. The margins of resection are free of neoplasm."* The final diagnosis is: *"Nodular malignant melanoma, maximum tumor thickness 3.9 mm."*

Clinical course: You attend a case review session several weeks later with pathology, surgery, dermatology, and oncology staff. Careful physical examination and multiple imaging studies show no enlarged lymph nodes or other evidence of metastasis.

The conference team recommends 1) wider excision of the original site to ensure a broad margin of normal-appearing tissue around the lesion, 2) further careful evalua-

tion to identify other similar lesions on her body, 3) chemotherapy, and 4) melanoma vaccine therapy. The patient is found to have dozens of moles at various locations. Four of these prove to be dysplastic nevi and are excised. Each shows melanocytic atypia, but there is no evidence of advancement to malignant melanoma. Further detailed medical history reveals that the first lesion was noticed by her husband, also a healthcare professional, after he attended a lecture on clinical recognition of early melanoma. Family history establishes that the patient had an uncle who died of malignant melanoma. Despite careful scrutiny and appropriate therapy, she died of metastatic melanoma 3 years later.

DISCUSSION

This patient clearly has **heritable melanoma syndrome**: multiple moles, dysplastic moles, and family history of malignant melanoma.

The "missing link" in this case is the primary care internist who had ample opportunity (three annual routine physical examinations) to find this lesion but didn't. *Inspection and assessment of all moles and pigmented lesions is an essential part of every history and physical examination.* Close inspection of the skin of white patients at the time of first visit is a vital part of responsible patient care, as essential as measuring blood pressure—initial diagnosis (or suspicion) of melanoma is in the hands of primary caregivers. Look for large (>1 cm) dark brown lesions with irregular borders and variegated pigmentation and keep in mind the mnemonic: **MMRISK**, which stands for:

- **M**oles: many common moles
- **M**oles: dysplastic or unusual moles
- **R**ed hair or freckles
- **I**nability to tan
- **S**unburns, especially as a child
- **K**indred: family history of melanoma

POINTS TO REMEMBER

- Inspection and assessment of all moles and pigmented lesions is an essential part of every history and physical examination.

CASE STUDY 24-1 *THE ROAD NOT TAKEN—AN ALTERNATIVE SCENARIO*

For all sad words of tongue or pen,
The saddest are these: "It might have been."
JOHN GREENLEAF WHITTIER (1807–1892),
AMERICAN QUAKER POET AND REFORMER, *MAUD MULLER*

THE CASE

With a bit of imagination, we can speculate how this case might have had a happier ending.

Setting: You are enrolled as a graduate student in a school of allied health sciences. In one of your clinical lectures a professor makes extended remarks about the frequency of skin disease, the ease of skin examination, and the peculiarities of the language of skin disease. She recommends that all students pay more attention to skin disease because it offers plentiful clues to other diseases and is an easy way ▶

[Case 24-1, continued] to become an expert in an aspect of medicine that students often disregard or is not emphasized in the curriculum.

Taking her advice to heart, you buy a used color atlas of dermatology and begin carrying it with you on your various clinical rotations. Soon you learn the truth of your instructor's advice and become the "go to" consultant among your classmates when they have patients with skin conditions.

Clinical history: At a class picnic celebrating your class's upcoming graduation, you share a table with a classmate and his wife. The weather is hot and sunny, and soon the conversation turns to her fair skin, red hair, and tendency to sunburn. You recall something you learned recently about dysplastic nevi and malignant melanoma. One remark leads to another and your classmate's wife invites you to look at some skin lesions on back, arms, and upper chest.

Physical examination and other data: She has multiple nevi, one of which on her upper back is much larger than the others; you estimate it to be about 15 mm in diameter. The center is raised and darker than the surrounding lesion and has somewhat irregular borders.

Clinical course: You discuss with her and her husband your concern that the lesion could be a dysplastic nevus and recommend that a dermatologist should examine it and the rest of her skin.

A few weeks later at a party after graduation, you see her and her husband and learn that the dermatologist excised the lesion on her back and several others. All was dysplastic nevi, but none was malignant. She was instructed to have annual dermatologic examinations.

Objectives Recap

1. *Differentiate between dermis, epidermis, and subcutis*: Epidermis is the surface squamous epithelium of skin; dermis is the fibrocollagenous layer of skin beneath the epidermis, which is separated from epidermis by the basement membrane and contains skin appendages such as sweat glands and hair follicles; subcutis is the layer of fat immediately beneath the dermis.

2. *Define eczema, and offer an example*: Eczema is dermatitis expressed as itchy, papulovesicular, oozing, crusted lesions. The most common type of eczema is allergic contact dermatitis; poison ivy, for example.

3. *List several systemic diseases with important skin findings*: Systemic lupus erythematosus, systemic sclerosis, AIDS, hyperthyroidism and hypothyroidism, hyperlipemia, diabetes, and neurofibromatosis.

4. *Explain the pathogenesis of psoriasis*: Psoriasis is caused by an over-proliferation of epidermal cells in genetically inclined persons. It is probably an autoimmune disease.

5. *Define lichen simplex chronicus*: It is a common pattern of skin reaction caused by chronic rubbing or scratching of skin affected by disease, usually allergic dermatitis, which stimulates epidermal growth and produces thick, rough skin with exaggerated normal skin lines.

6. *Name two characteristics of diseases of the basement membrane zone, and list several diseases*: Disease of the basement membrane zone usually produce vesicles or bullae, and most are autoimmune. Some diseases are epidermolysis bullosa, bullous pemphigoid, dermatitis herpetiformis, erythema multiforme, lupus erythematosus, and lichen planus.

7. *Explain the pathogenesis of allergic contact dermatitis, and give an example*: It is a type 4 delayed hypersensitivity (T-cell) reaction. The rash of poison ivy, which occurs a few days after skin contact with the plant, is an example.

8. *Explain the pathogenesis of atopic dermatitis, and name one characteristic of susceptible persons*: Atopic dermatitis is a very common allergic skin disease caused by type 1 (anaphylaxis), IgE dependent hypersensitivity reaction occurring in people with other allergic conditions such as hay fever or asthma.

9. *Explain how acne vulgaris differs from rosacea*: Acne vulgaris is a disease of teenagers with oily skin and comedos that lead to scarring. Rosacea is a disease most often found in fair-skinned women aged 30–50 of Northern European descent, and it usually does not cause scarring.

10. *Define impetigo*: Impetigo is a common superficial skin infection that forms pustules. It occurs most often in infants or children; usually caused by *Staphylococcus* or *Streptococcus* infection.

11. *Explain the pathogenesis of epidermoid cysts*: Epidermoid cysts are formed of epidermis trapped beneath the surface, often in association with a hair follicle; the cells continue to proliferate and produce a cyst filled with keratin debris.

12. *Name the cause of skin warts*: Infection by human papillomavirus.

13. *Name the skin cancer that may originate in a solar keratosis*: Squamous carcinoma.

14. *Name the most common skin cancer, and discuss the behavior of skin cancers*: Basal cell carcinoma is the most common skin cancer: The great majority of skin cancers are basal or squamous cell carcinoma. They almost never metastasize or cause death of the patient. Malignant melanoma, however, is highly malignant and frequently metastasizes and causes death.

15. *List several neoplasms or neoplasm-like lesions of the dermis*: Lipoma, dermatofibroma, angioma, xanthoma, keloid, Kaposi sarcoma, skin appendage tumors.

16. *Name the most common benign tumor of melanocytes*: Nevus (melanocytic nevus).

17. *List several clinical features of malignant melanoma that may be clues to early clinical diagnosis*: The most important clinical feature to look for is a change in the color or pigmentation of a preexisting pigmented lesion (for example, areas of increasing or decreasing pigmentation). Other warning signs are: enlargement of an existing pigmented lesion, a nodule in an otherwise flat pigmented lesion, itching or pain in a previously silent pigmented lesion, development of a new pigmented lesion in adult life, irregular borders, satellite areas of pigmentation, and varied coloration, especially areas of pink or gray discoloration or unusually dense black coloration.

18. *Explain the importance of accurate microscopic measurements of the thickness of a malignant melanoma*: Tumor thickness (depth of invasion) is a good guide to therapy and is closely correlated with survival.

Typical Test Questions

1. Which of the following is an epidermal stem cell?
   A. Keratinocyte
   B. Mast cell
   C. Basal cell
   D. Melanocyte
   E. None of the above

2. Which of the following is especially associated with pregnancy?
   A. Melasma
   B. Lentigo
   C. Ephelis
   D. Vitiligo
   E. None of the above

3. The pathogenesis of psoriasis is which one of the following?
   A. Allergic reaction to a hapten
   B. Reaction to a chemical irritant
   C. Epidermal over-proliferation
   D. Gene defect
   E. None of the above

4. Lichen simplex chronicus is caused by which one of the following?
   A. Genetic defect
   B. Autoimmunity
   C. Chronic rubbing or scratching
   D. Sun exposure
   E. None of the above

5. Which of the following is the most common malignancy of skin?
   A. Malignant melanoma
   B. Basal cell carcinoma
   C. Melanocytic nevus
   D. Squamous carcinoma
   E. None of the above

6. True or False? A papule is a small, solid, raised lesion less than 0.5 cm in diameter.

7. True or False? People exposed to relatively large amounts of sunlight in childhood are more likely to develop nevi.

8. True or False? Rosacea is most common is adolescent females.

9. True or False? Seborrheic keratoses are premalignant.

10. True or False? The underlying immune reaction is the same in systemic lupus and cutaneous discoid lupus.

Diseases of the Eye and Ear

This chapter begins with a review of the normal eye and the optics and physiology of vision, as well as the normal ear and the physiology of hearing and balance. Eye diseases and disorders discussed include refractive disorders, infections, cataract, glaucoma, chorioretinitis, and neoplasms. Ear diseases and disorders include acute otitis media, deafness, and vertigo.

Section 1: Diseases of the Eye

BACK TO BASICS
• The Anterior Segment
• The Posterior Segment
DISORDERS OF ALIGNMENT AND MOVEMENT
DISORDERS OF REFRACTION
DISORDERS OF THE ORBIT
DISORDERS OF THE EYELID, CONJUNCTIVA, SCLERA, AND
    LACRIMAL APPARATUS
DISORDERS OF THE CORNEA
CATARACT
DISORDERS OF THE UVEAL TRACT

DISORDERS OF THE RETINA AND VITREOUS HUMOR
DISORDERS OF THE OPTIC NERVE
GLAUCOMA
NEOPLASMS

Section 2: Diseases of the Ear

BACK TO BASICS
DISORDERS OF THE EXTERNAL EAR
DISORDERS OF THE MIDDLE EAR
DISORDERS OF THE INNER EAR
DEAFNESS

Learning Objectives

After studying this chapter you should be able to:
1. Describe the anterior and posterior segments of the globe and the anterior and posterior chambers of the anterior segment.
2. Trace the flow of aqueous humor
3. Name the layers of the posterior segment of the globe from the interior outward
4. Explain the cause of myopia, hyperopia, and presbyopia
5. Distinguish between blepharitis and conjunctivitis
6. Define keratitis
7. Explain keratoconus
8. Define cataract
9. Name the components of the uveal tract and several causes of uveitis
10. Explain the causes of retinal detachment
11. Name the two most common causes of retinal vascular disease
12. Explain the effect of age-related macular degeneration and why it is an important disease
13. Define papilledema, and explain its importance
14. Discuss the relationship of intraocular pressure to glaucoma
15. Distinguish between primary open-angle glaucoma and primary closed-angle glaucoma
16. Name the three anatomic divisions of the ear, and explain the hearing function of each
17. Characterize otitis media by the age of most patients, pathogenesis, and cause of inflammation
18. Name the three general categories of hearing loss

Key Terms and Concepts

DISEASES OF THE EYE

BACK TO BASICS
- anterior segment
- posterior segment
- anterior chamber
- posterior chamber
- macula
- uveal tract

DISORDERS OF REFRACTION
- myopia
- presbyopia
- hyperopia

DISORDERS OF THE ORBIT
- proptosis

DISORDERS OF THE CORNEA
- keratitis
- keratoconus

CATARACT
- cataract

DISORDERS OF THE UVEAL TRACT
- uveitis

DISORDERS OF THE RETINA
- hypertensive retinopathy
- diabetic retinopathy
- age-related macular degeneration

DISORDERS OF THE OPTIC NERVE
- papilledema

GLAUCOMA
- glaucoma

DISEASES OF THE EAR

BACK TO BASICS
- tympanic membrane
- tympanic cavity
- semicircular canals
- eustachian tube

DISORDERS OF THE MIDDLE EAR
- acute otitis media
- otosclerosis

Section 1: Diseases of the Eye

None so blind as those that will not see.

MATTHEW HENRY (1662–1714), NONCONFORMIST ENGLISH CLERGYMAN,

WHOSE MOST FAMOUS QUOTATION IS "BETTER LATE THAN NEVER."

BACK TO BASICS

The eye (Fig. 25-1) and related structures occupy a bony socket in the skull, the **orbit**, and are protected by cranial bone on all sides except anteriorly where the eyeball (the **globe**) is protected by the **eyelids** and by a film of fluid (tears).

The eyeball occupies most of the space in the orbit; however, in addition to the globe the orbit also contains:

- The external muscles of the eye: six small skeletal muscles that move the globe.
- The nasolacrimal apparatus, which consists of the lacrimal glands, one in the upper-outer edge of each orbit, which secrete tears, and the associated tear drainage ducts.
- Nerves, blood vessels, fat, loose fibrous tissue, and interstitial fluid.

The **eyelids** (palpebrae) are flaps of tissue covered externally by skin and lined internally by mucosa, called the **conjunctiva**, which is lined by a layer of epithelial cells and contains numerous mucous-secreting cells. The conjunctival mucosa extends deep under the eyelid where it connects with the outer covering of the eyeball, the **sclera**, a tough, fibrous membrane that anteriorly is the white of the eye. The epithelial cells of the sclera continue across front of the eye to cover the **cornea**—the anterior, domed, clear part of the globe—where they become flat (squamous) and clear to admit light.

The lids also contain other structures:

- The **tarsal plate**, a band of stiff, fibrous tissue that is especially dense along the lid edge and maintains the structure of the lid
- Fibers of skeletal muscle that move the lids (blinking)
- Eyelashes and hair follicles and their sebaceous glands

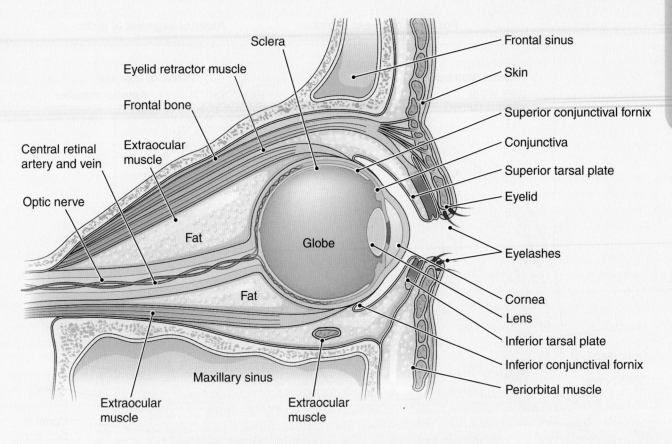

Sclera

Eyelid retractor muscle

Frontal bone

Extraocular muscle

Central retinal artery and vein

Optic nerve

Fat

Globe

Fat

Maxillary sinus

Extraocular muscle

Extraocular muscle

Frontal sinus

Skin

Superior conjunctival fornix

Conjunctiva

Superior tarsal plate

Eyelid

Eyelashes

Cornea

Lens

Inferior tarsal plate

Inferior conjunctival fornix

Periorbital muscle

Figure 25-1 **The orbit and its contents.** A sagittal section is shown here.

The *nasolacrimal apparatus* consists of the **lacrimal glands** and ducts and keeps the eye bathed in **tears** produced by lacrimal glands, one under the upper lateral edge of each orbit. Tears cross the eye to drain through tiny pores in the nasal margin of the upper and lower eyelids into short ducts that lead to a **lacrimal sac** in the wall of the nose. From there tears drain into the nose via the **nasolacrimal duct**.

The *globe* (Fig. 25-2) is divided by the posterior edge of the lens (the clear, round, pillow-shaped focusing organ) into the *anterior segment*, consisting of the lens and everything in front of it, and the *posterior segment*, which lies in back of the lens.

THE ANTERIOR SEGMENT

The **anterior segment**, illustrated in Figure 25-3, consists of the cornea, iris, lens, and related spaces and structures. The anterior segment is divided into two compartments: the **anterior chamber**, a fluid-filled space that lies behind the cornea and in front of the iris, and the **posterior chamber**, which lies behind the iris and in front of the lens. Note that the posterior chamber is in *front* of the lens. Light passing into the eye travels across the following structures and spaces, in order, before falling on the light-sensing layer (retina) at the

back of the eye: the cornea, anterior chamber, pupil, posterior chamber, lens, and vitreous humor (the fluid that fills the posterior segment).

The **cornea** is the domed, clear (it lacks blood vessels and lymphatics) anterior part of the eye, which has much more light-bending (focusing) power than the lens does. The cornea is covered by squamous epithelium that is an extension of the conjunctiva. Beneath this epithelium, the stroma of the lens is composed of fine, precisely aligned collagen fibers, which enhance transparency.

Encircling the anterior segment along its outer edge is the **ciliary body**, a highly vascular, doughnut-shaped organ to which the iris and lens are attached. The **iris** is a thin, pigmented membrane between the cornea and lens with a central opening (the **pupil**), which reacts to light and other stimuli by becoming larger or smaller to admit more or less light. The **lens** sits immediately behind the iris and is a flattened sphere attached by **suspensory ligaments** to a circular muscle, the **ciliary muscle**, which tugs on the suspensory ligaments and adjusts the thickness of the lens to focus on far or near objects.

The ciliary body secretes **aqueous humor**, a clear, watery fluid, into the posterior chamber. The aqueous humor flows out of the posterior chamber through the pupil and into the anterior chamber (Fig. 25-3). It then

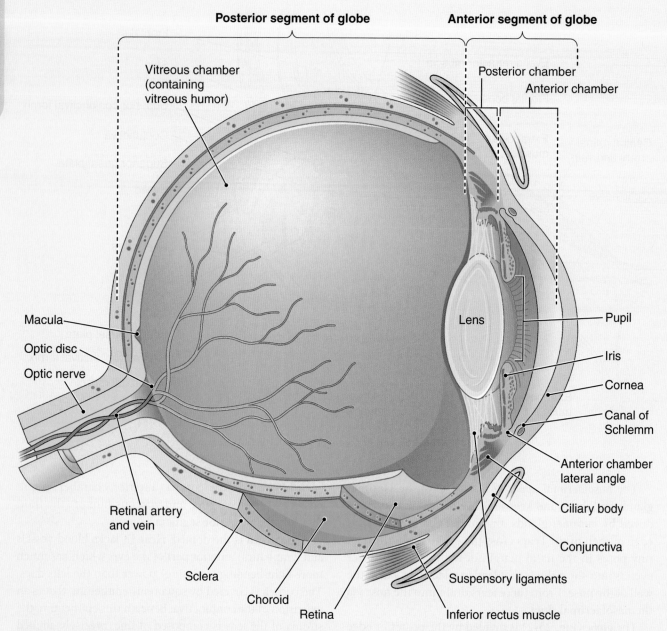

Posterior segment of globe   **Anterior segment of globe**

Vitreous chamber
(containing
vitreous humor)

Posterior chamber

Anterior chamber

Macula

Optic disc

Optic nerve

Lens

Pupil

Iris

Cornea

Canal of
Schlemm

Anterior chamber
lateral angle

Ciliary body

Conjunctiva

Retinal artery
and vein

Sclera

Choroid

Retina

Suspensory ligaments

Inferior rectus muscle

Figure 25-2 **Internal anatomy of the globe.** The two major divisions of the globe are shown here: the posterior segment and the anterior segment.

flows outward to the edge of the anterior chamber and enters **Schlemm's canal**, a tire-like duct in the ciliary body that encircles the anterior chamber, and is absorbed into blood. Production of aqueous humor creates and maintains **intraocular pressure**, which is transmitted from the anterior segment into the posterior segment, keeping the globe inflated to a uniform pressure.

THE POSTERIOR SEGMENT

The **posterior segment** consists of the entire globe behind the anterior segment—the globe, its large chamber, the **vitreous chamber**, and the clear gel that fills it (the **vitreous humor**), which is 99% water and 1% collagen.

The **retina** is the light-sensing layer that lines the inside of the globe. The innermost layer of the retina is a transparent layer of nerve fibers radiating outward from the optic nerve like spokes on a wheel. Beneath this nerve layer is light-sensing cells, the *rods* and *cones*. **Cones**, which sense color, are concentrated in the center of the retina. **Rods**, which are responsible for night vision, motion detection, and peripheral vision, are spread widely throughout the retina. The rods and cones convert light into nerve signals that are transmitted by the optic nerve to the brain.

Dead center in the retina, straight back from the cornea, is the **macula** (Fig. 25-4), a small and highly sensitive part of the retina responsible for detailed, cen-

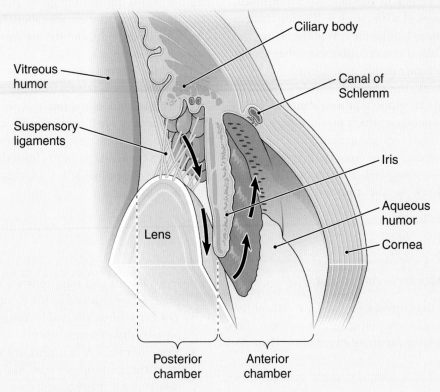

Figure 25-3 **Anatomy of the anterior segment of the eye.** The black arrows indicate the flow of aqueous humor.

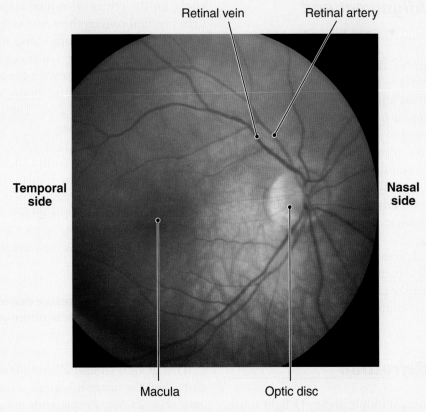

Figure 25-4 **The normal retina.** This funduscopic view is of the right retina.

tral vision. In the center of the macula is the **fovea**, which is densely packed with cones and is responsible for the sharpest vision. Unlike the rest of the retina, the fovea contains no blood vessels; otherwise, they would interfere with light transmission and vision.

The retina rests on the **choroid**, a richly vascular, pigmented layer of the globe that also contains collagen fibers and melanocytes, which produce pigment in proportion to the degree of pigmentation of the skin; that is, people with dark skin have dark retinas. The melanin produced by these cells absorbs light and prevents reflection back to the rods and cones. The

choroid wraps around the globe and extends into the anterior segment to form the ciliary body and iris. The choroid, ciliary body, and iris are called the **uveal tract** or **uvea**.

The **optic nerve** connects the eye to the brain. The retinal blood supply travels from the internal carotid artery with the optic nerve into the eye. Where the optic nerve enters the eye it forms the **optic disc** (Fig. 25-4), a coin-shaped white spot in the retina at which nerve fibers from the retina gather to form the optic nerve and branches of the retinal artery and vein radiate outward into the retina.

MAJOR DETERMINANTS OF DISEASE

- The shape of the cornea and globe are critical for clear vision.
- Older people have far more eye disease than do younger ones.
- Normal vision is a complex, multi-step process that involves the eye, optic nerve, and brain.
- Eye allergies and infections are common because the eyes are exposed to the environment.
- The eye is often affected by systemic disorders, especially diabetes and vascular diseases.
- Some normal eye antigens are masked (hidden) from the immune system; autoimmune disease may result if they become unmasked.

Disorders of Alignment and Movement

Normal vision requires that the eyes be precisely aligned and move together in strict coordination. **Strabismus** is an abnormal alignment of one eye (cross-eye) that may be caused by neurologic disease or by weakness or shortening of an ocular muscle. **Diplopia** (double vision) is the result. In children strabismus must be corrected promptly or the brain will permanently suppress the signal from the affected eye, which will have dim vision (**amblyopia**) or become blind despite having no pathologic abnormality other than deviation.

Nystagmus is rapid, involuntary repetitive motion of one or both eyes. Movement may be horizontal, vertical, or circular and may be caused by neurologic disease (especially of the cerebellum), disease of the inner ear, or drug toxicity.

Disorders of Refraction

Normal vision requires multiple steps: 1) light must pass uninterrupted from cornea to retina; 2) the cornea and lens must refract (bend) light to focus images pre-

cisely on the retina; 3) retinal cells must receive the light rays and convert them into nerve signals; 4) nerve signals must pass normally along the optic nerve and brain visual tracts to the visual cortex in the occipital lobes; and 5) the optical cortex must receive the image and, with other parts of the brain, assimilate it into a perception. The nearby box, The Clinical Side, discusses tests of eye function.

Refractive disorders (Fig. 25-5) are those in which images are blurred by failure of light rays to focus (converge) crisply on the retina. These abnormalities may be caused by abnormal shape of the cornea, elongation or shortening of the globe, or stiffening of the lens, which interferes with focus adjustment. Refractive disorders are not associated with other pathologic abnormalities.

> *All refraction errors are caused by abnormal shape of the globe or cornea or to stiffness of the lens.*

If the globe is elongated, rays converge in front of the retina, and the image is blurred, a condition called **myopia** (Fig. 25-5B). People with myopia are said to be *nearsighted* because the lens is usually able to overcome the defect for near objects. On the other hand, if the

THE CLINICAL SIDE

SEEING THE BIG E

The most common test of eye function is the familiar eye chart test, which tests visual acuity or sharpness.

The usual chart is a Snellen chart, named for a 19th-century Dutch ophthalmologist Hermann Snellen (1834–1908), who came up with the idea. It is imprinted with block letters that decrease in size from the top line to the bottom line. The top line ("the big E") is the 200 line, which can be read by a normal person standing 200 feet away. The bottom line is the 10 line, which can be read by a normal person standing 10 feet away.

The test is administered with the patient standing 20 feet away. Therefore, if a patient standing 20 feet away can only read the "big E" (the 200 line) as the top, the patient's vision is 20/200, which is very poor. On the other hand, if a patient standing at 20 feet can read the smallest line (the 10 line) at the bottom, the patient's vision is 20/10, which is excellent.

globe is foreshortened, the retina is too close to the cornea, the focal point is behind the retina, and the image is blurred, a condition called **hyperopia** (Fig. 25-5C). People with hyperopia are said to be *farsighted* because the lens is often able to overcome the defect for distant objects.

For focus on distant objects ciliary muscles tug at the edges of the lens and flatten it; for near objects the muscles relax and allow the lens to assume a thicker, more globular shape. Focusing power is gradually lost over the years and results in a slow decrease in the ability of the eye to focus on objects nearby, a condition called **presbyopia** (from Greek *presbus*, for old man, Fig. 25-5D). About age 40, people gradually notice an inability to focus on near objects as they find they need to hold reading materials further away. Presbyopia is a natural part of the aging process and affects everyone.

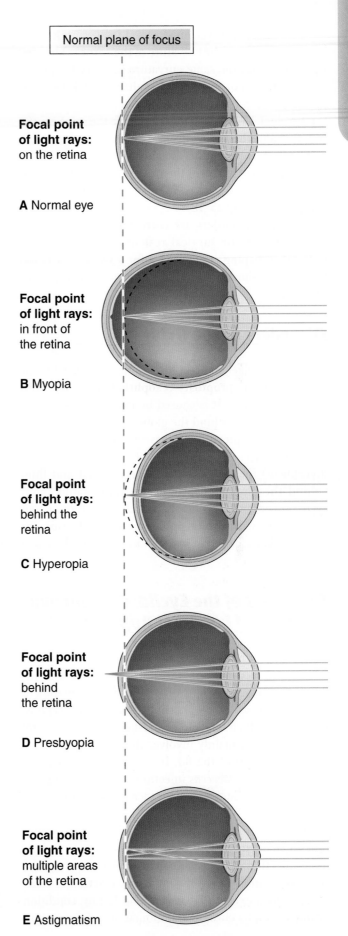

Figure 25-5 **Refractive disorders. A,** Normal. **B,** Myopia (nearsightedness). The globe is elongated: Rays from distant objects converge in front of the retina, and the retinal image is blurred. The lens is able to focus rays from near objects. **C,** Hyperopia (farsightedness). The globe is foreshortened: Rays from near objects converge behind the retina, and the retinal image is blurred. The lens is able to focus rays from distant objects. **D,** Presbyopia. With age, the lens stiffens and can no longer cause rays from near objects to converge on the retina. Rays converge behind the retina. **E,** Astigmatism. Irregular curvature of the cornea causes some areas of the image to converge on the retinal and others to converge in front of or behind the retina.

Normal plane of focus

Focal point of light rays: on the retina

A Normal eye

Focal point of light rays: in front of the retina

B Myopia

Focal point of light rays: behind the retina

C Hyperopia

Focal point of light rays: behind the retina

D Presbyopia

Focal point of light rays: multiple areas of the retina

E Astigmatism

Sometimes, however, misfocused images are caused by irregularities in the curvature of the cornea. The normal cornea has the same curvature in every imaginary cross-section. For example, visualize a clock face imposed on the cornea: the curvature across the cornea in the 1 o'clock to 7 o'clock line should be the same for the line through the cornea from 4 o'clock to 10 o'clock, and so on for every other line across the cornea. If the curvature is not uniform the image is properly focused in some areas and blurred in others, a condition called **astigmatism** (Fig. 25-5E).

Refractive disorders are correctable by eyeglasses, contact lenses, or surgical reshaping of the cornea. Corneal reshaping compensates for a globe that is too long or too short or for a lens that no longer focuses properly.

Disorders of the Orbit

Forward displacement of the globe in the orbit, or bulging eyes, is **proptosis** (**exophthalmos** when both eyes are affected). It is caused by increased tissue and fluid in the orbit behind the globe. An important cause of bilateral proptosis is Graves disease (Chapter 18), which is a type of over-activity of the thyroid (hyperthyroidism) that causes accumulation of fat and fluid behind the globe and produces a remarkable "bug-eyed" appearance. Proptosis is a clinical finding that also occurs with orbital inflammation, infection, or mass such as hemangioma, lymphoma, or lacrimal gland adenoma.

Disorders of the Eyelid, Conjunctiva, Sclera, and Lacrimal Apparatus

The most common disorders or the eyelid, conjunctiva, sclera, and lacrimal apparatus are infections and inflammatory disease (Fig. 25-6). Diffuse inflammation of the eyelids is called **blepharitis** (from Greek, *blefaros*, for eyelid), which tends to be most severe at the lateral lid margins and mainly involves the external, nonconjunctival margin of the lid. It is common and usually caused by *Staphylococcus* infection, seasonal allergy, or skin conditions such as acne rosacea or seborrheic dermatitis.

Sty (*hordeolum*) is localized inflammation, sometimes a small abscess, of the eyelid resulting from bacterial infection of the sebaceous glands in the lid. Like sty, **chalazion** is a local inflammatory reaction of sebaceous glands except that it is a long-lasting condition characterized by chronic granulomatous inflammation.

Tumors of the lids are rare; the most common is basal cell carcinoma of eyelid skin.

Inflammation of the conjunctiva (**conjunctivitis**) is common, mild, and usually bacterial or allergic. The sclera and the underside of the lids are affected. Newborn infants are especially vulnerable to conjunctivitis obtained by passage through an infected vaginal canal. The risk of neonatal conjunctivitis associated with maternal venereal infection with *Neisseria gonorrhoeae* or *Chlamydia trachomatis* is so great that all neonates receive prophylactic antibiotic eye drops immediately after delivery, which has almost completely eliminated the problem. In developed nations most adult conjunctivitis is caused by seasonal allergy. However, in developing nations chronic conjunctival infection with *Chlamydia trachomatis* (**trachoma**) is a major cause of blindness—conjunctival scarring and contraction turns the eyelids inward (*entropion*) so that with every blink the cornea is chronically scratched and becomes scarred.

Keratoconjunctivitis sicca is a clinical syndrome of chronic dry eyes that can usually be attributed to insufficient tear formation, but it may alternatively be caused by poor tear quality and excessive evaporation. It may be caused by dry, cold air and therapeutic drugs, but often the cause is not detectable. When combined with dry mouth (*xerostomia*) it is called *Sjögren syndrome* (Chapter 7), which is usually caused by autoimmune inflammation of lacrimal and salivary gland.

Subconjunctival hemorrhage, or bleeding under the conjunctiva, is very alarming to patients because it is so sudden and dramatic—the white sclera suddenly becomes blood red. It may occur at any age and often without apparent cause, but it most often occurs in association with trauma, sneezing, or coughing. It is rarely of much clinical significance.

Pinguecula and **pterygium** are lumps of yellowish fibrovascular tissue that grow in the sclera on either side of the cornea as a result of sun exposure. Pinguecula is the most common and is usually seen as a small lump on the nasal side of the cornea in an elderly person. Pterygium (from Greek *pterus* for wing) is less common, larger, and shaped like an insect wing; it becomes increasingly common with advancing age. It may grow over the outside edge of the cornea—pinguecula does not—but does not cross into the field of vision. Either pinguecula or pterygium may be excised for cosmetic reasons.

Neoplasms of the conjunctiva and sclera are very rare.

The **lacrimal apparatus** consists of the lacrimal (tear) glands, the lacrimal sac, and the nasolacrimal duct (tear duct), which carries tears from the conjunctiva into the

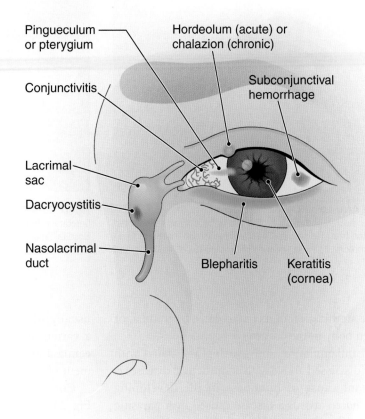

Pingueculum
or pterygium

Hordeolum (acute) or
chalazion (chronic)

Conjunctivitis

Subconjunctival
hemorrhage

Lacrimal
sac

Dacryocystitis

Nasolacrimal
duct

Blepharitis

Keratitis
(cornea)

Figure 25-6 **Disorders of the eyelid, conjunctiva, sclera, and lacrimal apparatus.** The most common infections are shown here.

nose. Inflammation of the lacrimal apparatus is called **dacryocystitis** (from Greek *dakryos* for tear) and may obstruct the flow of tears and predispose to infection. The duct may be obstructed congenitally, or it may become obstructed at its drainage point in the nose owing to nasal conditions such as polyps, allergic rhinitis, or nasal conditions. Unrelieved obstruction may lead to bacterial infection of the lacrimal sac, scarring and permanent ductal damage, or obstruction. Irrigation, probing, and antibiotics are usually effective but some cases may require surgery to reestablish normal flow.

Disorders of the Cornea

The most common problem of the cornea is abnormal shape, which is associated with the refractive abnormalities discussed above.

As the most anterior part of the globe, the cornea is more exposed to the environment than are other parts of the eye and therefore more subject to injury and other environmental influences. Corneal abrasions are common and usually heal without consequence, but corneal scarring may occur. Chemical burns are especially likely to cause scars and may require corneal transplantation.

Arcus senilis, illustrated in Figure 25-7, is a white arc of lipid deposited around the edge of the cornea. It is usually, but not invariably, seen in older persons who have abnormally high blood lipid levels.

Inflammation of the cornea is called **keratitis.** Virtually any type of infectious agent can cause it. Herpesvirus infection (with either herpes simplex virus or varicella-zoster virus) may cause particularly severe inflammation and ulceration, which, as with cold sores or shingles, may be recurrent.

In addition to herpes and shingles, **corneal ulcer** may be caused by bacterial infection (typically *Staphylococcus* or *Streptococcus*). It may also be caused by wearing a contact lens for an extended time without removal, by

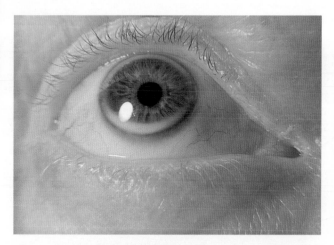

***Figure 25-7* Arcus senilis.** Whitish-yellow arcs at the edge of the cornea may indicate abnormally high levels of blood lipids. Reprinted with permission from Tasman W. The Willis Eye Hospital Atlas of Clinical Ophthalmology, 2nd Ed. Philadelphia. Lippincott Williams and Wilkins, 2001.

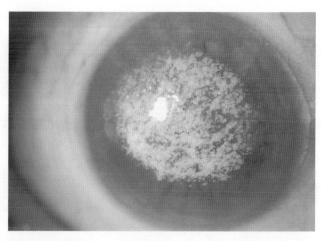

***Figure 25-9* Corneal dystrophy.** Most cases of this disorder are hereditary. Reprinted with permission from Tasman W. The Willis Eye Hospital Atlas of Clinical Ophthalmology, 2nd Ed. Philadelphia. Lippincott Williams and Wilkins, 2001.

inadequate sterilization of a contact lens, by trauma, or by a foreign body in the cornea.

Corneal inflammation and scarring associated with trachoma (discussed above with conjunctival disease) is an important cause of blindness in the developing world. *Onchocerciasis* is a disease caused by a parasitic worm spread by the bites of black flies in Africa and South America. Larval worms invade the cornea and other anterior segment tissues, causing inflammation and blindness.

Keratopathy is a noninflammatory disease of the cornea. *Band keratopathy* (Fig. 25-8) is an opaque, horizontal band of calcium deposits across the cornea that

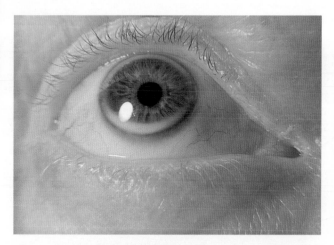

usually affects only one eye and may be associated with a variety of systemic conditions including hypercalcemia and inflammatory diseases of the anterior segment of the globe.

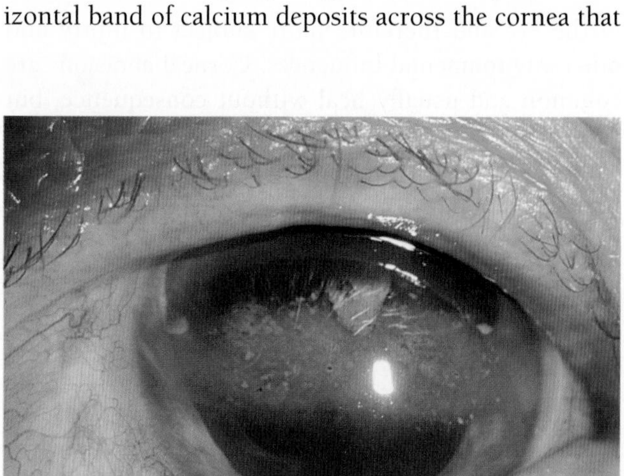

Corneal dystrophy (also called *stromal dystrophy*, Fig. 25-9) is a bilateral noninflammatory clouding of the cornea, usually as a result of a specific genetic defect. There are many varieties, and all affect one or more layers of the cornea. The result is gradual corneal clouding and loss of visual acuity, which may lead to blindness.

Keratoconus is a misshaped cornea that is conical instead of spherical. It affects about 1 in 2,000 persons, and about 10% of cases are hereditary. It is usually bilateral and characterized by progressive bulging and thinning of the cornea. The abnormal shape distorts vision and is difficult to correct with glasses. Rigid contact lenses may provide effective refractive relief. Corneal transplant is effective if contact lenses fail.

Cataract

A **cataract** (Fig. 25-10) is a clouding of the lens. Cataracts are a major cause of poor vision and blindness around the world. In the United States most cataracts are caused by age-related degeneration of lens fibers, which breaks the fibers into molecules small enough to exert an osmotic effect (Chapter 5), that attracts water into the lens, clouding the lens and interfering with light transmission.

Cataracts can be caused by a large variety of other conditions; foremost among them is diabetes, in which excessive blood sugar is converted in the lens into sor-

***Figure 25-8* Band keratopathy.** Corneal calcium deposits in sun-exposed cornea may be associated with many eye and systemic disorders. Reprinted with permission from Tasman W. The Willis Eye Hospital Atlas of Clinical Ophthalmology, 2nd Ed. Philadelphia. Lippincott Williams and Wilkins, 2001.

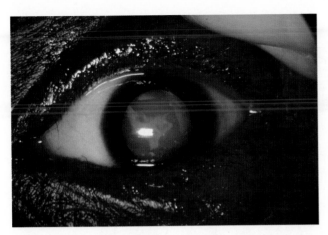

***Figure 25-10* Cataract.** The lens in this patient is completely opaque. Reprinted with permission from Rubin E. Pathology. 4th ed. Philadelphia. Lippincott Williams and Wilkins, 2005.

bitol, a molecule with high osmotic power that attracts water and clouds the lens. Other causes of cataracts include hereditary disease, glaucoma, chronic steroid therapy, congenital rubella infection, and many more. The Clinical Side box nearby describes surgery for cataracts as well as for refractive errors and glaucoma.

In neglected cases the cataractous lens may degenerate so markedly that debris escapes. Because lens proteins are normally sequestered from the immune system (Chapter 7), they are viewed as nonself once they have escaped the confines of the eye. An autoimmune inflammatory reaction may be incited, owing to the fact that the autoimmune antibodies thus created can attack both the affected eye and the opposite eye.

Disorders of the Uveal Tract

The **choroid** is the highly vascular, pigmented layer of the retina that wraps around the posterior segment of the globe and extends anteriorly to become the ciliary body and the iris in the anterior segment of the globe. The **uveal tract** consists of the choroid, the ciliary body, and the iris, all of which are richly vascular. Inflammation of the uvea is called **uveitis**. For practical purposes, uveitis is the only significant disorder of the uvea.

As is illustrated in Figure 25-11, uveitis may occur in any part of the uvea. **Iritis** is inflammation of the iris only; **iridocyclitis** is inflammation of the iris and ciliary body. **Choroiditis** is inflammation of the choroidal layer of the retina and may or may not be associated with iritis or iridocyclitis.

Lens or corneal surgery or trauma to the anterior segment may cause iritis or iridocyclitis. Uveitis is frequently associated with rheumatoid arthritis, juvenile rheumatoid arthritis, ankylosing spondylitis, and other autoimmune diseases (Chapter 22). Uveitis is also often caused by infectious agents, especially in patients with AIDS or other immune deficiency. *Toxoplasma*, syphilis, cytomegalovirus, and herpesvirus are the most common infectious agents. About one third of patients with sarcoidosis (Chapter 13) have uveitis.

THE CLINICAL SIDE

SURGERY FOR REFRACTIVE ERRORS, GLAUCOMA, AND CATARACTS

In the United States, refractive errors, cataracts, and glaucoma and are the most common disorders of the eye for which people seek professional help.

Refractive errors can be corrected in many people by surgical reshaping of the cornea by the *laser-assisted in-situ keratomileusis* (LASIK). In this procedure, a highly precise surgical instrument is used to cut a flap of tissue in the outer layer of the cornea. The flap is raised, and a computer-guided laser precisely shapes the middle layer of the cornea by burning away precisely enough tissue to correct the refractive error. The flap is folded back in place, and the wound heals quickly. The procedure takes only a few minutes, vision recovers quickly, and there is a minimum of postoperative pain.

Lasers can also be used in the treatment for glaucoma in patients whose intraocular pressure is not well controlled by eyedrops. In *laser trabeculoplasty* a laser beam is guided into the later angle to burn open holes so that aqueous humor can flow into the canal of Schlemm. This procedure, too, takes only a few minutes and is usually pain free.

Cataracts are typically removed by *phacoemulsification* (from Greek *phacos,* for bean). In this procedure a tiny (~3 mm) incision is made in the sclera near the edge of the cornea and an ultrasonic probe is inserted into the lens. The lens is liquefied by high frequency sound waves, sucked out, and replaced by an artificial lens. The procedure is associated with mild postoperative discomfort.

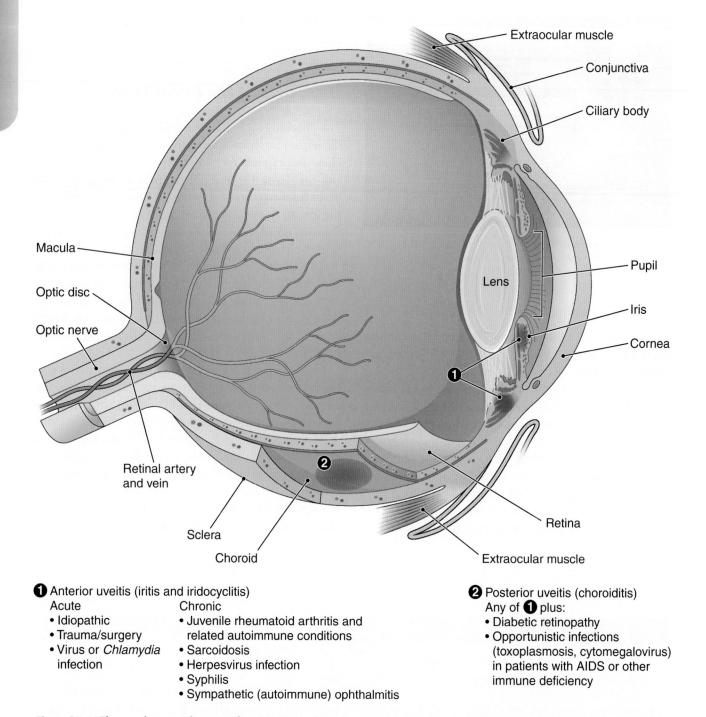

Extraocular muscle

Conjunctiva

Ciliary body

Macula

Optic disc

Optic nerve

Lens

Pupil

Iris

Cornea

Retinal artery and vein

Sclera

Choroid

Retina

Extraocular muscle

❶ Anterior uveitis (iritis and iridocyclitis)
  Acute
  • Idiopathic
  • Trauma/surgery
  • Virus or *Chlamydia* infection

  Chronic
  • Juvenile rheumatoid arthritis and related autoimmune conditions
  • Sarcoidosis
  • Herpesvirus infection
  • Syphilis
  • Sympathetic (autoimmune) ophthalmitis

❷ Posterior uveitis (choroiditis)
  Any of ❶ plus:
  • Diabetic retinopathy
  • Opportunistic infections (toxoplasmosis, cytomegalovirus) in patients with AIDS or other immune deficiency

Figure 25-11 **The uveal tract and causes of uveitis.** Types of anterior uveitis (1) and posterior uveitis (2) are illustrated and summarized here.

Uveitis may have severe consequences, including adhesions (**synechiae**) between the iris and the lens or cornea, obstruction to the flow of aqueous humor with resultant glaucoma, cataract, detached retina, and retinal neovascularization, any of which can cause blindness.

Sympathetic ophthalmitis is an autoimmune uveitis involving the entire uveal tract that occurs after a latent period (a few weeks, months, or years) in response to eye injury. The reaction is caused by traumatic liberation (unmasking) of retinal antigens not previously exposed to the immune system. The immune system reacts to these antigens as if they are alien, not native, and incites an autoimmune reaction (Chapter 7) in either or both eyes.

Disorders of the Retina and Vitreous Humor

Normally the vitreous humor is lightly but securely adherent to the retina, but with age the connection becomes less secure, and the vitreous can become detached, usually in the back of the eye. *Vitreous detachment* is not a problem and does not interfere with vision, but in some instances it can pull the retina away (*retinal detachment*), which is very serious. Sometimes vitreous protein may condense to form bits of condensed material that appear as "*floaters*" in the field of vision. Although floaters are not a threat to vision, they can be a forerunner of retinal detachment and call for careful examination of the retina by an eye specialist.

Vitreous hemorrhage is a consequence of some associated condition, most often diabetic retinopathy (discussed immediately below); other causes include trauma and retinal detachment. Blood in the vitreous humor impairs vision because it blocks light transmission; but more important is that blood is toxic to the retina and may cause permanent retinal damage with visual loss.

Retinal detachment is a peeling away of the retina from its attachment to the underlying layers of the globe. The separation occurs along the plane of tissue where the deep edge of the light-sensing neural (rod and cone) layer meets the choroid. *Retinal detachment is a medical emergency.* Separated retina is sightless; but sight can usually be restored with reattachment.

As is illustrated in Figure 25-12, there are two types of detachments: those associated with tears of the retina and those without. When no tear is present the retina may be pulled away from the wall of the globe by abnormalities that occur in the vitreous humor. For example, inflammatory conditions or infections in the vitreous may create adhesions to the retina that pull the retina away as the adhesions mature and retract. In other circumstances, inflammatory conditions deep in the retina or choroid may cause inflammatory fluid to seep into the potential space beneath the retina and lift the retina away.

Retinal tears are often caused by trauma or age-related shrinking of the vitreous, which may pull on the retina and tear it. Tears allow fluid from the vitreous humor to seep under the retina and lift it away from its attachment.

Surprisingly, full thickness traumatic penetrations of the wall of the globe are not associated with retinal detachment even though they can cause very large retinal tears.

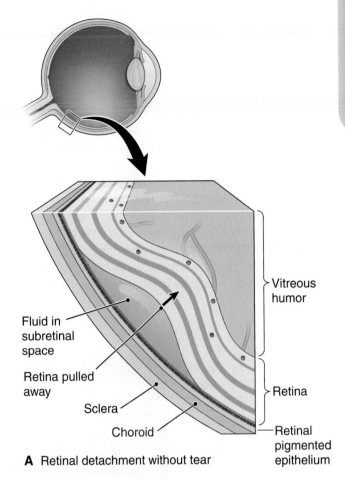

A Retinal detachment without tear

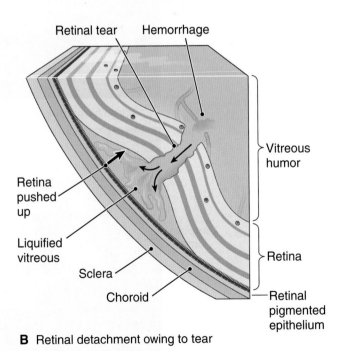

B Retinal detachment owing to tear

***Figure 25-12* Retinal detachment. A,** In a detachment without tear, the retina is pulled away by conditions in the vitreous humor. **B,** In a detachment with tear, a tear in the retina allows seepage through the tear of liquefied vitreous humor, which accumulates beneath the retina and pushes it away.

Retinal vascular disease is a frequent and serious complication of two of the most common diseases of humans: diabetes and hypertension. Changes are easily observable by visual examination of the retina.

The most basic form of retinal vascular abnormality is arteriolosclerosis (Chapter 11), illustrated in Figure 25-13. **Hypertensive retinopathy** occurs in direct proportion to the severity of hypertension (Chapter 12). Normal retinal arteries (actually arterioles) appear somewhat broad and red, but as retinal arteriolosclerosis progresses vessels changes from relatively broad and red to stiff, hard, shiny, narrow vessels that create a glossy "copper wire" (or "silver wire") effect visible in the retina by funduscopy. At points where these stiff arterioles cross veins, they narrow (nick) the veins (A-V nicking). Other findings include flame-shaped hemorrhages,

yellow exudates, and the white "cotton wool" spots of an ischemic retina. In malignant hypertension with cerebral edema the optic nerve may be pushed forward by the bulging brain, a condition known as **papilledema**, which is a feature common to any condition associated with markedly increased intracranial pressure.

Blockage of either the central retinal artery or vein (**retinal occlusive vascular disease**) may be caused by thrombosis, embolism, vasospasm, or external compression. Occlusion of the central retinal artery causes death of retinal light-sensing cells and permanent blindness unless the ischemia lasts less than a few minutes. Occlusion of the central retinal vein causes hemorrhage and edema in the retina and may produce obscured vision, but blindness rarely occurs despite the dramatic appearance of the retina. The ischemia produced by

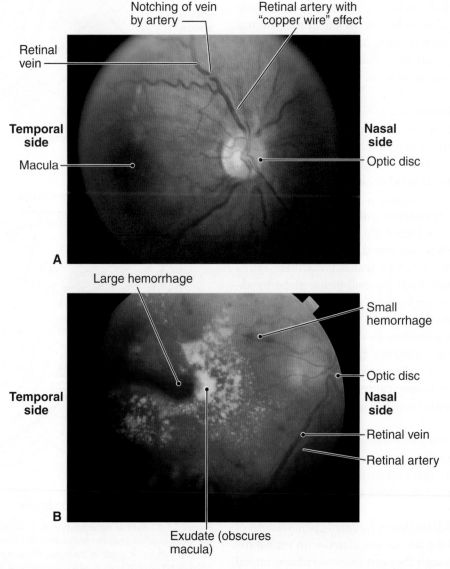

Figure 25-13 **The retina in hypertension. A,** Arteriolosclerosis of retinal arterioles creates a "copper wire" effect and notching of vein at points where arteries cross veins (A-V nicking). **B,** Hemorrhages and exudates are evident in this image.

retinal vein occlusion frequently causes glaucoma secondary to inflammation and scarring in the anterior chamber.

The most common and serious retinal vascular disease is associated with diabetes (Chapter 17). The eye is profoundly affected by diabetes—cataracts, glaucoma, retinal detachment, and choroiditis are common; however, virtually all patients with diabetes develop some form of **diabetic retinopathy** (Fig. 25-14) during the course of their disease. Diabetic retinal arteries develop microaneurysms and leak plasma or blood, creating retinal exudates and hemorrhages, which are the characteristic findings of *early diabetic retinopathy* (also called *background retinopathy* or *nonproliferative retinopathy*, Fig. 24-14A). Early retinopathy is present in about one third of patients with diabetes at the time diabetes is first diagnosed.

Virtually every patient with type 1 diabetes, and most with type 2 diabetes, will have detectable retinopathy within 10–15 years of diagnosis, even those patients who do not have retinopathy initially.

After many years background retinopathy progresses to *proliferative retinopathy*, a much more severe condi-tion (Fig. 25-14B). Delicate new blood vessels, which bleed easily and obscure vision, begin to sprout among the hemorrhages and exudates. They first appear at the optic nerve and grow on the surface of the retina and into the vitreous humor. A film of reactive gliosis (neural scar tissue, Chapter 23) develops in the retina and obscures vision. These scars may retract as they mature, causing retinal detachment and blindness. Blindness in a patient with diabetes is an ominous development because it usually indicates long-standing, severe, poorly controlled disease that is associated with high mortality from cardiovascular and renal disease.

> **The most widely accepted definition of blindness is visual acuity of less than 20/200 with correction, or a field of vision less than 20 degrees. More than 50% of blindness in Anglos is caused by age-related macular degeneration, while among African Americans, cataract and glaucoma account for more than 60% of blindness. Other common causes of blindness include glaucoma, optic nerve disease, and diabetic retinopathy.**

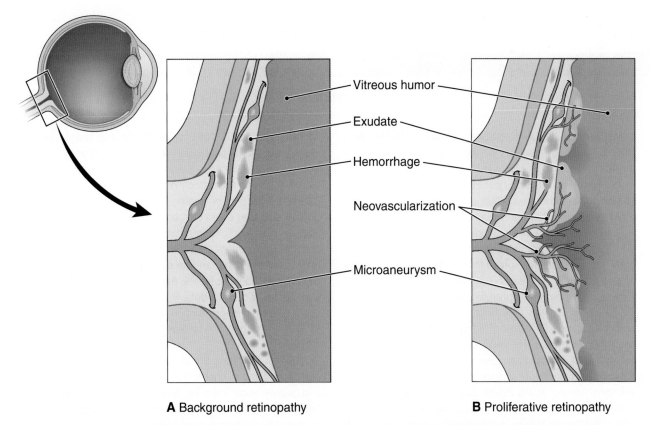

A Background retinopathy   **B** Proliferative retinopathy

Figure 25-14 **The retina in diabetes. A,** Background (early, nonproliferative) retinopathy is seen in most diabetics at the time of the original diagnosis. No new growth of blood vessels (neovascularization) is present. **B,** In proliferative retinopathy (a late complication of diabetes), new blood vessels sprout in areas of hemorrhage and exudate.

Degenerative disease of the retina is a common cause of blindness. Especially common is **age-related macular degeneration**, which robs patients of the most critical aspect of sight—central vision. Age-related macular degeneration is a deterioration of the macula, the central part of the retina with the greatest concentration of rods and cones, which provides sharp, central vision. The cause is unknown. It usually affects both eyes and is the leading cause of blindness in the United States. Patients are usually legally blind (vision <20/200) despite having good peripheral vision. Age-related macular degeneration is more common in smokers, and it is associated with distinct genetic tendencies; for example, it is more common in African Americans than other United States racial groups. (The nearby History of Medicine box provides information about the Braille system, which enables blind people to read with their fingers.)

Retinitis pigmentosa describes a group of related, inherited conditions that feature bilateral, progressive retinal degeneration resulting in night blindness (an inability to see clearly in dim light) and constricted visual fields (tunnel vision). Later the macula densa becomes involved, and complete blindness ensues. About half of patients have a positive family history for the disease. Multiple genetic defects have been identified in these patients. The name *retinitis pigmentosa* derives from the fact that as retinal cells are destroyed they release their melanin pigment, which migrates to the surface of the retina and discolors it a deep brown.

"Retrolental fibroplasia" is an old term applied to **retinopathy of prematurity**, a condition induced in premature infants by oxygen treatment after birth. Until the relationship to oxygen was discovered in the mid 20th century it was the leading cause of blindness in infants. High concentrations of oxygen destroy the immature blood vessels of the premature retina, prohibiting further retinal development. The name derives from the fact that the retina becomes scarred and detaches and shrinks into a ball of fibrous tissue behind the lens.

Disorders of the Optic Nerve

Papilledema is edema of the head of the optic nerve where it enters the globe at the optic disc. It may occur unilaterally following compression of the optic nerve, usually by a neoplasm or other mass, but most often it is bilateral and caused by increased intracranial pressure, which causes the optic nerve to bulge into the rear of the eye. Papilledema is not associated with visual loss, but it

---

History of Medicine

BRAILLE

The Braille system, which enables blind people to read with their fingers, is a product of the genius of Louis Braille (1809–1852), who was born to a saddle and harness maker in the French countryside near Paris. At the age of 3, while playing in his father's workshop, he accidentally punctured an eye with an awl, a sharp tool for making holes in leather. He quickly lost sight in the injured eye, and by the time he was four he was completely blind in both eyes. Most early accounts say "infection spread to the other eye" and caused him to go blind, but reason suggests he suffered from autoimmune sympathetic ophthalmitis.

Young Braille was very bright and kept up his studies orally in a standard classroom. At age 10 he was enrolled in the Royal Institution for Blind Youth in Paris, which also taught students orally; however the library contained a few volumes of bulky books written with very large, raised conventional letters, which Braille used for a while but abandoned as much too slow for practical use. Louis performed well in his regular studies but displayed exceptional musical talent at the piano, which honed his tactile skills.

Then one day in 1821, when Braille was but 12 years old, in one of those casual moments that change world history, he met Charles Barbier, a former French soldier who was visiting the school. While in the army, Barbier had invented a system of coding military messages in raised dots so that they could be read at night, without having to wait for dawn or lighting a flame, which might reveal their position to an enemy. Barbier recognized that his system might help the blind, and he discussed it with Braille, who quickly realized its potential. Barbier's system was phonetic and used a grid of 12 dots. Realizing that a grid of 6 dots could encode enough symbols, Braille reduced the 12 dots to 6 and changed the system from sounds to alphabetic letters.

The rest is history. Braille has been adopted worldwide and has evolved to enable the blind to write and read music and mathematical formulas, and to use computers. A skilled Braille reader can read a Braille version of this sentence almost as fast as you can read it visually.

is a sign of serious underlying disease that requires immediate diagnosis. Among the most common causes of papilledema are malignant hypertension (Chapter 11) and primary brain diseases such as brain tumor, hemorrhage, abscess, or encephalitis (Chapter 23).

Ischemic optic neuropathy is caused by diminished blood flow (ischemia) in the optic artery, which can be caused by atherosclerotic obstruction, arteritis, or embolism, and which can cause necrosis of part or all of the optic nerve, with permanent loss of vision.

In daily clinical language **optic neuritis** describes loss of vision owing to demyelinization of optic nerve fibers, preventing transmission of nerve signals from the retina to the brain. However, despite "itis" in the name, inflammation may not be present. The causes of optic neuritis are many and varied and include multiple sclerosis, syphilis, lead or methanol poisoning, vitamin deficiency (especially in alcoholics), viral infection, therapeutic drugs, and hereditary disease.

However, the most common cause of optic nerve disease is glaucoma.

Glaucoma

Glaucoma is a disease of the optic nerve that causes progressive visual loss. Glaucoma is usually, but not always, associated with *increased intraocular pressure* (ocular hypertension) caused by abnormalities of flow and absorption of aqueous humor in the anterior segment of the globe. However, some patients develop glaucomatous optic nerve damage but have normal intraocular pressure, presumably because they are unusually sensitive to even normal levels of intraocular pressure. Conversely, some patients with increased intraocular pressure do not develop optic nerve damage and, therefore, do not have glaucoma despite having ocular hypertension. It is common, but erroneous, to refer to patients with increased intraocular pressure as having glaucoma even if they do not have nerve damage.

Glaucoma is a common cause of blindness in the United States. About 2 million people in the United States have increased intraocular pressure and are at risk for glaucoma, but perhaps a third of them do not know it.

As is illustrated in Figure 25-15, the anterior segment of the globe encompasses the cornea, iris, lens, and related structures, and is divided into an anterior chamber between cornea and iris and a posterior chamber between iris and lens. Aqueous humor is secreted into the posterior chamber by the ciliary body, flows into the anterior chamber through the pupil, and flows

outward into the **lateral angle** of the anterior chamber, where it is absorbed into blood via the **canal of Schlemm**. The production of aqueous humor contributes to the maintenance of intraocular pressure, which normally is 11–21 mm Hg. However, as mentioned above, the eyes of some people are very sensitive to intraocular pressure and may be damaged by pressures that by definition are normal, and conversely there are others whose optic nerves remain healthy even though they have abnormally high intraocular pressure. Nevertheless, the primary risk factor for glaucoma is increased intraocular pressure.

Glaucoma can be divided into two subtypes according to the angle at which the peripheral edge of the iris meets the cornea. If the patient has glaucomatous optic nerve damage and the angle is normal, the disease is called **primary open-angle glaucoma**. On the other hand, if the angle is narrower than normal, the disease is called **primary closed-angle glaucoma**. Primary open-angle glaucoma is a chronic disease that is clinically asymptomatic and is discovered by an eye specialist during a patient visit for an unrelated problem. On the other hand, primary closed-angle glaucoma usually presents as an acute eye emergency.

Primary open-angle glaucoma (Fig. 25-15B) is a chronic disease that accounts for about two thirds of glaucoma and occurs in patients with no visible abnormality of the angle. Patients with primary open-angle glaucoma have increased intraocular pressure because of obstructed absorption of aqueous humor into the canal of Schlemm. However, about 15–20% of patients with glaucomatous damage to the optic nerve have an open (normal) angle and normal intraocular pressure.

Generally patients with primary open-angle glaucoma do not have pain, blurred vision, or other symptoms, despite progressive loss of peripheral vision. Diagnosis is usually made by an eye specialist in the course of a visit for an unrelated eye problem. By the time the patient becomes aware of visual field loss, optic nerve damage is severe, and the lost vision cannot be recovered.

As is illustrated in part 1 of Figure 25-15C, *primary closed-angle glaucoma* usually occurs in people over age 40, because the anterior chamber becomes shallower and the angle narrower with advancing age. In these patients there is anterior displacement of the peripheral iris with narrowing of the angle, which obstructs the flow of aqueous humor into the canal of Schlemm.

Primary closed-angle glaucoma usually presents as an acute disease. As is illustrated in part 2 of Figure 25-15C, dilation of the pupil, as occurs at night or in a darkened theater, accentuates the problem because as

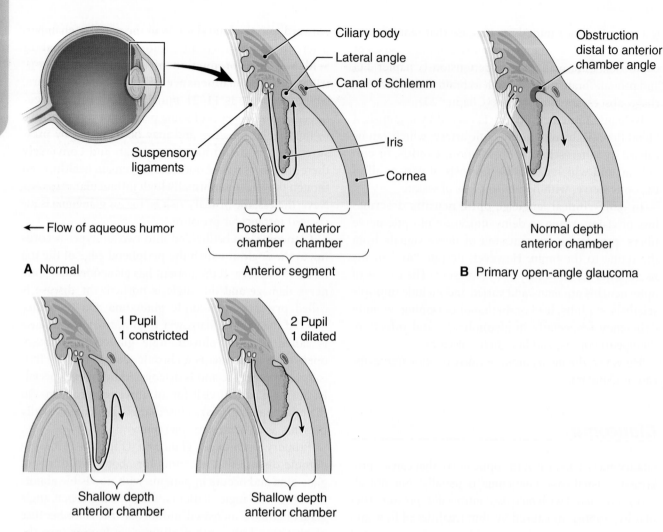

← Flow of aqueous humor

A Normal

B Primary open-angle glaucoma

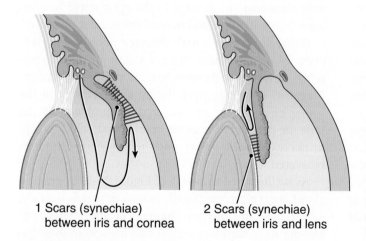

1 Pupil
1 constricted

2 Pupil
2 dilated

Shallow depth
anterior chamber

Shallow depth
anterior chamber

C Primary closed-angle glaucoma

1 Scars (synechiae)
between iris and cornea

2 Scars (synechiae)
between iris and lens

D Secondary glaucoma

Figure 25-15 **The eye in glaucoma. A,** Normal flow of aqueous humor. **B,** Primary open-angle glaucoma. The angle is wide. Flow is obstructed at the canal of Schlemm. **C,** Primary closed-angle glaucoma. In part 1 (left), the pupil is constricted, and the angle is narrow, slowing flow. In part 2 (right), the pupil is dilated. The iris retracts to open the pupil, and "piles up" in the angle, acutely obstructing flow. **D,** Secondary glaucoma. In part 1 (left), scars (synechiae) between the iris and cornea obstruct the flow of aqueous humor. In part 2 (right), scars between the iris and the lens obstruct flow.

the pupil dilates the iris gathers thickly around the edges and further obstructs flow of aqueous humor. An attack usually features severe pain in the eye (or forehead above the affected eye), tearing, redness, blurred vision, and puffy eyelids, and is an emergency requiring treatment within 24–48 hours if vision is to be maintained (see Case Study 25-1 at the end of this chapter). Acute medical therapy usually consists of eyedrops to constrict the pupil and restore flow. Primary closed-angle glaucoma may become symptomatic in one eye many years before the other eye is affected. Intraocular pressure may be normal between attacks. Longer term therapy may include lasering holes in the iris to restore free flow of the aqueous humor from the posterior chamber to the anterior chamber.

As is illustrated in Figure 25-15D, *secondary glaucoma* may be caused by almost any condition of the anterior chamber that produces inflammation and scar tissue: trauma, infection, hemorrhage, and so on, the result of which is obstructed flow of aqueous humor caused by fibrous bands (synechiae) between the iris and the cornea (part 1 of Fig. 25-15D) or lens (part 2).

In patients with glaucomatous damage to the optic nerve, the optic disc is enlarged, pale, and cupped (depressed). Other findings can include symptoms of an acute attack, as described above, and loss of peripheral vision.

Primary care screening for glaucoma by routine measurement of intraocular pressure is not recommended because about half of patients with glaucoma have normal pressure at a single measurement. Measurement of intraocular pressure, visual examination of the optic disc, and testing peripheral vision provide clues but are too difficult and expensive to be used widely in primary care settings. The job of detecting increased intraocular pressure and early glaucoma is best left in the hands of eye specialists, who can integrate these measurements into patient visits for eyeglasses, contact lenses, or other ocular needs with special attention to high risk people: African Americans older than 40, Anglos older than 65,

and patients with a family history of glaucoma or a personal history of diabetes or severe myopia. The nearby box, The Clinical Side, offers more information about diagnosing glaucoma.

Neoplasms

The eye contains a wide variety of tissues, any of which may become malignant. However, most ocular neoplasms arise from immature retinal neurons and melanocytes in the choroidal layer of the uvea.

The most common malignancy in the eye of an adult is metastatic cancer, which usually lodges in the rich vascularity of the choroid layer of the uveal tract. However, the most common primary ocular neoplasms are nevi and melanoma of the choroidal (uveal) melanocytes. As in skin, choroidal nevi are common and occur in about 10% of persons. Ocular **malignant melanoma** (MM), on the other hand, is very rare.

Retinoblastoma is the most common primary ocular malignancy in children. It is a tumor of primitive neuronal cells in the retina and may be an inherited genetic defect (40% of cases) or a spontaneous mutation (60% of cases). It may be unilateral or bilateral and may metastasize or invade the brain via the optic nerve; however, 90% of cases can be cured if detected while confined to the globe. Most patients are diagnosed at about age 3–4 years, when a parent catches a glimpse of something white in the pupil instead of the usual blackness.

THE CLINICAL SIDE

DIAGNOSING GLAUCOMA

Glaucoma is a clinical diagnosis based on detection of optic nerve damage. Supporting evidence includes increased intraocular pressure, lost (restricted) peripheral vision, changes in the appearance of the optic disc, and changes in the anatomy of the anterior segment of the globe.

Intraocular pressure can be measured in several ways and requires special equipment and training. A common method measures the force required to flatten a certain area of the cornea. Anesthetic drops are placed in the eye, and a probe is pressed against the cornea to measure the force required to flatten the cornea. If intraocular pressure is high, more force is required.

Peripheral vision can be tested (perimetry) by a simple clinical examination, but accurate assessment requires specialized equipment and training. A quick and basic perimetry exam can be performed without special equipment. The

examiner faces the patient, one of the patient's eyes is covered, and the other eye is tested. The patient is asked to stare at the examiner's nose while the examiner moves one hand from far to one side toward his nose. The patient is instructed to speak when he sees the examiner's hand. By moving his hand inward from various points to one side, above, and below, and by testing both eyes, the examiner can approximately map the patient's peripheral vision. Much more accurate perimetry can be performed using special equipment.

Clinical assessment of changes in the optic disc and anterior segment of the globe, such as a narrow angle, shallow anterior chamber, and synechiae (fibrous bands from one structure to another), requires a specialist's use of a sophisticated microscope, which is called a slit-lamp because the light beam used to illuminate the eye is focused on the eye as a narrow, vertical beam (as if the light has passed through a slit).

Section 2: Diseases of the Ear

Deafness: a malady affecting dogs when their person calls them and they want to stay out.

SOURCE: THE FIRST AND MOST COMMON DEFINITION FOUND IN AN INTERNET SEARCH FOR DEFINITIONS OF DEAFNESS, 2005

▶ BACK TO BASICS

The ear has two functions—hearing and balance (body equilibrium). As is illustrated in Figure 25-16, the ear is divided into three anatomic parts: the external, the middle, and the inner ear. Each part is involved in hearing; only the inner ear is involved in balance.

The **external ear** consists of the **auricle**, attached to the side of the head, and the external auditory canal. The auricle is covered by skin and is composed of elastic cartilage, fat, and fibrous tissue. The **external auditory canal** is lined by skin and leads from the auricle to the middle ear, which is embedded in the bone of the skull. The external half of the auditory canal is surrounded by soft tissue, and the internal half is encased in the temporal bone. The auricle collects sound waves and channels them into the canal, which conveys them to the tympanic membrane (eardrum) of the middle ear.

Hollowed out of bone at the end of the external auditory canal is the **middle ear**. Its outer wall is the **tympanic membrane** (eardrum), which vibrates in response to sound waves transmitted down the ear canal. On the inner side of the tympanic membrane is the **tympanic cavity**, an air-filled space in the temporal bone that is lined by simple cuboidal epithelium. Crossing the tym-

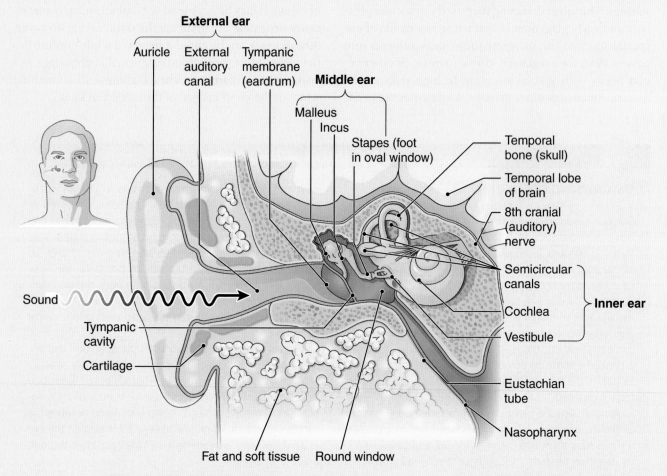

Figure 25-16 **The anatomy of the ear.** The diagram details the external ear, middle ear, and inner ear.

panic cavity from the eardrum, three tiny bones (**ossicles**)—the **malleus, incus**, and **stapes**—connect the ear drum to the **oval window** of the inner ear. The oval window is an opening between the middle ear and the inner ear into which the footplate of the stapes fits precisely. Vibrations of the eardrum vibrate the ossicles, which transmit the vibrations through the oval window and into the inner ear. The **facial nerve** (the 7th cranial nerve) passes through the temporal bone very near tympanic cavity and is separated from it only by a very thin layer of bone. Disease of the middle ear can, therefore, affect the facial nerve.

Deepest in the temporal bone is a cavity that contains the inner ear, which consists of the *cochlea* (for hearing) and the *semicircular canals* (for balance). Both are hollowed out of bone, filled by fluid, and lined by ciliated sensory cells that connect to the brain via the **auditory nerve** (the 8th cranial nerve). The **cochlea** is a hollow tube coiled upon itself like a snail shell. It joins the tympanic cavity of the middle ear via two openings—the *oval window* and the *round window*. Sound vibrations transmitted through the oval window are transformed into pressure waves in cochlear fluid, which radiate into the cochlear spiral and disturb the cilia, creating nerve signals in the 8th cranial (auditory) nerve. These pressure waves also radiate to the **round window**, which vibrates sympathetically much like one end of a drum vibrates in response to the other. The round window acts as a relief mechanism for vibrations that are transmitted to it by the ossicles. Without this mechanism it would be difficult to create pressure waves in the cochlear fluid.

The second element of the inner ear is three **semicircular canals**, collectively called the **labyrinth**. They are tubular arcs, each set at a 90° angle to one another, like the sides of a box corner, such that each is oriented in one major anatomic plane of the body—horizontal, sagittal (vertical through the nose), and coronal (vertical through the shoulders). The semicircular canals are also filled with fluid and lined by ciliated sensory cells connected to the 8th (auditory) cranial nerve. Just as sudden motion of a glass of water causes the water inside to slosh up one side, motion of the head disturbs canal fluid and agitates the cilia to create 8th nerve signals that are processed by the brain to maintain body equilibrium.

The tympanic cavity of the middle ear is indirectly connected to the air outside the body via the **eustachian tube**, which runs from space of the middle ear to the back of the nasal cavity (nasopharynx). This connection equalizes atmospheric pressure on both sides of the eardrum: pressure on the outside via the external auditory canal is matched by pressure on the inside via the eustachian tube. Unequal pressure on the eardrum, as can build up, for example, if a stuffy nose has occluded the nasal end of the eustachian tube during an elevator ride, creates tension on the eardrum that temporarily impairs hearing and can, in severe cases, be very painful or cause rupture of the eardrum.

MAJOR DETERMINANTS OF DISEASE

- Most diseases of the external ear are skin diseases similar to skin disease elsewhere.
- The tympanic membrane (eardrum) is directly open to the environment.
- Obstruction of the eustachian tube predisposes to middle ear infection, especially in children.
- Diseases of the inner ear can affect both hearing and balance.
- Most hearing loss occurs in older people and is caused by age-related changes in the middle and inner ear.
- Normal hearing is a complex, multi-step process that involves the external, middle, and internal ear, the 8th cranial nerve, and the brain.

Disorders of the External Ear

Most conditions affecting the auricle are diseases of skin (Chapter 24). Auricular skin may be affected by virtually any skin disease, particularly atopic dermatitis. The top of the auricle is exposed to direct sunlight and in older persons is frequently involved by **basal cell** and **squamous cell carcinomas**, which behave no differently on the ear than on skin elsewhere. In genetically susceptible persons (usually of African ancestry) the earlobe is a common site for **keloids** subsequent to cosmetic piercing.

The auditory canal is also lined by skin and it, too, may be affected by almost any skin disease or infection. Patient attempts to clean the canal with toothpicks or cotton swabs, for example, usually do more harm than good—earwax or debris is pushed further into the canal, the skin may be irritated or cut, or the eardrum may be perforated. **Otitis externa** is inflammation of the

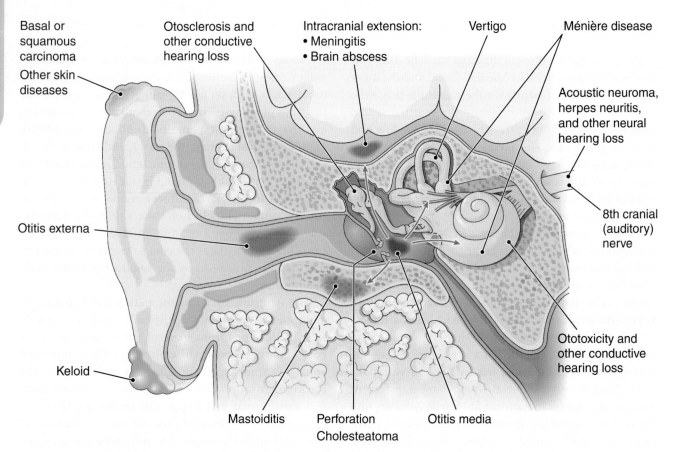

Figure 25-17 **Diseases of the ear.** Common diseases of both the external and internal ear are shown here.

external ear and usually comes to medical attention because of inflammation in the ear canal. The most common cause is bacterial infection, often associated with swimming and water in the ear canal (*swimmer's ear*). Otitis externa is also more common in people whose ears are affected by some skin condition such as psoriasis or atopic eczema, and it is usually caused by bacterial infection. Because the inner half of the canal is constricted by bone and has little room to swell, otitis externa may be extremely painful. Figure 25-17 shows diseases of both the external and internal ear.

Disorders of the Middle Ear

Because it is exposed to the environment, the tympanic membrane is subject to direct trauma, either from objects or from sound waves so strong that the membrane ruptures. Small perforations usually heal quickly and spontaneously, but larger ones may require surgery. **Acute otitis media**, acute inflammation of the middle ear, is a common affliction of children from 3 months to 3 years old—about 10% of children have three episodes before their first birthday. Acute otitis media is often

secondary to an upper respiratory infection that causes nasopharyngeal edema and blockage of the eustachian tube. Effusion fluid accumulates in the tympanic cavity (*serous otitis media,* or *otitis media with effusion*), which then becomes infected by bacteria from the eustachian tube. Most cases respond promptly to oral antibiotic therapy, but serous fluid can persist for 4–6 weeks. Patients in whom the fluid persists for a longer time are said to have *chronic otitis media.* No infection is present but the fluid can cause mild hearing loss that can impair language skills in children. These patients usually respond favorably to surgical insertion of drainage tubes in the tympanic membrane. Some otitis media infections can spread into the temporal bone to cause chronic osteomyelitis (Chapter 22) or into the cranial cavity to cause meningitis (Chapter 1, Case Study 1-1). Case Study 25-2 at the end of this chapter presents a typical case of acute otitis media.

Serous otitis media is usually painless and resolves without treatment unless it persists for several months and is associated with hearing loss. Most children in the United States have at least one episode of serous otitis media. A few have recurrent or continuous effusions that keep the middle ear filled with watery fluid, which can become infected. The fluid impairs motion of the drum and with time may become thick (*glue ear*) and cause hearing loss. Some cases require insertion of grommets or tubes in the eardrum to facilitate drainage.

Pain and fever are the usual symptoms of *acute purulent otitis media*. The eardrum is bulging, dull, and red. Antibiotics are the mainstay of treatment. In severe or neglected cases the eardrum may rupture and discharge pus into the ear canal. Complications of purulent otitis media can be severe: septicemia, meningitis, or invasion of the mastoid process of the temporal bone (*mastoiditis*). Chronic otitis media may cause widespread local damage, including osteomyelitis in the adjacent mastoid process of the temporal bone (**mastoiditis**) or destruction of the facial nerve and inner ear.

Cholesteatoma is an accumulation of keratin debris in the middle ear caused by ingrowth of squamous epithelium from the ear canal, associated with a defect in the tympanic membrane. Despite the name, it is not a neoplasm. The simple cuboidal epithelium lining the tympanic cavity is replaced by squamous epithelium that migrates into the middle ear from the ear canal through a hole in the eardrum. As squamous cells multiply, mature, and are shed, the dead cells have no place to go, and keratin debris accumulates in the closed space of the tympanic cavity. Cholesteatoma is usually associated with chronic middle ear infection (otitis media) and if untreated may result in deafness caused by damage to the middle ear's ability to transmit sound vibrations.

Otosclerosis is a major cause of hearing loss in adults. It is much more common in Anglos than in African Americans, and about twice as common in women as in men. Both ears are usually affected, and there is strong familial influence. The pathologic abnormality is deposition of bone in the oval window, which limits the ability of the ossicles to transfer sound vibrations to the inner ear from the eardrum. In advanced cases the entire stapes becomes encased in new bone and may require surgical excision with replacement by prosthesis.

Disorders of the Inner Ear

Inasmuch as the inner ear is composed of the cochlea, which senses sound, and the semicircular canals, which sense body orientation and movement, diseases of the inner ear produce either impaired hearing or dizziness (vertigo) or both. The most common example is **Ménière's disease**, a clinical triad of vertigo, hearing loss, and **tinnitus** (ringing in the ears). The etiology is unknown, but it is associated with increased fluid in the cochlea. It occurs in middle-aged adults and is marked by clustered episodes of vertigo, nausea, and vomiting for about 12–24 hours, followed by recovery. Vertigo becomes less frequent with time, but most often hearing is eventually permanently impaired. Low-salt diet and diuretics may have some beneficial effect by lowering the amount of fluid in the cochlea.

The inner ear may be affected by a number of other diseases, the cause of which is not clear. Viral infection of the 8th cranial nerve is believed to be responsible for a clinical condition known as *vestibular neuronitis*, which is characterized by severe, weeklong nausea and vertigo in adolescents and young adults. Multiple attacks occur over 12–18 months but eventually disappear. There is no associated tinnitus or hearing loss. Some patients suffer attacks of vertigo for which no cause is ever clearly determined. *Herpes zoster infection* of the 8th cranial nerve is associated with severe ear pain, hearing loss, vertigo, and facial nerve paralysis. Certain drugs produce **ototoxicity** by damaging the cochlea, but are nevertheless sometimes used if serious disease leaves no less risky choice. Notable ototoxic drugs include antibiotics (among them streptomycin, vancomycin, gentamicin), the diuretic furosemide, and the antimalarial quinine and related compounds. Large doses of aspirin may cause tinnitus and hearing loss that is usually temporary. Neuromas (Chapter 23) of the acoustic nerve account for about 7% of intracranial tumors and may be associated with vertigo and hearing loss.

Deafness

Hearing loss caused by disease in the ear canal or middle ear that interferes with transmission of sound waves is called **conductive hearing loss**. Hearing loss caused by cochlear disease is **sensory hearing loss**; loss caused by 8th cranial nerve disease is **neural hearing loss**.

Conductive hearing loss may result from something as simple as impacted cerumen (earwax) in the canal or as complex as otosclerosis or other diseases of the middle ear; in any case, the problem lies in conduction of sound vibrations down the canal and across the middle ear to the cochlea. *Sensory hearing loss* is a result of cochlear disease. Ototoxic drugs are an important cause of sensory loss; some elderly people have sensory loss for unknown reasons. *Neural hearing loss*, the least common type of hearing loss, occurs in association with lesions in the 8th cranial nerve or, less commonly, in the central nervous system. Perhaps the most important cause is neuroma of the 8th cranial nerve, because neuromas are benign and surgically curable, although lost hearing may not be recovered ■

CASE STUDY 25-1 *"I'M HAVING A DIFFERENT KIND OF MIGRAINE"*

TOPIC
Glaucoma

THE CASE

Setting: You are employed as a "front-line" caregiver in one of several neighborhood walk-in clinics operated by a multi-specialty group in a large metropolitan area.

Clinical history: Your next patient is Mrs. S., whom you find seated in the exam room holding an ice pack to her right forehead. She is a well-groomed, poised woman who looks younger than her stated age of 50.

You ask, "How may I help you, this evening?"

She replies, "I'm having a different kind of migraine."

On questioning, you learn she has been having headaches for many years. She has been taking pills prescribed by her family physician in a small town 2 hours away. She is in the city visiting her daughter, whose personal physician is a member of your medical group. This morning after breakfast she began having a severe headache while taking a stroll around the neighborhood with her daughter. They returned home where the patient vomited and her daughter called your clinic.

"When my headaches began 10 years ago, my doctor did a lot of tests and put me on this medicine," she says, showing you a vial of prescription migraine pills. "But this headache feels different," she continues, pointing to her forehead above her right eye. "It's in the front, not on the sides as usual, and it's on one side, not both."

As you prepare to examine her, she adds, "It may have something to do with my eye. It's been watering ever since this headache started, and my vision is blurry, too."

Physical examination: Vital signs are unremarkable, and physical exam reveals no abnormalities except for the right eye—it is mildly red and tearing, and the lids are a bit swollen.

Clinical course: Concluding that she has an acute eye disease, you ask a colleague on duty for her opinion; she agrees

with your thoughts, and you make an emergency referral of the patient to an ophthalmologist at the main clinic. Later in the day you call the ophthalmology department and speak to a nurse, who tells you the patient was diagnosed with acute closed-angle glaucoma, treated, and sent home with instructions to return the next day.

A fax of records from the ophthalmology department reveals that initial intraocular pressure in the right eye was 48 mm Hg (normal <21) and 18 in the left eye. Visual acuity was 20/60 in the right eye, 20/40 the left eye. Mild cataracts were present on both sides. In the right eye the conjunctiva was congested, the cornea was edematous, the pupil was dilated and fixed, and the anterior chamber angle was closed all the way around. In the left eye the angle was open but narrowed, and the anterior chamber was shallow. The right optic disc was mildly pale, enlarged, and cupped, and a visual field examination revealed normal peripheral vision.

DISCUSSION

The patient's long-standing migraine headaches were unrelated to her current complaint. Fortunately, she recognized that the different character of the current headache and the eye symptoms might mean something new was going on; and it was.

Acute angle closure glaucoma is easy to diagnose, and this patient had classic symptoms: headache or eye pain, redness, blurred vision or halos around lights at night, headache, nausea, and vomiting. This patient also had typical physical findings: tearing, puffy eyelids, cloudy cornea, fixed-dilated pupil, and conjunctival redness. Fortunately, rapid diagnosis and treatment meant a good prognosis; with therapy she is not likely to sustain visual loss.

Unfortunately, chronic glaucoma is much more common and more difficult to diagnose because it destroys vision while remaining clinically asymptomatic.

POINTS TO REMEMBER

• Acute closed-angle glaucoma has distinctive signs and symptoms and requires prompt and continuing therapy to avoid visual loss.

CASE STUDY 25-2 "JUJU HAS A FEVER"

TOPICS
Otitis media

THE CASE

Setting: You are employed in a pediatrician's office, where today you are assigned to see patients coming to the "isolation room," where children with fever are brought to keep them apart from the main waiting room in order to limit exposure to children with potentially contagious disease.

Clinical history: JuJu is a 6-month-old girl brought to the office by her mother, who says, "JuJu has a fever." On questioning, she says that the child has been irritable and "feverish" for several days because of "a cold." When you ask what she means by "a cold," she says she has "a cough and a runny nose." The mother says she became especially concerned the night before when the child became increasingly irritable, vomited, and began pulling at her left ear. Further questioning reveals that the pregnancy was normal and the child had no previous medical problems and had not been given any medicine other than acetaminophen.

Physical examination and other data: Physical examination reveals a healthy infant crying in her mother's arms. Temperature is 101.7 °F. Heart rate and respirations are rapid but not unusual for a child with fever. Crusted mucus is present around the nostrils and the child is mouth breathing. The chest is clear, and cardiac sounds are not remarkable. The neck is supple, and the anterior fontanelle is small, soft, and flat. The right ear is normal, but the left tympanic membrane is bulging and red.

Clinical course: You conclude the baby has acute otitis media and consult with the pediatrician, who agrees with your diagnosis and your recommendation of oral antibiotic therapy. You write a prescription for the antibiotic, instruct the mother to call you the next day, and schedule a follow-up visit for 2 weeks. The next day the mother reports that the fever is almost gone and the baby's appetite has improved. On follow-up at 2 weeks, JuJu is happy and asymptomatic, but she has serous effusions in both middle ears. You explain to the mother that effusions frequently occur but are not serious unless they persist for several months. You schedule a second follow-up in a month. When you see JuJu a month later the effusions have disappeared, and she seems perfectly happy and content.

DISCUSSION

This child had a classic case of acute otitis media: an acute middle ear infection, which occurs most often in young children and which usually arises as a complication of an otherwise unremarkable viral upper respiratory infection. Like most such patients, she responded well to oral antibiotics, but, as many children do, she developed bilateral serous otitis media in the aftermath of the acute infection. In addition, as most cases do, the serous otitis media resolved without further therapy.

POINTS TO REMEMBER

- Acute otitis media is a common childhood illness.
- Serous otitis media is a common consequence of acute otitis media.

Objectives Recap

1. *Describe the anterior and posterior segments of the globe and the anterior and posterior chambers of the anterior segment*: The anterior segment of the globe encompasses the cornea, iris, lens, and related structures. The posterior segment consists of the remainder of the globe and the vitreous humor. The anterior segment is divided into two compartments: the anterior chamber between the iris and cornea and the posterior chamber between the iris and lens.

2. *Trace the flow of aqueous humor*: The aqueous humor is secreted from the ciliary body and flows first into the posterior chamber. From there it flows through the pupil into the anterior chamber and moves laterally to the angle of the anterior chamber (where the iris meets the lateral edge of the cornea) and is absorbed into blood through Schlemm's canal.

3. *Name the layers of the posterior segment of the globe from the interior outward*: Innermost is the

neurosensory layer of the retina (the rods and cones); next outward is the choroid, which is highly vascular and pigmented; outermost is the tough, fibrous sclera.

4. *Explain the cause of myopia, hyperopia, and presbyopia*: In myopia (nearsightedness) the eyeball is elongated; images focus in front of the retina and are out of focus by the time they reach the retina. In hyperopia (farsightedness) the eyeball is foreshortened, and images are focused behind the retina so that when they reach the retina they are not yet in focus. In presbyopia the lens is stiffened and cannot accommodate to focus on near objects.

5. *Distinguish between blepharitis and conjunctivitis*: Blepharitis is inflammation of the lid margins and is most notable at the lateral lid edges; the conjunctiva is not involved. Conjunctivitis is inflammation of the epithelium lining of the conjunctival sac and involves the white sclera of the globe and the underside of the eyelids.

6. *Define keratitis*: Inflammation of the cornea.

7. *Explain keratoconus*: An abnormal bulging of the cornea, which is conical rather than spherical. It is associated with severe refractive problems.

8. *Define cataract*: A clouding of the lens.

9. *Name the components of the uveal tract and several causes of uveitis*: The uveal tract is composed of the choroid, ciliary body, and iris. Inflammation (uveitis) is the most common disorder of the uveal tract. Inflammation may involve the choroid (choroiditis), the iris (iritis), or the iris and ciliary body (iridocyclitis). Causes of uveitis include uveitis associated with juvenile rheumatoid arthritis, ankylosing spondylitis and other autoimmune disease, infections (especially in patients with AIDS or other immune deficiency), and trauma to or surgery on the lens, cornea, or iris.

10. *Explain the causes of retinal detachment*: The neurosensory layer of the retina may detach from the underlying layers of the wall of the globe because it is pulled inward by pathology in the vitreous, or it may be pushed upward after a tear in the retinal allows liquified vitreous fluid to seep into the potential space between the deep layer of the retina and the neurosensory layer.

11. *Name the two most common causes of retinal vascular disease*: Diabetes and hypertension.

12. *Explain the effect of age-related macular degeneration and why it is an important disease*: Age-related macular degeneration is a degenerative condition of the macula, that part of the central part of the retina with the greatest concentration of rods and cones, which provides sharp, central vision. Patients with age-related macular degeneration are severely debilitated by loss of central vision, although peripheral vision usually remains unimpaired. It is the most common cause of blindness in the United States.

13. *Define papilledema, and explain its importance*: It is edema of the head of the optic nerve as it enters they globe at the optic disc. It is a serious condition, often caused by increased intracranial pressure or tumor, and it signals the need for diagnostic evaluation.

14. *Discuss the relationship of intraocular pressure to glaucoma*: Strictly defined, glaucoma is a disease of the optic nerve that can severely impair vision. Most patients with glaucomatous damage to the optic nerve have increased intraocular pressure, but some have normal pressure. However, not all patients with increased intraocular pressure develop glaucomatous damage to the optic nerve.

15. *Distinguish between primary open-angle glaucoma and primary closed-angle glaucoma*: Primary open-angle glaucoma, the more common of the two, occurs in patients with a normal (open) angle between the iris and cornea and is caused by failure of the aqueous humor to be absorbed via the canal of Schlemm. On the other hand, primary closed-angle glaucoma is associated with narrowing of the angle, which obstructs aqueous flow into the canal of Schlemm.

16. *Name the three anatomic divisions of the ear, and explain the hearing function of each*: The ear is divided into outer, middle, and inner ears. The outer ear collects and channels sound waves down the ear canal to the tympanic membrane. The middle ear (the tympanic membrane and ossicles) converts sound into vibrations and conveys them across the tympanic cavity to the inner ear, where they are converted by the cochlea into nerve signals transmitted to the brain by the 8th cranial nerve.

17. *Characterize otitis media by the age of most patients, pathogenesis, and cause of inflammation*: Most otitis media occurs in children less than 4 years old and is usually associated with upper respiratory infections, which produce edema and obstruction of the eustachian tube and lead to accumulation of effusion fluid in the cavity of the middle ear. Secondary bacterial infection often supervenes and creates an acute, purulent inflammatory reaction.

18. *Name the three general categories of hearing loss*: Conductive, sensory, and neural.

Typical Test Questions

1. Which of the following forms the posterior side of the anterior chamber?
   A. Ciliary body
   B. Retina
   C. Choroid
   D. Iris

2. Blockage of absorption of aqueous humor is associated with:
   A. Retinal edema
   B. Papilledema
   C. Glaucoma
   D. Proptosis

3. In myopia and hyperopia the principal abnormality is:
   A. Abnormal opacification of the lens
   B. Abnormal shape of the cornea
   C. Keratoconus
   D. Abnormal shape of the globe

4. Iridocyclitis is inflammation of:
   A. Part of the uveal tract
   B. The cornea
   C. The retina
   D. The lacrimal apparatus

5. The main function of the eustachian tube is:
   A. To drain fluid from the middle ear
   B. To collect sound waves for conversion to nerve signals
   C. To equalize air pressure on both sides of the tympanic membrane
   D. To aid in maintaining body orientation and balance

6. True or false? Refractive disorders are not associated with pathologic change other than stiffness of the lens or abnormal shape of the globe or cornea.

7. True or false? Scleral pinguecula and pterygium can grow into the field of vision.

8. True or false? Papilledema is a common cause of loss of vision.

9. True or false? Almost all patients with diabetes suffer from diabetic retinopathy.

10. True or false? Conductive hearing loss is caused by cochlear disease.

Glossary

This glossary is intended to serve as a quick reference to many of the most important words and phrases commonly encountered in the study of pathology. It does not include all of the boldfaced terms in the text but instead focuses on terms that are often misunderstood or unfamiliar. It also includes some terms that are not boldfaced in the text, especially ones that may be unfamiliar. Definitions of boldfaced terms not included here can be located by referring to the comprehensive main index at the end of this book.

abnormal A measurement or observation not falling into the usual range

abortion Interruption of pregnancy before 20 weeks or 500 grams fetal weight

abrasion Injury to skin that scrapes away epidermis

acetylcholine A neurotransmitter; a molecule released at the ends of nerve fibers that carries the nerve signal across the synapse to cause action on the other side

achalasia Painful esophageal muscle spasms

acid-fast stain A laboratory dye to stain tuberculosis bacilli for diagnosis

acidosis Blood pH that is lower (more acid) than normal

ACTH See *adrenocorticotrophic hormone*

actin One of the two contractile proteins in muscle cells (the other: myosin)

acute A condition that arises rapidly, lasts a short time, and is accompanied by distinct symptoms

adenocarcinoma A malignant tumor of gland epithelium

adenohypophysis See *anterior pituitary*

adenoma A benign tumor of glandular epithelium

ADH See *antidiuretic hormone*

adhesion Fibrous scar tissue that binds together anatomic parts not normally joined

adnexa Accessory or adjoining anatomical parts, such as sweat glands and skin

adrenal cortex The outer layer of the adrenal; under control of the anterior pituitary; secretes cortisol, aldosterone, testosterone, and other steroid hormones

adrenal medulla The inner layer of the adrenal; connected to and controlled by the autonomic nervous system; secretes epinephrine and norepinephrine

adrenalin See *epinephrine*

adrenocorticotrophic hormone (ACTH) The hormone released by the pituitary that stimulates the adrenal cortex to produce and release cortisol and other hormones

aerobic Requiring oxygen for metabolism

afferent arteriole The arteriole bringing blood into the glomerulus

agammaglobulinemia Absence of plasma gamma globulins; an immunodeficiency

agent An infective bacterium, virus, prion, or other object that causes infectious disease

agglutinin Naturally occurring blood group antibodies; anti-A and anti-B

agranulocytosis Marked decrease in the number of blood granulocytes

AIDS Acquired immunodeficiency syndrome

albumin The most abundant blood protein, made by the liver; accounts for most plasma osmotic pressure

aldosterone An adrenocortical hormone that stimulates kidney retention of sodium and water, thereby increasing vascular volume and cardiac output; also stimulates kidney excretion of potassium

alkalosis Blood pH that is higher (more alkaline) than normal

allele One gene of a pair that controls a given trait; one allele inherited from the father, one from the mother

allergen A substance capable of causing an allergic reaction

allergic Exaggerated immune responses to environmental substances (allergens)

alopecia Abnormal hair loss

alpha fetoprotein A blood protein marker associated with some neoplasms and neural tube defects

alpha-1 antitrypsin A protein made by the liver that neutralizes digestive enzymes released in inflammatory reactions

alveoli Lung air sacs where gas exchange takes place between air and blood

amenorrhea Absence of menstruation

amino acid A small molecule that is the building block of proteins

aminoaciduria A disorder of protein metabolism in which excessive amounts of amino acids are excreted in the urine

amniocentesis Penetration of the amniotic sac to collect amniotic fluid

amylase A carbohydrate-digesting enzyme secreted by salivary glands and pancreas

amyloid Abnormal protein deposits with characteristic microscopic features, which appear in certain pathological conditions

anaerobic Requiring the absence of oxygen for metabolism

anaphylaxis Severe type 1 (immediate) hypersensitivity reaction

anasarca Generalized edema

anatomic pathology The study of structural changes caused by disease

anemia Abnormally low levels of blood hemoglobin, usually associated with decreased numbers of erythrocytes

anencephaly Congenital absence of most of the brain and skull

aneuploid Having an abnormal number of chromosomes (in humans, other than 46)

aneurysm A localized dilation of an artery or heart chamber

angioneogenesis (angiogenesis) Growth of new blood vessels

angiotensin A vasoconstrictor produced by the action of angiotensin-converting enzyme; increases vascular resistance and blood pressure

angiotensin-converting enzyme An enzyme that acts on angiotensinogen to produce angiotensin

anterior chamber In the eye, the space behind the cornea and in front of the iris

anterior pituitary The adenohypophysis; the anterior lobe of the pituitary, which secretes endocrine hormones

anterior segment In the eye, the cornea, iris, lens, and related structures

antibody A programmed immune system attack protein in blood made by B lymphocytes

anti-CA-125 An antibody to cancer antigen sometimes found in the blood of patients with ovarian cancer

antidiuretic hormone (ADH) The hormone secreted by the posterior pituitary that acts on renal tubules to stimulate retention of water by the kidney

antigen Any molecule capable of stimulating an immune reaction

antimicrobial susceptibility Laboratory estimation of the effectiveness of antibiotics against infective agents, usually bacteria

antinuclear antibodies Autoimmune antibodies to nuclear proteins DNA and RNA

anuria Little or no urine output

aortic valve The one-way valve that separates the left ventricle from the aorta

Apgar score Numerical assessment of newborn infant vigor

apoprotein The protein to which blood lipids are bound; the protein portion of a lipoprotein

apoptosis Natural, programmed cell death

appropriate for gestational age Infants weighing as much as predicted for gestational age

arachnoid granulations Arachnoid membrane bodies that resorb cerebrospinal fluid into blood

arrhythmia Irregular heartbeat

arteriolosclerosis A disease of small blood vessels mainly caused by hypertension and diabetes

ascaris One of a family of large intestinal parasitic roundworms

ascites Fluid accumulation in the peritoneal space

astigmatism Blurred vision caused by irregular curvature of the cornea

Astler-Coller staging A method for assessing the invasiveness and spread of carcinoma of the colon and thereby estimating prognosis

astrocyte A cell that provides the structural framework for all other cells in the central nervous system

atelectasis Collapse of lung tissue

atheroma A localized fatty deposit in atherosclerosis

atherosclerosis A lifestyle disease of arteries related to smoking, lack of exercise, obesity, and high fat diet, characterized by chronic inflammation, scarring, and cholesterol deposits in large and medium-sized vessels

atopy A hereditary predisposition toward developing certain allergic reactions

atresia Failure of a body opening or duct to develop

atrioventricular node A focus of specialized cardiac muscle fibers in the lower interatrial septum that receives heartbeat electrical impulses from the sinoatrial node and forwards them down the excitatory-conduction system to the ventricles

atrium One of the two upper, low-pressure chambers of the heart

atrophy Decreased size of a cell or organ

atypia Abnormal appearance of cell nuclei, usually an indication of malignancy or premalignancy

auditory ossicles Tiny bones of the middle ear that transmit sound vibrations from the tympanic membrane to the inner ear

autoimmune A condition in which the immune system attacks "self," the body's own proteins, instead of foreign ones

autosomal dominant A trait or disease requiring only one allele of an autosomal gene pair

autosomal recessive A trait or disease requiring two identical alleles in an autosomal gene pair

autosome A nonsex chromosome; in humans there are 22 sets of two, numbered 1 to 22

axon A long, thin cytoplasmic extension of a neuron; carries nerve signals

azotemia Renal failure detectable only by laboratory tests

B cell B lymphocyte; a lymphocyte that programs and secretes antibodies into blood to attack foreign substances (usually proteins)

bacillus A rod-shaped bacterium

bacterium A microscopic organism with a cell wall and DNA but no chromosomes or nucleus; can reproduce outside of cells

bacteriuria Bacteria in urine

band neutrophil A freshly made neutrophil with a banana-shaped nucleus

Barrett metaplasia Change of esophageal epithelium from squamous to gastric glandular

basal cell The stem cell of epidermis; located near the basement membrane

basement membrane A thin film of noncellular material that supports epithelium

basophils Leukocytes with large, blue-black granules that are important in some allergic reactions

Bence Jones protein Fragments of monoclonal protein in the urine of patients with multiple myeloma or other plasma cell dyscrasia

benign Usually not capable of causing death

bile A mixture of metabolic waste and bile acids secreted by the liver

bile acids Chemicals made by the liver from cholesterol and secreted via bile ducts into the intestine to emulsify fat for digestion

bile duct A duct that carries bile out of the liver

bilirubin An intensely yellow pigment produced from hemoglobin derived from dead erythrocytes

biopsy The collection of tissue for diagnosis

bleb A large, air-filled sac

blepharitis Inflammation of the eyelid

blood pressure See *hemodynamic pressure*

blood urea nitrogen (BUN) A laboratory measure of metabolic waste in blood that is due to be excreted by the kidneys

blood-brain barrier A function of cerebral capillaries that inhibits exchange of certain large molecules between blood and brain

body mass index Body weight in kilograms divided by the square of body height in meters

Bordetella pertussis A bacterium; the agent of whooping cough

Borrelia burgdorferi A bacterium; the agent of Lyme disease

Bowman space A space surrounding the glomerulus, into which the glomerular filtrate passes from blood; connects directly to a renal tubule

bronchiole The smallest airway in the lungs

bulla A large cystic space filled with air or fluid; in dermatology, a cystic space filled with fluid that is larger than a vesicle

BUN See *blood urea nitrogen*

burn Injury produced by fire, heat, radiation, electricity, or a caustic chemical

bursa A flat, closed fibrous sac filled with oily fluid; positioned between tendon and bone or skin and bone to smooth movement where tissues rub together

cachexia Physical wasting associated with disease

calculus Stone; usually of the biliary or renal tract

callus A mixture of blood vessels, fibrous (scar) tissue, and newly forming bone at a fracture site

Campylobacter jejuni A bacterium; an agent of bacterial diarrhea

cancellous bone Spongy bone in the medullary cavity of a bone

cancer Any kind of malignant neoplasm

Candida albicans A fungus; normally present on the skin and in the mouth, intestines, and vagina; may become pathogenic under some circumstance; the agent of candidiasis (moniliasis; thrush)

capillary The smallest blood vessel

carbohydrates A large class of organic chemical compounds that includes sugars, glycogen, starches, and cellulose; long chains of saccharides that can be digested into sugars

carbon monoxide A colorless, odorless gas produced by imperfectly burned fuel, which binds irreversibly to hemoglobin and prevents oxygen transport

carcinoembryonic antigen A blood protein marker associated with colon cancer and other conditions

carcinogenesis The transformation of benign cells into malignant ones

carcinoma A malignant neoplasm of epithelial cells

carcinoma in situ Carcinoma that has not penetrated below the basement membrane of the epithelium from which it arose

cardiac output The volume of blood pumped by the heart per unit of time

cardiac shunt A defect that diverts blood from one side of the heart or great vessels to the opposite side

cardiac troponin A protein originating only from cardiac muscle; normally exists in low concentration in blood

carrier An asymptomatic person or animal harboring an infective agent

caseous necrosis Necrosis caused by tuberculosis infection

catalyst A substance, usually used in small amounts relative to the reactants, that modifies and increases the rate of a reaction without being consumed in the process

cataract Opacity of the lens of the eye

catecholamines A group of related compounds including adrenal medullary hormones epinephrine and norepinephrine, which act to resist stress; also includes the neurotransmitter dopamine

CD antigens T-cell receptor antigens; different types of T cells have different CD antigens

cellular immunity See *delayed immunity*

chancre An ulcer that is the initial infection site in primary syphilis

chlamydia A type of common gram-negative microorganism causing chronic conjunctivitis (trachoma) and genital infections

Chlamydia trachomatis A bacterium; the agent of trachoma and most nongonococcal sexually transmitted disease

cholesterol A lipid found in animal tissue and some foods, synthesized by the liver; an important part of cell membranes and a precursor to steroid hormones; important in the development of atherosclerosis

chorionic gonadotropin One of the gonadotropins; a hormone produced by the placenta that has the same effect as luteinizing hormone

choroid In the eye, the dark-brown vascular layer of the retina immediately beneath the rods and cones; anteriorly is continuous with the ciliary body and iris

choroid plexus In the brain, specialized vascular projections in the ventricles that produce cerebrospinal fluid

chromosome In humans, one of 46 sets of DNA; the structural carrier of hereditary characteristics

chronic A condition that usually begins slowly, with signs and symptoms that are difficult to interpret, persists for a long time, and generally cannot be prevented by vaccines or cured by medication

cilia Hair-like processes extending from the surface of a cell; larger than microvilli; capable of rhythmical motion to move nearby fluid or objects

clinical pathology The study of the functional aspects of disease by laboratory study of tissue, blood, urine, or other bodily fluids

clone A set of identical cells descended from a single ancestor

clostridium One of a family of large, Gram-positive, anaerobic bacteria

Clostridium botulinum A bacterium; the agent of botulism and source of the cosmetic agent Botox©

Clostridium difficile A bacterium; the agent of pseudomembranous colitis

Clostridium perfringens A bacterium; the agent of gas gangrene

Clostridium tetani A bacterium; the agent of tetanus

clot A gelatinous mixture of fibrin, plasma, and trapped blood cells normally formed to stop hemorrhage

clotting system A set of proteins that interact with one another to cause blood to clot

coagulation Clotting; part of the normal response to hemorrhage; normally the production of a fibrin clot outside the vascular space by action of the coagulation system

coagulative necrosis A gel-like change in blocks of freshly dead cells in which cell outlines remain microscopically visible

Coccidioides immitis A fungus, the agent of coccidioidomycosis

coccus A round bacterium

colic Crampy pain

collagen A structural protein; a major component of scars, cartilage, bone, tendon, and connective tissue

complement system A set of proteins that interact with one another to promote inflammation and attack agents of infectious disease

complete blood count Laboratory assessment of the amount of blood hemoglobin and the number and types of blood cells and platelets

concussion A period of temporary brain dysfunction following head injury

condyloma acuminatum A wart-like growth of the anogenital region, caused by human papillomavirus

congenital Present at birth

congenital deformation Birth defect resulting from maternal mechanical factors

congenital malformation Birth defect resulting from abnormal embryologic development; usually genetic

congestion Passive vascular dilation resulting from hydrostatic forces

conjugated bilirubin Bilirubin soluble in water; bilirubin joined to glucuronide

consumptive coagulopathy Intravascular coagulation, which consumes clotting factors

contagion The spread of infection from one host to another

contusion   Blunt force injury that results in local hemorrhage

cornea   The clear, domed, anterior aspect of the eyeball

corpus luteum   The yellow endocrine body formed in the ovary from a ruptured graafian follicle; secretes estrogen and progesterone to prepare the endometrium for implantation of a fertilized ovum; disappears if pregnancy does not occur; persists if pregnancy occurs

cortex   The outermost layer of an organ

cortical bone   The dense, outer layer of bone

corticosteroids   Hormones secreted by the adrenal cortex: cortisol, aldosterone, testosterone, and others

cortisol (hydrocortisone)   An adrenocortical hormone that increases glucose production, inhibits peripheral glucose utilization, resists stress, suppresses immune reactions, and limits inflammation

Corynebacterium diphtheriae   A bacterium; the agent of diphtheria

C-reactive protein   A protein made by the liver in increased amounts in response to inflammation anywhere in the body

creatine kinase   A family of enzymes found in high concentration in myocardium

creatinine   A metabolic product formed in muscle that is one of the principal wastes in blood and urine

cross-eye   See *strabismus*

crust   In dermatology, a surface collection of dried serum and cell debris

Cryptococcus neoformans   A fungus; the agent of cryptococcosis

Cryptosporidium parvum   A protozoan; an opportunistic pathogen; a cause of severe diarrhea in AIDS

cul de sac   A cavity or pouch open at one end only; in female anatomy, the pouch of peritoneum posterior and inferior to the uterus

cyst   A rounded, closed space lined by a distinct layer of cells that contains fluid or semisolid material; in dermatology, a closed space beneath the epidermis that contains fluid or semisolid material

cystitis   Inflammation of the urinary bladder

cytogenetic   Relating to disease caused by extra or missing chromosomes, or abnormalities of large parts of chromosomes

cytology   The study of individual cells; usually collected for the assessment of potential malignancy

cytomegalovirus   A virus; one of the TORCH pathogens of fetal infection; an opportunistic pathogen in AIDS

cytoplasm   The fluid part of a cell inside the cell membrane and outside the nucleus; contains cell organelles

cytotoxic reaction   See *type 2 hypersensitivity*

cytotoxic T cell   Killer T cell; T cells programmed to attack foreign antigen

darkfield microscopy   A microscopic technique for clinical identification of syphilis bacteria and other spirochetes

dehiscence   Rupture of a healing wound

dehydration   Abnormally low water concentration in body fluids

delayed hypersensitivity   See *type 4 hypersensitivity*

delayed immunity   T-cell immunity; T cells directly attack antigen; no antibody is produced

dementia   A deterioration of mental abilities, such as memory, attention span, and reasoning, resulting from brain disease

demyelinating disease   Disease that affects the myelin sheath of nerve tracts or peripheral nerves

denervation   Loss of nerve supply

deoxyribonucleic acid (DNA)   A very large molecule that constitutes most of a cell nucleus and whose structure contains the genetic code; genes are composed of DNA

depressant   A drug with a depressive or sedative effect

dermis   The fibrous layer of skin beneath the epidermis

dexamethasone suppression test   A diagnostic test that depends on the ability of dexamethasone to suppress cortisol production in healthy patients; cortisol production is not affected in patients with Cushing syndrome

diaphysis   The center shaft of a long bone

diarrhea   An excessive number of liquid stools

diastole   Relaxation of cardiac muscle and refilling of chambers with blood

diffusion   Movement of molecules from an area of high concentration to a region of lower concentration

diploid   The number of chromosomes (46 in humans) resulting from the union of one sperm and one ovum

diplopia   Double vision

disease   An unhealthy state resulting from the effects of injury

dislocation   The displacement of one bone in a joint so that the articular surfaces no longer meet

diuresis   Increased urine output in response to therapy or change in physiologic condition

diverticulum   A blind pouch with a mouth opening onto the lumen of a space

DNA   See *deoxyribonucleic acid*

dominant   In genetics, a powerful gene in one chromosome of a pair of autosomes; can cause development of its trait without a matching allele in the companion chromosome

dose An amount of medicine or toxin

Down syndrome The clinical characteristics associated with having three copies (instead of two) of chromosome 21

duct A tubular canal, especially one carrying glandular secretions

duodenum The first part of the small bowel; attached to the stomach

dysentery Severe diarrhea with cramping and watery stools containing blood, pus, and mucus

dysmenorrhea Painful menstruation

dysphagia Difficult swallowing

dysplasia A premalignant hyperplasia of cells

dystrophic calcification Abnormal calcification occurring secondary to inflammation or necrosis

dystrophy A degenerative disorder, especially of nerve or muscle cells, in which cells become damaged or do not develop properly

dysuria Painful urination

ecchymosis Hemorrhage larger than 1 cm

ectocervix That portion of the female cervix that projects into the upper vagina

ectoparasite Small insect-like creatures that attach to or live in the skin

ectopic Out of place; misplaced

ectropion A rolling outward of the margin of a body part, especially the eyelid in trachoma, or with glandular metaplasia of the ectocervix

eczema Inflamed, crusted skin with vesicles

edema A collection of excess fluid in tissue or a body space

efferent arteriole The arteriole carrying blood away from the glomerulus

effusion Edema fluid collections in pleural, peritoneal, or pericardial space

electrocardiogram A record of the microvoltage transmitted to skin by each heartbeat

electrophoresis A laboratory method for separating substances according to molecular weight and electrical charge

embolus A mass that travels from one place to another inside the vascular system

empyema An accumulation of pus in a body space

emulsion A suspension of small globules of one liquid (fat) in a second liquid (water) in which the first would not otherwise mix

endemic The normal or expected rate of disease or infection in a population

endocardium Cells lining cardiac chambers

endocervical canal A channel from the external cervical os to the endometrium

endocrine Pertaining to ductless glands whose secretions (hormones) enter the bloodstream directly

endometrium The lining mucosa of the uterus

endoplasmic reticulum A network of membranes in cell cytoplasm; some contain ribosomes (rough ER) and synthesize protein; others contain no ribosomes (smooth ER) and synthesize steroids and break down drugs and other substances

endothelium The cellular lining of all blood vessels and the heart

endotoxin A toxin produced by some bacteria and released upon destruction of the bacterial cell wall

Entamoeba histolytica A protozoan intestinal parasite; the agent of amebiasis

Enterobius vermicularis A small intestinal roundworm parasite; the agent of pinworm infection

enterocolitis An inflammation of the bowel associated with diarrhea; almost always infectious

enterohepatic circulation Secretion by the liver of bile acids and other compounds, portions of which are reabsorbed into blood by the bowel and returned to the liver

enzyme A protein that increases the rate of a chemical reaction

eosinophilia Increased numbers of eosinophils in tissue or blood

eosinophils Leukocytes with large, red cytoplasmic granules that react to allergens and parasites

epicardium The external surface membrane covering the heart

epidemic More than the normal or expected rate of disease or infection in a population

epidermis A layer of epithelial cells that forms the skin surface

epinephrine (adrenalin) An adrenal medullary hormone stimulated by stress, which causes bronchial dilation; increases metabolic rate, heart rate, and respiratory rate; and increases blood pressure by vasoconstriction

epiphyseal growth plate A layer of cartilage near the end of long bones, from which bone growth occurs by forming cartilage on the advancing side, which is turned into bone on the trailing side

epiphysis A cap of dense bone at the end of a long bone

epithelium A sheet of cells that covers or lines a body surface

Epstein-Barr virus The agent of infectious mononucleosis; also associated with some malignancies, especially lymphoma

erythrocyte Red blood cell

erythrocyte sedimentation rate A laboratory test; the rate at which red blood cells settle in their own plasma; increased in response to inflammation anywhere in the body

erythrocytosis See *polycythemia*

erythropoietin A kidney hormone that stimulates erythrocyte production in the bone marrow

essential hypertension Abnormally high blood pressure of unknown cause

estrogen Any one of several steroid hormones produced chiefly by the ovaries; promotes growth of the endometrium and the development and maintenance of female secondary sex characteristics

ethanol (grain alcohol) The intoxicant in alcoholic drinks

etiology The cause of disease

euploid Having a normal set of chromosomes (in humans, 46)

eustachian tube An air-filled tube that connects the middle ear with the back of the nose and throat

euthyroid Normal thyroid metabolism

excitatory-conduction system A network of specialized cardiac muscle cells that transmit a wave of electrical impulse through the heart to cause contraction (systole)

exocrine Pertaining to glands whose secretions are excreted from the gland via a system of ducts

exocytosis The expulsion of large particles or packets from a cell; the opposite of phagocytosis

exophthalmos (proptosis) Abnormal protrusion of the eyeball

exotoxin A toxic substance secreted by a living bacterium and released into the medium in which it grows

extramedullary hematopoiesis The production of blood cells in organs other than the bone marrow

extrinsic coagulation pathway The combination of blood coagulation factors activated by blood contact with extravascular tissue

exudate High-protein edema fluid accumulation owing to inflammation

fallopian tubes Muscular tubes that extend from the uterus to the ovary; allow passage of sperm outward and fertilized or unfertilized ova inward to the endometrium

false negative An observation or measurement that incorrectly suggests the absence of disease

false positive An observation or measurement that incorrectly suggests the presence of disease

familial Referring to hereditary disease or genetic influence

fat (lipid) Any of various soft, solid, or semisolid organic compounds including triglyceride, cholesterol,

and related compounds that occur especially in the adipose tissue of animals and in the seeds, nuts, and fruits of plants

fecalith A small ball of dried fecal matter

ferritin An iron-protein complex that is a store of bone marrow iron

FEV₁ See *forced expiratory volume in one second*

fibrillation Fine, rapid twitching of individual muscle fibers without effective muscle function

fibroid A benign uterine smooth muscle tumor; a uterine leiomyoma

fibrosarcoma A malignant tumor of fibrous cells

fibrosis Fibrous repair; scarring; an accumulation of collagenous tissue in response to injury

fissure A groove or crack-like lesion

folic acid A vitamin necessary for normal blood cell production

follicle 1. A roughly spherical mass of cells usually containing a cavity; 2. A crypt, such as the skin depression from which hair sprouts

follicle-stimulating hormone A gonadotropin; the hormone released by the pituitary that in the ovary stimulates follicle maturation and ovulation and in the male stimulates sperm production

follicular lymphoma A type of lymphoma featuring microscopic lymphoid follicles

fomite An inanimate object that carries an infective agent

forced expiratory volume in one second (FEV₁) A rate measurement that is the volume of air expelled from maximum inspiration in the first second of effort

forced vital capacity (FVC) A volume measurement that is the amount of air expelled from maximum inspiration to maximum expiration, regardless of time

Frank-Starling law The fundamental principle of myocardial contraction: the force of contraction is proportional to initial fiber length

fructosamine A protein-glucose combination in plasma; formed in increased amounts in patients with diabetes

FSH See *follicle stimulating hormone*

full term A pregnancy of 38–40 full weeks

fungus A microorganism larger than a bacterium; has a nucleus and can reproduce outside of cells; grows as branching chains of filaments (hyphae) or round buds (yeast)

FVC See *forced vital capacity*

gamma globulin The fraction of plasma protein containing antibodies (immunoglobulins)

gastrin A hormone secreted by the stomach that promotes gastric acid secretion, pancreatic enzyme production, and intestinal peristalsis

gene A segment of DNA that codes for a specific protein to be made by a cell; chromosomes are formed of multiple genes

genotype The genetic characteristics of a condition

germ cell Specialized ovarian or testicular cells from which ova and sperm are derived by reduction division (meiosis)

German measles See *rubella*

gestational age Length of time in the womb

Ghon complex The initial lung lesion (Ghon tubercle) of arrested pulmonary tuberculosis and associated lesions in nearby lymph nodes

Giardia lamblia A protozoan intestinal parasite; the agent of giardiasis

Gleason score A microscopic method for grading the potential aggressiveness of cancer of the prostate

glia All neural cells in the central nervous system except neurons

globulin All blood proteins that are not albumin; especially gamma globulins

glomerular filtrate Fluid that passes from blood in the glomerulus into the Bowman space and then into renal tubules

glomerulus A tuft of capillary loops projecting into the Bowman space, where the glomerular filtrate is separated from blood

glucagon A hormone produced by alpha cells of the pancreatic islets of Langerhans; elevates blood glucose level by stimulating conversion of stored glycogen to glucose; promotes the breakdown of body fat for energy use

glucose tolerance test A diagnostic test for diabetes involving the measurement of blood glucose level before and several times after oral administration of a standard dose of glucose to a fasting patient

glycohemoglobin Hemoglobin with glucose attached; normally present in low levels; increased in diabetics

glycosuria Glucose in urine

goiter An enlarged thyroid

Golgi apparatus Hollow structures in cell cytoplasm that perform a "post office" function by accepting and packaging incoming and outgoing materials

gonad An organ that produces reproductive cells (gametes); the ovary or testis

gonadotropin A hormone that stimulates the gonads

graafian follicle A fluid-filled vesicle in the ovary that contains a maturing ovum

grading In the study of malignancies, microscopic estimation of the degree of malignancy

Gram stain A laboratory dye process that colors bacteria red or blue-black

gram-negative Red bacteria after Gram stain

gram-positive Blue-black bacteria after Gram stain

granulation tissue A highly vascular mix of capillaries, fibroblasts, edema, and leukocytes occurring as part of the repair process

granulocytes The leukocytes of acute inflammation, which contain large cytoplasmic granules

granulocytosis Increased numbers of granulocytes in blood

granulomatous inflammation A special type of chronic inflammation occurring in tuberculosis and other conditions; features inflammatory nodules (granulomas)

gray matter Collections of neuron cell bodies in the central nervous system

group B streptococcus A variety of streptococcus; a cause of neonatal and urinary tract infections

group D streptococcus A variety of streptococcus; a frequent cause of bacterial endocarditis

growth fraction The fraction of the cells in a tumor that are dividing at any moment

growth hormone (somatotropin) A hormone of the anterior pituitary that promotes growth of tissues

gynecomastia Enlargement of the male breast owing to an increased amount of breast gland tissue

hallucinogen A drug that distorts perceptions of reality

haploid The number of chromosomes (23 in humans) contributed by one sperm or one ovum

HDL cholesterol (high-density lipoprotein cholesterol) Cholesterol attached to high-density lipoprotein; so-called "good cholesterol"

healing A type of fibrous repair that occurs after injury when regeneration of normal anatomy and function is not possible

health The absence of disease

Helicobacter pylori A bacterium; a cause of chronic gastritis; the agent of most peptic ulcer disease

helminth A parasitic worm

helper T cells T cells that promote B-cell immunity

hemangioma A benign tumor of blood vessels

hemarthrosis Bleeding into a joint

hematemesis Vomiting blood

hematochezia Passage of red, unaltered blood in stool

hematocrit The percentage of blood volume occupied by erythrocytes

hematoma A localized mass of hemorrhaged blood

hematuria Intact red blood cells in urine

hemodynamic pressure Blood pressure; the force required to move blood through the vascular tree; the product of cardiac output and vascular resistance

hemoglobin The red, oxygen-binding protein of erythrocytes, which transports oxygen from lungs to tissue

hemoglobin A Molecularly normal hemoglobin

hemoglobin A1C See *glycohemoglobin*

hemoglobin S The molecularly abnormal hemoglobin of sickle cell disease

hemoglobinopathy A genetic disorder of hemoglobin synthesis

hemolysis Premature destruction of red blood cells

Haemophilus influenzae A bacterium; an agent of middle ear infections and meningitis in children, and pneumonia in adults

hemoptysis The coughing of blood or of blood-streaked sputum

hemorrhage The escape of blood from blood vessels

hemorrhagic diathesis Bleeding beyond the expected amount for a certain injury, or bleeding without obvious injury

hemostasis The collective blood vessel and blood coagulation response to prevent or stop hemorrhage

hepatic lobule The basic histologic unit of the liver, consisting of masses of liver cells arranged around a central vein (a terminal branch the hepatic vein), at the periphery are branches of the portal vein, hepatic artery, and bile duct

hepatitis virus One of a family of five viruses (A–E) that cause hepatic infection

hepatocyte The main functional (parenchymal) cell of the liver

hereditary Transmissible from parent to child by DNA carried in ova or sperm

hernia The protrusion of a bodily structure through the wall that normally contains it

herpesvirus A family of viruses causing common oral cold sores and genital infections; one of the TORCH pathogens of fetuses

heterophil antibody An antibody typically found in the blood of patients with infectious mononucleosis

heterozygous For a genetic characteristic, having nonidentical genes (alleles) at a particular site in a pair of chromosomes

high-density lipoprotein See *HDL cholesterol*

hirsutism The growth of dark, thick hair in women in locations where hair is normally minimal or absent

histologic Pertaining to the microscopic structure of the tissues of organisms

Histoplasma capsulatum A fungus; the agent of histoplasmosis

HIV See *human immunodeficiency virus*

homeostasis A balanced, steady state in the body; physiologic equilibrium

homozygous For a genetic characteristic, having identical genes (alleles) at a particular site in a pair of chromosomes

hookworm An intestinal roundworm parasite

hormone A chemical produced by a cell and capable of influencing cell function

host An infected person or animal

HPV See *human papillomavirus*

human immunodeficiency virus (HIV) A virus that causes failure of the immune system by infecting and killing T lymphocytes; the agent of AIDS

human papillomavirus (HPV) A family of viruses that cause skin and genital warts, and genital dysplasia or cancer

humoral immunity B-cell immunity

hydatidiform mole A benign tumor-like overgrowth of placental cells caused by abnormal combinations of ovum and sperm

hydrocephalus An excessive accumulation of cerebrospinal fluid in or around the brain

hydrocortisone See *cortisol*

hydrolysis Metabolic modification or breakup of a chemical compound by reaction with oxygen and hydrogen derived from water

hydropic change A reversible accumulation of excessive water in cells as a result of cell injury or stress

hydrostatic pressure The force exerted on blood vessel walls by the weight of a column of fluid blood

hyperemia Active vascular dilation owing to inflammation

hyperglycemia Abnormally high blood sugar

hyperopia Blurred vision caused by foreshortening of the globe; images focus behind the retina; farsightedness

hyperplasia Increased numbers of cells; increased size of an organ owing to increased numbers of cells

hypersensitivity An exaggerated immune reaction to certain antigens or other molecules

hypertension Abnormally high blood pressure

hyperthyroid Abnormally high thyroid metabolism

hypertrophy Increased size of a cell; increased size of an organ owing to increased cell size

hypoalbuminemia Low plasma albumin level

hypochromic Pertaining to an erythrocyte with low hemoglobin concentration

hypogammaglobulinemia Low plasma gamma globulin level

hypothalamus Part of the brain immediately above the pituitary, which controls the pituitary

hypothyroid Abnormally low thyroid metabolism

hypoxia Inadequate oxygenation

iatrogenic Caused by diagnostic procedure or treatment

idiopathic Of unknown cause

IgA antibodies Immunoglobulin A antibodies; a special class of antibodies heavily concentrated in breast milk and in respiratory tract and gastrointestinal mucus

IgG antibodies Immunoglobulin G antibodies; late-appearing antibodies that provide long-term immunity

IgM antibodies Immunoglobulin M antibodies; early-appearing antibodies that provide quick immune defense

ileum The final part of the small bowel; follows the ileum and attaches to the colon; absorbs digested foodstuffs, bile acids, and vitamin B_{12}

ileus Paralysis of intestinal peristalsis

immediate hypersensitivity See *type 1 hypersensitivity*

immune The special function of lymphocytes and macrophages that defends the body against foreign substances and infectious agents

immune complex See *type 3 hypersensitivity;* an antigen-antibody combination

immune surveillance The antineoplastic function of the immune system

immunodeficiency A condition of impaired immunity

immunoglobulin The class of proteins from which antibodies are made

impetigo A contagious, superficial skin infection of preschoolers, usually caused by streptococci

incidence The number of new cases of disease that appear per year

incubation period The time between invasion of an infective agent and appearance of signs or symptoms

infarct Pathologic death of a block of cells fed by a common vascular supply

infection Invasion of the body by an infectious agent that results in tissue injury and inflammation

infertility The inability of a couple to conceive after one year of regular intercourse

inflammation The combined response to injury by local blood vessels, blood cells, plasma proteins, and tissue

influenza virus One of several types of viruses that cause severe respiratory infections in humans and animals, especially birds

inhalant A substance other than air inhaled into the lungs; usually not beneficial

inoculation Invasion of the body by an infective agent

insulin A polypeptide hormone secreted by beta cells in the islets of Langerhans in the pancreas; promotes glucose uptake and utilization by cells, protein syn-

thesis, and the formation and storage of lipids in body fat

interatrial septum A fibrous wall separating the right and left atria

interstitial space The space between adjacent cells

interstitium A gap or space between functional units of an organ; usually contains blood vessels, nerves, lymphatics, and supporting tissue

interventricular septum A muscular wall separating the right and left ventricles

intrinsic coagulation pathway The combination of blood coagulation factors activated by blood contact with foreign surfaces such as glass, metal, or plastic

intrinsic factor A protein secreted by the stomach, which binds to vitamin B_{12} and enables B_{12} absorption in the ileum

introitus The vaginal opening

intussusception A reversible telescoping of bowel, in which the distal (downstream) segment swallows the proximal one

invasiveness The ability of a neoplasm to invade tissues, especially basement membrane, blood vessels, and lymphatics

iridocyclitis Inflammation of the iris and ciliary body

ischemia Hypoxia owing to poor arterial blood flow or low blood oxygen content

islets of Langerhans Clusters of endocrine cells scattered throughout the pancreas that secrete insulin, glucagon, and somatostatin

jaundice A yellow discoloration of skin owing to abnormally high blood bilirubin level

jejunum The second part of the small bowel; follows the duodenum; digests foodstuffs

joint A place where two bones meet

juxtaglomerular apparatus A cluster of cells in the wall of the afferent arteriole of the glomerulus that sense blood pressure and secrete renin to adjust it

karyotype Photographic display of all chromosomes arranged in numerical order

keloid A hyperplastic scar that contains excessive collagen

keratitis Inflammation of the cornea

keratopathy Any noninflammatory disease of the cornea

ketones Small, acidic molecules that are the product of fat metabolism in diabetic patients lacking sufficient insulin to burn glucose

killer T cell   See *cytotoxic T cell*

kinin system   A set of molecules that interact with one another to promote vasodilation and increase endothelial cell permeability

Kupffer cell   A liver macrophage

Kussmaul respirations   Deep, regular, driven breathing

kyphosis   An abnormal, forward curvature of the spine

labia majora   The two outer rounded, thick folds of skin and fat lateral to the vaginal orifice; form the outer margin of the vulva; the female counterpart of the scrotum

labia minora   The two delicate inner folds of mucosa medial to the labia majora, which frame the vaginal orifice

labile cells   Rapidly dividing cells with a short life span that continuously regenerate from stem cells

laceration   Tearing of tissue

lamellar bone   The layered design of normal adult bone; has a tree-ring-like pattern

Langerhans cell   Specialized immune-system macrophages of skin

LDL cholesterol (low-density lipoprotein cholesterol)   Cholesterol attached to low-density lipoprotein; so-called "bad cholesterol"

leiomyoma   A benign tumor of smooth muscle cells

lentigo   Pigmented, nonneoplastic, localized hyperplasia of melanocytes

leptin   An anti-obesity hormone secreted by fat cells

lesion   A structural abnormality caused by disease

leukemia   A malignant proliferation of leukocytes in which malignant cells appear in blood

leukocytes   White blood cells; the primary cells of the inflammatory response to injury

leukocytosis   Increased numbers of leukocytes in blood

leukopenia   Abnormally low numbers of leukocytes in blood

leukoplakia   A patch of white squamous mucosa

LH   See *luteinizing hormone*

lichenified   In dermatology, an area of skin with thickening of the epidermis and exaggeration of normal skin lines; caused by chronic rubbing or scratching

ligament   A fibrous strap joining two body parts

lipase   A fat-digesting enzyme

lipids   Complex organic chemicals, including the fats, oils, and triglycerides, that are insoluble in water and oily to the touch; together with carbohydrates and proteins, the most common material of cells

lipoprotein   Blood lipid attached to an apoprotein; usually classified by density (high or low)

liquefactive necrosis   Liquification of dead cells

lordosis   An abnormal, backward curvature of the spine

low-density lipoprotein   See *LDL cholesterol*

lower urinary tract   The ureters, bladder, and urethra

lupus anticoagulant   An antibody found in some patients with systemic lupus erythematosus, which interferes with laboratory coagulation tests and produces a false suggestion of coagulation deficiency

luteinizing hormone (LH)   A gonadotropin; the hormone released by the pituitary that in the ovary stimulates development of the corpus luteum after ovulation, and in the male stimulates testicular production of testosterone

lymphadenopathy   Abnormally enlarged lymph nodes

lymphedema   High-protein edema caused by lymphatic obstruction

lymphocytes   Leukocytes that mediate immune reactions; the principal cells of chronic inflammation

lymphocytosis   Increased numbers of lymphocytes in blood

lymphoid   Pertaining to lymphocytes

lymphoma   A malignant neoplasm of lymphoid cells in which no malignant cells appear in blood

lymphopenia   Abnormally low number of lymphocytes in blood

lysosomes   Cytoplasmic packets of digestive enzymes

macrocytic   Pertaining to an abnormally enlarged cell, usually an erythrocyte

macrophages   Large phagocytic leukocytes important in inflammation and immunity

macula   In the eye, a small and highly sensitive part of the retina directly in line with the line of sight; responsible for detailed, central vision

macule   In dermatology, a flat, discrete, discolored lesion less than 1 cm in diameter

major blood groups   Strong red cell antigens that determine A, B, and O blood groups

major histocompatibility complex (MHC)   Human lymphocyte antigen complex; a family of genes important in the immune system; responsible for most immune rejection of organ transplants

malignant   Capable of causing death

malignant hypertension   Extremely high blood pressure

malignant melanoma   A malignant tumor of melanocytes

malnutrition   Deficiency of calories or essential nutrients

mammography   Specialized breast x-rays

Mantoux test   A test for tuberculosis performed by injecting an extract of tuberculosis protein into skin and observing the reaction

marker In cancer biology: a substance produced by normal or neoplastic tissue that can appear in increased amounts in blood in association with malignancy and other conditions

mass effect The local, pressure, or size effect of a neoplasm on adjacent tissue or structures

MCHC See *mean cell hemoglobin concentration*

MCV See *mean cell volume*

mean The average of quantitative measurements

mean cell hemoglobin (MCH) The amount of hemoglobin in an average erythrocyte

mean cell hemoglobin concentration (MCHC) The average concentration (weight per volume) of hemoglobin in erythrocytes

mean cell volume (MCV) The size of an average erythrocyte

medullary cavity The hollow central part of a long bone that contains bone marrow

megakaryocyte The bone marrow cell that produces platelets

megaloblastic anemia An anemia characterized by enlarged erythrocytes

meiosis Reduction division; cell division in germ cells of the ovary or testis, during which in humans the number of chromosomes is reduced from 46 in the germ cell to 23 in the ovum or sperm

melanocyte The pigment-producing cell of epidermis

melanoma See *malignant melanoma*

melasma Facial skin darkening associated with pregnancy

melena Black, tarry stool containing blood from intestinal hemorrhage that has been altered by intestinal juices

membrane potential The electrical potential difference (voltage) across a cell membrane

memory cells Immune B or T cells programmed by prior antigen exposure to linger in the body and proliferate quickly on reexposure to antigen

Mendelian Referring to rules of genetic inheritance for monogenic (single gene) characteristics

meningococcus *Neisseria meningitidis*; a bacterium; the agent of epidemic bacterial meningitis

menopause The normal, age-related cessation of ovulation and menstruation

menorrhagia Excessive bleeding at the time of regular menstrual flow

mesentery A broad fold of peritoneum that attaches to bowel and encloses arteries, veins, and lymphatics to the bowel

metabolic rate Energy consumption per unit of time; varies with rest or exercise; influenced by thyroid and adrenal medullary hormones and activity of the autonomic nervous system

metaphysis The flared, wide, distal end of a long bone

metaplasia Change of one cell type into another

metastasis The ability of a tumor to spread from one place to another

metrorrhagia Irregular bleeding between periods

MHC See *major histocompatibility complex*

microbe A minute life form; especially a bacterium that causes disease

microbial culture Laboratory growth of microbes for identification

microcytic Pertaining to an abnormally small cell, usually an erythrocyte

microglia Macrophages of the central nervous system

microscopic hematuria See *occult hematuria*

microvascular disease Disease of small blood vessels, especially in diabetes

microvilli Tiny, parallel, hair-like projections of cell membrane; smaller than cilia

micturition Urination

minor blood groups Weak red cell antigens that are not part of the ABO group

mitochondria Small structures in the cell cytoplasm that produce cell energy

mitosis The division of one cell into two identical daughter cells

mitotic figure The appearance of the nucleus of a cell during mitosis

mitral valve The one-way valve that separates the left atrium from the left ventricle

mold A type of fungus that at normal body temperature grows as long, branching filaments (hyphae)

molecular mimicry The mechanism by which similarity of some foreign antigens to self-antigens is the cause of some autoimmune disease

monilia See *Candida albicans*

monoclonal protein Immunoglobulin made in excess in patients with multiple myeloma or other plasma cell disorder

monocytes Large phagocytic leukocytes important in chronic inflammation and immune reaction

monogenic Caused by a single gene

monosomy Having only one copy of an autosomal gene instead of two

motor unit The organizational unit of the neuromuscular system: a lower motor neuron, the motor end plate (neuromuscular junction), and skeletal muscle cell

M-protein See *monoclonal protein*

M-spike The appearance of an M-protein on protein electrophoresis

mucinous Thick, like mucus

mucosa A membrane lining all body passages that open directly to the environment and having cells or associated glands that secrete mucus

mutagenic Capable of causing DNA mutation

mutation An abnormal, permanent change in DNA

mycobacterium One of a family of bacteria that cause tuberculosis and leprosy

Mycobacterium avium A bacterium; the agent of avian (bird) tuberculosis; an opportunistic pathogen in AIDS

Mycobacterium leprae A bacterium; the agent of leprosy

Mycobacterium tuberculosis A bacterium; the agent of human tuberculosis

mycoplasma The smallest bacteria; can exist without oxygen

myelin A fatty, white substance made by Schwann cells, which sheaths axons

myeloid Pertaining to erythrocytes, monocytes, megakaryocytes, and granulocytes

myelophthisis Bone marrow scarring or destruction

myocardium Cardiac muscle

myoglobin An iron-containing molecule in skeletal muscle similar to hemoglobin, binds oxygen in muscle

myometrium The thick, muscular wall of the uterus

myopathy Any generalized noninflammatory disease of muscle that is not muscular dystrophy

myopia Blurred vision caused by elongation of the globe; images focus in front of the retina; nearsightedness

myosin One of the two contractile proteins in muscle cells (the other: actin)

myxedema 1. A clinical term for hypothyroidism; 2. A type of hard edema of skin most often seen in patients with hypothyroidism but sometimes in patients with normal thyroid function

narcotic Any one of several physically and mentally addictive drugs derived from the opium poppy, the cocoa plant, and synthetic drugs with similar effect; reduce pain and induce euphoria and either stimulation or sedation

necrosis Pathologic death of cells owing to disease

negative feedback Activity by the target organ of an endocrine hormone that opposes activity of the gland that produced the hormone

Neisseria gonorrhoeae A bacterium; the agent of gonorrhea

Neisseria meningitidis See *meningococcus*

neonatal The first month after birth

neoplasia The formation of a neoplasm

neoplasm An uncontrolled growth of new cells, benign or malignant

nephrolithiasis Stones in the kidney

nephron unit A glomerulus and its associated renal tubule

nephropathy Disease of the kidney

nephrosclerosis Disease of kidney small blood vessels related to blood pressure or diabetes

nephrosis Childhood renal disease that in adults is called nephrotic syndrome; characterized by marked proteinuria (albuminuria), hypoalbuminemia, and generalized edema

neuron The main parenchymal (functional) cell of the brain

neuropathy Disease of peripheral nerves

neutropenia Abnormally low number of neutrophils in blood

neutrophilia Increased number of neutrophils in blood

neutrophils Leukocytes with large, tan granules that are the principal cells of acute inflammation

nevus A benign tumor of melanocytes

nicotine A chemical stimulant in tobacco, responsible for the addictive quality of smoking

nocturia Urination at night

nodule A discrete, solid mass; in dermatology, a firm, raised lesion that is larger and deeper than a papule

norepinephrine An adrenal medullary hormone stimulated by stress, which increases blood pressure by powerful vasoconstriction

normal A measurement or observation falling into the usual range in a healthy person

normal range An established span for quantitative tests that have numerical results

normochromic Pertaining to an erythrocyte with normal hemoglobin concentration

normocytic Pertaining to a cell of normal size, usually an erythrocyte

nosocomial Referring to hospital-acquired infection

nucleotide base One of several small molecules that is a building block for DNA and RNA

nucleus The largest cell organelle, which contains DNA and controls all cell function; in the brain: a collection of neurons

nystagmus Rapid, involuntary repetitive motion of one or both eyes

occult bleeding Undetected bleeding; usually intestinal

occult hematuria Blood in urine not visible to the naked eye

occult proteinuria An excessive amount of protein in urine without clinical signs or symptoms

occupational disease Work-related disorders

oligodendrocyte A cell of the central nervous system that wraps around axons and makes myelin

oligomenorrhea Prolonged menstrual cycles

oliguria Less than normal urine output

omentum A fold of peritoneum between stomach and colon that serves as a store of fat and hangs in front of the small bowel like an apron

oncogene A gene that causes the transformation of normal cells into tumor cells

oncology The study of neoplasms

oocyte An ovarian germ cell; develops into an ovum

opportunistic pathogen Infectious agents that rarely cause disease in patients with healthy immune systems; most often infect patient with immune deficiency

optic disc A coin-shaped, pale spot on the retina where the optic nerve joins the eye

organelle A small, specialized structure in a cell

organic Pertaining to carbon-containing compounds that are the constituents of all living things

os Mouth; an anatomic opening

osmosis Movement of solvent (in biology: water) across a semipermeable membrane from the high-solvent concentration side to the low-solvent concentration side

osmotic edema See *transudate*

osmotic pressure Pertaining to solvents (in biology, water) separated by a semipermeable membrane: the amount of hydrostatic pressure that must be applied to a solution on the side with low-concentration of solvent (water) to prevent solvent from the high-concentration of solvent side from crossing the membrane

osteoblast Bone-forming cells

osteoclast Bone-dissolving cells

osteoid Bone protein, which is mineralized to form bone

osteomalacia A qualitative defect of bone structure characterized by defective mineralization (calcification) of bone protein (osteoid)

osteoporosis A quantitative defect of bone structure characterized by increased bone porousness and decreased bone mass

ovulation Ejection of an ovum from a ruptured graafian follicle

ovum The female reproductive cell or gamete

oxytocin A hormone secreted by the posterior pituitary that stimulates uterine contractions in labor

panniculitis Inflammation of subcutaneous fat

pannus A pathologic vascular membrane; especially over the cornea or a joint surface

Papanicolaou smear (Pap smear) Cells collected from the cervix for microscopic examination, especially as a screen for dysplasia or cancer

papilledema Edema of the head of the optic nerve where it enters the globe at the optic disc

papilloma An epithelial tumor with cauliflower or fern-like fronds that protrudes from an epithelial surface

papule In dermatology, a firm, raised lesion less than 0.5 cm in diameter

paraneoplastic syndrome A far-reaching set of effects of a neoplasm; usually caused by hormone production

parasite A disease-causing organism that lives on or in a human or animal and derives nourishment from its host

parathormone (PTH) The hormone produced by the parathyroid gland; increases blood calcium by mobilizing bone calcium, increasing intestinal calcium absorption, and decreasing kidney calcium excretion

parenchyma The specialized cells that perform the main functions of an organ

patch In dermatology, a flat, discrete, discolored lesion larger than a macule

pathogenesis The natural history and development of disease

pathology The study of changes in bodily structure and function that occur as a result of disease

pedunculated Attached by a long, thin base

peptic ulcer An intestinal ulcer associated with gastric secretions; usually in the stomach or duodenum

peptide A compound containing two or more linked amino acids

pericardium The sac in which the heart sits

perinatal The period of time from the 28th week of pregnancy to the seventh day after birth

periosteum A tough, fibrous outer membrane covering all bones

peristalsis Waves of smooth muscle contraction that move intestinal contents down the bowel

peritoneum The lining layer of cells in the abdominal cavity, which covers the bowel and parts of other viscera

permanent cells Cells that cannot regenerate and must last a lifetime

petechiae Tiny hemorrhages; usually resulting from platelet abnormality

phagocytosis The ingestion of bacteria and other large particles into a cell; the opposite of exocytosis

phenotype The physical expression of a genetic condition

photoaging Excessive wrinkling and sagging of skin owing to chronic sun overexposure

photosensitivity An exaggerated skin reaction to sunlight

pituitary stalk A bundle of nerves and blood vessels that connects the pituitary gland to the brain

placenta accreta Placenta implanted abnormally deeply in the uterine wall

placenta previa Abnormal implantation of the placenta in the lower part of the uterus

plaque 1. In dermatology, a raised, flat-topped, superficial lesion larger than a papule; 2. On teeth, an accumulation of bacteria, dead cells, and mucus; 3. In arteries, an accumulation of atheromatous fat

plasma The liquid part of blood

plasma cell A characteristic-appearing B cell actively making antibodies

plasma cell dyscrasia An abnormal proliferation of plasma cells

plasma membrane A specialized layer of molecules that forms the outer surface of a cell and mediates exchange of material into and out of the cell

plasmodium A protozoan parasite that infects erythrocytes; the agent of malaria

platelet A minute, nonnucleated fragment of megakaryocyte cytoplasm that circulates in blood to promote clotting

pneumoconiosis One of a group of lung diseases caused by inhaled substances (inhalants)

Pneumocystis jiroveci A fungus; an opportunistic pathogen; frequently the cause of pneumonia in AIDS patients

pneumocytes Cells forming pulmonary alveoli

pneumonia Inflammation of the lung

pollutant A substance in air or water that can injure those exposed to it

polycythemia (erythrocytosis) Abnormally high numbers of erythrocytes in blood

polydipsia Unusually high volume of water intake, especially when associated with diabetes or other disease

polygenic Caused by multiple genes

polymenorrhea Short menstrual cycles

polyp A mass protruding from the epithelial lining of an organ

polypeptide A long chain of peptides forming a small protein or part of a large protein molecule

polyphagia Unusually high volume of food intake, especially when associated with diabetes or other disease

polyuria More than normal urine output

poorly differentiated Referring to a neoplasm having few recognizable microscopic features of the tissue of origin

portal vein The vein that carries blood from the intestine to the liver

posterior chamber In the eye, the space behind the iris and in front of the lens

posterior pituitary The neurohypophysis; the posterior lobe of the pituitary, which secretes antidiuretic hormone

posterior segment In the eye, the entire globe behind the cornea, iris and lens

post-term Infants born after 42 weeks

predictive value In medical testing, the ability of a test to correctly indicate the presence or absence of disease

premalignant A state of tissue capable of becoming malignant

premature Born before the end of the 37th week of pregnancy

presbyopia Age-related loss of lens ability to focus on nearby objects

prevalence The number of people who have a disease at any given moment

prion A transmissible (infective) protein without DNA or RNA but capable of causing disease; no metabolism; not a living thing

progesterone A steroid hormone, mainly secreted by the corpus luteum of the ovary and placenta; stimulates development of secretory endometrium to prepare it for implantation of the fertilized ovum; sustains pregnancy and promotes development of the breasts

prognosis The likelihood of recovery from a disease

prolactin The pituitary hormone that stimulates milk production by the breast

prolapse A sagging or slipping out of place; in the heart, a turning inside-out of valve leaflets; for the uterus, a sagging into the vagina

proptosis Bulging eye; exophthalmos

prostate-specific antigen A protein made by the normal prostate that circulates in blood at low levels and which is increased in blood in various prostate conditions, especially carcinoma of the prostate

protease A protein-digesting enzyme

protein A very large polypeptide; a complex organic molecule that is a very long chain of amino acids; together with lipids and carbohydrates, the most common material of cells

proteinuria An abnormal amount of protein in urine

proto-oncogene A gene that stimulates cell growth and has the potential to change into an oncogene

protozoa Motile, single-cell microorganisms with a nucleus

pseudocyst A localized collection of fluid without an organized cell lining

Pseudomonas aeruginosa A bacterium; an opportunistic pathogen; a cause of infections in debilitated or hospitalized patients

PTH See *parathormone*

pulmonary valve The one way valve separating the right ventricle from the pulmonary artery

purpura Hemorrhage less than 1 cm in diameter

purulent Relating to the accumulation of pus in acute, severe inflammation

pus In acute inflammation, an accumulation of thick, creamy fluid composed of liquefied cell debris

pustule In dermatology, a small, superficial abscess

pyogenic Relating to acute, purulent inflammation

pyogenic granuloma Persistent granulation tissue

pyuria White blood cells in urine

radioactive iodine uptake A diagnostic test that determines the rate of thyroid uptake of a test dose of radioactive iodine

rapid plasma reagin (RPR) test A simple blood test for syphilis antibodies

Raynaud phenomenon An exaggeration in fingers or toes of normal vasoconstriction and vasodilation (vasomotor) reactivity to cold or emotional stress

receptor A protein molecule designed to attach and hold other proteins

recessive In genetics, a weak gene that for expression of its trait requires an identical gene (allele) at the same point in its companion chromosome

red cell Erythrocyte

red cell indices Measures of the size and hemoglobin content of the average erythrocyte

red infarct A bloody block of necrotic tissue caused by venous or arterial obstruction in loose, spongy tissue or tissue with a dual blood supply, especially the lung

Reed-Sternberg cell A cell characteristic of Hodgkin disease

reflux Backwards flow

regeneration The complete or nearly complete restoration of normal anatomy and function by the regrowth of functional cells

renal tubules Tubes formed of kidney epithelial cells, which adjust the glomerular filtrate to form urine by absorbing more or less water and other substances

renin A kidney hormone important in blood pressure regulation

repair The collective attempt to restore normal structure and function after injury

reservoir A place or animal from which infective agents spread

respiratory syncytial virus (RSV) The agent of bronchiolitis

reticulocyte A freshly made red blood cell

retinopathy Any disorder of the retina

rhabdomyolysis Sudden necrosis of skeletal muscle with release of large amounts of myoglobin into blood

rheumatoid factor An antigen-antibody complex in blood usually associated with rheumatoid arthritis

rhinovirus One of a group of viruses responsible for many upper respiratory infections

Rh negative Red cells not carrying Rh D antigen

Rh positive Red cells carrying Rh D antigen

ribonucleic acid (RNA) A large molecule, formed by imprint from DNA, that carries genetic commands to the cell cytoplasm

ribosomes Small structures in the cell cytoplasm that produce proteins by instruction from DNA

rickettsia Tiny gram-negative bacteria that cannot live outside of cells

RNA See *ribonucleic acid*

RPR test See *rapid plasma reagin test*

RSV See *respiratory syncytial virus*

rubella A virus; one of the TORCH pathogens of fetal infection; the agent of rubella (German measles)

saccharides The basic building block of sugars and other carbohydrates

salmonella A bacterium; one of several salmonella species that cause bacterial diarrhea

salpingitis Inflammation of the fallopian tube

sarcoma A malignant neoplasm of mesenchymal tissue

scale In dermatology, a superficial, thin, plate-like flaking of shedding epidermal cells

schistosome One of a family of worms (helminths); an agent of schistosomiasis

scoliosis An abnormal lateral bending of the spine

secondary hypertension Abnormally high blood pressure owing to a specific cause

sella turcica A bony cradle at the base of the skull that contains the pituitary

semicircular canals Fluid-filled, arced tubules of the inner ear that sense motion

semipermeable membrane A membrane allowing free passage of solvent (in biology: water) but not of dissolved substances

sensitivity In medical testing, the ability of a test to be positive in the presence of disease

sepsis Systemic bacterial infection

septicemia Severe blood infection, usually by bacteria

serous Watery

serum The fluid remaining after blood clots; differs from plasma in that serum contains no fibrinogen

sessile Attached by a broad base

sex chromosome A chromosome that determines sex and influences other characteristics; in humans there are two: X and Y

sex-linked recessive A trait or disease requiring only a single copy of a recessive gene on the X chromosome

sexually transmitted disease Any of various diseases usually obtained via sexual intercourse or other sexual contact

shigella A bacterium; one of several shigella species that cause shigellosis, a bacterial diarrhea

shock Circulatory collapse; a state of systemic low blood flow

sickle cell disease A disorder of hemoglobin synthesis caused by having two copies of the hemoglobin S gene; homozygous hemoglobin S genotype

sickle cell trait The condition of having a single copy of the hemoglobin S gene; heterozygous hemoglobin S genotype

signs Direct observations by an examiner

sinoatrial (SA) node A focus of specialized cardiac muscle in the right atrium that originates the electrical signal causing each heartbeat

sinusoid A venous cavity through which blood passes in various glands and organs

small for gestational age Infants weighing less than predicted for gestational age

soft tissue Nonepithelial tissue that is not bone, cartilage, brain or nerve, meninges, bone marrow, or lymphoid tissue; mainly fat, skeletal and smooth muscle, and fibrous tissue

solid joint A joint where bones are connected by dense, fibrous tissue, have no joint cavity, and provide little movement

somatic cell Cells that are not germ cells; form all organs except parts of the testis and ovary

somatotropin See *growth hormone*

specificity In medical testing, the ability of a test to be negative in the absence of the disease

sperm The male reproductive cell or gamete

spirochete Corkscrew-shaped bacterium

spirometry The process of measuring the lung capacities and volumes

sprain A stretch injury to a ligament

sprue Passage of excessively fatty stools

squamocolumnar junction A point where glandular and squamous epithelium meet; especially in the cervix and gastroesophageal junction

stable cells Slowly dividing cells with a long lifespan that regenerate quickly from stem cells after injury

staging In the study of malignancies, a clinical assessment of the extent of tumor spread

stalk effect Interference by a pituitary mass on normal hypothalamic inhibition of pituitary prolactin secretion, thereby allowing abnormal prolactin production

standard deviation A statistical measure of the degree of natural variability of quantitative results

staphylococcus One of a family of gram-positive cocci (round bacteria) that causes purulent infection that localizes into an abscess

Staphylococcus aureus A bacterium; one of the most virulent and common of staphylococci

statin A drug that reduces serum cholesterol by inhibiting liver synthesis of cholesterol

statistical Relating to the mathematics of the collection, organization, and interpretation of numerical data, especially the analysis of data by sampling a specific population

stem cells Primitive cells capable of quickly evolving into functional cells

stenosis Obstruction of a tubular structure, such as coronary artery, valve, or gland duct

steroids Chemical compounds that include cholesterol, bile acids, adrenal corticosteroids

stimulant A drug that produces enhanced awareness and euphoria

strabismus An abnormal alignment of one eye ("cross-eye")

strain A stretch injury to a tendon

streptococcus One of a family of gram-positive cocci (round bacteria) that cause purulent infections that tend to spread along superficial surfaces or tissue planes

Streptococcus pneumoniae A bacterium; the pneumococcus; the agent of lobar pneumonia

subluxation A minor joint dislocation

sugars Molecules with sweet taste that are composed of one or more saccharide molecules; names end in −ose

suppressor T cells T cells that suppress B-cell immune reaction

surfactant In human physiology, a soapy fluid secreted by pneumocytes that makes the lungs more easily expandable

symptoms Complaints reported by the patient or by someone else on behalf of the patient

synapse The junction across which a nerve impulse passes from nerve to nerve, or from nerve to muscle cell or epithelial cell

syndrome A collection of clinical signs, symptoms, and data

synechiae Fibrous adhesions between the iris and the lens or cornea

synovial cells Cells lining the joint space of synovial joints

synovial joint A joint where bones are connected by ligaments across a space lined by synovial cells, and which provides for a wide range of movement

systole Contraction of cardiac muscle and the ejection of blood from atria and ventricles

T cell T lymphocyte; a lymphocyte that is programmed to directly attack foreign substances (usually proteins)

T lymphocyte See *T cell*

T$_3$ See *triiodothyronine*

T$_4$ See *thyroxine*

tachycardia Rapid heartbeat

tapeworm An intestinal parasitic worm

tartar On teeth, calcified plaque

TBG See *thyroxine-binding globulin*

teratogen An agent capable of inducing congenital malformation

teratoma A tumor of ovarian or testicular germ cells that contains tissues not normally found in the ovary or testis, such as skin or brain

thrombocytopenia Abnormally low blood platelet count

thromboembolism The intravascular movement (embolization) of a thrombus from the site of its formation to another site

thrombophlebitis Formation of venous thrombi in response to local injury or abnormal blood flow

thrombus An intravascular pathologic accumulation of the solid elements of blood—platelets, leukocytes, and red cells—which forms owing to local factors and attaches to the lining of large blood vessels or inside the heart

thyroglobulin The protein in thyroid follicles that binds and stores thyroid hormones

thyroid-stimulating hormone (TSH) The hormone released by the pituitary that stimulates thyroid production and release of thyroxine (T$_4$) and triiodothyronine (T$_3$)

thyroid-stimulating immunoglobulin An autoimmune antibody that stimulates excessive production of thyroid hormones

thyroxine (T$_4$; tetraiodothyronine) A hormone produced by the thyroid gland that contains three iodine molecules; increases the rate of metabolism; less potent than triiodothyronine

thyroxine-binding globulin (TBG) A plasma protein to which circulating thyroid hormones are attached

tinnitus Ringing in the ears

TNM system A standardized method of cancer staging: <u>T</u>umor size, lymph <u>N</u>ode metastasis, distant <u>M</u>etastasis

TORCH complex Congenital fetal malformations induced by one of the TORCH teratogens

TORCH teratogens A group of infectious teratogens

toxin Any substance injurious to health or dangerous to life

Toxoplasma gondii A protozoan; one of the TORCH pathogens of fetal infection and an agent of retinitis in AIDS

transferrin A plasma iron-transport protein

transudate Low-protein edema fluid accumulation caused by hydrostatic or osmotic forces

trauma Injury to the body caused by violence or accident

Treponema pallidum A bacterium; the agent of syphilis

Trichinella spiralis A roundworm parasite that infects muscle; the agent of trichinosis

Trichomonas vaginalis A parasitic protozoan; the agent of trichomoniasis of the vagina and urethra in women and the prostate and urethra in men

tricuspid valve The one-way valve that separates the left atrium from the left ventricle

triglyceride A type of blood lipid; the chief constituent of body fat and dietary oils

triiodothyronine (T$_3$) A hormone produced by the thyroid gland that contains three iodine molecules; increases the rate of metabolism; more potent than thyroxine

trisomy Having three copies of an autosome instead of two

true negative An observation or measurement that correctly suggests the absence of disease

true positive An observation or measurement that correctly suggests the presence of disease

TSH See *thyroid-stimulating hormone*

tumor A mass; in everyday language, a neoplasm

tumor suppressor gene A gene that suppresses cell growth

tympanic cavity The hollow space of the middle ear; contains air and the auditory ossicles

tympanic membrane The eardrum; separates the external auditory canal from the middle ear

type 1 hypersensitivity Immediate hypersensitivity; a B-cell immune reaction between free antigen and preformed antibody

type 1 muscle fibers Slow twitch fibers

type 2 hypersensitivity Cytotoxic hypersensitivity; a B-cell immune reaction between antibody and antigen that is part of a cell

type 2 muscle fibers   Fast twitch fibers

type 3 hypersensitivity   Immune complex hypersensitivity; a B-cell immune reaction in which an antigen-antibody combination circulates and damages tissue where deposited

type 4 hypersensitivity   Delayed (or cellular) hypersensitivity; the only T-cell immune reaction

ulcer   A crater-like defect of skin or mucous membrane; usually slow to heal; in dermatology, a cavity not covered by epidermis

unconjugated bilirubin   Bilirubin not soluble in water; bilirubin not joined to glucuronide

urea   A metabolic product containing nitrogen that is the principal waste in blood and urine

uremia   Renal failure with clinical signs and symptoms

ureterovesical junction   The juncture of ureter and bladder

ureterovesical valve   The one-way valve effect of the anatomy of the ureterovesical junction, where the ureter enters the bladder

urinalysis   Laboratory analysis of urine

urinary tract   The kidneys, renal pelves, ureters, bladder, and urethra

urobilinogen   A metabolic product produced in the bowel from bilirubin excreted by the liver; gives stool its brown color

urolithiasis   Stones in the urinary tract

urticaria   A localized, acute allergic reaction that causes local vasodilation and increased vascular permeability featuring transient, pale or pink, firm, itchy streaks and papules

uveal tract (uvea)   The choroid, ciliary body, and iris

valvular insufficiency   Failure of a cardiac valve to maintain one-way flow

valvular stenosis   Constriction of a cardiac valve that impedes blood flow

varicosity (varicose vein)   An abnormally dilated vein

vascular resistance   The resistance to flow that must be overcome for blood to circulate

vasculitis   Inflammation of blood vessels, especially arteries

vasodilation   Dilation of blood vessels

vector   An intermediate carrier of infectious disease

venereal disease   Sexually transmitted disease

ventricle   One of the two anatomically lower, high-pressure chambers of the heart

vesicle   A small cystic space, especially one containing fluid; in dermatology, a fluid-filled cystic space less than 0.5 cm in diameter

Vibrio cholera   A bacterium; the agent of cholera

villous   Having small finger-like projections

virus   A submicroscopic parasite composed of a central core of DNA or RNA coated by protein; no metabolism; not usually considered a living thing

vitamin B$_{12}$ A vitamin necessary for normal blood cell production

vitiligo   Macules of white, depigmented skin

vitreous chamber   The large, spherical chamber of the eyeball

vitreous humor   The gelatinous fluid that fills the eyeball

volvulus   A twisting of a segment of bowel on its vascular stalk

vulva   The external female genitalia

wart   See *Verruca vulgaris*

watershed infarct   A brain infarct that occurs in a borderland area of the brain where two blood supplies meet

well differentiated   Referring to a neoplasm having recognizable features of the tissue of origin

wheal   A smooth, slightly elevated lesion that is reddish or pale and usually itchy

white cell   Leukocyte

white cell differential   Laboratory assessment of the number and type of white cells in circulating blood

white infarct   A bloodless block of necrotic tissue caused by arterial obstruction in dense, solid tissue

white matter   Myelinated axons (extensions) of neurons

wound   An injury resulting from short-term injury at a discrete site

woven bone   An interlaced pattern of bone fetal bone growth that is always pathologic in adults

xerostomia   Dry mouth

yeast   A type of fungus that at normal body temperature grows by rounded buds

Yersinia pestis   A bacterium; the agent of plague

zymogen   An enzyme precursor

Index of Case Studies

The table below is a quick-reference key to the common diseases and disorders discussed in the case studies that appear at the end of each chapter. It is arranged alphabetically by disorder, with cross-references to the case studies that contain information about the condition.

Disease/Disorder	Related Case Study		Page
AIDS	Case 8-1,	"I'm Afraid I Have AIDS"	173
Amniotic fluid embolism	Case 5-1,	"She's Gone"	83
Angina pectoris	Case 10-1,	"My Chest Feels Funny"	229
Barrett metaplasia of the esophagus	Case 2-1,	"This Heartburn is Killing Me"	31
Blood glucose testing	Case 1-2,	How High Is Up?	12
Bronchopneumonia	Case 9-1,	"I Knew She was Sick when She Didn't Want a Cigarette"	201
Cancer of the cervix	Case 21-1,	"I Can't Get Pregnant"	576
Carcinoma of the breast	Case 21-2,	"I Have a Lump in my Breast"	578
Carcinoma of the colon	Case 15-1,	"I'm in Great Shape"	384
Cholelithiasis	Case 17-1,	"He Drinks; I Don't"	443
Chronic obstructive pulmonary disease	Case 14-1,	Cigarette Asthma	349
Chronic salpingitis	Case 21-1,	"I Can't Get Pregnant"	576
Cigarette smoking, effects of	Case 9-1,	"I Knew She was Sick when She Didn't Want a Cigarette"	201
	Case 14-1,	Cigarette Asthma	349
Colon cancer	Case 11-1,	"I'm Tired and Short of Breath All the Time"	266
Diabetes mellitus	Case 4-1,	"You'd Think I'd Know Better"	62
	Case 1-2,	How High Is Up?	12
Dysplasia	Case 2-1,	"This Heartburn is Killing Me"	31
Fibromyalgia	Case 22-1,	"The Doctor Told Me I was Being Poisoned"	609
Glaucoma	Case 25-1,	"I'm Having a Different Kind of Migraine"	700
Glomerulonephritis, acute	Case 19-1,	"His Water Looks Like Coca-Cola"	506
Hepatitis C infection	Case 16-1,	"I Didn't Give it a Second Thought"	418
Hostility, patient	Case 3-1,	"My Doctor Thinks I'm Crazy"	48
Hypertension	Case 12-1,	A Man Found Dead in His Office	288
Hypothyroidism	Case 18-1,	"I'm Running Out of Gas"	475
Infant small for gestational age	Case 7-1,	"I Thought it Would Go Away"	140
Infertility	Case 21-1,	"I Can't Get Pregnant"	576
Influenza	Case 9-1,	"I Knew She was Sick when She Didn't Want a Cigarette"	201
Intestinal bleeding	Case 11-1,	"I'm Tired and Short of Breath All the Time"	266
Iron deficiency anemia	Case 11-1,	"I'm Tired and Short of Breath All the Time"	266
Lung cancer	Case 6-1,	"I Have a Chest Cold That Won't Go Away"	106
Melanoma, malignant	Case 24-1,	"She Fries Easier Than Bacon"	673
Meningitis, acute	Case 1-1,	A Diagnosis Missed and a Diagnosis Made	11
Metabolic syndrome	Case 10-1,	"My Chest Feels Funny"	229
Metaplasia	Case 2-1,	"This Heartburn is Killing Me"	31
Myocardial infarction, acute	Case 13-1,	"He's Been Having a Lot of Heartburn Lately"	319

Disease/Disorder	Related Case Study	Page
Nosocomial infection	Case 14-1, Cigarette Asthma	349
Obesity	Case 10-1, "My Chest Feels Funny"	229
Opportunistic infections	Case 8-1, "I'm Afraid I Have AIDS"	173
Otitis media, acute	Case 1-1, A Diagnosis Missed and a Diagnosis Made	11
	Case 25-2, "JuJu has a Fever"	701
Pancreatitis, acute	Case 17-1, "He Drinks; I Don't"	443
Paraneoplastic syndrome	Case 6-1, "I Have a Chest Cold That Won't Go Away"	106
Patient compliance	Case 12-1, A Man Found Dead in His Office	288
Pneumonia	Case 14-1, Cigarette Asthma	349
Polymyalgia rheumatica	Case 3-1, "My Doctor Thinks I'm Crazy"	48
Premature birth	Case 7-1, "I Thought it Would Go Away"	140
Respiratory distress syndrome of the newborn	Case 7-1, "I Thought it Would Go Away"	140
Sexually transmitted disease	Case 21-1, "I Can't Get Pregnant"	576
Shock	Case 5-1, "She's Gone"	83
Streptococcal pharyngitis	Case 19-1, "His Water Looks Like Coca-Cola"	506
Stroke	Case 12-1, A Man Found Dead in His Office	288
Stroke	Case 23-1, "Something Doesn't Seem Right in My Head"	644
Syphilis	Case 20-1, "A Spider Bit Me"	532
Test sensitivity and specificity	Case 1-1, A Diagnosis Missed and a Diagnosis Made	11
	Case 1-2, How High Is Up?	12
Uterine infection	Case 7-1, "I Thought it Would Go Away"	140
Vascular disease, peripheral	Case 4-1, "You'd Think I'd Know Better"	62
Wound healing	Case 4-1, "You'd Think I'd Know Better"	62

Index

Page numbers in *italics* indicate figures. Page numbers followed by "t" indicate tables. Words in bold indicate diseases or conditions.

A

Abdominal aortic aneurysm, *285*
Abdominal obesity, 225
Abortion, 565
Abrasion, 207
Abscess, 44, 313
Absolute risk, relative risk, distinguished, 571
Absorption, 355
Abuse, 217, 366
Accumulated secretions, 340
Accumulation of neutrophils, 42
Acetaminophen, 215
Acetylcholine, 622
Achalasia, 358, 365
Acidosis, 300, 436
Acids, 25
Acne, 177, 663
Acne rosacea, 663
Acne vulgaris, 663
Acoustic neuroma, 642
Acquired immunodeficiency syndrome, 168, 173
　infections, *194*
　pathologic features of, *171*
　phases of, *170*
Acromegaly, 456, *456–457*
ACTH adenoma, 457
Actin, 603
Actinic keratoses, 667, *667*
Addiction, 217
Addison disease, 473, *474*
　bronze skin pigmentation, *475*
Aden, 88–89
Adenocarcinoma, 89, 348, 366
Adenohypophysis, 450
Adenoma, 88, 455, 670
Adenomatous polyp, 380
Adenomyosis, 556, *557*
ADH. *See* Antidiuretic hormone
Adhesions, 379
Adrenal cortex, 284, 454
Adrenal gland, *454*
Adrenal hyperplasia, 471, *471*
Adrenal medulla, 454 chromaffin cells, 454
Adrenergic effect, 620
Adrenocortical adenoma, 469, *469*
Adrenocortical atrophy, 469
Adrenocortical hyperplasia, 468
Adrenocortical insufficiency, 472
Adrenogenital syndrome, 471, *471*, 472
Adult polycystic disease, 493
Adult respiratory distress syndrome, 338, *338*
Adventitia, 272

Afferent arteriole, 480, 483
African trypanosomiasis, 197
Age-related macular degeneration, 692
Agglutinins, 152–152t
Agranulocytosis, 249
Agriculture chemicals, 212
Agyria, 624
AIDS. *See* Acquired immunodeficiency syndrome
Air pollution, 210
Airflow, 328
Airway hyperreactivity, 332
Aktin, 667
Albinism, 657
Alcohol abuse, 398, 409, 427, 429
　cerebellar atrophy, *219*
　cirrhosis, 410
　effects of, *218*
　fatty liver of, *219*
　hepatitis, 410
　hypoglycemia, 442
　liver, *410*
　Mallory's alcoholic hyaline, 409
Aldosterone, 274, 454
Alkaline phosphatase, 585
Alkalis, 25
Alleles, 119
Allergens, 153, 159
Allergic alveolitis, 336
Allergic conjunctivitis, 159
Allergic contact dermatitis, 661
　eczema, *662*
Allergic rhinitis, 330
Allergy, 153, 159
Alopecia, 654
Alopecia areata, 654, *654*
Alopecia totalis, 654
Alopecia universalis, 654
Alpha-1 antitrypsin, 123, 333, 412
Alpha-1 antitrypsin deficiency, 123, 412
Alpha-fetoprotein, 106
Alveolar pneumonia, 339, *339*
Alveoli, 325
Alzheimer disease, 637, *638*
Amblyopia, 682
Amebiasis, 197, *198*
Amebic dysentery, 181, 374
Amenorrhea, 456, 555
Amino acids, 357
Aminoaciduria, 485
Amniocentesis, 130
Amniotic fluid, 79, *80*, 83
Amphetamines, 220
Ampulla of Vater, 358, 392, 423

Amyloid, 167
Amyloidosis, 167, *167*
Amyotrophic lateral sclerosis, 638, *638*
ANA. *See* Antinuclear antibodies
Anaerobic infection, 47, 177, 191, 359
Anagen phase, 652
Anal fissures, 378
Analgesic nephropathy, 503
Anaphylaxis, 154, 159
Anaplastic carcinoma, 465
Anasarca, 72
Anatomic pathology, defined, 4
Androgenic steroids, 454
Anemia, 240, 242–243, *244*, 246–247, 490
Anencephaly, 113–114, 624, *624*
Aneurysm, 277, 280, *629*
Aneurysmal bone cyst, 594
Angina, 281, 304
Angina pectoris, 229
Angiodysplasia, 370
Angioedema, 661
Angioma, 669, *669*
Angioneogenesis, 40, 44, 57, *58*, 97, 439
Angiosarcoma, 287, 572
Angiotensin, 274
Angiotensin-converting enzyme, 274
Ankylosing spondylitis, 164, 599, *599*
Annular pancreas, 427
Anorexia nervosa, 221
Anti-CCP. *See* Anticyclic citrullinated peptide
Anti-HAV antibodies, 403
Anti-phospholipid antibody, 266
Antibiotic sensitivity testing, *200*
Antibiotics, discovery of, 184
Antibody, 149, 404, 565
Anticyclic citrullinated peptide, 599
Antidiuretic hormone, 459
Antigen-anti-HBs, 404
Antigen-antibody complex, 152
Antigen exposure, antibody response to, *151*
Antigens, 148, 404
Antimicrobial protective mechanisms, *147*
Antimicrobial susceptibility, 200
Antimitochondrial antibody, 413
Antinuclear antibodies, 161
Antireagin antibodies, 529–530
Antitreponemal antibody, 529
Aorta
　misplaced, 317
　normal, *280*
Aortic aneurysm, thrombus, *280*
Aortic insufficiency, *310*
Aortic stenosis, *310*
Aortic valve disease, 294

Apgar score, 134
Aphthous ulcers, 363
Aplastic anemia, 247, *247*
Apnea, 283
Apoplexy, 627
Apoproteins, 275
Apoptosis, 24, 29
Appendicitis, 384, *384*
Aqueous humor, 679
Arachnoid granulations, 614
Arbovirus encephalitis, 637
Arcus senilis, 685, *686*
Arrhythmia, 297
Arteries, 271
Arteriole, *274*
Arteriolosclerosis, 277
Arteritis, 286
Arthritis, 162, 310
    joint changes in, *597*
    rheumatoid, *598*
Articular cartilage, 595
Asbestos, 210
Asbestosis, 336
Ascariasis, 196
Ascaris species, 196
Ascending cholangitis, 413, 417
Ascites, 72, 396, 398, *400*
Aseptic meningitis, 634
Aseptic necrosis, 589
Askos, 398
Aspergillus species, 92, 181
Aspiration pneumonia, 341
Aspirin, 214
Asterixis, 397
Asthma, 331, *332,* 349–350
Asthmatic bronchitis, 332, 334
Astigmatism, 684
Astler-Coller staging, 382–382t, *383*
Astrocytes, 622
Astrocytoma, 641, *642*
Asymptomatic hepatitis, 402
Atelectasis, 330, *331*
Atheroma, 277, *278*
Atherosclerosis, 277, *281,* 298, 303
Atherosclerotic debris, 79
Athletes' foot, 518
Atom, defined, 15
Atopic dermatitis, 159, *662*
Atopy, 159, 332
Atresia, 370
Atrial fibrillation, 298, 300
Atrial flutter, 298
Atrial septal defect, 316
Atrioventricular node, 295
Atrophic gastritis, 247, *368*
Atrophy, 28
Auditory nerve, 697
Auricle, 696
Autoimmune antibodies, 162
Autoimmune destruction, 434
Autoimmune disease, 160t
Autoimmune hepatitis, 407
Autoimmune reaction, 159
Autoimmune vasculitis, 243
Autoimmunity, 149, 153–154, 159, 309, 494,
    655
Autonomic nervous system, 613, 619, *621*
Autopsy, 4

Autosomal dominant, 119
Autosomal recessive, 119
Autosomes, 116
Avascular necrosis, 589
Avulsion, 601
Axons, 603, 620
Azoospermia, 517
Azotemia, 487, 490

B

B cells, 148–149. *See also* B lymphocytes
B lymphocytes, 45
Bacillary dysentery, 372
Back pain, 601
Bacteria, 47, 177, 181t, 187, 520.
    See also under specific bacteria
Bacterial culture, *200*
Bacterial cystitis, 515
Bacterial endocarditis, 312–313, *313*
Bacterial enterocolitis, 372, *373*
Bacterial pneumonia, *340*
Bacterial prostatitis, 520
Balanitis, 517
Balding, 397
Band keratopathy, 686, *686*
Band neutrophil, 251
Barbiturates, 220
Barrett esophagus, *366. See also* Barrett
    metaplasia
Barrett metaplasia, 31, 358, 366
Barrier effect, 484
Bartholin abscess, 545
Bartholin glands, 538
Bartonella henselae, 252
Basal cell carcinoma, 668, *668,* 697
Basal cells, 649
Basal ganglia, 637–638
Basement membrane, 16, 55, *55,* 272, 649
Basophils, 36, 38, 236
Becker muscular dystrophy, 606
Bell's palsy, 643
Bence Jones protein, 253
Bends. *See* Decompression sickness
Benign nephrosclerosis, 284, *498,* 498–499
Benign tumors, characteristics of, 93t
Benzodiazepines, 220
Beriberi, 222
Berry aneurysm, 629
Bicuspid aortic valve, 310
Bile, 392
Bile acids, 394
Bile duct, *391, 392*
Biliary atresia, 412, 417
Biliary cirrhosis, 397–398, 413, *413*
Biliary obstruction, 395
Biliary tract, 389–421
Bilirubin, 392
Bilirubinuria, 488
Biologic false positives, 530
Biopsy specimen, defined, 4
Birth defects, preventing, 114
Blackheads, 663
Bladder, 480
Bleb, 333
Bleeding/coagulation defects, 490
Bleeding disorders, 260–284, 397
    See also under specific disorder
    lab tests, 262

Bleeding time, 263
Blefaros, 684
Blepharitis, 684
Blindness, 691
Blood, composition of, *237*
Blood amylase, laboratory tests for, 430
Blood BUN, 486
Blood cells
    diseases, 235–260
    normal reference ranges, 236t
Blood circulation, 272, 316, 392
Blood coagulation, 234–269
Blood corpuscles, 39
Blood flow, disorders of, 65–85
Blood glucose testing, 12
Blood lipid abnormalities, 655
Blood pressure, 66, 282–283t
    functions, 67
    measuring, 282
    regulation of, *274*
Blood transfusion, *165*
Blood typing, 165
Blood urea nitrogen, 485
Blood vessels, 270–292
    anatomy of, *273*
BMI. *See* Body mass index
Body mass index, 224–225t
Bone, diseases of, 582–594
Bone anatomy, *584*
Bone infarcts, 589
Bone marrow malignancies, *250*
Bone tumors, primary, common sites of, *592*
Bony callus, 587
Borderline malignant, 561
Borrelia species, 137, 182, 187, 195, 600
Botulism, 193
Bowel obstruction, *362*
Bowen disease, 518, *518*
Bowman space, 481, 484
Brachial plexus, 619
Brain, 135, 162, *616*
    arterial blood supply to, *619*
    functional anatomy of, *617*
    lymphoma, 642
Brain abscess, 636, *636*
Brain edema, 626
Brain herniations, *625*
Breast, 303
    anatomy, *569*
    diseases of, 568–581
    fibrocystic change, *570*
    phyllodes tumor, *572*
Breathing, rapid, deep, 436
Brittle bone disease, 585
Broad ligament, 538
Broad-spectrum antibiotic therapy, 372
Bronchial dysplasia, 136
Bronchial epithelium, 340
Bronchiectasis, 335
Bronchiole, 325
Bronchiolitis, 137
Bronchitis, 333–334
    emphysema, relationship, *334*
Bronchogenic carcinoma, 347
    types of, *347*
Bronchopneumonia, 201, 339
Bronchus, 325
Brush border, 358

Bruton disease, 167
Budd-Chiari syndrome, 414
Bulimia, 221
Bulla, 333
Bullous pemphigoid, 659
Bundle of HIS, 296
Bunion deformity, 596
Burns, *209*
Bursitis, 601

C

C-reactive protein, 46, 280
Cachexia, 101
    of malignancy, *99*
Calcific aortic stenosis, 310, *312*
Calcitonin, 465
Calcium stone, renal pelvis, *504*
Calculi, 503
Calymmatobacterium granulomatis, 532
Campylobacter species, 164, 189, 372, 599
Canal of Schlemm, 693
Cancellous bone, 583
Cancer. *See also under* specific type
    causes of, *91*
    genetic inheritance, 100t
    treatments, 104t
Cancer of bladder, *516*
Cancer of breast, 105, 572t, *573, 575,* 578
Cancer of cervix, 105, 532, 545, *550,* 552,
    555, 576
Cancer of colon, 105, 266, 381, 382, 384–385
    Astler-Coller staging system, *383*
    clinical stages, 382t
Cancer of esophagus, 366
Cancer of larynx, 330
Cancer of lung, 105–106
    smoking, relationship, *217*
Cancer of pancreas, 431, *432*
Cancer of prostate, 105, *524*
Cancer of skin, 652
Cancer of testis, 520
Cancer of thyroid, 465
Cancer of uterus, 557
Candida species, 168, 181, 193, 345–346,
    363–364, 545, 568, 654
Candidiasis, 193, 346, 364, 545
Capillaries, 39
Capillary hemangioma, 287, 669
Caput medusa, 398
Carbohydrates, 357
Carbon monoxide poisoning, 210, *210*
Carbon particles, 27
Carbon pigment, intracellular accumulation
    of, *27*
Carcinoembryonic antigen, 106, 382, 576
Carcinogenesis, 91
Carcinogenic, 118
Carcinoma, 88, 571–572t
Carcinoma *in situ,* 94, *94,* 572
Carcinoma of bladder, *516*
Carcinoma of breast, 105, *573, 575,* 578
Carcinoma of cervix, 105, 532, 545, *550,* 552,
    555, 576
Carcinoma of colon, 105, 266, 381, *382,*
    384–385
    Astler-Coller staging system, *383*
    clinical stages, 382t
Carcinoma of esophagus, 366

Carcinoma of kidney
Carcinoma of larynx, 330
Carcinoma of liver
Carcinoma of lung, 105–106
    smoking, relationship, *217*
Carcinoma of ovary
Carcinoma of pancreas, 431, *432*
Carcinoma of prostate, 105, *524*
Carcinoma of skin, 652
Carcinoma of stomach, 359
Carcinoma of testis, 520
Carcinoma of thyroid, 465
Carcinoma of uterus, 557
Cardiac chambers, valves, *295*
Cardiac output, 273
Cardiac shunt, 315
Cardiac troponin, 307
Cardiac valves, 294
Cardiogenic shock, 81
Cardiomyopathy, 314–315
    dilated, *314*
Caries, 361
Carotid artery, *631*
Carpel tunnel syndrome, 602
Carrier state, 402, 407
Carriers, 184, 242
Cat scratch fever, 252
Catagen phase, 652
Cataract, 439, 686, *687*
    surgery for, 687
Catecholamines, 274, 454
Cavernous hemangioma, 287, 414
CBC. *See* Complete blood count
CEA. *See* Carcinoembryonic antigen
Celiac sprue, 374, 659
Cell death, 24
Cell repair, 51–64
Cellular hypersensitivity, *158*
Cellular immunity, 45, 158
Central nervous system, 613, *614*
Cerebellar tonsillar herniation, pontine
    hemorrhage secondary, *626*
Cerebellum, 613
Cerebral cortex, 637
    vascular malformation, *630*
Cerebral hemispheres, 613
Cerebral palsy, 136, 624, *624*
Cerebrospinal fluid, 614, *615*
    laboratory examination of, 635
Cerebrovascular accident, 627
Cerebrum, 613, *632*
Ceruloplasmin, 412
Cervical cancer, 532
Cervical epithelium, changes with age, *547*
Cervical erosion, 548
Cervical intraepithelial neoplasia, 549
Cervical plexus, 619
Cervicitis, 548–549
Cervix, 538, 550t, 552t
    ectropion, *548*
    Pap smear, 102, *102,* 549, *551,* 552–553,
    554
    squamocolumnar junction, *548*
Cestodes, 196
Chagas disease, 197
Chalazion, 684
Chancre, 189, 527, *527*

Chancroid, 532, 544
Charcot-Bouchard microaneurysms, 630
Charcot joint, 440
Chemical, 92, 275
Chemokines, 41
Chemotaxis, 41
Chest cold, 106–107
Chest pain, 229
Chickenpox, 137
Chimney sweeps' cancer, 211
Chlamydia, 181, 189–190, 195, 200, 340,
    515–516, 530–532, 545, 560, 568, 599,
    684
Cholangiocarcinoma, 415, 417
Cholangitis, 416, *416,* 417, *417*
Cholecystitis
Cholelithiasis, 415, *416–417*
Cholera, 189, 372
Cholestasis, 396
Cholesteatoma, 699
Cholesterol, 275–276, 279, 357
Cholesterol gallstones, 415, *416*
Cholinergics, 620
Cholinesterase, 603, 622
Chondrosarcoma, 593, *593*
Choriocarcinoma, 520, 566–567
Chorionic gonadotropin, 542
Choristoma, 139
Choroid, 682, 687
Choroiditis, 687
Christmas disease, 264
Chromosome, 17
    subdivisions of, *19*
Chronic disease, defined, 3
Chronic non-specific lymphadenitis, 252
Chronic nonbacterial prostatitis, 520
Chronic obstructive pulmonary disease, 332,
    349
Cigarette asthma, 349–350
Cigarette smoking, 279, 333, 349
    effects of, 201, *216*
    lung cancer, relationship, *217*
Cilia, 20
Ciliary body, 679
Ciliary muscle, 679
Circulating antigen-antibody complexes, 494
Circulation of blood, *272,* 316, 392
Circumcision, 511
Cirrhosis, 365, 394, 397, *397,* 398–398t,
    399–400, 413
CJD. *See* Creutzfeldt-Jacob Disease
CK-MB, 307
Classic hemophilia, 124
Clear cell carcinoma, 505
Cleft lip, 361
Cleft palate, 361
Clinical pathology, defined, 4
Clitoris, 537
Clone, 96, 252
Closed-angle glaucoma, 693
Closed fracture, 586
Clostridium, 193
Clostridium botulinum, 186
Clostridium difficile, 193, 372
Clostridium perfringens, 47, 193, 607
Clostridium tetani, 193, 607
Clotting system, 40, 76
CMV. *See* Cytomegalovirus

Coagulation, 30, 75, 78, 260
Coagulation factors, 262
Coagulative necrosis, 30, *30*
Coarctation of aorta, 318
Cocaine, 220
Coccidioides species, 188, 346
Coccidioidomycosis, 188, 346
Cochlea, 697
Cold sore, 191, 363, 664, *665*
Collecting systems, 480, 510
Colloid, 452, 463
Colon, 380, *381*
Colon cancer, 381
Colonic adenoma, 380
    dysplastic change in, *381*
Colonic adenomas, *380*
Comedo, 663
Comminuted fracture, 586
Common bile duct, 392, 423
Common colds, 187
Community-acquired pneumonia, 340
Compensated heart failure, 299
Complement system, 40, 154
Complete blood count, 237
Complete fracture, 586
Complete resolution, 44
Complex hyperplasia, 557
Components of blood, 38t
Compression atelectasis, 331, *331*
Compression fracture, 586
Concussion, 633
Conductive hearing loss, 699
Condyloma acuminatum, 189, 531, 544,
    546, 666
Condyloma lata, 528, *528*, 531, 545–546
Cones, 680
Confabulation, 218
Congenital abnormalities, 111, 114–115,
    139, 310, 370, 377, 471, *471*, *502*,
    517, 529
Congestive heart failure, 74, 298, *301*, 314
Congestive splenomegaly, cirrhosis, *399*
Conjugated bilirubin, 392, 396
Conjunctiva, 678, *685*
Conjunctivitis, 365, 684
Conn syndrome, 470
Consumptive coagulopathy, 76, 265
Contact dermatitis, 661
Contagion, 184
Contraction atelectasis, 331
Contrecoup injury, 633, *634*
Convalescence, 197, 402
Coombs tests, 165–166
COPD. *See* Chronic obstructive pulmonary
    disease
Cor pulmonale, 300, 335, 338
Cornea, 678–679, 682
Corneal dystrophy, 686, *686*
Corneal ulcer, 685
Coronary artery
    atherosclerosis, 298
    thrombosis, *304*
Coronary occlusion, 281
Coronary sinus, 295
Coronary thrombosis, 304
Coronary vasospasm, 304
Coronary veins, 295
Corpus albicans, 542

Corpus cavernosum, 510
Corpus luteum, 542
Corpus spongiosum, 510
Cortex, 454, 468, 614
Cortical hormones, 474
Cortisol, 454
Corynebacterium diphtheriae, 137, 187
Councilman bodies, 394, 409
Coup-contrecoup injury, 633, *634*
Coxsackie A or B, 314
Cradle cap, 658
Cranial nerves, 618
Craniopharyngioma, 455
Creatine kinase, 307, 606
Creatinine, 485–486
Crepitus, 596
Crescentic glomerulonephritis, *496*
Cretinism, 463
Creutzfeldt-Jakob disease, 181, 637
Crohn disease, 374, *375*, 375t, *376*
Croup, 137
Cryptococcosis species, 193, 346, 634
Cryptorchidism, 518, *518*
Cryptosporidiosis, 197
Cryptosporidium parvum, 193
CSF. *See* Cerebrospinal fluid
Cushing syndrome, 458, 468, *470–471*
    laboratory diagnosis of, 472
    pathogenesis of, *469*
Cutaneous lupus erythematosus, 660
Cyanosis, 316
Cystadenocarcinoma, 561
Cystic disease, 493, 561
Cystic fibrosis, 124, 431
    laboratory testing for, 139
    lungs in, *139*
Cystic hyperplasia, 557
Cystic medial degeneration, 285
Cystic serous tumor, ovary, *563*
Cysticercosis, 197
Cystitis, 515, *515*
Cystocele, 515, 560
Cytogenetic disease, 26, 117, 125, *129*
Cytokines, 41, 149
Cytomegalic inclusion disease, 193
Cytomegalovirus, 170, 193, 346
Cytoplasmic organelles, 19
Cytotoxic edema, 626
Cytotoxic hypersensitivity, *156*
Cytotoxic T cells, 149, 152, 158
Cytoxicity, 159

D

Dacryocystitis, 685
Dandruff, 658
Darkfield microscopy, 527
De Quervain thyroiditis, 464
Deafness, 677–703, *696*, 696–703, *698*
Decompression sickness, 79
Decreased cough reflex, 340
Deep mycoses, 346
Defective liver processing, 395
Deformations, 111
Degenerative disc disease, 601
Degenerative joint disease, 595
Degranulation, 37
Dehiscence, 61
Dehydration, 71, *371*

Delayed hypersensitivity, 158
Delayed immunity, 152
Dementia, 637
Dendrites, 620
Denervation, 605
Deoxyribonucleic acid. *See* DNA
Depressants, 220
Dermatitis, *658*, 662
Dermatitis herpetiformis, 659
Dermatofibroma, 669, *669*
Dermatomyositis, 607
Dermatophytes, 191, 665
Dermatophytosis, 664
Dermis, 651, 665
Dermoid cyst, *564*
Desmoid tumors, 608
Detectable, defined, 6
Developmental abnormalities, 111–115
Diabetes, 164, 277, 279, 433–434, *434–435*,
    654
    derivation of word, 434
    laboratory diagnosis, 441
    long-term complications of, *438*
    type 1, type 2, compared, 433
Diabetes insipidus, 459
Diabetes mellitus, 12, 433
Diabetic coma, 436, *437*
Diabetic glomerulosclerosis, 498
Diabetic nephropathy, 439
Diabetic nephrosclerosis, 439, *439*
Diabetic nodular glomerulosclerosis, 439
Diabetic peripheral neuropathy, 605, 643
Diabetic retinopathy, 439, *440*, 691
Diabetic ulcer, *656*
Diagnosis
    defined, 11
    tests in, usefulness of, 10–12
Dialysis, 486
Diaphysis, 583
Diarrhea, 188, 371
Diastole, 271, 297
Diet, 205–232
Dietary sodium, 283
Differentiated teratoma, 519
Diffuse axonal injury, 633
Diffuse lymphoma, 256
Diffusion capacity, 328
DiGeorge syndrome, 168
Digestive system, 355, *356–357*
Dilated capillaries, 42
Dilated cardiomyopathy, 308, 314, *314*
Dilutional anemia, 240
Dimorphic fungi, 346
Dioxin, 212
Diphtheria, 137
Diplopia, 17, 682
Direct contact, 184
Discoid lupus erythematosus, 660
Disease
    defined, 3
Dislocation, 601
Dissecting hematoma, 285
Disseminated intravascular coagulation,
    76, 243
Disuse atrophy, 605
Diverticulitis of colon, 377, *379*
Diverticulosis of colon, 377, *379*
Diverticulum, 377

DNA, 17, *22, 118*
repair system, 91
Dominant genes, 119
Donor plasma, 165
Donor RBCs, 165
Dopamine, 638
Down syndrome, 127, *128*
chromosomes in, *126*
Droplets, 184
Drug abuse, *220*
Dubin-Johnson syndrome, 396
Duchenne muscular dystrophy, 606
Ductal carcinoma, 572–573
Ducts, 423
Duodenum, 358, 368
Dura mater, 614
Dust cells, 328
Dyscrasia, 252
Dysentery, 189, 371
Dysfunctional uterine bleeding, 555
Dysmenorrhea, 555
Dysphagia, 330, 358, 365
Dysplasia, 29, 31, 94–95, 545, 549, *550–551*
Dysplastic nevus, 671
Dystrophic calcification, 31

E

Ear, 677–703, *698*
anatomy of, *696*
diseases of, 696–703, *698*
Ear lobe, keloid, *61*
Early diabetic retinopathy, 691
EBV, 170, 251
Ecchymosis, 75, *76*
Echinococcosis, 197
Eclampsia, 568
Ectocervix, 538
Ectoderm, 15
Ectoparasites, 182
Ectopic pancreas, 427
Ectopic pregnancy, 560, 565
fallopian tube, *566*
Ectropion, 548
Eczema, 662, *662*
Edema, 72, 490
Efferent arteriole, 480, 483
Effusions, 72, 300
Eggs, 197
Ejection fraction, 299
Electrical activity of heart, *296*
Electrocardiogram, 297
Embolus, 78–79
Embryonal carcinoma, 519–520
Emergency salt water therapy, 72
Emphysema, 333
bronchitis, relationship, *334*
microscopic development, *334*
Empyema, 416
cholecystitis with, *416*
Enchondroma, 593
End-stage renal disease, 492, 498
Endocardium, 294
Endocervical canal, 538
Endocervical polyp, 548, *548*
Endochondral ossification, 583
Endocrine system, 423–424, 448–478, *450*
Endoderm, 16

Endometrial adenocarcinoma, 557
Endometrial carcinoma, *559*
Endometrial cycle, *542*
Endometrial hyperplasia, 556, *558*
Endometriosis, 555, *556–557*, 560
Endometrium, 538
Endometrioid tumors, 561
Endomyocardial fibrosis, 315
Endoplasmic reticulum, 20
Endosteum, 583
Endothelial cell, 39, 69, 272, 278, 484
Endothelium, 272
Endotoxins, 81, 186
Entamoeba histolytica, 197, 374, 408
Enteritis, 188
Enterobius vermicularis, 196
Enterococcus, 313
Enterocolitis, 372
Enterohepatic circulation, 282, 392, *393*, 394
Entropion, 684
Enzymes, 122, 423, 622
Eosinophilia, 36, 38, 47, 196, 236, 251
Ependymal cells, 622
Ependymomas, 641–642
Epicardium, 293
Epidemic typhus, 195
Epidemics, 184, 402
Epidemiology, 100
Epidermal growth factor, 56
Epidermis, 648–673
neoplasms of, 665–677
normal, *650–651*
pigmentation, 657
Epidermoid cyst, 665, *666*
Epidermolysis bullosa, 659
Epididymis, 511
Epididymitis, 519
Epidural, 627
Epidural hematoma, 627, *628*
Epiglottitis, 137
Epinephrine, 454
Epiphyseal growth plate, 583
Epispadias, 517
Epithelial cells, 484, 561
Epithelial hyperplasia, 570
Epithelial malignancy, *94*
Epithelium, 16, 556
Epstein-Barr virus, 136–137, 170, 251
Equilibrium, 372
Erectile dysfunction, 517
Erection, 510
Erosions, 367
Eruptive xanthomas, 655
Erysipelas, 191, 664, *664*
Erythema migrans, 600
Erythema multiforme, 660
Erythema nodosum, 663
Erythrocyte sedimentation rate, 46, 48
Erythrocytes, 236
Erythrocytosis, 248
Erythropoietin, 236, 248, 480, 483
Escherichia coli, 183, 185, 191, 193, 340–341, 372, 502, 515, 520, 634
Esophageal hiatus, 358
Esophageal varices, 287, 365, *366*, 398
ESR. *See* Erythrocyte sedimentation rate
Essential hypertension, 283
Essential thrombocythemia, 259

Esterase, 487
Estrogen replacement therapy, 543
Ethanol, 217, 220
Etiology, defined, 4
Eunuch, 523
Euploid, 17
Eustachian tube, 697
Euthyroid, 452
Ewing sarcoma of bone, 594
Excess granulation tissue, 61
Exchange transfusion, 135
Excitatory-conduction system, 295
Excretory failure, 400
Exocrine, 423
Exocytosis, 20
Exophthalmos, 459, 684
Expansion defects, 315
Experimental evidence, 348
Exstrophy, 514
External auditory canal, 696
External ear, 696
External hemorrhoids, *371*
External hydrocephalus, 626
External respiration, 325
External urethral orifice, 537
Extracellular matrix, 55–56
Extrahepatic biliary obstruction, *418*
Extramedullary hematopoiesis, 258
Extraparenchymal, 627
Extravascularly, 76
Extrinsic coagulation pathway, 262
Exudate, 72, 349
Eye
anterior segment of, *681*
diseases of, 678–695
glaucoma, *694*
Eyelid, 678, *685*

F

Facial nerve, 697
Facies, Down syndrome, *128*
Factor V Leiden, 266, 337
Fallopian tube, 538, *539, 566*
False negative, 6
False positive, 6
Falx cerebri, 614
Familial hypercholesterolemia, 124
Familial polyposis, 381
Farmer's lung, 158
Fat necrosis, 31, 569
Fat solubility, 221
Fatigue, 266–267
Fatty heart syndrome, 227
Fatty liver of alcoholism, *219*, 409
Faulty meiosis, 129
Fecalith, 384
Female genitalia, 536–580, *538, 540*, 544t
Femur, osteoarthritis, *596*
Ferritin, 27
Fetal alcohol syndrome, 114, 134, 219
Fetal blood circulation, 316
Fetor hepaticus, 396
Fever blister, 363
Fibrillation, ventricular, 298, 309
Fibrinogen, 46
Fibrinous inflammation, 43, *43*
Fibroadenoma of breast, 571
Fibrocystic change of breast, 569–570, *570*

Fibrocyte migration, 57
Fibroepithelial polyp, *665*
Fibroid tumor of uterus, 558
Fibromatosis, 608
Fibromyalgia, 602, 609
Fibrosarcoma, 89, 594, 608
Fibrosis, 44
Fibrous cortical defect of bone, 593
Fibrous dysplasia of bone, 593
Fibrous histiocytoma
Fibrous joints, 594
Fibrous repair, 57, *57*
Fibrous xanthoma, atypical, 608
Filariasis, 196
Filum, 196
Fimbriated extremity, 538
Fine needle aspiration, 103
Fixed macrophages, 392
Flat bones, 583
Flatworms, 196
Floaters, 689
Fluid balance, disorders of, 65–85
Fluid flow, microcirculation, *69*
Foam cells, 279
Focal segmental glomerulosclerosis, 494
Folate, 246
Folic acid, 114, 246
Follicle, 540
Follicle cysts, 560
Follicle stimulating hormone, 458, 540
Follicles, 452
Follicular carcinoma, 465
Follicular lymphoma, 256
Food allergy, 159
Foot drop, 601
Foramen magnum, 618
Foramina of Luschka and Magendie, 614
Forced expiratory volume, 328
Forced vital capacity, 328
Fournier gangrene, 193
Fovea, 682
Fracture, 586
    complete, 586
    healing of, *588*
    types of, *587*
Frank-Starling curve, *299*
Frank-Starling Law, 299
Freckle, 657
Frostbite, 209
Frostnip, 209
Fructosamine, 439
FSH. *See* Follicle stimulating hormone
Fulminant hepatic failure, 402
Fulminant hepatitis, 402
Function, defined, 3
Functional disorder, defined, 5
Functioning adenoma, 455–456
Fundus, 358, 538
Fungi, 181, 188
Fusiform, 177, 285

G

Gallstones, 415, 427
Gamma globulin, 151
Ganglia, 620, 622
Ganglion cyst, 602, *602*
Ganglioneuroma, 643
Gas gangrene, 193, 607

Gastric stress ulcers, *368*
Gastrin, 358
Gastrinomas, 442
Gastritis, 189, 367, *367*
Gastroenteritis, 372, 490
Gastroesophageal junction, 358
Gastrointestinal bleeding, 359
Gastrointestinal infection, *188*
Gastrointestinal tract, 354–388
Gastroschisis, 370
Gaucher disease, 122
Gene inheritance, 17, 111, 117, *120–121*, 279
Genetic disease, 117t
    laboratory diagnosis in, 132
Genetic disorders, 116–132
Genetic enzyme deficiency, 395 –396
Genital herpes, 531
Genital ulcer, 527
Genitalia
    female, 536–580, *538, 540*, 544t
    male, 509–535, *512*
Genitourinary infections, *190*
Genotypes, 116, 152
Germ cells, 116, 561
    division of, 127
Gestational age, 133
Gestational diabetes, 436, 440
Ghon complex, 342
Ghon tubercle, 342
Giant cell arteritis, 286, 600–601
Giant cell tumor of tendon sheath, 602
Giardia species, 47, 181, 197, 372, 374
Giardiasis, 197, 374
Gigantism, 456
Gilbert syndrome, 395
Gingivitis, 363
Glaucoma, 439, 693, *694, 695,* 700
    surgery for, 687
Gleason score, 523
Glia, 622
Glioblastoma multiforme, 641, *642*
Glioma, 641
Global hypoxia of brain, 632
Global ischemia, *632*
Globe, 678–679
    internal anatomy of, *680*
Glomerular filtrate, 481, 483–484
    rate, 484
    tubular processing, *485*
Glomeruli, 481
Glomerulonephritis, 162, 491, 494–495, *495,* 497, 506
Glomerulus, 480, *492*
    anatomy of, *483*
Glucagon, 424
    metabolism of, *426*
Glucose, *426*
    production of, 454
Glucose-6-phosphate dehydrogenase
    deficiency, 242
Glucose tolerance test, 440, *441*
Glue ear, 699
Glutamic acid, 118
Gluten-sensitive enteropathy, 374
Glycogen metabolism, *426*
Glycogen storage disease, 123
Glycohemoglobin, 439
Glycosuria, 436, 489

Glycosylation, 438
Goblet, 358
Goiter, 459, 463, *463*
Golgi apparatus, 20
Gonadotropin-releasing hormone, 540
Gonococcus, 530
Gonorrhea, 189, 530, *531*
Gout, 600
Graafian follicle, 540, 560
Graft-*versus*-host reaction, 165
Gram negative, 177
Gram positive, 177
Gram stain, 177, *180,* 199, *531*
Granular endoplasmic reticulum, 20
Granulation tissue, 58, *59*
Granulocyte, 36, 236, 257
Granulocytosis, 251
Granuloma annulare, 661
Granuloma inguinale, 532, 544
Granulomas, 45, 159
Granulomatous enteritis, 374
Granulomatous inflammation, 45, *45,* 335, 341, 344
Granulomatous thyroiditis, 464
Granulosa cells, 539
Granulosatheca cell tumor, 563
Graves disease, 459
Gray matter, 614, 620, 637
Greenstick fracture, 586
Gross examination, defined, 4
Gross hematuria, 487
Growth factors, 56
Growth hormone, 456
Gunshot wound, *208*
Gynecomastia, 397

H

Haemophilus ducreyi, 532
Haemophilus influenzae, 137, 340, 634
Hallucinogen, 221
Hamartoma, 139, 347
Haploid, 17
Haptens, 149
Hashimoto thyroiditis, 464, *464*
Haversian canals, 583
Hay fever, 159
Hazardous materials, 212t
HbsAg, 404
HCV-RNA, 406
HDL cholesterol, 275
Healing by first intention, *60*
Healing by second intention, *60*
Health, defined, 6
Heart
    anterior view, *294*
    electrical activity of, *296*
Heart block, 298
Heart disease, 292–324
Heart failure, 74, 298, *301*
    compensated, 299
Heartburn, 31–32, 319–321
Heat cramps, 209
Heat exhaustion, 209
Heat stroke, 210
Heavy chain disease, 151, 253
Heberden nodes, 596
Helicobacter pylori, 47, 189, 367–369, 442
Helminths, 181, 195

Helper T cells, 152, 160
Hemangioma, 139, 287, 669, *669*
Hemarthrosis, 264
Hematemesis, 359, 367
Hematochezia, 359, 371
Hematocrit, 239
Hematologic diseases, 656
Hematomas, 75
    subdural, *629*
Hematopoiesis, *238*
Hematoxylin, 37
Hematuria, 489
Hemochromatosis, 243, 398, 410–411, *411*
    complications of, *411*
    primary, 410
    secondary, 411
Hemodynamic edema, 337
Hemodynamic pressure, 66
Hemoglobin, 237, 239, 241–242, 439
Hemoglobinopathies, 242
Hemoglobinuria, 489
Hemolysis, 237, 241, 243
Hemolytic anemia, 265
Hemolytic disease of newborn, 137
Hemopericardium, 319
Hemophilia, 124, 264
Hemoptysis, 330
Hemorrhage, 75, 247, 265
Hemorrhagic diathesis, 76, 263
Hemorrhagic gastritis, 367
Hemorrhagic pancreatitis, 427, 429, *429*
Hemorrhoids, 287, 370, *371*, 378, 398
Hemosiderin, 27
Hemostasis, 260, *261–262*, 263
Hemothorax, 349
Hepatic duct, 392
Hepatic encephalopathy, 397, 639
Hepatic failure, 396
Hepatic lobule, 392
Hepatic malfunction, 395
Hepatic sinusoids, 392
Hepatitis, 394, 401–401t, 402, *403*, 404,
    404–405, 406, *406*, 407, *407*, 418–419
Hepatocellular carcinoma, 414, *414*
Hepatocytes, 392
Hepatorenal syndrome, 397
Hereditary nonpolyposis colorectal carcinoma
    syndrome, 381
Hereditary polycystic kidney disease, *493*
Hereditary spherocytosis, 242
Heritable melanoma syndrome, 671
Hernia, 370
Herniated intervertebral disc, 601, *601*
Heroin, 221
Herpes virus infection of genitalia, 136, 190,
    363, 531, 544, 699
Herpetiformis, 659
Heterophil antibodies, 137, 251
Heterosexual, 191
Heterozygous, 119
Hiatal hernia, 358, 365
High-grade tumors, 516, 641
Highly sensitive tests, defined, 8
Highly specific tests, defined, 8
Hirschsprung disease, 370
Hirsutism, 654
Histamine, 38, 41
Histoplasma capsulatum, 181, 188, 346

Histoplasmosis, 188, 346
HIV. *See* Human immunodeficiency virus
HLA. *See* Human lymphocyte antigens
HNPCC. *See* Hereditary nonpolyposis
    colorectal carcinoma syndrome
Hodgkin lymphoma, 255, *256*
Homeostasis, 23, 449
Homocysteine, 279
Homoios, 23
Homozygous, 119
Hookworms, 196
Hordeolum, 684
Hormones, 23, *23*, 424, 449–450, 523
Horseshoe kidney, 493
Hostile patient, 48
HPV. *See* Human papillomavirus
Human immunodeficiency virus, 168, *169,*
    191, 654
    phases of, *170*
    T lymphocytes in, *169*
Human lymphocyte antigens, 149
Human papillomavirus, 189, 518, 531, 544,
    546, 549, 551
Humoral immune system, 45, 149
Hunner ulcers, 516
Hyaline arteriolosclerosis, 277, 284, *284*, 439
Hydatid disease, 197
Hydatidiform mole, 197, 566, *567*
Hydatis, 566
Hydrocele, 518
Hydrocephalus, 626, *626*, 627
Hydrochloric acid, 358
Hydrocortisone, 454
Hydrolysis, 357
Hydronephrosis, 500, *502*
Hydropericardium, 72
Hydropic change, 26
Hydrops fetalis, 138, *138*
Hydrostatic edema, 67, 72
Hydrostatic pressure, 67
Hydrothorax, 72
Hyperacute organ rejection, 164
Hyperaldosteronism, 470–471
Hyperammonemia, 397
Hypercalcemia, 466, 468
Hypercholesterolemia, *124*
Hyperchromatism, 93
Hyperemia, 74
Hyperglycemia, 433
Hyperkeratosis, 364
Hyperlipidemia, 492
Hypernephroma, 505
Hyperopia, 683
Hyperosmolar coma, 436
Hyperparathyroidism, 466, *466*, 467, *467*
Hyperplasia, 28, *29,* 557
Hyperplastic arteriolitis, 284
Hyperplastic arteriolosclerosis, 277
Hyperplastic polyp, 380
Hypersensitivity disease, 153, 158, 336
Hypersplenism, 260
Hypertension, 277, 279, 282–283, 288, 398,
    399, 400, 490
Hypertensive encephalopathy, 284
Hypertensive retinopathy, 284, 690
Hyperthyroidism, 452, 459, *460–461*
Hypertrophic cardiomyopathy, 314
Hypertrophy, 28, *28*

Hypoalbuminemia, 74, 397, 491
Hypogammaglobulinemia, 253
Hypoglycemia, 397, 442
Hypospadias, 517
Hypothalamus, 450, *451*
Hypothermia, 209
Hypothyroidism, 452, 460, *461*, 462, 475
Hypovolemic shock, 81
Hypoxia, 300

I

Iatrogenic, defined, 4
Iatros, defined, 4
Icterus, 392, 395
Idiopathic, defined, 4
Idiopathic dilated cardiomyopathy, 314
Idiopathic pulmonary fibrosis, 336
Ileitis, 374–375
Ileum, 358
Ileus, 361, 370
Immediate hypersensitivity, *155*
Immune cell neoplasms, 670
Immune complex, 154
Immune-complex hypersensitivity, *157*
Immune paint, 149, 328
Immune surveillance, 100
Immune system, 144–175, *148*, 154, *155–157,*
    158, *158,* 665
    sequence of, *150*
Immune thrombocytopenic purpura, 264
Immunodeficiency, 153, 167
Immunoglobulins, 45, 151, 168, 497
Impacted fracture, 586
Impaired fasting glucose, 435, 440
Impaired glucose tolerance, 440
Impetigo, 191, 664, *664*
Impotence, 517
Inadequate bone marrow red cell production,
    245
Incarcerated hernia, 361, *363*
Incidence, defined, 10
Increased blood bilirubin, 242
Increased intraocular pressure, 693
Incubation period, 197, 402
Incus, 697
Indicator-dilution principle, 71
Indirect contact, 184
Indivisible, defined, 15
Indoor pollutants, 210
Ineffective RBC production, 260
Inefficient pumping stroke, 298
Infarction, 30, *30, 80,* 313, 458
Infection, 182, 243, 247, 335, 342, 404, 500,
    567
    blood markers of, *403*
    natural course of, *199*
Infectious disease, 176–204
    agents of, *178*
    history of fight against, 183
    mortality from, 182t
Infectious mononucleosis, 136, 251, *251*
Infective endocarditis, 312–313
Infertility, 517, 561, 576
Inflammation, 34–50, *43, 44, 44,* 159, 279,
    517, 519, 643
    chain of events in, 37
    laboratory indicators, 47
    sequence of events in, 42

Inflammatory bowel disease, 374
Inflammatory carcinoma, 574
Inflammatory cells, 39, 45
Inflammatory edema, 72, 74
Inflammatory events, timing of, *41*
Inflammatory exudate, 42
Inflammatory myopathies, 164
Inflammatory response, elements of, *36*
Inflammatory state, 224
Influenza, 187, 201
Inguinal hernia, 361, 518
Initial functional disorder, defined, *5*
Initial structural disorder, defined, *5*
Initiating phase, 499
Injured cells, 42
Insulin, 424, *426*
Insulinomas, 442
Interatrial septum, 294
Intermittent claudication, 281
Internal hemorrhoids, *371*
Internal hydrocephalus, 626
Internal respiration, 325
Interstitial cystitis, 516
Interstitial fibrosis, *335*
Interstitial fluid, 69
Interstitial nephritis, 503
Interstitial pneumonia, 339
Interstitial space, 70
Interstitial tissue, 511
Interventricular septal defect, 294
Intervertebral disc disease, 601
Intestinal bleeding, 266, *360*
Intestinal phase malabsorption, 374
Intracardiac mural thrombus, *307*
Intracardiac thrombus, *78*
Intracranial tumors, *641*
Intraductal papilloma, 571
Intraductal papillomatosis, 571
Intramembranous ossification, 583
Intraocular pressure, 680
Intrauterine growth restriction, 134
Intravascular coagulation, 76
Intravenously injected illegal drugs, effects of, *220*
Intrinsic coagulation pathway, 262
Intrinsic factor, 247
Introitus, 537–538
Intussusception, 361
Ionizing radiation, 92, 465
Iridocyclitis, 687
Iritis, 687
Iron deficiency anemia, 241, 245–246, *246,* 266
Irritable bowel syndrome, 371
Irritant contact dermatitis, 662
Ischemia, 25, *80,* 499, 630
Ischemic cardiomyopathy, 307, 314
Ischemic heart disease, 302–303, 308
Ischemic optic neuropathy, 693
Islets of Langerhans, 424
Isosporidiosis, 197
IUGR. *See* Intrauterine growth restriction

J

Jaundice, 135, 392, 395, *395,* 396, *396,* 402, 412
Jeel-bear, 395
Jejunum, 358, *370*

Jock itch, 518
Joint diseases, 594–602
Joint spurs, 596
Juvenile polyps, 380
Juvenile rheumatoid arthritis, 163, 599
Juxtaglomerular apparatus, 480, 483–484

K

Kaposi sarcoma, 287, *656,* 670
Karyotype, *116, 125*
Keloid, 61, *61,* 669
Keratin, 364
Keratinocytes, 649
Keratitis, 685
Keratoacanthoma, 668, *668*
Keratoconjunctivitis sicca, 684
Keratoconus, 686
Keratopathy of cornea, 686
Kern, 395
Kernicterus, *135,* 138, 395
Ketones, 436
Ketonuria, 436
Kidney, 479–508
    anatomy of, *482*
    cyst of, *493*
    fatty change in, *27*
Kinin system, 41
Klinefelter syndrome, 129–130, *130*
Korsakoff psychosis, 218
Krukenberg tumor, 563
Kupffer cells, 39, 392
Kussmaul respiration, 436
Kwashiorkor, 222, *222*
Kyphosis, 585

L

Labia majora, 537
Labia minora, 537
Labile cells, 21, 52
Laboratory findings, 199
Lacerations, 207, 365
Lacrimal apparatus, 684, *685*
Lacrimal glands, 679
Lacrimal sac, 679
Lactation, 456
Lacunae, 583
Lamellar bone, 583
Laminar cortical necrosis of brain, 633, *633*
Langerhan cells, 649
Lanugo hairs, 652
Large cell carcinomas, 348
Laryngeal papillomas, 330
LDL cholesterol, 275
Lead toxicity, 212–213, *214*
Left circumflex coronary artery, 294
Left coronary artery, 294
Left-heart failure, 299, *299,* 300
Left-to-right congenital cardiac shunts, *317*
Left-to-right shunt, 315
Left ventricle, 293
Left ventricular dilation, 309
Left ventricular hypertrophy, *309*
Legionella pneumophila, 340
Leiomyoma, 558, 608
Leiomyosarcoma, 559, 608
Leishmaniasis, 197
Lentigo, 657, *657*
Leprosy, 195

Leptin, 225
Lesion, defined, 4
Leukemia, 139, 249, *252, 260*
Leukemoid reaction, 251
Leukocyte esterase, 487
Leukocytes, 36, 236
Leukocytosis, 46, 249
Leukodystrophy, 639
Leukopenia, 47, 248
Leukoplakia, 364, 545
Leukorrhea, 549
Lewy bodies, 638
Leydig cells, 514, 520
LGV. *See* Lymphogranuloma venereum
Lichen planus, 660, *660*
Lichen sclerosus of vulva, 545–546
Lichen simplex chronicus, 545, 658, *659*
Lid lag, 460
Light chain disease, 151, 253
Lines of Zahn, 76
Lipase, 423, 430
Lipids, 275
Lipiduria, 492
Lipofuscin, 27
Lipoid nephrosis, 497
Lipoma, 608, *608,* 669
Lipoprotein, 275
Liposarcomas, 608
Liquefactive necrosis, 30
Lissencephaly, 624
Listhesis, 601
Liver, 135, 391. *See also* Alcohol abuse
    alcoholic, *410*
    metastatic carcinoma in, *414*
Liver cells
    adenoma, 414
    fatty change in, *27*
    hydropic change, *26*
Liver function, 393t
Liver function tests, 395
Liver infarcts, 414
Lobar pneumonia, 339
Lobular carcinoma, 572
Long bones, 583
Lordosis, 585
Lou Gehrig disease, 638, *638*
Low birth weight, 133–134
Low blood haptoglobin, 242
Low body temperature, 25
Low-grade tumors, 516
Low-protein edema, formation of, *73*
Lower esophageal sphincter, 358
Lower gastrointestinal bleeding, 361
Lower limit of normal, defined, 7
Lower respiratory tract, 325
Lower urinary system, 480, 510, *511*
Ludwig angina, 607
Lumbar puncture, *635*
Lumbosacral plexus, 619
Lumen, 272
Luminal phase malabsorption, 374
Lung abscess, 341
Lupus erythematosus, 266, 530
Luteal cysts, 561
Luteinizing hormone, 458, 514, 540
Lyme disease, 47, 182, 195
Lymph nodes, malignant lymphoma, *255*
Lymphadenitis, 46, 251–252

Lymphadenopathy, 46, 251
Lymphangiomas, 287
Lymphangitis, 46, 185
Lymphatic system, 46, *98*
Lymphedema, 72, 74
Lymphocytes, 38, 45–45t, 149t, 236
Lymphocytes-B cells, 149
Lymphocytic leukemia, 172, 249, 252, *253*, 256
Lymphocytosis, 47, 251
Lymphogranuloma venereum, 190, 532, 544
Lymphoid cells, 236, 249
Lymphoma, 89, 172, 249
Lymphopenia, 249
Lysosomes, 20

M

M-protein, 253
M-spike, 253
Macrocytic anemia, 246
Macroglobulin, 151
Macrophages, 39, 45, 149
Macular degeneration, 680
Mad cow disease, 181
Mainstream smoke, 210
Major blood groups, 152
Major crossmatch, 165
Major histocompatibility complex, 149
Mala aria, 243
Malabsorption syndrome, 374
Malar "butterfly" rash, *163*
Malaria, 181, 195, 197, 243, *245*
Male genital system, 509–535, *512*
Male urinary tract, *481*
Malignancy, 153, 561
    clinical hallmark of, 99
    grading, *102, 104*
    staging of, *102*
Malignant fibrous histiocytoma, 608
Malignant hypertension, 284, 498
Malignant melanoma, 670–671, *672, 673,* 695
Malignant nephrosclerosis, 284, 498
Malignant thrombocythemia, 258–259
Malignant tumors, characteristics of, 93t
Malleus, 697
Mallory bodies, 27, 409
Mallory-Weiss syndrome, 365, *365*
Mallory's alcoholic hyaline, 409
Malnutrition, 221
Malrotation defects, 315
Mammography, 573
Mantoux skin test, 342, 345
Marasmus, 222
Marfan syndrome, 124, *125–126*
Marie-Strümpell disease, 599
Marijuana, 221
Marked generalized edema, 491
Marrow fat, 79
Mastoiditis, 699
mDNA. *See* Mitochondrial DNA
Mean cell hemoglobin, 239
Mean cell volume, 239
Mean deviation, 7
Measles, 136
Measurements, defined, 6
Mechanical bowel obstruction, causes of, *362*
Meckel diverticulum, 369, *370*
Meconium ileus, 138

Medulla, 454, 468
Medulla oblongata, 613, 618
Medullary carcinoma, 465
Medullary cavity, 583
Medulloblastoma, 642
Megacolon, 370
Megakaryocytes, 236
Megaloblastic anemia, 246
Meiosis, 23, 127
Melanin, 649
Melanocytes, 665
Melanoma, 671
Melasma of pregnancy, 652, 657
Melena, 359, 367, 371
Meleney synergistic bacterial gangrene, 193
Membrane factors, 41
Membrane potential, 622
Membranous glomerulonephritis, 496, *496–497*
Memory B cells, 149
Memory T cells, 152, 158
MEN syndromes. *See* Multiple endocrine neoplasia syndromes
Meninges, 614
Meningioma, 642, *642*
Meningitis, 11, 634
Meningocele, 624
Meningomyelocele, 624
Menorrhagia, 555
Menses, 542
Mesangial cells, 484
Mesentery, 358
Mesoderm, 16
Mesothelioma, 349
Messenger RNA, 17, 19
Metabolic processes, 19
Metabolic rate, 452
Metabolic syndrome, 225, 229
Metachromatic leukodystrophy, 639
Metals, 212
Metaphysis, 583
Metaplasia, 29, *29,* 31
Metastasis, 98, 347
    by seeding, *99*
Metrorrhagia, 555
MHC. *See* Major histocompatibility complex
Microbes, 160, 182
Microbial culture, 199
Microcephaly, 624
Microcytic hypochromic, 243
Microglia, 39, 622
Microorganisms, 177
Microscopic examination, defined, 4
Microscopic findings, 494
Microscopic hematuria, 487
Microstaging, 673
Microvascular disease, 439
Microvascular injury, 337
Microvilli, 20, 358
Micturition, 510
Midbrain, 613
Middle ear, 696
Migraine, 700
Miliary tuberculosis, 343
Minimal change glomerulonephritis, 496
Minor blood groups, 153
Minor crossmatch, 165
Minor transfusion reaction, 167

Miscarriage, 565
Misplaced aorta, 317
Mitochondria, 18–19
Mitochondrial DNA, 20
Mitosis, 20, 23
Mitotic figures, 93
Mitral valve disease, 294, 312, *313*
Mixed tumor, 365
Mixed with stool, 359
Molds, 181
Molecular defenses, 146
Molecular density, 275
Molecular mimicry, 160, *161,* 310
Molecularly defective, 242
Molecules, 181
Moles, 566–567, *671*
Molluscum contagiosum, 532, 545
Moniliasis, 364
Monoclonal gammopathy, 172, 253
Monoclonal spike, 253
Monocytes, 39, 45, 236
Monogenic, 117
Mononuclear cells, 45
Monosomy, 126
Monostotic, 594
Mons pubis, 537
Morbid obesity, 226
Motor unit, 603, *604*
Mucinous cystadenocarcinoma, ovary, *563*
Mucinous tumors, 561
Mucosa, 538
Mucosa-associated lymphoid tissue, 328, 359
Multifocal leukoencephalopathy, 637
Multinucleated giant cells, 45
Multiple endocrine neoplasia syndromes, 475
Multiple myeloma, 172, 253, *254,* 594
Multiple sclerosis, 164
Mumps, 136, 365
Mural thrombus, 305
Muscle, normal, *605*
Muscle wasting, 400
Muscular dystrophy, 606, *606*
Musculoskeletal disease, 598t
Myasthenia gravis, 260, 607
Mycobacterium avium, 172, 194, 341
Mycobacterium leprae, 195
Mycobacterium tuberculosis, 44, 158, 172, 194, 341–342, *343,* 345, 589
Mycoplasma, 515–516, 560
Mycoplasma hominis, 531
Mycoplasma pneumoniae, 243, 340
Mycoplasma species, 181, 200, 340
Mycosis fungoides, 670
Myelin, 616, 639
Myelocytic leukemia, 249, 257, *258,* 259
Myelodysplasia, 260
Myelofibrosis, 258, *258,* 259
Myelogenous leukemia, 257
Myeloid cells, 236, 249
Myeloid leukemia, *258*
Myelophthisis, 247
Myeloproliferative disorder, 248, 257
Myocardial infarct, 281, 304, *305–306, 308,* 319
Myocarditis, 162, 310, 314
Myocardium, 297
Myometrium, 538
Myopia, 682

Myosin, 603
Myxedema, 460, 462
Myxomatous degeneration of mitral valve,
    309

N

Narcotic, 220
Narkosis, 220
Nasolacrimal apparatus, 679
Nasolacrimal duct, 679
Nature of disease, 3–6
Nearsightedness, 683
Necrosis, 24, 47
Necrotizing arteriolitis, 284
Necrotizing enterocolitis, 136, 373
Necrotizing fasciitis, 193
Necrotizing vasculitis, 162, 286
Negative feedback loop, 449, 451
Negative tests results, 9
Neisseria gonorrhoeae, 189, 516, 525,
    530–531, 544, 600, 684
Neisseria meningitidis, 634
Nematodes, 196
Neonatal cholestasis, 412, 417
Neonatal hepatitis, 412
Neonatal mortality risk, *133*
Neoplasms, 86–109, 518, 561
    gross structure of, *92*
Nephritic syndrome, 487, 491
Nephrolithiasis, 487, 493, 503, *504*
Nephron unit, 481
Nephrosclerosis, 283, *499*
Nephrosis, 492
Nephrotic syndrome, 487, 491, *492*
Nephrotoxic syndrome, 499
Nerve tracts, 613–614
Nervous system, 612–647, *623*
Neural hearing loss, 699
Neural tube defect, *113*, 624
Neuroblastoma, 475, 643
Neurocutaneous syndromes, 656
Neuroendocrine cells, 454
Neurofibroma, 643, 670
Neurofibromatosis, 124
Neurofibrosarcoma, 643
Neurogenic atrophy, 605
Neurohypophysis, 450
Neuromuscular apparatus, *604*
Neuromuscular junction, 603
Neuron, 614
Neurosyphilis, 529
Neurotransmitter, 622
Neutropenia, 249
Neutrophilia, 47, 251
Neutrophils, 36–37, 236
Nevus, 670
Nevus flammeus, 670
New bone formation, 524
Nicotine, 217. *See also* Smoking
Nitrates, 487
Nitric oxide, 41, 275
Nitrogen, 79
Nodular fasciitis, 608
Nodular goiter, 459, 463
Nodular hyperplasia, 521
Nodular lymphoma, 257
Nodular melanoma, 673, *673*
Nodular sclerosis Hodgkin lymphoma, 255

Nodular xanthomas, 655
Non-Hodgkin lymphoma, 255–256
Nonbacterial cystitis, 516
Nonbacterial thrombotic endocarditis, *313*
Nonendocrine organs, tissues, 451
Nongonococcal infections, 545
Nongonococcal urethritis, 189, 531
Nonimmune antimicrobial protective
    mechanisms, *147*
Noninfective thrombotic endocarditis, 312
Nonneoplastic diseases, 651–665
Nonossifying fibroma of bone, 593
Nonproliferative fibrocystic change, 570
Nonproliferative retinopathy, 691
Nontoxic goiter, 463
Nontropical sprue, 374
Norepinephrine, 454
Normal birth weight, 133
Normal cell, *16*
Normal distribution curve, 7
Norwalk virus, 188, 372
Nosocomial infection, 184, 349
Nosomial infection, 341
Nuclear atypia, malignant neoplasms, *93*
Nuclear DNA, 18
Nucleotide bases, 17
Nucleus pulposus, 601
Null cell adenoma, 458
Nummular dermatitis, 662
Nystagmus, 682

O

Obesity, 222, 224, 229, 435
Obstruction of small blood vessels, 243
Obstructive chronic bronchitis, 334
Obstructive lung disease, 328–329, 331
Obstructive nephropathy, 500
Obstructive sleep apnea, 283
Occult bleeding, 359
Occult blood test, 360
Occult hematuria, 492
Occult proteinuria, 487, 492
Occupational disease, 211
Occupational toxic exposure, 211t
Oligodendrocytes, 622, 639
Oligodendroglioma, 641–642
Oligomenorrhea, 555
Oliguria, 490
Omentum, 358
Omphalocele, 370
Onchocerciasis, 686
Oncogenes, 21, 90
Oncology, 87
Oocyte, 539–540
Open-angle glaucoma, 693
Opportunistic infections, 171
Opportunistic pathogens, 172, 193
Optic disc, 682
Optic nerve, 682
Optic neuritis, 693
Oral contraceptives, 214
Oral herpesvirus, *665*
Oral hypoglycemic drugs, 442
Orbit, 678, *679*
Organ rejection, 164
Organogenesis, 113
Organophosphates, 212
Orthostatic, 490

Osmolality, 485
Osmosis, 67, *68*
Osmotic diuresis, 436
Osmotic edema, 72, 74
Osmotic pressure, 67, 74
Ossicles, 697
Osteitis deformans, 585
Osteoarthritis, 595
    cartilage damage in, *596*
    femur head, *596*
Osteoblasts, 583
Osteochondroma, 593, *593*
Osteoclastoma, 594
Osteocytes, 583
Osteogenesis imperfecta, 585
Osteogenic sarcoma, 593
Osteomalacia, 587, 589, 591
Osteomyelitis, 587
Osteon, 583
Osteophytes, 596
Osteoporosis, 587, *590*
    causes, consequences of, *590*
Osteosarcoma, 585, 593
Otitis externa, 697
Otitis media, 3, 11, 137, 698, 701
Otosclerosis, 699
Ototoxicity, 699
Ovarian cycle, 542
Ovarian cystic teratoma, *564*
Ovarian fibroma, *564*
Ovarian hormones, *542*
Ovarian ligament, 538
Ovarian stromal cell tumors, 563
Ovarian teratomas, 562
Ovarian tumors, 562, 564t
Ovaries, 116, 538, *539*, 563
    bilateral serous cystadenocarcinoma, *563*
    cystic serous tumor, *563*
    endometriosis, *556*
    mucinous cystadenocarcinoma, *563*
Overhydration, 71
Ovulatory bleeding, 555
Oxygen, 273
Oxygen superoxide, 41
Oxytocin, 459

P

Paget disease, 574, 585
Palmar erythema, 397
Pancreas, 422–447, *424–425*
Pancreatic carcinoma, 432
Pancreatic duct, 423
Pancreatic juice, 426t
Pancreatic pseudocyst, 428
Pancreatitis, 427, *428*, 429, *431*
    complications of, *432*
    laboratory tests, 430
    pathogenesis of, *428*
Panniculitis, 663
Pannus, 597
Pap smear, 102, *102*, 549, *551*, 552–553, *554*
Papillary carcinomas, 465
Papillary dermis, 651
Papillary transitional cell carcinoma, 516
Papilledema, 626, 690, 692
Papilloma, 93
Papillomavirus, 189, 518, 531, 544, 546, 549,
    551

Paragangliomas, 474
Paraganglionic system, 454
Paraneoplastic syndromes, 101, 106, 348
Paraphimosis, 517
Parasitic disease, 47, 189, 195–196t, 251, 372
Parasitos, 195
Parasympathetic system, 619–620
Parathormone, 453
Parenchyma, 16, 93, 392
Paresis, 529, *529*
Parkinsonism, 637–638
Partial thromboplastin time, 262
Passive congestion, 74, 414
Passive immunity, 151
Patent ductus arteriosus, 316
Patent foramen ovale, 316
Pathogenesis, defined, 4
Pathologic fracture, 586
Pathologic uterine bleeding, 555
Pathophysiology, defined, 4
Patient compliance, 288
Peau d'orange, 74
Pediatric disease, 110–234
Pedunculated tubular adenomas, colon, *381*
Pelvic inflammatory disease, 560
Pelvic relaxation syndrome, 560
Pelvis, *540*
Pemphigoid, 659
Pemphigus, 659, *659*
Pemphix, 659
Penetrance, 120
Penis, 510
    Bowen disease, *518*
    chancre, *527*
Pepsin, 358
Pepsinogen, 358
Peptic ulcer, 189, 367–368, *368*
Peptides, 357
Perforated peptic ulcer, stomach, *369*
Periapical abscess, 363
Pericardial effusion, 319
Pericarditis, 310, 319, 490
Periodontitis, 363
Periosteum, 583
Peripheral nervous system, 490, 613, 618, *620*
Peripheral neuropathy, 440
Peripheral vascular insufficiency, 281
Peristalsis, 355
Peritoneal effusions, 302
Peritonitis, 379
Permanent cells, 54
Pernicious anemia, 247
Persistent chronic inflammation, 45
Persistent proteinuria, 490
Petechiae, 75, 314
Petroleum products, 212
Peyer patches, 359
Peyronie disease, 517–518
Phagocytes, 45
Phagocytosis, 20, 37, *40*
Pharyngitis, 330
Phenotype, 116
Pheochromocytoma, 101, 284, 474
Phimosis, 517
Photoaging of skin, 652, 660, *661*
Photosensitivity, 652

Phototherapy, 135
Phylaxis, 154
Phyllodes tumor of breast, 571, *572*
Physiologic jaundice, 135, 412
Physiologic proteinuria, 490
Pia mater, 614
Pickwickian syndrome, 227
PID. *See* Pelvic inflammatory disease
Pigment gallstones, 415
Pigment stones, *416*
Pigmented villonodular synovitis, 602
Pinguecula, 683
Pinworm, 196
Pitting, low-protein edema, *73*
Pituitary adenoma, 455, *455*
Pituitary gland, *451*, 456t
Pituitary hormones, 452t, *542*
Pituitary stalk, 450
Placenta, 134
Placenta accreta, 566
Placenta previa, 566
Plague, 195
Plaque, 304, 363
Plasma, 89, 235
Plasma cell diseases, 39, 252
Plasma cells, 45, 149, 252
Plasma-derived, 40
Plasma lipids, 275
Plasma membrane, 20, *21*
Plasma proteins, 40
Plasmodium falciparum, 242, 245
Plasmodium species, 195, 245
Platelet abnormalities, 76
Platelet count, 263
Platelet function analysis, 263
Platelets, 236, 312
Pleomorphic adenoma, 365
Pleural effusion, 302, 349
Pleurisy, 341, 349
Pleuritis, 349
Pnein, 283
Pneumoconiosis, 215, 336
Pneumocystis, 193
Pneumocystis jiroveci, 172, *172*, 181, *193*, 346, *347*
Pneumocystis pneumonia, 346
Pneumocytes, 327
Pneumonia, 339–340, 349
Pneumothorax, 349
Podagra, 600
Point mutation, 118
Poisoning
Pollutants, 210
Polyarteritis nodosa, 164, 286
Polycystic disease, 493
Polycystic ovary syndrome, 561
Polycythemia vera, 248, 257, 259
Polydactyly, 114
Polydipsia, 436
Polygenics, 117–118
Polyhydramnios, 624
Polymenorrhea, 555
Polymorphonuclear leukocytes, 37
Polymyalgia rheumatica, 48, 600
Polymyositis, 607, *607*
Polyphagia, 436
Polyps, 93
Polyuria, 436

Pontine hemorrhage, *626*
Portal cirrhosis, 397–398
Portal hypertension, 398, *399,* 400
Portal triads, 392
Portal venous system, 390, *391*
Positive test results, defined, 7
Postadolescent acne, 663
Posterior descending coronary artery, 294
Postinflammatory pigmentation, 658
Poststreptococcal glomerulonephritis, 494
Postural hypotension, 440
Postural proteinuria, 490
Potassium hydroxide test, 665
Pre-eclampsia, 568
Prehepatic jaundice, 395
Preleukemia, 260
Premalignant conditions, 92, 95, 549
Premature atrial contractions, 298
Premature birth, 134, 140
Premature ventricular contractions, 298
Prenatal specimen collection, genetic diagnosis, *131*
Prepuce, 510
Presbus, 683
Presbyopia, 683
Presumably healthy, defined, 7
Pretibial myxedema, 459, 654
Priapism, 518
Priapus, 518
Primary progressive tuberculosis, 342–343
Primary sclerosing cholangitis, 413
Proctitis, 193
Prodromal period, 197
Produces sputum, 333
Progeria, 24
Programmable, 147
Prolactinoma, 456
Proliferative breast disease, 570–571
Proliferative fibrocystic change, 570
Proliferative phase, 542
Proliferative retinopathy, 691
Proliferative synovitis, 597
Propionibacterium acnes, 177, 663
Proprioceptive sense, 613
Proptosis, 684
Prostate, 514
    anatomy, *521*
    nodular hyperplasia of, *522*
Prostate-specific antigen, 106, 524
Prostatic adenocarcinoma, 521
Prostatitis, 520
Proteases, 423
Protein, 17, 222, 357
Protein electrophoresis, 253, *254*
Protein-energy malnutrition, 222
Protein synthesis, *19,* 399
Proteinuria, 486, 490–491
Prothrombin time, 262
Proto-oncogenes, 21, 56, 90, 124
Protozoa, 197, 372
Pseudarthrosis, 587
Pseudofolliculitis barbae, 654
Pseudomembranous colitis, 193, 372
Pseudomonas, 193–194, 340
Psoriasis, 658, *658*
Psoriatic arthritis, 600
Pterygium, 684
PTT. *See* Partial thromboplastin time

Pulmonary arteriole, pulmonary hypertension, *338*
Pulmonary artery, rechanneled, *79*
Pulmonary atresia, 319
Pulmonary congestion, 340
Pulmonary edema, 74, 299–300, 337
Pulmonary hyaline membranes, *135*
Pulmonary hypertension, 337, *338*
Pulmonary infarct, *337*
Pulmonary interstitium, 328
Pulmonary membrane, 328
Pulmonary surfactant, 327
Pulmonary thromboembolism, *79*, 337
Pulmonary tuberculosis, *346*
Pulmonary valve, 294
Pulmonary valve stenosis, 317
Pupil, 679
Pure cholesterol stones, 415
Purpura, 75
Purulent meningitis, 634
Purulent otitis media, 699
Pyelonephritis, 502–503, *503*
Pyloric sphincter, 358
Pylorus, 358
Pyogenic granuloma, 61, 669

Q

Qualitative defect, 591
Quantitative defect, 589

R

Radial growth phase, 673
Radiant energy spectrum, 215t
Radiation, ionizing, 465
Radioactive bone scan, *525*
Radioactive iodine uptake, 461
Radon, 210
Rapidly progressive glomerulonephritis, 495
Raynaud phenomenon, 164
RDS. *See* Respiratory distress syndrome
Reactant proteins, 46
Reactive arthritis, 599
Reactive hyperplasia, 46, 251
Reactive hypoglycemia, 442
Reactive lymphadenitis, 251
Reactive oxygen compounds, 41
Reagins, 529
Receptors, 123, 149
Recessive genes, 119
Recipient RBC, 165
Recovery from injury, 51–64
Rectocele, 560
Red blood cell antigens, and agglutinins, 152t
Red blood cells, 236, 239, *239, 241,* 259
Red marrow, 583
Red stroke, 627, 630
Reed-Sternberg cell, 255
Reflux esophagitis, 366
Reflux nephropathy, 500
Refractive disorders, 682, *683*
Refractive errors, 682, 687
Refractory anemia, 260
Regeneration, 52, 57
Regional enteritis, 374
Reiter syndrome, 190
Relative risk, absolute risk, distinguished, 571
Renal ablation glomerulopathy, 498, 500
Renal adenocarcinoma, 505

Renal agenesis, 493
Renal cell carcinoma, 505, *506*
Renal colic, 493
Renal disease, 284
Renal dysplasia, 493
Renal failure, 486–487, 492, 591
Renal pelvis, 480, *504*
Renal tubules, 480, 483
Renin, 274, 480–481, 483–484
Renin-angiotensin-aldosterone system, 300, 469, 484
Renovascular hypertension, 499
Renovascular insufficiency, 281
Reservoir, 184
Resorption atelectasis, 331
Respiration, 325, 436
Respiratory distress syndrome of adults, 135
Respiratory distress syndrome of neonates, 140
Respiratory infections, *187,* 330
Respiratory syncytial virus, 136–137
Respiratory system, 324–353, *326*
Restrictive disease, 328–329
Restrictive lung disease, 335
Retention polyps, 380
Reticular dermis, 651
Reticulocytes, 239
Retina, 680
    in diabetes, *691*
    in hypertension, *690*
    normal, *681*
Retinal detachment, 689, *689*
Retinal occlusive vascular disease, 690
Retinal vascular disease, 690
Retinitis pigmentosa, 692
Retinoblastoma, 100, 695
Retinopathy, 136, 692
    background, 691
Retrograde ejaculation, 517
Retroperitoneum, 510
Retropharyngeal abscess, 607
Reye syndrome, 214
Rhabdomyolysis, 607
Rhabdomyoma, 608
Rhabdomyosarcoma, 608
Rheumatic fever, 309–310
Rheumatic heart disease, 309, *311*
Rheumatic valvulitis, 310, *312*
Rheumatoid arthritis, 163, 596–597, *598,* 599
Rheumatoid factor, 163, 597
Rheumatoid nodules, 163, 597, *598*
Rheumatoid spondylitis, 599
Rhinovirus, 187
Ribosomal RNA, 17, 19
Ribosomes, 19
Rickets, 222, 591
Rickettsia species, 181, 195, 200, 340
Right atria, 293
Right coronary artery, 294
Right-heart failure, 300
Right middle lobe syndrome, 331
Right-to-left shunts, 315–316
Right ventricle, 293
Right ventricular heart failure, 300
Right ventricular hypertrophy, 317
Ringworm, 518
RNA synthesis, 17, *18,* 19
Rocky Mountain spotted fever, 195

Rods, 680
Rosacea, 663
Rotavirus, 188, 372
Rough endoplasmic reticulum, 20
Round ligament, 538
Round window, 697
Roundworms, 196
RSV. *See* Respiratory syncytial virus
Rubella, 136
Rule of nines, 208
Ruptured mitral valve chordae tendineae, 309

S

Saccharides, 357
Saccular aneurysm, 629, *629*
Saddle embolus, 337
Salicylism, 214
Salmonella species, 164, 189, 200, 243, 372
Salmonellosis, 372
Salpingitis, 560, 576
Salt wasting, 472
Salt water therapy, 72
Sarcoidosis, 656
Sarcomas, 88–89, 572, 608
Saturation, 245
Scar development, 44–45, 47, 57, *57*
Scarlatina, 191
Scarlet fever, 191
Schistosoma, 196
Schistosomiasis, 182, 196
Schlemm's canal, 680
Schwann cells, 622
Schwannomas, 643
Sciatica, 601
SCID. *See* Severe combined immunodeficiency
Sclera, 678, *685*
Scleral icterus of jaundice, 395
Scleroderma, 164, *164,* 660
Sclerosing cholangitis, 376–377, 398
Sclerosing panencephalitis, 637
Sclerosis, 164, *164,* 277, 639
Scrotum, 513
Seborrheic dermatitis, 658, *658*
Seborrheic keratosis, 666, *667*
Secondhand smoke, 210. *See also* Smoking
Seeding, 98, *99*
Sella turcica, 450
Semen, 513
Semicircular canals, 697
Seminal vesicles, 511
Seminiferous tubules, 511
Seminoma, 519, *520*
Semipermeable membrane, 67–68
Sensitive tests, 10
Sensitivity, 307
    defined, 8
    specificity, distinguished, 9
Sensory hearing, 699
Septal defects, 315
Septic arthritis, 600
Septic shock, 81
Septicemia, 191, 199
Septum, 315
Serologic tests, 530
Seronegative spondyloarthropathies, 164, 599
Serous cystadenocarcinoma, *563*
Serous effusions, 162
Serous inflammation, 42

Serous otitis media, 698
Serous tumors, 561
Sertoli cells, 511
Severe combined immunodeficiency, 168
Sex chromosomes, 116
Sex-linked recessive, 119
Sexually transmitted disease, 189, 525–526t, 544–544t, 576
    prevention of, 525
Sheehan syndrome, 458, *458*
Shigella species, 164, 189, 200, 372, 599
Shock, 83
    stages of, *82*
Short bones, 583
Shortness of breath, 266–267
Sialadenitis, 365
Sickle cell disease, 242, *242, 243, 244*
Sickle cell trait, 242
Sickness, defined, 6
Sidestream smoke, 210
SIDS. *See* Sudden infant death syndrome
Signs, defined, 5
Silicosis, 336
Simple cysts, 493
Simple fracture, 586
Simple hyperplasia, 557
Singer's nodes. *See* Vocal cord nodules
Single gene, 117
Sinoatrial node, 295
Sjögren syndrome, 164, 365, 684
Skeletal muscle, 581–650
Skin, 648–673
    neoplasms of, 665–677
    normal, *650–651*
    pigmentation, 657
Skin burns, pathology of, *209*
Skin lesions, 162
    types of, *653*
Skin tag, 665, *665*
Skin wart, 666
Skull fracture, 627
SLE. *See* Systemic lupus erythematosus
Small bowel, Crohn disease, *376*
Small cell carcinomas, 347–348
Small cell lymphocytic lymphoma, 252, 256
Small pulmonary artery, 317
Small vessels, 286, 439
Smoking, 279, 333, 349
    effects of, 201, *216*
    lung cancer, relationship, *217*
Smoldering leukemia, 260
Smooth endoplasmic reticulum, 20
Smooth muscle cells, 273, 279
Soft callus, 587
Solar keratosis, 667, *667*
Somatic cells, 116, 118
Somatostatin, 358, 424, 426
Somatotropin adenoma, 456
Specificity, defined, 8
Sperm, 514
Spermatic cord, 511
Spermatocele, 518
Spermatocyte, 511
Spermatogenesis, *513*
Spermatozoa, 513
Spider angiomas, 652, 670
Spider angiomata, 397
Spider bite, 532–533

Spina bifida, 113, 624
Spinal cord, 618
Spinal curvature, abnormalities of, *585*
Spinal nerves, 618
Spine, osteoporosis, *590*
Spiral fracture, 586
Spirochetes, 177
Spirography, *329*
Spirometry, 328, 333, 335
Spleen, 260
Splenomegaly, 260, 398
Spondylitis, rheumatoid, 599
Spondyloarthropathy, 163–164, 599
Spondylolisthesis, 601
Spondylos, 599, 601
Spongiform encephalitides, 637
Spontaneous subarachnoid hemorrhage, *629*
Sporadic goiter, 463
Sprain, 601
Sprue, 374
Squama, 16, 649
Squamocolumnar junction, 538, 546
Squamous cell carcinoma, 16, 348, 364, 366, 544–545, 552, 669, 697
Stable angina, 304
Stable cells, 52
Staghorn calculus, *504*
Stalk effect, 455
Standard deviation, 7
Stapes, 697
Staphylococcus species, 26, 43, 177, 185, 191, 193, 340–341, 587, 664
Stasis dermatitis, 287, 660, *661*
Statin drugs, 281
Statistical evidence, 347
Status asthmaticus, 332
Stein-Leventhal syndrome, 561
Stem cells, 29, 52–53, *54*
Stenosis, 370
Sterile peritonitis, 379
Sternum, chondrosarcoma of, *593*
Steroid therapy, 659
Stevens-Johnson syndrome, 660
Still disease, 163
Stimulants, 220
Stokes-Adams seizure, 298
Stomach, peptic ulcer, *368–369*
Stones, 415, *416, 504*
Stool occult blood test, 360, 382
Strabismus, 682
Strain, 601
Strangulated hernia, 361
Stratum corneum, 649
Streptococcal diseases, *192*
Streptococcal pharyngitis, 191, 506
Streptococcus species, 137, 186, 191, 313, 339–340, 634
Stress fracture, 586
Stress ulcers, 367
Striae, 652
Stroke, 281, 288, 627, 631, 644
Stromal dystrophy, 686
Structural disorder, defined, 5
Structure, defined, 3
Sty, 684
Subacute sclerosing panencephalitis, 637
Subarachnoid hemorrhage, 627–628

Subarachnoid space, 614
Subconjunctival hemorrhage, 684
Subcutaneous tissue, 651
Subdivisions of chromosome, *17*
Subdural hematoma, 627, *628–629*
Subendocardial infarct, 305
Subluxation, 601
Sudden infant death syndrome, 137
Sugars, 357
Sunburn, 652
Superficial spreading melanoma, 673
Superficial ulcers, 367
Superior sagittal sinus, 614
Suppressor T cells, 152, 160
Suppurative inflammation, 43
Surface epithelial cells, 538
Suspensory ligaments, 679
Sweat chloride test, 138
Swimmer's ear, 698
Sympathetic chain, 620
Sympathetic fibers, 620
Sympathetic ophthalmitis, 688
Symptoms, defined, 5
Synapse, 603, 622
Synaptic space, 603, 622
Syndactyly, 114
Synechiae, 688
Synovial joint, 594, *595*
Synovial sarcoma, 608
Syphilis, 47, 189, 525, 527–530, 544
    condyloma lata of, *528*
    serologic tests for, 530
Syphilitic aneurysm, 285
Syphilitic aortitis, 309, *528*
Syphilitic meningitis, 634–636
Systemic anaphylaxis, 159
Systemic lupus erythematosus, 160, *163, 656,* 660
Systemic sclerosis, 164, *164*

T

T-cell receptor, 152
T cells, 148t–149t, 152, 160
Tabes dorsalis, 529
Tachycardia, 297
Takayasu aortitis, 286
Tapeworms, 196
Tarsal plate, 678
Tartar, 363
TB. *See* Tuberculosis
TBG. *See* Thyroxine binding globulin
Telangiectasis, 670, *670*
Telogen effluvium, 654
Telogen phase, 652
Temporal arteritis, 286, 601
Tendinitis, 602
Tendon, 601
Tenosynovitis, 602
Tentorial herniation, 625
Tentorium, 614
Teras, 114
Teratogen, 114
Teratoid, 114
Teratoma, 562
Terminal ileitis, 374–375
Tertiary hyperparathyroidism, 467
Test results, positive, defined, 9
Test sensitivity, specificity, 11–12

Test usefulness, effect of disease prevalence on, 10
Testicular atrophy, 397
Testicular cancer, 520
Testicular neoplasms, *519*
Testis, 116, 511, 513, 518, *518*
  seminoma, *520*
  undescended, 518
Testosterone, 511, 513–514
Tests
  in diagnosis, usefulness of, 8–12
  highly sensitive, defined, 10
  highly specific, defined, 10
  sensitive, 12
Tetanus, 193, 607
Tetraiodothyronine, 452
Tetralogy of Fallot, 317, *318*
Thalassemia, 242–243
Thalassemia major, 243
Thalassemia minor, 243
Theca cells, 539
Thromboangiitis obliterans, 286
Thrombocythemia, essential, 259
Thrombocytopenia, 75–76, 264
Thrombocytosis, 259
Thromboembolism, 78–79
Thrombophlebitis, 78, 287
Thrombosis, 265, 304, *304*
Thrombotic endocarditis, nonbacterial, *313*
Thrombus formation, 76, 77–78, 79, *280*
Thrush, 346, 364
Thymic hypoplasia, 168
Thymus, 260
Thyroglobulin, 452
Thyroglossal duct cyst, 114
Thyroid adenoma, 464
Thyroid cancer, 465
Thyroid function, 462t, 654
Thyroid gland, *463*
  hyperthyroidism, *460*
Thyroid hormone, *453*
Thyroid-stimulating hormone, 460
Thyroid stimulating hormone adenoma, 458
Thyroid-stimulating immunoglobulin, 459
Thyroiditis, 462–463
Thyrotoxicosis, 459
Thyrotropin-releasing hormone, 450
Thyroxine, 452
Thyroxine binding globulin, 453
TIBC. *See* Total iron binding capacity
Tics, 47, 182, 195
Tinnitus, 699
Tissue organization, 17–18
Tobacco smoking, 201, *216*, 279, 333, 349
  lung cancer, relationship, *217*
Tonsillar herniation, 625
Topical steroid therapy, 659
TORCH syndrome, 115, *115*
TORCH teratogens, 114
Total blood volume, 71
Total cholesterol, 275
Total iron binding capacity, 245
Total plasma cholesterol, 276
Total red cell mass, measurement of, 248
Toxemia, 568
Toxic epidermal necrolysis, 660
Toxic goiter, 463

Toxic megacolon, 377
Toxoplasma gondii, 193, 687
Toxoplasmosis, 193
Trachoma, 195, 684
Transfer RNA, 17, 19
Transferrin, 245
Transformation zone, 548
Transfusion reaction, 165–166
Transient ischemic attack of brain, 632
Transitional cell carcinoma, 506, 516
Transitional cells, 510
Transitional epithelium, 516
Transmural infarct, 305
Transplant rejection, 164
Transport proteins, 123
Transposition of great vessels, 318
Transudate, 72, 349
Trauma, 207, 643
  mortality, U.S., *207*
Trematodes, 196
Treponema pallidum, 44, 527–529, 531
Trichina species, 196
Trichinella, 606
Trichinosis, 196, 606
Trichomonas vaginalis, 47, 181, 197, 531, 545
Trichomoniasis, 191, 197, 545
Tricuspid valve, 294
Triglyceride, 275
Trisomy, 127
Tropical diseases, 194
Tropical sprue, 374
True negative, 6
True positive, 6
Trypanosomiasis, 197
Tuberculin skin test, 345
Tuberculosis, 341–342, *343*, 344, *346*.
  See also Mycobacterium tuberculosis
  atypical, 194
  natural history of, *343*
  secondary, 344
Tuboovarian abscess, 560, *560*
Tubular adenoma of colon, 380
Tubular epithelium, 483
Tubular necrosis of kidney, 492, 499, *499*
Tubular processing, glomerular filtrate, *485*
Tubulointerstitial nephritis, 493–494, 500, *500*
Tumor cell heterogeneity, 98
Tumor-cell heterogeneity, 97
Tumor doubling time, *96*
Tumor growth fraction, 96
Tumor suppressor genes, 21, 91, 124
Tunica albuginea, 518
Tunica vaginalis, 513
Turner syndrome, 130–131, *131*, 555
Tuskegee syphilis experiment, 529
Tympanic cavity, 696
Tympanic membrane, 696
Typhoid fever, 189, 372

U

Ulcerative colitis, 164, 374, *375*, 376
  colon in, *376–377*
  complications of, *378*
  Crohn disease, 375t
Uncompensated failure, 299
Unconjugated bilirubin, 392, 395

Undescended testis, 518, *518*
Unstable angina, 304
Upper gastrointestinal bleeding, 359–361
Upper respiratory tract, 187, 325
Upper urinary tract, 480, 510
Urea, 485
Uremia, 487, 490
Ureterovesical junction, *502, 510, 515*
Ureterovesical urine reflux, *515*
Ureters, 480
Urethral exudate, gonorrhea, *531*
Urethritis, 516
Urinalysis, 487, *489*
Urinary obstruction, 500, *501, 522*
Urinary reflux, 500
Urinary sediment, *489*
Urinary space, 484
Urinary tract syndromes, 487, 491t, 492
  male, *481*
  neoplasms of, *505*
Urine, 481, 483, 485
  dark, 506–507
Urobilinogen, 392
Urolithiasis, 493
Urticaria, 159, 661
Urticarial wheals, *661*
Uterine infection, 140
Uterine prolapse, 560
Utero obstruction, urinary flow, 493
Uterosacral ligament, 538
Uterus, 538, *539, 558, 560*
Uveal tract, 682, 687, *688*
Uveitis, 687, *688*

V

Vagina, 538, *539*
Vaginal speculum, *551*
Vaginitis, 545
Valine, 118
Valley fever, 346
Valve disease, 310
Valvular insufficiency, 309, 313
Valvular stenosis, 309
Valvulitis, 310
Varicella-zoster virus, 137
Varicocele, 517–518
Varicose vein, 74
Varix, 365
Vas deferens, 511
Vascular endothelial growth factor, 56
Vascular malformation, 629–630
Vascular resistance, 273
Vasculitis, 286
Vasoactive amines, 41
Vasoconstriction, 273
Vasodilation, 81, 273
Vasogenic edema, 626
Vellus hairs, 652
Ventricles, 614
Ventricular fibrillation, 298, 309
Ventricular septal defect, 316–317, *318*
Ventricular tachycardia, 298
Verruca vulgaris, 666, *666*
Vertebral body, collapse fracture of, *591*
Vertical growth phase, 673
Vestibular neuronitis, 699
Vibrio cholerae, 189, 372

Villi, 358
Villonodular synovitis, 602
Villous adenoma, 380
Viral encephalitis, 637
Viral hepatitis, 398, 401–402
Viral meningitis, 634
Visceral epithelial cells, 484
Vitamin B$_{12}$, 246, *246*
Vitiligo, 657, *657*
Vitreous chamber, 680
Vitreous detachment, 689
Vitreous hemorrhage, 689
Vitreous humor, 680
Vocal cord nodules, 330
Volatile organic compounds, 212
Volume depletion, 436
Volvulus, 361, 370, *370*
Vomit, 359
Von Recklinghausen disease, 124, 643, *644*
Von Willebrand disease, 264
VSD. *See* Ventricular septal defect
Vulvar dysplasia, 546
Vulvar intraepithelial neoplasia, 546
Vulvar squamous dysplasia and malignancy, 546

W

Waldenstrom macroglobulinemia, 253
Wart, 191, 531, 666, *666*
Waterhouse-Friderichsen syndrome, 472
Weber-Christian disease, 663
Wegener granulomatosis, 286
Wens, 665
Werner syndrome, 24
Wernicke encephalopathy, 218
Western Equine fever, 637
Wheals, urticarial, *661*
White blood cells, 36, 236–239
White matter, 616, 622
White stroke, 627, 630, *632*
Whiteheads, 663
Whole chromosomes, 117
Whooping cough, 137
Wilson disease, 412
Woven bone, 583

X

X chromosome, *122*
X-linked agammaglobulinemia, 167
X-linked recessive gene inheritance, 122, *123*

X-rays, discovery of, 586
Xanthelasma, 655
Xanthomas, 396, 655
  eruptive, 655
  fibrous, 608
  nodular, 655
Xeroderma pigmentosa, 91
Xerostomia, 365, 684
Xerotica obliterans, balanitis, 517

Y

Yeast, 181
Yeast-like fungi, 346
Yellow marrow, 583
Yersinia enterocolitica, 372
Yersinia pestis, 195
Yolk sac carcinoma, 520

Z

Z deformity, 597
Zahn, lines of, 76
Zollinger-Ellison syndrome, 369, 442
Zymogens, 423